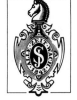

E. Faist   J. L. Meakins
F. W. Schildberg (Eds.)

Host Defense Dysfunction in Trauma, Shock and Sepsis

Mechanisms and Therapeutic Approaches

With 416 Figures and 153 Tables

Springer-Verlag

Berlin Heidelberg New York
London Paris Tokyo
Hong Kong Barcelona Budapest

Editors

Priv.-Doz. Dr. med. Eugen Faist
Prof. Dr. Friedrich W. Schildberg
Dept. of Surgery,
Ludwig-Maximilians-University Munich
Klinikum Großhadern
Marchioninistr. 15, 8000 Munich 70, FRG

Jonathan L. Meakins M.D., D.Sc.
Dept. of Surgery, McGill University
Room 510.34 687 Pine Avenue West
Montreal, Quebec, H3A 1A1, Canada

ISBN 3-540-55329-0 Springer-Verlag Berlin Heidelberg New York
ISBN 0-387-55329-0 Springer-Verlag New York Berlin Heidelberg

Library of Congress Cataloging-in-Publication Data
Host defense dysfunctions in trauma, shock, and sepsis: mechanisms and therapeutic approaches /
Eugen Faist, Jonathan L. Meakins, F. W. Schildberg, (eds.).
Includes index.
ISBN 3-540-55329-0 (alk. paper). – ISBN 0-387-55329-0 (alk. paper)
1. Septic shock – Immunological aspects. 2. Multiple organ failure – Immunological aspects.
3. Traumatism – Immunological aspects. 4. Immunosuppression. 5. Wounds and Injuries –
immunology. I. Faist, E. (Eugen) II. Meakins, Jonathan L. III. Schildberg, F.W. (Friedrich W.)
[DNLM: 1. Immunity – physiology. 2. Infection – immunology, 3. Shock – immunology. QW
504 H831] RB150. S5H67 1992 616.07'9–dc20

Typesetting: Macmillan India Ltd., Bangalore-25
Printing: Saladruck, Berlin, Binding: Lüderitz & Bauer, Berlin
24/3020-543210—Printed on acid-free paper

CID 5186 90005252

Preface

This book presents a unique overview of all aspects of host defense alterations under stressful conditions. It is based on the most important contributions given at the "2nd International Congress on the Immune Consequences of Trauma, Shock, and Sepsis—Mechanisms and Therapeutic Approaches," which was held in Munich under the auspices of the most distinguished scientific societies involved in this field (Society of Critical Care Medicine, European Society of Intensive Care Medicine, Société Internationale de Chirurgie, Surgical Infection Society, Surgical Infection Society Europe, European Society for Surgical Research, International Society for Burn Injury, American Association for the Surgery of Trauma, and National Institutes of Health). Since the first conference of this kind in 1988, new information from basic studies and clinical trials has provided exciting and novel insights into the immune dysfunctions accompanying trauma, shock, and sepsis.

The volume is divided into 18 parts presenting the structural background of trauma-induced alterations of immune and imflammatory mechanisms as well as the currently discussed therapeutic interventions designed to restore or maintain normal host defenses following major injury.

Introducing the general theme of the book is a summary of the essential keystones of trauma and sepsis-related immune deficits. Discussions of the progress in trauma care brought through better understanding of the cell biology of injury and of the major clinical factors that influence host defense integrity in operative medicine provide a setting for understanding the wide array of detailed information that is presented thereafter. The sequential steps of host defense impairment following trauma, a phenomenon which starts within the immediate post-trauma phase and ultimately leads to the development of multiple organ failure (MOF) with subsequent death, are then outlined. In dissecting the genesis of MOF, we have somewhat arbitrarily distinguished between the phase of shock and ischemia, an intermediate inflammatory phase, and a phase of manifest sepsis syndrome. Subsequent chapters go into the immune pathways for controlling infection under physiologic and stressful conditions and the inflammatory mechanisms in traumatic and septic injury, and four parts of the book then consider the characteristics of various cytokines and their pleiotropic functions in acute-phase states, trauma, and sepsis and approaches to modulate cytokine actions.

This volume also brings up-to-date information on the effects of endotoxins, including the massive impact of bacterial translocation on endocytosis, and on the most recent regimens for endotoxin shock protection, including neutralization with intravenous immunoglobulins and monoclonal anti-endotoxin antibodies. Additional chapters consider the most recent promising immunomodulatory approaches to both prevention and treatment of septic shock.

Updates on the mechanisms of wound healing, the role of nutrition in host defense, clinical aspects of MOF, and antibiotic interactions with host defenses represent further exciting topics that receive extensive discussion within this book.

The editors are grateful to the many distinguished basic and clinical scientists who have contributed to this book, enabling us to offer an unparalleled breadth and depth of scientific information about the cellular mechanisms and therapeutic approaches of host defense dysfunction in trauma, shock, and sepsis. Only this form of integrated approach involving the many disciplines of theoretical and clinical medicine will bring a sound conceptual basis for the management and prevention of sepsis syndrome in the immunocompromised host. We hope that this book will encourage and further promote this approach.

Finally, the editors gratefully acknowledge the cooperation, tremendous efforts, and invaluable work of three individuals who have put all their energy into the creation of this complex book. Christian Schinkel and Svenja Zimmer, as assistant editors, were in charge of the proofreading and the preparation of the subject index, while Evi Gerstmeyr was responsible for the secretarial organization related to this book and the previous congress. The editors are also indebted to the editorial staff of Springer-Verlag for their willingness and terrific support in preparing this book. Finally, they would like to thank Erika Hanesch for the cover design.

Munich, October 1992   Eugen Faist
                                                        Jonathan L. Meakins
                                                    Friedrich W. Schildberg

Table of Contents

Section 3

**From Injury to Multiple Organ Failure:
Sequential Steps of Host Defense Impairment**

3.1 Shock and Ischemia

3.2 Intermediate Inflammatory Phase

Section 4

**Immune Mechanisms for the Control of Infection Under Physiologic
and Stressful Conditions**

Section 5

Inflammatory Mechanisms in Traumatic and Septic Injury

Section 6

Hepatocellular Injury in Ischemia, Trauma and Sepsis

Section 7

Cytokines and Modulation of Cytokine Action

Section 8

Cytokines in Acute Phase States and Trauma

Section 9

The Mediator Role of TNF in Sepsis

Section 10

Endotoxin—Mechanisms of Action and Protection from Shock

Section 11

Clinical Aspects of Multiple Organ Failure

Section 12

**The Pathophysiologic Impact of Bacterial Translocation
and Strategies for Its Prevention**

Section 13

Antibiotic Interactions with Host Defenses

Section 14

The Role of Nutrition in Host Defense

Section 15

New Insights into the Mechanisms of Wound Healing

Section 18

Interventional Strategies in the Therapy of Septic Shock

Section 1

General Aspects/Perspectives

Progress in Trauma Care Through Understanding the Cell Biology of Injury

A. E. Baue

Great progress has been and is being made in trauma care. I will use the broad definition of trauma to include accidental injury, purposeful injury, and operations of an emergency or elective nature. The setting and the magnitude or dose of injury may vary, but the biologic response is similar. Much of the progress in recent years has been of an organizational and educational nature. Centers and systems have been developed so that facilities, transportation, communications, personnel, education, and training for the care of the injured and operated patient are extensive and impressive. This has been reviewed most recently by Dr. Lewis Flint in the February issue of *The American Journal of Surgery* [2]. Dr. Flint points out something that many know: the job of organization of trauma care in the United States is far from complete. The contributions from Switzerland, Austria, Germany, and Great Britain to these developments were reviewed by Dr. Martin Allgower in the same issue of this journal [3]. He describes particularly the early fixation of fractures, stressing the immobilization of fractures to mobilize the patient, and the development of the *Unfallkrankenhaus*—the Accident Hospital.

Much has also been accomplished in diagnosis and therapy, the computed tomography (CT) scanner, intensive care monitoring, and organ support. Much progress has been made, with even greater headway anticipated. There are many real, and even more potential, benefits. The problems of trauma can be divided into five categories, from immediate death to complete survival (Table 1). The only answer for patients in groups A and B is prevention of injury or better protection against injury. I will focus attention on patients in categories C and D, where what we know and what we do make the difference.

This is a period of great excitement. The wonderful world of cytokines and cell and molecular biology show promise in revolutionizing our care of patients. Our understanding of the cell biology of injury has just begun. New mediators are being discovered continually. For example, another novel family of cytokines called macrophage inflammatory proteins 1 and 2 has been identified but as yet has no recognized function [4]. Although this exciting information has greatly increased our understanding of injury, inflammation, and infection, we are not yet able to do much about it. Molecular and cellular biology is leading us

---

Department of Surgery, Saint Louis University Medical Center, 3635 Vista Avenue at Grand Boulevard, St. Louis, MO 63110-0250, USA

Host Defense Dysfunction
in Trauma, Shock and Sepsis
Eds. Faist/Meakins/Schildberg
© Springer-Verlag, Berlin Heidelberg 1993

Table 1. Possible results after injury

Group	Trauma	Possible result
A	Ruptured aorta	Immediate death
B	Irreversible central nervous system injury	Early death
C	Severe multisystem injury	ISS Survival
D	Severe multisystem injury	Should survive unless disaster strikes or Iatrogenic problems develop
E	All survive	

ISS,

Table 2. The biologic systems involved with injury, infection, and inflammation

1. Neuroendocrine response-integrative
2. Cellular mediator response-local with systemic activation[a]
3. Cell-cell and cell matrix response (adherence molecules, receptors)[a]
4. Intracellular response-(heat-shock proteins, etc.)
5. Biologic control mechanisms (feedback loops for control of these responses)
6. Interrelationships and influences of 1, 2, 3, 4 and 5 on each other

[a] Part of the inflammatory response

into an age of understanding from which better care of our patients will come. The world of cytokines will soon be translated into practical approaches.

The contributions in this book emphasize the complexities of injury, infection, and inflammation. Not only must we deal now with the neuroendocrine response to injury and the cellular mediators but also the cell-to-cell and cell-to-matrix responses, the intracellular responses, the biologic control mechanisms of inflammation, and the interrelationships of all of these (Table 2).

Other contributions demonstrate the importance and extent of the local mediators of inflammation that produce the calor, rubor, dolor, and tumor of injury and infection (Table 3). The sequences of clinical events and the interrelationships of systems and organs after injury or operation or illness are complex, as shown in this branching and domino chain of events leading to multiple organ failure (MOF); (Fig. 1).

I will now digress for a moment and use an historic observation to raise a most important question. Paul Ehrlich was a nineteenth century German pioneer in immunology and chemotherapy. As a histochemist he developed the aniline dyes and discovered mast cells. As an immunologist he studied antibodies and complement and developed the side chain theory, for which he received the Nobel Prize in 1908. In later life as a chemotherapist, he developed the arsenicals, the initial chemotherapeutic treatment for syphilis.

In 1901, Ehrlich, along with Morgenroth, wrote in the *Berliner Klinische Wochenschrift* about the "horror autotoxicus" [5]. We read from Ehrlich.

Table 3. Local mediators of acute inflammation

A. Increased microvascular permeability
    Mast cells, basophils → histamine, vasoactive amines
    Kallikrein-kinin system: bradykinin, kallidin
    Eicosanoids, (prostaglandins, prostacyclin and leukotrienes;
    acidic lipids)

B. Leukocyte infiltration: diapedesis, chemotaxis
    Complement system: C5a, C3a
    Leukotriene B_4
    Lysosomal products

C. Tissue damage
    Lysosomal enzymes
    Cachectin
    Other cytokines

D. Vasodilatation
    Prostacyclin
    Serotonin
    Bradykinin

E. Coagulation activation

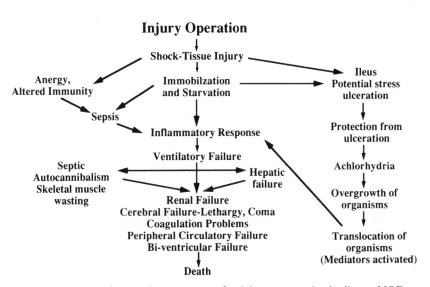

Fig 1. The sequence of events that may occur after injury or operation leading to MOF

In the third communication on isolysins, we pointed out that the organism possesses certain contrivances by means of which the immunity reaction, so easily produced by all kinds of cells, is prevented from acting against the organism's own elements and so giving rise to autotoxins. Further investigations made by us have confirmed this view so that one might be justified in speaking of a "horror autotoxicus" of the organism. The formation of tissue autotoxins would, therefore, constitute a danger threatening the organism.

Ehrlich thought that these regulating contrivances were the disappearance of receptors or the presence of autoantitoxins such as autoanticomplement.

Ehrlich used the term "horror autotoxicus" in 1901 to express his concern for the destruction that an autoimmune reaction could produce. Today, we are learning that patients after operation or with severe injury may be threatened by the very mechanisms that should protect them. Inflammatory reactions or responses to infection so necessary for survival, if overwhelming, could be self-destructive and set in motion the chain of events leading to MOF.

Binz and Wizgell [6] indicated that immunocompetent T lymphocytes do react against self-determinants and that there could be positive consequences of induced autoimmunity to induce specific immune tolerances and for other purposes. Thus there could be a "gaudium autotoxicum" [6].

In another contribution, I address the following theme: "Clinical-Mediator Correlations of MOF and Preventive/Therapeutic Strategies: To Block, Stimulate, or Replace? That is the Question." Several strategies are presently being evaluated in great detail, including the blockade of mediators, particularly if their levels or effects become excessive and threaten the individual. Unfortunately, many of the approaches of blockade prevent production of the mediator and/or require intervention before the insult. Such interventions provide valuable information about mechanisms but little help with treatment. Another approach would be to stimulate lost factors or mediators which could be strengthened. An example of this is the present multi-institutional evaluation of surfactant for the treatment of the adult respiratory distress syndrome (ARDS).

The third approach is to stimulate various biologic activities through the use of growth factors or other mediators that may control some of the toxic factors. A fourth area of activity which has become quite exciting is the study of those natural biologic control mechanisms or feedback loops that try to keep inflammation under control. The approach to decrease or prevent systemic activation of inflammation while maintaining the necessary local effect at the site of injury could be fruitful.

Certainly a form of Ehrlich's horror autotoxicus seems to occur in injured and operated patients, but it is not the concern that Ehrlich had about autoimmunity. Although autoimmunity may develop in injured patients because of the breakdown of proteins, the process is not well understood. It seems that the very mechanisms of inflammation and host defense which are meant to protect the individual from invasion by bacteria, foreign antigens, and foreign materials and from tissue injury may become overactive with severe injury and damage organs and tissues. Does man self-destruct if the injury is severe or the response is overwhelming? The answer seems to be yes. This is shown in a branching logic fashion with injury (Fig. 2). Most patients survive. Some will die of an inadequate host response and some from an overwhelming response.

An example of this biologic conundrum can be provided by the cell adhesion receptors or molecules which are so important in injury and inflammation for

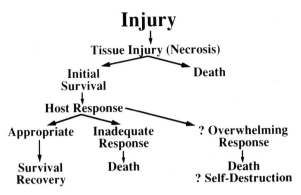

Fig 2. Sequences of events that can occur after injury

Table 4. Cell adhesion molecules and receptors

1. Integrins
   LFA-1
   Fibronectin
   Platelet glycoprotein
2. AM of immunoglobulins
3. Cadherins
4. LEC, CAM, ELAM-1
5. Lymphocyte homing receptors

cell-to-cell and cell-to-matrix attachment (Table 4). They have also been implicated in this self-destruction with overwhelming injury. A monoclonal antibody
to an adherence molecule, CD18, will protect animals from the effects of
hemorrhagic shock [7]. This group has more recently found that this same
monoclonal antibody increases the incidence and severity of abscesses after
Staphylococcus aureus injection in rabbits [8]. In addition, there are congenital
abnormalities of adherence molecules, such as an endothelial leukocyte adhesion molecule (ELAM) deficiency, in which children die of infection at a young
age [9]. Other examples are a lactic acid dehydrogenase (LAD)–integrin B
deficiency which leads to infection and a bleeding disorder is known as
Glanzmann's thrombasthenia. Thus, if excessive activation of these receptors
leads to tissue and organ damage but a deficiency or blockade leads to infection,
can we interfere with these molecules in the injured patient? This presents, then,
a biologic conundrum because the question which must follow is: If inflammation threatens the injured person, can we fool Mother Nature by blocking this
response, or can we block only the excessive portions of it?

Another example is tumor necrosis factor (TNF), which produces the
symptoms of illness with gram negative bacterial infection and endotoxin
injection. In excessive amounts, TNF is destructive; however, in small or

regulated amounts it can protect the host. This presents a great dilemma in the use of blocking factors, particularly in the complex multisystem-injured patient.

I would like to review now the hypotheses of factors that contribute to the development of MOF. These were reviewed some time ago at a symposium led by Dr. James Carrico and published in *Archives of Surgery* [10]:

1. Altered gastrointestinal barrier function in injured patients seems to be an important factor in initiating mediator activation and toxicity, with bacterial translocation.
2. Bacterial invasion, whether involving the lung, the liver, the kidney, the peritoneal cavity, or the pleural space, is an important ingredient in the development of MOF.
3. Systemic immune activation or host defense inflammatory mediator activation that is greater than needed for local control of the injury seems also to be a factor in the production of ARDS and other organ damage.
4. It has been shown by a number of workers, including Goris et al. [11], that inflammation alone with no evidence of bacterial invasion can produce organ damage. This very likely occurs through the same mechanisms as systemic host defense activation from an infectious focus.
5. This hypothesis is a composite of all the previous mechanisms with an emphasis on ischemia. Injury, shock, and sepsis contribute to inadequate blood flow to organs and cells, which combine or contribute to altered gastrointestinal function, mediator activation, and infection. This initiates a cycle of cell and organ injury. I propose that ischemia plays a larger role in the development of MOF than has been thought [12].

This is supported by a study carried out some years ago by Dr. Christopher Baker and our group at Yale [13], in which it was found that the important risk factors or predictors of a fatal outcome following major trauma were, first of all, the age of the patient, secondly, the total injury severity score; and thirdly, the presence of shock (a systolic blood pressure below 80 mm Hg) and the length of time in shock. These patients were resuscitated and operated upon, only to die later of MOF in the intensive care unit. Others have confirmed this observation. Why should the presence and duration of shock in the early injury phase be a predictor of morbidity and mortality at a later time? Does the ischemia-reperfusion injury that occurs at the time of wounding, which is not totally corrected during operation and the immediate postoperative period, contribute to ischemic cell and organ damage, thus adding to the burden and setting the stage for the problems that develop later?

What, then, are specific contributions of cell and molecular biology to the care of the wounded? All of the advances and contributions that I will cite may not have been used as yet in trauma patients; however, that potential exists, and very likely such studies will be forthcoming. I will limit my review to those contributions made in patients, generally through carefully controlled and randomized trials. A large number of animal studies also suggest great benefits from various molecular and cell factors. Other contributions to this book review many of them. I will cite here only those reports which indicate a clinical contribution to the care of patients.

Important studies have investigated the use of monoclonal antibodies against endotoxin. Ziegler et al. [14] reported a randomized, double-blind, placebo-controlled trial of an HA-1A human monoclonal antibody to endotoxin in patients with gram-negative bacteremia. The mortality was 49% for those receiving the placebo and 30% for those receiving the antibody—a significant reduction. Deaths in septic shock patients were reduced from 57% in the placebo group to 33% in those treated with the antibody, also a significant improvement. This antibody was found to be safe and effective for the treatment of patients with sepsis and gram-negative bacteremia.

A similar study has been reported by Bernard et al. [15] using another monoclonal endotoxin antibody called Xoma-E5. It, too, was found to be effective. This approach promises to be an exciting one for the control of gram-negative infection.

There is also considerable excitement in promoting wound healing by the use of various growth factors. Brown et al [16] found that epidermal growth factor accelerated the healing of partial thickness skin wounds (skin graft donor sites), and recommended further studies to determine the clinical importance of their finding.

Recombinant human growth hormone has been found by Herndon et al. [17] to significantly shorten the donor-site healing times in severely burned children. Atri et al. [18] used homologous platelet factors to achieve total healing of recalcitrant skin ulcers in patients. These were chronic, nonhealing skin ulcers in which healing progressed satisfactorily using this substance.

Recombinant human granulocyte colony-stimulating factor (rG-CSF) has been used in several studies. It has been used in patients with congenital agranulocytosis and led to a large increase in the number of functional neutrophils [19].

In another study, cyclic neutropenia was treated with granulocyte cell-stimulating factor (GCSF) in patients and found to be effective [20]. The therapy reduced the frequency of oropharyngeal inflammation, fever, and infections in these patients.

A study by Moore et al. [21] found that patients with major torso trauma had inadequate granulopoiesis and colony-stimulating factor was deficient. The impairment of granulocytes in burn patients in the generation of mediators such as platelet-activating factor and leukotriene B_4 identified by Schonfeld et al. [22] may be amenable to such an approach. Cioffi et al. [23] gave granulocyte-macrophage colony-stimulating factor (GM-CSF) to a group of patients with burns and compared them with controls. White cell counts improved in those treated, increasing significantly after a lag time of about 1 week. In these patients, GM-CSF "primed" the cells for increased oxidative function. This study demonstrated the safety of giving this substance to patients with 20%–70% body burns. However, whether the administration of this growth factor was beneficial or not could not be determined from this nonrandomized study.

Chronic granulomatous disease is an uncommon inherited disorder in which there is defective production by white cells of the reactive intermediates of oxygen. These patients have recurrent and severe pyogenic infections. A controlled trial of interferon-γ by an international cooperative study group was recently reported to prevent infection in such patients [24]. They found that interferon-γ therapy was an effective and well-tolerated treatment that reduced the frequency and severity of infection.

This study also indicates the biologic conundrum with which we must deal. If excess superoxide production is bad, but not having enough is a disaster, can we ever block superoxide production or its effects in the multi-system injured patient without increasing the likelihood of infection and other problems?

Manson et al. [25] found that recombinant human growth hormone promoted nitrogen retention and protein synthesis in malnourished patients receiving only hypocaloric parenteral nutrition. These and other investigators are now evaluating whether this effect will occur in severely stressed injured patients and whether these changes will make any difference in their outcome.

Gore et al. [26] studied isolated limbs of burn patients and found that human growth hormone (HGH) decreased breakdown and increased protein synthesis. This will require further confirmation. Septic patients, however, failed to respond to biosynthetic HGH, according to Dahn et al. [27]. Their patients, in contrast to normal controls, failed to reduce nitrogen losses and increase insulinlike growth factor 1 (IGF-1) production with HGH administration. It is known that IGF-1 is inhibited in such patients and this may be the reason why HGH was ineffective. Whether or not the use of insulinlike growth factor itself will make a difference in injured or septic patients remains to be determined.

Gottardis et al. [28] reported on the administration of recombinant HGH to 20 patients with sepsis. IGF-1 increased significantly after the administration of HGH. Nitrogen balance did not become positive, but urea production could be reduced. The results indicate this treatment might improve the nitrogen intake but had no influence on the course of sepsis.

There has been considerable interest in enteral feeding in injured patients because of its potential additional effect on the mucosal integrity of the gastrointestinal tract and reduction in bacterial translocation. Enteral feeding soon after injury was found to be safe and effective in delivering nutritional support to burn patients by McDonald et al. [29]. One positive feature of this study was that the enteral feedings prevented upper gastrointestinal bleeding and eliminated the need for antacids of H_2-blockers. Whether these patients benefited further from this approach could not be determined.

Enteral nutrition was compared with parental nutrition in patients following major abdominal trauma by Moore et al. [30] They found that enteral nutrition was well tolerated in these severely injured patients and that the incidence of septic complications seemed to be reduced. There was a significant decrease in major septic morbidity in the treated patients. Obviously this work requires confirmation in larger and multiple studies.

Interesting work continues on the alterations in host resistance that develop with injury. Recent clinical reports indicate that patients with major burns have inadequate IL-2 production, which seems to underlie the defects in cell-mediated immunity seen in these patients [31]. Faist et al. [32] have again confirmed that indomethacin administration (cyclooxygenase inhibition) in patients with major surgical trauma provided considerable alleviation of post-operative monocytosis and improved delayed type hypersensitivity, but IL-2 synthesis was not increased over the control group. There seemed to be a lower rate of early opportunistic infections in the treated patients. Prolonged use of indomethacin could improve these results.

The importance of oxygen delivery and consumption in injured and septic patients has been emphasized by Shoemaker and his group [33]. Bihari et al. [34] evaluated a 30-min infusion of the vasodilator prostacyclin to 27 critically ill patients with acute respiratory failure. They found increases in oxygen delivery and oxygen consumption. The oxygen uptake increase was greater in patients who died. This suggested a substantial oxygen debt in those patients and emphasizes the potential importance of promoting a higher than normal oxygen transport and consumption in patients before MOF develops.

Arginine has been used as a dietary supplement in normal human volunteers and was found to increase lymphocyte mitogenesis and enhance the amount of collagen deposited into a standardized wound [35]. Wilmore's observation, presented elsewhere in this volume, that glutamine given to patients having bone marrow transplants decreased the number of infections suggests potential clinical application in the injured patient.

Dominioni et al. [36] from Varese, Italy gave high-dose immunoglobulin G (IgG) to a number of septic surgical patients in a randomized study. The IgG-treated group had a significantly lower mortality (38% compared to 67%). Septic shock was the cause of death in 7% of the IgG-treated patients and in 33% of the controls. This is most interesting and stimulating and also requires confirmation and more detailed evaluation.

Part of the biologic conundrum facing us consists of the differences between various experimental models and complex clinical situations. The sequential pattern of eicosanoid, platelet, and neutrophil activation and interaction has been described by Rivkind et al. [37] in multiply injured trauma patients. The production by neutrophils of leukotriene B_4 in surgical patients at risk for the development of ARDS was found to be greatly increased at the same time that there was complement activation. Davis et al. [38] believed that this is a predictor of subsequent ARDS. In contrast to this, Girotti et al. [39] found no evidence of oxygen-induced membrane damage as manifested by increased plasma levels of conjugated dienes or malondialdehyde within 2–6 h of blunt injury. Could it be occurring later?

There is no doubt that the inflammatory mediators play a role such as that of histamine, complement, and xanthine oxidase in thermal injury of skin as shown by Friedl et al. [40]. However, nonspecific macrophage stimulation by glucan in

Table 5. Relationships of clinical problems, therapy, and the underlying mechanisms

Clinical	Treatment	Pathophysiology	Cellular-molecular
Shock	Resuscitation	Ischemia-reperfusion Altered host resistance	Leukotrienes Thromboxane
CNS injury	Decompression	Edema Blood, Vascular spasm	
Aortic rupture Crushed chest Liver lacerations Dirty wounds	 Repair Support Debridement	 Tissue Necrosis, Inflammation	Cytokines WBC's activated Macrophages Histamine Kallikreins

Colon-GI
    injuries
	Repair
	Exteriorization
	Delayed primary
	    closure of wounds
		Contamination
		Sepsis
			TNF
			Interleukins
			complement
			other mediators

Fractures	Immobilization	Injury	Mediators
Burns	Wound excision, Coverage	Hyper metabolism Infection	Mediators
Crushed extremities	Debridement amputation	Tissue Necrosis	Mediators

WBC, white blood cells; TNF, tumor necrosis factor; GI, gastrointestinal

trauma patients was associated with a lower mortality in general but not that due to sepsis [41]. Serum IL-1 but not TNF was greater in the glucan group.

Available treatment seems so simple compared to what is being learned about pathophysiology and the cellular-molecular mediators. The challenge is to move this information over into the therapy list. How do we approach these cellular-molecular complexities in the multisystem-injured patient? If we compare clinical abnormalities and their presently available treatments for these abnormalities with the pathophysiologic abnormalities that develop and the cellular or molecular mediators produced, we recognize the difficulty of the situation (Table 5).

We return then to the principles of prevention of MOF in 1991. The following seven major areas seem to be worthy of note:

1. Improving microcirculatory blood flow early after injury to decrease ischemia-reperfusion injury
2. Stopping or controlling the injury by early definitive operation
3. Removing as much necrotic tissue as soon as possible
4. Promoting a higher than normal oxygen transport and consumption
5. Supporting metabolism and the gut
6. Preventing infection by maintaining adequate host defenses, appropriate antibiotic use, and wound and body cavity care
7. Treating infection early and adequately if it develops

Table 6. Terms used to describe problems related to
multiple organ failure

- Multi-organ instability (MOI)
- Malignant intravascular inflammation
- Hyperemic hypoxia
- Biologic cyanide capsule
- The septic hypermetabolic state
- Septic syndrome
- Posttraumatic organ-system infection
  syndrome (PTOSIS)

In summary, progress is being made in the care of the injured and operated
patient. There is great promise that cell and molecular biology will make
immense contributions not only to our understanding of injury but to our
therapeutic capability as well, and along with these possibilities and successes,
new terms, expressions, or acronyms will be added to our list of names and
responses: (Table 6) shows some of those presently used and debated. Multiorgan instability occurs with injury and may lead to MOF. I suggest that posttraumatic organ system infection syndrome not only covers it all but provides a
useful acronym: ptosis

References

1. Faist E, Baue AE, Ditmer H, Heberer G (1983) Multiple organ failure in polytrauma patients.
   J Trauma 23:775–787
2. Flint L (1991) Achievements, present-day problems, and some solutions for trauma care,
   surgical critical care and surgical education. Am J Surg 161:207–212
3. Allgower M (1991) Trauma systems in Europe. Am J Surg 161:226–229
4. Wolpe SD, Cerami A (1989) Macrophage inflammatory proteins 1 and 2: members of a novel
   superfamily of cytokines. FASEB J 3:2565–2573
5. Ehrlich P, Morganroth J (1901) II. Ueber Hamylysine. Fünfte Mitteilung. Berl Klin Wochenschr
   38:251–257
6. Binz H, Wigzell H (1978) Horror autotoxicus. Fed Proc 37:2365–2369
7. Vedder NB, Fouty BW, Winn RK, Harlan JM, Rice CL (1989) Role of neutrophilis in
   generalized reperfusion injury associated with resuscitation from shock. Surgery 106:509–516
8. Sharar SR, Winn RK, Harlan JM, Rice CL (1991) Anti-CD 18 antibody increases the incidence
   and severity of subsutaneous abscess formation after high dose *S. aureus* injection in rabbits.
   Surgery (in press)
9. Albelda SM, Buck CA (1990) Integrins and other cell adhesion molecules. FASEB J
   4:2868–2880
10. Carrico CJ, Meakins J, Marshall JC et al. (1986) Multiple organ failure syndrome. Arch Surg
    121:196–208
11. Goris RJA, teBoekhorst TPA, Nuytinek JKS (1985) Multiple organ failure: generalized auto-
    destructive inflammation? Arch Surg 120:1109–1115
12. Baue AE (1990) Theories and common threads in multiple organ failure. In: Baue AE (ed)
    Multiple organ failure: patient care and prevention. Mosby, St Louis, pp 473–486
13. Baker CE, Degutis LC (1986) Predicting outcome in multiple trauma patients. Infect Surg
    5:243–245
14. Ziegler EJ et al. (1991) Treatment of gram-negative bacteremia and septic shock with HA-1A
    human monoclonal antibody against endotoxin. N Engl J Med 324:429–436

15. Bernard GR, Grossman JE, Campbell GD, Gorelich RP, Xomas Sepsis Study Group (1989) Multicenter trial of monoclonal anti-endotoxin antibody (Xoma-E5) in gram-negative sepsis. Chest 98:137
16. Brown GL et al. (1989) Enhancement of wound healing by topical treatment with epidermal growth factor. N Engl J Med 321:75–79
17. Herndon DN et al. (1990) Effects of recombinant human growth hormone on donor-site healing in severely burned children. Ann Surg 212:424–431
18. Atri SC, Misra J, Bisht D, Misra K (1990) Use of homologous platelet factors in achieving total healing of recalcitrant skin ulcers. Surgery 108:508–512
19. Bonilla MA et al. (1989) Effects of recombinant human granulocyte colony-stimulating factor on neutropenia in patients with congenital agranulocytois. N Engl J Med 320:1574–1580
20. Hammond WP et al. (1989) Treatment of cyclic neutropenia with granulocyte colony-stimulating factor. N Engl J Med 320:1306–1316
21. Moore FA et al. (1990) Inadequate granulopoiesis after major torso trauma: a hematopoietic regulatory paradox. Surgery 108:667–674
22. Schonfeld W et al. (1990) Metabolism of platelet activating factor (PAF) and lyso-PAF in polymorphonuclear granulocytes from severly burned patients. J Trauma 30:1554–1561
23. Cioffi WG et al. (1991) Effects of granulocyte-macrophage colony-stimulating factor in burn patients. Arch Surg 126:74–79
24. Gallin JI et al. (1991) Controlled trial of interferon gamma to prevent infection in chronic granulomatous disease. N Engl J Med 324:509–516
25. Manson JM, Smith RJ, Wilmore DW (1988) Growth hormone stimulates protein synthesis during hypocaloric parenteral nutrition. Ann Surg 208:136–149
26. Gore DC et al. (1991) Effects of exogenous growth hormone on whole-body and isolated-limb protein kinetics in burned patients. Arch Surg 126:38–43
27. Dahn MS, Lange MP, Jacobs LA (1988) Insulin-like growth factor 1 production is inhibited in human sepsis. Arch Surg 123:1409–1414
28. Gottardis M et al. (1991) Improvement of septic syndrome after administration of recombinant human growth hormone (rhGH). J Trauma 31:81
29. McDonald WS, Sharp CW, Deitch EA (1991) Immediate enteral feeding in burn patients is safe and effective. Ann Surg 213:177–183
30. Moore FA et al. (1989) TEN versus TPN following major abdominal trauma-reduced septic morbidity. J Trauma 29:916–923
31. Wood JJ et al. (1984) Inadequate interleukin-2 production: a fundamental immunological deficiency in patients with major burns. Ann Surg 200:311–319
32. Faist E et al. (1991) Immunoprotective effects of cyclooxygenase inhibition in patients with major surgical trauma. J Trauma 30:8–18
33. Shoemaker WC et al. (1988) Prospective trial of supranormal values of survivors as therapeutic goals in high risk surgical patients. Chest 94:1176–1186
34. Bihari D et al. (1987) The effects of vasodilation with prostacyclin on oxygen delivery and uptake in critically ill patients. N Engl J Med 317:397–403
35. Barbul A et al. (1990) Arginine enhances wound healing and lymphocyte immune responses in humans. Surgery 108:331–337
36. Dominioni L et al. (1991) Effects of high-dose IgG on survival of surgical patients with sepsis scores of 20 or greater. Arch Surg 126:236–240
37. Rivkind A et al. (1989) Sequential patterns of eicosanoid, platelet, and neutrophil interactions in the evolution of the fulminant post-traumatic adult respiratory distress syndrome. Ann Surg 210:355–373
38. Davis JM et al. (1990) Elevated production of neutrophil leukotriene B_4 precedes pulmonary failure in critically ill surgical patients. Surgery 170:495–500
39. Girotti MJ et al. (1991) Early measurement of systemic lipid peroxidation products in the plasma of major blunt trauma patients. J Trauma 31:32–35
40. Friedl HP, Till GO, Trentz O, Ward PA (1989) Roles of histamine, complement and xanthine oxidase in thermal injury of skin. Am J Pathol 135:203–217
41. Browder W et al. (1990) Beneficial effect of enhanced macrophage function in the trauma patient. Ann Surg 211:605–613
42. Baue AE (ed) (1990) Multiple organ failure: patient care and prevention. Mosby, St Louis

Trauma, Sepsis, and Immune Defects

J. A. Mannick

Traumatic injury and burns remain a major cause of morbidity and mortality in the United States and despite modern techniques of resuscitation and intensive care and an ever increasing number of powerful and effective antibiotics nearly 80% of deaths that occur in trauma and burn patients more than 7 days after injury are caused by sepsis [1]. During the past 10 years the longstanding clinical assumption that host defenses against invading microorganisms were impaired following severe injury has become grounded in fact through the study of injured patients and appropriate animal models. Abnormalities in both specific and nonspecific mechanisms of defense against microorganisms have been described by a number of laboratories, including our own. Nonspecific mechanisms include function of polymorphonuclear [2–4] and mononuclear phagocytes [5–6], natural killer cells [7–9], and products of complement activation [10–13]. Specific defense mechanisms include antibody formation by B lymphocytes [14–16], direct microbial killing by T lymphocytes, and T lymphocyte activation of mononuclear phagocytes [17–19].

It has become apparent over the past 5 years that serious injury is accompanied by alterations in the secretion of cytokines by cells of the immune system [6, 19–22] as well as by increases in circulating "stress" hormones including cortisol, epinephrine, and glucagon [23]. Alterations in the synthesis of prostanoids also occur [6, 24–26].

It is clear that the cells involved in the specific and nonspecific defense against microorganisms communicate with one another by means of cytokines and other molecular mediators and that alterations in cytokine secretion are likely to play a major role in producing the perturbation of host responses against microorganisms found after injury [19, 20, 22, 27]. It is also clear that the stress hormones released in response to injury influence the behavior of the immune system [28, 29] and that cytokines released by immunocompetent cells have a number of important metabolic actions [30]. Thus the interplay of various cytokines and hormones is not only reflected in the metabolic abnormalities known to accompany serious injury, but also in the immunologic derangements which are noted under the same circumstances.

Recent attention has focused on cells of the monocyte/macrophage lineage as playing a central role in abnormalities of host defense following injury.

Harvard Medical School, Department of Surgery, Brigham and Women's Hospital, 75 Francis St., Boston, MA 02115, USA

Host Defense Dysfunction
in Trauma, Shock and Sepsis
Eds. Faist/Meakins/Schildberg
© Springer-Verlag, Berlin Heidelberg 1993

Several investigators have observed an increase in the secretion of tumor necrosis factor α (TNF), interleukin-1 (IL-1), and interleukin-6 (IL-6) [6, 20–22] by this family of mononuclear cells in response to injury. The same cells have been shown to produce increased quantities of prostaglandin E_2 (PGE_2) [6, 25, 26], a powerful inhibitor of lymphocyte activation. Thus, modulation of cytokine and prostanoid secretion by monocytes and macrophages may be an important mechanism for controlling the abnormalities of host defenses following injury. Recent studies from our laboratory and from others have shown that polymorphonuclear leukocytes (PMN) are not simply phagocytic cells, but are also important sources of cytokines, responding in the same fashion as monocytes or macrophages with the elaboration of IL-1, TNF and IL-6 [31–33] (Rodrick, unpublished observations). Thus the interaction of these cells with cells of the immune system is also likely to be important in altering host defenses in injured patients.

In the current immunologic literature, considerable attention has been given to evidence that under certain conditions T-helper lymphocytes can be subdivided into two functionally distinct subsets, T-helper 1 (Th1) and T-helper 2 (Th2) [34, 35]. Th1 cells are believed to play a primary role in cellular immunity including delayed hypersensitivity and secrete principally IL-2 and interferon-γ (IFN-γ). Th2 cells are believed to act principally in inducing antibody formation and secrete predominantly IL-4, IL-5, and the recently characterized IL-10 [36]. In some studies IFN-γ has been shown to downregulate Th2 proliferation and IL-10 has been found to decrease Th1 cytokine production. Although the classification of T-helper cells into these subsets is based largely on analyses of mouse clones, recent data suggest that even in humans different diseases are associated with development of cells of the Th1 and Th2 phenotypes. Thus these two subsets may represent differentiated helper T-cells and their development may reflect particular types of antigenic stimulation. The clinical relevance of these observations is unknown. However, since critically injured patients and animals are known to lack delayed hypersensitivity and to manifest impaired IL-2 production, both Th1 activities, it seems appropriate now to look for increased Th2 activity in such individuals and in relevant animal models.

Suppression of lymphocyte activation by serum or serum fractions from seriously injured patients has also been reported by our laboratory and by others [37–40]. Our group was perhaps the first to suggest that serum factors played a role in the immune deficiency seen in trauma and burn patients [37]. The serum suppressive activity is chiefly found in a low molecular weight polypeptide-containing fraction which has recently been purified to apparent homogeneity. This fraction, which is nontoxic to cells, is inhibitory of T lymphocyte activation by mitogens and of T cell-dependent antibody formation in vitro. This fraction is also suppressive of IL-2 synthesis by normal human peripheral blood lymphocytes [41]. The source of the serum suppressive peptide fraction remains unknown at this point, but its activities clearly resemble some of those described for IL-10 [36] and for transforming growth factor-β (TGF-β) [42], and the possible identity of the serum suppressive fraction recovered in our laboratory and these known cytokines needs to be explored. Circulating suppressor substances have also been described by other investigators in a variety of disease states. A low molecular weight suppressor peptide has been found in burn serum Ninneman, Ozkan, and their associates [40]. These investigators have attributed the activity of their peptide to its ability to bind prostaglandins, particularly PGE_2, though recently this idea apparently has been discarded. We have been unable to demonstrate PGE_2 in our serum suppressive peptide fractions. However, the in vivo activity of our suppressive peptide fraction can be abrogated by cyclooxygenase inhibitors [43] thus suggesting that the material acts, at least in part, by altering prostaglandin synthesis.

Abnormalities of PMN function noted after serious injury, and once believed to be signs of unresponsiveness of this cell population, now appear to be clearly the result of hyperactivation of these cells [44, 45]. Impaired PMN chemotaxis has been documented by several groups following major thermal or traumatic injury. Studies from our own and other laboratories suggest that after major burn injury there is a temporary impairment of PMN chemotaxis to the C5a in zymosan-activated serum [4, 17, 44]. This recovers promptly and does not appear to be related to sepsis. However, septic trauma and burn patients, as well as septic patients in general, characteristically manifest impairment of PMN chemotaxis to C5a though not consistently to F-Met-Leu-Phe (FMLP) [44]. However, we have found that phagocytosis and bactericidal activity of PMNs from trauma, burn, and other septic patients are normal or increased as compared with simultaneously studied controls [46], a finding at variance with reports from other investigators and possibly related to the timing of the studies [3]. We, in collaboration with Dr. Francis Moore Jr [44], have shown that major injury is followed by a marked increase in the expression of CR1 and CR3 receptors on PMN as determined by the monoclonal antibody technique of Fearon and Collins. Sepsis is also associated with the same findings. These results suggest that diminished chemotaxis to zymosan-activated serum may represent a downregulation of responsiveness to C5a because of prior exposure to high concentrations of this material. The increased expression of CR3 receptors (i.e., the CD11, CD18 complex) on circulating PMN increases the ability of these cells to adhere to intercellular adhesion molecule 1 (ICAM-1) induced by inflammatory cytokines on endothelial cells [47]. This may play a major role in producing the pulmonary capillary damage and the resultant interstitial pulmonary edema observed in traumatized and septic patients.

Antibody formation was once believed to be normal in trauma and burn patients, but recent reports suggest that, following serious injury, antibody formation to common protein antigens is impaired [14–16], and that this impairment is accompanied by a marked increase in nonspecific polyclonal immunoglobulin synthesis by circulating B lymphocytes in the same patients, a situation analogous to that reported for individuals with acquired immunodeficiency syndrome (AIDS). However, the antibody response to bacterial polysaccharide antigens remains intact. Work from our laboratory has shown that impaired responsiveness to tetanus toxoid in burn patients is associated with markedly diminished IL-2 production by the peripheral blood mononuclear cells (PBMC) of the same patients [48], thus suggesting, but not proving, a casual relationship between deficient T helper cell activity and depression of antibody response to protein antigens.

While the immunologic abnormalities associated with injury have been described in considerable detail, mechanisms are less well understood and potential therapies are just now beginning to be put forward. One likely trigger mechanism for a number of the alterations in host defenses noted after serious injury is endotoxin leak from the gut or translocation of endotoxin-producing bacteria from the gut, both of which have been well described by a number of investigators [49, 50]. With this in mind, our laboratory and others have made detailed observations on the effect of the infusion of small amounts of endotoxin into human volunteers [51–54]. Studies in our laboratory revealed that a number of the immunologic abnormalities associated with traumatic injury can be duplicated by endotoxin infusion [51]. These include depression of both T lymphocyte proliferation and secretion of IL-2 and an initial depression followed by subsequent overshoot of the production of IL-1, TNF, and IL-6 by circulating monocytes. Increased secretion of PGE_2 by the latter cells has also been detected. No complement activation was noted with the dose of endotoxin used in these studies. However, increased complement receptor expression on PMNs was observed as an endotoxin effect [54].

The work of other groups, specifically Cannon et al. [52] and Fong et al [53], on similarly treated normal volunteers has shown that IL-1, IL-6, and TNF levels in the plasma or serum all may be increased after endotoxin challenge. Our results on cytokine secretion by in vitro stimulated adherent cells suggest a negative regulation of IL-1 and TNF secretion shortly after endotoxin infusion, which could be due to a negative feedback by cytokines already secreted in vivo and detected in the blood. Increased circulating levels of these inflammatory cytokines could clearly account for a number of the physiologic and immunologic abnormalities noted after endotoxin infusion or after serious injury.

Thus an explanation for many if not all of the immunologic abnormalities associated with major injury which fits the known facts is that the trigger is release of endotoxin from the gut directly or by bacteria which have translocated from the gut. This stimulus in turn could induce secretion of prostaglandins of the E series, particularly PGE_2, by monocytes, macrophages, and possibly by PMNs, and could further induce these cells to produce inflammatory cytokines, particularly TNF. Increased TNF production can account for most of the observed metabolic and physiologic derangements associated with major injury or the septic state. Increased PGE_2 production can clearly explain the inhibition of lymphocyte activation and deficient IL-2 production noted under the same circumstances. Alterations of PMN function can be explained as a response to cytokines (e.g., TNF and IL-8), to prostaglandins, and to complement activation, which in turn may be caused by endotoxin directly or by antibody interactions with the translocated bacteria themselves. It is also clear that endotoxin alone can activate PMNs [46].

Most aspects of this hypothetical explanation for the perturbations of host defenses associated with serious injury and sepsis are now being tested or will be tested in the near future in a number of laboratories throughout the world. Current and future knowledge of mechanisms underlying the observed perturbations will clearly direct attempts at therapy, some of which are already undergoing testing in animals and, in a few instances, in man. An incomplete list includes anti-endotoxin antibodies, cyclooxygenase inhibitors, low dose IL-2, endotoxin binding by low-dose polymyxin, granulocyte–macrophage colony-stimulating factor (GM-CSF), and anti-TNF-α antibodies.

We have good reason to be optimistic that within 5 years we will have in hand safe and effective therapeutic measures to prevent and counteract the defective resistance to invading microorganisms paradoxically manifested by seriously injured and septic patients.

References

1. Baker CC, Oppenheimer L, Stephens B, Lewis FR, Trunkey DD (1980) Epidemiology of trauma deaths. Am J Surg 140:144–150
2. Grogan JB, Miller RC (1975) Impaired function of polymorphonuclear leukocytes in patients with burns and other trauma. Surgery 78:316
3. Alexander JW, Ogle CK, Stinnett JD, MacMillan BG (1978) A sequential, prospective analysis of immunologic abnormalities and infection following severe thermal injury. Ann Surg 188:809
4. Maderazo E, Albano SD, Wornick CL, Drezner AD, Quercia R (1983) Polymorphonuclear leukocyte migration abnormalities and their significance in severely traumatized patients. Ann Surg. 198:736
5. Stephan RN, Ayala A, Harkema JM, Dean RE, Border JR, Chaudry IH (1989) Mechanism of immunosuppression following hemorrhage: defective antigen presentation by macrophages. J Surg Res 46:553–556
6. Takayama TK, Miller C, Szabo G (1990) Elevated tumor necrosis factor α production concomitant to elevated prostaglandin E_2 production by trauma patients' monocytes. Arch Surg 125:29–35
7. Stein MD, Gamble DV, Klempel DH, Herdon DH, Klempel GR (1984) Natural killer cell defects resulting from thermal injury. Cell Immunol 86:551–556
8. Blazar BA, Rodrick ML, O'Mahony JB, Wood JJ, Bessey PQ, Wilmore DW, Mannick JA (1986) Suppression of natural killer cell function in man following thermal and traumatic injury. J Clin Immunol 6:26–36
9. Garcia-Penarrubia P, Bankhurst AD, Koster FT (1989) Experimental and theoretical kinetics study of antibacterial killing mediated by human natural killer cells. J. Immunol 142:1310–1317
10. Gelfand JA, Donelan M, Burke JF (1983) Preferential activation and depletion of the alternative complement pathway by burn injury. Ann Surg 198:58
11. Fearon DT, Collins LA (1983) Increased expression of C3b receptors on polymorphonuclear leukocytes induced by chemotactic factors and by purification procedures. J Immunol 130:370
12. Solomkin JS, Cotta LA, Ogle JD, Brodt JK, Ogle CK, Satoh PS, Hurst JM, Alexander JW (1984) Complement-induced expression of cryptic receptors on the neutrophil surface: a mechanism for regulation of acute inflammation in trauma. Surgery 96:336
13. Morgan EL, Thoman ML, Weigle WO, Hugli TE (1985) Human C3a-mediated suppression of the immune response. I. Suppression of murine in vitro antibody responses occurs through the generation of non-specific Lyt-2 T cell. Immunology 134:51

14. Nohr CW, Christou NV, Rode H, Gordon J, Meakins JL (1984) Abnormal in vitro immunoglobulin production in surgical patients. Surg Forum 35:146–148
15. Wood JJ, O'Mahony JB, Rodrick ML, Mannick JA (1984) Immunoglobulin production and suppressor T cells after thermal injury. Surg Forum 35:619–621
16. Nohr CW, Christou NV, Rode H, Gordon J, Meakins JL (1984) In vivo and in vitro humoral immunity in surgical patients. Ann. Surg 200:373–380
17. Meakins JL, Pietsch JB, Bubenick O, Kelly R, Rode H, Gordon J, Maclean LD (1977) Delayed hypersensitivity: indicator of acquired failure of host defenses in sepsis and trauma. Ann Surg 182:207–217
18. Organ BC, Antonacci AC, Chiao J, Kumar A, de Riesthal HF, Yuan L, Black D, Calvano SE (1989) Changes in lymphocyte number and phenotype in seven lymphoid compartments after thermal injury. Ann Surg 210:78–89
19. Wood JJ, Rodrick MD, O'Mahony JB, Palder SB, Saporoschetz I, d'Eon P, Mannick JA (1984) Inadequate interleukin-2 production: a fundamental immunological deficiency in patients with major burns. Ann Surg 311–320
20. Marano MA, Fong Y, Moldawer LL, Wei H, Calvano SE, Tracey KJ, Barie PS, Manogue K, Cerami A, Shires GT, Lowry SF (1990) Serum cachetin/tumor necrosis factor in critically ill patients with burns correlates with infection and mortality. Surg. Gynecol Obstet 170:32–38
21. Grzelak I, Olszewski WL, Rowinski W (1989) Blood mononuclear cell production of IL-1 and IL-2 following moderate surgical trauma. Eur Surg Res 21:114–122
22. Guo Y, Dickerson C, Chrest FJ, Adler WH, Munster AM, Winchurch RA (1990) Increased levels of circulating interleukin-6 in burn patients. Clin Immunol Immunopathol 54:361–371
23. Bessey PQ, Watters JM, Aoki TT, Wilmore DW (1984) Combined hormonal infusion stimulates the metabolic response to injury. Ann Surg 200:264–681
24. Ninnemann JL, Stockland AE (1984) Participation of prostaglandin E in immunosuppression following thermal injury. J Trauma 24:201–207
25. Goodwin JS, Bromberg S, Staszak C, Kaszubowski PA, Messner RP, Neal JF (1981) Effect of physical stress on sensitivity of lymphocytes to inhibition by prostaglandin E_2. J Immunol 127:518–522
26. Faist E, Ertel W, Cohnert T, Huber P, Inthorn D, Heberer G (1990) Immunoprotective effects of cyclooxygenase inhibition in patients with major surgical trauma. J Trauma 30:8–17
27. Mayoral JL, Schweich CJ, Dunn DL (1990) Decreased tumor necrosis factor production during the initial stages of infection correlates with survival during murine gram-negative sepsis. Arch Surg 125:24–28
28. Richardson RP, Rhyne CD, Fong Y, Hesse DG, Tracey KJ, Marano MA, Lowry SF, Antonacci AC, Calvano SE (1984) Peripheral blood leukocyte kinetics following in vivo lipopolysaccharide (LPS) administration to normal human subjects. Influence of elicited hormones and cytokines. Ann Surg 210:239–245
29. Michie HR, Wilmore DW (1990) Sepsis, signals, and surgical sequelae (hypothesis). Arch Surg 125:531–536
30. Mealy K, van Lanschot JJB, Robinson BG, Rounds J, Wilmore WD (1990) Are the catabolic effects of tumor necrosis factor mediated by glucocorticoids? Arch Surg 125:42–48
31. Dubravec D, Grbic J, Horgan P, Rodrick M, Collins K, Ellwanger K, Mannick JA (1988) Interleukin-1 (IL-1) production by polymorphonuclear neutrophils (PMN) is regulated by the endogenous cyclooxygenase pathway. Fed Proc 47:A1602
32. Tiku K, Tiku ML, Skosey JL (1986) Interleukin-1 production by human polymorphonuclear neutrophils J Immunol 136:3677–3685
33. Dubravec D, Spriggs DR, Mannick JA, Rodrick ML (1990) Circulating human peripheral granulocytes synthesize and secrete tumor necrosis factor alpha. Proc Natl Acad Sci USA 87:6758–6761
34. Daynes RA, Araneo BA, Dowell TA, Huang K, Donald D (1990) Regulation of murine lymphokine production in vivo. III. The lymphoid tissue microenvironment exerts regulatory influences over T helper cell function. J Exp Med 171:979–996
35. Mosmann TR, Coffman RL (1989) Th1 and Th2 cells: different patterns of lymphokine secretion lead to different functional properties. Annu Rev Immunol 7:145
36. Moore KW, Vieira P, Fiorentino DF, Trounstine ML, Khan TA, Mosmann TR (1990) Homology of cytokine synthesis inhibitory factor (IL-10) to the Epstein-Barr virus gene BCRFI. Science 248:1230–1243
37. Constantian MB, Menzoian JO, Nimberg RB, Schmid K, Mannick JA (1977) Association of a

circulating immunosuppressive polypeptide with operative and accidental trauma. Ann Surg 185:73–79

38. McLoughlin GA, Wu AV, Saporochetz I, Nimberg R, Mannick JA (1979) Correlation between anergy and a circulating immunosuppressive factor following major surgical trauma. Ann Surg 190(3):297–304

39. Wolfe JHN, Wu AVO, O'Connor NE, Saporoschetz I, Mannick JA (1982) Anergy, immunosuppressive serum, and impaired lymphocyte blastogenesis in burn patients. Arch Surg 117:1266–1271

40. Ozkan AN, Ninnemann JL (1985) Suppression of in vitro lymphocyte and neutrophil responses by a low molecular suppressor active peptide from burn-patient sera. J Clin Immunol 5:172–179

41. Rodrick ML, Saporoschetz I, Wood JJ, Grbic JT, Palder SB, Mannick JA (1985) Inhibition of human interleukin-2 (IL-2) production and action by human serum. Cell Mol Biol Lymphokines 761:765

42. Espervik T, Waage A, Faxvaag A, Shalaby M (1990) Regulation of interleukin-2 and interleukin-6 production from T cells: involvement of interleukin-1 β and transforming growth factor β. Cell Immuno 126:47–56

43. Horgan PG, Rodrick ML, Ellwanger K, Collins KC, Dubravec D, Mannick JA (1988) In vivo effects of an inmmunosuppressive factor isolated from patients following thermal injury. Surg Forum 44:96–99

44. Moore FD, Davis CF, Rodrick M, Mannick JA, Fearon DT (1986) Neutrophil activation in thermal injury as assessed by complement receptor upregulation. N Engl J Med 314: 948–953

45. Christou NV, Tellado JM (1989) In vitro polymorphonuclear neutrophil function in surgical patients does not correlate with anergy but with "activating" processes such as sepsis or trauma. Surgery 106:718–724

46. Davis CF, Moore FD, Jr, Rodrick ML, Fearon DT, Mannick JA (1987) Neutrophil activation after burn injury: contributions of the classic complement pathway and of endotoxin. Surgery 102:477–484

47. Smith C, Marlin SD, Rothlein R, Toman C, Anderson D (1989) Cooperative interactions of LFA-1 and Mac-1 with intercellular adhesion molecule-1 in facilitating adherence and transendothelial migration of human neutrophils in vitro. J Clin Invest 83:2008–2017

48. Wood JJ, O'Mahony JB, Rodrick ML, Eaton R, Demling R, Mannick JA (1986) Abnormalities of antibody production following thermal injury: an association with reduced interleukin-2 production. Arch Surg 121:108–115

49. Deitch E (1990) Intestinal permeability is increased in burn patients shortly after injury. Surgery 107:411–416

50. Jones WG, Minei JP, Barber AE, Rayburn JL, Fahey TJ, Shires GT (1990) Bacterial translocation and intestinal atrophy after thermal injury and burn wound sepsis. Ann Surg 211: 399–405

51. Rodrick ML, Michie HR, Moss NM, Grbic JT, Revhaug A, O'Dwyer ST, Gough DB, Dubravec D, McK. Manson J, Wilmore DW, Mannick JA (1989) In vivo infusion of a single dose of endotoxin in healthy humans causes in vitro alterations of both T-cell and adherent cell functions. In: Faist E, Ninnemann JL, Green DR (eds) Immune consequences of trauma, shock and sepsis. Springer, Berlin, Heidelberg New York

52. Cannon JG, Tompkins RG, Gelfand JA, Michie HR, Stanford GG, van der Meer JWM, Enders S, Lonemann G, Corsetti J, Chernow B, Wilmore D, Wolff SM, Burke JF, Dinarello CA (1990) Circulating interleukin-1 and tumor necrosis factor in septic shock and experimental endotoxin fever. J Infect Dis 161:79–84

53. Fong Y, Moldawer LL, Marano M, Wei H, Tatter SB, Clarick RH, Santhanam U, Sherris D, May LT, Sehgal PB, Lowry SF (1989) Endotoxemia elicits increased circulating β-IFN/IL-6 in man. J Immunol 142:2321–2324

54. Moore FD Jr, Moss NM, Revhaug AV, Wilmore D, Mannick JA, Rodrick ML (1987) A single dose of endotoxin activates neutrophils without activating complement. Surgery 102:200–205

Clinical Factors Influencing Host Defense Integrity

J. L. Meakins

Introduction

The stress response (neuroendocrine, lymphokine-cytokine) is thought to be inevitable following surgery or trauma, and little consideration is given by clinicians to its control, limitation or elimination. Can we, by clinical behaviour, reduce the cost to the patient of an injury or an operation? In 1987, at the First Conference in Munich, the data were limited and somewhat indirect; however, today there is increasing evidence that blunting these responses decreases morbidity. The biology is not clear at present, but it is quite apparent that afferent blockade, postoperative pain control, surgical technique, transfusions, nutrition, speed of resuscitation, the products of modern biotechnology and surgical approaches can all dramatically influence the cost of surgery and trauma to a patient. The patient-based factors are acute and chronic state of health, fitness, medications, magnitude of injury, etc. The surgeon controls are pre- as well as intra-operative decision making, anaesthetic techniques, and a host of ancillary therapeutic manoeuvres. The differences in clinical evolution between laparoscopic and open cholecystectomy suffice to indicate that clinical approaches can influence the stress response. The relative ease of liver transplantation and modern results in burn care all indicate that clinical care profoundly influences biology and patients' clinical evolution.

Clinical Factors: Non-operative

The "anergic patient" represents the compromised surgical patient, and Fig. 1 depicts the clinical challenge. Specifically, it is to take a patient with a high probability of infection and to care effectively for this problem without infection as a process or sepsis as a response. The years of discussion on the importance of anergy have indeed changed behaviour, yet the biological entity is not completely understood. The clinical goal is to move the region in Fig. 1 indicating increased susceptibility to infection to the right, allowing the patient to cope

Department of Surgery, McGill University, 687 Pine Avenue West, Montreal, Quebec H3A 1A1, Canada

Host Defense Dysfunction
in Trauma, Shock and Sepsis
Eds. Faist/Meakins/Schildberg
© Springer-Verlag, Berlin Heidelberg 1993

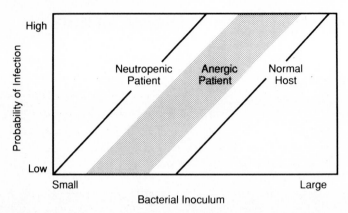

Fig. 1. The anergic patient represents the surgical patient and increased risk of infection. As host defences approach normal, resistance to infection increases, and a larger inoculation can be tolerated with a low incidence of infection

with a larger inoculum of bacteria while having the same or a lower incidence of infection. The first step is a non-operative approach to modulating the host.

There have been significant changes in the approach to preoperative assessment in recent years. The approach to the cardiovascular system has changed radically since Goldman et al. [1] clearly defined risk factors and further since Del Guercio's studies [2]. The maintenance or restoration of normal physiology, here as blood volume, oxygenation, perfusion, becomes the key to preventing complications. Hunt's work demonstrating the importance of PaO_2 and tissue oxygen levels in wound healing and resistance to infection extend the importance of maintaining and supporting physiology [3].

In the traumatized or bleeding patient, rapid resuscitation, control of blood loss and restoration of blood volume are the key elements to avoidance of late ischaemic effects such as acute tubular necrosis, peripheral ischaemia, stroke, myocardial infarction, intestinal ischaemia with ulcers, adult respiratory distress syndrome (ARDS) and multiple organ failure [4]. There is clear evidence that specific resistance to infection is altered at the time of shock and for up to 5 days after shock [5, 6]. In both time frames, there is an inoculum effect; that is, infection rates are markedly altered by numbers of bacteria. The shocked animals require many fewer organisms to generate infection compared to normal animals [5]. These results would be expected in the short term because altered perfusion decreases the inflammatory response and resistance to infection at the time of contamination [5–7]. Of great significance is that for up to 5 days after shock the resistance to infection is reduced. This can only be mediated through a significantly altered systemic immune response as all local perfusion defects will have long been corrected. These observations are further supported by Rush's group who have shown in man and animals the role of shock in the development of systemic infection [8, 9]. Haemorrhage has also been shown, as a function of volume of blood loss and transfusion requirements, to be associated with anergy [10].

The implications for care are clear. Bleeding and trauma, the basic causes of shock, are surgical diseases. Resuscitation and management of bleeding source with speed and efficacy are critical to reducing the late systemic effects of shock. Prevention and control of haemorrhage in the operating room is crucial both for early and late effects. Once shock has occurred, behaviour must be as if the patient is immunocompromised with alterations of both local and systemic host resistance.

The incidence of postoperative infections, wound, urinary, pulmonary, have been substantially reduced over the past 15 years [11–13]. Antibiotics are a part of the improvement but the totality of pre- and postoperative care has improved significantly. The literature abounds with reports of major operations carried out in the past with major infectious morbidity and mortality now being performed with vastly improved results and much reduced rates of infection [13, 14]. These aspects of care include better fluid management, maintenance of tissue perfusion and oxygenation, early mobilization, a better understanding of metabolism and preoperative preparation.

A fine example of the efficacy of total care is seen in the management of Crohn's disease by Hill's group [15]. Integrating preoperative preparation, drainage, details of care, control of inflammation, and nutritional support with eventual surgical repair, their results are excellent. Crohn's disease patients, when ill, are known to have major abnormalities in their immune system which correct themselves following control of the disease by either medical or surgical therapy (Table 1). Clinical factors and appropriate treatment modulate the immune response and should be thought of as biological response modification. Controlling the disease controls its expression, one aspect of which is immunosuppression.

Control of the stress response, the inevitable reaction to trauma, surgery and infection, has been shown recently to be feasible [16–18]. While this may be a two-edged sword, as manipulating biology always is, the benefits may be

Table 1. Therapy of crohn's disease: effect on immunity

	Before	After
Severity of disease (CDAI)	341.2 ± 33	63.7 ± 223.1
Skin tests		
Reactive	–	10
Relative anergy	7	–
Anergy	3	–
Neutrophil chemotaxis	103.7 ± 3.2	126.6 ± 2.3
Neutrophil delivery to skin windows × 10^5		
6 h	0.5 ± 0.2	11.4 ± 2.0
12 h	25.2 ± 12.5	144.4 ± 23.1

CDAI, Crohn's Disease Activity Index

significant for patients with respect to improved control of infection, decreased catabolism and earlier return to function. Nutrition [18–21], prostaglandin inhibitors [22] and regional anaesthesia [17] can all influence the stress response, as indeed can control of infection.

The role of nutrition as an immune modulator has been responsible for cutting down many trees. It is a believed in but is a yet not completely proven immunotherapy [19–21]. There can be no doubt of its importance in supportive care of the critically ill and in the maintenance or restoration of body composition. It has recently been shown that preoperative total parenteral nutrition reduces infectious complications in the severely malnourished yet there is an increase in mild and moderate malnutrition. The use of specific amino acids are showing promise, specifically glutamine [23] and arginine [24]. While data remain promising, and maintenance of fuel and energy requirements [19] are essential, the exact role of nutrition per se and specific nutrients as an immunomodulator is uncertain and requires further exploration [21].

Clinical Factors: Surgery

The surgical act modifies the immune response. There is a wealth of data to show that surgery, as a function of its length, complexity and magnitude, directly influences the immune reactions [25–29]. Surgery is immunosuppressive. In this context, the quality of surgery can significantly influence development of infections and other complications in either a positive or a negative fashion.

The importance of the surgeon and technique can best be seen in the interplay between the determinants of infection and the surgeon's role in prevention of wound infection [30]. The surgeon can, by preoperative care, give his patient the best chance to resist infection by improving host variables and diminishing potential bacterial contamination. In the operating room, bacteria can be controlled; the operation perfectly performed leaves a wound best able to resist infection. For example, a patient with 12 h of fecal peritonitis should not have the wound closed primarily. Infection rates are 50%–70% and entail important sequelae. Cruse [11] and Olson et al. [12] have shown that keeping individual surgeons informed of their wound infection rates keeps them low. The technical importance of haemostasis has been shown by Polk and Lopes-Mayor to be critical to the number of bacteria required to infect a wound [31]. Poor haemostasis reduces by two to three orders of magnitude (10 000 to 10–100) the number of bacteria required for a 20% wound infection rate in a contaminated wound without antibiotics.

There are many variables under the surgeon's control which impact on the determinants of infections [30], and those factors which influence wound infection also influence the development of deep, operative site infection and therefore the results of major surgery [31]. However, rather than a simple wound infection, the resulting infection or complication will be more serious and mortality may increase. The principles of gentle tissue handling, atraumatic anatomic dissection, careful haemostasis, preservation of blood supply and anastomoses without tension improves results. In addition, modern anaesthesia and monitoring techniques have eliminated the demand for speed, which was once a measure of skill. The surgeon's persona no longer needs to be linked to the length of the procedure; results count.

In published series, there is considerable variation in infectious morbidity after hepatic resection [14, 32, 33]. Subphrenic abscesses remain common in published reports and therefore in unpublished series, yet it is possible to carry out resectional surgery of the liver with very low (1%) mortality and infection rates [14]. Cameron's group has recently compared results over time and shown that pancreato-duodenectomy can be performed with very low morbidity and mortality rates [13]. Therefore, excellence of surgical technique and the preservation of local and systemic host responses by gentle, non-traumatic surgery has a major role as a potential immunomodulator.

Can the operation itself restore immune responses? Unequivocally yes, resection of pathology or inflammatory foci and drainage of abscesses can return altered host defences to normal [34]. Specifically, complement components [35], fibronectin [36], neutrophil chemotaxis [37], skin tests [38], amongst others, show clear improvement. There is no immunomodulator as effective as the drainage of infection. Resection therapy can similarly have a profound effect upon the immune system.

The presence of ascites uncontrolled by salt restriction, bed rest and diuretics is invariably associated with a serious state of malnutrition and altered immune competence [39]. If ascites cannot be controlled, prognosis is dismal. Peritoneovenous shunting, when performed in a meticulous manner [40, 41], permits cirrhotic patients to recover body composition [42] and immunocompetence via a number of mechanisms [39]. The shunt must be placed with zero mortality and low morbidity to have validity. The act, however, allows immune modulation as control of ascites is associated with recovery of appetite, sense of health, and other imponderables, leading to some recovery of liver function.

Summary: Clinical Factors and Host Response

There is a sense that little progress has been made in the modulation of the immune response in surgical or traumatized patients. While no magic bullets have yet been found, the evolving complexity of the stress response and the immune system suggest that no single agent will work and that the search for the magic bullet is an alchemist's dream. The support of these compromised patients must therefore be multi-factorial: clinical, pharmacological, biotechnological.

Has any progress been made? This brief review demonstrates that our clinical behaviour can and does modify and benefit patients. Biological insights have been translated into changed clinical practice, and traditional clinical activities have been shown to positively influence biology.

The development of laparoscopic surgery has taken the surgical world by storm. Cholecystectomy is now almost an out-patient procedure. The stress response has been virtually eliminated [43]. While the two procedures have not yet been properly compared, interim analysis of the McGill-Toronto gallstone study show dramatic differences in favour of the laparoscopic approach (unpublished observation, McGill-Toronto Gallstone study, 1991).

Clinical factors, operative and non-operative, influence the host response to surgery and trauma. The upcoming introduction of specific biological immunomodulation should enhance the progress already defined and provide much improved outcome to our patients and to society.

References

1. Goldman L, Caldera DL, Nussbaum SB et al. (1977) Multifactorial index of cardiac risk in noncardiac surgical procedures. N Engl J Med 297:845–850
2. Savino JA, del Guercio LRM (1988) Hemodynamic monitoring in the elderly. In: Meakins JL, McClaran JC (eds) Surgical care of the elderly. Year Book Medical Publisher, Chicago, Chap 16
3. Hunt TK (1987) Surgical wound infection: an overview. Am J Med 70:712–717
4. Faist E, Baue AE, Dittmer H et al. (1983) Multiple organ failure in polytrauma patients. J Trauma 23:775
5. Livingstone DH, Malangoni MA (1988) An experimental study of susceptibility to infection after hemorrhagic shock. Surg Gynecol Obstet 168:138–142
6. Miles AA (1980) The inflammatory response in relation to local infections. Surg Clin North Am 60:93–105
7. Nichols RL, Smith JW, Klein DB et al. (1954) Risk of infection after penetrating abdominal trauma. N Engl J Med 311:1065
8. Sori AJ, Rush BJ, Lysz TW et al. (1988) The gut as a source of sepsis after hemorrhagic shock. Am J Surg 155:187–192
9. Rush BF, Redan JA, Flanagan JJ et al. (1989) Does bacteremia observed in hemorrhagic shock have clinical significance? A study in germ free animals. Ann Surg 210:342–347
10. Christou NV, Meakins JL, Gotto D, MacLean LD (1979) Influence of gastrointestinal bleeding on host defence and susceptibility to infection. Surg Forum 30:46–47
11. Cruse PJE (1987) Wound infections: epidemiology and clinical characteristics. In: Howard RJ, Simmons RL (eds) Surgical infectious diseases. Appleton and Lange, Norwalk
12. Olsen M, Connor M, Schwartz ML (1984) Surgical wound infections: a 5-year prospective study of 20, 193 wounds at the Minneapolis VA Medical Center. Ann Surg 199:253–265
13. Crist DW, Sitzmann JV, Cameron JL (1987) Improved hospital morbidity, mortality and survival after the Whipple procedure. Ann Surg 206:258–265
14. Franco D, Smadja C, Meakins JL et al. (1989) The operative risk of elective hepatic resection for liver tumours: results of a series of one hundred consecutive hepatectomies in cirrhotic and noncirrhotic patients. Arch Surg 124:1033–1037
15. Hill GL, Bouchier RG, Whitney GB (1988) Surgical and metabolic management of patients with external fistulas of the small intestine associated with Crohn's disease. World J Surg 12:191–197
16. Kehlet H (1989) The stress response to surgery: release mechanisms and the modifying effect of pain relief. Acta Chir Scand [Suppl] 550:22–28
17. Kehlet H (1989) Anesthetic technique and surgical convalescence. Acta Chir Scand [Suppl] 550:182–187
18. Mochizuki H, Trocki O, Dominioni L et al. (1984) Mechanism of hypermetabolism and catabolism by early enteral feeding. Ann Surg 200:297–303

19. Bartlett RH, Dechert RE, Mault JR et al. (1982) Measurement of metabolism in multiple organ failure. Surgery 92:771–779
20. Muller JM, Brenner U, Daoust C et al. (1982) Preoperative parenteral feeding in patients with gastrointestinal carcinoma. Lancet i:68–73
21. Dempsey DT, Mullen JL, Buzby GP (1988) The link between nutritional status and clinical outcome: can nutritional intervention modify it? Am J Clin Nutr 47:352–356
22. Holcroft JW, Vassar MJ, Weber CJ (1986) Prostaglandin E, and survival in patients with the adult respiratory distress syndrome. Ann Surg 203:371–378
23. Wilmore DW, Smith RJ, O'Dwyer ST et al. (1988) The gut: a central organ after surgical stress. Surgery 104:917–923
24. Barbul A, Fishel RS, Shimazu S et al. (1985) Intravenous hyperalimentation with high arginine level improves wound healing and immune function. J Surg Res 38:328–334
25. Meakins JL (1988) Host defense mechanisms in surgical patients: effect of surgery and trauma. Acta Chir Scand [Suppl] 550:43–53
26. Slade MS, Simmons RL, Yunis EJ, Greenberg LJ (1975) Immunodepression after major surgery in normal patients. Surgery 78:363
27. Akiyoshi T, Koba S, Arinaga S et al. (1985) Impaired production of interleukin-2 after surgery. Clin Exp Immunol 59:45–49
28. Lennard TWJ, Shenton BK, Borzotta A et al. (1985) The influence of surgical operations on components of the human immune system. Br J Surg 72:771–776
29. McLoughlin GA, Wu AV, Saporoschetz I et al. (1979) Correlation between anergy and circulating immunosuppressive factor following major surgical trauma. Ann Surg 190:297–304
30. Meakins JL (1988) Guidelines for the prevention of wound infection. In: Wilmore DD, Brennan M, Harken A, Holcroft J, Meakins JL (eds) The care of the surgical patient. Scientific American, New York, Chap 6
31. Polk HC Jr, Lopez-Mayor JF (1969) Postoperative wound infection: a prospective study of determinant factors and prevention. Surgery 66:97–103
32. Pachter JL, Spencer FC, Hofstetter SR et al. (1983) Experience with finger fracture technique to achieve intra-hepatic hemostasis in 75 patients with severe injuries of the liver. Ann Surg 197:771–778
33. Schwartz SI (1983) In discussion of Pachter (43). Ann Surg 197:777
34. Meakins JL (1981) Clinical importance of host resistance to infection in surgical patients. Adv Surg 15:225–255
35. Heichmann M, Saravis C, Clowes GHA (1982) Effect of non viable tissue and abscesses on complement depletion and development of bacteremia. J Trauma 22:527–532
36. Richards WO, Scovill WA, Shin B (1983) Opsonic fibronectin deficiency in patients with intraabdominal infection. Surgery 94:210–217
37. Solomkin JS, Bauman MP, Nelson RD et al. (1981) Neutrophils dysfunction during the course of intraabdominal infection. Ann Surg 194:9–17
38. Meakins JL, Christou NV, Shizgal HM, MacLean LD (1979) Therapeutic approaches to anergy in surgical patients: surgery and levamisole. Ann Surg 190:285–296
39. Franco D, Charra M, Jeambrun P et al. (1983) Nutrition and immunity after peritoneovenous drainage of ascites in cirrhotic patients. Am J Surg 146:652–657
40. Smadja C, Franco D (1985) The leVeen shunt in the elective treatment of intractable ascites in cirrhosis. A prospective study on 140 patients. Ann Surg 201:488–493
41. Meakins JL, Hillaire S, Vons C, Smadja C, Franco D (1988) Perioperative antibiotics (2 doses) control early but not late infectious complications of peritoneovenous shunts (PVS). Surg Res Commun 3:51–54
42. Blendis LM, Harrison JE, Russel DM et al. (1987) Effects of peritoneovenous shunting on body composition. Gastroenterology 90:127–134
43. The Southern Surgeons Club (1991) A prospective analysis of 1518 laparoscopic cholecystectomies. N Engl J Med 324:1073–1078

The Intensive Care Unit of Tomorrow

H. J. Dieterich and K. Peter

Introduction

Next to medical progress structural considerations will help to optimize intensive care cost-benefit ratio as well as the quality of patient care today and in future. Investments in today's clinical practice and in basic as well as clinical research will also improve the quality of intensive care medicine. All these factors are strongly interacting and dependent on each other: the intensive care unit (ICU) of tomorrow is a very sensitive and complex network.

Current State

In 1990, nearly 1350 out of 1850 acute hospitals in West Germany had an ICU. The total number of beds available in these ICUs was approximately 14000. This represents an increase of 30% within the last decade. In 1988, 1.2 million patients were admitted to ICUs. Only 25% of these patients died during their stay on the ICU, although most of them suffered from severe impairment of vital functions. This impressive result was only attained by a high level of expenditure on this part of the health care system.

The cost of installing a new bed in an ICU in West Germany lies between 700 000 and 1.4 million deutsche marks (DM). The daily cost of stay in the ICU is at least 1500–2000 DM per bed. More specialized units, for example for burn injuries or sterile units for bone marrow transplant patients, are several times more expensive. Not only in Germany is intensive care responsible for a very significant proportion of the growing cost of medical care: total expenditure on health care in the United States has reached between 11% and 12% of the gross national product. Experts estimate that about 20% of all hospital costs are generated in ICUs [1].

There is currently a significant number of beds that are not in use due to a great lack of nurses, but even if all the beds already established can be used, the number will be too small to meet future needs in this high-technology field of medicine.

Institute of Anesthesiology, Ludwig-Maximilians University of Munich, Munich, FRG

Host Defense Dysfunction
in Trauma, Shock and Sepsis
Eds. Faist/Meakins/Schildberg
© Springer-Verlag, Berlin Heidelberg 1993

Future Trends

Plans for building or renewing a hospital in Germany should be based on the guidelines of the German Interdisciplinary Society of Intensive Care and Emergency Medicine (DIVI). The guidelines lay out the size, the equipment required, and the ratio of intensive care beds to the total number of beds within the hospital or department [2].

Taking the number of patients with vital function impairments, size of the hospital, duration of stay, and other factors into account, it is recommended that in orthopedics at least 1% of the total number of beds be dedicated to Intensive Care, in surgery, internal medicine, and pediatrics each about 10%, in heart surgery 15%–20%, and in neurosurgery 20%.

The increasing average age of the population and the much more agressive and extensive therapeutic procedures in operative and nonoperative medicine are making care of the patient during or after therapy and operation more complex. In the United States not long ago the national recommendation was to have 5% of the hospital beds reserved for intensive care. This limit has now been exceeded, especially in major teaching hospitals. At the Presbyterian University Hospital in Pittsburgh, for example, the tenth ICU will be opened this year, 15% of the total number of hospital beds now being in ICUs [3].

Multidisciplinary ICU

The early critical care units evolved as specialized units for postoperative care, for the management of neurosurgical patients, for respiratory care, and subsequently for cardiac, renal, and pediatric care. However, in the early 1960s it was already apparent that there were no fundamental differences between medical and surgical patients in the monitoring and the life-support interventions required. The same hemodynamic and respiratory monitoring techniques were employed, as well as the same supplies and equipment for respiratory care. In brief, there was substantial impetus to combine rather than to split resources and thereby make substantial gains in efficiency of operation. This development is continuing and is leading to larger multidisciplinary ICUs as subspecialties of the primary specialties like anesthesiology, surgery, internal medicine, and pediatrics. Nevertheless, some specialized units at major teaching hospitals or university departments are still having success focusing on intensive care in specific specialties.

Two examples will show that multidisciplinary intensive care can indeed improve the survival rate and the quality of a surviver's life:

The APACHE II score (acute physiology and chronic health evaluation) is used worldwide to predict the prognosis of patients on the basis of their current physical state [4]. Our own data from 78 patients with more than 25 points out

Table 1. APACHE II score and mortality

Score	Mortality (%)	
	Knaus et al. (1985) [4] (n = 5815)	Institute of Anesthesiology, Munich (1988) (n = 78)
25–29	46	28
30–34	74	25
35	85	45

of a total of 1064 intensive care patients of all categories show an impressive decrease in mortality (Table 1), particularly in the high-risk group with more than 34 points of the APACHE score, where mortality decreased from about 88% to 45%. Similar increases in survival rates were achieved in the other two groups as well.

We also analyzed the mortality of patients after simultaneous transplantation of kidney and pancreas in two 4-year periods. From 1980 to 1984, five of 23 patients (21.7%) died after simultaneous transplantation. In the next period, from 1985 to 1989, only 1 out of 80 patients died (1.3%).

These results were achieved due to an increase in clinical research and acquisition of knowledge and experience in all disciplines sharing in the intensive care of these patients.

Cost-Benefit Ratio

It is important to bear in mind that the research and increased knowledge needed to improve survival were made possible only by investing enormous sums of money. However, as we can see, the investment in one generation of patients soon brings advantages to the next generation.

The financial investment in intensive care is not only in the patients' interest, it also makes sense from a general socio-economic point of view. For instance, a patient with end-stage liver disease who cannot be given a transplant, for whatever reason, consumes on average health care costs of more than US $ 45000 within the last year of his life. In some cases the amount exceeds US $ 100000. In addition to these personal costs, the costs of relief for dependents, the loss of in income tax revenue, and other costs must be included.

In June 1983 the Consensus Development Conference on Liver Transplantation in Washington declared liver transplantation for clinical routine [5]. A not exactly known amount of money had been spent to bring the whole program from the stage of trial to clinical application. Currents costs for a single liver transplantation are about US$ 92000, and US$ 5000–6000 are required per year after transplantation, mostly for immunosupressive drugs. The 1-year-survival of these patients is at least 70%–80%, while the further survival is similar to that of the normal population. Again, 80% of these survivers in the United State can be fully rehabilitated. These patients need no annuity, they pay tax and contribute to the gross national product by their ability to work.

Research

The costs mentioned above may seem extremely high, but compared with industrial investments they are really not excessive. For example, the automobile industry has to calculate several billion DM for planning and developing a new car. Even expenditure before starting the assembly line is a few hundred million DM. To obtain an optimal result in the future, most of the money has to be invested now in basic research: medical progress is very similar to a successful industrial project (Table 2).

We have to be aware that adult respiratory distress syndrome (ARDS), sepsis and multiple organ failure, the classical fields of clinical research in intensive care, are limited. Progress will only be achieved by integrating basic research areas like immunology and molecular biology. In fact, the analysis of molecular mechanisms of cellular and organ function is of growing importance in clinical medicine. This means that the development of diseases will be better understood on a molecular basis.

With regard to basic clinical research, a wide spectrum of cell- and molecular-biological methods must be combined with studies on the pathogenesis and therapy of diseases. At the same time, diseases can be seen as an "experiment of nature" and provided the possibility to understand molecular and cellular mechanisms of normal and pathological function of the human body. Thus, basic research as well as clinical research must come together more frequently, by inspiring each other and by using molecular biological methods in both areas.

The ICU is not a laboratory with patients, but in the ICU of tomorrow the patient must be closer to the lab, closer to research than nowadays.

Table 2. Equivalence of industrial projects and medicine

Automobile Industry	Medicine
Investment	Investment
Planning	Basic Research
Development	Clinical Research
Expenditure	Expenditure
Before assembly line start	Clinical research/trials
After assembly line start	Clinical routine

Conclusion

The ICU of tomorrow will be a factor of ever more growing importance in medicine. We must therefore, increase the quantity and quality of intensive care. For both goals we must generate resources. Financial resources are needed for investment in equipment and personnel. Furthermore, we must invest in manpower and brainpower in clinical and basic research, to achieve a higher level of scientific quality in intensive care. Only if we succeed in this we will meet the challenge of the ICU of tomorrow.

References

1. Weil MH, von Planta M, Rackow EC (1989) Critical care medicine: introduction and historical perspective. In: Shoemaker WC, Ayres S, Grenvik A, Holbrook PR, Thompson WL (eds) Textbook of critical care. Saunders, Philadelphia
2. Association News/Information (1990) Empfehlungen zur baulichen Gestaltung und Einrichtung von Intensivbehandlungseinheiten. Anasth Intensivmed 31:356
3. Grenvik A (1991) From blood pressure to cellular function: 40 years intensive care medicine. In: Lawin P, Peter K, Prien (eds) Intensivmedizin 1991. Thieme, Stuttgart (Intensivmedizin, Notfallmedizin, Anaesthesiologie, vol 77)
4. Knaus WA, Draper EA, Wagner DP et al. (1985) APACHE II: a severity of disease classification system for acutely ill patients. Crit Care Med. 13:818
5. National Institute of Health (1984) Consensus development conference on liver transplantation. Hepatology 4 (1) [Suppl Jan/Feb]

Section 2

Host Defense Integrity–Response and Stress

How the Immune System Discriminates Infectious Nonself from Noninfectious Self*

C.A. Janeway Jr.

Introduction

It is abundantly clear that the complex of host defense systems now known as the immune system arose in evolution to provide the host with defense against infectious agents. All host defense reactions involve three components. First, the foreign material must be recognized by some mechanism that discriminates it from self. Second, a response must be initiated. Third, that response must lead to the removal of the foreign material from the body. In this paper, I wish to make three points about the host system of defense. First, the removal or final effector system are the same for both innate and adaptive immune responses. Second, I argue that the adaptive immune response arose through the development of clonally distributed receptors encoded in rearranging genes and utilizes these receptors to regulate existing innate defense mechanisms. Third, I want to show that these two classes of responses are also linked at the recognition and response phase, in that adaptive immunity utilizes an older, nonclonal system of recognition to discriminate the infectious from the noninfectious, as well as its clonally distributed receptor to discriminate nonself from self. Thus, one can see that the immune response discriminates infectious nonself from noninfectious self. Without both of these types of recognition event, responses fail to occur. This has important consequences both for host defense and for the avoidance of autoreactivity [1].

The basic paradigm of adaptive immunity is the clonal selection hypothesis [2]. All aspects of the clonal selection hypothesis have been thoroughly and convincingly documented by modern experimental approaches to basic immunology. However, there are two modifications that need to be incorporated into the clonal selection hypothesis to account for host defense in its broader sense. First, the immune response actually occurs in three phases, all important to host defense, and only the last phase involves clonal selection. The immediate phase of host defense is completely lacking in specificity, is noninducible, and cannot show immunological memory. This phase is fairly rapidly succeeded by a second phase which is largely nonclonal but differs from the first phase in that it

* Supported by Grants NIH AI-26810 and the Howard Hughes Medical Institute
Section of Immunobiology, Howard Hughes Medical Institute, Yale University School of Medicine, New Haven, CT 06511, USA

Host Defense Dysfunction
in Trauma, Shock and Sepsis
Eds. Faist/Meakins/Schildberg
© Springer-Verlag, Berlin Heidelberg 1993

is inducible. This phase also does not generate immunological memory. If one divides the body into different compartments, each of which can be attacked by a distinct class of pathogen, and then examines the effector mechanisms active at each phase of the response in each compartment, it becomes evident that the same basic effector mechanisms are required for removal of the infectious agent in each phase. This is illustrated in Table 1. What differs in each phase of the immune response is the mechanism by which self is discriminated from nonself. This can be readily documented by examining the activation of the complement cascade at different phases of the immune response. The immediate phase of the immune response is mediated by the alternative pathway of complement activation, in which complement derived from C3b tickover in the serum is deposited on bacteria as well as host cells. Host cells are protected by complement regulatory proteins such as decay accelerating factor, allowing self to be discriminated from nonself at all times. Shortly after this, the complement cascade can be initiated by the binding of mannose binding protein to bacteria with mannans in their cell walls. Mannose binding protein, an acute phase protein produced in the liver, is strongly induced by the production of interleukin-6 by macrophages, in turn triggered by bacterial constituents such as lipopolysaccharide. Subsequently, T-independent protection of immunoglobulin M(IgM) antibodies can activate the classical complement pathway. Finally, after about 4–5 days, T-dependent antibody responses of the IgM and IgG isotype are made and activate complement through the classical pathway. Thus, complement activation passes from an unspecific but nevertheless discriminatory mechanism of activation in the immediate phase of the response, to a specific but not clonally distributed mechanism in the early inducible phase of the response, to a highly specific and clonally distributed recognition system in the late phase of the response. It is only this last component of the response that can provide long-lasting immunological memory.

Viewed in this way, it becomes apparent that effector mechanisms utilizing recognition systems that respond to a wide range of pathogens comprise the early phase of any immune response and play a very important role in the early containment of infection. The crucial importance of these early phase reactants can be seen from their rare deficiency diseases. However, the final removal mechanisms utilized in all phases of the response are the same. If ontogeny really recapitulates phylogeny, then it seems likely that the immune system originated as a nonclonal system, and that adaptive immunity arose through the development of genes that rearrange to encode receptors in somatic cells. Here again, evolution and ontogeny provide clues as to the origins of clonally distributed recognition systems. Studies of antibody gene rearrangement in a wide range of vertebrate species have demonstrated that rearrangement always regulates transcription of receptor genes in two ways, first by forming a complete coding unit by joining V to D and J elements, and second by initiating transcription from promoters by bringing them under the regulation of C gene-associated enhancer elements. Interestingly, elasmobranch fishes, birds, and mammals all share this mechanism, but differ radically in the means by which they generate

Table 1. The three phases of host defense in different body compartments

Phase of the immune response	Barrier functions	Extracellular forms	Intracellular bacteria	Virus-infected cells
Immediate (0–4 h) Nonspecific Innate No memory No specific T cells	Skin epithelia	Phagocytes, alternative complement pathway	Macrophages	Natural killer cells
Early (4–96 h) Nonspecific and specific Inducible No memory No specific T cells	Local inflammation (C5a) Local TNF-α	C-reactive protein, TI-B cell antibody plus complement	TI macrophage activation, IL-1, IL-6, TNF-α, TGF-β	Interferons-α and interferon-activated natural killer cells
Late (after 96 h) Specific Inducible Memory Specific T cells	IgA antibody in luminal spaces IgE antibody on mast cells	IgG antibody and Fc receptor bearing cells IgG, IgM antibody plus classical complement pathway	T cell activation of macrophages by interferon-γ	Cytolytic T cells, interferon-γ

diversity. Thus, gene rearrangement apparently arose to control gene expression, and its use to generate diversity came later.

In mammalian ontogeny, the earliest T cells to arise have $\gamma\delta$T cell receptors and home to specific epithelia. Furthermore, within an epithelium only a single T cell receptor specificity is observable. Thus, the first cells of adaptive immune responses to use rearranging receptors appear not to behave according to clonal selection, since all cells in a given tissue have the same receptor. Nevertheless, it seems certain that the receptor is used to mount a response. Thus, $\gamma\delta$T cells must respond either to an invariant component of pathogens or an invariant component of host cells. CD5 B lymphocytes appear to be quite similar, arise early in ontogeny, and have relatively nondiverse immunoglobulin receptors utilizing proximal V genes in their formation. As the animal matures, $\gamma\delta$T cell receptor bearing T cells and conventional B cells appear with highly diverse receptors utilizing all V gene segments and having extensive junctional diversity.

The second crucial modification to the clonal selection theory was originally proposed by Bretscher and Cohn [3]. They suggested that lymphocyte activation would require two signals, one delivered through the clonally distributed antigen binding receptor, which they termed signal one, and the other deriving from some other source. Bretscher and Cohn focused on the antibody response, and proposed that the second signal was derived from a helper T cell providing a second antibody specific for the same antigen. We now know that help is derived in the form of lymphokines coming from helper T cells, and that lymphokines provide the essential second signal for B cell clonal expansion and differentiation to antibody production. Interestingly, helper T cell-derived interleukin-6 appears to play a critical role in the production of specific antibody just as it does in the production of the protoantibodies mannose-binding protein and C reactive protein produced in hepatocytes. However, for B cells to be activated helper T cells must be primed; what is the nature of the second signals that lead to helper T cell priming? This issue is just now being examined. It appears that the major receptor for second signals on CD4 T cells is the molecule CD28, and that ligation of CD3:T cell receptor and CD28 is required for activation of T cells to clonally expand and differentiate to effector function [4]. The natural ligand for CD28 appears to be the inducible B cell surface molecule B7/BB1. This molecule is not present on normal B cells but is inducible with a variety of bacterial and viral substances, such as lipopolysaccharide, double-stranded RNA, and mannans. Interestingly, all B cells express this product when stimulated with these microbial substances. This must involve some kind of non-clonally distributed receptor that recognizes common microbial constituents and makes the response in the form of expression of costimulatory molecules. As both signals are required for T cell activation, this means that antigens not associated with infectious agents will not induce immunity. Indeed, most soluble protein antigens are only immunogenic when they are mixed in an insoluble form with bacterial constituents. Although it has not been formally proven, it seems highly likely that the essential function fulfilled by the microbial constituents is to induce the expression of second signals or costimulatory activity on antigen presenting cells (Fig. 1) [1, 5].

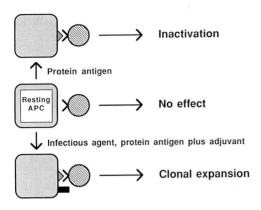

D   **Specific Antigen**

■   **Signal 2**

Fig. 1. The immune response depends on T cell activation, which in turn requires two signals, one in the form of a specific peptide MHC complex recognized by the T cell receptor and the other in the form of a cell-associated stimulus known as signal two or costimulator. Pure protein antigens induce signal one and not signal two, while infectious agents induce both signal one and signal two. Signal one alone leads to clonal inactivation, while signal two alone has no known effect. The two signals together lead to clonal expansion and differentiation to effector function (*APC*, antigen presenting cell)

One cell that appears to violate this paradigm of the requirement for inducible second signals is the dendritic cell of Steinman, which he has shown is the only significant stimulator of mixed lymphocyte reactions [6]. The dendritic cell appears to have constitutive expression of costimulatory activity, allowing it to induce T cell proliferation in the absence of microbial stimulation. Such a cell might appear to be highly dangerous as it might present self constituents to the immune system. However, studies of Matzinger and Guerder [7] have shown that the dendritic cell is also the most potent cell at inducing clonal deletion of T cells during development. Thus, any antigen of self that the dendritic cell might present has already been presented to developing T cells in the thymus, and all T cells potentially autoreactive to the dendritic cell have been clonally deleted. Furthermore, the dendritic cell appears to be quite inefficient at acquiring antigen. Unlike the B cell, it cannot use a specific clonally distributed receptor to internalize antigens, and unlike the macrophage it cannot ingest particulate antigens, clearly the most important form of extracellular antigen. Given this relative inability to internalize antigens, what possible utility could the dendritic cell have? One possibility, not yet fully tested, is that dendritic cells could exist to present viral antigens which can enter the cell in the form of infectious virus. Whether dendritic cells are uniquely susceptible to viral infection remains to be determined, but virally infected dendritic cells can activate naive T cells in vitro [8].

It is known from studies of transplantation that antigen presenting cells found within solid tissues are the inducers of graft injection. This raises the question of whether a T cell in a tissue simultaneously in contact with a tissue cell bearing a tissue-specific autoantigen that would not be expressed in the thymus and also with a costimulator-positive antigen presenting cell could become activated. To examine this, we have deliberately mixed cells that can deliver signal one without signal two and cells that can deliver signal two without signal one and asked whether they can induce T cell proliferative responses in naive CD4 T cells [9]. Using two different systems, we find that both the ligand and the costimulator must be presented to naive CD4 T cells by the same antigen presenting cell (Fig. 2). Thus, the presence of antigen presenting cells in tissues does not appear to pose a threat to the host. Such cells must be important in presenting antigens derived from tissue-specific infectious agents to the immune system. Indeed, Steinman et al. [6] have proposed that precursors of lymphoid dendritic cells exist in the tissues and actively ingest antigens, after which they migrate to the lymphoid organs and acquire their costimulatory activity. Their role in taking up and presenting self antigens has not yet been elucidated.

Once T cells are activated to proliferate and differentiate into effector cells, they have an obvious need to be able to mediate their effector functions in the tissues. For instance, a T cell primed by a competent antigen presenting cell to become an active cytolytic effector T cell must be able to enter the tissues and

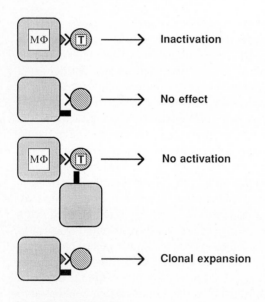

▷   Specific Antigen

■   Signal 2

Fig. 2. Signal one and signal two need to be delivered by a single cell. If a cell expressing signal one is mixed with a cell expressing signal two, clonal expansion is not observed, while the two signals on one cell do lead to clonal expansion and differentiation to effector function (*MØ*, macrophage)

kill virally infected tissue cells. Thus, T cell effector function should not require signal two, and has never been shown to do so. Nevertheless, this arrangement also poses risks to the host. Should a T cell become activated by an infectious agent and have cross-reactive activity against a tissue-specific autoantigen, that cell might be able to destroy the entire tissue. In fact, this is unlikely to occur. A number of experimental systems have shown recently that T cells responding in vivo are short-lived [10, 11]. We have examined this question in a model system utilizing a cloned T cell line that has cytolytic potential [12]. When this cloned T cell line is activated in the presence of competent antigen presenting cells, it proliferates and differentiates into an activated killer cell. By contrast, when it is activated in the absence of a functional antigen presenting cell, most of the cells die rapidly, and the remainder become immunologically inert or anergic. The activated cells die through a two signal mechanism, one signal again being delivered through the receptor and the second signal being delivered in the form of interferon-γ (Fig. 3). Thus, even when effector cells become inadvertently activated against host tissue, they are unlikely to produce sustained damage. This raises the interesting and important question of how damage against self tissues is sustained in autoimmune disease. The most likely explanation is that local inflammatory responses lead to the induction of high levels of major histocompatibility complex (MHC) antigens on tissue cells as well as the induction of costimulatory activity. Recent experiments appear to show that interferon-γ can activate tissue cells to express costimulatory activity. Thus, local viral or bacterial infection might trigger autoimmune processes through stimulating the release of interferon-γ in local tissues.

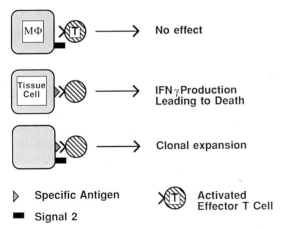

Fig. 3. When activated effector cells recognize antigen in the absence of signal two, death of the effector cell can occur. In the systems we have studied, interferon-γ ($IFN\gamma$) plays a critical role, in that cell death can be blocked by anti-interferon-γ. In the presence of signal two, clonal expansion is observed even in the presence of abundant interferon-γ. This mechanism may protect tissues from effector cells activated by infectious agents that cross-react with host tissues

It is interesting to note that the innate and early inducible phases of the immune response have essentially no associated autoimmune type diseases. This is likely to be the case because the receptors that regulate the innate defense systems arose over evolutionary time, and those that coded for self recognition that was damaging to the host would clearly be eliminated by evolutionary processes. Indeed, the problem of self/nonself discrimination as we know it today arose simultaneously with the appearance of highly diverse clonally distributed receptors. The price paid for having a completely open repertoire of receptors is the potential for autoreactivity that is always present. Given the adequacy of the innate and early inducible immune responses in protecting the host from many different infectious agents, what is the utility of the adaptive immune response, and why has it been retained in all vertebrates studied? There appear to be two major benefits to the host of having clonally distributed highly diverse receptors encoded in rearranging genes. First, this system of adaptive immunity allows the host to make a vast array of different receptors out of a small amount of DNA, and to select them for utility and harmlessness in somatic cells. This system imposes a low evolutionary burden in the form of few inherited receptors with a very high gain in terms of breadth of recognition. It appears to be extremely rare for the adaptive immune response to fail because there is no recognition of foreign materials or infectious agents. The second great benefit of adaptive immunity is that it allows for immunological memory, the specific protection against any infectious agent previously encountered by the host. In a long-lived species like man in which intergenerational time is great, the ability to repeatedly resist the same infection is tremendously important. Only through clonally distributed receptor systems in which stimulation leads to clonal expansion and differentiation to memory cells can immunological memory be developed. It is for this, perhaps more than anything else, that clonally distributed receptor systems arose and have persisted throughout the vertebrate kingdom.

Thus, the immune system appears to have arisen from a series of host defense mechanisms triggered by the recognition of common pathogenic patterns. The recognition systems of this innate immune system have mainly not been discovered, but they are highly specific and they appear to be directed at constituents of microorganisms that are fundamental to their biology and therefore relatively immutable. In a complex organism like a vertebrate, this type of host defense mediated by evolutionarily selected nonclonally distributed receptors did not provide optimal protection, especially over long generational times. Clonally distributed highly diverse receptors encoded in rearranging gene families provide a great range of recognitive capabilities and allow the organism to develop immunological memory. However, they also carry the risk of responsiveness to self. The immune system appears to have retained its ancient ability to discriminate the infectious from the noninfectious using microbial pattern reecognition receptors, and to utilize antigen presenting cells as a translator mechanism that allows the immune system to simultaneously discriminate the infectious from the noninfectious and self from nonself. Only when the immune system receives both the antigenic message of foreignness and the pattern induced stimulus that an infectious agent is present can an immune response ensue. Receipt of signal one only, for instance from host cells, leads either to cell death or cell inactivation. Thus, even in the presence of an open repertoire, failure to respond to self is maintained.

References

1. Janeway CA Jr (1989) Approaching the asymptote? Evolution and revolution in immunology. Cold Spring Harbor Symp Quant Biol 54:1–13
2. Burnet FM (1959) The clonal selection theory of immunity. Vanderbilt University Press, Nashville
3. Bretscher PA, Cohn M (1970) The theory of self-nonself discrimination. Science 169:1042
4. Linsley PS, Brady W, Grosmaire L, Aruffo A, Damle NK, Ledbetter JA (1991) Binding of the B cells activation antigen B7 to CD28 costimulates T cell proliferation and IL-2 mRNA accumulation. J Exp Med (in press)
5. Liu Y, Janeway CA Jr (1991) Microbial induction of co-stimulatory activity for CD4 T cell growth. Int Immunol (in press)
6. Steinman RM, Metlay J, Bhardwaj N, Freudenthal P, Langhoff E, Crowley M, Lau L, Witmer-Pack M, Young JW, Pure E, Romani N, Inaba K (1989) Dentritic cells: nature's adjuvant. In: Janeway CA et al. (eds) Immunogenicity. Liss, New York
7. Matzinger P, Guerder S (1989) Does T cell tolerance require a dedicated antigen-presenting cell? Nature 338:74–76
8. Macatonia SE, Taylor PM, Knight SC, Askonas BA (1989) Primary stimulation by dendritic cells induces anti-viral proliferative and cytoxic T cell responses in vitro. J Exp Med 169:1255
9. Liu Y, Janeway CA Jr Clonal expansion of normal CD4 T cells requires expression of both ligand and co-stimulator on one cell. (submitted)
10. Webb S, Morris C, Sprent J (1990) Extrathymic tolerance of mature T cells: clonal elimination as a consequence of immunity. Cell 63:1249–1256
11. Kawabe Y, Ochi A (1990) Programmed cell death and extrathymic reduction of $V\beta 8^+$, $CD4^+$ T cells in Staphylococcus enterotoxin B-specific tolerance. Nature (in press)
12. Liu Y, Janeway CA Jr (1990) Interferon γ plays a critical role in induced cell death of effector T cell: a possible third mechanism of self-tolerance. J Exp Med 172:1735–1739

Signal Transduction Mechanisms: Pathophysiologic Alterations

M.M. Sayeed

Introduction

To transmit their messages, water-soluble extracellular messenger molecules (e.g., endo- para-, or autocrine agents, neurotransmitters, growth factors) reversibly combine with specific receptors in the plasma membrane of their target cells. In certain cases the messenger-receptor combination results in the activation of an enzyme or an ion channel which is an integral part of the receptor's molecular structure, e.g., insulin receptor–tyrosine protein kinase [1], and acetylcholine receptor – cation channel [2]. Thus the activation of the enzyme or the ion channel by the messenger directly contributes to a cellular response. In many other cases, the reversible combination of the messenger with the receptor leads to a sequential activation of (a) an enzyme or an ion channel regulatory protein (the guanine nucleotide binding protein, G protein) and (b) an intracellular messenger-generating enzyme or ion channel. The latter step then results in the generation of one or more intracellular messengers (e.g., cyclic adenosine monophosphate, AMP, Ca^{2+}, inositol 1,4,5-triphosphate, IP_3, 1,2-diacyl glycerol, DAG). The intracellular messenger(s) in turn elicit(s) the specific cellular response(s). This last step often involves a reversible adenosine triphosphate (ATP)-linked phosphorylation of a "response protein" by a protein kinase. The covalent modification of the intracellular protein appears to be the final common pathway of the signal transduction processes. The sequelae of events involving the regulatory G protein, the intracellular messenger-generating enzyme, and the intracellular messenger(s) constitute the "signal transduction pathway (Fig. 1). Since the intracellular messenger-generating enzyme or ion channel serves to amplify the message, it is depicted as the "amplifying protein".

The Regulatory G Protein

A number of studies have provided detailed information on the mechanisms by which beta-adrenergic receptor activation is coupled to the regulation of the

Department of Physiology, Loyola University of Chicago, Stritch School of Medicine, Maywood, IL 60153, USA

Host Defense Dysfunction
in Trauma, Shock and Sepsis
Eds. Faist/Meakins/Schildberg
© Springer-Verlag, Berlin Heidelberg 1993

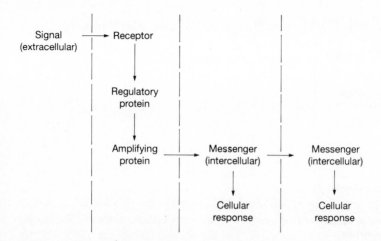

Fig. 1. Signal transduction pathway

guanine nucleotide-binding G proteins and the actenylate cyclase system, both of which reside within the plasma membrane [3]. Figure 2 represents inter-actions among the beta-adrenergic hormone, the receptor, G protein, and the enzyme adenylate cyclase. The reversible binding of the hormone to the receptor initiates the communication of the message to the G protein. The hormone-receptor complex initially binds to the inactive form of the G protein (G protein with guanosine diphosphate, GDP, tightly bound to it, G-GDP) [4]. Once the ternary hormone-receptor-G-GDP complex is formed, the presence of guano-sine triphosphate (GTP) promotes the replacement of G protein's GDP with GTP. The GTP-bound G protein (active form of G protein) then dissociates from the hormone-receptor complex. The active G-GTP complex also effects a dissociation of an alpha subunit of G protein (G_α)—with GTP attached to it—from the part of G protein made up of the beta and gamma subunits ($G_{\beta,\gamma}$). The GTP-bound subunit (G_α-GTP) in turn interacts with the adenylate cyclase system. Both a stimulatory G protein (G_s) and an inhibitory G protein (G_i) have been characterized and are known to respectively up- and down-regulate the enzyme adenylate cyclase. The interaction of G_α-GTP with the enzyme, resulting in the stimulation or inhibition of the enzyme, also causes the hydrolysis of GTP to GDP and thus the deactivation of the G_α-GTP to G_α-GDP. As shown in the diagram of generalized G protein interactions (Fig. 2), G_α-GDP recombines with the $G_{\beta,\gamma}$ portion and this leads to the restoration of the inactive form of the G protein. The stimulation and inhibition of the enzyme adenylate cyclase can lead to an increase or decrease, respectively, in the generation of the intracellular messenger cyclic AMP.

Recent investigations have identified G proteins which regulate other mem-brane-amplifying proteins such as the enzymes phospholipase C (PLC), phos-pholipase A_2 (PLA_2), and cyclic guanosine monophosphate (GMP) phospho-

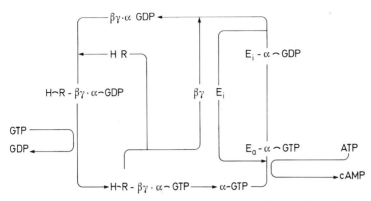

Fig. 2. Interactions among beta-receptor, G protein and adenylate kinase. *HR*, hormone receptor complex; $\alpha\beta\gamma$, α and $\beta\gamma$ subunits of G proteins; E_i inactive amplifying enzyme (adenylate cyclase): E_a, active amplifying enzyme

Table 1. Properties of regulatory G proteins

G Proteins	Amplifying proteins
1. G_s (M_r 44–46 × 10³)	Activates adenylate cyclase Activates Ca^{2+} channel
2. G_i (M_r 41 × 10³)	Inhibits adenylate cyclase
3. G_p (M_r 40 × 10³), and G_o (M_r 40 × 10³	Activates phospholipase C Activates phospholipase A_2 Activates Ca^{2+} channel
4. G_1 (M_r 40 × 10³)	Activates cyclic GMP phosphodiesterase

diesterase (cGMPD) [5]. The latter enzyme activation would lead to a decrease in cyclic GMP which may serve as an intracellular signal for vasodilation in the vascular system. Table 1 lists some properties of the various G proteins that have been identified in different tissues or cell types.

The Cyclic AMP-Linked Ca^{2+} Signalling: Alterations with Isoproterenol Toxicity

Figure 3 shows a flow diagram of the signal transduction pathway which is turned on through the activation of the beta-adrenergic receptors in the cardiac muscle cells. This pathway leads to an enhancement of the sarcolemmal slow inward Ca^{2+} channel (L type) activity by either a direct effect of the G protein on the channel or an indirect effect through an increase in the generation of intracellular messenger cyclic AMP and the ensuing increase in the cyclic AMP-dependent protein kinase (PKA) [6]. The latter enzyme phosphorylates the

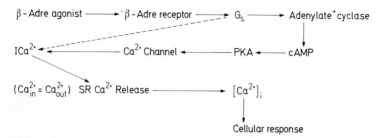

Fig. 3. Signal pathway in cardiomyocytes involving cyclic AMP-linked Ca^{2+} messenger system. *, activated enzyme. See text for symbols

voltage-dependent Ca^{2+} channel and thus enhances the inward Ca^{2+} current ($I_{Ca^{2+}}$) through it. The increased $I_{Ca^{2+}}$ triggers a larger release of Ca^{2+} from I_{Ca}^{2+} sarcoplasmic reticulum (SR) to result in a higher elevation in cystolic Ca^{2+} levels ($[Ca^{2+}]_i$) and a higher contractile force development. Because the SR rapidly resequesters the released Ca^{2+} and the Ca^{2+} entering the cell through the Ca^{2+} channel is extruded via the sarcolemmal $3Na^+/Ca^{2+}$ exchanger, the elevation in $[Ca^{2+}]_i$ is transient, and is referred to as the intracellular Ca^{2+} transient. A notable feature of the beta-adrenergic signal transduction pathway is a direct relationship between the magnitude and the duration of Ca^{2+} transient and the contractile response.

The treatment of rats with large doses of a beta-adrenergic agonist (isoproterenol toxicity) results in a disturbance in myocardial function characterized by inadequate relaxation of the heart [7]. This disturbance can be traced to alterations in the signal transduction mechanisms. The increase in cyclic AMP with beta-adrenergic stimulation of the heart produces both an increase in contractile force and an increase in heart rate. The increase in heart rate is effected through the activation of the Ca^{2+} channel coupled to a pacemaker current activation which augments the rate of diastolic depolarization in the conducting cardiac cells. The consequence of a higher rate of activation of cardiomyocytes is a greater shortening of the diastolic phase than the systolic phase of the cardiac cycle. This leads to an imbalance of Ca^{2+} fluxes into and out of the cytosolic compartments. With the increased heart rate, "systolic Ca^{2+} fluxes" (viz. influx through the Ca^{2+} channel and Ca^{2+} release from the SR) are less attenuated than the "diastolic Ca^{2+} fluxes" (viz. efflux via the $3NA^+/Ca^{2+}$ exchanger and SR Ca^{2+} uptake). This type of imbalance in Ca^{2+} fluxes would be expected to lead to a net accumulation of Ca^{2+} in the cytosolic compartment. Such an intracellular Ca^{2+} accumulation may be prevented by a pathophysiologic uptake of Ca^{2+} by SR and mitochondria. In the case of isoproterenol toxicity, the intracellular accumulation of Ca^{2+} presumably exceeds the Ca^{2+}-buffering capacity of SR and mitochondria and causes a sustained elevation of $[Ca^{2+}]_i$ (intracellular Ca^{2+} overload). Thus the interference with "diastolic Ca^{2+} fluxes" impairs relaxation and produces a myocardial dysfunction. Treatment of rats simultaneously with isoproterenol and the Ca^{2+} channel blocker verapamil resulted in the prevention of intracellular Ca^{2+} overload and the associated myocardial dysfunction [8].

The Phosphoinositide-Linked Ca^{2+} Signalling

Whereas there is a direct relationship between the intracellular Ca^{2+} transient and the cellular response in the cyclic AMP-linked signal transduction pathway such as is found in the cardiomyocytes, a number of other cell types (e.g., pituitary cells, adrenal cortical glomerulose cells, and pancreatic exocrine cells) show a cellular response which is dependent on an elevation in $[Ca^{2+}]_i$ but the duration of cellular response is not related to the duration of the Ca^{2+} transient [9]. In these cell types intracellular Ca^{2+} signalling is linked with the turnover and metabolism of phosphoinositides within the plasma membranes. Figure 4 shows a flow diagram of the signal transduction pathways involving phosphoinositides. In this system, stimulation of receptors (e.g., alpha-adrenergic, m-cholinergic, v_1-vasopressin, and angiotensin II) is coupled to activation of a G protein (G_p) which in turn activates the plasma membrane enzyme phospholipase C (PLC) [10]. This enzyme catalyzes the cleavage of phosphatidylinositol 4,5-bisphosphate into inositol 1,4,5-triphosphate (IP_3) and 1,2-diacylglycerol (DAG). DAG, a lipophilic molecule, is retained in the plasma membrane and there it serves as a second messenger which activates the plasma membrane enzyme protein kinase C (PKC). IP_3, a hydrophilic molecule, serves as a second messenger in the cytosol to promote the release of Ca^{2+} from the endoplasmic reticulum (ER) and transiently elevates cytosolic free Ca^{2+} concentration. The generation of the Ca^{2+} transient initiates the cellular response (e.g., secretion in the above-mentioned cell systems). The response, however, continues after the cessation of the Ca^{2+} transient. The sustenance of the cellular response beyond the duration of the Ca^{2+} transient is presumably mediated by the second messenger DAG and its activation of PKC. This latter enzyme phosphorylates protein, which may play a role in providing a sustained elicitation of the

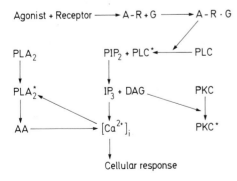

Fig. 4. Signal pathway involving phosphoinositide-linked Ca^{2+} messenger system.* activated enzyme. See text for symbols

response beyond the duration of the Ca^{2+} transient. In some cell systems, the Ca^{2+} transient may serve not only as an initiator of the cellular response but also as a signal for the activation of another amplifying enzyme in the plasma membrane, e.g., phospholipase A_2, which catalyzes the hydrolysis of phospholipids (PL) to yield arachidonic acid (AA) [11]. The latter fatty acid is the key precursor of prostaglandin and leukotriene compounds. The AA-derived compounds may also act as second messengers to produce cellular responses such as vasoconstriction and vasodilation in the vascular system or chemoattraction of inflammatory/immune system cells to sites of inflammation.

Signal Transduction Pathways in Inflammatory Cells

Inflammatory cells, neutrophils, macrophages, and lymphocytes provide for a vertebrate host's defense against exogenous and endogenous toxins, or harmful invading microorganisms. In these cells, a variety of receptors for ligands and the F_c portion of the antibodies (bound to antigens) have been recognized. The mechanisms of signal transductions in the inflammatory cells are at present under active investigation. A number of neutrophil and macrophage functions such as phagocytosis, O_2^- production, and the release of cytokines evidently depend on the activation of these cells via signal pathways involving a variety of signal regulating and amplifying proteins, and second messenger systems.

Figure 5 shows components of the signal transduction pathway implicated in the activation of neutrophil production of the free radical superoxide O_2^- by a chemotactic peptide, f-Met-Leu-Phe (f-MLP). Much evidence has been presented to show the involvement of the phosphoinositide-specific enzyme phospholipase C, the subsequent mobilization of Ca^{2+} from an intracellular site, and the activation of PKC [12]. An interesting finding reported is that when

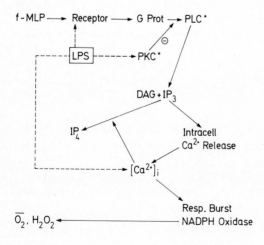

Fig. 5. Lipopolysaccharide-induced alterations in neutrophil signal pathway. *, activated enzyme. See text for symbols

neutrophils are "primed" with lipopolysaccharide (LPS) by incubating them with LPS, the f-MLP-mediated elevation of cytosolic Ca^{2+} is much greater. Accompanying the increase in cytosolic $[Ca^{2+}]_i$ is an increase in O_2^- production with its tissue/cell-damaging potential. This lends support to the concept that the gram-negative septic mediator lipopolysaccharide (LPS) enhances neutrophil activation via hypersensitization of the signal transduction mechanism. Thus, LPS mediator increased O_2^- production could serve not only to augment the nonspecific inflammatory response to contain invading bacteria but also potentially pose a hazard to host tissues. The site of action of LPS (in the signal transduction pathway) appears to be the mobilization of Ca^{2+} from an intracellular store rather than f-MLP interaction with its receptor or the activation of the enzyme PKC [13]. While $[Ca^{2+}]_i$ is implicated as a second messenger in the neutrophil superoxide-producing response, its role is not certain in the endocytic response in neutrophils [14].

The various inflammatory and immune responses elicited by macrophages are ascribed to their ability to release cytokines. Interleukin-1 (IL-1α or IL-1β) and tumor necrosis factor (TNFα) are the two most extensively studied cytokines. A variety of stimuli or messengers, such as LPS, IL-2, interferon-γ, and prostaglandins modulate the release of these cytokines from the macrophages [15]. The signal transduction pathways involving these messengers have been elucidated by the use of activators or inhibitors of various potential second messengers that may be involved. These studies have centered around the use of (a) phorbol esters as activators of PKC, (b) H7 as a PKC inhibitor, (c) W7 as an inhibitor of Ca^{2+} and calmodulin-dependent kinase, and (d) HT1004 as a blocker of cyclic AMP and cyclic GMP. Although the interpretations of these studies have not unequivocally shown the operation of specific signal pathways during the activation of macrophages by LPS, it is generally accepted that both IL-1 and TNFα release involves PKC. Recent studies have shown that whereas PKC inhibition alone abolishes induction of TNFα messenger ribonucleic acid (mRNA), both PKC and calmodulin-dependent kinase are required for IL-1 mRNA induction [16]. The PKC pathway also appears to be involved in the IL-1-mRNA induction by IL-2 [17]. Since HT1004 did not inhibit IL-1 or TNFα production by macrophages, it is suggested that the cyclic AMP pathway may not play a significant role.

Figure 6 shows components of the signal transduction pathways that appear to be operative in the activation of macrophages by the immune complexes through the macrophage F_c receptors [12]. Three separate signal pathways are shown. One of the two F_c receptors interacts with immune complex 2a (Ia-IgG2a) to activate an enzyme casein kinase II (CKII), which in turn activates the enzyme adenylate cyclase, resulting in the generation of cyclic AMP. Cyclic AMP seems to participate in the O_2^- production and phagocytosis by macrophages. A second F_c receptor interacting with Ib antigen IgG2B complexes apparently results in the activation of membrane enzyme phospholipase A_2 which leads to the formation of arachidonic acid (AA) and prostaglandin E_2 (PGE$_2$). Experiments have also supported the presence of a PGE$_2$ receptor on

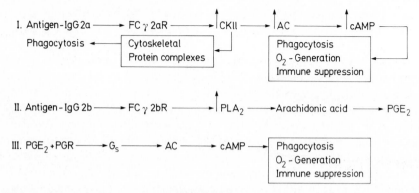

Fig. 6. Signal pathways in macrophages. See text for symbols

macrophages [12]. PGE receptor activation, as shown in Fig. 6, could contribute to generation of second messenger cyclic AMP. Also, a role of cyclic AMP in immune suppression may be mediated through these signal transduction pathways.

References

1. Rosen OM (1987) After insulin binds. Science 237:1452–1458
2. Aldrich RW, Dionne VE et al. (1986) Ion transport through ligand-gated channels. In: Andrioli TE et al. (eds) Membrane transport processes in organized systems. Plenum, New York, pp 107–132
3. Casperson GF, Bourne HR (1987) Biochemical and molecular genetic analysis of hormone-sensitive adenylyl cyclase. Annu Rev Pharmacol Toxicol 27:371–384
4. Gilman AG (1990) Regulation of adenylyl cyclase by G proteins. In: Nishizuka Y et al. (eds) The biology of medicine of signal transduction. Raven, New York, pp 51–57
5. Stryer L, Bourne HR (1986) G proteins: a family of signal transducers. Annu Rev Cell Biol 2:391–419
6. Pilkis SJ, El-Maghrabi MR, Claus TH (1988) Hormonal regulation of hepatic gluconeogenesis. Annu Rev Biochem 57:755–783
7. Bloom S, Concilla PA (1969) Myocytolysis and mitochondrial calcification in rat myocardium after low doses of isoproterenol. Am J Physiol 54:373–391
8. Rasmussen H, Barret P, et al. (1990) Calcium ion as intracellular messenger and cellular toxin. Environ Health Perspect 84:17–25
9. Barrett PQ, Kojima IK et al. (1990) Short term memory in the calcium messenger system. Biochem J 238:905–912
10. Berridge MJ (1987) Inositol lipids and calcium signalling. Proc R Soc Lond [Biol] 234:359–378
11. Volpe P, Krause KH, et al. (1988) Calciosome, a cytoplasmic organelle: the inositol 1,4,5-trisphosphate-sensitive Ca^{2+} store of nonmuscle cells. Proc Natl Acad Sci USA 85:1091–1095
12. Nishizuke Y (1986) Studies and perspectives of protein kinase C. Science 233:305–312
13. Forehand JR, et al. (1989) Lipopolysaccharide priming of human neutrophils for an enhanced burst. J Clin Invest 83:74–83
14. Stossel TP (1988) The mechanical response of white blood cells. In: Gallin JI et al. (eds) Inflammation: basic principles and clinical correlates. Raven, New York, pp 325–342
15. Kovacs EJ (1991) Control of IL-1 and TNFα production at the level of second messenger pathways In: Kimball ES (ed) Cytokines in inflammatory diseases. CRC Press, Boca Raton, pp 89–107

16. Hamilton TA, Adams DO (1987) Molecular mechanisms of signal transduction in macrophages. Immunol Today 8:151–158
17. Kunkel SL, Scales WE, et al. (1988) Dynamics and regulation of macrophage tumor necrosis factor-α (TNF), interleukin-1α (IL-1α) and interleukin-1β (IL-1β) gene expression by arachidonate metabolites, monokines. In: Powanda MC et al. (eds) Monokines and other non-lymphocytic cytokines. Liss, New York, pp 61–66

Neuroendocrine Regulation of Immune Function

J. W. Holaday[1], J. R. Kenner[2], P. F. Smith[3], H. U. Bryant[4], and E. W. Bernton[5]

Introduction

The body's global responses to stress, injury, and disease involve an orchestrated communication among the brain, endocrine and immune systems. Within the past decade, a newly emerging field of biomedical research has established many of the mechanisms of communication within this "neuroendocrine-immune axis." This review will focus on the role of this axis in the body's physiological and pharmacological responses to the severe stress of shock, trauma, and sepsis.

The body's reaction to chronic stress (which may differ from acute stress) includes marked changes in the regulation of neuroendocrine function within the brain, pituitary, and target glands. For example, chronic stress results in the sustained elevation of circulating glucocorticoids and the reduced secretion of gonadotropins, thyroid stimulating hormone (TSH), prolactin, and growth hormone (GH) in the plasma [1]. All of these neuroendocrine hormones affect survival of the organism via their important roles in the regulation of growth, reproduction, metabolism, and immunity.

Although the suppressive effects of endogenous or pharmacologically administered glucocorticoids on immune responses have been known for some time [2], other steroid and peptide hormones have more recently been shown to affect immunity. Current research reviewed herein indicates that pituitary- or lymphocyte- derived prolactin may function as an immunopermissive hormone. Evidence is also accumulating to indicate that these brain/endocrine/immune interactions, are not unidirectional. For example, the release of monokines such as interleukin-1 (IL-1), interleukin-6 (IL-6) or tumor necrosis factor (TNF) from macrophages as part of immunological responses to infection or inflammation may also affect brain and neuroendocrine function by stimulating or inhibiting the release of many pituitary hormones [3–7].

[1] Medicis Pharmaceutical Corporation, 100 E. 42nd St., New York, NY 10017, USA
[2] George Washington University, School of Medicine, Washington, DC 20037, USA
[3] Department of Anatomy, Uniformed Services University of the Health Sciences, Bethesda, MD 20814, USA
[4] Department of Immunology, Pulmonary & Leukotriene Research, Eli Lilly and Co., Lilly Corporate Center, Indianapolis, IN 46285, USA
[5] Department of Medical Neurosciences, Division of Neuropsychiatry, Walter Reed Army Institute of Research, Washington, DC 20307, USA

Host Defense Dysfunction
in Trauma, Shock and Sepsis
Eds. Faist/Meakins/Schildberg
© Springer-Verlag, Berlin Heidelberg 1993

Endocrine Substances Affecting Immune Responses

Elevations in glucocorticoids, e.g., cortisol, in response to stress depend upon a sequence of actions in the neuroendocrine network, including the hypothalamic release of corticotropin-releasing hormone (CRH) which activates the anterior pituitary gland to result in the release of adrenocorticotropic hormone (ACTH). In turn, ACTH stimulates the release of adrenal glucocorticoids. The physiological release or pharmacological administration of glucocorticoids feeds back upon the brain and pituitary glands to inhibit the further release of CRH, ACTH, and cortisol. In homeostatic conditions, circulating cortisol levels are maintained within physiological levels by this feedback network; circadian oscillations result in increased cortisol in the morning, with cortisol levels declining throughout the day and night. Disruption of circadian cortisol rhythms brought about by critical illnesses or by its chronic management may contribute to temporal changes in lymphocyte counts and other measures of immune function.

Among their many biological actions, glucocorticoids are known to result in a reduction in spleen and thymus size, as well as impaired cellular and humoral immunity. At the leukocyte level, glucocorticoids block macrophage IL-1 and TNF release, block the inflammatory actions of IL-1 and decrease gamma-interferon and interleukin-2 (IL-2) release by T lymphocytes. In the practice of critical care medicine, patients are known to experience sustained glucocorticoid levels either due to chronic stress or due to the pharmacological use of "steroids" for the treatment of disorders such as sepsis, stroke, or inflammation. The cascade of immunological responses brought about by glucocorticoids may contribute to impaired host defenses in these individuals.

Prolactin is one member of a superfamily of related hormones, including GH, proliferin, and placental lactogen, that share some structural similarities and biological actions [8]. Although prolactin is classically associated with lactation, prolactin subserves several additional physiological functions, including its profound effects upon the immune system (see [8] for review).

As with glucocorticoids, the physiological release of prolactin from the pituitary fluctuates in a pulsatile circadian fashion and is further modulated by behavioral and environmental stimuli, the reproductive cycle, steroid hormones, neurotransmitters, immunoregulatory cytokines, and various drugs. Prolactin secretion is tonically inhibited by the release of the neurotransmitter dopamine from the hypothalamus that acts upon dopamine-2 (DA-2) receptors located on lactotroph cells of the anterior pituitary. The opposite effect occurs when dopamine antagonists such as metoclopramide or haloperidol are used; the tonic inhibition of prolactin release is removed, resulting in prompt prolactin secretion.

Early evidence indicated the potential importance of prolactin in immune function. Either hypophysectomy or the drug bromocryptine, a DA-2 agonist that inhibits prolactin secretion, were shown to suppress antibody formation in a prolactin-reversible manner [9]. Our laboratories have extended these early findings by studies demonstrating that bromocryptine-induced hypoprolactin-emia in mice results in a variety of immunological effects, including: (a) increased lethality of an infectious challenge with *Listeria monocytogenes*; (b) abrogation of T-lymphocyte-dependent activation of macrophages, as well as the production of lymphocyte-derived macrophage - activating factor (gamma - interferon) following inoculation with Listeria or mycobacteria; and (c) suppression of T-lymphocyte proliferation without affecting the production of IL-2 [10]. All of the changes produced by bromocryptine were prevented by coincident administration of ovine prolactin.

Unlike hypoprolactinemia, the stimulation of prolactin release by the administration of dopamine antagonists such as metoclopramide (a drug commonly used in managing the critically ill) reverses many measures of immunosuppression brought about by cyclosporine, glucocorticoids, or chronic morphine treatment in mice. Although collective evidence such as this strongly indicates that prolactin stimulates immune function, prolactin cannot be considered to serve as an immunostimulant per se since hyperprolactinemia does not further enhance immune function if it is already functioning adequately [7, 8]. Instead, prolactin may be an important counter-regulatory immunotrophic hormone that can oppose the immunosuppressive actions of drugs such as cyclosporine, morphine, or glucocorticoids.

Prolactin-like Protein in Lymphocytes: A New Autocrine Cytokine?

Perhaps one of the most interesting developments in the newly evolving discipline of neuroendocrine immunology has been the discovery that leukocytes are capable of producing many of the hormones usually associated with an anterior pituitary origin, including GH, TSH, and ACTH [11]. We have added to this list of "pituitary hormones" found in lymphocytes with our evidence that lymphocytes also produce a prolactin-like protein [12]. In fact, we have proposed that lymphocyte-derived prolactin-like protein may function as an autocrine cytokine that facilitates lymphocyte proliferation.

Using immunocytochemical techniques with antibodies specific to pituitary prolactin, it was demonstrated that 48 h following mitogenic stimulation with concanavalin A (Con-A), phytohemagglutinin, or antibody to the T3 receptor, a large subpopulation of human or murine T and B lymphocytes contain prolactin immunoreactivity [12]. The T-cell mitogen Con-A increased the expression of lymphocytic prolactin more that 2.5-fold [12]. In a manner uncharacteristic of most secreted proteins, electron microscopic studies indicated that lymphocyte prolactin was localized in discrete cytoplasmic avesicular foci (Fig. 1). Control studies demonstrated the specificity of these antiprolactin antibodies for prolactin and confirmed that the prolactin within the lymphocytes did not derive from the media or from the pituitary [12]. From these

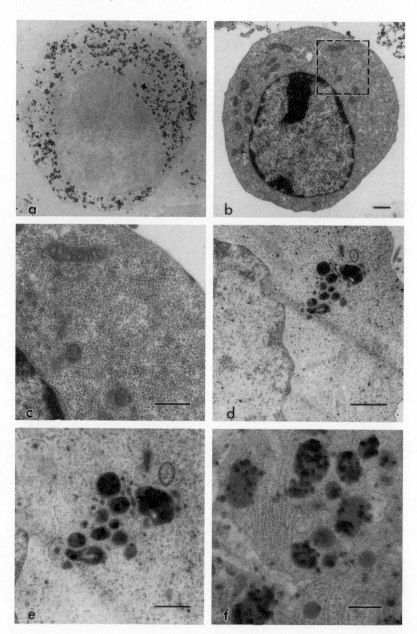

Fig. 1a–f. Electron micrographs of splenocytes grown in serum-free medium and stimulated 48 h with the mitogen Con-A. Cells were labeled with anti-prolactin antiserum. **a** Photomicrograph of a lymphocyte demonstrating dark granular cytoplasmic staining for prolactin immunoreactivity. **b** A serial section of the same lymphocyte stained with uranyl acetate and lead citrate, enlarged in **c** (scale bar 1 μm). On rare occasion, prolactin-like immunoreactivity was observed in a few, large secretory granules (**d** scale bar 1 μm; **e** scale bar 0.5μm), reminiscent of prolactin granules in pituitary lactotropes (**f** scale bar 0.5μm). (Reprinted with permission from [12])

results, it remains unclear as to whether lymphocyte prolactin is secreted by lymphocytes or acts within the lymphocyte.

Estimates of molecular weight for lymphocyte prolactin-like protein using western blot analysis indicated that this polypeptide had a molecular weight of 48 000, approximately twice as large as pituitary prolactin [12]. Furthermore, the lymphocyte-derived prolactin-like protein was shown to function in cell proliferation in studies demonstrating that the addition of antiprolactin antibodies to mitogen-stimulated lymphocytes inhibited their proliferation in a prolactin reversible manner [13].

Interleukin-1: Effects on Anterior Pituitary Hormone Release

Following inflammation, endotoxemia, or infectious stimuli, (IL-1) is rapidly secreted by mononuclear phagocytes, e.g., macrophages, to achieve detectable levels in the circulation. In addition to amplifying T-cell responses to antigens, this monokine has numerous hormone-like systemic effects and pharmacologic actions within the brain. For example, the central injection of IL-1 induces sleep, fever, and the synthesis of acute-phase proteins by the liver. Many of these signs and symptoms typically occur in critically ill patients suffering from septic shock.

We were interested in determining whether IL-1, by direct actions on the anterior pituitary, could play a role in orchestrating acute neuroendocrine adaptations to infectious stressors [3, 4]. The application of subnanomolar concentrations of human recombinant IL-1 beta or mouse recombinant IL-1 alpha to 72 h monolayer cultures of dispersed rat pituitary cells was shown to result in significant increases in the secretion of ACTH, GH, TSH and luteinizing hormone (LH). By contrast, prolactin secretion was slightly decreased [3]. The initial studies using primary pituitary cell cultures were reinforced by data obtained from perfusion of hemipituitaries; these experiments were performed to study the time course of IL-1 actions and to more closely approximate physiological tissue [4]. Results indicated that human IL-1 beta stimulated almost immediate release of ACTH, GH, TSH, and LH into the perfusate. When compared across time, prolactin release in response to IL-1 differed in that fresh hemipituitary perfusates demonstrated increased prolactin release, whereas prolactin levels (but not ACTH, GH, TSH, or LH) in response to IL-1 in pituitary sections incubated for 72 h were significantly blunted [4].

While other investigators have shown that the stimulation of ACTH release in rats injected with IL-1 seemed to be mediated by stimulation of CRF via hypothalamic actions [5], our studies suggest that physiological concentrations of IL-1 may also function as a direct and relatively nonspecific anterior pituitary secretagogue; these suggestions are reinforced by recent data demonstrating IL-1-immunoreactive innervation of the hypothalamus, including the median eminence [14], as well as by recent evidence indicating the presence of IL-1 receptors in the brain and pituitary. Thus, we suggest that IL-1 appears to be another hypophysiotropic factor having actions upon the brain or directly on the pituitary to affect endocrine or behavioral responses to infection or injury. Abnormal endocrine responses in the critically ill, including the "sick euthyroid" syndrome, may well be a direct or indirect consequence of IL-1 or other cytokine actions on the neuroendocrine axis.

Summary

In this review, some important functional interactions among the brain, endocrine, and immune systems are summarized, with particular relevance to the practice of critical care medicine. The neuroendocrine axis regulates the production of hormones that modify immune function, including ACTH and adrenal glucocorticoids, as well as prolactin. Prolactin levels are profoundly affected by dopaminergic drugs commonly used in the intensive care setting. We have demonstrated that the immunosuppressive effects of hypoprolactinemia, chronic morphine treatment, and glucocorticoids are reversed by prolactin or by drugs that stimulate endogenous prolactin release. Evidence was also reviewed to indicate that cytokine products of the orchestrated immune response to infection or inflammation, such as IL-1, can feed back upon the neuroendocrine system to affect the spectrum of hormones released during critical illnesses.

Although much of this research reflects animal experimentation, there are several clinical correlates to indicate that dopamine agonists do indeed play a role in suppressing human immune responses via suppression of prolactin release. It was noted that the use of bromocryptine for the treatment of Parkinson's disease also improved autoimmune uveitis in a small population of patients with this coincident condition [15]. The response was attributed to the decrease in circulating prolactin. The combined use of cyclosporine and bromocryptine to prevent rejection of transplanted organs has also been suggested based upon the immunosuppressive effects of hypoprolactinemia.

Many drugs commonly found in the intensive care setting may have beneficial or detrimental actions well beyond their intended purpose. For example, dopamine drips used to maintain renal perfusion in septic shock patients may contribute to the anergy of critical illnesses by depriving the organism of the immunopermissive actions of prolactin. Future clinical research based upon animal and in vitro studies, such as those reviewed above, may reveal that therapy with prolactin, GH, or drugs such as metoclopramide, might reconstitute immune host defenses. Thus, our increasing knowledge of the functional role of the neuroendocrine-immune axis may well improve our knowledge of how to care for the critically ill patient.

References

1. Tache Y, Du Ruisseau P, Ducharme JR, Collu R (1978) Pattern of adenohypophyseal hormone changes in male rats following chronic stress. Neuroendocrinology 26:208–219
2. Parrillo JE, Fauci AS (1979) Mechanisms of glucocorticoid action on immune process. Annu Rev Pharmacol Toxicol 19:129–201
3. Bernton E, Beach J, Holaday JW, Smallridge R, Fein H (1987) Release of multiple hormones by a direct action of interleukin-1 on pituitary cells. Science 238:519–521
4. Beach JE, Smallridge RC, Kinzer CA, Bernton EW, Holaday JW, Fein HG (1989) Interleukin-1 releases multiple hormones from perifused rat pituitaries. Life Sci 44:1–8
5. Berkenbosch F, van Oert J, Del Ray A, Tilders F, Besedovsky H (1987) CRF-producing neurons in the rat are activated by interleukin-1. Science 238:524–526
6. Dubuis JM, Dayer JM, Siegrist-Kaiser CA, Burger AG (1988) Human recombinant interleukin-1 beta decreases plasma thyroid hormone and thyroid-stimulating hormone levels in rats. Endocrinology 123:2175–2181
7. Holaday JW, Bryant HU, Kenner JR, Bernton EW (1988) Pharmacologic manipulations of the endocrine/immune axis. Prog Neuroendocrin Immunol 1:6–8
8. Bernton EW (1989) Prolactin and immune host defenses. Prog Neuroendocrin Immunol 2:21–29
9. Nagy E, Berczi I, Wren GE, Asa SL, Kovacs K (1983) Immunomodulation by bromocryptine. Immunopharmacology 6:231–243
10. Bernton EW, Meltzer MS, Holaday JW (1988) Suppression of macrophage activation and T-lymphocyte function in hypoprolactinemic mice. Science 239:401–403
11. Weigent DA, Blalock JE (1987) Interactions between the neuroendocrine and immune systems: Common hormones and receptors. Immunol Rev 100:79–96
12. Kenner JR, Holaday JW, Bernton EW, Smith PF (1990) Prolactin in murine lymphocytes: morphologic and biochemical evidence. Prog Neuroendocrin Immunol 3:188–195
13. Hartmann DP, Holaday JW, Bernton EW (1989) Inhibition of lymphocyte proliferation by antibodies to prolactin. FASEB J 3:2194–2202
14. Breder C, Dinarello C, Saper C (1988) Interleukin-1 immunoreactive innervation of the human hypothalamus. Science 240:321–323
15. Palestine AG, Nussenblatt RB (1988) The effect of bromocriptine on anterior uveitis. Am J Ophthalmol 104(4):488–489

Beneficial Effects of Stress Response Blockade on Patients Undergoing Surgery

H. Kehlet

Predictable and well-described physiological and metabolic changes occur in response to anaesthesia and surgery [1, 2]. The physiological significance of these alterations characterized by hypermetabolism, substrate mobilization and altered immune function is usually considered to confer an advantage for survival, being a homeostatic defense mechanism to help the body to heal tissue and adapt to injury. Although some components of the stress response undoubtedly are of value, the necessity for the global stress response, and in particular the classical catabolic hormonal response, has been questioned in modern anaesthesiologic and surgical settings [3, 4]. Furthermore, concern about detrimental effects such as myocardial infarction, pulmonary complications, thromboembolism and postoperative fatigue, which may not be directly related to imperfection of surgical technique, has led to the hypothesis that the injury response may be an important pathogenetic factor. Subsequently, strategies have been developed to alter the responses in such a way that functions supposed to be beneficial and to promote recovery should be stimulated, while others, which may enhance catabolism and lead to organ dysfunction, should be suppressed.

An improved understanding of the release mechanisms of the surgical injury response to be afferent and efferent neural reflex responses as well as various humoral mediators (arachidonic cascade metabolites, cytokines etc.) has subsequently led to modifying techniques to alter the neurohumoral response to surgery (Fig. 1) in the hope that such manipulation will improve outcome.

This paper briefly summarizes the modifying effect of general anaesthesia, pain relief and humoral mediator blockade on the stress response and potential effects on surgical outcome, while the effect of hormonal manipulation and nutrition will be covered in other chapters in this volume.

The modifying effect of *general anaesthetic techniques* on the surgical stress response is minimal except for high-dose opioid anaesthesia, hypothermic anaesthesia and etomidate [3, 5]. No data have been published from controlled studies to demonstrate beneficial or detrimental effects of a modification of the surgical stress response by these techniques. However, no important clinical effect should be expected, since these techniques only inhibit the stress response during the operation without prolonged effects into the postoperative period.

Department of Surgical Gastroenterology, Hvidovre University Hospital, 2650 Hvidovre, Denmark

Host Defense Dysfunction
in Trauma, Shock and Sepsis
Eds. Faist/Meakins/Schildberg
© Springer-Verlag, Berlin Heidelberg 1993

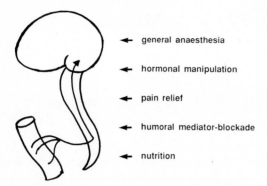

general anaesthesia

hormonal manipulation

pain relief

humoral mediator-blockade

nutrition

Fig. 1. Modifying factors of the neurohumoral response to injury

The effect of *pain relief* on the surgical stress response has been reviewed recently [4–6], and can be summarized as follows: Pain relief with antagonists to peripheral mediators of pain (prostaglandins, histamine, serotonin, substance P etc.) has not been demonstrated to be very effective when used alone [3, 6], except for the nonsteroidal anti-inflammatory drugs (NSAIDs) who, besides their pain releiving effect, also reduce the hyperthermic response, improve nitrogen balance and improve cardiovascular stability, although the overall effect is only moderate [4–7]. Ibuprofen has also been demonstrated to reduce the hypermetabolic and endocrine response, tachycardia and fever, but not leucocytosis and acute phase protein response following endotoxin administration [8]. The clinical effect of the NSAIDs on postoperative morbidity, besides pain relief, has not been clarified [9], but probably the effect will be minor. However, further studies with the NSAIDs on different stress responses to surgery and organ function should be performed including new arachidonic cascade blockers such as lipooxygenase inhibitors etc. The effect of local anaesthetics in the wound, intrapleurally, intraperitoneally or on the skin is a variable degree of pain relief, but without important effects on the surgical stress response or outcome [4–6].

The effect of nociceptive blockade and pain relief with central neural blockade with spinal or epidural analgesia with local anaesthetics, opioids or alpha agonists is well described [3–6, 10]. These studies have demonstrated intrathecal or epidural local anaesthetics to be the most effective technique to inhibit the surgical stress response by reducing hypermetabolism and catabolism, but without major influence on immunological alterations. Protein economy is improved and organ function preserved. However, these effects are mostly observed in procedures in the lower part of the abdomen (gynaecological procedures, major orthopaedic and urological surgery) while the technique is less effective in major abdominal and thoracic procedures, probably because of insufficient afferent blockade [4–6]. pain relief with epidural opioids is a selective nociceptive blockade, without major effects on the surgical stress response [4, 5], and similar findings have been observed using epidural alpha agonists [4–6]. Recent observations (unpublished) suggest that increasing the

Table 1. Effect of neural blockade by regional anaesthesia on the surgical stress response and postoperative morbidity, based upon cumulated data from [3–6]

Cumulated experience	Stress response/morbidity
Data conclusive of a beneficial effect of neural blockade	Inhibition of the catabolic response to lower body procedures Reduction in intraoperative blood loss Reduction in thromboembolic complications Reduction in postoperative gastrointestinal ileus Reduction in early postoperative mortality in acute hip surgery
Data suggestive of a beneficial effect of neural blockade	Moderate inhibition of the catabolic response to major abdominal surgery Reduction in postoperative pulmonary complications Decreased hospital stay following lower body procedures
No proven effect or too few data	Postoperative mental dysfunction Cardiac complications
Detrimental effects of neural blockade	No data from controlled studies

volume of epidural local anaesthetic or using a combination of epidural and spinal local anaesthetics will improve the afferent blockade and thereby enhance the inhibitory effect of these techniques on the stress response, even to major abdominal operation.

The clinical effects of neural blockade techniques on postoperative outcome is quite well described by plenty of controlled studies [5, 11, 12]. These effects are summarized in Table 1 and clearly represents a clinical advantage since similar all-over effects cannot be obtained by other techniques. However, although these techniques may alter the surgical stress response and positively influence outcome, there is still no final proof of a causal relationship. Nevertheless, these two lines of research strongly suggest that inhibition of surgically induced nociceptive stimuli and thereby various aspects of the stress response, may actually improve postoperative outcome.

The effect of humoral mediator blockade (arachidonic cascade metabolites, cytokines etc.) on the surgical stress response and postoperative outcome has not been clarified except for the effect of NSAIDs as mentioned above. Blockade of cytokine responses by specific release inhibitors or peripheral antagonists have not been done in surgical patients. Pharmacological doses of glucocorticoids represent a possibility for an overall inhibition of various humoral mediators (all arachidonic cascade metabolites, cytokines etc.). The limited data from the use of high-dose glucocorticoids preoperatively suggest an inhibition of the hyperthermic interleukin-6 (IL-6) and prostaglandin E_2 (PGE_2) responses as well as pain relief, pulmonary function and postoperative fatigue may be improved when used in combination with epidural techniques and indomethacin [12, 13]. However, the potential side effects of such single, high-dose glucocorticoid therapy in surgical patients on immunofunction, and resistance to infection and wound healing obviously need to be investigated.

Conclusion

As to the important question of whether the surgical stress response should be prevented, the literature unfortunately contains a limited amount of postoperative data from controlled studies compared with the rather extensive amount of data on the effect of various modifying techniques on biochemical parameters of the stress response. However, the data obtained from surgical patients operated on during neural blockade with local anaesthetics with or without combinations with other drugs (opioids, systemic NSAID), have clearly demonstrated this to be our most effective technique to inhibit the surgically induced endocrine metabolic changes. It shall be emphasized that the technique is not optimal, especially during major procedures. Nevertheless, several controlled clinical studies suggest these neural blockade techniques to reduce various aspects of postoperative morbidity. Therefore, these data should stimulate further research to improve afferent neural blockade and inhibition of the surgical stress response followed by well-designed clinical studies on outcome. In addition, techniques which may modify the stress response may be combined with techniques to stimulate anabolism such as various growth factors as well as nutrition in order to enhance recovery. Such investigations may hopefully in the near future provide a breakthrough in the treatment of major surgery and to give an answer to the question whether "stress-free anaesthesia in surgery" is just an attractive working hypothesis or an instrument to improve surgical outcome. Finally, such knowledge may help us to improve outcome when applied in trauma patients and other severely ill patients.

References

1. Weissman C (1990) The metabolic response of stress, an overview and update. Anesthesiology 73:308–327
2. Bevan DR (ed) (1989) Metabolic response of surgery. Clin Anaesth 3:295–450
3. Kehlet H (1987) Modification of responses to surgery by neural blockade: clinical implications. In: Cousins MJ, Bridenbaugh PO (eds) Neural blockade in clinical anesthesia and management of pain, 2nd edn. Lippincott, Philadelphia, pp 145–188
4. Kehlet H (1989) Surgical stress. The role of pain and analgesia. Br J Anaesth 63:189–195
5. Kehlet H (1991) Differential effects of regional versus general anaesthesia: responses to surgery and postoperative outcome. In: Rogers M, Tinker J, Covino B (eds) Principals and practice of anesthesiology. Mosby, St. Louis (in press)
6. Kehlet H (1990) Neural release mechanisms in the response to injury. In: Aasen AO, Risberg B (eds) Surgical pathophysiology. Harwood Academic, New York, pp 77–90
7. Dahl JB, Kehlet H (1991) Non-steroidal antiinflammatory drugs: rationale for use in severe postoperative pain. Br J Anaesth (in press)

8. Revhaug A, Mitchie HR, Manson Mc J et al. (1988) Inhibition of cyclooxygenase attenuates the metabolic response to endotoxin in humans. Arch Surg 123:162–170
9. Schulze S, Roikjær O, Hasselstrøm L, Jensen NH, Kehlet H (1988) Epidural bupivacaine and morphine plus systemic indomethacin eliminates pain but not systemic response and convalescense after cholecystectomy. Surgery 103:321–327
10. Scott NB, Kehlet H (1988) Regional anaesthesia and surgical morbidity. Br J Surg 75:299–304
11. Kehlet H (1990) Epidural anaesthesia in surgical practice. Curr Pract Surg 2:223–226
12. Schulze S, Møller IW, Bang U, Rye B, Kehlet H (1990) Effect of combined prednisolone, epidural analgesia and indomethacin on pain, systemic response and convalescence after cholecystectomy. Acta Chir Scand 156:203–209
13. Schulze S, Summer P, Bigler D et al. (1991) Effect of combined prednisolone, epidural analgesia and indomethacin on the systemic response after colonic surgery (submitted)

The Impact of Preexisting Disease Conditions for Host Defense Integrity in Traumatized and Critically Ill Patients

N. V. Christou[1] and J. M. Tellado[2]

Trauma affects both components of host defense in that specific immunity is altered as well as nonspecific immunity. The question remains whether these changes are beneficial or detrimental for the host. Preexisting disease conditions such as cancer, inflammatory diseases, nutritional deficits, infection, and immunosuppressive drugs are all associated with alterations in host defense that may influence changes in host immunocompetence seen following trauma [1]. There are several methods for testing the host defense capacity of trauma victims. Some of these use single in vitro measurements such as lymphocyte responses to phytohemaglutinin (PHA). Others use in vitro multiple measures such as measurement of the cytokines tumor necrosis factor (TNF), interleukin-1 (IL-1), IL-2, IL-6, IL-8 or several of the immunoglobulins. Lastly, there are in vivo measurements such as response to skin test antigens [2].

All of these have their own inherent advantages and disadvantages. For example, Munster et al. [3], have reported that lymphocyte stimulation ratio after exposure to PHA or to streptokinase-streptodornase (SKSD) predicted the development of "sepsis" (Fig. 1). SKSD stimulation of lymphocytes produced a "dip" by the second day after burn which returned to normal by the 21st day after burn. This alteration of lymphocyte responses to the antigen SKSD was felt to be a good predictor of sepsis. More recently, Moore et al. [4] have shown that the cytokine response in trauma is altered and this alteration is very rapid. They demonstrated a very rapid rise in granulocyte colony stimulating factor (G-CSF) followed by a rapid decline in G-CSF by the 24th hour post-trauma. Il-6 was detected within hours of trauma and then declined slowly, detectable at 1.2 pg/ml serum for many days post-trauma. Faist et al. [5] have also demonstrated that trauma is associated with decreased secretion of IL-1, IL-6, and IL-8 secretion up to the 7th day post-trauma (Fig. 2). Septic patients also demonstrated a decrease of cytokine release following treatment of their monocytes with lipopolysaccharide (LPS). Neopterin levels were, on the contrary, slightly increased following trauma and sepsis, indicating macrophage activation.

A means of globally assessing host defense response is the delayed-type hypersensitivity (DTH) response to ubiquitous antigens (Fig. 3). This is an objective measurement which is easily performed. There are extensive data in

[1] Department of Surgery, McGill University, 687 Pine Avenue West, Montreal, Quebec, Canada H3A 1A1
[2] Cirugia General III, Hospital Gregorio Maranon, c/Dr. Esquerdo 46, 28007 Madrid, Spain

Host Defense Dysfunction
in Trauma, Shock and Sepsis
Eds. Faist/Meakins/Schildberg
© Springer-Verlag, Berlin Heidelberg 1993

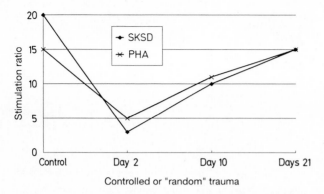

Fig. 1. The stimulation ratio of lymphocytes from trauma patients exposed to antigens (SKSD) or mitogens (PHA) at various times after trauma. (Adapted from [3])

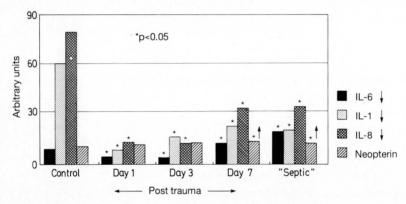

Fig. 2. The cytokine response after trauma correlated with macrophage activation (neopterin levels). (Adapted from [5])

the literature and this method is applicable in trauma patients. This response depends on prior sensitization where a nonimmune lymphocyte having antigen presented on the surface of macrophage becomes an immune lymphocyte. The second step involves recognition, where an immune lymphocyte encounters the antigen injected in the skin and then sets up a cytokine and lymphokine response which involves nonspecific inflammation and thus detection of a "bump" in the skin. In our experience with this technique we determined that, if patients are found to be *anergic* (no DTH skin test response to five ubiquitous antigens) upon admission to hospital, they had a 33% mortality rate, compared to 4% for reactive patients (those who responded to two or more antigens). Over 80% of the deaths in these anergic patients were related to an infectious complication, either present at admission, or evolved while in hospital [6]. Many other laboratories concur with these findings.

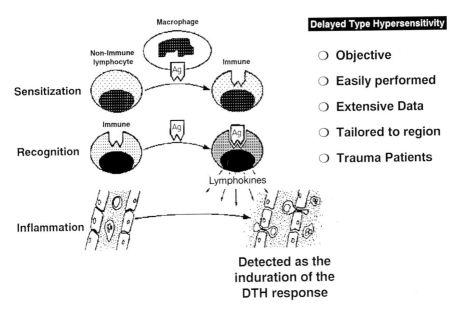

Fig. 3. The immunology of the delayed-type hypersensitivity skin test response

The various components of the immune system are elegantly integrated in vivo in order to control bacterial infections. We have used logistic regression analysis of immune and nonimmune variables, and demonstrated that serum albumin, the DTH response, and patient age are significantly and independently correlated with the probability of mortality, as given by the equation:

$$P(\text{death}) = 1/\{1 + \exp[-1.343 + 1.372 \times (\text{albumin}) + 0.173$$
$$\times \ln(\text{DTH score})] - 0.026(\text{age})\}$$

We have also demonstrated [2] that the incidence of anergy following trauma increases with the severity of the trauma. All patients with an injury severity score (ISS) of > 25 are usually anergic upon admission and this anergy can last up to 40 days depending on the degree of injury, varying from 3–4 days with an ISS of 10 or less to more than 40 days with an ISS of 40 or greater. The clinical implication of anergy after trauma is well demonstrated in the literature and is, basically, that infection occurs more readily in anergic patients than in reactive patients after trauma. What is extremely interesting, however, is that a higher percentage of the infected anergic patients who go on to die compared to the infected reactive patients. It would appear that patients having an intact DTH skin test response after trauma respond appropriately to their infection, do not develop multiple organ failure, and survive, whereas the anergic patients either fail to control their infections, leading to dissemination of the infection and death, or "overreact" to their infection or the signal(s) triggered by their infection, develop multiple organ failure, and die.

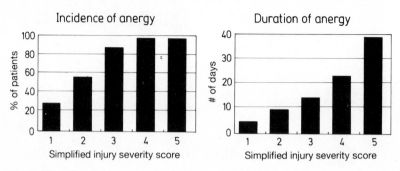

Fig. 4. The effect of the magnitude of trauma on the incidence and duration of anergy

In some cases, over 75% of anergic patients who develop an infection (defined as intra-abdominal infection or positive blood culture) go on to die from this infection during their hospital stay. One hypothesis, thus, is that anergy indicates a state of immunosuppression and an inability to control infection, leading to death. If this hypothesis were correct, one should detect abnormalities in the various components of host defense. Interestingly, the humoral immune response after trauma appears to be suppressed for protein antigens [7]. We have demonstrated that tetanus toxoid immunization of anergic patients with trauma leads to a much weaker antitetanus antibody response compared to reactive patients after similar degrees of trauma. On the other hand, the antibody response to polysaccharide antigens such as pneum-ovax appears to be intact after trauma, with no differentiation between those who are reactive and those who are anergic. We have also demonstrated that pokeweed mitogenstimulated immunoglobulin G synthesis is suppressed by the fifth day after trauma and returns back to normal by 14 days after trauma.

Cell mediated immunity after trauma can be summarized as follows. There is a "anergic environment" operating within severely traumatized patients. This anergic environment leads to a block of in vivo T cell function which appears to be overcome when T cell stimulation and function are assessed in vitro.

The nonspecific immune system after trauma is more interesting. Poly-morphonuclear neutrophil (PMN) adherence increases proportionally as one proceeds from normal laboratory controls to severely traumatized patients (Fig. 5). This difference, however, between reactive and anergic patients is not statistically significant (though both are significantly higher then controls) and varies in the order of approximately 8%–10%. Polymorphonuclear chemotaxis demonstrates an opposite response in trauma in that reactive and anergic patients demonstrate marked diminution of cell migration compared to controls (Fig. 5). Again, anergic patients show a slightly lower chemotactive response than reactive patients but this difference is not statistically significant (using pooled zymosan activated serum as chemoattractant). When PMN surface membrane receptor expression is analyzed, the data tend to support this increased adherence and decreased chemotactic tendency (Fig. 6). F-actin

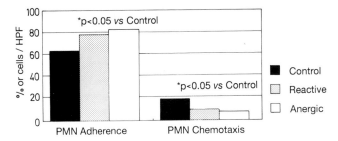

Fig. 5. The effect of trauma on PMN adherence and chemotaxis

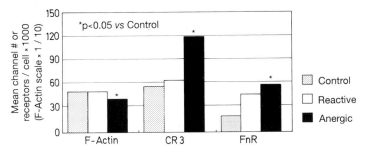

Fig. 6. F-actin content and complement (CR3) and fibronectin (FnR) receptor expression in PMN in relation to the DTH response

receptors are significantly reduced in anergic patients and CR3 receptor is significantly increased, as is the fibronectin receptor. The CR3 and fibronectin receptors would tend to make the cells stickier, whereas the F-actin may lead to decreased microtubule formation within the PMN which might influence their chemotactic ability.

The key measurement is PMN exudation to inflammatory sites after trauma. In other words, are the adherence and chemotactic variations seen after trauma clinically significant in that they influence the ability of the host to deliver PMNs to the inflammatory site? We have examined this question in traumatized patients and have found some interesting data (Fig. 7). The reactive patients, who demonstrate increased adherence and decreased chemotaxis very close to that seen in the anergic patients but much different from control subjects, deliver more neutrophils, almost 100% more, to inflammatory skin windows compared to laboratory controls. In anergic patients, PMN exudation numbers are less than reactive patients by 1 000 000 cells/ml but significantly higher than reactive patients. These exuded PMNs appears to be primed for superoxide production following phorbol myristate acetate (PMA) stimulation. There is a trend of more superoxide production as one studies exudate neutrophils from control subjects to reactive patients to anergic patients [8]. In addition, there is evidence of intravascular activation of PMNs after trauma in that plasma lactoferin levels

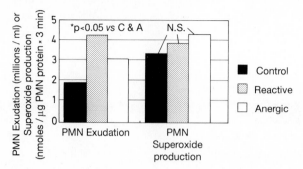

Fig. 7. PMN exudation and function in critically ill trauma patients in relation to their DTH response

are increased in those patients who are anergic and the total intracellular PMN lactoferin content is decreased in the anergic patients compared to the reactive patients, indicating an intravascular degranulation of the neutrophils.

Anergy in patients before suffering multiple trauma is also associated with a higher mortality from infection. If there are preexisting disease conditions such as cancer, inflammatory diseases, nutritional deficits, infection, or immunosuppression in patients sustaining trauma, these may influence the development of anergy and thus increased mortality after trauma. We have examined the relationship of cancer and anergy found no correlation between the extent of the malignancy as graded by the Dukes' classification and the DTH skin test response [9]. B-cell function in relation to anergy is the same before trauma as that after trauma. Similarly, cell mediated immunity before trauma appears to demonstrate an "anergic environment" within some patients, in that there is a block of in vivo T cell function. This block can be overcome by stimulating the cells outside of the anergic environment, i.e. an in vitro situation.

Nonspecific immunity before trauma is interesting in that there are no differences whatsoever between the adherence and chemotactic migration of PMNs [10]. It would appear that trauma specifically activates (or deactivates) the nonspecific immune system demonstrating the changes described above. PMN exudation and function prior to trauma is also interesting and surprising. There is no difference in the delivery of neutrophils to inflammatory skin windows within the reactive and the control patients (Fig. 9). The anergic patients, however, demonstrate a marked increase in the delivery of neutrophils to inflammatory sites by at least 300% compared to the reactive and anergic patients. Also, there is a slight increase in PMN superoxide production from anergic patients following exudation, but this difference is not statistically significant.

It would appear then that the specific side of host defense is similar before and after trauma. Trauma, however, leads to a priming of the primitive but very effective PMN host defense mechanism against bacterial infections. Is this "activation" of the PMN, especially the intravascular activation of these cells

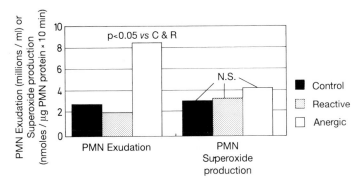

Fig. 8. PMN exudation and function in nontraumatized patients in relation to their DTH response

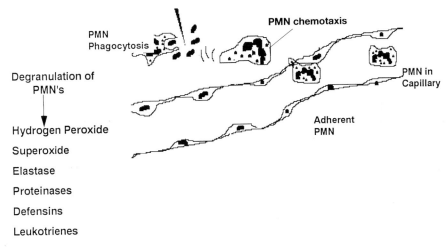

Fig. 9. Most defense against bacteria: primitive but effective

and the potential polymorphonuclear endothelial cell intractions that can ensue, beneficial or detrimental to the host? This is an important question. It can be put in perspective if one assesses host defense against bacteria which is a very primitive but effective defense, as shown in Fig. 9. If a thorn introduces bacteria into the skin, PMNs detect this signal, adhere to the capillary endothelial wall, migrate through this, and then they follow chemotactic gradients to reach the site of the bacterial invasion, arriving in sufficient numbers to phagocytose appropriately opsonized bacteria and kill them by various mechanisms. These involve degranulation of the PMNs, releasing hydrogen peroxide, superoxide, elastase, proteinases, defensins, leukotrienes, etc. This is a very primitive but very effective defense.

It would appear that if we look at control subjects vs all patients after trauma, there is an upregulation of this response in terms of PMNs delivered since all patients taken together deliver twice the number of cells compared to controls (Fig. 10) [11]. In addition to this host defense against tissue trauma/infection, there is a "host response" to tissue trauma/infection, which is primarily mediated by the macrophage (Fig. 11). A trigger can be lipopolysaccharide or antigen-antibody complexes, or bacteria or complement breakdown products such as C5a which converts resting macrophages to activated macrophages. The activated macrophages produce a cytokine response which at nonlethal injury levels is beneficial and may upregulate the primitive host defense against tissue trauma/infection. We propose that this host response is appropriate and beneficial up to a certain "level" of activation signals generated by the tissue destruction of nonlethal trauma or a nonlethal infection.

When does this response become detrimental? When the injury is of sufficient magnitude to generate this response to an excessive and inappropriate degree. For example, consider the situation shown by Fig. 12. During human evolution when a prehistoric hunter was only "bumped" by a mastodon, resulting in an open arm fracture, a sufficient cytokine response was produced to repair the injury and combat possible infection while the hunter would lie in a cave taking only water until the fracture healed. If the mastodon ran over him and broke both his femurs, crushed his chest, ruptured his spleen and caused minor head injury, there would be no question as to the outcome. The hunter would die, there being no trauma center to resuscitate him. The degree of injury

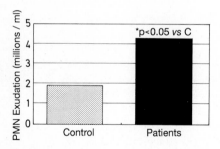

Fig. 10. PMN exudation after trauma in all patients regardless of their DTH response

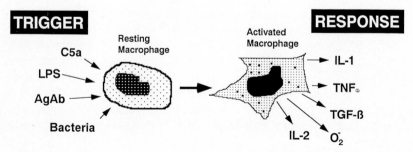

Fig. 11. Host response to tissue trauma/bacteria: if uncontrolled it can lead to multiple organ failure and death

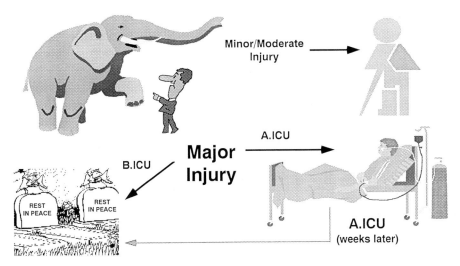

Fig. 12. Possible outcomes of an unfortunate accident

sustained would produce a "trigger" of sufficient magnitude to produce an exaggerated cytokine response. This excessive cytokine response would be detrimental to host survival due to a dysregulated primitive host defense (e.g. excessive PMN–endothelial cell interactions and the consequences thereof). Since our prehistoric hunter was not meant to survive this degree of injury, the excessive cytokine "side effect" was not detrimental to the continuation of the species. Modern day man sustaining the injuries described above would be resuscitated in an intensive care unit. He would be kept alive long enough for the "side effect" of a dysregulated or exaggerated cytokine response to manifest itself. The final outcome might be the same, i.e. death after several weeks in the intensive care unit where he would succumb to multiple organ failure and death. Some patients manage to "turn off" this cytokine response and survive. The key to survival is the effective but primitive host defense against infection initiated by the cytokine response. Learning how to maintain this response appropriately until healing of massive injury (or control of life threatening infection) takes place, then turning it off, is the challenge of the 1990s.

References

1. Christou NV (1985) Host defense mechanisms in surgical patients: a correlative study of the delayed hypersensitivity skin test response, granulocyte function and sepsis in 2202 patients. Can J Surg 28:39–49
2. Christou NV, McLean APH, Meakins JL (1980) Host defense in blunt trauma: interrelationships of kinetics of anergy and depressed neutrophil function, nutritional status, and sepsis, J Trauma 20:833–841

3. Munster AM, Winchurch RA, Keane RM, Shatney CH, Ernst CB, Zuidema GD (1981) The "in vitro skin test: a reliable and repeatable assay of immune competence in the surgical patient. Ann Surg 194:345–352
4. Moore FA, Poggetti RS, Moore EE, Renick M, Bennett L, Parsons P, Peterson VM (1990) Postinjury cytokine response: a selective depression of G-CSF in the face of elevated interleukin-6. Surg Forum 41:107–109
5. Faist E et al. (1990) Functional analysis of monocyte activity via synthesis patterns of interleukin 1.6.8 and neopterin in surgical intensive care patients. 10th SIS Annual Meeting
6. Christou NV, Meakins JL, MacLean LD (1981) The predictive role of delayed hypersensitivity in preoperative patients. Surg Gynecol Obstet 152:297–301
7. Nohr CW, Christou NV, Rode H, Gordon J, Meakins JL (1984) In vivo and in vitro humoral immunity in surgical patients. Ann Surg 200:373–380
8. Tellado J, Christou NV (1991) J Leukocyte Biol (in press)
9. Meakins JL, Christou NV, Halle C, MacLean LD (1979) Influence of cancer on hostdefense and susceptibility to infection. Surg Forum 30:115–117
10. Christou NV, Tellado JM (1989) In vitro polymorphonuclear function in surgical patients does not correlate with anergy but with "activating" processes such as sepsis or trauma. Surgery 106:718–724
11. Tellado JM, Giannias B, Kapadia B, Chartrand L, de Santis M, Christou NV (1990) Anergic patients before elective surgery have enhanced nonspecific host-defense capacity. Arch Surg 125:49–53

Section 3

**From Injury to Multiple Organ Failure:
Sequential Steps
of Host Defense Impairment**

3.1 Shock and Ischemia

Oxygen Radical-Mediated Endothelial Cell Injury

G. O. Till and P. A. Ward

Acute inflammatory processes are frequently accompanied by injury to vascular endothelial cells. It is well recognized that endothelial cells can be damaged in vitro by toxic oxygen metabolites of activated neutrophils. More than a decade ago, Sacks et al. [1] demonstrated that complement (C5a)-activated neutrophils induce chromium release from ^{51}Cr-labeled human umbilical vein endothelial cells in vitro. Because addition of catalase was protective, it has been concluded that the endothelial cell injury was mediated primarily by oxidants (hydrogen peroxide) produced by the activated granulocytes. Since then, the mechanisms of the killing of endothelial cells either by activated neutrophils or by the addition of reactive oxygen species has been extensively studied. Clearly, a better understanding of the mechanisms involved should ultimately lead to more effective therapeutic interventions. In the present communication we review briefly some recent studies on mechanisms of oxidant-mediated endothelial cell injury in vitro and, secondly, compare these findings with observations of endothelial cell injury in vivo.

Mechanisms of Endothelial Cell Injury In Vitro

Role for Hydroxyl Radical

Activated neutrophils release a number of different products including proteolytic enzymes and reactive oxygen metabolites [2–4] which may be responsible for damage to vascular endothelial cells [5]. As mentioned above, a toxic role for oxygen metabolites in the in vitro injury to endothelial cells was first suggested by Sacks et al. [1] and subsequently confirmed by others [6, 7]. Because in vivo studies had suggested an involvement of hydroxyl radical (–OH) in neutrophil-dependent cell and tissue injury associated with systemic activation of the complement system [8] or immune complex deposition in the skin [9], studies were performed to determine whether –OH plays a role in the endothelial cell damage produced in vitro by activated neutrophils.

Department of Pathology, University of Michigan Medical School, 1301 Catherine Road, Ann Arbor, MI 48109-0602, USA

Host Defense Dysfunction
in Trauma, Shock and Sepsis
Eds. Faist/Meakins/Schildberg
© Springer-Verlag, Berlin Heidelberg 1993

When bovine pulmonary artery endothelial cells were exposed to phorbol ester(12-O-tetradecanoyl phorbol-13-acetate, TPA)-stimulated human neutrophils, there was a significant ^{51}Cr release from prelabeled endothelial cells at an effector-to-target ratio as low as 2:1 [10]. In addition, similar killing of endothelial cells was observed when neutrophils were stimulated with immune complexes or complement-opsonized zymosan particles which, like TPA, induced in a dose-dependent fashion the release of ^{51}Cr from the target cells. Neutrophils stimulated with TPA, immune complexes, or zymosan produced large amounts of H_2O_2, whereas stimulation with a chemotactic tripeptide formyl-methionyl-leucyl-phenylalanine, (fMLP) or platelet-activating factor (PAF) resulted in very limited production of H_2O_2. Accordingly, fMLP- or PAF-stimulated neutrophils showed poor killing of endothelial cells [10].

In order to further define the principle involved in endothelial cell killing by activated neutrophils, various inhibitors were employed, including antioxidant enzymes (superoxide dismutase, catalase), hydroxyl radical scavengers (mannitol, dimethyl sulfoxide), an iron chelator (deferoxamine), a proteinase inhibitor (soybean trypsin inhibitor, SBTI), and a myeloperoxidase inhibitor (sodium azide). When these inhibitors were added to cultures containing TPA-stimulated human neutrophils and bovine pulmonary artery endothelial cells, it was observed that catalase, the hydroxyl radical scavengers, and the iron chelator (but not iron-saturated deferoxamine) provided significant protection against injury, whereas superoxide dismutase, SBTI, and sodium azide were ineffective in blocking endothelial cell damage [10]. Based on these observations, it appears most likely that the in vitro killing of endothelial cells by activated neutrophils is brought about by the hydroxyl radical (–OH), which may be generated by the iron-catalyzed Haber-Weiss reaction and/or by the peroxynitrite pathway.

The iron-catalyzed Haber-Weiss reaction:

$$Fe^{3+} + O_2^- \rightarrow Fe^{2+} + O_2 \tag{1}$$

$$Fe^{2+} + H_2O_2 \rightarrow Fe^{3+} + -OH + OH^- \tag{2}$$

The peroxynitrite pathway:

$$O_2^- + -NO \rightarrow ONOO^- + H^+ \rightarrow ONOOH \tag{3}$$

$$ONOOH \rightarrow -OH + -NO_2 \rightarrow NO_3^- + H^+ \tag{4}$$

As depicted in reactions 1 and 2, the reduction of ferric ion to ferrous ion by superoxide is followed by the hydrogen peroxide-mediated oxidation of ferrous ion back to ferric ion (redox system) resulting in the production of hydroxyl radical which appears to be the ultimate toxic product generated from this iron-dependent pathway. Recently, a second pathway for the generation of hydroxyl radical has been described, in which –OH is generated from an iron-independent reaction involving nitric oxide and superoxide (reactions 3 and 4). As suggested by Beckman et al. [11]. nitric oxide (–NO) can react with superoxide (O_2^-) to form peroxynitrite anion ($ONOO^-$) which decays rapidly once protonated to form nitric dioxide ($-NO_2$) and the highly reactive hydroxyl radical ($-OH$).

Presently it is not clear which of the two pathways predominates in oxidant-mediated killing of endothelial cells by activated neutrophils. As mentioned above, the presence of the iron chelator deferoxamine, which interacts with Fe^{3+} and thus interferes with $-OH$ production in the Haber-Weiss reaction, is highly protective against neutrophil-mediated killing of endothelial cells [10]. On the other hand, Beckman et al. [11] have shown that deferoxamine reacts with peroxynitrite to block the formation of $-OH$. Clearly, generation of $-NO$ has been demonstrated in cytokine-stimulated endothelial cells [12] as well as neutrophils, macrophages, and other cell types [13, 14]. Varani et al. [15] have recently demonstrated that pretreatment of endothelial cells with tumor necrosis factor-α or interleukin-1 increases in a time- and dose-dependent fashion the sensitivity of these cells to killing by neutrophils stimulated by phorbol myristate acetate (PMA) or C5a. Whether this increase in cytotoxicity is due to increased production of $-NO$ by endothelial cells and/or improved adherence interactions between endothelial cells and neutrophils remains to be elucidated.

Role for Iron and Superoxide Anion

As described above, activated neutrophils can cause injury to endothelial cells in vitro which can be prevented by the presence of catalase, hydroxyl radical scavengers, and iron chelators such as deferoxamine and apolactoferrin. These interventional studies have shown that there is a critical requirement for hydrogen peroxide and iron, suggesting that the hydroxyl radical plays a major role in endothelial cell killing by neutrophils [10], and that $-OH$ is probably being generated via the iron-catalyzed Haber-Weiss reaction. If iron is essential for the cytotoxic process, two important questions are to be asked: (a) what is the source of iron, and (b) what is the mechanism that makes ferrous iron available for $-OH$ production by hydrogen peroxide?

In order to determine the source of iron in neutrophil-mediated killing of endothelial cells, Gannon et al. [16] pretreated neutrophils with protective concentrations of deferoxamine (5–20 mM) for 1 h. The treatment with the iron chelator had no effect on the neutrophils' ability to kill endothelial cells or to generate hydrogen peroxide or superoxide. However, when endothelial cells were pretreated with the same amounts of deferoxamine, their susceptibility to subsequent cytotoxicity by PMA-stimulated neutrophils was significantly reduced. The protection was dependent upon the concentration of the chelator employed and the duration of pretreatment with deferoxamine, and it was also observed when endothelial cells were washed following exposure to the chelator [16]. These observations suggest that the endothelial or target cell provides the iron necessary to mediate its killing by the effector cells (neutrophils). Similar observations were made by Starke and Farber [17] who demonstrated significant in vitro protection of hepatocytes from $-OH$-mediated killing (following exposure to glucose oxidase-generated hydrogen peroxide) when the hepatocytes were pretreated with deferoxamine.

What are the effects of deferoxamine on the target cell iron? When endothelial cells were preloaded with ^{59}Fe and then incubated with deferoxamine, no significant reduction in ^{59}Fe content occurred during the first 4 h of deferoxamine treatment [16], the time in which maximal protection against neutrophil-mediated cytotoxicity is afforded. Reverse-phase HPLC analysis revealed that the iron chelator remained associated with the cells after washing since it could be detected as iron-saturated deferoxamine in extracts of chelator-treated endothelial cells. Spectrophotometric analyses of cell extracts provided similar data, and it was determined that the cell extract contained 15.1 µM Fe-deferoxamine or 14 fmol per cell [16]. These observations suggest that deferoxamine becomes associated with endothelial cells following exposure of the cells to the iron chelator, and that the protective effects of deferoxamine are due to chelation of intracellular iron and not to physical removal of iron from the target cells.

Clearly, iron appears to play a crucial role in neutrophil-dependent and oxygen radical-mediated injury of endothelial cells. If, as shown above, the iron is derived from the endothelial cell, an important question is the mechanism by which the intracellular iron is made available for the generation of the cytotoxic hydroxyl radical. It has been shown that endothelial cells can produce O_2^- and H_2O_2 [18, 19], and that the introduction into cells of superoxide dismutase (SOD) or catalase increases the resistance of these cells against oxidant-induced injury [20, 21]. Since O_2^- plays a role in the iron-catalyzed Haber-Weiss reaction by reducing ferric to ferrous ion, Markey et al. [22] examined SOD-supplemented rat pulmonary artery endothelial cells for their susceptibility to oxidant-induced injury to determine whether intracellular O_2^- plays a role in H_2O_2 and neutrophil-induced endothelial cell injury.

Incubation for 16–18 h of endothelial cells with increasing amounts of bovine CuZn-SOD resulted in a more than 17-fold increase in intracellular SOD activity, which was resistant to trypsinization of the incubated cells, suggesting an intracellular localization of the antioxidant enzyme [22]. Incubation of SOD-loaded cells in culture medium for 4 h (the standard time period for H_2O_2 or neutrophil-dependent cytotoxicity reactions) resulted in some loss of intracellular SOD activity, but the remaining activity was still about six-fold the endogenous level in nonsupplemented cells. When SOD-loaded endothelial cells were exposed to cytotoxic levels of H_2O_2 (0.1 mM), they showed significant protection from cytotoxicity that was dependent on the amount of intracellular SOD activity present. No protection was observed when the H_2O_2 concentration reached levels of 0.5 mM and higher [22]. Similarly, SOD-supplemented endothelial cells were also protected from injury when exposed to PMA-stimulated neutrophils, but the magnitude of protection decreased with increasing numbers of neutrophils. These observations demonstrate that H_2O_2 or neutrophil-mediated killing of vascular endothelial cells is inversely related to the amount of SOD present in the endothelial cell, thus providing support for the conclusion that intracellular O_2^- (in the target cell) plays a significant role in endothelial cell killing by H_2O_2 or activated neutrophils. Whether intracellularly generated O_2^- is involved in the reduction of Fe^{3+} to Fe^{2+}, which can then interact with H_2O_2 (diffusing into the endothelial cell) to result in the formation of the highly reactive –OH, remains to be determined.

Activation of Xanthine Oxidase

Vascular endothelial cells have been shown to produce O_2^- in vitro [18, 19] although these cells, unlike the neutrophil, do not contain nicotinamide adenine dinucleotide phosphate, reduced form, oxidase—the O_2^- generating enzyme in the neutrophil. One possible source for O_2^- generation in endothelial cells is xanthine oxidase (XO), which has been demonstrated in endothelial cells [23, 24], and which in the presence of its substrate xanthine reduces O_2 to O_2^- [25]. In endothelial cells, this enzyme is usually present predominantly in the dehydrogenase form, which uses nicotinamide adenine dinucleotide instead of O_2 as the electron acceptor [26]. Conversion of xanthine dehydrogenase (XD) to XO has been observed in vitro during purification procedures under nonreducing conditions [27, 28] or after mild proteolysis [27, 29]. Whether similar mechanisms apply to in vivo situations is not clear, but conversion of XD to XO has been observed under conditions of ischemia followed by reperfusion or reoxygenation [30, 31].

Since cultured rat pulmonary artery endothelial cells have also been shown to possess XO and XD activity [32], the question was asked whether activated neutrophils can affect endothelial XO levels, and whether XO might play a role in neutrophil-mediated killing of endothelial cells in vitro. When PMA-activated human neutrophils (which contain no detectable levels of XO) were added to rat pulmonary artery endothelial cells, a significant rise in XO activity in the endothelial cells was observed, accompanied by an equivalent reduction in XD activity [32]. This conversion of XD to XO occurred fairly rapidly (within 10 min after PMA addition) and was dependent on the activation of neutrophils since nonactivated neutrophils failed to cause any significant alteration in endothelial XD/XO activities. Likewise, the addition of culture supernatants of activated neutrophils to endothelial cells or exposure of endothelial cells to PMA in the absence of neutrophils did not cause conversion of XD to XO.

Additional experiments revealed that both the neutrophil-mediated conversion of XD to XO and the cytotoxic effect of neutrophils on endothelial cells [32]. Although the ultimate killing of endothelial cells by activated neutrophils is related to H_2O_2 production by neutrophils [10], addition of H_2O_2 to endothelial cells failed to induce conversion of XD to XO [32]. As to be expected, the XO inhibitors allopurinol and oxypurinol inhibited XD and XO activity in endothelial cells. However, these inhibitors also protected endothelial cells from neutrophil-mediated cytotoxicity. On the other hand, catalase or deferoxamine, known to protect endothelial cells from injury by activated neutrophils, failed to interfere with the conversion of XD to XO [32]. These observations suggest that the endothelial increase in XO activity is important for the neutrophil-induced killing process of endothelial cells probably by providing a source for O_2^-. The protective effects of catalase or deferoxamine may be related to their intervening with the iron-catalyzed Haber-Weiss reaction which provides the cytotoxic hydroxyl radical.

Recent data suggest that inflammatory mediators are also able to cause activation of XO in endothelial cells (i.e., the conversion of XD to XO). Incubation of rat pulmonary artery endothelial cells with human recombinant C5a resulted in a pronounced conversion of XD to XO which was dose- and time-dependent [33]. Similar effects on endothelial cells were observed following incubation with human recombinant tumor necrosis factor-α and the chemotactic peptide N-fMLP. This process appeared to be mediator-specific because C3a, bradykinin, recombinant human interleukin-1β, or PMA lacked converting activity. The conversion of XD to XO in endothelial cells following exposure to the inflammatory mediators occurred with 5–10 min and required intact endothelial cells [33], similar to what had been observed when endothelial cells were incubated with activated neutrophils [32].

In spite of the fact that endothelial XO can be activated by both inflammatory mediators and activated neutrophils, only the neutrophil is able to cause injury to the endothelial cell. While XO can generate O_2^- which may function in the reduction of Fe^{3+} to Fe^{2+}, exogenous, neutrophil-derived H_2O_2 appears to be necessary to facilitate the oxidation of ferrous ion resulting in the reduction of H_2O_2 to –OH. However, neutrophil-derived H_2O_2 may play an additional role in injury to endothelial cells, namely by initiating the intracellular generation of hypoxanthine and xanthine, the substrates for XO. When rat pulmonary artery endothelial cells were exposed to reagent H_2O_2, the resulting injury was time dependent and related to the concentration of H_2O_2 added, and, as observed in neutrophil-mediated killing of endothelial cells, addition of catalase, deferoxamine or the XO inhibitors allopurinol and oxypurinol provided significant protection [34]. More importantly, the exposure of endothelial cells to cytotoxic concentrations of H_2O_2 resulted in a rapid fall in intracellular ATP levels, which was accompanied by the simultaneous appearance of purine degradation products including hypoxanthine and xanthine. Strikingly, the breakdown of ATP could not be prevented by the addition of deferoxamine or allopurinol and was essentially of the same magnitude as in unprotected, H_2O_2-treated endothelial cells [34]. These observations are consistent with findings from previous studies in which ATP depletion was found to be dissociable from cytotoxicity [35–37]. Although the ATP breakdown does not appear to be directly accountable for the cell injury, it might very well participate in H_2O_2 or neutrophil-mediated endothelial cell injury by providing substrate (hypoxanthine, xanthine) for XO.

Endothelial Cell Injury In Vivo

Over the past several years, our group has been studying the pathomechanisms of acute microvascular lung injury in the rat following systemic complement activation. This animal model, characterized by oxidant-mediated injury to vascular endothelial cells, may serve as an example by which features of in vivo endothelial cell injury can be compared with the above-described processes of oxidant-dependent endothelial cell damage in vitro.

Intravenous injection into rats of cobra venom factor (CVF) has been shown to result in rapid complement activation with appearance of C5-derived chemotactic activity in the plasma, sequestration of blood neutrophils in pulmonary vessels, and the rapid development of pulmonary microvascular injury as evidenced by extravasation of radiolabeled (^{125}I) bovine serum albumin from the pulmonary vessels into lung interstitium [38]. Electron microscopic examinations revealed large numbers of neutrophils in close contact with vascular endothelium, focal destruction of endothelial cells and basement membrane of pulmonary capillaries, and evidence of fibrin deposits and erythrocytes in alveolar spaces. Depletion of experimental animals of complement or of circulating blood neutrophils resulted in significant protection from acute pulmonary injury [38], demonstrating the existence of a relationship between systemic complement activation, blood neutrophils, and lung damage. It may be assumed that intravascular activation of complement leads to C5a-mediated stimulation of blood neutrophils, their sequestration within pulmonary capillaries, and subsequent microvascular injury by products from these complement-activated neutrophils. Studies in C5-deficient mice have indicated that C5 is required for the development of acute lung microvascular injury following intravenous injection of CVF [39]. Similarly, an absolute requirement for C5 in the induction and the development of CVF-induced lung injury has also been observed in rats [40], suggesting that an activation product of C5 (most likely C5a) plays a key role in complement and neutrophil-mediated acute pulmonary injury. Furthermore, treatment of experimental animals with catalase or (SOD) also significantly attenuated CVF-induced acute lung injury, suggesting participation of H_2O_2 and O_2^- in this process. These in vivo observations support previous findings by Sacks et al. [1] who provided in vitro evidence that activation of neutrophils with complement-derived chemotactic products can result in oxidant-mediated injury of endothelial cells.

Additional studies revealed that pretreatment of experimental animals with the hydroxyl radical scavenger dimethyl sulfoxide or with iron chelators such as deferoxamine or apolactoferrin (but not iron-saturated chelators) provided significant protection against complement and neutrophil-mediated lung injury [8]. These observations suggest that an iron-catalyzed conversion of neutrophil-generated hydrogen peroxide into the hydroxyl radical may be a critical step in the process leading to microvascular endothelial cell injury in lungs secondary to systemic complement activation. Again, these in vivo findings are supported by in vitro studies demonstrating that hydroxyl radical scavengers or the iron chelator deferoxamine can provide significant protection from neutrophil-mediated endothelial cell injury [10].

Finally, there is experimental evidence to suggest that XO contributes to neutrophil-dependent endothelial cell injury in vivo as well. Treatment of experimental animals with XO inhibitors (allopurinol, lodoxamide) has recently been shown to provide significant protection from CVF-induced acute lung injury [41]. These in vivo observations may appertain to similar in vitro findings demonstrating that neutrophil-dependent injury to endothelial cells could be attenuated by the application of XO inhibitors including allopurinol, oxypurinol, and lodoxamide [32].

Conclusion

Although it has been known for more than a decade that endothelial cells can be damaged in vitro by toxic oxygen metabolites of activated neutrophils, it is only now that enough additional information has accumulated that allows for a more detailed evaluation of the killing process. Somewhat surprisingly, the neutrophil-mediated killing of endothelial cells in vitro appears to depend also on an active role of the endothelial target cell. Following increased adhesive interactions with the endothelial cell, activated neutrophils may release a "converting factor" that causes activation of XO in endothelial cells. Furthermore, by providing H_2O_2, which easily penetrates the endothelial cell, the neutrophil may also contribute to ATP breakdown resulting in the endothelial generation of xanthine and hypoxanthine, the substrates for XO. In addition, neutrophil-derived H_2O_2 may participate in the iron-catalyzed Haber-Weiss reaction to bring about the generation of $-OH$, which appears to be the most likely oxidant directly involved in the killing process of endothelial cells. The endothelial cell appears to provide O_2^- (by the reaction of XO with xanthine/hypoxanthine) as well as iron, both of which appear to be necessary for the killing process involving the Fenton reaction. Alternatively, endothelial cell-derived O_2^- may react with endothelial nitric oxide to bring about the generation of $-OH$ via the peroxynitrite pathway, but there is currently no evidence that this pathway is relevant in the in vitro killing of endothelial cells by neutrophils. Treatment with catalase, iron chelators, XO inhibitors, or $-OH$ scavengers, interventional measures which protect the endothelial cell from the cytotoxic effects of activated neutrophils in vitro, have also been demonstrated to attenuate the development of endothelial cell injury in vivo. Taken together, these observations suggest that events leading to neutrophil-dependent endothelial cell damage in vitro can be linked to the development in vivo of acute vascular injury by activated neutrophils.

References

1. Sacks T, Moldow CF, Craddock PR, Bowers TK, Jacob HS (1978) Oxygen radical mediated endothelial cell damage by complement-stimulated granulocytes. An in vitro model of immune vascular damage. J Clin Invest 61:1161
2. Janoff A (1975) At least three human neutrophil lysosomal proteases are capable of degrading joint connective tissues. Ann NY Acad Sci 256:402
3. Babior BM (1978) Oxygen-dependent microbial killing by phagocytes. N Engl J Med 298:659
4. Klebanoff SJ (1980) Oxygen metabolism and the toxic properties of phagocytes. Ann Intern Med 93:480
5. Fantone JC, Ward PA (1983) Mechanism of neutrophil-dependent lung injury. In: Ward PA Immunology of inflammation. Elsevier, Amsterdam, p 89 (Handbook of inflammation, vol 4)
6. Weiss SJ, Young J, LoBuglio AF, Slivka A, Nimeh NF (1981) Role of hydrogen peroxide in neutrophil-mediated destruction of cultured endothelial cells. J Clin Invest 68:714
7. Martin WJ (1984) Neutrophils kill pulmonary endothelial cells by a hydrogen peroxide-dependent pathway: an in vitro model of neutrophil-mediated lung injury. Am Rev Respir Dis 130:209
8. Ward PA, Till GO, Kunkel R, Beauchamp C (1983) Evidence for a role of hydroxyl radical in complement and neutrophil-dependent tissue injury. J Clin Invest 72:789
9. Fligiel SEG, Ward PA, Johnson KJ, Till GO (1984) Evidence for a role of hydroxyl radical in immune complex-induced vasculitis. Am J Pathol 115:375
10. Varani J, Fligiel SEG, Till GO, Kunkel RG, Ryan US, Ward PA (1985) Pulmonary endothelial cell killing by human neutrophils. Possible involvement of hydroxyl radical. Lab invest 53:656
11. Beckman JS, Beckman TW, Chen J, Marshall PA, Freeman BA (1990) Apparent hydroxyl radical production by peroxynitrite: implications for endothelial injury form nitric oxide and superoxide. Proc Natl Acad Sci USA 87:1620
12. Kilbourn RG, Belloni P (1990) Endothelial cell production of nitrogen oxides in response to interferon gamma in combination with tumor necrosis factor, interleukin-1, or endotoxin. J Natl Cancer Inst 82:772
13. Hibbs JB, Taintor RR, Vavrin Z, Rachlin EM (1987) Nitric oxide: a cytotoxic activated macrophage effector molecule. Biochem Biophys Res Commun 157:87
14. Wright DC, Mulsch A, Busse R, Osswald H (1989) Generation of nitric oxide by human neutrophils. Biochem Biophys Res Commun 160:813
15. Varani J, Bendelow MJ, Sealey DE, Kunkel SL, Gannon DE, Ryan US, Ward PA (1988) Tumor necrosis factor enhances susceptibility of vascular endothelial cells to neutrophil-mediated killing. Lab Invest 59:292
16. Gannon DE, Varani J, Phan SH, Ward JH, Kaplan J, Till GO, Simon RH, Ryan US, Ward PA (1987) Source of iron in neutrophil-mediated killing of endothelial cells. Lab Invest 57:37
17. Starke PE, Farber JL (1985) Ferric iron and superoxide ions are required for the killing of cultured hepatocytes by hydrogen peroxide: evidence for the participation of hydroxyl radicals formed by iron-catalyzed Haber-Weiss reaction. J Biol Chem 260:10099
18. Freeman BA, Jackson RM, Matalon S, Harding SM (1988) Biochemical and functional aspects of oxygen-mediated injury to vascular endothelium. In: Ryan US (ed) Endothelial cells, vol III. CRC Press, Boca Raton, p 13
19. Rosen GM, Freeman BA (1984) Detection of superoxide generated by endothelial cells. Proc Natl Acad Sci USA 23:7269
20. Freeman BA, Young SL, Crapo JD (1983) Liposome-mediated augmentation of superoxide dismutase in endothelial cells prevents oxygen injury. J Biol Chem 258:12534
21. Beckman JS, Minor RL, Freeman BA (1986) Augmentation of antioxidant enzymes in vascular endothelium. Free Radic Biol Med 2:359
22. Markey BA, Phan SH, Varani J, Ryan US, Ward PA (1990) Inhibition of cytotoxicity by intracellular superoxide dismutase supplementation. Free Radic Biol Med 9:307
23. Ratych RE, Chuknyiska RS, Bulkley GB (1987) The primary localization of free radical generation after anoxia/reoxygenation in isolated endothelial cells. Surgery 102:122
24. Jarasch ED, Grund C, Bruder G, Heid HW, Keenan TW, Franke WW (1981) Localization of xanthine oxidase in mammary gland epithelium and capillary endothelium. Cell 25:67
25. McCord JM, Fridovich I (1968) The reduction of cytochrome c by milk xanthine oxidase. J Biol Chem 243:5753

26. Parks DA, Granger DN (1986) Xanthine oxidase: biochemistry, distribution and physiology. Acta Physiol Scand 548 [Suppl]:87
27. Batelli MG, Lorenzini E, Stirpe F (1973) Milk xanthine oxidase type D (dehydrogenase) and type O (oxidase): purification, interconversion, and some properties. Biochem J 131:191
28. Della Corte E, Stirpe F (1972) The regulation of rat liver xanthine oxidase. Involvement of thiol groups in the conversion of the enzyme activity from dehydrogenase (type D) into oxidase (type O) and purification of the enzyme. Biochem J 126:739
29. Waud WR, Rajagopalan KV (1976) Purification and properties of the NAD$^+$-dependent (type D) and O$_2$-dependent (type O) form of rat liver xanthine dehydrogenase. Arch Biochem Biophys 172:354
30. Batelli MG, Della Corte E, Stirpe F (1972) Xanthine oxidase type D (dehydrogenase) in the intestine and other organs of the rat. Biochem J 126:747
31. Engerson TD, McKelvey TG, Rhyne DB, Boggio EB, Snyder SJ, Jones HP (1987) Conversion of xanthine dehydrogenase to oxidase in ischemic rat tissues. J Clin Invest 79:1564
32. Phan SH, Gannon DE, Varani J, Ryan US, Ward PA (1989) Xanthine oxidase activity in rat pulmonary artery endothelial cells and its alteration by activated neutrophils. Am J Pathol 134:1201
33. Friedl HP, Till GO, Ryan US, Ward PA (1989) Mediator-induced activation of xanthine oxidase in endothelial cells FASEB J. 3:2512
34. Varani J, Phan SH, Gibbs DF, Ryan US, Ward PA (1990) H$_2$O$_2$-mediated cytotoxicity of rat pulmonary endothelial cells. Changes in adenosine triphosphate and purine products and effects of protective interventions. Lab Invest 63:683
35. Jennings RB, Hawkins HK, Lowe JE, Hill ML, Klotman S, Reimer KA (1987) Relation between high energy phosphate and lethal injury in myocardial ischemia in dogs. Am J Pathol 92:187
36. Kristensen SR (1989) A critical appraisal of the association between energy charge and cell damage. Biochim Biophys Acta 1012:272
37. Wysolmerski RB, Lagunoff D (1988) Inhibition of endothelia cell retraction by ATP depletion. Am J Pathol 132:28
38. Till GO, Johnson KJ, Kunkel R, Ward PA (1982) Intravascular activation of complement and acute lung injury. Dependency on neutrophils and toxic oxygen metabolites. J Clin Invest 69:1126
39. Tvedten HW, Till GO, Ward PA (1985) Mediators of lung injury in mice following systemic activation of complement. Am J Pathol 119:92
40. Till GO, Morganroth ML, Kunkel R, Ward PA (1987) Activation of C5 by cobra venom factor is required in neutrophil-mediated lung injury in the rat. Am J Pathol 129:44
41. Till GO, Friedl HP, Ward AP (1991) Lung injury and complement activation: role of neutrophils and xanthine oxidase. Free Radic Biol Med 10:379

Characteristics of Neutrophil Dysfunction*

G. F. Babcock, C. L. White-Owen, J. W. Alexander, and G. D. Warden

Introduction

Overwhelming sepsis is a major source of morbidity and mortality in patients following severe thermal injury or other traumatic injury. Despite this fact, the mechanisms underlying these potentially fatal complications have not been elucidated. It is likely that at least some of these altered immunological parameters are associated with infections and sepsis. Several lines of investigation have implicated neutrophil dysfunction as one of the major causes of increased infection rates in groups of patients. Since that time several reports have established a relationship between abnormal neutrophil functions and the development of life-threatening infections [1], whereas other investigators have failed to find high correlations between the defects and patient mortality [2, 3]. However, several laboratories, including our own, have found a significant correlation between the degree of the neutrophil dysfunction and the morbidity of the patient [4, 5].

Neutrophil dysfunction could be the product of the environmental influences or some defect in cellular regulation. It is not yet clear if one or both of these mechanisms explain the changes observed in neutrophils following major traumatic injury. In addition, altered cellular regulation could be the product of altered cytokine production, either too much or too little, or an as yet undefined intrinsic abnormality in the cellular function. Whatever the mechanism, most investigators have clearly demonstrated that neutrophil function is altered following severe injury.

Early studies by Warden and others [6–8] demonstrated a decrease in both random migration and chemotaxis following severe burn injury. In addition, impaired bactericidal activity has been reported by several groups [9–11]. The mechanism(s) for this loss of activity is probably very complex, with many cellular parameters related to the killing of microorganisms being altered. Several investigators reported a decrease in neutrophil phagocytic activity [12, 13], while Bjerknes et al. [14] reported an initial increase in phagocytic activity of severely burned patients upon admission. This was accompanied by a

* Supported in part by a grant from the Shriners of North America.

University of Cincinnati Medical Center, Department of Surgery, and Shriners Burns Institute, Cincinnati, Ohio, USA

reduction of 25%–35% in intracellular killing of both bacteria and yeast. In relation to this, a relatively large number of cellular parameters were found to be altered, including decreased glucose oxidation and oxygen consumption [15], reduced H_2O_2 production [14, 16, 17], alterations of phagolysosomal acidification [18], and loss of or defect in lysosomal enzymes [5, 19, 20]. Koller et al. [21] reported lower leukotriene (LT) generation from neutrophils of severely burned patients including LTB_4, and the metabolites 20-OH-LTB_4 and 20-COOH-LTB_4. This could account for some of the chemotactic and chemokinetic alterations reported by other investigators. Rothe et al. [22] used flow cytometry to distinguish the effects of trauma and trauma plus sepsis on neutrophil phagocytosis. These investigators found that severe trauma caused hyperergic phagocytosis while sepsis following trauma caused hypoergic phagocytosis.

Serum-related defects or suppressor substances have also been found in patients following severe thermal or traumatic injury. The original report by Warden et al. [23] demonstrated a serum-related chemotactic defect which was independent of drug effects and reversed after incubation of neutrophils with normal serum, and Bjorson et al. [24] observed serum-mediated defective phagocytic and bactericidal activity but did not measure chemotaxis. Grogan [7] was able to show chemotactic defects in neutrophils isolated from thermally injured patients, but could not produce the same effect on normal neutrophils with burn serum. Similarly, other groups were unable to show serum-mediated defects in chemotaxis with either serum or blister fluid [25]. Jeyapaul et al. [26] identified a serum-mediated reduction in the receptor expression of normal neutrophils. Alexander et al. [5] found a decrease in the level of serum opsonins, decreased immunoglobulin G (IgG) levels, and depressed levels of C3. Of all these serum-related parameters only low levels of serum opsonins appeared to be a predisposing factor only when associated with a co-existing abnormality of neutrophils to kill bacteria.

Although these studies indicate that neutrophil function is altered following thermal or traumatic injury and that these changes may be related to infection, information is lacking as to the exact mechanism(s) causing this neutrophil dysfunction. All studies reported to date have used heterogeneous populations of neutrophils. Other investigators have found changes in neutrophil subpopulations but did not examine the function of these cells or their relationship to infection [19]. If altered neutrophil cell population(s) can be well characterized rather than a heterogeneous population of functional and non-functional cells, then a more rational basis for developing the proper methodology to correct these defects can be developed.

The focus of our investigations have centered on changes which occur in neutrophil phenotype and cellular function following major thermal and non-thermal injury. A strong correlation has been shown to exist between these changes and the onset of infections and sepsis. The significance of these studies may have diagnostic as well as therapeutic implications in the early recognition and successful management of infections in high risk trauma patients.

Materials and Methods

Subjects. Patients selected for the study included those with severe blunt or penetrating trauma ($n = 20$) and severe thermal injury ($n = 85$) admitted to University Hospital and Shriners Burns Institute in Cincinnati, Ohio, USA. All nonthermal trauma patients presented with an initial APACHE II score [31] of ≥ 10. They were divided into two groups based on their initial APACHE II score: group A with an APACHE II of 10–18 ($n = 11$), and group B with an APACHE II of 19–25 ($n = 9$). Thermal trauma patients had a mean burn size of 55% (range 29%–99%) of the total body surface area (TBSA) and a mean full thickness burn size of 39%. Informed written consent was obtained from all individuals according to the guidelines set by the University of Cincinnati Medical Center Institutional Review Board on Human Experimentation. The control group consisted of 50 healthy age-matched volunteers.

Sample Preparation. Blood samples were drawn within 48 h of admission and 3 days following the initial sample. Further blood samples were drawn at weekly intervals for the duration of the patient's acute hospital course. Blood was collected in sodium ethylenediaminetetraacetate (EDTA) and stored at room temperature for no more than 24 h prior to processing. When functional studies were to be performed the blood was processed within 6 h. A complete blood count (CBC) and differential count were performed on each sample using standard clinical methods.

Monoclonal Antibodies. Monoclonal antibodies were purchased from Becton-Dickinson Immunocytometry Systems (Mountain View, California), Gen Trak (Plymouth Meeting, Pennsylvania), or Medarex (West Lebanon, New Hampshire). Antibodies were conjugated with fluorescein isothiocynate (FITC), phycoerythrin (PE), or biotin, or in some cases used unconjugated. Allo-phycocyanine-strepavidin (APC) was used as a second-step reagent with biotin-labeled antibodies while FITC-labeled goat anti-mouse was used as a second-step reagent when unlabeled monoclonal antibodies were used. A list of the reagents used appears in Table 1.

Flow Cytometry. Flow cytometry was performed on a dual laser Coulter 753 flow cytometer (Coulter Electronics, Hileah, Florida) as previously described [28, 29]. FITC and PE were excited with an argon ion laser (488-nm line) while APC was excited with a tuneable dye laser (595 nm). Fluorescence emission for FITC, PE, and APC was detected by selectively collecting 530 ± 15 nm, 575 ± 12.5 nm, and 660 ± 12.5 nm, respectively. Two electronic gates are set for each sample based on forward angle (FALS) and $90°$ light scattering ($90°$). One gate is set to include granulocytes, while platelets, debris, dead cells, and remaining erythrocytes are excluded from both gates. The gates of the population to be analyzed are adjusted such that $> 95\%$ of the cells enclosed within

Table 1. Specificity of monoclonal antibodies

Cluster designation	Specificity
CD10	CALLA
CD11a	LFA-1
CD11b	CR3-iC3b receptor
CD11c	gp150/95
CD14	Adherent monocytes
CD15	Fucosyl N acetyllactosamine
CD16	FcRIII for IgG
CD18	Beta chain of CD11a,b,c
CD32	FcRII for IgG
CD33	Immature neutrophils
CD35	CR1 receptor for C3b, C4
CD45	Common leukocyte antigen

the gated region stained positive with CD45. In addition, neutrophils were gated to exclude CD14 positive cells. At least 20 000 events within the gated region were counted. Histograms were analyzed using Easy 2 software (Coulter Electronics).

Phagocytosis. This assay is performed as previously described [30]. FITC-labeled *Staphylococcus aureus* were mixed with neutrophils at a ratio of 20:1 (bacteria:neutrophils) for 2, 5, and 8 min at 37 °C, followed by dilution in cold phosphate-buffered saline (PBS), and held at 4 °C until analyzed by flow cytometry. The fluorescence of extracellular bacteria is quenched with Immunolyse (Coulter Electronics).

Intracellular H_2O_2 Assay. This assay was performed by a modification of the method described by Bass et al. [31]. Neutrophils are loaded with 2'-7'-dichlorofluorescin (DCFH) followed by activation with N-formylmethionylleucyl phenyl alanine (FMLP). The green fluorescence produced is proportional to the amount of H_2O_2. Conversion of the DCFH to 2'-7'-dichlorofluorescein (DCF) if monitored using flow cytometry.

Results

In our previous studies we reported on the correlation between changes in the $CD11b^+CD16^+$ neutrophil populations and bacterial infections following severe thermal injuries [29]. In order to analyze the data in terms of infections the hospital stay was divided into five periods: noninfected, presepsis, septic, postseptic, and never septic. The period from admission to presepsis was classified as noninfected, the period from 3 to 7 days prior to the first positive blood culture was defined as presepsis, the septic period was 3 days prior to the first positive blood culture until 2 weeks after the last positive blood culture, and the postseptic period began 2 weeks after the last positive blood culture. Patients who remained asymptomatic and culture negative were classified as never septic.

A summary of the flow cytometric analysis of $CD11b^+CD16^+$ neutrophils from severely burned patients experiencing bacteremic infections appears in Fig. 1. As the patients go from the preseptic period to confirmed sepsis, the percentage of $CD11^+CD16^+$ neutrophils decreases significantly ($p < 0.05$). As the patients enter the postseptic period the percentage of $CD11b^+CD16^+$ significantly ($p < 0.05$) increases to preseptic levels. An almost identical pattern was observed when the absolute number of these neutrophils were examined (data not shown). The percentage and absolute number of neutrophils expressing CD35 did not correlate with infections. The actual value or number of neutrophils expressing CD11b and CD16 did not appear to be important as essentially all patients had below normal values. The changes which occur following burn injury appear to be much more important than the actual values.

Patients undergoing severe blunt or penetrating trauma were examined for CD11b and CD16 expression to determine if changes were similar to those seen following thermal injury [32]. A summary of the results obtained from an examination of 20 patients appears in Fig. 2. The patients were divided into two groups based upon the initial APACHE II score; group A (10–18) and group B (19–25). It can be seen that all patients had a reduced percentage of $CD11b^+CD16^+$ following injury. An analysis of the data indicated that at week 0 all groups were significantly different from each other. At week 0.5 group B was different from group A and the control group but group A did not differ significantly from the controls. At week 1 both groups were different from the control group but not significantly different from each other. At week 2 only

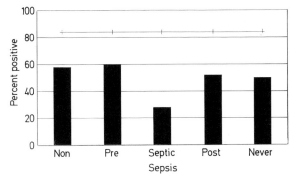

Fig. 1. The mean percent ± standard error $CD11b^+CD16^+$ neutrophils from thermal trauma patients. Three groups of individuals are shown. Those patients who eventually displayed septic or infectious complications, those patients remaining infection free (never), and normal individuals. The time course for sepsis appears in the text. *NON*, noninfected; *PRE*, presepsis; *POST*, postseptic; *NEVER*, never septic; ——+——, normal

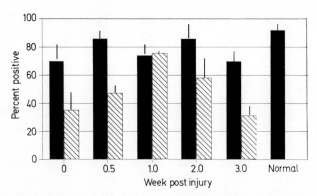

Fig. 2. The mean percent ± standard error CD11b⁺CD16⁺ neutrophils from blunt or penetrating trauma patients over time post injury. The patients were divided into two groups according to their APACHE II scores. *Filled bars*, APACHE II of 10–18; *hatched bars*, APACHE II of 19–25

group B was different from the controls while at week 3 all groups were again significantly different from each other.

It is interesting to note that patients in group A suffered an average of 0.8 late septic or infectious complications per patient, whereas those in group B had an average of 3.3 septic complications. Only 4 of the 20 patients did not have significant infections or septic complications. All four of these patients had near normal percentages of CD11b⁺CD16⁺ neutrophils upon admission. These results suggest that an decrease in the CD11b⁺CD16⁺ neutrophils may be prognostic of later septic or infectious complications.

A further characterization of neutrophils following thermal injury is currently underway. Emphasis has been placed on determining the phenotype and functional properties of the neutrophils which are not CD11b⁺CD16⁺ [33, 34]. We examined these cells to determine the major phenotype present following injury (Fig. 3). It can be seen that following thermal injuries the predominant neutrophil subpopulation is CD11b⁻CD16⁻, while following blunt or penetrating trauma the CD11b⁺CD16⁻ phenotype predominates. The significance or reason for these differences is not yet understood.

A comparison of the phagocytic properties of the various neutrophil subpopulations isolated from burn patients appears in Fig. 4. It can be seen that most of the neutrophils from normal individuals are phagocytic. CD11b⁻CD16⁻ cells are significantly less phagocytic, with 40% phagocytizing *S. aureus* in the presence of normal serum and only 23% phagocytizing bacteria in the presence of their own serum. The CD11b⁺CD16⁻ subpopulation displayed a slightly reduced but significant reduction in phagocytosis (74%) while the double positive cells essentially matched normal values.

The oxidative metabolic burst was examined using CD11b⁻CD16⁻ and CD11b⁺CD16⁻ neutrophils obtained from burn patients. The mean channel fluorescence of the patient cells was compared to that obtained from normal individuals. The normal values were set at 100%. It can be seen in Fig. 5 that the

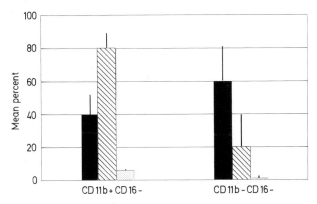

Fig. 3. The mean percent ± standard error of CD11b⁺CD16⁻ and CD11b⁻CD16⁻ neutrophils from trauma and burn patients. The data represent the mean values obtained during the first 3 weeks post injury. *Filled bars,* burns; *hatched bars,* trauma; *stippled bars,* normal

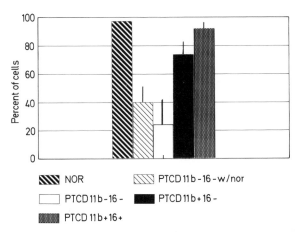

Fig. 4. The percentage ± standard error of neutrophils capable of phagocytosis following thermal injury. All cells were tested using autologous serum unless marked otherwise

CD11b⁺CD16⁺ neutrophils from patients displayed a nearly normal metabolic response while CD11b⁻CD16⁻ neutrophils from the same patients displayed a response 60% of normal.

Additional studies have been performed to examine the neutrophils from burn and trauma patients for the presence or absence of a number of important receptors. Expression of CD35 (CR1) is slightly higher or unchanged following either burns or trauma. The expression of CD10 was variable (usually negative) in contrast to reports by other investigators. In addition, only a very small percentage of the neutrophils expressed CD33 indicating that most of the cells were differentiated.

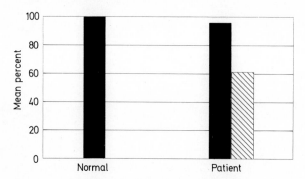

Fig. 5. The oxidative burst response of neutrophils subpopulations from burn patients following activation. Values obtained using neutrophils from normal individuals were set at 100%. *Filled bars,* CD11$^+$CD16$^+$; *hatched bars,* CD11$^-$CD16$^-$

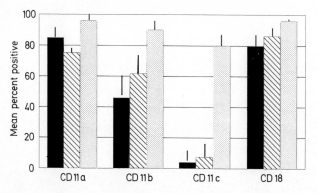

Fig. 6. The mean percentage $\pm$ standard error of neutrophils expressing β_2-integrins. *Filled bars,* burns; *hatched bars,* trauma; *stippled bars,* normal

Two major groups of receptors on neutrophils with a defined function have been examined following trauma or thermal injury. These include the β_2-integrin group, CD11a,b,c and CD18, and the Fc receptors, CD16 and CD32. It can be seen in Fig. 6 that the expression of these molecules following burns or trauma varies greatly. The expression of CD11a on neutrophils is only slightly lower in burn patients and trauma patients, while the expression of CD11b and CD11c is greatly reduced, especially in burn patients. The expression of CD18 is essentially normal or very slightly reduced following thermal or traumatic injury. The expressing of Fc receptors on neutrophils is shown in Fig. 7. Both CD16 and CD32 are expressed at a signficantly lower percentage following both thermal and traumatic injuries. Patients with thermal injury express a significantly lower percentage of both receptors on neutrophils when compared to trauma or normal individual.

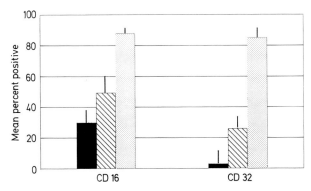

Fig. 7. The mean percentage ± standard error of neutrophils expressing FcRII and FcRIII follow-ing burns or other trauma. *Filled bars*, burns; *hatched bars*, trauma; *stippled bars*, normal

Discussion

Infections in burn and trauma patients continue to be a major problem and one of the leading causes of death. Our results demonstrate a strong correlation between neutrophil dysfunction and the onset of infections or sepsis. It is important to note that the patients must be compared to themselves rather than to each other or to predetermined normal values. It appears that the change in the CD11b⁺CD16⁺ neutrophil population rather than any particular value is the important value. The magnitude of this change appears to be more related to the severity of the injury in trauma patients than in burn patients. Trauma patients with higher initial APACHE II scores display a greater reduction in CD11⁺CD16⁺ neutrophils than patients with lower initial APACHE II scores. In burn patients the reduction in CD11b⁺CD16⁺ neutrophils varies only slightly with burn size in patients with 35% or greater TBSA injuries.

The functional capabilities of neutrophils lacking CD11b and/or CD16 is markedly reduced as accessed by phagocytosis or the production of H_2O_2. This is to be expected as CD11b and CD16 have been shown to play an important role in neutrophil phagocytosis [35, 36]. The CD32 molecule, which was also found to be significantly reduced following burns or trauma, also appears to be important for normal phagocytic function [37].

Although the neutrophils from both burn and trauma patients display altered expression of CD11b and CD16 there appears to be subtle differences in the expression of these two receptors. Burn patients often have a significantly higher percentage of CD11b⁻CD16⁻ neutrophils compared to trauma patients. The biological significance of this observation is unknown but this sub-population of neutrophils is less phagocytic in vitro.

The processes or mechanisms which explain the reduction in CD11b, CD11c, CD16, or CD32 are unknown. Several plausible explanations exist, all of which may play some role. These include the release of very immature myeloid cells from the bone marrow which do not yet express these receptors, or a blockade of these molecules preventing detection. Another possibly is that thermal injury or trauma in some way affects normal differentiation and/or maturation of neutrophils such that these receptors are not inserted into the cell membrane or are improperly transcribed.

It is felt, however, that patients displaying a large reduction in neutrophils expressing CD11b or CD16 should be monitored closely for the onset of septic complications. Clearly, more extensive investigations into the clinical significance of these changes are indicated.

References

1. Alexander JW, Ogle CK, Stinnett J, MacMillan BG (1978) A sequential prospective analysis of immunological abnormalities and infection following severe thermal injury. Ann Surg 188:809–816
2. Deitch E. McDonald J (1982) Influence of serum on impaired neutrophil chemotaxis after thermal injury. J Surg Res 33:251–257
3. Christou NV, Tellado JM (1989) In vitro polymorphonuclear neutrophil function in surgical patients does not correlate with anergy but with "activating" processes such as sepsis or trauma. Surgery 106:718–724
4. Alexander JW, Stinnett JD, Ogle C, Ogle JD, Morris M (1979) A comparison of immunologic profiles and their influence on bacteremia in surgical patients with a high risk of infection. Surgery 86:94–104
5. Alexander JW, Ogle CK, Stinnett JD, White M, Morris M, MacMillan BG (1979) Relationship between host defence variables and infection in severe thermal injury. Burns 5:248–254
6. Warden G, Mason A, Pruitt B (1974) Evaluation of leukocyte chemotaxis in vitro in thermally injured patients. J Clin Invest 54:1001–1004
7. Grogan J (1976) Suppressed in vitro chemotaxis of burn neutrophils. J Trauma 16:985–988
8. Davis J, Dineen P, Gallin J (1980) Neutrophil degranulation and abnormal chemotaxis after thermal injury. Annu Rev Med 124:1467–1471
9. Alexander JW, Wixson J (1970) Neutrophil dysfunction and sepsis in burn injury. Surg Gynecol Obstet 130:431
10. Curreri PW, Heck E, Browne L, Baxter C (1973) Stimulated nitro blue tetrazolium test to assess neutrophil antibacterial function: prediction of wound sepsis in burned patients. Surgery 74:6–13
11. Ogle C, Alexander JW, Nagy H, Wood S, Palkert D, Carey M, Ogle J, Warden G (1990) A long-term study and correlation of lymphocyte and neutrophil function in the patient with burns. J Burn Care Rehabil 11:105
12. Grogan J (1976) Altered neutrophil phagocytic function in burn patients. J Trauma 16:734–738
13. Heck E, Edgar M, Hunt J, Baxter C (1980) A comparison of leukocyte function and burn mortality. J Trauma 20:75–77
14. Bjerknes R, Vindenes H, Pitkanen J, Winneman J, Laerum OD, Abyholm F (1989) Altered polymorphonuclear neutrophilic granulocyte functions in patients with large burns. J Trauma 29:847–855
15. Heck E, Browne L, Curreri PW, Baxter C (1975) Evaluation of leukocyte function in burned individuals by in vitro oxygen consumption. J Trauma 15:486–488
16. Duque R, Phan S, Hudson J, Till G, Ward P (1985) Functional defects in phagocytic cells following thermal injury. Am J Pathol 118:116–127
17. Gadd M, Hansbrough J (1989) The effect of thermal injury on murine neutrophil oxidative metabolism. J Burn Care Rehabil 10:125–130
18. Bjerknes R, Vindenes H (1989) Neutrophil dysfunction after thermal injury: alteration of phagolysosomal acidification in patients with large burns. Burns 15:77–81

19. Gallin J (1985) Neutrophil specific granule deficiency. Annu Rev Med 36:263–274
20. Piller N (1976) A comparison of the effect of benzopyrones and other drugs with anti-inflammatory properties on acid and neutral protease activity levels in various tissues after thermal injury. Br J Exp Pathol 57:411–418
21. Koller M, Konig W, Brom J, Erbs G, Muller F (1989) Studies on the mechanisms of granulocyte dysfunctions in severely burned patients – evidence for altered leukotriene generation. J Trauma 29:435–445
22. Rothe G, Kellerman W, Valet G (1990) Flow cytometric parameters of neutrophil function as early indicators of sepsis- or trauma-related pulmonary or cardiovascular organ failure. J Lab Clin Med 115:52–61
23. Warden G, Mason A, Pruitt B (1975) Suppression of leukocyte chemotaxis in vitro by chemotherapeutic agents used in the management of thermal injuries. Ann Surg 181:863–869
24. Bjornson A, Bjornson HS, Altemeier W (1981) Serum-mediated inhibition polymorphonuclear leukocyte function following burn injury. Ann Surg 194:568–575
25. Deitch E, Gelder F, McDonald J (1982) Prognostic significance of abnormal neutrophil chemotaxis after thermal injury. J Trauma 22:199–204
26. Jeyapaul J, Mehta N, Arora S, Antia N (1984) Fc and complement receptor integrity of polymorphonuclear (PMN) cells following thermal injury. Burns 10:387–395
27. Alexander JW (1967) Serum and leukocyte lysosomal enzyme derangements following severe thermal injury. Arch Surg 95:482–490
28. Babcock GF, Taylor AF, Hynd B, Sramkoski RM, Alexander JW (1987) Flow cytometric analysis of lymphocyte subset phenotypes comparing normal children and adults. Diagn Clin Immunol 5:175–179
29. Babcock GF, Alexander JW, Warden GD (1990) Flow cytometric analysis of neutrophil subsets in thermally injured patients developing infection. J Clin Immunol Immunopathol 54:117–125
30. White-Owen C, Babcock GF, Sramkoski RM, Alexander JW (1991) A rapid whole blood microassay for human neutrophil phagocytosis of FITC-labeled *Staphylococcus aureus* using flow cytometry. (submitted for publication)
31. Bass D, Parce J, Dechatelet L, Szejda P, Seeds M, Thomas M (1983) Flow cytometric studies of oxidative product formation by neutrophils: a graded response to membrane stimulation. J Immunol 130:1910–1917
32. White-Owen C, Alexander JW, Babcock GF (1991) Reduced expression of neutrophil CD11b and CD16 after severe trauma. J Surg Res (in Press)
33. White-Owen C, Babcock GF, Alexander JW (1990) Identification of a subpopulation of human neutrophils with altered phagocytic capacity in patients suffering severe thermal or traumatic injury. 6th International Symposium on Infections in the Immunocompromised Host 6:175 (Abstract)
34. White-Owen C, Alexander JW, Babcock GF (1990) Phagocytosis by CD11b-CD16- neutrophils. J Leukocyte Biol 1 [Suppl]:48
35. Smith CL, Baker CJ, Anderson DC, Edwards MS (1990) Role of complement receptors in opsonophagocytosis of group B streptococci by adult and neonatal neutrophils. J Infect Dis 162:489–495
36. Graham I, Brown E (1991) Extracellular calcium results in a conformational change in Mac-1 (CD11b/CD18) on neutrophils: differentiation of adhesion and phagocytosis function of Mac-1. J Immunol 146:685–691
37. Salmon J, Brogle N, Edberg J, Kimberly R (1991) Fc$_\gamma$ receptor III induces actin polymerication in human neutrophils and primes phagocytosis mediated by Fc$_\gamma$ receptor II. J Immunol 146:997–1004

Endothelial Dysfunction as an Early Critical Event in Ischemia and Shock

A. M. Lefer and X. Ma

Introduction

Splanchnic artery occlusion (SAO) followed by reperfusion (R) of the ischemic splanchnic visceral organs results in precipitous decline in systemic blood pressure, leading to a circulatory shock state [1]. SAO + R shock is a very severe form of shock with a characteristic high mortality rate (i.e., 80%–95%). The pathogenesis of SAO + R shock is complex and involves multiple mechanisms including (a) capillary leakage and hypovolemia, (b) loss of vascular control mechanisms (e.g., tendency towards poor splanchnic perfusion, vasospasm), and (c) depression of myocardial contractility [2]. Recently, neutrophils have been implicated in contributing to SAO + R shock [3, 4]. Neutrophil accumulation in tissues may lead to the release of a variety of humoral mediators of shock including (a) oxygen derived free radicals (e.g., superoxide radical), (b) cytokines (e.g., tumor necrosis factor, TNF), and (c) proteolytic enzymes (e.g., elastase). Additionally neutrophils may accumulate in small blood vessels and physically obstruct blood flow there, thus contributing to the perpetuation of the ischemic state [5]. Similar effects occur during myocardial ischemia and reperfusion (MI + R) [5, 6] except that a lethal form of shock does not develop.

One of the important early significant events in the pathophysiology of ischemia and reperfusion is endothelial dysfunction, characterized by a loss of ability to release endothelium-derived relaxing factor (EDRF). This decline in EDRF occurs within 2.5 min after reperfusion in both rats and cats subjected to MI + R [6, 7], but does not occur prior to reperfusion despite 90 min of ischemia. These findings indicate that loss of EDRF is a sensitive and early marker of vascular dysfunction following reperfusion of a previously ischemic vascular bed. Previous experiments have shown that superoxide radicals contribute significantly to the postreperfusion endothelial dysfunction [6, 7]. Moreover, the major source of the early superoxide generation appears to be the vascular endothelium itself [7, 8].

Department of Physiology, Jefferson Medical College, Thomas Jefferson University, Philadelphia, PA 19107, USA

Host Defense Dysfunction
in Trauma, Shock and Sepsis
Eds. Faist/Meakins/Schildberg
© Springer-Verlag, Berlin Heidelberg 1993

Endothelial Dysfunction in Shock States

Endothelial dysfunction as assessed by markedly decreased EDRF release is a very significant occurrence, since EDRF exerts many important biological effects [9], and since reduced EDRF probably contributes to enhanced capillary leakiness and reduced release of prostacyclin (PGI_2), a cytoprotective eicosanoid produced largely by endothelial cells. EDRF exerts a variety of important biological effects, as shown in Fig. 1. In addition to mediating the vasorelaxation induced by endothelial-dependent dilators (i.e., the endothelial-dependent relaxation, EDR, EDRF also inhibits platelet aggregation, inactivates superoxide radicals, decreases neutrophil (PMN) adherence to endothelium, and may preserve cardiac myocytes [9, 10]. All of these effects would also be useful in SAO + R. Indeed, infusion of the substance thought to be EDRF (i.e., nitric oxide, NO) in SAO + R significantly protects against splanchnic injury and death occurring in SAO + R in cats [11].

Since splanchnic ischemia is a cardinal feature of all forms of circulatory shock (e.g., hemorrhagic, endotoxemic, traumatic, and SAO shock), endothelial dysfunction in the mesenteric vasculature could be an important common pathophysiologic event in circulatory shock. The major purposes of this paper is to (a) review the status of mesenteric vascular endothelial integrity in a variety of forms of circulatory shock and (b) discuss the time course and mechanisms of endothelial dysfunction in these shock states.

Table 1 summarizes endothelial-dependent (i.e., to acetylcholine) and endothelium-independent (i.e., to acidified $NaNO_2$) responses of superior mesenteric artery rings in untreated control or shock rats. It is evident that endothelial

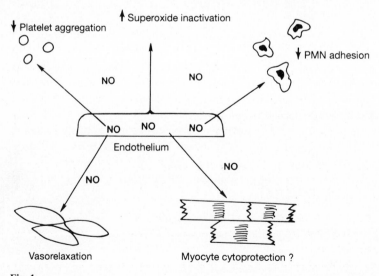

Fig. 1

Table 1. Endothelial dysfunction in isolated superior mesenteric artery rings in rats subjected to circulatory shock

Type of shock	Vasorelaxation to acetylcholine (%)	Vasorelaxation to $NaNO_2$ (%)
Sham shock	82 ± 5 (8)	97 ± 5 (8)
Endotoxic	27 ± 5* (10)	95 ± 4 (10)
SAO + R	29 ± 4* (10)	96 ± 5 (10)
Traumatic	13 ± 4* (9)	91 ± 2 (9)

All values are means ± SEM (n in parentheses taken from superior mesenteric artery rings isolated 60–90 min after induction of shock.
*$p < 0.001$ from sham shock control values.
SAO + R, splanchnic artery occlusion + reperfusion

dysfunction occurs in all three forms of circulatory shock, but not in sham shock control rats. These findings thus indicate that endothelial dysfunction is a prominent feature in the splanchnic vasculature during a variety of types of circulatory shock.

Not only is splanchnic vascular endothelial dysfunction an important event in shock states, the dysfunction occurs very early after reperfusion in the case of SAO + R, and at a comparable time in the other forms of shock. SAO for 90 min without reperfusion (i.e., 0 min reperfusion) does not result in any significant degree of EDR, similar to that situation occurring in MI + R [6]. However, reperfusion for a period as short as 2.5 min produces a significant degree of endothelial dysfunction. This degree of impairment of EDR continues to progress at 10 and 20 min postreperfusion and reaches a maximal degree of dysfunction at 60 min postreperfusion. Thus, endothelial dysfunction is a very early marker for vascular injury in shock and coincides with a peak of superoxide generation in the ischemic heart 1.5–2 min postreperfusion [7]. In types of shock in which the ischemia and reperfusion occur more gradually (i.e., endotoxic shock), the onset of endothelial dysfunction may be somewhat delayed (i.e., 20–40 min postendotoxemia [12]).

Mechanisms of Endothelial Dysfunction

A myriad of experiments have been conducted in recent years concerning the mechanisms of endothelial dysfunction and injury under a variety of experimental conditions and in a wide diversity of experimental preparations. Basically, endothelial dysfunction can be attributed to three major classes of effects. These are: (1) direct intrinsic effects or changes within endothelial cells, (e.g., free radicals generated by endothelial cells); (2) effects induced by humoral mediators produced near endothelial cells (e.g., TNF, leukotriene B_4 [LTB_4], platelet activating factor [PAF]) [13]; and (3) effects produced by other cells adhering to endothelial cells (e.g., neutrophils binding to adhesive proteins on endothelial cells). Of course, there can be combinations of effects since neutrophils also generate superoxide radicals, TNF, and other mediators, as well as some of the mediators which are chemoattractant (e.g., LTB_4, PAF) and recruit additional PMNs to the endothelium.

Figure 2 illustrates some of these principles in cat coronary artery rings isolated from isolated cat hearts that were perfused under constant flow for 110 min with Krebs-Henseleit solution without blood or blood cells. The top panel illustrates typical responses to coronary artery rings isolated from a cat heart perfused for 110 min of normal flow (i.e., 40–50 ml/min). The bottom panel illustrates coronary rings isolated from a cat heart perfused for 90 min of ischemia (i.e., at 15% of control) followed by reperfusion at normal flow for an additional 20 min. When autologous neutrophils (PMN) or F-methionyl-leucyl-phenylalanine (fMLP) were added alone, no contraction occurred. However, when fMLP + PMNs were added (i.e., activation of the neutrophils occurred), a significant contraction occurred. Moreover, this contraction was greater in the arterial rings from the ischemic-reperfused heart. This suggests a sensitization of the coronary vascular rings as a result of ischemia and reperfusion. Additionally, when endothelial-dependent vasodilators (e.g., acetylcholine, A23187) were tested following washout of the neutrophils, the rings from the ischemic reperfused hearts showed almost a total endothelial dysfunction, whereas the rings from the control heart showed only a 30%–35% endothelial dysfunction. These findings strongly implicate endothelial dysfunction as a key event following reperfusion of an ischemic vascular bed and a compounding of the insult by neutrophils. Additional experiments have shown that this PMN-induced endothelial dysfunction is due to superoxide radicals released from the activated neutrophils inactivating EDRF and thus opposing its vasodilator effect, hence resulting in a vasoconstriction. The response does not occur in a vascular ring having an injured or denuded endothelium.

Figure 3 illustrates the role of LTB_4-activated neutrophils interacting with the endothelium of superior mesenteric arteries to produce endothelial dysfunc-

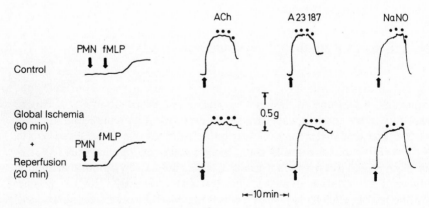

Fig. 2

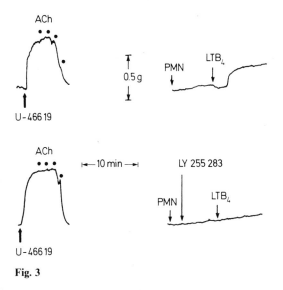

Fig. 3

tion in a manner comparable to that observed by fMLP-activated PMNs in coronary artery rings. In rat superior mesenteric artery rings shown to have an intact endothelium (i.e., responding with a nearly complete vasorelaxation to acetylcholine), addition of 1×10^{-6} PMNs/ml and subsequent activation of the PMNs with LTB_4 produces a marked vasoconstriction indicative of superoxide release [14]. Subsequently, these SMA rings failed to relax to acetylcholine but relaxed fully to acidified $NaNO_2$. This endothelial dysfunction is prevented by addition of LY-255283, an LTB_4 receptor antagonist. Additional experiments have also shown that the addition of an antibody to CD-18, the common β-chain of the integrin family of adhesive proteins, also prevents this endothelial dysfunction [14, 15]. The mechanism of this latter effect is not clear, but it may involve cooperation among inducers of adhesive proteins and rapidly inducible or constitutively present adhesive receptors.

Summary

Endothelial dysfunction is thus an early and critical event in ischemia and reperfusion injury, including a variety of types of circulatory shock and trauma. This dysfunction can serve as an early marker for subsequent tissue injury. A variety of approaches to prevent the early endothelial dysfunction and later tissue injury have been found to be useful, including scavenging superoxide radicals (e.g., hSOD) [6], infusion of TGF-β, which also inactivates or prevents formation of free radicals as well as of TNF [16], LTB_4 receptor antagonists [17], antibodies to adhesive proteins [15] which prevent PMN adherence to endothelial cells, and infusion of EDRF (i.e., NO or NO donors) itself [11]. Future work is necessary to sort out these provocative mechanisms and to evolve the best strategy with which to deal with reperfusion injury.

References

1. Milliken J, Nahor A, Fine J (1965) A study of the factors involved in the development of peripheral vascular collapse following release of the occluded superior mesenteric artery. Br J Surg 52:699–704
2. Lefer AM, Barenholz Y (1972) Pancreatic hydrolases and the formation of a myocardial depressant factor in shock. Am J Physiol 223:1103–1109
3. Grisham MB, Hernandez LA, Granger DN (1986) Xanthine oxidase and neutrophil infiltration in intestinal ischemia. Am J Physiol 251:G567–G574
4. Hernandez LA, Grisham MB, Granger DN (1987) A role for iron in oxidant-mediated ischemic injury to intestinal mikcrovasculature. Am J Physiol 253:G49–G53
5. Engler RL, Dahlgren MD, Peterson MA, Dobbs A, Schmid-Schonbein GW (1986) Accumulation of polymorphonuclear leukocytes during 3-h experimental myocardial ischemia. Am J Physiol 251:H93–H100
6. Tsao PS, Aoki N, Lefer DJ, Johnson G. III, Lefer AM (1990) Time course of endothelial dysfunction and myocardial injury during myocardial ischemia and reperfusion in the cat. Circulation 82:1402–1412
7. Tsao PS, Lefer AM (1990) Time course and mechanism of endothelial dysfunction in isolated ischemic and hypoxic perfused rat hearts. Am J Physiol 259:H1660–H1666
8. Zweier JL (1988) Measurement of superoxide-derived free radicals in the reperfused heart. Evidence for a free radical mechanism of reperfusion injury. J Biol Chem 263:1353–1357
9. Moncada S, Palmer RMJ, Higgs EA (1990) Discovery and biological relevance of the L-arginine: nitric oxide pathway. In: Rubanyi GM, Vanhoutte PM (eds) Endothelium-Derived Relaxing Factors. Karger, Basel, pp 55–63
10. Johnson G. III, Tsao PS, Lefer AM (1991) Cardioprotective effects of authentic nitric oxide in myocardial ischemia with reperfusion. Crit. Care Med. (in press)
11. Aoki N, Johnson G. III, Lefer AM (1990) Beneficial effects of two forms of NO administration in feline splanchnic artery occlusion shock. Am J Physiol 258:G275–G281
12. Siegfried MR, Ma X-I, Erhardt J, Lefer AM (1991) Role of intravenous superoxide dismutase in the protection of vascular endothelial function in rat endotoxic shock. 2nd international conference on shock, Vienna, 2–6 June 1991 (in press)
13. Aoki N, Siegfried M, Lefer AM (1989) Anti-EDRF effect of tumor necrosis factor in isolated perfused cat carotid arteries. Am J Physiol 256:H1509–H1512
14. Ma X-I, Tsao PS, Viehman GE, Lefer AM, Neutrophil-mediated vasoconstriction and endothelial dysfunction in ischemic-reperfused cat coronary artery (submitted for publication)
15. Ma X-I, Tsao PS, Lefer AM (1990) Antibody to CD-18 exerts endothelial and cardiac protective effects in myocardial ischemia and reperfusion. J Clin Invest 88:1237–1243
16. Lefer AM, Tsao P, Aoki N, Palladino MA Jr, (1990) Mediation of cardioprotection by transforming growth factor-β. Science 249:61–64
17. Karasawa A, Guo J-P, Ma X-I, Tsao PS, Lefer AM (1991) Protective actions of a leukotriene B$_4$ antagonist in splanchnic ischemia and reperfusion in rats. Am J Physiol 261:G191–G198

Role of Oxidants, Proinflammatory Agents, and Granulocytes in the Post Ischemic Intestine*

P. Kubes and D. N. Granger

In 1981, it was first postulated that xanthine oxidase (XO)-derived oxidants play an integral role in the microvascular injury associated with the reperfusion of ischemic tissue [1]. Since that time much work has been done to substantiate this hypothesis and to further expand on the pathophysiological alterations associated with ischemia-reperfusion (I/R). Figure 1 illustrates that during ischemia, cellular adenosine triphosphate (ATP) is converted to the catabolic substrate hypoxanthine while the enzyme xanthine dehydrogenase (XD) is converted to XO. Following reperfusion, oxygen reacts with hypoxanthine and XO to produce superoxide and hydrogen peroxide. These reactive oxygen metabolites may then be converted to the highly cytotoxic hydroxyl radical by the ironcatalyzed Haber-Weiss reaction. This initiates the process of lipid peroxidation which may stimulate the release of chemoattractants and the subsequent activation and recruitment of granulocytes. The objective of this chapter is to summarize supportive evidence regarding each component of the scheme presented in Fig. 1.

The mechanisms underlying I/R-related tissue injury have been studied in many organ systems, but the focus of this discussion will largely be confined to the small intestine. In our intestine model, microvascular permeability to plasma proteins has been a useful index for the assessment of the microvascular alterations produced by brief (1 h) periods of ischemia [2], whereas morphological alterations in the mucosal region of the small intestine serve as an index of the tissue injury produced by prolonged (3 h) periods of ischemia [3]. Of particular interest has been the observation that if the blood flow is reduced to approximately 20% of control for 1 h (ischemia) a twofold increase in microvascular permeability is noted (Fig. 2a). However, if an hour of reperfusion follows the ischemic episode, the increment in microvascular permeability is much larger (fivefold). A similar pattern is observed in mucosal permeability (an index of barrier dysfunction) in the postischemic gut (Fig. 2b). Crissinger et al. [4]. have demonstrated significantly greater mucosal dysfunction during the reperfusion period than during the ischemic episode. Additionally, it has been reported that the mucosal injury produced by 3 h of ischemia and 1 h of reperfusion is significantly greater than that produced by 4 h of ischemia alone

* The work summarized in this chapter was supported by a grant from the National Institutes of Health (DK 33594)
Department of Physiology, Louisiana State University Medical Center, Shreveport, LA 71130, USA

Host Defense Dysfunction
in Trauma, Shock and Sepsis
Eds. Faist/Meakins/Schildberg
© Springer-Verlag, Berlin Heidelberg 1993

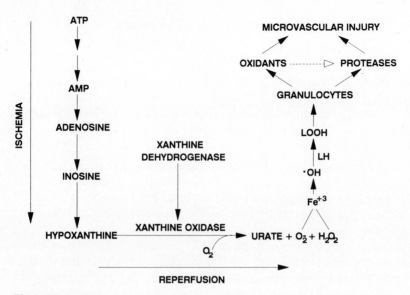

Fig. 1. Mechanism proposed to explain the involvement of xanthine derived oxidants, proinflammatory agents, and leukocytes in I/R-induced microvascular dysfunction. (Modified from [1])

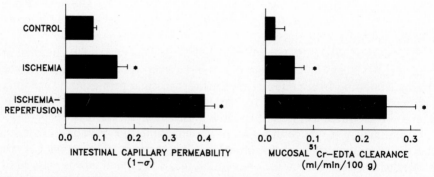

Fig. 2. *Left*, Effects of 1 h ischemia and 1 h I/R on intestinal microvascular permeability. σ, Osmotic reflection coefficient of intestinal capillaries to total plasma proteins. *Right*, Effect of 3 h ischemia and 3 h ischemia + 1 h reperfusion on mucosal permeability to ^{51}Cr-EDTA [4]. *$P < 0.05$ versus control

[3]. It is clearly during the reperfusion phase, rather than the ischemic phase, that the largest increment in permeability occurs.

It is now believed that it is the reintroduction of oxygen, resulting in the production of oxyradicals, that may be the primary source of tissue injury. Reperfusion of intestine with a nitrogenated electrolyte solution after 3 h of ischemia produced significantly less injury than that observed with whole blood [3]. Furthermore, Korthuis et al. [5] demonstrated that the increased microvascular permeability and injury associated with I/R was greatly attenuated in skeletal muscle if it is reperfused with anoxic rather than oxygenated blood. Evidence to suggest that oxygen radicals were involved was based on the finding that antioxidants and inhibitors of oxy-radical formation offer protection against vascular and mucosal injury. This protection was as effective if the antioxidants were given just prior to reperfusion as when the agents were administered before ischemia [6]. Therefore the overall pattern and time course of injury in these studies is consistent with the view that the reintroduction of oxygen during reperfusion is largely responsible for the initiation of the injury process.

Role of Xanthine Oxidase

The first component of our working hypothesis is that XO is an important source of oxidants such as hydrogen peroxide and superoxide anion in post ischemic tissue. It is widely distributed among tissues, the small intestine being the richest source [7, 8]. Its activity is found mainly in the mucosal layer with an increasing gradient from villus base to tip, where levels of XO have been reported to exceed 100 mU/g wet weight of tissue [9]. This finding is consistent with reports that the villus tip is most susceptible to ischemic injury. The cytotoxic potential of the XO activity in intestinal mucosa is exemplified by the observation in vitro that isolated cells are injured when exposed to XO levels as low as 2 mU/ml [10]. Under normal conditions XO exists in the cell as an oxidized form of nicotinamide adenine dinucleotide (NAD^+)-reducing XD and not the oxy-radical producing oxidase XO. However, conversion of XD to XO (D-O conversion) can be induced by I/R [11]. Parks et al. [12] have reported that D-O conversion was a relatively constant and slow process (13% per hour) over the 3 h of ischemia in the rat intestine. Although D-O conversion in the feline postischemic intestine has not been measured, Parks et al. [12] have alluded to the possibility that this conversion may be even slower in the small bowel of the cat than the rat.

The contention that XO is the primary source of oxygen radicals in ischemic tissues was for some time based solely on the observation that allopurinol, a competitive inhibitor of this enzyme, greatly reduced the injury observed following I/R (Table 1). Although allopurinol is a fairly specific XO inhibitor it does produce metabolic and physiologic responses beyond its inhibition of XO [13]. Direct free radical scavenging properties have been implicated in this drug's ability to protect against I/R injury in vitro [14]. However, concentrations well above those that afforded protection are required to induce radical scavenging. Nevertheless, to address this controversy, other XO inhibitors were tested for their ability to protect against microvascular injury associated with reperfusion of the ischemic small intestine. Pterin aldehyde (a potent inhibitor of intestinal XO) also attenuated the increased vascular permeability produced by reperfusion of the ischemic small bowel [15, 16]. XO can also be inactivated if

Table 1. Modulation of I/R-induced increase in microvascular permeability

Condition	Microvascular permeability $(1-\sigma)$
Control	0.08 ± 0.01
I/R	0.41 ± 0.02
I/R + treatment with:	
Allopurinol	0.18 ± 0.01
SOD	0.14 ± 0.01
Catalase	0.19 ± 0.01
Deferoxamine	0.15 ± 0.01
Apotransferrin	0.17 ± 0.01
DMSO	0.19 ± 0.02
Antineutrophil serum	0.13 ± 0.01
Monoclonal Antibody 60.3	0.12 ± 0.01

Values are means $\pm$ SE. SOD, superoxide dismutase; DMSO, dimethyl sulfoxide; σ, osmotic reflection coefficient to total plasma protein.

tungsten replaces molybdenum, at the active site of the enzyme. It has been demonstrated that a molybdenum-deficient, tungsten-supplemented diet decreased XO activity to approximately 10% of control in rat small intestine [17]. This regimen in cats greatly attenuated the increase in vascular permeability associated with I/R [18]. An important observation is that conversion of XD to XO can be prevented by the administration of protease inhibitors such as soybean trypsin inhibitor [11]. The I/R-induced increase in vascular permeability (1 h I/R) and mucosal lesion formation (3 h I/R) were largely prevented in soybean trypsin inhibitor-treated animals [19]. This suggests that the D-O conversion itself may be a very important biochemical step in the initiation of postischemic injury. Further, normal intestinal levels of XO are probably not of sufficient quantity to produce the postischemic injury. Taken as a whole, these results support the claim that XO is the major source of oxy-radicals in the ischemic small intestine.

Role of Reactive Oxygen Metabolites

Having established that I/R increases vascular permeability in the small intestine, attention was focused on factors that may mediate this response. Since XO was implicated in our model of I/R, reactive oxygen metabolites including superoxide anion and hydrogen peroxide were considered as strong candidates for the mediator of the I/R-induced increase in vascular permeability. Pretreatment with superoxide dismutase (SOD), a superoxide radical scavenging enzyme, significantly attenuated the permeability changes induced by regional ischemia (Table 1). Furthermore, a small lipophilic compound that is known to have SOD-like activity, Cu (II)-3,5-diisopropylsalicylic acid (CuDIPS), also attenuates the I/R-induced increase in capillary permeability [20]. Finally, when oxygen radicals are generated experimentally, by infusing XO and hypoxanthine into nonischemic intestine, the resulting increase in microvascular permeability mimics that observed following I/R. This permeability increase is largely prevented if SOD is infused along with XO and hypoxanthine [21]. The bulk of these data implicates superoxide in the I/R-induced increase in microvascular permeability.

Although the SOD studies provided strong evidence for the involvement of oxygen radicals in I/R-induced microvascular injury, the superoxide anion per se is a relatively weak oxidant. The low reactivity of this compound suggests that it is unlikely to be the final mediator of I/R injury but it may be a precursor to a more potent oxidant that eventually mediates reperfusion damage. While superoxide is formed by XO, nearly 80% of the O_2 consumed by the enzyme is divalently reduced to H_2O_2. Furthermore, the superoxide generated by XO spontaneously and rapidly dismutates to produce hydrogen peroxide and O_2. Similar to data with SOD, catalase, a hydrogen peroxide detoxifying agent, also reduced the vascular dysfunction induced by I/R, as noted in Table 1 [22]. Although H_2O_2 is rather innocuous in the absence of trace metals and a sluggish oxidant in its reactivity towards biological compounds, in the presence of certain transition metals, particularly iron, it yields (Haber-Weiss reaction) the hydroxyl radical OH, a potent oxidizing agent. Normally, iron is stored in enterocytes in the form of ferritin micelles. However, superoxide can react with Fe^{3+} in ferritin to liberate Fe^{2+} [23, 24]. Thus, XO-generated superoxide provides ferrous iron, which together would then react with H_2O_2 to form OH in the postischemic intestine. To evaluate the role of iron in I/R-induced hydroxyl radical production an iron chelator (deferoxamine) and an iron-binding protein (apotransferrin) were tested to determine whether they afford protection against the increased intestinal microvascular permeability produced by I/R [25]. Table 1 clearly demonstrates that both deferoxamine and apotransferrin provided significant protection in our I/R model. However, if deferoxamine or transferrin were iron-loaded prior to administration, then no protection was observed, suggesting that iron binding accounts for the beneficial effects of these substances [25].

The hydroxyl radical, considered to be the most reactive free radical produced in vivo, is capable of damaging many biological compounds [26, 27] including proteins, lipids, carbohydrates, and nucleotides [28]. The principal mechanism proposed to explain radical-mediated increases in permeability involves peroxidation of lipid components of cellular membranes. The formation of lipid-derived free radicals such as conjugated dienes, lipid hydroperoxide radicals, and fragmentation products, (e.g., malondialdehydes), alters the structural integrity and biological function of cell membranes [29]. Evidence for reperfusion-induced lipid peroxidation in the intestinal mucosa was reported by Younes et al. [30], who observed a 100% increase in the tissue levels of conjugated dienes 10 min after reperfusion of the ischemic bowel. Furthermore, the assumption that the hydroxyl radical plays a critical role in I/R injury is supported by studies in which cats were treated with dimethylsulfoxide (DMSO), a hydroxyl radical scavenger (Table 1). Microvascular permeability was greatly attenuated in these animals [31]. Therefore the protective effects of DMSO, deferoxamine and transferrin, and elevated levels of conjugated dienes are consistent with the view that the cytotoxic hydroxyl radical is formed during reperfusion by the Haber-Weiss reaction and that it plays a role in the injury to intestinal cells induced by I/R. It should be mentioned that the same therapeutic interventions also protect the mucosa against I/R-induced dysfunction [3, 22].

Role of Neutrophils

Work in our laboratory indicates that neutrophils accumulate in both the vasculature [32] and mucosa [33] during reperfusion of the ischemic bowel (Fig. 3). The former observation was based on intravital microscopy experiments (visualization of the microvasculature), which produce a quantitative assessment of the number of cells that adhere and extravasate under control, ischemic, and reperfusion conditions. Prior to ischemia the number of adherent leukocytes per 100 μm length of mesenteric venules was 4.0 ± 0.8. There was a rapid sevenfold increase in adherent leukocytes within the first 10 min of reperfusion and this level was maintained for the next 60 min (Fig. 3a). Leukocyte emigration out of the vasculature can also be quantitated using this technique (Fig. 3b). There was a dramatic rise in the number of leukocytes observed in the interstitium from 8.6 ± 1.5 under control conditions to 68.6 ± 5.6 during 60 min of reperfusion. In comparative studies of the mucosa (Fig. 3c), the biochemical myeloperoxidase assay [33] was used to demonstrate that the number of infiltrating leukocytes

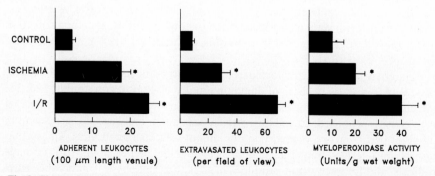

Fig. 3. The number of adherent (*left*) and extravasted leukocytes (*middle*) during control conditions, ischemia (1 h) and I/R in the feline mesentery using intravital microscopy *Right*, Myeloperoxidase activity (index of neutrophil infiltration) of the small intestinal mucosa during control conditions, ischemia (3 h), and I/R P. *$P < 0.05$ versus control

into this tissue was greatly increased at the time of reperfusion. These findings raised the important question of whether neutrophils are a cause or an effect of the I/R-induced increase in microvascular and mucosal permeability.

A role for neutrophils in oxy-radical production after I/R was first proposed by Romson and coworkers [34] in studies of the myocardium. Neutrophil depletion was observed to reduce infarct size to the same extent as pretreatment with oxy-radical scavengers. We have used two approaches to assess the role of neutrophils in the I/R-induced increase in intestinal capillary permeability, i.e., neutrophil depletion and prevention of neutrophil adherence with monoclonal antibodies (MoAb 60.3 and IB_4) directed against specific membrane-associated glycoproteins that modulate adherence to endothelium [35]. Table 1 illustrates the ability of these immunologic techniques to attenuate the I/R-induced permeability increases in the small intestine. These results indicate that neutrophils are the major mediators of I/R-induced microvascular injury. The observation that neutrophil depletion and prevention of neutrophil adherence are equally effective in attenuating the microvascular injury suggests that neutrophil adherence is the rate-limiting step in reperfusion-induced, neutrophil-mediated microvascular injury. This same approach, however, was not effective at preventing the I/R-induced mucosal dysfunction. Administration of MoAb IB_4 immediately before I/R failed to reduce the mucosal dysfunction observed [36]. Myeloperoxidase (MBO) measurements in these animals suggested that although MoAb IB_4 prevented leukocyte infiltration into the postischemic intestine, there was already a substantial number (10^7 g wet weight mucosa) of interstitial leukocytes present prior to I/R that may have been responsible for the tissue injury. Chronic MoAb IB_4 administration over a number of days, however, depleted the number of mucosal leukocytes and greatly reduced the mucosal dysfunction. Based on these data we propose that intravascular leukocytes mediate the I/R-induced microvascular injury whereas interstitial leukocytes are more important in the immediate mucosal alterations.

Link Between Oxidants and Leukocytes

There is a substantial body of evidence to link XO-derived reactive oxygen metabolites to the neutrophil infiltration observed in the postischemic intestinal mucosa [33]. We have observed that pretreatment with either the XO inhibitor allopurinol or SOD dramatically decreased the extent of neutrophil infiltration into the reperfused mucosa. Moreover, catalase, the hydroxyl radical scavenger dimethyl thiourea (DMTU), and deferoxamine all attenuated the reperfusion-induced neutrophil infiltration comparably to that observed with allopurinol and SOD. These data suggest that the superoxide anion, hydrogen peroxide, the hydroxyl radical formed by the iron-catalyzed Haber-Weiss reaction, or iron-centered radicals such as ferryl ion produced at the time of reperfusion may directly or indirectly attract and activate neutrophils. Additional support for this idea was derived from intravital microscopy data which demonstrated that allopurinol- and SOD both attenuated the increase in leukocyte adherence observed at both 10 and 60 min of reperfusion [32]. In addition, the migration of leukocytes out of the vasculature and into the interstitium was also attenuated in allopurinol- and SOD-pretreated animals, corresponding well with the mucosal leukocyte infiltration data. These results are consistent with the hypothesis that XO-derived oxidants produced at the moment of reperfusion mediate the leukocyte adherence and extravasation.

It is presently not known whether oxygen radicals per se or in combination with some plasmogen cause the recruitment of neutrophils. The chemotactic potential of feline plasma exposed to oxy-radical-producing substrates (hypoxanthine and XO) was examined, and both in vivo and in vitro studies indicate that the chemotactic potential of feline extracellular fluid was not enhanced by exposure to these agents [37]. Therefore, we were unable to obtain evidence in cats implicating plasma-based superoxide-dependent chemoattractants in I/R injury. In contrast other investigators have reported that human plasma exposed to these superoxide-generating substrates becomes potently chemotactic to human neutrophils in vitro [38, 39]. Furthermore, intradermal injection of this plasma caused heavy infiltration of neutrophils at the injection site [38]. In both studies SOD was able to inhibit the neutrophil migration, suggesting that oxy-radicals react with certain molecules in the extracellular fluid to produce a potent chemoattractant. It still remains to be resolved where other oxidants such as hydrogen peroxide can interact with extracellular fluid to form a chemoattractant.

There is some evidence which supports the possibility that XO-derived oxidants produced at the time of reperfusion may initiate the formation and release of proinflammatory agents from endothelial cells which subsequently attract and activate leukocytes. It is known that the intestinal mucosa is capable of metabolizing arachidonic acid to a variety of lipoxygenase products [40, 41] including the potent chemoattractant leukotriene B_4 (LTB_4) which is frequently implicated as a mediator of reperfusion-induced neutrophil infiltration. Several studies have demonstrated an increase in the amount of LTB_4 produced by the intestine during an inflammatory insult [42–44], including a report by Mangino et al. [45] which demonstrated a significant increase in LTB_4 production by dog ileal mucosa subjected to 3 h of ischemia and 1 h reperfusion. Although granulocyte accumulation was not monitored in the study, it was concluded that LTB_4 is a likely mediator of the massive neutrophil infiltration observed following reperfusion of the ischemic small intestine. More recently, Zimmerman et al. [46], showed that animals pretreated with either a lipoxygenase inhibitor (L663, 536) or the LTB_4 antagonist (SC-41930), decreased the magnitude of the reperfusion-induced granulocyte infiltration, providing the first direct evidence that LTB_4 accumulation in the intestinal mucosa is a cause, rather than an effect, of reperfusion-induced granulocyte infiltration. The mechanisms responsible for the enhanced LTB_4 production following reperfusion of the ischemic bowel have not been clearly defined. Recent studies demonstrated that both exposure of cells to oxidants [47] and reperfusion of ischemic intestine [48] lead to phospholipase A_2 activation, whereas inhibitors of phospholipase A_2 attenuate I/R-induced polymorpho-nuclear-neutrophil (PMN) infiltration in intestinal mucosa [49]. This would suggest that production of oxygen-derived free radicals result in the activation of phospholipase A_2 which consequently leads to the generation of LTB_4.

There is accumulating evidence supporting a role for platelet-activating factor (PAF) in ischemia-induced damage in the gastrointestinal tract. Firstly, it has recently been reported that the concentration of PAF increases 14-fold and 4-fold at 5 and 60 min after reperfusion of the canine intestine, following 2 h of complete superior mesenteric artery occlusion [50]. In that study, pretreatment of animals with the PAF antagonist BN 52021 prevented the functional impairments induced by the ischemia, indicating a major role for PAF in this system. Tagesson et al. [51] have shown that the increase in lysosomal enzyme release, intestinal permeability, and lipid peroxidation following I/R of the rat distal ileum were all significantly reduced with BN 52021. Interestingly, in that study, BN 52021 had no effect on reperfusion-induced infiltration of neutrophils in the intestinal mucosa. These findings suggest that PAF plays a role in the activation but not the attraction of neutrophils in the postischemic intestine. In contrast, more recent intravital microscopy data suggests a very important role for PAF during I/R [52]. When animals were pretreated with WEB 2086, a PAF receptor antagonist, a dramatic reduction in the number of adherent and extravasated leukocytes was observed during both ischemia and reperfusion. Of particular interest in that study was the observation that WEB 2086 also reduced the proportion of adherent leukocytes that ultimately extravasate during reperfusion by 80%. This suggests that the PAF receptor antagonist interferes with leukocyte extravasation by a process that is at least in part independent of adherence. Although it remains unclear exactly how WEB 2086 alters leukocyte extravasation, based on in vitro data, it is conceivable that the phospholipid participates in the extravasation process by promoting the limited release of neutrophil proteases (e.g., elastase) that in turn facilitate the migration of phagocytic cells across restrictive barriers such as the basement membrane [53, 54]. Interestingly, in the study of Kubes et al. [52], BN 52021 was much less effective than WEB 2086 at reducing the number of emigrating leukocytes, possibly explaining the negative data of Tagesson et al. [51]. In another study, SOD, allopurinol, and PAF antagonists were equally effective in protecting against postischemic mucosal damage in the rat stomach [55]. These investigators proposed a possible pathologic role of oxy-radicals and PAF in I/R-induced gastric mucosal ulcerations. It is quite possible that hydrogen peroxide induces PAF production to mediate these leukocyte events; in vitro data have suggested that O_2 metabolites (H_2O_2) stimulate cultured endothelial cells to produce PAF and consequently promote an adhesive interaction between leukocytes and endothelial monolayers [47].

Like PAF, tumor necrosis factor (TNF) has been shown to enhance neutrophil superoxide production and adherence [56]. While it appears that,

TNF per se possesses proinflammatory properties, recent studies suggest that the relationship between TNF and PAF is very important, particularly in mediating endothelial cell damage [57]. TNF can prime PAF-induced superoxide generation by human neutrophils and this effect is completely abolished by a number of structurally different PAF antagonists [58, 59]. Apart from inducing vascular damage via infiltration and degranulation of neutrophils, both TNF and PAF exert a direct effect on endothelial cells, causing them to retract in vitro [57]. However, no direct evidence has to date been provided to implicate TNF as a mediator of I/R injury. In fact, in the feline 3 h ischemia and 1 h reperfusion model, no detectable levels of TNF were observed (unpublished data from our laboratory).

Numerous vasoactive substances including histamine, prostaglandins, and lysosomal enzymes have also been proposed as potential mediators in the pathogenesis of intestinal ischemia. This contention is based on indirect evidence that these substances are released from the ischemic small bowel and increase microvascular permeability when infused into the normally perfused small intestine [60, 61]. However, pretreatment with either antihistamines (benadryl + cimetidine), indomethacin, or methylprednisolone did not significantly alter the permeability increase induced by regional ischemia, suggesting that neither histamine, lysosomal enzymes, nor prostaglandins are involved in the I/R-induced increase in capillary permeability [1]. Another possible mediator, bacterial endotoxin, was shown to increase capillary permeability [62]. However, since lethal doses of this substance are required to increase permeability and the magnitude of the increase in permeability produced by the endotoxin is small relative to I/R, it appears unlikely that endotoxins play a role in the I/R-induced vascular permeability changes [1]. The possibility nevertheless exists that these mediators may play a role in the postischemic mucosal dysfuncion and perhaps in other organ systems.

Although the results provide strong evidence that neutrophil infiltration is necessary for I/R-induced microvascular damage, the mechanism by which damage occurs is not fully understood. Several in vitro studies indicate that adherent leukocytes are capable of degrading various structural components of the basement memberane [53, 63, 64]. Furthermore, it has been demonstrated that neutrophil-mediated degradation of endothelial basement membrane can be prevented by inhibitors of elastase activity. These observations have led to the proposal that limited release of elastase is a prerequisite for the neutrophil extravasation associated with acute and chronic forms of inflammation. Recently, two structurally dissimilar elastase inhibitors, Eglin C and L658, 758, were used to determine whether elastase plays a role in the leukocyte infiltration observed following I/R [65]. The data suggest that the reperfusion-induced increase in mucosal MPO activity is significantly attenuated in animals pretreated with either Eglin C (which inhibits both elastase and cathepsin G) or L658, 758 (a specific elastase inhibitor). These results indicate that the rate of accumulation of neutrophils in postischemic intestinal mucosa is dependent upon the release of elastase from activated phagocytes. Consistent with this hypothesis is the observation that L658, 758 dramatically reduced the number of adherent leukocytes that ultimately extravasate to the extravascular compartment. This supports the contention that elastase plays a role in the I/R-induced process of extravasation.

Neutrophils are also capable of producing superoxide by the membrane-associated enzyme NADPH oxidase [66]. Activated neutrophils also secrete MPO, an enzyme which catalyzes the formation of hypochlorous acid (HOCl) from H_2O_2 and chloride ions. The hydrogen peroxide which fuels this reaction is derived from the spontaneous dismutation of neutrophil-derived superoxide. Hypochlorous acid is a potent oxidizing and chlorinating agent which can react with primary amines to yield N-chloramines. These substances cause extensive damage to a variety of proteins, including hemoproteins and cytochromes, and deoxyribonucleic acid (DNA). Until recently, it was impossible to dissect the role of XO-derived oxidants and neutrophil-derived oxidants. However, with the advent of inhibitors of the NADPH oxidase enzyme such as diphenyleneiodonium [67], it may now be possible to assess the role of neutrophil-derived oxidants in I/R-induced tissue injury.

Clearly there are many questions that remain unanswered regarding the hypothesis proposed in Fig. 1. The complexity of our scheme continues to grow, particularly in the area of neutrophil recruitment and activation. Future progress in this field, particularly from a therapeutic viewpoint, will depend on the development of new techniques for monitoring granulocyte function in vivo and the identification of new compounds that selectively interfere with one or more of the many granulocyte processes.

References

1. Granger DN, Rutili G, McCord JM (1981) Superoxide radicals in feline intestinal ischemia. Gastroenterology 81:22–29
2. Granger DN, Sennett M, McElearney PM, Taylor AE (1980) Effect of local arterial hypotension on cat intestinal capillary permeability. Gastroenterology 79:474–480
3. Parks DA, Granger DN (1986) Contributions of ischemia and reperfusion to mucosal lesion formation. Am J Physiol 250:G749–G753
4. Crissinger KD, Granger DN (1989) Mucosal injury induced by ischemia and reperfusion in the piglet intestine: influences of age and feeding. Gastroenterology 97:920–926
5. Korthuis RJ, Smith JK, Carden DL (1989) Hypoxic reperfusion attenuates post-ischemic microvascular injury. Am J Physiol 256:H315–H319
6. Morris JB, Bulkley GB, Haglund U, Cardenas E, Sies H (1987) The direct, real-time demonstration of oxygen free radical generation at reperfusion following ischemia in rat small intestine. Gastroenterology 92:1541
7. Krenitsky TA, Tuttle JV, Cattau EL, Wang PA (1974) A comparison of the distribution and electron acceptor specificities of xanthine oxidase and aldehyde oxidase. Comp Biochem Physiol 181:177–182
8. Batelli MG, Dellacorte E, Stirpe F (1972) Xanthine oxidase type D (dehydrogenase) in the intestine and other organs of the rat. Biochem J 126:747–749
9. Parks DA, Granger DN (1986) Xanthine oxidase: biochemistry, distribution and physiology. Acta Physiol Scand [Suppl] 548:87–99

10. Simon RH, Scoggin CH, Patterson D (1981) Hydrogen peroxide causes the fatal injury to human fibroblasts exposed to oxygen radicals. J Biol Chem 256:7181–7186

11. Roy RS, McCord JM (1983) Superoxide and ischemia: conversion of xanthine dehydrogenase to xanthine oxidase. In: Greenwald RA, Cohen RA, Cohen G (ed) Oxy radicals and their scavenger systems, vol II: cellular and medical aspects. Elsevier/North Holland Biomedical, New york, pp 143–153

12. Parks DA, Williams TK, Beckman JS (1988) Conversion of xanthine dehydrogenase to oxidase in ischemic rat intestine: a reevaluation. Am J Physiol 254:G768–G774

13. Gilman AG, Goodman LS, Gilman A (1980) The pharmacological basis of therapeutics, 6th edn. MacMillan, New York

14. Moorhouse PC, Grootveld G, Halliwell B, Quinlan JG, Gutteridge JMC (1987) Allopurinol and oxypurinol are hydroxy radical scavengers. FEBS Lett 213:23–28

15. Spector, T, Ferone R (1984) Folic acid does not inactivate xanthine oxidase. J Biol Chem 259:10784–10786

16. Granger DN, McCord JM, Parks DA, Hollwarth ME (1986b) Xanthine oxidase inhibitors attenuate ischemia-induced vascular permeability changes in the cat intestine. Gastroenterology 90:80–84

17. Topham RW, Walker MC, Calisch MP, Williams RW (1982) Evidence for the participation of intestinal xanthine oxidase in the mucosal processing of iron. Biochemistry 21:4529–4535

18. Parks DA, Henson JL, Granger DN (1986) Effect of xanthine oxidase inactivation on ischemic injury to the small intestine (abstract) Physiologist 29:101

19. Parks DA, Granger DN, Bulkley GB, Shah AK (1985) Soybean trypsin inhibitor attenuates ischemic injury to the feline small intestine. Gastroenterology 89:6–12

20. Hernandez LA, Grisham MB, Granger DN (1987) Effects of Cu-DIPS on ischemia-reperfusion injury. In: Sorenson JRJ (ed) Biology of copper complexes. Humana, Clifton, pp 201–210

21. Parks DA, Shah AK, Granger DN (1984) Oxygen radicals: effects on intestinal vascular permeability. Am J Physiol 247:G167–G170

22. Granger DN, Hollwarth ME, Parks DA (1986) Ischemia-reperfusion injury: role of oxygen-derived free radicals. Acta Physiol Scand [Suppl] 548:47–64

23. Thomas CE, Morehouse LA, Aust SD (1985) Ferritin and superoxide-dependent lipid peroxidation. J Biol Chem 260:3275–3280

24. Weiss SJ (1986) Oxygen, ischemia, and inflamation. Acta Physiol Scand [Suppl] 548:9–38

25. Hernandez LA, Grisham MB, Granger DN (1987) A role for iron in oxidant-mediated ischemic injury to intestinal microvasculature. Am J Physiol 253:G49–G53

26. Bielski BHJ, Shiue GG (1979) Reaction rates of superoxide radicals with the essential amino acids. In: Ciba Found (ed) Oxygen free radicals and tissue damage. Elsevier, New York, pp 43–56

27. Jennings RB, Reimer KA, Hill ML, Mayer SE (1981) Total ischemia in dog hearts in vitro. Circ Res 49:892–899

28. Buege JA, Aust SD (1976) Lactoperoxidase-catalyzed lipid peroxidation of microsomal and artificial membranes. Biochim Biophys Acta 444:192–201

29. Freeman BA, Crapo JD (1982) Free radicals and tissue injury. Lab Invest 47:412–426

30. Younes M, Mohr A, Schoenberg MH, Schildberg FW (1987) Inhibition of lipid peroxidation by superoxide dismutase following regional intestinal ischemia and reperfusion. Res Exp Med (Berl) 187:9–17

31. Parks DA, Granger DN (1983) Ischemia-induced vascular changes: role of xanthine oxidase and hydroxyl radicals. Am J Physiol 245:G285–G289

32. Granger DN, Benoit JN, Suzuki M, Grisham MB (1989) Leukocyte adherance to venular endothelium during ischemia reperfusion. Am J Physiol 257:G683–G688

33. Grisham MB, Hernandez LA, Granger DN (1986) Xanthine oxidase and neutrophil infiltration in intestinal ischemia. Am J Physiol 25J:G567–G574

34. Romson JL, Hook BG, Kunkel SL, Abrams GD, Schork A, Lucchesi BR (1983) Reduction of the extent of ischemic myocardial injury by neutrophil depletion in the dog. Circulation 67:1016–1023

35. Hernandez LA, Grisham MB, Twohig B, Arfors KE, Harlan JM, Granger DN (1987) Role of neutrophils in ischemia-reperfusion induced microvascular injury. Am J Physiol 253:H699–H703

36. Kubes PK, Hunter JA, Granger ND (1991) Chronic but not acute treatment with a CD-18 specific antibody protects the intestine against ischemia/reperfusion (I/R)-induced mucosal dysfunction (abstract). Gastroenterology (in press)

37. Zimmerman BJ, Grisham MB, Granger DN (1990) Role of oxidants in ischemia/reperfusion-induced granulocyte infiltration. Am J Physiol 258:G185
38. Petrone WF, English DK, Wong K, McCord JM (1980) Free radicals and inflammation: Superoxide dependent activation of a neutrophil chemotactic factor in plasma. Proc Natl Acad Sci USA 77:1159
39. Perez HD, Weksler BB, Goldstein IM (1980) Generation of a chemotactic lipid from arachidonic acid by exposure to a superoxide-generating system. Inflammation 4:313
40. Dreyling KW, Hoppe U, Peskar BA, Morgenroth K, Kozuschek W, Peskar BM (1986) Leukotriene synthesis by human gastrointestinal tissues. Biochim Biophys Acta 878:184
41. Boughton-Smith NK, Hawkey CJ, Whittle BJR (1983) Biosynthesis of lipoxygenase and cyclooxygenase products from [14C]-arachidonic acid by human colonic mucosa. Gut 4:1176
42. Lauritsen K, Laursen LS, Bukhave K, Rask-Madsen J (1988) In vivo profiles of eicosanoids in ulcerative colitis, Crohn's colitis, and clostridium difficile colitis. Gastroenterology 95:11
43. Mullane K, Read N, Salmon JA, Moncada S (1984) Role of leukocytes in acute myocardial infarction in anesthetized dogs: relationship to myocardial salvage by anti-inflammatory drugs. J Pharm Exp Ther 228:510 (1984)
44. Sharon P, Stenson WF (1984) Enhanced synthesis of leukotriene B4 by colonic mucosa in inflammatory bowel disease. Gastroenterology 86:453
45. Mangino MJ, Anderson CB, Murphy MK, Brunt E, Turk J (1989) Mucosal arachidonate metabolism and intestinal ischemia-reperfusion injury. Am J Physiol 257:G299
46. Zimmerman BJ, Granger DN (1990) Role of leukotriene B in ischemia/reperfusion-induced granulocyte infiltration. Gastroenterology (1990) 99:1358–1363
47. Lewis MS, Whatley RE, Cain P, McIntyre TM, Prescot SM, Zimmerman GA (1988) Hydrogen peroxide stimulates the synthesis of platelet-activating factor by endothelium and induces endothelial cell-dependent neutrophil adhesion, J Clin Invest 82:2045
48. Otamiri T, Lindmark D, Franzen L, Tagesson C (1988) Increased phospholipase A$_2$ and decreased lysophospholipase activity in the small intestinal mucosa after ischaemia and revascularisation. Gut 28:1445
49. Otamiri T, Lindahl M, Tagesson C (1988) Phospholipase A$_2$ inhibition prevents mucosal damage associated with small intestinal ischaemia in rats. Gut 29:489.
50. Filep J, Herman F, Braquet P, Mozes T (1989) Increased levels of platelet activating factor in blood following intestinal ischemia in the dog. Biochem Biophys Res Commun 158:353–359
51. Tagesson C, Lindahl M, Otamiri T (1988) BN 52021 ameliorates mucosal damage associated with small intestinal ischaemia in rats. In: Braquet P (ed) Ginkgolides: chemistry, biology, pharmacology and clinical perspectives. Prous, Barcelona, pp 553–561 (1990)
52. Kubes P, Ibbotson G, Russell J, Wallace JL, Granger DN (1990) Role of platelet-activating factor in reperfusion-induced leukocyte adherence. Am J Physiol 259:G300–G305
53. Weiss SJ, Curnutte JT, Regiani S (1986) Neutrophil-mediated solubilization of the subendothelial matrix: oxidative and nonoxidative mechanisms of proteolysis used by normal and chronic granulomatous disease phagocytes. J Immunol 136:636
54. Pipoly DJ, Crouch EC (1987) Degradation of native type IV procollagen by human neutrophil elastase. Implications for leukocyte-mediated degradation of basement membranes. Biochemistry 26:5748
55. Droy-Lefaix M, Drouet Y, Geraud G, Braquet P (1988) Involvement of platelet-activating factor in rat ischemia reperfusion gastric damage. In: Braquet P (ed) Ginkgolides: chemistry, biology, pharmacology and clinical perspectives. Prous, Barcelona, pp 563–574
56. Berkaw RL, Wang D, Larrich JW, Howard TH (1986) Recombinant necrosis factor augments human neutrophil superoxide production (abstract). Blood 68:80
57. Braquet P, Paubert-Braquet M, Koltai M, Bourgain R, Bussolino F, Hosford D (1989) Is there a case for PAF antagonists in the treatment of ischemic states TIPS 10:23–30
58. Paubert-Braquet M, Longchampt MO, Koltz P, Guilbaud J (1988) Tumor necrosis factor (TNF) primes human neutrophils (PMN) platelet activating factor (PAF)-induced superoxide generation. Consequences in promoting PMN-mediated endothelial cell (EC) damages (abstract). Prostaglandins 35:803
59. Braquet P, Hosford D, Braquet M, Bourgain R, Bussolino F (1989) Role of cytokines and platelet-activating factor in microvascular immune injury. Int Arch Allergy Appl Immunol 88:88–100
60. Kobold EE, Thal AP (1963) Quantitation and identification of vasoactive substances liberated during various types of experimental and clinical intestinal ischemia. Surg Gynecol Obstet 117:315–322

61. Haglund U, Lundholm K, Lundgren O, Shersten T (1977) Intestinal lysosomal enzyme activity in regional simulated shock: influence of methylprednisolone and albumin. Circ Shook 4:27–34
62. Ballin HM, Meyer MW (1960) Intestinal lymph flow in dogs after endotoxin. Proc Soc Exp Biol Med 103:93–95
63. Weiss SJ, Regiani S (1984) Neutrophils degrade subendothelial matrices in the presence of alpha-1-proteinase inhibitor. J Clin Invest 73:1297
64. Weitz JI, Huang AJ, Landman SL, Nicholson SC, Silverstein SC (1987) Elastase-mediated fibrinogenolysis by chemoattractant-stimulated neutrophils occurs in the presence of physiologic concentrations of antiproteinases. J Exp Med 166:1836
65. Zimmerman BJ, Granger DN (1990) Reperfusion-induced leukocyte infiltration: role of elastase. Am J Physiol 259:H390–H394
66. Rossi F (1986) The superoxide forming NADPH oxidase of phagocytes: nature, mechanisms of activation and function. Biochim Biophys Acta 853:65–89
67. Cross AR, Jones ATG (1987) The inhibition by diphenyleneiodonium and its analogues of superoxide generation by macrophages. Bioch J 242:103–107

Hepatic Parenchymal and Nonparenchymal Cells in Hemorrhage and Ischemia*

M. G. Clemens

Although it is widely accepted that ischemia can make a major contribution to organ dysfunction in trauma, shock, and sepsis, the exact mechanisms remain unclear. Since ischemia is, by definition, an imbalance between blood (or oxygen) supply and demand one might predict that susceptibility to ischemia damage might be well modeled by anoxia to parenchymal cells. However, in intact organs, the presence of multiple cell types complicates the response to an ischemic insult. This response is even more complicated when ischemia is followed by reperfusion which exacerbates the injury in intact organs. For instance, vascular endothelial cells have been shown to contain large quantities of xanthine dehydrogenase that can be converted to xanthine oxidase and anoxic stress resulting in the production of oxygen-derived free radicals during reoxygenation [1]. Indeed, in organs such as the heart, such "oxyradicals" of endothelial origin are likely to be major contributors to reperfusion injury [2]. In the liver the situation is further complicated by the presence of a substantial number of macrophages, the hepatic Kupffer cells, and during in vivo reperfusion infiltration by neutrophils which can then constitute a significant population of nonparenchymal cells. Thus, the purpose of this paper is to review the relative susceptibility to ischemic or anoxic injury of hepatocytes and the intact liver.

When studied as an isolated cell the hepatocyte shows considerable tolerance to hypoxic conditions. Using an oxystat system to control the extracellular partial pressure of oxygen (PO_2) surrounding isolated hepatocytes very precisely, Noll et al. [3] found that the half-maximal rate of cellular respiration occurred at a PO_2 of approximately 0.5–0.7 mmHg. Of more functional importance, the same group subsequently found that adenosine triphosphate (ATP)/adenosine diphosphate (ADP) ratio was maintained at half-maximal levels when the extracellular PO_2 is approximately 1.4 mmHg over the course of a 15-min incubation [4]. Even with virtual anoxia, however, isolated hepatocytes remain resilient even in the face of severely inhibited oxidative ATP production. When hepatocytes isolated from fed rats are incubated under anaerobic conditions for up to 3 h a slow decrease in cell viability occurs. This rate of loss of cell viability is not substantially different from what would be

*This work was supported by USPHS grant DK38201 and the Robert Garrett Fund.
Division of Pediatric Surgery, Johns Hopkins University School of Medicine, Baltimore, Maryland, USA

expected under normoxic conditions. Moreover, during this 3-h incubation, reoxygenation of the hepatocytes resulted in no further loss of cell viability indicating that reoxygenation injury did not occur. Only after the 3-h period did a significant increase in the rate of loss of cell viability occur along with exacerbation of cell injury with reoxygenation [4]. This phenomenon of the rapid reversibility of anoxic injury with reoxygenation in isolated hepatocytes was graphically demonstrated by Herman et al. [5], who showed that progressive anoxia is associated with the formation of hepatocyte plasma membrane blebs. Bleb formation preceded an increase in cytoplasmic free calcium [6] and the uptake of vital dyes such as propidium iodide [5, 6]. Rupture of the membrane blebs resulted in immediate loss of viability but reoxygenation prior to the rupture of blebs, rather than causing exacerbation of the injury (reoxygenation injury), was associated with resorption of the blebs and prevention of cell death [5]. Thus these studies would suggest that even with severely hypoxic conditions which are capable of severely depleting cellular energy stores, isolated hepatocytes are relatively resistant to irreversible cell injury. Moreover, reoxygenation injury which is observed in intact organs does not occur in isolated hepatocytes prior to the onset of significant cell death from the anoxic insult itself.

The question then arises, how closely does the isolated hepatocyte model duplicate in vivo situations? One obvious difference is that isolated hepatocyte studies are performed using hypoxia while in vivo, hypoxic hypoxia rarely occurs and the more common cause of inadequate oxygen is ischemia. By definition ischemia is blood flow inadequate to meet the needs of the tissue. During hemorrhage the inadequacy of blood flow results from systemic hypotension and is effectively a low-flow ischemic state. In contrast, no-flow ischemia results from local obstruction of blood vessels and in the case of the liver is most often the result of cross-clamping of the portal vein and hepatic artery during surgical procedures following trauma or transplantation. During no-flow ischemia, the hepatocytes very quickly become uniformly anoxic. These conditions of severe anoxia are reasonably well mimicked by the isolated hepatocytes of deGroot's group in which PO_2 is homogeneously set at a level far below the K_m for mitochondrial respiration [3, 4].

During the low-flow ischemia that accompanies hemorrhage shock, on the other hand, the situation is more complicated. It is well-known that splanchnic vasoconstriction accompanies hemorrhagic hypotension and, as a result, hepatic microvascular (sinusoidal) blood flow decreases as a linear function of the decrease in blood pressure [7]. However, the decrease in hepatic blood flow is primarily the result of decreasing portal flow which is low in oxygen content and less so with respect to the oxygen rich hepatic artery blood flow. As a result, the ratio of hepatic artery to portal vein blood supply to the hepatic microcirculation is increased, thus attenuating the decrease in oxygen supply [8]. In spite of this hepatic artery buffer system, as it has been termed [8], ischemia is of sufficient severity in hemorrhagic shock to result in depletion of high-energy phosphates. Pearce and Drucker [9] have reported a decrease in liver ATP levels to 35% of control in the late stages of hemorrhagic shock, while Chaudry et al. [10] showed a decrease to 13% of control immediately following resuscitation with blood. Although these results would suggest that the ischemic insult to the liver during hemorrhagic shock is significantly less severe than that which occurs during no-flow ischemia, the low-flow conditions of hemorrhage produce heterogeneous conditions for the hepatocytes. Because of the acinar architecture of the liver, microvascular blood flow is essentially unidirectional with no opportunity for counter current exchange. As a result, even under normal conditions, relatively steep gradients of oxygen and other metabolites are established between the periportal inflow and pericentral outflow regions of the acinus [11]. This is exacerbated during low flow. Thus low-flow ischemia sets up three functional zones in the hepatic acinus: the periportal region where oxygen supply is adequate, a midzonal region where moderate hypoxia occurs, and a pericentral region which is exposed to severe hypoxia [12]. The relative size of these zones depends upon the severity of blood flow decrease and the metabolic demands of the tissue. As a result, during hemorrhagic shock, only a relatively small portion of the liver (the pericentral zone) is exposed to anoxia comparable to that which is imposed in isolated hepatocyte studies as described above.

The above information would suggest that, in spite of the equal or lesser severity of anoxic insult imposed upon the hepatocyte during no-flow or low-flow ischemia in vivo compared to isolated hepatocytes, the severity of outcome is greater in vivo. Table 1 shows a comparison of the approximate time durations of livers or isolated hepatocytes exposed to ischemic or anoxic conditions. These comparisons must be viewed with the caveat that these models differ by more than isolated cell vs intact organ. Particularly important is the nutritional state of the cell or organ particularly with respect to glycogen stores [13, 14]. Nevertheless, under approximately similar conditions, intact livers appear to be more susceptible to injury than are isolated hepatocytes [15]. This is especially true in the case of in vivo ischemia which is accompanied by fairly severe acidosis which has been shown to be protective in isolated hepatocytes [16]. A possible explanation for the increased susceptibility of the intact liver compared to isolated hepatocytes is the presence of a large number of nonparenchymal cells which may amplify the ischemia-induced injury. Another difference is that in the intact organ continued function is vitally dependent upon structural integrity [17, 18]. Especially important is the maintenance of

Table 1. Tolerance to hypoxia/reoxygenation

	Time	Mortality (%)	Reference
Isolated hepatocytes	Up to 3 h	0–10[a] (fed)	4
	2 h	$\sim$ 40[a] (fasted, pH 6.8)	16
Hemorrhagic shock	1.5–2 h	$\sim$ 90	10
No-flow ischemia	1.5–2 h	75–100	15, 18

[a]Adjusted for rate of cell death at $PO_2 = 70$ mmHg

the integrity of the microcirculation. Since the major nonparenchymal cells line in sinusoids, microvascular failure may, at least in part, also be the result of ischemic effects on hepatic nonparenchymal cells. Under normal conditions, the nonparenchymal cells of the liver comprise primarily the endothelial cells and Kupffer cells, plus a smaller contribution of Ito (fat-storing) cells [19]. In addition, marginated neutrophils reside in the liver in relatively small numbers under normal conditions but may be recruited to the liver during pathological states such that they constitute a major population of nonparenchymal cells [20]. The major focus of this discussion will be the potential contributions of the Kupffer cell and the neutrophil in augmenting hepatic injury following hemorrhage or ischemia.

The Kupffer cells constitute greater than 80%–90% of the total body tissue macrophages and, as such, are a major contributor to the clearance of particulate material from the blood stream. Moreover, in terms of cell numbers, they make up a substantial portion of the liver although, because of their relatively small size, they contribute 10% or less to the total hepatic mass [21]. Nonetheless, the Kupffer cells, because of their close proximity to blood endothelial cell and hepatocyte, are strategically located to allow them to interact with all constituents of the liver. When activated, Kupffer cells are capable of releasing a number of mediators such as prostaglandins [22, 23], leukotrienes [24], cytokines [25], and oxyradicals [23]. Finally, there is a growing body of literature showing that activated Kupffer cells are capable of modulating a number of metabolic [26–28] and microvascular parameters in the liver [29, 30]; however, their role in modulating the effects of hypoxia or ischemia are much less well documented.

The recent study by Jaeschke and Farhood [31] has provided evidence for reactive oxidant formation by Kupffer cells during the early stages of reperfusion following 45–120 min of hepatic ischemia. In these studies, the oxidation of extracellular glutathione suggested that oxidant production during early reperfusion was an extracellular event. Since prior inactivation of the Kupffer cells with either gadolinium chloride or methylpalmitate resulted in approximately a 60% decrease in both oxidation of glutathione and plasma alanine transaminase levels (indicating hepatocellular damage), the authors concluded that the Kupffer cell was the source of the oxidant stress [31]. Kobayashi and Clemens [32] have also shown that the presence of Kupffer cells in coculture with hepatocytes exacerbates the release of lactic dehydrogenase in response to hypoxia/reoxygenation injury; however, in these studies the Kupffer cell-dependent injury was not prevented by addition to the medium of superoxide dismutase and catalase in quantities effective in scavenging extracellularly generated free radicals [33]. This would suggest that mechanisms other than reactive oxidant production might also be operative in the Kupffer cell-induced injury.

The role of Kupffer cells in modulating hepatic injury during low-flow ischemia, such as occurs during hemorrhagic shock, is even less well documented; however, the work of Ayala et al. [34] has indicated a central role for the Kupffer cell in the suppressed immune response following simple nonlethal hemorrhage. These studies have focused primarily upon functions such as antigen presentation by the hepatic macrophage, but their most recent study [35] presented at this meeting shows that the cytotoxic activity of Kupffer cells against certain tumor cell lines is markedly enhanced following simple hemorrhage. This increased cytotoxicity correlated with increased expression of tumor necrosis factor (TNF), suggesting that the cytotoxicity may be specific to TNF-sensitive cell lines [35]. Whether such effects are also exerted against non-neoplastic cells such as hepatocytes or hepatic vascular endothelial cells remains to be determined.

Although neutrophils are not normally considered to be hepatic cells, marginated neutrophils do reside in the liver under normal circumstances and the number of neutrophils marginated in the liver can increase dramatically following ischemic episodes [31, 36, 37] and in nonsurvivors following liver transplantation [38]. Thus during reperfusion or resuscitation neutrophils can become a functionally very important nonparenchymal cell population in the liver. Using histochemical techniques, Jaeschke and Farhood [37] have found that neutrophil accumulation in the liver following no-flow ischemia with reperfusion is only moderate within the first hour of reperfusion, but progressively increases until 24 h, at which time neutrophils in liver tissue are approximately 100 times that found at the end of ischemia. In these studies, however, the methodology used did not allow spatial localization of the neutrophils to specific areas of the acinus or to vessel type. Using in vivo videomicroscopic techniques with fluorescent labeling of all white blood cells, studies from our laboratory [39] have shown that the accumulation in different orders of vessel, particularly sinusoids vs terminal hepatic venules in the liver, is distinctly heterogeneous during early reperfusion. The studies showed that although white cells did not accumulate in substantial numbers in sinusoid fields early in reperfusion, the number of white cells adhering to the walls of the terminal hepatic venules increased by a factor of approximately 40 fold within the first 15 min of reperfusion. This biphasic influx of white cells into the liver microcirculation with discret localization during the two phases suggests that differential mechanisms may be operative to stimulate adherence of the neutrophils to the two populations of vascular endothelium. Although in vivo labeling techniques do not allow differentiation of types of white cell, it is likely that the adherent cells observed are neutrophils.

In addition to accumulating in the liver during reperfusion, there is evidence that neutrophils may contribute to hepatic injury. There are data in a number of tissues showing that depletion of neutrophils results in attenuation of injury [e.g., 37, 40, 41]. In the liver we have previously shown that the presence of white cell-containing blood compared to washed red blood cells in the liver during ischemia markedly exacerbates the microvascular injury that occurs during reperfusion [42]. Moreover, Jaeschke et al. [37] have shown that treatment of rats with monoclonal antibodies directed against neutrophils in sufficient quantities to produce neutropenia significantly attenuates the hepatocyte necrosis that occurs with ischemia/reperfusion. These results would strongly suggest that neutrophils are indeed significant contributors to hepatic failure following ischemia. Several possible mechanisms have been proposed to explain neutrophil-mediated tissue injury during reperfusion. These include plugging of capillaries (or sinusoids) [43] and damage to vascular endothelium resulting in permeability increase [41]. Our studies have shown that the magnitude of total white cell accumulation in the liver during reperfusion is approximately proportional to the overall loss of perfused sinusoid density [44]. These results are consistent with the notion of sinusoid plugging by neutrophils and, indeed, in viewing the liver microcirculation during reperfusion, white cells are periodically observed to stick in sinusoids and obstruct flow. However, this appears to be a relatively infrequent event and cannot account for the large number of sinusoids failing to conduct flow. The notion of neutrophil plugging as an important mechanism is further reflected by the fact that, when a spatial correlation analysis was performed between areas of white cell accumulation vs integrity of the microcirculation as indicated by the number of sinusoids conducting flow and by red blood cell velocity in the sinusuoids, little correlation was found [44]. With respect to the number of sinusoids conducting flow, the number of accumulated white cells were increased to an equal number in areas with flow vs areas without flow. In order to test whether neutrophil accumulation caused a graded flow reduction rather than an overt plugging, we measured red blood cell velocities in the sinusoids. When red blood cell velocity was plotted as a function of the number of white cells accumulated in a microscopic field there was no correlation in normal animals, which is to be expected from the overall low number of white cells found in the liver; however, inspite of the marked increase in the number of accumulated white cells following ischemia/reperfusion, only a relatively small correlation ($r = -0.4$) was found. Although this correlation was found to be statistically significant, it does not establish a strict cause and effect relationship between neutrophil accumulation and microvascular injury. However, it must be stressed that these correlations were done within the first 2 h of reperfusion and, thus, the portion of microvascular injury dependent upon accumulation of neutrophils in sinusoid areas may occur later in the reperfusion process. Further studies are needed to resolve this matter.

The work of Kubes et al. [45] in the intestinal microcirculation has emphasized the relationship between neutrophil adhesion to venular endothelium and increases in vascular permeability. If these results could be extrapolated to the liver, it would suggest that the early portion of microvascular injury may be the result of neutrophil adhesion to the endothelium of the terminal hepatic venules resulting in permeability changes. While this is an attractive comparison to make and fits very well with the biphasic accumulation of neutrophils first in the terminal hepatic venule followed by a much later accumulation in sinusoids, it may not be valid because of the vastly different permeability characteristics of the liver compared to the intestine. While the intestinal vessels are only very slightly permeable to colloids such as albumin, the fenestrated endothelium of the hepatic sinusoid is highly permeable to colloids [46]. As a result, even under normal conditions, the hepatic micro-circulation is more permeable to protein than are the intestinal microvessels during reperfusion. Thus the exact functional role of neutrophil adherence to venular endothelium in the liver during reperfusion, with respect to the genesis of hepatic injury, remains to be determined.

During low-flow ischemia to the liver, such as occurs during hemorrhagic shock, the role of neutrophil accumulation in the liver is less clear. Barroso-Aranda et al. [43] showed that neutrophils accumulate in increased numbers in capillaries of heart, kidney, pancreas, and skeletal muscle during a severe hemorrhagic shock model; this increase in tissue neutrophils correlated with the loss of perfused capillaries. Although these investigators did not specifically study the changes in liver, they did report in a subsequent study that the level of activation of circulating neutrophils, as indicated by the nitro blue tetrazolium test, was an excellent predictor of survival from hemorrhagic shock. These results would suggest that neutrophil activation is a generalized phenom-enon and may thus be expected to have an effect in the liver. The studies of Marzi et al. [47] and also preliminary studies in our laboratory, however, indicate that white cell kinetics in the liver during hemorrhagic shock are markedly different from that seen following no-flow ischemia. Most notably, the adherence of white cells to terminal hepatic venules which is markedly increased during reperfusion following no-flow ischemia is rarely observed during re-suscitation following hemorrhagic shock. There are two possible reasons for this discrepancy between no-flow ischemia and hemorrhagic shock. First, it is possible that adhesiveness is not increased during hemorrhagic shock to nearly the extent that it is following no-flow ischemia. This possibility seems relatively unlikely to fully explain these observations since both models impose a severe ischemic stress upon the liver and result in activation of circulating neutrophils. The other possible mechanism is related to the relative flow velocities and resultant shear stresses that occur in the terminal hepatic venules following no-flow vs low-flow ischemia. The recovery of blood flow during reperfusion following no-flow ischemia can best be described as a "slow-flow" phenomenon. As a result of the very low red cell flow velocities during the early stages of reperfusion, the shear stresses in the terminal hepatic venules are sufficiently low that a moderate increase in adhesiveness can overcome the dispersive forces resulting in adherence. In contrast, during resuscitation from hemorrhagic shock initial flow is extremely brisk resulting in markedly augmented dispersive forces on the neutrophils. Such an increase in wall shear rate produced by elevated red blood cell velocity has been shown to be an important modulator of CD18-dependent neutrophil adherence to venular endothelium in the cat mesentery [48]. Thus, even in the presence of moderately elevated adhesive forces exerted by increased expression of adhesion proteins on the surface of neutrophils and venular endothelium during resuscitation from hemorrhagic shock, the markedly elevated wall shear stress would be predicted to largely prevent adherence of neutrophils to the venules. This would suggest that even in the absence of demonstrable adherence of neutrophils to venular endothelium in the liver during resuscitation from hemorrhagic shock, significant activation of the neutrophils may occur (e.g., via interaction with activated Kupffer cells) followed by reentry of the activated neutrophil into the circulation. Such a scenario is consistent with the findings of Barroso-Aranda and Schmidt-Schönbein [49] that the level of activation of circulating neutrophils in the blood following hemorrhagic shock is an excellent indicator of the severity of shock and predictor of ultimate mortality.

The above-described kinetics of neutrophil adherence and activation in the liver following either no-flow or low-flow hepatic ischemia lead us to propose the following generalized sequence of events resulting in both local injury to the liver and remote effects which may contribute to multiple organ failure. This can be divided into an acute response and a chronic response. The acute response outlined in Fig. 1 is initiated by activation of Kupffer cells and vascular endothelium, especially that of the terminal hepatic venules during ischemia. Through elaboration of various mediators and expression of adhesion molecules, the Kupffer cells and vascular endothelium respectively interact with the neutrophils resulting in activation. Under relatively low shear conditions, such as occurs during reperfusion following no-flow ischemia, neutrophils adhere to the terminal hepatic venular endothelium resulting in local effects. Although the exact nature of these local effects in these vessels has not been elucidated, possibilities include injury to a vascular endothelium producing increased permeability [40], and release of vasoactive substances such as leukotriene D4 [24] or other prostanoids [22], which may cause constriction of post-sinusoidal sites of resistance. In contrast, under high-shear conditions such as occurs during resuscitation from hemorrhagic shock, while activation almost certainly occurs, little adherence has been demonstrated. In such a case the activated neutrophils reenter the circulation where they may exert toxic effects on remote organs, especially the lung. Such effects have been recently reported following hepatic [50] ischemia.

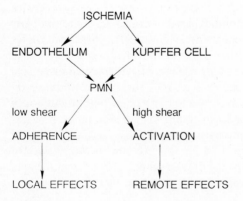

Fig. 1. Proposed schema for role of non-parenchymal cells in liver and remote organ injury during the early phase of reperfusion following hepatic ischemia or hemorrhagic shock. *PMN*, polymorphonuclear neutrophil leukocytes

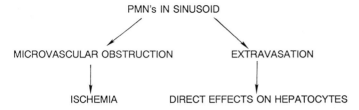

Fig. 2. Proposed schema for role of nonparenchymal cells, especially infiltrating neutrophils, in liver injury during the chronic phase of reperfusion. *PMN*, polymorphonuclear neutrophil leukocytes

The acute response which occurs almost immediately during reperfusion or resuscitation is followed by a chronic response which occurs over the course of 2–24 + h of reperfusion. During this chronic phase (Fig. 2), neutrophil adherence in sinusoids is observed followed by rapid extravasation into the perisinusoidal space [36]. During the period of adherence inside the lumen of the sinusoid, the neutrophils do obstruct flow. As a result further ischemia occurs to the hepatocytes fed by that sinusoid. However, in our videomicroscopy studies, this period of sinusoid obstruction is transient, and there is little evidence of obstruction of sinusoidal flow by neutrophils which have moved outside the sinusoidal lumen. The studies of Jaeschke et al. [37] have shown that treatment with a monoclonal antibody directed against rat neutrophils, in addition to preventing the late infiltration of neutrophils into the liver tissue, also markedly attenuate areas of hepatic necrosis. This would suggest that extravasated neutrophils during the chronic phase of infiltration might directly cause hepatocyte injury. It is not known, however, what effect these neutrophils infiltrating into sinusoidal areas during the chronic phase have on microvascular integrity late in reperfusion (> 2 h). Thus, it is still not possible to differentiate mechanistically between a direct hepatotoxic effect of infiltrating neutrophils vs an indirect effect via damage to the hepatic microcirculation followed by sustained ischemic effects on the hepatocytes.

In summary, considerable evidence suggests that the response of the intact liver to ischemia and reperfusion is considerably more complex than is anoxia reoxygenation injury in isolated hepatocytes. The additional mechanisms for hepatic injury in the intact liver are the result of the presence of nonparenchymal cells, particularly Kupffer cells and infiltrating neutrophils, that can exert hepatotoxic effects when activated during ischemia and reperfusion and the absolute dependence of the whole organ on intact microcirculation for its continued functioning. Moreover, the interaction between the parenchymal and nonparenchymal cells following ischemic stress may not only exacerbate hepatocyte injury but, via activation of neutrophils in transit through the liver, can contribute to multiple organ failure by providing a population of activated circulating neutrophils.

Acknowledgements. The author wishes to express his thanks to Mrs. Jackwalyn Beam for her assistance in the preparation of the manuscript and to Dr. George T. Drugas, Dr. Karen Chun, and Dr. Donald Jones for their comments on the manuscript.

References

1. Ratych RE, Chuknyiska RS, Bulkley GB (1987) The primary localization of free radical generation after anoxia/reoxygenation in isolated endothelial cells. Surgery 102:122–131
2. Jarasch ED, Bruder G, Heid HW (1986) Significance of xanthine oxidase in capillary endothelial cells. Acta Physiol Scand 548:39–46
3. Noll T, deGroot H, Wisseman P (1986) A computer-supported oxystat system maintaining steady-state O_2 partial pressures and simultaneously monitoring O_2 uptake in biological systems. Biochem J 236:765–769
4. DeGroot H, Littauer A (1989) Hypoxia, reactive oxygen, and cell injury. Free Radic Biol Med 6:541–551
5. Herman B, Nieminen A-L, Gores GJ, Lemasters JJ (1988) Irreversible injury in anoxic hepatocytes precipitated by an abrupt increase in plasma membrane permeability. FASEB J 2:146–151
6. Lemaster JJ, DiGuiseppi J, Nieminen A-L, Herman B (1987) Blebbing, free Ca^{2+} and mitochondrial membrane potential preceding cell death in hepatocytes. Nature 325:78–81
7. Koo A, Liang IYS (1977) Blood flow in hepatic sinusoids in experimental hemorrhagic shock in the rat. Microvasc Res 13:315–325
8. Lautt WW, McQuaker JE (1989) Maintenance of hepatic arterial blood flow during hemorrhage is mediated by adenosine. Can J Physiol Pharmacol 67:1023–1028
9. Pearce FJ, Drucker WR (1986) Relationship of portal flow and hepatic arterial flow to ATP content during hemorrhagic shock. Surg Forum 37:81–83
10. Chaudry IH, Sayeed MM, Baue AE (1974) Depletion and restoration of tissue ATP in hemorrhagic shock. Arch Surg 108:208
11. Jungermann K, Katz N (1989) Functional specialization of different hepatocyte populations. Physiol Rev 69:708–764
12. Marotto ME, Thurman RG, Lemasters JJ (1988) Early midzonal cell death during low-flow hypoxia in the isolated, perfused rat liver: protection by allopurinol. Hepatology 8: 585–590
13. Anundi I, deGroot H (1989) Hypoxic liver cell death: critical PO_2 and dependence of viability on glycolysis. Am J Physiol 257:G58–G64
14. Bradford BU, Marotto M, Lemasters JJ, Thurman RG (1986) New, simple models to evaluate zone-specific damage due to hypoxia in the perfused rat liver: time course and effect of nutritional state. J Pharmacol Exp Ther 236:263–268
15. Hirawasa H, Chaudry IH, Baue AE (1978) Improved hepatic function and survival with adenosine triphosphate-magnesium chloride after hepatic ischemia. Surgery 83:655–662
16. Gores GJ, Nieminen A-L, Fleishman KE, Dawson TL, Herman B, Lemaster JJ (1988) Extracellular acidosis delays onset of cell death in ATP-depleted hepatocytes. Am J Physiol 255:C315–C322
17. Clemens MG, McDonagh PF, Chaudry IH, Baue AE (1985) Hepatic microcirculatory failure following ischemia and reperfusion: improvement with ATP-$MgCl_2$ treatment. Am J Physiol H804–H811
18. Drugas GT, Paidas CN, Yahanda AM, Ferguson D, Clemens MG (1991) Conjugated desferoxamine attenuates hepatic microvascular injury following ischemia/reperfusion. Circ Shock (in Press)
19. Bouwens L, Geerts A, van Bossuyt H, Wisse E (1987) Recent insights into the function of hepatic sinusoidal cells. Neth J Med 31:129–148
20. Meszaros K, Bojta J, Bautista AP, Lang CH, Spitzer JJ (1991) Glucose utilization by Kupffer cells, endothelial cells, and granulocytes in endotoxemic rat liver. Am J Physiol 260:G7–G12
21. Jones EA, Summerfield JA (1988) Kupffer cells. In Arias IM, Popper H, Jakoby WB, Schachter D, Shafritz DA (eds) The liver. Biology and pathobiology, 2nd edn. Raven, New York, pp 683–704
22. Birmelin M, Decker K (1984) Synthesis of prostanoids and cyclic nucleotides by phagocytosing rat Kupffer cells. Eur J Biochem 142:219–225
23. Dieter P, Schulze-Specking A, Decker K (1986) Differential inhibition of prostaglandin and superoxide production by dexamethasone in primary cultures of rat Kupffer cells. Eur J Biochem 159:451–457
24. Ouwendyk RJTH, Zijlstra FJ, van der Broek AMWC, Brouwer A, Wilson JHP, Vincent JE (1988) Comparison of the production of eicosanoids by human and rat peritoneal macrophages and rat Kupffer cells. Prostaglandins 35:437–446

25. Braciak TA, Gauldie J, Fey GH, Northemann W (1991) The expression of interleukin-6 by a rat macrophage-derived cell line. FEBS Lett 280:277–280
26. Dieter P, Altin JG, Decker K, Bygrave FL (1987) Possible involvement of eicosanoids in the zymosan and arachidonic-acid-induced oxygen uptake, glycogenolysis and Ca^{2+} mobilization in the perfused rat liver. Eur J Biochem 165:455–460
27. Buxton DB, Fisher RA, Briseno DL, Hanahan DJ, Olson MS (1987) Glycogenolytic and haemodynamic responses to heat-aggregated immunoglobulin G and prostaglandin E_2 in the perfused rat liver. Biochem J 243:493–498
28. West MA, Keller GA, Hyland BJ, Cerra FB, Simmons RL (1986) Further characterization of Kupffer cell/macrophage-mediated alterations in hepatocyte protein synthesis. Surgery 100:416–423
29. Dieter P, Altin JG, Bygrave FL (1987) Possible involvement of prostaglandins in vasoconstriction induced by zymosan and arachidonic acid in the perfused rat liver. FEBS Lett 213:174–178
30. McCuskey RS, Urbaschek R, McCuskey PA, Urbaschek B (1983) In vivo microscopic observations of the responses of Kupffer cells and the hepatic microcirculation to mycobacterium bovis BCG alone and in combination with endotoxin. Infect Immunol 142:362–368
31. Jaeschke H, Farhood A (1991) Neutrophil and Kupffer cell-induced oxidant stress and ischemia-reperfusion injury in rat liver. Am J Physiol 260:G355–G362
32. Kobayashi S, Clemens MG (1989) Exacerbation of hepatocyte reoxygenation injury by Kupffer cells. FASEB J 1:A711
33. Kobayashi S, Clemens MG (1989) Role of free radicals in Kupffer cell exacerbation of hepatocyte reoxygenation injury. Circ Shock 98:331–332
34. Ayala A, Perrin MM, Chaudry IH (1990) Increased susceptibility to sepsis following hemorrhage: defective Kupffer cell-midiated antigen presentation. Surg Forum 40:102
35. Ayala A, Perrin MM, Wang P, Ertel W, Chaudry IH (1991) Enhanced Kupffer cell cytotoxic activity following hemorrhage: a potential cause of hepatocellular injury. (this volume)
36. Clemens MG, Paidas C, Wright J, McDonagh P (1989) Lack of evidence for leukocyte plugging of liver microvessels during reperfusion following ischemia. FASEB J 2:A1382
37. Jaeschke H, Farhood A, Smith CW (1990) Neutrophils contribute to ischemia/reperfusion injury in rat liver in vivo. FASEB J 4:3355–3359
38. Takei Y, Marzi I, Gao W, Gores GJ, Lemasters JJ, Thurman RG (1991) Leukocyte adhesion and cell death following orthotopic liver transplantation in the rat. Transplantation 51:959–965
39. Miescher E, Drugas GT, Biewer J, Clemens MG (1990) Distribution of white blood cell accumulation in rat liver during post-ischemic reperfusion. Circ Shock 31:79
40. Harlan JM (1987) Neutrophil-mediated vascular injury. Acta Med Scand 715:123–129
41. Hernandez LA, Grisham MB, Twohig B, Arfors KE, Harlan JM, Granger DN (1987) Role of neutrophils in ischemia-reperfusion-induced microvascular injury. Am J Physiol 253:H699–H703
42. Clemens MG, McDonagh PF, Reynolds JM (1986) Leukocyte/platelet dependence of ischemia-induced hepatic microvascular damage. Fed Proc 46:1524
43. Barroso-Aranda J, Schmidt-Schönbein GW, Zweifach BW, Engler RL (1988) Granulocytes and no reflow phenomenon in irreversible hemorrhagic shock. Circ Res 63:437–447
44. Ferguson D, Biewer J, Clemens MG (1990) Spatial correlation between leukocyte accumulation and red cell velocity during reperfusion after hepatic ischemia. FASEB J:A1251
45. Kubes P, Suzuki M, Granger DN (1990) Modulation of PAF-induced leukocyte adherence and increased microvascular permeability. Am J Physiol 259:G859–G864
46. Stock RJ, Cilento EV, McCuskey RS (1989) A quantitative study of fluorescein isothiocyanate-dextran transport in the microcirculation of the isolated perfused rat liver. Hepatology 9:75–82
47. Marzi I, Bauer C, Hower R, Menger M, Trentz O, Bühren V (1991) Deleterious effect of dexamethansone on hepatic microcirculation and leukocyte–endothelial interaction in hemorrhagic shock. (this volume)
48. Perry MA, Granger DN (1991) Role of CD11/CD18 in shear rate-dependent leukocyte-endothelial cell interaction in cat mesenteric venules. J Clin Invest 87:1798–1804
49. Barroso-Aranda J, Schmidt-Schönbein GW (1989) Transformation of neutrophils as indicator of irreversibility in hemorrhagic shock. Am J Physiol 257:H846–H852
50. Colletti LM, Burtch GD, Remick DG, Kunkel SL, Strieter RM, Guice KS, Oldham KT, Campbell DA Jr (1990) The production of tumor necrosis factor alpha and the development of a pulmonary capillary injury following hepatic ischemia/reperfusion. Transplantation 49:268–272

Acute Lung Injury Following Shock and Major Trauma

G. Schlag and H. Redl

Introduction

Acute respiratory failure has been described as a complex sequence of clinical events that eventually result in massive lung injury [1–3]. Acute respiratory failure progresses in several stages that are detectable by light and electron microscopy, leading from a reversible (early stage of "organ in shock" within hours) to an irreversible stage (from the early organ failure lung to the late organ failure, the typical adult respiratory distress syndrome—ARDS).

The sequence of acute lung failure associated with trauma depends on the type of injury, i.e., whether lung injury is direct or indirect.

Direct Lung Injury

A typical example of direct injury is lung contusion, the result of blunt thorax trauma with or without rib fractures. The prevalent morphologic manifestations are interstitial edema and hemorrhage, including the intraalveolar space, secondary to damage of pulmonary capillaries. There is fast sequestration of polymorphonuclear neutrophils (PMN) into the capillaries of the alveolar septa as a consequence of increased chemotaxis of PMN. This results in a localized inflammatory process quite similar to the indirect damage caused by PMN in shock. Edema and hemorrhage produce a collapse of the terminal airways in the form of microatelectasis and atelectasis. Bronchoscopy reveals hemorrhage in the large bronchi within minutes after trauma.

A major symptom associated with contusion is posttraumatic hypoxemia [4], leading to the rapid appearance of interstitial and intraalveolar hemorrhage and to edema formation. As a consequence of edema and hemorrhage the functional residual capacity (FRC) decreases; this in turn decreases the closing volume and blocks the terminal airways in association with a peripheral collapse of the alveoli. The shunt volume increases due to the ventilation/perfusion imbalance and results in hypoxemia, which may appear very rapidly.

Ludwig Boltzmann Institute for Experimental and Clinical Traumatology, Donaueschingenstr 13, 1200 Vienna, Austria

Host Defense Dysfunction
in Trauma, Shock and Sepsis
Eds. Faist/Meakins/Schildberg
© Springer-Verlag, Berlin Heidelberg 1993

This may be paralleled by an increase of pulmonary vascular resistance (PVR) due to reflectory vascular constriction in the pulmonary arteries with simultaneous decrease of the "compliance" (C), which is partly due to the rapid development of interstitial edema as well as hemorrhage in the presence of large contusion areas. The subsequent ventilation/perfusion disturbances (V/Q) may be caused by hypoventilation, by destruction of the surfactant in the alveolar region as a consequence of flooding with blood and fibrin together with the formation of massive atelectasis. This, in turn, gives rise to further ventilation/perfusion disturbances and thus creates the prerequisite for hypoxemia, which characterizes the clinical picture of severe lung contusion.

Lung contusion may lead to bacterial infection of the lung, which may seriously impair the clearance function, especially in the posttraumatic course, and is thus of decisive importance for the patient's prognosis (development of multiple organ failure, MOF).

The combination of traumatic shock and lung contusion causes a marked decrease of the clearance function [5], and pneumonia may be the result. In this setting, the indirect lung damage due to leukostasis of the lung with release of tissue-toxic mediators plays and important pathogenetic role.

The combination of contusion and traumatic shock may rapidly (within 24 h) transform the "organ in shock" into the "early organ failure lung." In this case, direct trauma is aggravated by the generalized nonbacterial inflammation.

Regel et al. [6] found that in their patient collective lung contusion was associated with a high incidence of subsequent ARDS (4 of 8 patients versus 1 of 8 patients without lung contusion). ARDS as a late organ failure appears as a frequent complication of lung contusions (59%). Putensen et al. [7] observed direct lung damage secondary to contusion in 77% of trauma patients with acute lung failure.

According to Putensen et al. [7], direct lung damage seems to be the predominant mechanism activating the early manifestation (< 72 h) of posttraumatic acute lung failure, which in our terminology either corresponds to the early organ failure lung or may already appear as typical ARDS (late organ failure) in the presence of infection (Fig. 1).

In addition, direct lung damage includes the consequences of aspiration and inhalation damage sustained during burns. Aspiration and inhalation damage primarily involves not only the proximal branches of the tracheobronchial tree but also the alveolar area (especially in aspiration injury), and thus the gas exchange surface directly [8].

We have studied aspiration trauma in an experimental setting in rabbits by intratracheal administration of a betaine hydrochloride pepsin. In this model we could demonstrate the alveolar damage histologically and by static compliance measurement. The compliance had already significantly deteriorated 6 h after injury [9].

Inhalation damage is often associated with early pulmonary edema resulting in severe ARDS [10–12].

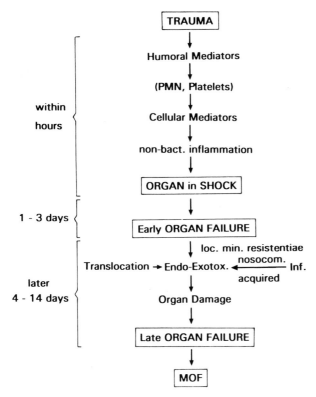

Fig. 1. Mechanisms leading to posttraumatic organ failure (*MOF*, multiple organ failure)

These types of direct lung damage may occur very early and may eventually lead to the early organ failure lung, irrespective of a traumatic shock event. This early organ damage lung constitutes a specific place of least resistance towards an infectious component (bacteremia, endotoxemia), which may very rapidly give rise to late (septic) organ failure, the typical ARDS.

Mutz et al. [13] have published very interesting data on this aspect. They measured extravascular lung water (EVLW) and observed that patients with severe multiple trauma and concomitant thoracic trauma revealed a typical biphasic course of extravascular lung water data on days 3 and 7 posttrauma, while the EVLW was in the pathological range for 10 days during the entire observation period. The EVLW increase on day 3 corresponds to the typical early organ failure lung, which is in a morphologically reversible stage. The EVLW data remain in the pathological range and continue to demonstrate maximum tissue damage, especially in the late stage of a septic event. In this case there is a second rise of the EVLW, which is commonly seen 7–10 days posttrauma.

Indirect Lung Injury

Indirect lung damage is related to the different effects of a multitude of mediators released via activation of humoral and cellular systems. These activation processes take place during trauma and include fat embolism caused by large bone fractures in the immediate posttraumatic course.

Soft tissue trauma associated with polytrauma as well as intraoperative events rapidly trigger activation of the complement and coagulation systems. Smashed muscle tissue and ischemic tissue cause massive complement activation, resulting in elevated levels of the important anaphylatoxins C3a and C5a. The pathogenesis of acute respiratory failure and the role of anaphylatoxins (C3a, C5a) is still controversial [14, 15]. Nuytinck [16] has demonstrated that a hypoxic component with complement activation induces a syndrome similar to the early phase of lung failure. In polytraumatized patients a hypoxic component may often be encountered.

Trauma results in an activation of the coagulation cascade via the exogenous and endogenous pathways. Activation via the release of thromboplastin caused by trauma and intravasation of bone marrow and fat globuli results in thrombin activation and excess thrombin formation, expressed by fibrin formation (e.g., fibrin monomers). Fibrin monomers may impair surfactant function.

The activation products of these humoral systems play an important role in the activation of the cellular systems, such as platelets and PMN.

In previous lung biopsies performed in polytraumatized patients there was repeated evidence of fat in the alveolar capillaries. We feel that fat plays no major role, except for its mechanical effects such as blockade of the capillaries. Bosch et al. [17] found intracellular fat in 91% of 80 patients, mostly in the macrophages, already 9 h after trauma. In our own lung biopsies performed 24 h after trauma we also noted fat in the alveolar space and in the alveolar macrophages. Hypothetically, intraalveolar fat could play a role in the activation of macrophages. The earlier fat appears in the alveolar space, the earlier the activation process of the macrophages may start. We may thus conclude that intraalveolar fat plays a role in the pathogenetic course.

As a result of complement activation and anaphylatoxin formation (C3a, C5a), activation of PMN is observed. Activated PMN sequestrate and marginate in the venules of the microcirculation of the lung. In addition, platelets may play a role in the vascular microaggregation process. Platelets may interact with PMN, resulting in PMN aggregation [18].

Leukostasis of the lung, which is observed within hours, constitutes the substrate for the early organ failure lung, also referred to as "organ in shock," as the consequence of nonbacterial inflammation. Leukostasis in the lung is the morphological hallmark of shock and is always associated with severe PMN degranulation. Leukostasis was determined quantitatively by using ^{111}In-oxine-labeled neutrophils in animals (dogs) [19] and in humans with a special esterase staining method for morphometric evaluation. Patients ($n = 6$) who died within

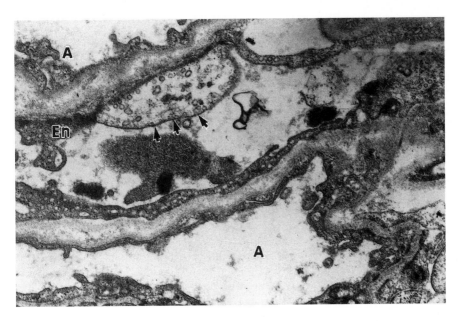

Fig. 2. Typical focal endothelial (*En*) swelling (*arrows*) in a lung capillary after polytrauma (A, alveoli)

48 h after polytrauma showed 8% ± 2.3% of the alveolar septa filled with PMN, compared with 2.4% ± 0.9% in controls ($p < 0.001$) [20]. These autopsies were performed in patients who died within 48 h after trauma without evidence of direct lung damage.

The endothelial cell (EC)—especially in the lung—is a major target in shock and thus represents the substrate for generalized tissue damage (Fig. 2).

In traumatic shock the EC are involved in PMN adherence, synthesis of eicosanoids and the platelet activating factor (PAF), and lipid peroxidation, and contribute to the permeability increase, which leads to perivascular and later to interstitial edema.

The prerequisite for EC damage by activated PMN is their adherence to the endothelial cell. An increased adherence, in turn, is probably the prerequisite for the release of tissue-damaging mediators from PMN and for PMN migration. In traumatic shock adherence appears to be due to a neutrophil-dependent mechanism. With direct PMN stimulation, e.g., complement fragments, this neutrophil-dependent mechanism may be activated, while the expression of adherence proteins takes place within minutes. We may depart from the assumption that the EC at that time (within 1 h) have not yet been activated.

The CD11/CD18 molecules are able to mediate transient adhesion of PMN to EC in vivo [21]. Vedder et al. [22] have attempted to block the neutrophil adherence function by monoclonal antibodies (MAb 60.3) directed to the adherence glycoproteins CD18. They were able to preclude organ injury in hemorrhagic shock (as compared to controls) without any lung involvement. The damage encountered was similar to the damage seen in control animals. These results suggest either an alternative ligand on the CD11/18 complex or a different molecule for PMN adherence in the lung.

The assumption that EC have not yet been stimulated at an early stage of shock was also suggested by the fact that expression of the endothelial leukocyte adhesion molecule-1 (ELAM-1) could not be confirmed by immunohistochemistry, while in animals (baboon) with septic shock there was widespread expression of ELAM-1 in various organ systems. At this early stage we may assume that translocation of bacteria/endotoxin via the gut, which eventually triggers cytokine release and thus contributes to EC activation, has not yet taken place.

ELAM-1 expression is commonly detectable after 3–6 h. During this period we were able to demonstrate the incipient extravasation of PMN into the interstitium of the lung by way of electron microscopic sections. Degranulation of PMN in the lung capillaries, a morphological proof of PMN activation, may be detected very early.

Oxygen products that appear within the first stage (up to 4 h) are mainly responsible for damage to the EC per se, while proteases appear to contribute insignificantly to the early phase of injury [23].

PMN extravasation (migration) may occur either via the junctions of the EC or via the EC directly (Fig. 3). In the interstitium of the lung there may be further degranulation and thus release of mediators (protease, collagenase). At this point in time it is unclear if the PMN play a role in the fibrogenetic process. More likely, there is a platelet–fibroblast interaction with the release of the platelet-derived growth factor (PDGF) via activation of intrapulmonary platelets [24]. We know that interstitial fibrosis in the lung may occur very early (within a week) [25, 26]. Interstitial fibrosis is frequently associated with intraalveolar fibrosis, which commonly becomes manifest in the second week and is responsible for the impairment of gas exchange.

In the further course of events associated with indirect lung damage (1–3 days posttrauma) the alveolar space is also affected. Before this, the events are predominantly due to nonbacterial inflammation. The alveolar space demonstrates a shift of the intraalveolar cells in favor of PMN versus macrophages at a very early stage, i.e. up to 50% neutrophils in the first 2 days versus a decrease in the macrophage count [27]. This invasion of the alveolar space by PMN in the first 2–3 days can be explained by a chemotactic gradient. Parsons et al. [28] have investigated the lavage fluid of lungs affected by ARDS and have noted marked accumulation of PMN (up to 85%) as well as two chemotactic factors. Alveolar macrophages produce chemotactic factors for PMN, such as leukotriene B_4 (LTB_4), IL-8, and other peptides. The activation of macrophages commonly occurs in the later course of events, i.e., when infection (bacteremia, endotoxemia) becomes manifest.

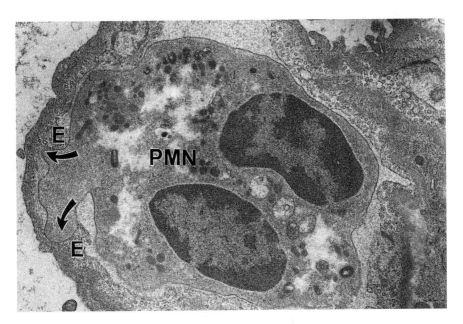

Fig. 3. A granulocyte (PMN) is starting to migrate (*arrows*) in between two endothelial cells (*E*) of a lung capillary.

Joka et al. [29] have encountered complement split products (C3a) in the lavage fluid of patients without direct lung damage within the first few hours after trauma. These complement split products may be released secondary to activation of macrophages, in the same way as other substances that may rapidly transport neutrophils into the alveolar space and/or into the interstitium of the lung via the chemotactic route. The activation of macrophages immediately after trauma could be related to hypoxic periods during trauma.

The mechanisms of PMN migration and extravasation are highly complex, on the one hand, as already stated, due to chemotactic factors, without any infectious stimulus, and on the other hand by specific macrophage activation via, for example endotoxin. The latter, however, appears to become manifest only in connection with the early organ failure lung. This stage of early organ failure is a place of least resistance for infection. The infection may either be preexistent, acquired (wound infection, peritonitis, nosocomial infection), or occur in association with generalized endotoxemia or bacteremia via gut translocation. The trigger mediators in this stage are endotoxin and/or bacterial wall products, which further activate humoral cellular systems that release numerous toxic mediators (eicosanoids, PAF, free oxygen radicals, proteinases, cytokines, procoagulative substances, etc.) from, for example, PMN, EC, monocytes–macrophages, platelets, and mast cells. This causes further tissue damage, which may lead to massive organ damage and thus to the late (or septic) organ failure lung (typical ARDS).

This presentation addresses only the early stages of the organ damage lung via the "organ in shock" and early organ failure, excluding late damage sustained during septic or septiform events.

References

1. Ashbaugh DG, Bigelow DB, Petty TL (1967) Acute respiratory distress in adults. Lancet 2:319–323
2. Schlag G, Regele H (1972) Lungenbiopsien bei hypovolämisch-traumatischem Schock. Med Welt 23:1755–1758
3. Andreadis N, Petty TL (1985) Adult respiratory distress syndrome: problems and progress. Am Rev Respir Dis 132:1344–1346
4. Buchinger W, Schlag G, Redl H, Thurnher M (1990) Tierexperimentelle Untersuchungen zum Ablauf der Lungenkontusion. Hefte Unfallheilkd (in press)
5. Richardson JD, Woods D, Johanson WG Jr, Trinkle JK (1979) Lung bacterial clearance following pulmonary contusion. Surgery 86:730–735
6. Regel G, Sturm, JA, Friedl HP, Nerlich M, Bosch U, Tscherne H (1988) Die Bedeutung der Lungenkontusion für die Letalität nach Polytrauma. Möglichkeiten der therapeutischen Beeinflussung. Chirurg 59:771–776
7. Putensen C, Waibel U, Koller W, Putensen-Himmer G, Beck E, Benzer H (1990) Das akute Lungenversagen nach Thoraxtrauma. Anaesthesist 39:530–534
8. Glause FL, Millen JE, Falls R (1979) Increased alveolar epithelial permeability with acid aspiration: the effects of high dose steroids. Am Rev Respir Dis 120:1110–1123
9. Strohmaier W, Redl H, Schlag G (1990) Studies of the potential role of a semisynthetic surfactant preparation in an experimental aspiration trauma in rabbits. Exp Lung Res 16:101–110
10. Tranbaugh RF, Elings VB, Christensen JM, Lewis FR (1983) Effect of inhalation injury on lung water accumulation. J Trauma 23:597–604
11. Herndon DN, Traber DL, Niehaus GD, Linares HA, Traber LD (1984) The pathophysiology of smoke inhalation injury in a sheep model. J Trauma 24:1044–1051
12. Traber DL, Schlag G, Redl H, Traber LD (1985) Pulmonary edema and compliance changes following smoke inhalation. J Burn Care Res 6:490–494
13. Mutz N, Neumann M, Hörmann C, Koller W, Putensen C, Putz G, Benzer H (1990) Verlauf des extravaskulären Lungenwassers (EVLW) bei schwerverletzten Intensivpatienten mit und ohne Thoraxtrauma. Anaesthesist 39:535–539
14. Maunder RJ (1985) Clinical prediction of the adult respiratory distress syndrome. Clin Chest Med 6:413–426
15. Solomkin JS, Cotta LA, Satoh PS, Hurst JM, Nelson RD (1985) Complement activation and clearance in acute illness and injury; evidence of C5a as a cell directed mediator of the adult respiratory distress syndrome in man. Surgery 97:668–678
16. Nuytinck JKS (1985) The adult respiratory distress syndrome and multiple organ failure. The role of complement activation and granulocytes. Thesis, Catholic University of Nijmegen
17. Bosch U, Reisser S, Regel G, Windus G, Kleemann WJ, Nerlich ML (1989) Pulmonary fat embolism – an epiphenomenon of shock or a proper mediator mechanism? 701–706
18. Redl H, Hammerschmidt DE, Schlag G (1983) Augmentation by platelets of granulocyte aggregation in response to chemotaxins: studies utilizing an improved cell preparation technique. Blood 61:125–131
19. Schlag G, Redl H (1985) Morphology of the microvascular system in shock: lung, liver and skeletal muscles. Crit Care Med 13:1045–1049
20. Redl H, Dinges HP, Schlag G (1987) Quantitative estimation of leukostasis in the posttraumatic lung-canine and human autopsy. 165–173
21. Lo SK, Detmers PA, Levin SM, Wright SD (1989) Transient adhesion of neutrophils to endothelium. J Exp Med 169:1779–1793
22. Vedder NB, Fouty BW, Winn RK, Harlan JM, Rice CL (1989) Role of neutrophils in generalized reperfusion injury associated with resuscitation from shock. Surgery 106:509–516

23. Varani J, Ginsburg I, Schuger L, Gibbs DF, Bromberg J, Johnson KJ, Ryan US, Ward PA (1989) Endothelial cell killing by neutrophils. Synergistic interaction of oxygen products and proteases. Am J Pathol 135:435–438
24. Heffner JE, Sahn SA, Repine JE (1987) The role of platelets in the adult respiratory distress syndrome. Culprits or bystanders? Am Rev Respir Dis 135:482–492
25. Hassenstein J, Riede UN, Mittermayer C, Sandritter W (1980) Zur Frage der Reversibilität der schockinduzierten Lungenfibrose. Anaesth Intensivther Notfallmed 15:340–349
26. Auler JOC Jr, Calheiros DF, Brentani MM, Santello JL, Lemos PCP, Saldiva PHN (1986) Adult respiratory distress syndrome: evidence of early fibrogenesis and absence of glucocorticoid receptors. Eur J Respir Dis 69:261–269
27. Pison U, Brand M, Joka T, Obertacke U, Bruch J (1988) Distribution and function of alveolar cells in multiply injured patients with trauma induced ARDS. Intensive Care Med 14:602–609
28. Parsons PE, Fowler AA, Hyers TM, Henson PM (1985) Chemotactic activity in bronchoalveolar lavage fluid from patients with adult respiratory distress syndrome. Am Rev Respir Dis 132:490–493
29. Joka T, Obertacke U, Sturm J, Jochum M, Kirschfink M, Schramm W, Dwenger A, Bartels H (1990) Startreaktionen des traumatischen Schocks: zelluläre Reaktionen. Hefte Unfallheilkd 212:45–53

Hemorrhage-Induced Alterations in Cell-Mediated Immune Function

I. H. Chaudry[1,2], A. Ayala[1,3], D. Meldrum[1], and W. Ertel[1]

Introduction

Hemorrhage resulting from trauma is a major problem facing many clinicians on a daily basis, and the resulting sepsis and multiple organ failure [1–6] is responsible for 60% of the deaths in the surgical intensive care units [7]. Although the improved resuscitation of such patients has resulted in increased short-term survival, the fact remains that late septic complications continue to prevail [2]. It is encouraging, however, that the complex pathophysiology of hemorrhagic shock is becoming better understood as more studies are being reported [8–15]. Through such studies, information might be forthcoming that would lead to the better management of trauma victims.

A large number of investigators have examined and continue to examine the effects of various forms of trauma on the immune system [16–23]; the current details of those are provided elsewhere in this book. The primary emphasis of this article, therefore, will not be to describe the immune consequences of trauma per se, but to examine the alterations in cell-mediated immunity which occur following simple hemorrhage and hemorrhagic shock. In addition, since trauma victims are usually resuscitated with blood and/or fluids, we will also discuss whether the immunological abnormalities following hemorrhage can be corrected by fluid resuscitation alone, or whether additional measures, such as pharmacological interventions, are needed following severe hemorrhage.

Hemorrhage is a prevalent complication in trauma victims arising from soft-tissue and bone injuries causing life-threatening blood loss. Hemorrhage is also frequently encountered during complex surgical procedures. Since there exists a close temporal relationship between hemorrhage and other injuries, such as soft-tissue destruction, this frequent association makes it difficult to dissociate the ef whether additional measures, such as pharmacological interventions, are needed following severe hemorrhage.

Hemorrhage is a prevalent complication in trauma victims arising from soft-tissue and bone injuries causing life-threatening blood loss. Hemorrhage is also frequently encountered during complex surgical procedures. Since there exists a

[1] Shock and Trauma Research Laboratories, Department of Surgery, Michigan State University, East Lansing, MI 48824, USA
[2] Department of Physiology, Michigan State University, East Lansing, MI 48824 USA
[3] Department of Microbiology, Michigan State University, East Lansing, MI 48824, USA

Host Defense Dysfunction
in Trauma, Shock and Sepsis
Eds. Faist/Meakins/Schildberg
© Springer-Verlag, Berlin Heidelberg 1993

close temporal relationship between hemorrhage and other injuries, such as soft-tissue destruction, this frequent association makes it difficult to dissociate the effects of pure hemorrhage on immunity in a clinical setting. Thus, there is a need to utilize experimental models in other mammals which allow an in-depth evaluation of the effects of simple hemorrhage on the immune function in the absence of the above complications. In this regard, although various species have been used, the immune function in rodents, particularly rats and mice, has been more extensively studied.

Effect of Hemorrhage on Lymphocytes and Lymphokines

Using a rat model, Abraham and Chang [24] found that after a fixed 30% withdrawal of total blood volume, mitogen-induced proliferation of blood lymphocytes were depressed as early as 30 min, but returned to normal by 48 h posthemorrhage. Additional studies indicated that interleukin-2 (IL-2) production by peripheral blood lymphocytes of rats was reduced by greater than 90% 2 h after blood loss; however, it was 50% normal on day 1 and it returned to normal 48 h after hemorrhage [24]. In this regard, it should be pointed out that the secretion of IL-2, primarily by T-cells, plays an important role in the activation of both helper and cytotoxic T cells following the activation by antigen [25]. Although these studies indicate that the loss of 30% of intravascular blood volume produces a marked defect in peripheral blood lymphocyte proliferation and the capacity to produce IL-2 remains depressed for at least 24 h after the insult, the fact remains that the hemorrhaged animals were not resuscitated with fluids following hemorrhage. Thus, it remained unknown whether this depression would persist after resuscitation. Moreover, the lack of well-defined immunological assays and agents for rats limit the depth to which the effects of hemorrhage on the immune function can be examined in this species. Because of these limitations at present, it would be advantageous to use a mouse model of hemorrhage, since standardized immunological assays using lymphoid cell lines for mice are more readily available than for the rat. Thus, the use of a mouse hemorrhage model would allow an in-depth evaluation of different aspects of immunological function in a systematic and reliable manner.

We have developed and used a mouse (C3H/HeN, endotoxin sensitive and CeH/HeJ, endotoxin tolerant, ∼ 20 g body wt) model of hemorrhagic shock and resuscitation which is nonlethal in nature [26–29]. Using this model, our results indicate that the proliferative responses of spleen cells to concanavalin A stimulation was markedly impaired on day 1 posthemorrhage. A slow and steady increase, however, was observed on subsequent days and the responses returned to normal by day 10 after hemorrhage and resuscitation [26]. More recent studies not only confirm the earlier data that IL-2 production is depressed after hemorrhage [30], but were extended to include depressed IL-3, IL-6, and interferon-γ (IFN-γ) production by splenocytes [31]. It should be pointed out that the depression of IL-3 has a direct effect on a variety of different cellular components involved in cell-mediated immunity, including the recruitment and maturation of a variety of immune cell types, (i.e., monocytes, T cells, thymocytes, etc.). Since IL-6 plays an important role in B-Cell activation, the depression in this lymphokine may have important implications for the development of a competent humoral response. In this regard, studies have indeed indicated that B-cell responsiveness is depressed after hemorrhage [32]. Moreover, the changes in IL-6 production may also have an effect on inflammatory responses associated with hemorrhage. Similarly, the marked decline in the capacity of T cells to elaborate IFN-γ after hemorrhage would be expected to lead to the impairment of macrophage activation [33], activation of cytotoxic T cells, as well as natural killer cell function [34]. Studies have, in fact, indicated that processes, such as macrophage major histocompatibility complex (MHC) class II expression [28], as well as natural killer cell function [35], are significantly depressed after hemorrhage. Livingston et al. [36] have shown that after trauma in humans, there is a significant drop in IFN-γ production by peripheral blood mononuclear cells. The decrease in IFN-γ production, therefore, appears to be an important event in the development of immune dysfunction associated with hemorrhage. These studies, taken together, would suggest that both cellular and humoral immunity is compromised after hemorrhage and resuscitation.

Effect of Hemorrhage on Splenic and Peritoneal Macrophage Functions

One of the important functions of the macrophage is its ability to activate resting T-cell lymphocytes by the processing and presentation of foreign antigens in an MHC class II (Ia)-restricted fashion. In order to perform this function, the macrophage must not only process and present the antigen, but also elaborate the appropriate costimulatory cytokines, such as IL-1, IL-6, and tumor necrosis factor (TNF), etc. [37–39]. In response to these interactions, the T-helper lymphocyte undergoes a series of events that induce clonal differentiation and elaboration of a variety of lymphokines, which provide T-cell "help" to both T-cell antibody response and various cell-mediated responses. This function of the macrophage, i.e., antigen presentation, is therefore critical in the stimulation of competent T-cell-mediated immune responses. The capacity of macrophages to present antigen was determined by assessing the macrophages' ability to present antigen, (e.g., conalbumin), to an antigen-reactive cloned T-helper cell line (D1O.G4.1) which responds by proliferation [40].

Our results demonstrated that antigen presentation by peritoneal macrophages and splenic adherent cells from hemorrhaged animals was markedly depressed immediately after hemorrhage and resuscitation [41]. Additional studies by Ayala et al. [28] indicated that a minimal drop in blood pressure to ~ 50 mm Hg for 1 h was sufficient to depress macrophage antigen presentation. Moreover, studies indicated that even a transient hypotensive episode of 15 min duration at 35 mm Hg was enough to produce a pronounced decline in antigen presentation [28]. The results also indicated that the depressed antigen presentation, while seen immediately after hemorrhage and resuscitation, remained detectable for at least 120 h thereafter. The process of defective antigen-presenting capability may be due to derangement in the Ia expression on the surface of the macrophage and may lead to the depressed macrophage function [27]. In this regard, studies using fluorescence-conjugated anti-Ia antisera indicated a significant decrease in the percentages of Ia-antigen positive cells after hemorrhage. This finding leads to the suggestion that the reduced antigen presentation after hemorrhage may be associated with the inability of these cells to express Ia [27]. Studies have also demonstrated that the depression in antigen presentation after hemorrhage and resuscitation was not due to changes in the capacity of these cells to either produce and/or express costimulatory cytokines such as IL-1 or membrane bound IL-1 [26]. However, more recent studies have indicated that hemorrhage-induced suppression of antigen presentation is not due to a reduced macrophage capacity to associate antigenic peptides with the MHC class II molecules, but to decreased antigen lysosomal catabolism by macrophages [42]. Since macrophage functions are depressed after trauma [43–45], it could be postulated that if significant blood loss is coupled with tissue injury, then a more pronounced depression in macrophage function would be expected to occur.

Kupffer Cell-Mediated Antigen Presentation and Cytokine Release

Kupffer cells, by virtue of their anatomical location in the mainstream of the splanchnic blood flow, are strategically positioned to have a constant exposure to antigens and potentially immunomodulating agents [46]. Their function consists of phagocytosis, clearing of toxins, and processing of enterically derived antigens [47]. Recently, however, the Kupffer cells have received increased attention as a macrophage which plays an important role in the development of antigen-specific immunity [48–49]. Studies have indeed shown that Kupffer cell antigen presentation is depressed after hemorrhage and remains depressed for 3–5 days despite adequate resuscitation [50]. The results also indicated that the depression in Kupffer cell antigen presentation was associated with the loss of MHC class II (Ia) antigens [51]. Since peritoneal, splenic, as well as Kupffer cell, antigen presentation was depressed after hemorrhage and resuscitation, it could be concluded that the depression of antigen presentation is of a global nature. Of interest to note is that, although macrophage (splenic, peritoneal, and Kupffer cell) antigen presentation was depressed after hemorrhage, Kupffer cells, but not the other two macrophage populations, exhibited an increased capacity to release inflammatory cytokines, IL-1, IL-6, and TNF-α [50, 51]. Although the reason for the increased cytokine production by Kupffer cells is unclear at present, it is possible that bacterial translocation across the gut [12, 14] and its delivery to the liver via the portal system is responsible for the enhanced cytokine production by the Kupffer cells.

   More recent studies from our laboratory have shown that Kupffer cells from hemorrhaged animals exhibited enhanced cytotoxicity, as opposed to reduced cytotoxicity by peritoneal macrophages [52]. This correlates well with studies which demonstrated that the Kupffer cells' capacity to release inflammatory cytokines is increased following hemorrhage [51]. In the light of these observations, it could be speculated that while the enhanced Kupffer cell cytotoxicity may be beneficial in the destruction of pathogens seen in the liver due to bacterial translocation, this same activity may also contribute directly or indirectly to hepatocellular dysfunction following hemorrhagic shock [53]. Thus, the enhanced inflammatory cytokine production by Kupffer cells implies that these cells play an important role in initiating various alterations in cell and organ function and may contribute to the host's enhanced mortality in the face of a septic challenge after hemorrhage and resuscitation [26].

Potential Causes of Immunodepression

A number of elegant studies have clearly demonstrated translocation of bacteria from the gut in a number of pathological conditions [12, 14, 54–56]. However, while translocation/ endotoxemia occurs after severe hemorrhage, endotoxin may not be solely responsible for the immunodepression after hemorrhage. This is due to the fact that the depression in macrophage and lymphocyte functions after hemorrhage was quantitatively similar irrespective of whether endotoxin-tolerant or endotoxin-sensitive mice were used [27, 28, 41, 57]. Further support for this notion comes from the studies of Rush et al. [58] which indicated that while 3-day mortality in germ-free animal can be reduced (by $\sim 10\%-15\%$ versus conventional rats), a significant number of animals (80%) still succumb after hemorrhage. These studies, therefore, suggest that endotoxin may not account for all the effects produced by hemorrhage on immune or organ function that occur following hemorrhage and resucitation. In addition, our studies indicated that there was no significant elevation of systemic endotoxin levels observed in the serum of C3H/HeN (endotoxin sensitive) mice after hemorrhage [27, 59]. It is possible, however, that the increases in endotoxin were not detected because portal blood was not sampled, thus leaving the possibility that endotoxin was cleared by the Kupffer cells. This may indeed be the reason why Kupffer cells, and not other macrophages, release inflammatory cytokines after hemorrhage [50–51]. Studies have also suggested that the elevated levels of prostaglandin $E_2(PGE_2)$ following hemorrhage [60] could be responsible for perturbations in cell-mediated immunity, since the blockade of prostaglandin synthesis with ibuprofen prevented the depression in macrophage functions following hemorrhage [61]. This occurred despite enhanced TNF synthesis. Additional studies indicated that alterations in calcium homeostasis following hemorrhage may also play a role in inducing immunosuppression [31].

TNF has been implicated as one of the primary mediators responsible for producing various alterations in both immune and organ function [62–64]. Although our studies demonstrate a marked increase in plasma TNF and IL-6 after hemorrhage [59], it remains to be determined whether TNF and/or IL-6, directly or indirectly via the production of other mediator(s), is/are responsible for producing the immunosuppression. Nonetheless, our recent studies have shown that antibodies against TNF could prevent the immunosuppressive effects of hemorrhage on Kupffer cell functions [65].

A common feature of all forms of shock is an inadequate circulation with a diminution of blood flow to tissues. Since a major portion of the oxygen required in tissue metabolism is used for the generation of high energy phosphate by the process of oxidative phosphorylation, the levels of compounds, such as adenosine triphosphate (ATP), should decrease as tissue hypoxia develops [66]. In this regard, our recent studies have indicated that ATP levels, as measured by ^{31}P nuclear magnetic resonance (NMR), in splenocytes were barely detectable after hemorrhage and remain depressed even 12 h after resuscitation [67]. Furthermore, such studies indicate that there is an association between decreased splenocyte ATP levels and depressed immune functions.

Additional support for this suggestion comes from our preliminary experiments which indicated that 2 h after exposure of animals to hypoxic gas mixtures (without blood loss), macrophage antigen presentation was depressed, while the production of TNF and PGE$_2$ was significantly increased.

Since hemorrhage is a potent stimulator of catecholamine and corticosteroid secretion [68, 69], it is possible that the transient elevation of these mediators may be sufficient to induce the prolonged state of immunodepression. However, the levels of these agents in the mouse model of hemorrhage and resuscitation remains to be determined.

It should be pointed out that while all of the above agents alone might induce changes in immune function, their combined effects may be equal or even more significant. Moreover, while many of the mediators are short-lived during or following hemorrhage, it is possible that they initiate a cascade of intracellular events leading to long-term immunodepression.

Potential Therapeutic Interventions

The studies of Livingston et al. [36] suggest that the capacity of rats to ward of infections after fixed pressure hemorrhagic shock is enhanced by combined rat IFN-γ and antibiotic therapy. The work of Ertel et al. [70] has demonstrated that the depressed Ia expression and antigen presentation capacity of mouse macrophages can be restored by the administration of murine IFN-γ following hemorrhage. In addition, Ertel et al. [71] utilized an alternative approach in which the blockade of cytokine production after shock was the target. The results demonstrated that chloroquine, an antimalarial drug thought to have lysosomotropic effects, when administered after hemorrhage in mice can block the release of TNF and IL-6. Work by Meldrum et al. [31] and Ertel et al. [29] indicated that the water soluble calcium channel blocker, diltiazem, has various salutary effects on immune functions following hemorrhage. Their studies indicated that animals treated with this agent during resuscitaton after hemorrhage showed a marked restoration of the capacity to produce various T-cell lymphokines (IL-2, IL-3, IL-6, and IFN-γ). This study, therefore, suggests that massive calcium influx may be occurring during hemorrhage/resuscitation which induces cellular dysfunction and damage. Work by Ertel et al. [29] further extended these observations and demonstrated that posttreatment of hemorrhaged mice with diltiazem can restore macrophage-antigen-presenting capacity and Ia expression. In addition, restoration of splenocyte IL-2 productive capacities after hemorrhage have also been reported by utilizing ATP-MgCl$_2$ treatment during resuscitation [30]. More recent studies indicated that the depressed macorphage antigen presentation functions can also be restored following hemorrhage by using ATP-MgCl$_2$ as an adjuvant to resuscitation. In addition to improving various immune functions, the use of chloroquine, diltiazem or IFN-γ also decreased the enhanced mortality rates following hemorrhage and sepsis.

Hypothesis

Based on the work of several investigative units and our own, we have developed a hypothesis of the cascade of events following hemorrhage leading to the depressed macrophage and lymphocyte functions, immunodepression, and subsequently to increased susceptibility to fatal outcome following a septic challenge. Our hypothesis, as shown in Fig. 1, is that following hemorrhage, there is

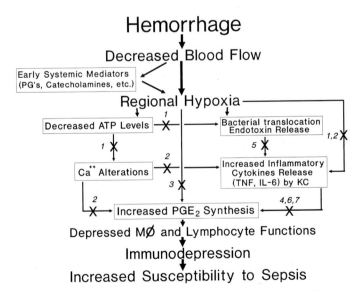

Fig. 1. Hypothesis of the cascade of events following hemorrhage leading to immunodepression and increased susceptibility to sepsis. Cascade inhibitors: *1*, ATP-MgCl$_2$; *2*, Ca^{2+} antagonists; *3*, cyclooxygenase inhibitors; *4*, chloroquine. Antibodies against: *5*, lipopolysaccharides; *6*, tumor necrosis factor (*TNF*); *7*, interleukin-6 (*IL-6*). *PG's* prostaglandins; *KC*, Kupffer cells; *MØ*, macrophage; *ATP*, adenosine triphosphate

decreased blood flow leading to regional hypoxia which causes decreased cellular ATP levels. The decreased ATP levels cause calcium alterations. In addition, the regional hypoxia and/or decreased ATP levels may produce bacterial translocation (and/or endotoxin release into the portal vein) across the gut wall. Moreover, regional hypoxia, as well as bacterial translocation, may cause increased inflammatory cytokine (TNF, IL-6) release by Kupffer cells which can in turn cause increased PGE_2 synthesis. It is also plausible that the calcium alterations, directly and/or indirectly via increased inflammatory cytokine release, might also stimulate increased PGE_2 synthesis. Thus, regional hypoxia, singularly or collectively because of decreased ATP, altered calcium and bacterial translocation and increased inflammatory cytokine release, eventually leading to a sustained increase in PGE_2 production which mediates the depression of macrophage and lymphocyte functions, thereby enhancing mortality in the face of septic insult.

Summary and Conclusions

The available information indicates that hemorrhage produces a marked depression in cell-mediated immunity which persists despite fluid resuscitation and decreases host survival to a septic challenge. This was evidenced by the depression of lymphocyte function and antigen presentation by peritoneal and splenic macrophages, as well as by Kupffer cells. While the dysfunctions in Kupffer cell antigen presentation and Ia expression were comparable to those found in peritoneal and splenic macrophages, the increases in inflammatory cytokine production appear to be specific to Kupffer cells. The depression in macrophage antigen presentation does not seem to be due to the elevation in serum endotoxin levels during or after hemorrhage. Hemorrhage-induced depression of antigen presentation does not appear to be due to the reduction in the macrophage capacity to associate antigenic peptides with the MHC class II molecules, but to decreased antigen lysosomal catabolism by the macrophages. Studies have indicated that the decreased cellular ATP levels and alterations in calcium homeostasis following hemorrhage may play an important role in inducing host immunosuppression. Additional studies have suggested that the elevated levels of PGE_2 following hemorrhage could be responsible for the perturbations in cell-mediated immunity. The results also demonstrate that the depressed macrophage and splenocyte functions were significantly improved by the posttreatment of animals with either IFN-γ, diltiazem, chloroquine, or ATP-$MgCl_2$ following hemorrhage. Furthermore, these agents also decreased the susceptibility to septic challenge following hemorrhage. Thus, the use of diltiazem, IFN-γ, chloroquine, or ATP-$MgCl_2$, offer new therapeutic modalities in the treatment of immunodepression and for decreasing the susceptibility to sepsis following severe hemorrhage.

Acknowledgements. The authors wish to express their thanks to Renee Ziobron for her skill, patience, and editorial assistance in typing this manuscript. This work was supported by USPHS grant RO1 GM 37127.

References

1. Baue AE (1990) Multiple organ failure. In: Baue AE (ed) Multiple organ failure. Mosby St Louis, pp 421–437
2. Cerra FB (1989) Multiple organ failure syndrome. In: Bihari DJ, Cerra FB (eds) Multiple organ failure. Society of Critical Care Medicine, Fullerton, pp 1–24
3. Faist E, Baue AE, Dittmer H et al. (1983) Multiple organ failure in polytrauma patients. J Trauma 23:775–787
4. Polk HC Jr, Shields CL (1977) Reomte organ failure: a valid sign of occult intra-abdominal infection. Surgery 81:310–313
5. DeCamp MM, Demling RH (1988) Posttraumatic multisystem organ failure. JAMA 260:530–534
6. Deitch EA (1990) Multiple organ failure: summary and overview. In: Deitch EA (ed) Multiple organ failure. Thieme, New York, pp 285–299
7. Goris RJ (1989) Multiple organ failure: whole body inflammation? Schweiz Med Wochenschr 119:347–353
8. Demling RH, Niehaus G, Will JA (1979) Pulmonary microvascular response to hemorrhagic shock, resuscitation, and recovery. J Appl Physiol 46:498–503
9. Wang P, Hauptman JG, Chaudry IH (1990) Hepatocellular dysfunction occurs early after hemorrhage and persists despite fluid resuscitation. J Surg Res 48:464–470
10. Livingston DH, Malangoni MA (1989) An experimental study of susceptibility to infection after hemorrhagic shock. Surg Gynecol Obstet 168:138–142
11. Lefer AM, Araki H, Okamatsu S (1981) Beneficial actions of a free radical scavenger in traumatic shock and myocardial ischemia. Circ Shock 8:272–282
12. Deitch EA, Bridges W, Baker J et al. (1988) Hemorrhagic shock-induced bacterial translocation is reduced by xanthine oxidase inhibition or inactivation. Surgery 104:191–198
13. Abraham E, Freitas AA (1989) Hemorrhage produces abnormalities in lymphocyte function and lymphokine generation. J Immunol 142:899–906
14. Rush BF, Sori AJ, Murphy TF et al. (1988) Endotoxemia and bacteremia during hemorrhagic shock. The link between trauma and sepsis? Ann Surg 207:549–554
15. Chaudry IH, Ayala A, Ertel W, Stephan RN (1990) Editorial review. Hemorrhage and resuscitation: immunological aspects. Am J Physiol 259:R663–R678
16. Antonacci A, Reaves L, Calvano S, Amad R, DeRiesthal H, Shires GT (1984) Flow cytometric analysis of lymphocyte subpopulations after thermal injury in human beings. Surg Gynecol Obstet 159:1–8
17. Ertel W, Faist E (1989) The influence of mechanical trauma on the B-cell system: phenotypes, terminal B-cell maturation, immunoglobulin synthesis and influence of lymphokines. In: Faist E, Ninnemann J, Green D (eds) Immune consequences of trauma, shock and sepsis, springer, Berlin Heidelberg New York, pp 143–156
18. Faist E, Kupper TS, Baker CC, Chaudry IH, Dwyer J, Baue AE. (1986) Depression of cellular immunity after major injury: its association with post-traumatic complications and its restoration with immunomodulating agents. Arch Surg 121:1000–1005
19. Faist E, Ninnemann J, Green D (eds) (1989) Immune consequences of trauma, shock and sepsis. Springer, Berlin Heidelberg New York, pp 1–564
20. Keane RM, Birmingham W, Shatney CM, Winchurch RA, Munster AM (1983) Prediction of sepsis in the multi-traumatic patients by assays of lymphocyte dysfunction. Surg Gynecol Obstet 156:163–167
21. Kupper TS, Green DR, Chaudry IH, Fox A, Baue AE (1984) A cyclophospamide-sensitive suppressor T-cell circuit induced by thermal trauma. Surgery 95:699–706
22. Alexander JW, Stinnett JD, Ogle CK, Ogle JK, Morris MJ (1979) A comparison of immunologic

profiles and their influence on bacteremia in surgical patients with a high risk of infections. Surgery 86:94–101

23. Ninnemann JL, Stockland AE (1984) Participation of prostaglandin E in immunosuppression following thermal injury. J Trauma 24:201–207

24. Abraham E, Chang YH (1986) Cellular and humoral bases of hemorrhage-induced depression of lymphocyte function. Crit Care Med 14:81–86

25. Smith KA (1988) Interleukin-2: inception, impact and implications. Science 240:1169–1176

26. Stephan RN, Kupper TS, Geha AS, Baue AE, Chaudry IH (1987) Hemorrhage without tissue trauma produces immunosuppression and enhances susceptibility to sepsis. Arch Surg 122:62–68

27. Ayala A, Walsh MM, Wagner PA, Chaudry IH (1990) Enhanced susceptibility to sepsis following simple hemorrhage: Depression of Fc and C3b receptor-mediated phagocytosis. Arch Surg 125:70–75

28. Ayala A, Perrin MM, Chaudry IH (1990) Defective macrophage antigen presentation following hemorrhage is associated with the loss of MHC Class II (Ia) antigens. Immunology 70:33–39

29. Ertel W, Meldrum D, Morrison M, Ayala A, Chaudry IH (1990) Immuno-protective effect of a calcium channel blocker on macrophage antigen presentation function, major histocompatibility class II antigen expression and interleukin-1 synthesis after hemorrhage. Surgery 108:154–160

30. Stephan RN, Janeway CA, Dean RE, Chaudry IH (1987) Decreased interleukin-2 production following simple hemorrhage and its restoration with ATP-MgCl$_2$ treatment. Magnesium 6:163

31. Meldrum D, Ayala A, Perrin MM, Ertel W, Chaudry IH (1991) Diltiazem restores IL-2, IL-3, IL-6, and IFN-γ synthesis and decreases host susceptibility to sepsis following hemorrhage. J Surg Res 51:158–164

32. Abraham E, Freitas AA (1989) Hemorrhage in mice induced alteration in immunoglobulin-secreting B cells. Crit Care Med 17:1015–1019

33. Hamilton TA, Adams DO (1987) Molecular mechanisms of signal transduction in macrophages. Immunol Today 8:151–158

34. Vilcek J, Kelker HD, Le J, Yip YK (1985) Structure and function of human interferon-gamma. In: Ford RJ, Maizel AL (eds) Mediators in cell growth and differentiation. Raven, New York, pp 299–313

35. Stephan RN, Poo WJ, Janeway CA, Zoghbi SS, Dean RE, Geha AS, Chaudry IH (1987) Prolonged impairment of natural killer (NK) cell activity following simple hemorrhage. Circ Shock 21:312–313

36. Livingston DH, Apel SH, Wellhausen SR, Sonnenfeld G, Polk HC (1988) Depressed interferon-gamma production and monocyte HLA—DR expression after severe injury. Arch Surg 123:1309–1312

37. Unanue ER (1984) Textbook of immunology. Williams and Wilkins, Baltimore, p 109

38. Unanue ER, Beller DI, Lu CT, Allen PM (1984) Antigen presentation: comments on its regulation and mechanism. J Immunol 132:1–5

39. Weaver CT, Unanue ER (1990) The costimulatory function of antigen-presenting cells. Immunol Today 11:49–55

40. Kaye J, Gillis S, Mizel SB, Shevach EM, Malek TR, Dinarello CA, Lachman LB, Janeway CA (1984) Growth of cloned helper T-cell line induced by a monoclonal antibody specific antigen receptor: interleukin-1 is required for expression of receptors for interleukin-2. J Immunol 133:1339–1345

41. Stephan RN, Ayala A, Harkema JM, Dean RE, Border JR, Chaudry IH (1989) "Mechanism of immunosuppression following hemorrhage: defective antigen presentation by macrophages. J Surg Res 46:553–556

42. Ertel W, Morrison MH, Ayala A, Chaudry IH (1991) Insights into the mechanism of defective antigen presentation following hemorrhage. Surgery 110:440–447

43. Cheadle WG, Hershman MJ, Wellhausen SR, Polk HS Jr (1989) Role of monocyte HLA-DR expression following trauma in predicting clinical outcome. In: Faist E, Ninnemann J, Green D (eds) Immune consequences of trauma, shock and sepsis. Springer, Berlin Heidelberg New York, pp 199–122

44. Miller CL, Baker CC (1976) Changes in lymphocyte activation after thermal injury: the role of suppressor cells. J Clin Invest 63:202–210

45. Miller CL, Fink MP, Wu JY, Sabo G, Kodys K (1988) Mechanisms of altered monocyte prostaglandin E$_2$ production in severely injured patients. Arch Surg 123:293–299

46. Paul WE (ed) (1989) Fundamental Immunology, 2nd edn. Raven, New York
47. Rogoff TM, Lipsky PE (1981) Role of Kupffer cells in local and systemic immune responses. Gastroenterology 80:854–860
48. Rogoff TM, Lipsky PE (1980) Antigen presentation by isolated guinea pig Kupffer cells. J Immunol 124:1740–1744
49. Shivaton Y, Okano K, Madsumoto K, Murao S (1984) antigen presentation of Kupffer cells in the rat. Scand J Gastroenterology 19:737–739
50. Ayala A, Perrin MM, Chaudry IH (1989) Increased susceptibility to sepsis following hemorrhage: defective Kupffer cell-mediated antigen presentation. Surg Forum 40:102–104
51. Ayala A, Perrin MM, Ertel W, Chaudry IH (1990) The effect of hemorrhage on Kupffer cell antigen presentation and those processes associated with it. FASEB J 28:A1020
52. Perrin MM, Ayala A, Wang P, Ertel W, Chaudry IH (1991) Differential effects of hemorrhage on macrophage cytotoxic capacity and TNF release/expression. FASEB J 5:A1619
53. Wang P, Hauptman JG Chaudry IH (1990) Hepatocellular dysfunction occurs early after hemorrhage and persists despite fluid resuscitation. J Surg Res 48:464–470
54. Border JR, Hassett J, LaDuca J et al. (1987) The gut origin septic states in blunt multiple trauma (ISS = 40) in the ICU. Ann Surg 206:427–448
55. Inoue S, Wirman JA, Alexander JW et al. (1988) *Candida albicans* translocation across the gut mucosa following burn injury. J Surg Res 44:479–492
56. Deitch EA, Ma W-J, Ma L et al. (1989) Endotoxin-induced bacterial translocation: A study of mechanisms. Surgery 106:292–299
57. Ayala A, Perrin MM, Chaudry IH (1989) Does endotoxin play a major role in the suppression of macrophage antigen presentation following hemorrhage? Circ Shock 27:317–318
58. Rush BF, Redan JA, Flanagan JJ et al. (1989) Does the bacteremia observed in hemorrhagic shock have clinical significance? A study in germ-free animals. Ann Surg 210:342–345
59. Ayala A, Perrin MM, Meldrum DR, Ertel W, Chaudry IH (1990) Hemorrhage induces an increase in serum TNF which is not associated with elevated levels of endotoxin. Cytokine 2:170–174
60. Lefer AM (1983) Role of prostaglandins and thromboxanes in shock states. In: Altura BM, Lefer AM, Schumer W (eds) Handbook of shock and trauma vol 1. Raven, New York, pp 355–376
61. Ertel W, Morrison MH, Ayala A, Perrin MM, Chaudry IH (1991) Blockade of prostaglandin production increases cachectin synthesis and prevents depression of macrophage functions following hemorrhagic shock. Ann Surg 213:265–271
62. Beutler B, Tkacenko V, Milsark I et al. (1989) The biology of cachectin/TNF - a primary mediator of the host response. Annu Rev Immunol 7:625–655
63. Nuytinck HK, Offermans XJ, Kubat K et al. (1988) Whole-body inflammation in trauma patients. An autopsy study. Arch Surg 123:1519–1524
64. Smith MR, Munger WE, Kung HF et al. (1990) Direct evidence for an intracellular role for tumor necrosis factor-alpha. J Immunology 144:162–169
65. Ertel W, Morrison MH, Ayala A, Perrin MM, Chaudry IH (1990) Passive immunization against cachectin (TNF-α) prevents hemorrhage-induced suppression of Kupffer cell functions. Surg Forum 41:91–93
66. Chaudry IH (1983) Cellular mechanisms in shock and ischemia and their correction. Am J Physiol 245:R117–R134
67. Meldrum DR, Ayala A, Wang P, Ertel W, Chaudry IH (1991) The decreased splenic ATP levels and immunodepression associated with hemorrhage is ameliorated with ATP-MgCl$_2$. FASEB J 5:A1501
68. Hume DM, Nelson DH (1954) Adrenal cortical function in Surgical shock. Surg Form 5:568–574
69. Beck L, Dontas AS (1955) Vasomotor activity in hemorrhagic shock. Fed Proc 14:318
70. Ertel W, Morrison MH, Ayala A, Dean RE, Chaudry IH (1991) Interferon-gamma attenuates hemorrhage-induced suppression of macrophage and splenocyte functions and decreases susceptibility to sepsis. Surgery (in press)
71. Ertel W, Ayala A, Morrison M, Perrin MM, Chaudry IH (1990) Chloroquine inhibits TNF and IL-6 synthesis but not IL-1 production. FASEB J 28:A1035

3.2 Intermediate Inflammatory Phase

Sepsis and Multiple Organ Failure: The Result of Whole Body Inflammation

R. J. A. Goris

Introduction

The adult respiratory distress syndrome (ARDS) still carries a mortality of 30%, despite intensive treatment. When followed by the sequential failure of multiple organ functions (MOF) and sepsis, mortality reaches 60%. Evidence is slowly gathering that excessively activated endogenous inflammatory cells are responsible for structural damage and functional deterioration in remote vital organ systems and for the syndrome of "clinical" sepsis in these patients [1].

MOF has been defined as a syndrome consisting of the sequential failure of two or more organ systems in patients with clinical signs of sepsis [2]. Respiratory dysfunction usually is the first apparent organ failure [3]. The other organ systems involved are the hepatic, renal, cardiovascular, nervous, hematologic, and gastrointestinal systems. We presently utilize the "MOF score" to define and grade (0 = not present, 1 = present, 2 = severe) the severity of failure in each of these seven organ systems (maximum score = 14) [3]. A MOF score of 5 or above indicates severe MOF. All studies available have shown a strong correlation between the number and severity of organ dysfunctions and mortality [3, 4].

Sepsis has been defined as a clinical syndrome of serious bacterial infection with a concurrent deleterious systemic response. For reasons to be discussed later this definition is not practicable in MOF patients.

Clinical Signs and Symptoms Including Organ Dysfunction

It is clear that MOF is not a specific clinical illness but a complication of a severe event such as major injury or infection. Thus, MOF is always preceded by a trigger. Clinicians are well aware of the nature of such triggers, as in some studies in selected patients at risk, the actual incidence of ARDS was 80% [5]. In trauma patients, the risk of ARDS increases with the severity of injury [6, 7].

In trauma patients, the early signs of incipient ARDS may be found within hours after injury and consist of tachypnea and respiratory alkalosis, followed

Department of Surgery, University Hospital, 6500 HB Nijmegen, The Netherlands

Host Defense Dysfunction
in Trauma, Shock and Sepsis
Eds. Faist/Meakins/Schildberg
© Springer-Verlag, Berlin Heidelberg 1993

by a decrease in arterial pO_2 ("early" ARDS). These signs may increase in severity (or in other patients first appear) after 4 or 5 days, when the patient becomes febrile and develops the clinical syndrome of sepsis ("late" or "septic" ARDS) [8].

In ARDS, lung capillary permeability to water and protein is increased, resulting in pulmonary edema, which is easily diagnosed on roentgenography and may be accurately measured by the thermo-dye method. Less attention has been given to the fact that these patients have a generalized increase in capillary permeability resulting in a positive fluid balance, *generalized permeability edema* [3, 9, 10], reduced plasma oncotic pressure [10], increased organ weights on post-mortem examination [11], and a protein-rich glomerular filtrate in the kidney [11].

Furthermore, these patients progressively develop *generalized vasodilatation*, with decreased peripheral resistance and increased cardiac output, together with moderately high fever ("clinical" sepsis). Though less obvious than the pulmonary symptoms, already at a very early stage functional disturbances are found in other organs such as the kidney and the liver [3, 12].

The clinical signs may thus be summarized as generalized inflammation: "rubor" (generalized vasodilatation), "calor" (fever), "tumor" (generalized permeability edema), and "function laesa" of several organ systems.

Morphology

The morphology of the lung is experimental and human ARDS has been well characterized with aggregation and margination of polymorphonuclear leukocytes (PMNs) ("lung in shock") and subsequent damage to the pulmonary capillary endothelium and alveolocapillary membrane ("shock-lung") [8, 11, 13, 14].

Surprisingly little attention has been given to the early morphological changes in other organs in experimental and human conditions leading to ARDS, sepsis, and MOF, but the available evidence indicates that the above alterations are also present in the liver, kidney, heart, and spleen [8, 11, 13–17]. Again these changes are indicative of a generalized inflammatory response.

Biochemal Changes

Though inflammation is intended to be a local process, it is obvious that in patients with severe trauma a systemic activation of inflammatory cells and a systemic spillover of inflammatory products and mediators may be expected. The "abnormal" systemic presence of any inflammatory mediator would then be a marker of systematic inflammation and the change from normal should

Table 1. Schematic presentation of the events and time range leading to multiple organ failure

Events		Time
Risk factors – – – – – – – – – – – – –➤ Markers		Day 0
Severity score ➘		
➘➤ Mediators		
⬋ P		
Early ARDS – – – – – – – – – – – – –	Markers	Day 1–2
Severity score ➘		
➘➤ Mediators		
⬋ P		
Late ARDS – – – – – – – – – – –➤	Markers	Day ± 7
MOF, "sepsis"		
Severity score		
➤ Survival		
Outcome ⬅ P		
➤ Death		

P, positive predictive value; ARDS, acute respiratory distress syndrome; MOF, multiple organ failure

correlate with its severity. However, if these compounds are themselves causing damage to otherwise healthy tissues and their specific functions, their detection in abnormal amounts in the systemic circulation should predict ARDS and MOF (Table 1).

Of the different cascade systems possibly involved in MOF, only the complement system has been well studied. In this respect, trauma patients are of special interest, as the primary stimulus is nonbacterial. Low plasma levels of the complement components C3 and C4 have been found in ARDS patients [18, 19]. Elevated plasma levels of C3a desArg have been found prior to the development of ARDS by several authors [18–23]. However, in most studies elevated levels of anaphylatoxins could only be found at an early stage of disease. In patients with sepsis or acute limb ischemia, elevated plasma levels of cytolytic terminal complement complexes were found, normalizing in successfully treated patients, or further increasing in patients developing ARDS [24].

Studying the number and function of circulating PMNs in MOF may not be relevant, since biologically active PMNs aggregate and stick to endothelial cells, while peripheral-blood PMNs may not be representative of the activated population [25]. At the site of inflammation, PMNs release numerous active substances, such as proteolytic enzymes (e.g., elastase) and toxic oxygen radicals, vasoactive substances (platelet activating factor, PAF; leukotrienes; prostaglandin E_2, PGE_2) and wound hormones (macrophage activating factor, MAF; granulocyte-macrophage colony-stimulating factor, GM-CSF). Actually it might be more appropriate to measure these substances as an index of PMN activity. Presently, the measurement of most of these substances in clinical patients is either impossible, impractical, or has barely been done.

Increasing data are available on elastase. Elastase is a serine protease, essential for PMN-mediated endothelial injury [26, 27] and is measured as the complex with its inhibitor α_1-antiprotease. All studies available have shown a positive relation between elastase and severity of ARDS, sepsis, and MOF in major trauma [19, 28–31], peritonitis [32], and sepsis [33–35]. A few studies found elastase to predict MOF [19, 28, 31, 34]. One study could demonstrate that the rise in extravascular lung water in trauma patients occurred subsequent to an increase in elastase and C3a [36]. The present evidence thus suggests an important role for elastase as a marker of PMN activity, and possibly as a predictor of ARDS and MOF, though specific plasma levels and time courses have yet to be set for optimizing the positive predictive value.

The involvement of free radicals in patients prone to ARDS and MOF is still poorly documented, due to the difficulty of demonstrating their presence or effects in vivo. Malondialdehyde, a stable end product of lipid peroxidation, is elevated in pulmonary tissue of trauma patients dying of ARDS and sepsis [37]. The MDA method, however, is subject to criticism, and more studies are urgently needed utilizing newer methods such as lipofuscin and hydroxynonenal.

Macrophages, as well as PMNs, exert their activities locally. Monitoring macrophage activity thus requires measuring their monokines (tumor necrosis factor, TNF; interleukin-1, IL-1) or metabolic products (e.g., neopterin). In some studies, sustained high plasma TNF levels correlated well with lactate levels, severity of illness, and mortality, not with positive blood cultures, endotoxin levels, or with subsequent septic shock [38–40]. Other studies found no such correlation with subsequent ARDS or mortality [41–43]. Plasma neopterin could accurately predict nonsurvivors several days before the event [31, 34, 44].

Bacteriology

Since the first authors to describe ARDS noticed that these patients subsequently die of sepsis [45], consensus has almost been reached that bacterial overgrowth is the cause of late ARDS and MOF. However, the evidence for such a causal relationship is poor, as an identical MOF syndrome develops in patients with primarily bacterial (peritonitis) and nonbacterial problems (severe trauma before bacterial invasion is obvious) [3]. No single study could reliably demonstrate positive blood cultures or elevated levels of circulating endotoxin preceding MOF (for review see [1]). Furthermore, there are no clinical, biochemical, or morphological differences between patients with the "clinical" sepsis syndrome (no bacteremia, no focus) and patients with the "classical" sepsis syndrome (bacteremia, septic focus) [3, 31, 46].

On the other hand, it is obvious that these patients demonstrate an important immunological dysfunction, a severely impaired host defense to bacterial invasion, and consequently are highly sensitive to nosocomial infections. Bacterial translocation from the gut may contribute to the pathogenesis or the perpetuation of the sepsis syndrome, but it has not yet been demonstrated that "septic" ARDS and MOF can be prevented by the administration of antibiotics or by selective decontamination of the gastrointestinal tract.

Oxygenation

The disturbed oxygenation of venous blood in the lung, and the resulting venous-arterial admixture and hypoxemia in ARDS, are well documented. This situation results from maldistribution of the pulmonary microcirculation and/or from impaired oxygen diffusion through the alveolocapillary membrane. Recently, it has been demonstrated that, in ARDS patients, oxygen consumption depends on oxygen supply over a much wider range of supply than normal (pathologic supply dependency), and high serum-lactate levels are found despite an adequate arterial oxygen supply (for review see [47, 48]). In fact, ARDS patients are unable to increase their oxygen extraction ratio (OER) above 0.30 in the presence of tissue hypoxia, while normally maximal OER is 0.80 when arterial oxygen supply is insufficient to meet tissue demands.

The same phenomenon has been described in septic and MOF patients, with another terminology: "high output failure." As very low tissue pO_2 values were found [49] in this condition, supply dependency is not caused by an impaired utilization of oxygen, but indicates disturbed diffusion of oxygen from the erythrocytes to the mitochondria. Thus in MOF the diffusion of oxygen is impaired in the lung as well as in peripheral tissues. A review of the literature on oxygen utilization indicated that a severe decrease in OER is ubiquitous phenomenon in severe inflammation [49]. Present therapeutic efforts in ARDS, MOF, and sepsis are aimed at increasing arterial oxygen transport, while the correct therapy should aim at increasing OER.

Pathophysiology

The sequence of events in inflammation, e.g., after local tissue trauma, begins with the local activation of the different cascade systems (complement, arachidonic acid, coagulation, fibrinolytic, and kinin-kallikrein), generating mediators from circulating proteins. Some of these mediators (anaphylatoxins: C3a, C5a) have strong chemotactic effects on circulating inflammatory cells (PMNs, monocytes) and activate these cells to produce proteolytic enzymes and toxic oxygen radicals.

In the next phase, cellular mediators have an important role. The wound PMNs and macrophages release systemic signals (e.g., GM-CSF, PGE_2, TNF, IL-1, IL-6) to adapt the organism to the local requirements of the local problem. These mediators, however, may have deleterious effects.

Experimental infusion of complement-activated plasma in rabbits induces tachypnea, leukopenia, and PMN-aggregation and sequestration in the lung, liver, kidney, and heart [13] resembling the early morphological changes in ARDS and MOF [11]. These alterations, however, are not severe and largely reversible. Only with an additional stimulus such as hypoxia can severe morphological changes be induced [13]. This indicates a strong synergism between complement activation and hypoxemia in inducing these changes ("two hit theory"). In complement-depleted or complement-deficient experimental animals, the pulmonary response to inflammatory stimuli is significantly diminished [50, 51].

The role of PMNs in inflammation and in increased microvascular permeability has been well defined [52], while in this process PMNs may injure otherwise healthy cells [52–55]. PMN depletion prevents pulmonary inflammation following intravascular complement activation [56, 57] and endotoxemia [58].

Experimental administration of elastase results in elevated pulmonary vascular resistance, decreased cardiac output, pulmonary leukostasis, disseminated intravascular coagulopathy (DIC), and increased venous admixture of oxygen [59]. However, in elastase-deficient mice, complement-induced lung injury and zymosan-induced MOF were not prevented [57, 60].

Free radicals are potent inflammatory agents. Experimental administration of (agents inducing) free radicals closely mimics ARDS and MOF [61]. In zymosan-induced MOF, increased PMN superoxide production and plasma and tissue malondialdehyde levels were observed, but pretreatment with various oxygen-radical scavengers could not prevent MOF [60].

Circulating monocytes are attracted to the site of inflammation and differentiate locally into macrophages. Macrophages are activated by C5a, hypoxia, and a score of signals from PMNs such as GM-CSF, low-molecular MSF, and PMN-IL-1-like activity [62]. Apparently it takes several days after activation for the full inflammatory reaction of macrophages to develop. Upon stimulation, macrophages may release some 53 different classes of secretory products, of whom some are proinflammatory (proteolytic enzymes, oxygen radicals, IL-1, TNF), while others are anti-inflammatory (PGE_2), immunosuppressive (IL-2), or procoagulatory [63].

Prolonged activation of macrophages by intraperitoneal administration of zymosan in rats induces the full clinical, morphological, biochemical, and bacteriological syndrome of ARDS, MOF, and sepsis, including bacterial translocation [14, 64–66]. Except for the bacteriological alterations, the same syndrome may be elicited in this way in germ-free rats [14]. We could prevent these alterations in conventional mice by macrophage depletion.

Experimental administration of IL-1 in rabbits results in hypotension, decreased peripheral resistance, increased heart rate and cardiac output, leukopenia, and thrombocytopenia [67]. Pretreatment and treatment with an IL-1 receptor antagonist significantly reduced mortality from endotoxin shock [68].

Experimental administration of TNF results in fever, diarrhea, tachypnea, hypotension, metabolic acidosis, elevated lactate levels, lethargy, ARDS-like changes in the lung, hemorrhagic necrosis of the kidneys and adrenals, and finally death [69]. These effects can be blocked by monoclonal antibodies against TNF [70].

Conclusions

Inventorying their inflammatory capacities, PMNs and macrophages seem able to induce a lethal reaction, characterized by clinical, morphological, and biochemical signs of whole body inflammation, bacterial overgrowth, impaired oxygen diffusion, and the consequent failure of organ functions. This whole body inflammation has hitherto largely escaped our attention, since in clinical studies inappropriate methods have been used such as counting peripheral leukocytes, and since monitoring key mediators (IL-1, TNF, PGE_2, leukotrienes) and key cells (activated PMNs, macrophages) was impossible until recently.

Today, a new set of methods allowing a closer look at this whole body inflammation are available, such as elastase (monitoring PMN activity), neopterin (monitoring macrophage activity), and clinical methods to monitor cytokines and endotoxin levels. Only after such comprehensive studies have been performed might it be concluded that—as in the experimental animal—sepsis and MOF may not necessarily be caused by bacteria or their endotoxins, but by an untoward autodestructive and self-sustaining activation of our own inflammatory cells.

References

1. Goris RJA (1989) Multiple organ failure: whole body inflammation? Schweiz Med Wochenschrift 199:347–353
2. Baue AE (1975) Multiple progressive or sequential systems failure. Arch Surg 110:779–781
3. Goris RJA, te Boekhorst TPA, Nuytinck JKS, Gimbrère JSP (1985) Multiple organ failure. Generalized autodestructive inflammation? Arch Surg 120:1109–1115
4. Knaus WA, Draper EA, Wagner DP, Zimmerman JE (1985) Prognosis in acute organ-system failure. Ann Surg 202:685–693
5. Pepe PE, Potkin RT, Holtman RD, Hudson LD, Carrico CJ (1982) Clinical predictors of the adult respiratory distress syndrome. Am J Surg 1444:124–130
6. Goris RJA (1987) Prevention of ARDS and MOF in trauma patients by prophylactic mechanical ventilation and early fracture stabilisation. In: Schlag G, Redl H (eds) First Vienna shock forum. Liss, New York, pp 163–173
7. Johnson KD, Cadambi A, Seibert GV (1985) Incidence of adult respiratory musculoskeletal injuries: effect of early operative stabilization of fractures. J Trauma 25:375–384
8. Schlag G, Redl H (1982) Neue Aspekte zur Shocklunge. Anaesth Intensivther Notfallmed 17:86–91

9. Kreuzfelder E, Joka T, Keinecke HO et al. (1988) Adult respiratory distress syndrome as a specific manifestation of a general permeability defect in trauma patients. Am Rev Respir Dis 137:95–99

10. Lucas CE, Ledgerwood AM, Rachwal WJ, Grabow D, Saxe JM (1991) Colloid oncotic pressure and body water dynamics in septic and injured patients. J Trauma 31:927–933

11. Nuytinck JKS, Offermans XJ, Kubat K, Goris RJA (1988) Whole body inflammation in trauma patients. An autopsy study. Arch Surg 123:1519–1524

12. Lobenhoffer HP, Oestern HJ, Sturm J, Maghsudi M (1984) Changes in laboratory profile in patients with multiple organ failure after major trauma. Langenbecks Arch Chir [Suppl] Chir Forum 15–19

13. Nuytinck JKS, Goris RJA, Weerts JGE (1986) Acute generalised microvascular injury by activated complement and hypoxia: the basis of ARDS and MOF? Br J Exp Pathol 67:537–548

14. Goris RJA, Boekholtz WKF, van Bebber IPT, Nuytinck JKS, Schillings PHM (1986) Multiple organ failure and sepsis without bacteria. An experimental model. Arch Surg 121:897–901

15. Caruana JA, Montes M, Camara DS, Ummer A, Potmesil SH, Gage AA (1982) Functional and histopathologic changes in the liver during sepsis. Surg Gynecol Obstet 154:653–656

16. Ruchti C (1986) Pathomorphologische Befunde nach Intensivtherapie. Schweiz Med Wochenschr 116:694–698

17. Mizer LA, Weisbrode SE, Dorinsky PM (1989) Neutrophil accumulation and structural changes in nonpulmonary organs after acute lung injury induced by phorbol myristate acetate. Am Rev Respir Dis 139:1017–1026

18. Heideman M, Hugli T (1984) Anaphylatoxin generation in multiple system organ failure. J Trauma 24:1038–1043

19. Nuytinck JKS, Goris RJA, Redl H, Schlag G, van Munster PJJ (1986) Posttraumatic complications and inflammatory mediators. Arch Surg 121:886–890

20. Solomkin JS, Cotta LA, Satoh PS, Hurst JM, Nelson RD (1985) Complement activation and clearance in acute illness and injury: evidence for C5a as a cell-directed mediator of ARDs in man. Surgery 97:668–678

21. Slotman GJ, Burchard KW, Yelling SA, Williams JJ (1986) Prostaglandin and complement interaction in clinical acute respiratory failure. Arch Surg 121:271–274

22. Tennenberg SD, Jacobs MP, Solomkin JS (1987) Complement-mediated neutrophil activation in sepsis- and trauma-related adult respiratory distress syndrome. Arch Surg 122:26–32

23. Howard RJ, Crain C, Franzini DA, Hood CI, Hugli TE (1988) Effects of cardiopulmonary bypass on pulmonary leukostasis and complement activation. Arch Surg 123:1496–1501

24. Heideman M, Norder-Hanssen B, Bengtson A, Mollnes TE (1988) Terminal complement complexes and anaphylatoxins in septic and ischemic patients. Arch Surg 123:188–192

25. Russel Martin R (1987) In host defense, leucocytes that are counted may not count. J Lab Clin Med 109:378–379

26. Smedley LA, Tonnessen RA, Sandhaus RA, Haslett C, Guthrie LA, Johnston RB, Henson PM, Worthen GS (1986) Neutrophil-mediated injury to endothelial cells. J Clin Invest 77:1233–1243

27. Henson PM, Johnston RB (1987) Tissue injury in inflammation. J Clin Invest 79:669–674

28. Redl H, Pacher R, Woloszczuk W (1987) Acute pulmonary failure-comparison of neopterin and granulocyte elastase in septic and non-septic patients. In: Pfeiderer W (Ed) Biochemical and clinical aspects of pteridines, vol. 5, de Gruyter, New York

29. Dittmer H, Jochum M, Fritz H (1986) Freisetzung von granulozytarer Elastase und Plasmaproteinveränderungen nach trauma-tisch-haemorrhagischem Schock. Unfallchirurg 89:160–169

30. Zheutlin LM, Thonar EJ, Jacobs ER, Hanley ME, Balk RA, Bone RC (1986) Plasma elastase in ARDS. J Crit Care 1:39

31. Nast-Kolb D, Jochum M, Waydhas C, Schweiberer L (1991) Die klinische Wertigkeit biochemischer Faktoren beim Polytrauma. Springer, Berlin Heidelberg New York (Hefte Zur Unffallheilkunde, vol 215, supplement)

32. Duswald KH, Jochum M, Schramm W, Fritz H (1985) Released granulocytic elastase: an indicator of pathobiochemical alterations in septicemia after abdominal surgery. Surgery 98:892–899

33. Schoeffel U, Lausen M, Ruf G, Specht von BU, Freudenberg N (1989) The overwhelming inflammatory response and the role of endotoxin in sepsis. In: Schlag G, Redl H (eds) Second Vienna shock forum. Liss, New York, pp 371–376

34. Pacher R, Redl H, Frass M, Petzl DH, Schuster E, Woloszczuk W (1989) Relationship between neopterin and granulocyte elastase plasma levels and severity of multiple organ failure. Crit Care Med 17:221–226

35. Tanaka H, Sugimoto H, Yoshioka T, Sugimoto T (1991) Role of granulocyte elastase in tissue injury in patients with septic shock complicated by multiple-organ failure. Ann Surg 213:81–85
36. Nerlich ML, Seidel J, Regel G, Nerlich AG, Sturm AJ (1986) Oxidative membrane damage in severe trauma: a clinical-experimental study. In: Streicher HJ, Schwaiger M (ed) Chirurgisches forum. Springer, Berlin Heidelberg New York
37. Nerlich ML, Seidel J, Regel G, Nerlich AG, Sturm AJ (1986) Klinische experimentelle Untersuchungen zum oxidativen Membranschaden nach schwerem Trauma. Langenbecks Arch Chir [Suppl]:217–222
38. Damas P, Reuter A, Gijzen P et al. (1989) Tumor necrosis factor-α and interleukin-1 serum levels during sepsis in humans. Crit Care Med 17:975–978
39. Offner F, Phillipe J, Vogelaers D et al. (1990) Serum tumor necrosis factor levels in patients with infectious disease and septic shock. J Lab Clin Med 116:100–105
40. Marks JD, Marks CB, Luce JM et al. (1990) Plasma tumor necrosis factor in patients with septic shock. Am Rev Respir Dis 141:94–97
41. Roten R, Markert M, Feihl F, Schaller MD, Tagan MC, Perret C (1991) Plasma levels of tumor necrosis factor in the adult respiratory distress syndrome. Am Rev Respir Dis 143:590–592
42. Calandra T, Baumgartner J-D, Grau GE et al. (1990) Prognostic values of tumor necrosis factor/cachectin, interleukin-1, interferon-α and interferon-γ in the serum of patients with septic shock. JID 161:982–987
43. Hyers TM, Tricomi SM, Dettenmeier PA, Fowler AA (1991) Tumor necrosis factor levels in serum and bronchoalveolar lavage fluid of patients with the adult respiratory distress syndrome. Am Rev Respir Dis 144:268–271
44. Strohmaier W, Redl H, Schlag G, Inthorn D (1987) D-Erythro-neopterin plasma levels in intensive care patients with and without septic complications. Crit Care Med 15:757–760
45. Ashbaugh DG, Petty TL (1972) Sepsis complicating the acture respiratory distress syndrome. Surg Gynecol Obstet 15:865–869
46. Nerlich ML (1989) The trigger for posttraumatic multiple organ failure: surgical sepsis or inflammation. In: Schlag G, Redl H (eds) Second Vienna shock forum. Liss, New York, pp 413–417
47. Cain SM (1984) Review: supply dependency of oxygen uptake in ARDS: myth or reality? Am J Med Sci 288:119–124
48. Goris RJA (1991a) Impaired oxygen extraction, an ubiquitous phenomenon in severe inflammation. In: Gutierrez G, Vincent JL (eds). Tissue oxygen utilization. Springer, Berlin Heidelberg New York, pp 350–369
49. Beerthuizen GIJM, Goris RJA, Kreuzer FJA (1989a) Early detection of shock in critically ill patients by skeletal muscle PO_2 assessment. Arch Surg 124:853–855
50. Dehring DJ, Steinberg SJ, Wismar BL, Lowery BD, Carey LC, Cloutier CT (1987) Complement depletion in a porcine model of septic acute respiratory distress. J Trauma 27:615–625
51. Hsueh W, Sun X, Rioja LN, Gonzales-Crussi F (1990) The role of the complement system in shock and tissue injury induced by tumour necrosis factor and endotoxin. Immunology 70:309–314
52. Wedmore CV, Williams TJ (1981) Control of vascular permeability of polymorphonuclear leukocytes in inflammation. Nature 89:646–650
53. Smedley LA, Tonnessen RA, Sandhaus RA et al. (1986) Neutrophil-mediated injury to endothelial cells. J Clin Invest 77:1233–1243
54. Henson PM, Johnston RB (1987) Tissue injury in inflammation. J Clin Invest 79:669–674
55. Anderson BO, Brown JM, Harken AH (1991) Mechanisms of neutrophil-mediated tissue injury. J Surg Res 51:170–179
56. Till GO, Johnson KJ, Kunkel R, Ward PA (1982) Intravascular activation of complement and acute lung injury. J Clin Invest 69:1126–1135
57. Tveden HW, Till GO, Ward PA (1985) Mediators of lung injury in mice following systemic activation of complement. Am J Pathol 119:92–100
58. Heflin AC, Brigham KL (1981) Prevention by granulocyte depletion of increased vascular permeability of sheep lung following endotoxemia. J Clin Invest 68:1253–1260
59. Stokke T, Bachardi H, Hensel I, Kostering H, Kathner T, Rahlf G (1986) Continuous intravenous infusion of elastase in normal and agranulocytic minipigs—effects on the lungs and the blood coagulation system. Resuscitation 14:61–79
60. van Bebber IPT, Goris RJA (1990) Experimental induction of whole body inflammation leads to ARDS, MOF and sepsis. The ZIGI-model in rats and mice. Schlag G, Redl H, Siegel JH (eds) First Wiggers-Bernard conference. Springer, Berlin Heidelberg New York, pp 461–485

61. Brigham KL (1986) Role of free radicals in lung injury. Chest 89:859–863
62. West MA (1987) Macrophage effector function in sepsis. Arch Surg 122:242–247
63. Nathan C (1987) Secretory products of macrophages. J Clin Invest 79:319–326
64. Goris RJA, van Bebber IPT, Hendriks T (1991b) Role of bacterial translocation and selective gut decontamination in the development of multiple organ failure. In: Schlag G, Redl H, Siegel JH, Traber DL (eds) Second Wiggers-Bernard conference. Springer, Berlin, Heidelberg New York, pp 133–146
65. Steinberg S, Flynn W, Kelley K et al. (1989) Development of a bacteria-independent model of the multiple organ syndrome. Arch Surg 124:1390–1395
66. Mainous MR, Tso P, Berg RD, Deitch EA (1991) Studies of the route, magnitude, and time course of bacterial translocation in a model of systemic inflammation. Arch Surg 126:33–37
67. Okusawa S, Gelfland JA, Ikejima T, Connolly RJ, Dinarello CA (1988) Interleukin 1 induces a shock-like state in rabbits. J Clin Invest 81:1162–1172
68. Ohlsson K, Bjoerk P, Bergenfeldt M, Hageman R, Thompson RC (1990) Interleukin-1 receptor antagonist reduces mortality from endotoxin shock. Nature 348:550–552
69. Gaskill HV (1988) Continuous infusion of TNF: mechanisms of toxicity in the rat. J Surg Res 44:664–671
70. Tracey KJ, Fong Y, Hesse DG et al. (1987) Anti-cachectin/TNF monoclonal antibodies prevent septic shock during lethal bacteremia. Nature 330:662–664

Multiple Organ Failure (MOF), and Whole Body Inflammation After Multiple Trauma

G. Regel, H.C. Pape, F. Koopmann, and J.A. Sturm

Introduction

Multiple organ failure (MOF) is a cumulative sequelae of organ failures seen in association with multiple trauma. The exact pathomechanisms of this syndrome are still not known. A common etiology for the different organ function disturbances however has been suggested. As a possible mechanism for lung injury acute respiratory distress syndrome (ARDS), the activation of poly-morphonuclear leukocytes (PMNL), and the release of toxic oxygen radicals and intracellular destructing enzymes (f.e. elastase) at the vascular endothelium have been discussed [2, 3, 5]. This leads to an increase in permeability, to interstitial edema, and consequently to respiratory dysfunction. Other organs are supposed to be injured by similar mechanisms, causing a generalized inflammatory reaction [1, 3, 4].

The morphologic characteristics of MOF are only described in a limited number of autopsy studies, with an inhomogeneous patient population (3). In order to elucidate possible pathomechanisms, this morphologic study was designed to clarify the following questions:
1. Do we see signs of a generalized inflammatory process after multiple trauma?
2. Which pathomechanisms are responsible for this development, with special emphasize on inflammatory cells (i.e., PMNL)?
3. Does permeability damage and interstitial edema lead to the organ dysfunction?
4. Do these pathomechanisms explain the variability of sequential organ failure?

Material and Methods

We reviewed all autopsy reports and histologic sections of 59 patients dying after multiple trauma during 1983 and 1990. The patients were divided into three groups. Group 1 included multiple trauma patients dying from brain injury in the first 58 h. Group 2 consisted of the patients dying between the third

Department of Trauma Surgery, Hanover Medical School, 3000 Hanover 61, FRG

Host Defense Dysfunction
in Trauma, Shock and Sepsis
Eds. Faist/Meakins/Schildberg
© Springer-Verlag, Berlin Heidelberg 1993

and sixth day after trauma (excluding all patients with severe head injury). Finally group 3 summarizes all patients dying of organ failure after more than 1 week (after the seventh day). Group 1 functioned as a control group, showing early morphologic changes not associated with increasing organ failure.

Histologic specimens were evaluated independently by two physicians. Particular criteria for evalution were all signs associated with capillary damage (that means interstitial and cellular edema), cell infiltration (PMNL, macrophages), and all signs of increasing tissue destruction (necrosis, hemorrhage). All data were scored according to mild (grade 1), moderate (grade 2), and severe changes (grade 3). Three histologic sections per organ were scored. The percentages compared to the total number of specimens are listed in the results. Pathologic findings that were probably preexisting were recorded in addition. The organ weights were reviewed additionally and compared to those of a normal patient population.

Results

Fifteen multiple trauma patients died of severe head injury in the first 24 h (Fig. 1). However, the majority showed early morphologic changes in all organs. PMNL, for instance, were seen in all organs initially. This cell infiltration was highest in group 2, where up to 58% of the specimens showed PMNL invasion (Fig. 2). These changes were seen especially in the lung, where neutrophils were found both in the interstitial and in the alveolar space.

Parallel to the cell infiltration a permeability edema was seen in all organs, again, with a maximum in group 2, i.e., between the second and sixth day. In group 3, both the percentage of neutrophil influx and edema were less severe. Edema was more pronounced in the lung and heart (Figs. 2 and 3). In the other

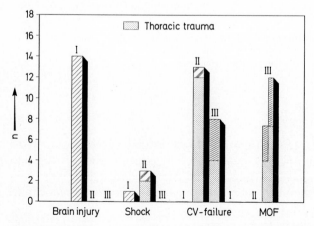

Fig. 1. Cause of death in the three groups studied. *CV*, cardiovascular

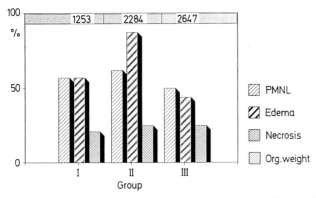

Fig. 2. Organ weight and presence of polymorphonuclear leukocytes (*PMNL*), edema, and necrosis in the lung

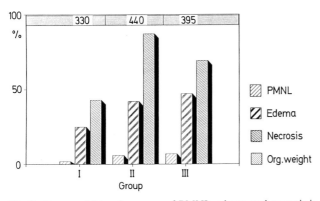

Fig. 3. Organ weight and presence of PMNL, edema, and necrosis in the heart

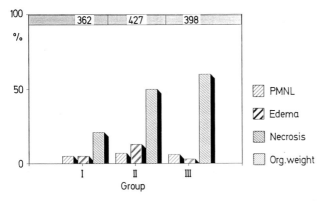

Fig. 4. Organ weight and presence of PMNL, edema, and necrosis in the kidney

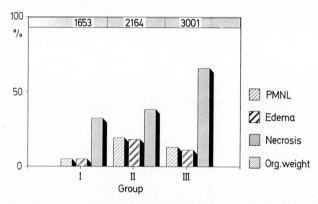

Fig. 5. Organ weight and presence of PMNL, edema, and necrosis in the liver

organs we saw more necrosis formation (Figs. 4 and 5). Necrosis was seen in all organs with a maximum in group 3 (death >7 days after trauma; $n = 28$).

Parallel to tissue destruction (necrosis) a continuous increase in organ weight is noted from group 1–3. The extent of weight increase is similar to other autopsy studies of multiple trauma [3].

Discussion

MOF is said to result from a whole-body inflammatory reaction [2–4]. This reaction is supposed to be the consequence of a "host injury" mechanism induced by activated PMNL adhering to the vascular endothelium following multiple trauma [5]. Recent morphologic studies, however, could not prove the independency of this "inflammation" from other posttraumatic complications (pneumonia, systemic infections) [3].

In our study PMNL infiltration was seen in all organs immediately after trauma (group 1), suggesting the independency of this pathomechanism from an infectious origin. A maximum was seen in those patients dying before the sixth day (group 2). Obviously initial trauma and here especially the resorption of debris into the blood circulation leads to a systemic activation of these cells followed by a generalized interstitial and cellular edema. Complement activation, for example, is one possible factor that can initiate this systemic reaction [2–4].

The degree of cell infiltration in the different organs is paralleled by a similar degree of interstitial edema, supporting the idea that the development of inflammation and permeability change in the microvasculature have the same pathomechanism in all organs.

In group 2 the fulminant onset of edema formation probably leads to an early organ dysfunction of the lung, which is often associated with the clinical

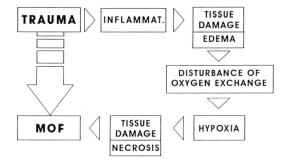

Fig. 6. Sequence of events leading to multiogan failure (*MOF*)

diagnosis ARDS (group 2:8/16 have an ARDS). In this group necrosis was seen particularly in the heart. This is thought to be the consequence of an oxygen mismatch in the microvasculature of the myocardium. Oxygen uptake and utilization could be disturbed because of an altered blood flow distribution in the capillary bed following edema formation, or could be the consequence of a decreased systemic gas exchange resulting from the described alterations in respiratory function (ARDS). Clinically this imposes a so-called "hypoxic cardiovascular failure" (group 2 12 out of 16 patients), (Fig. 1).

Late death, following a prolonged course (> 7 days) is mainly caused by sequential failure of all organs [1–4]. In these patients (group 3) an increase in necrosis formation in all organs was demonstrated (compared to group 2). Different etiologies for this tissue destruction have been discussed. Some authors believe that a considerable part of the morphologic abnormalities that are found in this series of patients may be explained by the toxic effects of the activated granulocytes [3, 4]. On the other hand ongoing hypoxia and ischemia in the capillary bed might also be the cause of the observed destruction [1]. From our results we believe, that a prolonged onset of edema formation may first lead to a compensatory oxygen mismatch. Only long-term disturbances (remaining tissue injury, hematoma, prolonged shock, etc.) aggravate cell activation and edema, leading to an increasing necrosis of all organs. The extent of tissue destruction is the morphologic predictor of MOF (Fig. 6). The sequence of organ dysfunction is dependent upon the sensitivity of the single organ to edema and necrosis formation.

References

1. Dorinsky PM, Gadek JE (1989) Mechanisms of multiple nonpulmonary organ failure in ARDS. Chest 96:885–892
2. Goris JA, te Boekhorst TP, Nuytinck JK (1985) Multiple organ failure: generalized auto-destructive inflammation? Arch Surg 120:1109–1115
3. Nuytinck HK, Xavier JM, Offermanns W, Kubat K, Goris JA (1988) Whole-body inflammation in trauma patients. Arch Surg 123:1519–1524

4. Nuytinck JK, Goris JA, Redl H, Schlag G, van Munster PJ (1986) Posttraumatic complications and inflammatory mediators. Arch Surg 121:886–890
5. Sacks T, Moldow CF, Craddock PR, Bowers TK, Jacob HS (1978) Oxygen radicals mediate endothelial cell damage by complement-stimulated granulocytes. J Clin Invest 22:1161–1167

Neutrophils, Cytokines, Oxygen Radicals, and Lung Injury

P. A. Ward, M. S. Mulligan, and J. S. Warren

Acute lung injury is a common feature of the adult respiratory distress syndrome in which there is cellular injury involving both pulmonary microvascular endothelial cells and alveolar epithelial cells. In an attempt to define in greater detail the pathophysiological events that underlie the development of acute lung injury, we have employed the rat model of acute lung injury following intraalveolar deposition of immunoglobulin G (IgG) immune complexes. In this model, injury involves both microvascular endothelial cells as well as alveolar epithelial cells in a manner that is complement dependent, neutrophil dependent, and related to the formation of toxic oxygen species, inasmuch as interventions involving catalase, superoxide dismutase, and scavengers of HO· are all protective [1–3]. It is now becoming evident that products of both neutrophils and lung macrophages are involved in the processes leading to injury.

The evidence that products of neutrophils are critical for the full development of injury is based primarily on the finding that neutrophil depletion by the use of polyclonal antibody has a highly protective effect on the outcome of lung injury. Injury, as defined by leakage of ^{125}I-albumin into lung parenchyma, is reduced by $> 70\%$. The protective effects of antibody to neutrophils have been confirmed by morphological analysis, which reveals the virtual absence of intraalveolar hemorrhage and fibrin deposition in neutrophil-depleted animals [1].

What is a bit surprising is the accumulating evidence in this model that products of lung macrophages play a key role in the ultimate process leading to lung injury. Evidence for macrophage involvement is not from macrophage-depletion procedures (which are difficult, uncertain, and subject to concerns of antibody specificity) but rather from experiments detailing the vital role of products uniquely derived from macrophages. One of the most important macrophage-related factors appears to be tumor necrosis factor α (TNF-α). This cytokine is present in relatively high concentrations in bronchoalveolar fluids (BAL) of rats developing injury following intraalveolar deposition of immune complexes [4]. Not surprisingly, direct stimulation in vitro of alveolar macrophages with IgG immune complexes will induce production and release of TNF-α as well as generation of oxygen products such as superoxide anion (O_2^-) and H_2O_2 [4, 5]. Formation and release of these products appears to be

Department of Pathology, The University of Michigan Medical School, 1301 Catherine Street, Ann Arbor, Michigan, USA

Host Defense Dysfunction
in Trauma, Shock and Sepsis
Eds. Faist/Meakins/Schildberg
© Springer-Verlag, Berlin Heidelberg 1993

facilitated by immune complexes that have been opsonized with complement. The fact that macrophages can contribute to the burden of toxic oxygen products in these lung inflammatory reactions may, in part, explain the contribution of macrophage products to injury. However, relatively simple calculations suggest that probably not more than 20% of the total burden of oxygen products is derived from macrophages in the model of IgG immune complex-induced injury.

The most compelling evidence for the role of lung macrophages in the model of IgG immune complex-induced injury comes from the finding that, in the presence of antibody that blocks the biological activity of TNF-α, there is a dramatic attenuation of the lung injury (> 80% reduction in increased vascular permeability) [4]. The most remarkable feature of the protective effects of antibody to TNF-α is the fact that, in the absence of available TNF-α, there is a profound reduction in the numbers of neutrophils accumulating in the lung following deposition of immune complexes. Not surprisingly, this is reflected morphologically by greatly diminished hemorrhage and deposition of fibrin within the alveolar compartment. By extraction from lung tissue of myeloperoxidase (a quantitative inductor of neutrophils), there is a > 60% reduction in lung accumulation of neutrophils. More impressively, there are few, if any, neutrophils within the alveolar compartment on the basis of morphological analysis.

These findings have led us to consider the manner by which TNF-α facilitates recruitment of neutrophils. Although there is some evidence that TNF-α may have chemotactic activity for neutrophils, the more obvious possibility is that TNF-α can activate endothelial cells in a manner that leads to upregulation on the surface of the endothelial cell of a molecule that has adhesive properties for neutrophils. This molecule, ELAM-1 (endothelial cell leukocyte adhesion molecule), reacts with a carbohydrate moiety on the neutrophil via a sial-Lew-x ligand attached to an unidentified protein backbone on the neutrophil [6]. ELAM is slowly upregulated in endothelial cells which have been incubated with TNF-α, reaching a peak at 4 h and subsequently disappearing from the surface of the endothelial cell [7–10]. Its upregulation requires active protein synthesis in the endothelial cell and can be blocked by cyclohexamide. The functional expression of ELAM can be detected by increased adherence of neutrophils to the TNF-α-exposed endothelial cells. Although ELAM is only one of many adhesion molecules expressed on endothelial cells, we have obtained preliminary evidence that its expression may be linked to the requirement for TNF-α in neutrophil recruitment into lung following deposition of immune complexes. *Firstly*, during the course of immune complex deposition in lung, immunoperoxidase staining for ELAM reveals a greatly increased reactivity of the lung vasculature with this antibody. Several hours after initiation of immune complex deposition, the immunoreactivity is found in venules and in what appear to be septal capillaries. At no time is vascular reactivity with anti-ELAM found in any other organ in the rat. *Secondly*, as indicated above, treatment in vivo of rats with anti-TNF-α greatly protects against injury following intrapulmonary deposition of immune complexes. This protection is associated with diminished recruitment into lungs of neutrophils. *Thirdly*, in rats pretreated with antibody to TNF-α, immunoperoxidase analysis of lung tissue reveals that treatment of rats with antibody to TNF-α virtually abolishes the upregulation of the pulmonary vasculature ELAM reactivity.

Thus, while incomplete, the accumulating evidence suggests the scheme of events outlined in Fig. 1. Following intraalveolar deposition of IgG immune complexes, there ensues both complement activation and stimulation of lung macrophages. The former yields the chemotactic peptide C5a, which is relatively nonfunctional until macrophage products "condition" the microenvironment. Activation of lung macrophages results in the release of TNF-α, which interacts with nearby endothelial cells to cause upregulation of ELAM (and probably other adhesion molecules). Increased expression of ELAM then permits adhesive interactions of endothelial cells with neutrophils, which can than respond to the chemotactic signal, C5a. The accumulating neutrophils are then stimulated by the tissue deposits of immune complexes to release toxic oxygen products as well as proteases, the combination of which will lead to damage of microvascular endothelial cells as well as alveolar epithelial cells.

The extent to which this pathway can be generalized to other inflammatory conditions associated with lung injury as well as to inflammatory mechanisms in

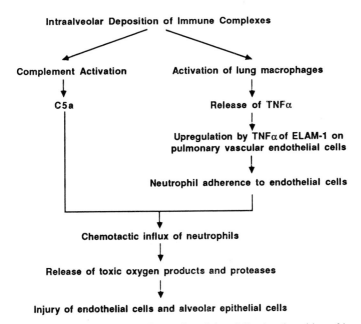

Fig. 1. Proposed pathways of acute lung injury following deposition of immune complexes. The ultimate injury, which can be ascribed to toxic oxygen products from phagocytic cells, is due to the combined effects of activated neutrophils and macrophages.

other organs is not known. However, with the increasing availability of antibodies to detect these molecules both in biological fluids as well as in tissues, it should be possible to resolve these important questions.

References

1. Johnson KJ, Ward PA (1974) Acute immunologic pulmonary alveolitis. J Clin Invest 54:349–356
2. Johnson KJ, Fantone JC, Kaplan J, Ward PA (1981) In vivo damage of rat lungs by oxygen metabolites. J Clin Invest 67:983–991
3. Johnson KJ, Ward PA (1981) Role of oxygen metabolites in immune complex injury of lung. J Immunol 126:1365–1369
4. Warren JS, Yabroff KR, Remick DG, Kunkel SL, Chensue SW, Kunkel RG, Johnson KJ, Ward PA (1989) Tumor necrosis factor participates in the pathogenesis of acute immune complex alveolitis in the rat. J Clin Invest 84:1873–1882
5. Ward PA, Duque RE, Sulavik MC, Johnson KJ (1983) In vitro and in vivo stimulation of rat neutrophils and alveolar macrophages by immune complexes. Production of O_2^- and H_2O_2. Am J Pathol 110:297–310
6. Lowe JB, Stoolman LM, Nair RP, Larsen RD, Berhend TL, Marks RM (1990) ELAM-1-dependent cell adhesion to vascular endothelium determined by a transfected human fucosyl-transferase cDNA. Cell 63:475–484
7. Gamble JR, Harlan JM, Klebanoff SJ, Vadas MA (1985) Stimulation of the adherence of neutrophils to umbilical vein endothelium by human recombinant tumor necrosis factor. Proc Natl Acad Sci USA 82:8667–8674
8. Pohlman TH, Stanness KA, Beatty PG, Ochs HD, Harlan JM (1986) An endothelial cell surface factor (2) induced in vitro by lipopolysaccharide interleukin 1, and tumor necrosis factor-α increases neutrophil adherence by a CDw18-dependent mechanism. J Immunol 136:4548–4553
9. Pober JS, Bevilacqua MP, Mendrick DL, Lapierre LA, Fiers W, Gimbrone MA Jr (1986) Two distinct monokines, interleukin 1 and tumor necrosis factor, each independently induce biosynthesis and transient expression of the same antigen on the surface of cultured human vascular endothelial cells. J Immunol 136:1680–1687
10. Bevilacqua MP, Pober JS, Mendrick DL, Cotran RS, Gimbrone MA Jr (1987) Identification of an inducible endothelial leukocyte adhesion molecule, ELAM-1. Proc Natl Acad Sci USA 84:9238–9242

The Role of β_2-Leukocyte Integrins In Vivo

S. R. Sharar, N. B. Vedder, W. J. Mileski, C. L. Rice, J. M. Harlan,
and R. K. Winn

Introduction

The acute inflammatory response is characterized by the destructive activity of leukocytes against foreign pathogens and/or host tissue. In the event of bacterial invasion, leukocytes are directed to the site of infection by the release of soluble chemotactic agents. Leukocyte localization to the appropriate endothelium results from adherence to endothelial cells, followed by subsequent migration to the site of infection. Leukocytes phagocytose the invading bacteria and release toxic products (e.g., oxygen radicals, proteases) into phagosomes to act against the invading pathogens to protect the host. In noninfectious conditions such as ischemia-reperfusion injury, leukocytes may release these same substances into surrounding tissue causing destruction to the host. This process can occur when activated leukocytes becoming adherent to endothelial cells form a protected microenvironment at the cell-cell interface. This region is relatively inaccessible to plasma inhibitors of toxic leukocyte products (e.g., antioxidants and antiproteases), resulting in direct endothelial cell injury by these leukocyte products, loss of vascular integrity, tissue edema, and thrombosis.

The key initial event in both of these examples of leukocyte-mediated destruction, one providing host defense and the other host destruction, is the adherence of leukocytes to endothelial cells. This cell-cell adherence is mediated by the interaction of a variety of leukocyte-cell surface-adherence receptors with cospecific counterstructures on endothelial cells. Functionally these receptors and counterstructures are either present in small numbers or totally absent on normal, unstimulated cells. However, with activation (e.g., infection, ischemia-reperfusion injury) these molecules are activated and/or upregulated, resulting in increased leukocyte adherence.

These adherence molecules are in general members of one of three families: immunoglobulins, selectins, or integrins. The integrins play the primary role in the adherence of neutrophils to endothelial cells. This review will focus on the β_2-integrin subfamily, and particularly on in vivo studies of neutrophil adhesion blockade.

Departments of Anesthesiology, Surgery, Medicine, and Physiology-Biophysics, University of Washington, Harborview Medical Center, Seattle, WA 98104, USA

Host Defense Dysfunction
in Trauma, Shock and Sepsis
Eds. Faist/Meakins/Schildberg
© Springer-Verlag, Berlin Heidelberg 1993

The β_2-Integrins

The integrin family consists of at least 14 heterodimers of paired α- and β-subunits (reviewed in [1, 2]). There are at least six distinct β-subunits and 11 α-subunits that in specific combination define different subfamilies. The β_2-subfamily of integrins consists of three leukocyte adhesion complexes designated CD11a/CD18, CD11b/CD18, and CD11c/CD18 (commonly called LFA-1, MAC-1, and GP150, 95, respectively). The complexes are each comprised of a common β-chain (CD18) and a distinct α-chain (CD11a, CD11b, or CD11c). CD11a/CD18 is expressed on lymphocytes and is involved with virtually every immune phenomenon requiring T-lymphocyte adhesion. It is also important in monocyte-endothelial cell interactions, but less involved in neutrophil adherence. CD11b/CD18, on the other hand, is found on monocytes and some lymphocytes, but is of primary importance in mediating neutrophil adhesion and aggregation. Little is known about CD11c/CD18, although it has been implicated in both monocyte and neutrophil adhesion to endothelium, and has been identified on some activated T-cell lines.

The β_2-integrins are normally expressed on leukocytes and can be up-regulated by exposure to chemotaxins such as formylated peptides, complement C5a, and phorbol esters. The mechanism of this increased surface expression appears to be the release of integrins from intracellular storage sites in peroxidase-negative granules. Under normal conditions these molecules are generally not activated and the activation process is poorly understood.

The importance of the β_2-integrins in the leukocyte inflammatory response became more clear with the development of specific monoclonal antibodies (MAbs) to each of the receptor complexes. The MAb of primary interest in our laboratory has been MAb 60.3 [3], a murine IgG_{2a} that recognizes a functional epitope on the CD18 subunit. This antibody has been shown in vitro to inhibit neutrophil aggregation, neutrophil adherence to endothelium, and endothelial disruption by activated neutrophils [4, 5]. In preliminary in vivo experiments, MAb 60.3 was found to inhibit neutrophil adherence and migration towards intradermal chemotaxins such as formylated peptides and leukotriene B_4 [6].

Endothelial Ligands of the β_2 Integrins

Leukocyte adherence molecules interact with cospecific receptors on the endothelial cell surface (reviewed ion [7]. β_2-integrins on neutrophils interact with intercellular adhesion molecule-1 (ICAM-1) on endothelial cells, with iC3b, and with fibrinogen as well as other yet to be identified molecules. ICAM-1 is expressed at low levels on human umbilical vein endothelium in vitro and on endothelium from a variety of vascular beds in vivo. Surface expression of ICAM-1 is increased with exposure to tumor necrosis factor (TNF), lipopolysaccharide (LPS), interleukin-1 (IL-1), and interferon-γ, resulting in increased neutrophil adherence. This upregulation is protein synthesis dependent, as it requires several hours and can be inhibited by the protein-synthesis inhibitors cyclohexamide or actinomycin-D. ICAM-2 is a truncated form of ICAM-1 and is involved in lymphocyte adherence to endothelium via CD11a/CD18 as well.

A large number of MAbs have been developed that block β_2-integrin-dependent leukocyte adherence and/or aggregation. These antibodies are either directed to one of the distinct α-chains or to the common β-chain. Antibodies directed to particular proteins in the CD11/CD18 complex may attach at different locations and result in slightly different actions. However, in general the anti-CD18 MAbs block the function of CD11a, CD11b, and CD11c. The effects of antibodies directed to α-chains may be more variable. The majority of MAbs recognize human molecules and many (especially anti-CD18 MAbs) cross react with other species.

In Vivo Studies of β_2-Adhesion Blockade

The in vitro data showing inhibition of neutrophil adherence with the use of MAbs against β_2-integrins has led numerous investigators to examine the potential beneficial effects of inhibiting adherence in vivo. The experimental protocols reviewed below primarily address ischemia-reperfusion injury; however, two additional studies examine bacterial meningitis and severe cold injury. In all but one of these investigations, anti-CD11/CD18 therapy showed benefit in terms of either animal mortality or morbidity.

Hernandez et al. [8] examined intestinal microvascular permeability in cats following 1 h of hypoperfusion (blood flows of 15%–20% of baseline) followed by subsequent reperfusion. Plasma protein permeability index, a measure of organ function, was measured in normal intestine prior to injury and then following ischemia-reperfusion. The protein permeability index for these experiments was determined from the lymph flow-independent lymph-to-plasma protein ratio (C_L/C_p). This C_L/C_p is theoretically equal to one minus the reflection coefficient and is used as the permeability index. Permeability index following ischemia-reperfusion was increased fourfold over baseline levels. However, pretreatment with MAb 60.3 or antineutrophil serum attenuated the increased protein permeability following ischemia and reperfusion. Hernandez et al. concluded that neutrophils mediate the oxygen radical-dependent injury associated with ischemic bowel.

Simpson et al. [9] examined myocardial ischemia-reperfusion injury in open chest anesthetized dogs using the anti-CD11b MAb 904. Ischemia was produced by occluding the left circumflex coronary artery for 90 min prior to reperfusion for 6 h. Antibody treatment was given after 45 min of ischemia. The infarct size as a percent of the region at risk was reduced from 47.6% $\pm$ 5.5% to 28.5% $\pm$ 5.7% in the MAb 904-treated group. These data demonstrated a reduction in infarct size with inhibition of neutrophil adherence when antibody was given after induction of ischemia but 45 min prior to reperfusion.

Vedder et al. [10] used two similar protocols of hemorrhagic shock to compare the morbidity and mortality of rabbits treated with MAb 60.3 to those treated with saline. In the first series of experiments rabbits were pretreated with MAb 60.3, then blood withdrawn until the cardiac output was at 30% of baseline values. Hypotension was maintained for 1 h before animals were resuscitated with their shed blood and lactated Ringer's solution to restore cardiac output to baseline levels. Survival at 5 days in the MAb 60.3-treated animals was 100% compared to only 29% in saline-treated animals. In addition, there was necropsy evidence of hepatic and gastric edema, hemorrhage, and necrosis in the control animals that was either absent or markedly attenuated in the antibody-treated rabbits.

In a second set of experiments, hemorrhage was again produced to 30% of baseline cardiac output but was sustained for 2 h [11]. In these experiments, MAb 60.3 was given at the time of resuscitation (i.e., at a clinically relevant time) and resulted in similar attenuation of both mortality and evidence of injury at necropsy similar to the pretreatment study. Survival at 5 days was 71% in the antibody-treated group compared to 0% in the control group. Pathologic tissue findings were similarly attenuated as in the pretreatment study. These data suggest that leukocyte adhesion plays a critical role in organ injury and survival after severe shock and resuscitation, and that a substantial portion of the injury occurs at the time of reperfusion. The degree of injury in this second set of experiments was more severe than in the first due to a longer duration of ischemia; however, administration of MAb 60.3 at the time of resuscitation appeared to provide equivalent protection to that seen with antibody pretreatment.

Regional ischemia-reperfusion injury was examined in the same laboratory using rabbit ears made ischemic for 10 h [12]. The ear was first transected leaving only the central artery and vein intact. It was then reattached and its volume measured by displacement. Animals were divided into four groups. Two groups were given MAb 60.3 (either before ischemia or at the time of reperfusion) and one was given normal saline as a control. A clip was placed on both artery and vein for 10 h for these three groups. The last group was prepared identically to the treatment groups but was not subjected to ischemia. The saline-treated group has significant edema following ischemia-reperfusion (Fig. 1), which was significantly reduced in the animals given MAb 60.3. MAb 60.3 was effective at preventing injury when administered prior to ischemia and equally effective when administered following ischemia but prior to reperfusion. The small difference between nonischemic control animals and MAb 60.3-treated animals was not statistically significant. Tissue necrosis at the end of the experiment was 23.8% $\pm$ 11.1% in saline-treated and 3.0% $\pm$ 2.0% in the MAb 60.3-treated animals. There was no necrosis in nonischemic animals. These experiments show that neutrophil adhesion causes much of the injury in this

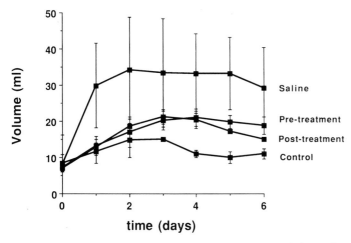

Fig. 1. Ear volume (Mean ± SE) is shown as an indicator of tissue edema following ischemia-reperfusion injury in four groups of rabbits: saline-treated animals sustaining ischemia-reperfusion injury ($n = 8$); pre-treatment with monoclonal antibody (MAb) 60.3 prior to ischemia and again prior to reperfusion ($n = 5$); post-treatment with MAb 60.3 immediately prior to reperfusion ($n = 5$); control animals undergoing identical surgical procedure but not made ischemic ($n = 3$). Injury protocol is described in text. (Adapted from [12])

type of regional ischemia-reperfusion injury, and that injury is primarily a consequence of reperfusion.

Different species may respond to hemorrhage differently; thus, it is important to examine the responses to shock and antibody treatment in another species. Mileski et al. induced hemorrhagic shock in a series of rhesus monkeys and gave MAb 60.3 at the time of resuscitation [13]. Cardiac output was reduced to 30% of baseline for 90 min, and then treatment was given with either saline ($n = 7$) or the anti-CD18 MAbs 60.3 ($n = 5$) or R 15.7 ($n = 1$). Monkeys were resuscitated with their shed blood. An infusion of 4 ml/kg per h of lactated Ringer's solution was started in all animals following return of shed blood, with additional volume being given as necessary to maintain cardiac output at preshock values. Two of five control monkeys died at 72 h, whereas none of the five antibody-treated animals died. Fluid requirements are shown in Fig. 2 for both groups of animals. The MAb 60.3-treated animals required less resuscitation fluid in the initial 24 h, gained less weight (0.08 + 0.11 kg vs 0.70 + 0.37 kg), and had no endoscopic evidence of gastritis compared to controls. Mileski et al. [13] concluded from these data that the protective effect of MAb 60.3 is not species specific and that the protective effect can be shown in a clinically relevant resuscitation protocol.

Tissue loss following severe cold injury was investigated in a series of experiments by W. J. Mileski (personal communication). The hind legs of rabbits were shaved and immersed in a salt water bath at -15 °C for 30 min then

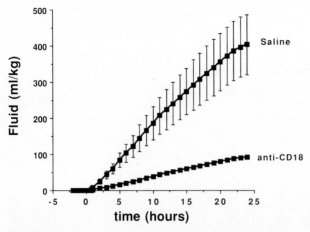

Fig. 2. Comparison of cumulative 24 h fluid resuscitation requirements (Mean $\pm$ SD) for two groups of rhesus monkeys following hemorrhagic shock: saline treatment after shock but prior to resuscitation ($n = 5$); anti-CD18 treatment after shock but prior to resuscitation ($n = 5$). Hemorrhagic shock and resuscitation protocol are described in text

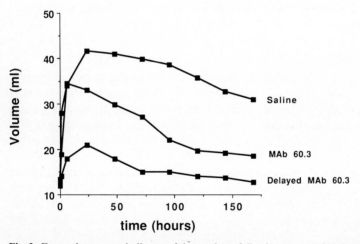

Fig. 3. Foot volume as an indicator of tissue edema following severe cold injury in three groups of rabbits: saline-treated animals ($n = 6$); monoclonal antibody (MAb) 60.3-treated animals ($n = 8$); delayed MAb 60.3-treated animals ($n = 5$). Injury protocol is described in text. (From W. J. Mileski, Personal communication)

rewarmed in a water bath at 42 ° for 30 min. Treatment was given with saline or MAb 60.3 at the time of reperfusion. A second treatment group received MAb 60.3 after rewarming was completed. Tissue edema and necrosis were measured and there was a significant reduction in tissue edema in animals treated with MAb 60.3 (Fig. 3). Limb blood flow was present immediately after rewarming in the antibody-treated group, and exceeded baseline by 350% at 60 min. In contrast perfusion did not return to control rabbit limbs until 30 min after rewarming, and never increased above baseline levels throughout the 3-day study period. Blood flow was not measured in the group treated at the time of rewarming. These studies indicate that a substantial component of severe cold injury occurs following rewarming, appears to be neutrophil mediated, and can be attenuated by treatment with MAb 60.3. The pattern of blood flow in the control and MAb-treated groups suggest that much of the injury might be due to a lack of perfusion.

In experiments examining a completely different class of injury, Tuomanen et al. described the effects of β_2-integrin blockade on the morbidity associated with experimental bacterial meningitis in rabbits [14]. With the administration of the anti-CD18 MAb, IB4, prior to intracisternal injection of live *Streptococcus pneumoniae*, the authors observed decreases in brain edema, time to development of bacteremia, and animal mortality compared to controls. These results are intriguing and somewhat unexpected, since normal leukocyte adherence appears to be a crucial initial event in host defense against bacterial pathogens. Interference with this adherence using MAbs to β_2-integrins would theoretically increase the morbidity associated with bacterial infections such as meningitis.

Thornton et al. have reported on the use of MAb 60.3 in rabbits following renal ischemia and 48 h of reperfusion [15]. Bilateral renal artery occlusion was produced after either pretreatment with saline or MAb 60.3. There was no difference between groups in the subsequent renal injury as assessed by histology, blood urea nitrogen, plasma creatinine concentrations at 24 and 48 h after the insult. These experiments lead to the conclusion that the neutrophil is not a critical participant in renal ischemia-reperfusion injury.

Conclusions

Late deaths in trauma patients frequently occur as a result of multiple organ failure syndrome (MOFS), which is accompanied by a generalized inflammatory response manifest by either leukocytosis or leukopenia, fever, tachacardia, and a hyperdynamic state. The generalized inflammation may result from a septic or nonseptic origin with approximately 50% of the cases having no known source of infection at autopsy [16, 17]. MOFS in trauma patients may account for some 25 000–40 000 deaths each year with an additional 25 000–40 000 patients having extended hospital stays as a result of MOFS. It is our hypothesis that the generalized inflammation occurs prior to any organ injury and that activated neutrophils through their attachment to endothelial cells cause the injury.

The events leading to generalized inflammation following trauma, particularly those of noninfectious origin, are postulated to results from maldistribution of perfusion leading to ischemic vascular beds followed by reperfusion at the time of resuscitation. The maldistribution of perfusion can occur even in the absence of severe hemorrhage but is more clearly defined if the hypovolemia is severe. Thus we propose that resuscitation from trauma results in an ischemia-reperfusion injury that can be treated with MAbs directed to β_2-leukocyte integrins.

The importance of leukocyte adherence molecules, in particular the β_2-integrins, in the development of microvascular and tissue injury following ischemia and reperfusion has been clearly demonstrated in the in vivo studies reviewed here. Ischemia-reperfusion injury is clearly caused by neutrophils using a pathway that involves the CD11/CD18 glycoprotein complex in cat gut, dog heart, rabbit ear, and whole body of both monkeys and rabbits. Ischemia and reperfusion of the kidney is not dependent on CD11/CD18 and probably is not due to neutrophils, since neutrophil depletion in rats did not alter outcome [15]. The extent that other organs are affected remains to be determined.

Acknowledgements. This work was supported by HL 43141, GM 42686, GM 07037, HL 30542, and a grant from The American Heart Association of Washington.

References

1. Larson RS, Springer TA (1990) Structure and function of leukocyte integrins. Immunol Rev 114:181–217
2. Albelda SM, Buck CA (1990) Integrins and other cell adhesion molecules. FASEB J 4:2868–2880
3. Patarroyo M, Beatty PG, Serhan CN, Gahmberg CG (1985) Identification of a cell-surface glycoprotein mediating adhesion in human granulocytes. Scand J Immunol 22:619–623
4. Diener AM, Beatty PG, Ochs HD, Harlan JM (1985) The role of neutrophil membrane glycoprotein 150 (GP-150) in neutrophil-mediated endothelial cell injury in vitro. J Immunol 135:537–543
5. Harlan JM, Schwartz BR, Reidy MA, Schwartz SM, Ochs HD, Harker LA (1985) Activated neutrophils disrupt endothelial monolayer integrity by an oxygen radical-independent mechanism. Lab Invest 52:141–150
6. Arfors KE, Lundberg C, Lindbom L, Lunderg K, Beatty PG, Harlan JM (1987) a monoclonal antibody to the membrane glycoprotein complex CD18 inhibits polymorphonuclear leukocyte accumulation and plasma leakage in vivo. Blood 69:338–340
7. Carlos TM, Harlan JM (1990) Membrane proteins involved in phagocyte adherence to endothelium. Immunol Rev 114:5–28
8. Hernandez LA, Grisham MB, Twohig B, Arfors KE, Harlan JM, Granger DN (1987) Role of neutrophils in ischemia-reperfusion-induced microvascular injury. Am J Physiol 253:H699–H703
9. Simpson PJ, Todd RF III, Fantone JC, Mickelson JK, Griffin JD, Lucchesi BR (1988) Reduction of experimental canine myocardial reperfusion injury by a monoclonal antibody (anti-Mol, anti-CD11b) that inhibits leukocyte adhesion. J Clin Invest 81:624–629
10. Vedder NB, Winn RK, Rice CL, Chi EY, Arfors KE, Harlan JM (19988) A monoclonal antibody to the adherence promoting leukocyte glycoprotein CD18 reduces organ injury and improves survival from hemorrhagic shock and resuscitation in rabbits. J Clin Invest 81:939–944
11. Vedder NB, Fouty BW, Winn RK, Harlan JM, Rice CL (1989) Role of neutrophils in generalized reperfusion injury associated with resuscitation from shock. Surgery 106:509–516
12. Vedder NB, Winn RK, Rice CL, Chi EY, Arfors KE, Harlan JM (1990) Inhibition of leukocyte adherence by anti-CD18 monoclonal antibody attenuates reperfusion injury in the rabbit ear. Proc Natl Acad Sci USA 87:2643–2646

13. Mileski WJ, Winn RK, Vedder NB, Pohlaman TH, Harlan JM, Rice CL (1990) Inhibition of CD18-dependent neutrophil adherence reduces organ injury after hemorrhagic shock in primates. Surgery 108:206–212
14. Tuomanen EI, Saukkonen Kirsi, Sande S, Cioffe C, Wright SD (1989) Reduction of inflammation, tissue damage, and mortality in bacterial meningitis in rabbits treated with monoclonal antibodies against adhesion-promoting receptors of leukocytes. J Exp Med 170:959–968
15. Thornton MA, Winn R, Alpers CE, Zager RA (1989) An evaluation of the neutrophil as a mediator of in vivo renal ischemic-reperfusion injury. Am J Pathol 135:509–515
16. Faist E, Bauer AE, Dittmer H, Heberer G (1983) Multiple organ failure in polytrauma patients. J Trauma 23:775–787
17. Goris RJA, te Boekhorst TPA, Nuytinck JKS, Gimbrere JSF (1985) Multiple organ failure. Generalized autodestructive inflammation? Arch Surg 120:1109–1115

The "Angry" Macrophage and Its Impact on Host Response Mechanisms

R.V. Maier

The severely injured or critically ill surgical patient in the intensive care unit (ICU) is at high risk for immune dysfunction. This immune dysfunction is thought to be caused by an uncontrolled, unfocused, disseminated activation of the host's normally protective inflammatory cascades. This resultant "malignant systemic inflammation" produces an immunologic dichotomy. The nondiscriminant systemic activation of the inflammatory process produces diffuse multiple organ bystander injury leading to progressive organ dysfunction and organ failure as seen in the multiple organ failure syndrome (MOFS) [1]. Concomitantly, this excessive activation and consumption plus a simultaneous endogenous attempt to downregulate or suppress this inflammatory response leads to a loss of normal immune responsiveness. This immunosuppression inhibits the ability to mount a focused immune response to contain areas of acute inflammation and early invasive infections. Thus, loss of local homeostasis occurs while simultaneous diffuse systemic organ injury and subsequent dysfunction occur.

Although this malignant systemic inflammation is most commonly caused by a disseminated infectious process, i.e., "sepsis," it has become well recognized that other massive inflammatory stimuli can also induce a similar host response, i.e., the "sepsis syndrome" [2, 3]. Massive soft tissue injury, hypovolemia-induced total body ischemia with subsequent reperfusion, fat embolization, multiple blood transfusions, and other events that lead to disseminated activation of the inflammatory cascades can produce the sepsis syndrome. The sepsis syndrome is defined as clinical evidence of systemic inflammatory activation with a concomitant hemodynamic impact. The important factor underlying the risk for MOFS is the development of malignant systemic inflammation. Studies investigating the adult respiratory distress syndrome (ARDS) and MOFS have shown that bacteremia per se is a low risk etiologic factor while a systemic host response to infection or other inflammatory stimulus produces a 30%–40% risk of ARDS and MOFS [4]. Thus, it is the host response to the inflammatory stimuli rather than the type or etiology of the inflammatory stimuli that produce the subsequent immunologic-induced dysfunction seen in the critically ill patient.

Systemic malignant inflammation represents nondiscriminant diffuse activation of both the humoral and cellular components of the host immune response

University of Washington, Northwest Regional Trauma Center, Harborview Medical Center, Seattle, WA, 98104, USA

Host Defense Dysfunction
in Trauma, Shock and Sepsis
Eds. Faist/Meakins/Schildberg
© Springer-Verlag, Berlin Heidelberg 1993

Table 1. Macrophage-derived inflammatory mediators

Mediators

Chemoattractants
  C5a
  Leukotriene B_4 (LTB_4)
  Interleukin-8 (IL-8)
Vasoactive Agents
  C3a
  Prostacycline (PGI_2)
  Leukotriene (LT) C_4; D_4
Thrombotic Factors
  Thromboxane A_2 (TXA_2)
  Procoagulant activity (PCA)
  Plasminogen activator inhibitor (PAI)
"Metabolic" Agents
  Interleukin-1 (IL-1)
  Interleukin-6 (IL-6)
Pathophysiologic Agents
  Tumor necrosis factor (TNF)
  Platelet activating factor (PAF)
Immunosuppressors
  Prostaglandin E_2 (PGE_2)
  Interferon gamma depressed

[1]. All of the inflammatory humoral cascades and a multitude of cellular components of the immune system have been identified as contributing to this uncontrolled inflammatory response. The humoral systems involved include the coagulation cascade (intrinsic and extrinsic pathways), complement activation, arachidonic acid metabolism, and multiple soluble mediators that function as cell-cell proinflammatory communicators. These include the interleukins (particularly IL-1, IL-6, and IL-8), interferon-γ, tumor necrosis factor, and platelet activating factor (Table 1). The cellular components of this inflammatory response involve neutrophil, platelet, monocyte/tissue-fixed macrophage, mass cell, basophil, and endothelial cell activation. While the neutrophil has been most studied and is known to be central to diffuse organ toxicity through activation and release of potent proteases and oxidants, the neutrophil is only one component of a multiply interlinked, highly complex response [5].

The tissue-fixed macrophage (Mø) is ideally located in each of the various injured organs of MOFS and the highly metabolic, long-lived Mø is recognized as a central regulator controlling the extent and dissemination of the inflammatory process [1, 6]. The Mø is an extremely active cell capable of producing not only directly cytotoxic agents similar to the neutrophil, but also multiple other cytokines and central mediators that regulate and augment the inflammatory response (Table 1). The Mø is the major source of (a) chemotactic agents for neutrophils, other monocytes, and other inflammatory cells, (b) production and release of vasoactive arachidonic acid metabolites, (c) complement components,

(d) thrombotic agents, (e) metabolic mediators, (f) physiologic modulators, and (g) immunosuppressive agents. Each of these products of macrophage metabolism is highly effective in enhancing and augmenting the local inflammatory response to invasive organisms or focal tissue damage. However, the disseminated activation of the Mø with diffuse production and activation of the subsequent inflammatory cascades and cells becomes deleterious and leads to multiple organ injury and subsequent MOFS.

The Mø is capable of producing essentially all of the toxic agents involved in activated neutrophil-induced injury [6]. The Mø through a nicotinamide adenine dinucleotide, reduced (NADH)-dependent oxidative burst produces toxic oxygen radicals including superoxide, hydrogen peroxide, and hydroxyl radical. Myeloperoxidase is not present in the Mø, and thus, production of hypochlorous and other halide acids does not occur. These toxic oxygen radicals are present in elevated concentrations during inflammation leading to MOFS. Bronchoalveolar lavage samples from patients with ARDS have increased levels of oxidants and the byproducts of oxidation, including lipid peroxides along with inactivated protective antioxidants and antiproteases [7]. In addition, the Mø, similar to the neutrophil, produces large quantities of multiple potent proteases including elastase, collagenase, β-glucuronidase, acid hydrolase, lysozyme, and other proteases. These proteases are capable of remodeling an area of injury or infection, and thus create a contained abscess or remodel a wound for healing. However, with nondiscriminant diffuse activation, significant injury to the structural substance and cellular content of the various organs occurs [7]. Diffuse destruction of the basement membrane and endothelial lining of the microcirculation leads to leakage and edema formation with subsequent thrombosis and parenchymal ischemia [8]. The location of the tissue-fixed Mø throughout the various organs that are seen to fail during MOFS and concomitant diffuse parenchymal injuries support the contribution of the Mø to this deleterious process.

The Mø is a major of chemotactic agents that activate, attract, and induce emigration and subsequent bystander cell injury by neutrophils. These chemotactic agents include C5a, LTB4, and interleukin-8 (IL-8) [9]. In addition to activation of the complement cascade with production of anaphylatoxins, C5a and C3a, the Mø is also capable of directly producing and releasing activated C5a and C3a [6]. In addition, the lipoxygenase-dependent arachidonic acid metabolite leukotriene B4 (LTB4) is produced by the tissue-fixed Mø. LTB4 produced by the alveolar Mø is thought to be the major chemotactic agent involved in attracting neutrophils to the lung [10]. In addition, increased production of interleukin-8 (IL-8) has been shown in inflammatory lung injury with an increase in messenger RNA and IL-8 protein in bronchoalveolar lavage and pulmonary tissue samples. The localized production and release of these chemotactic agents to create a gradient to attract neutrophils to areas of infection and tissue injury is appropriate while the diffuse production and nondiscriminant activation and attraction of neutrophils leads to deleterious injury to the microcirculation throughout the body.

During the inflammatory respone, once the neutrophil is activated and attracted to the area of inflammation, other mediators are released to enhance the emigration of the neutrophil from the intravascular space. This places the neutrophil in the interstitial space where the infectious process and tissue destructive process is occurring. The Mø contributes to this process by releasing vasoactive mediators that both cause vasodilation in the area of inflammation and increase microvascular permeability. The major mediators released by the Mø include C3a, leukotrienes C4 and D4, and the prostanoid PGI_2 or prostacyclin. Each of these agents causes significant vasodilation and increase in microvascular permeability allowing humoral and formed cellular elements to extravasate and migrate from the intravascular space to the interstitial space. The disseminated activation of this process again contributes to the marked microvascular permeability and massive third spacing and edema underlying subsequent organ dysfunction, particularly in the lung leading to the increased A-a gradient in ARDS [5].

Concomitant with the release of vasoactive mediators increasing microvascular permeability, the Mø simultaneously produces agents capable of enhancing the thrombotic process [11]. This process isolates the inflammatory or infectious process for both optimal resolution of the process and to prevent systemic dissemination. The Mø releases large quantities of thromboxane A_2 (TXA_2). TXA_2 is a potent vasoconstrictor leading to microvascular stasis which enhances thrombus formation. Production of procoagulants by both the Mø and the underlying injured, proinflammatory endothelial cell support this thrombic process. The Mø produces enormous quantities of procoagulant activity (PCA; similar to tissue factor) which initiates coagulation, particularly in the face of the microvascular stasis induced by the TXA_2 [11]. TXA_2, in addition, causes activation and aggregation of platelets leading to platelet plugging of the microcirculation. Other mediators released by the Mø including IL-1 and tumor necrosis factor (TNF) stimulate the production of procoagulant activity by the normally thrombotic-resistant endothelial lining. Finally, the Mø, in response to inflammatory stimuli, produces plasminogen activator inhibitor (PAI). PAI counteracts the activation of plasminogen to plasmin and retards lysis of clot in areas of inflammation. The combination of increased permeability in the areas of inflammation with thrombosis of surrounding microvasculature leads to an effective mechanism at focusing defense mechanisms while preventing systemic dissemination. The systemic occurrence of this process produces diffuse microvascular permeability and simultaneous thrombosis. As a result, repeated episodes of ischemia/reperfusion injury occur throughout the microcirculation of various organ beds leading to organ injury, dysfunction, and failure [1, 8].

The Mø produces major "metabolic" mediators with significant affects on metabolism, particularly catabolism. The major metabolic mediators produced in large quantities by the Mø include the interleukins, predominately IL-1 and IL-6, and TNF [12, 13]. IL-1, previously known as endogenous pyrogen, causes much of the catabolism during the response to inflammation. Endogenous pyrogen is responsible for resetting the thermostat of the hypothalamus via activation of arachidonic acid metabolism leading to pyrexia. In addition, IL-1 is a major stimulant for maturation and release of neutrophils from the bone marrow leading to the neutrophilia seen during inflammation. An IL-1 by-product is also known to be a major effector of the catabolism of peripheral skeletal muscle leading to release of amino acids for shunting into gluconeogenesis as an alternative energy source [12]. IL-6 is a major mediator of the acute-phase response. Production of protein C and other acute-phase reactants in response to stress is induced in large part by IL-6 released from hepatic macrophages (Kuppfer's cells). These combined events lead to a catabolic state with redistribution of amino acids to gluconeogenesis to maintain circulating glucose levels, and also in the production of acute-phase reactants by the liver in response to inflammation.

The physiologic derangements seen during the malignant systemic inflammation process are largely directed by by-products of Mø activation and directly mediated by arachidonic acid metabolites at the target-cell level. The major mediators produced include tumor necrosis factor (TNF) and platelet activating factor (PAF) [13, 14]. Both of these agents are potent central mediators of the pathophysiologic response to systemic inflammation from endotoxin, bacteria, and multiple other stimuli. TNF, first recognized for its ability to lyse certain tumor cell lines, has been found to be identical to the metabolic mediator, cachectin [13]. Cachectin is a major mediator of the cachectic wasting state seen in animal models and presumably in humans secondary to chronic infections with parasitic diseases and other wasting diseases including tumor burden. Direct infusion of recombinant TNF reproduces most of the pathophysiologic sequences seen following endotoxin injection and during sepsis [13]. In addition, antibody to TNF ameliorates the host response to endotoxemia and improves survival to lethal endotoxin infusion. Similarly, PAF reproduces many of the pathophysiologic responses to endotoxin in the systemic inflammatory process [14]. PAF is a by-product in most cells of arachidonic acid metabolism which releases a three carbon phosphorylated and acylated glycine compound from the lipid membrane. PAF originally was described as a small lipid molecule capable of activating platelets, leading to aggregation and microembolization. PAF is also a major activator of neutrophil function. PAF also augments and primes the Mø for subsequent enhanced reactivity to inflammatory stimuli [15]. PAF alone stimulates the release of minimal levels of inflammatory mediators such as TNF by the Mø. However, PAF primes the Mø to subsequent stimulation with endotoxin or other cytokines to produce and release enormous levels of TNF, PCA, and other mediators. Similar to TNF, PAF antagonists that compete for the PAF membrane receptor ameliorate the pathophysiologic response to endotoxin and enhance survival to lethal doses of endotoxin [14]. Thus, these potent central mediators of the inflammatory response are responsible for much of the physiologic alteration seen during endotoxemia and the malignant systemic inflammation reaction.

Finally, the Mø is also responsible for much of the immunosuppressive state seen subsequent to massive disseminated inflammation. The normal response to inflammatory stimuli is a subsequent release to mediators to downregulate the inflammatory response to protect the organism against an overreaction and potential deleterious effect. However, during the malignant systemic inflammation process, the immunosuppressive response becomes systemic and subsequently leads to an enhanced susceptibility to infection and infectious complications. The major mediator identified is the prostanoid PGE_2, which has diffuse immunosuppressive activities [16]. This agent appears to function similarly to a weak corticosteroid with diffuse effects throughout the immune system. A major impact of PGE_2 is to downregulate the production of many mediators by the Mø. PGE_2 is known to function through a cell membrane receptor which increases intracellular cyclic AMP and cause a downregulation of production and release of multiple mediators including TNF. In addition, PGE_2 downregulates the functional state of the T cell immune response with decreased expression of IL-2 receptor and decreased production of interferon-γ (IFN-γ). Decreased levels of IFN-γ subsequently lead to a decrease in expression of HLA-Dr antigen by the Mø/monocyte [17]. This antigen is necessary for presentation of antigen to the T cell for a normal cellular immune response. The downregulation of this antigen on the surface of the macrophage leads to paralysis of the cellular immune system and potential enhanced susceptibility to infection, particularly with nonbacterial agents. This response can be ameliorated by exogenous addition of IFN-γ or through inhibition of production of PGE_2 [17]. In the normal sequence, an inflammatory response occurs locally while PGE_2 and other downregulating agents prevent the dissemination, overproduction, or continued production of potentially deleterious products. However, the systemic production and release of PGE_2 over prolonged periods of time has been shown in numerous animal and clinical studies to depress the ability of the normal host response and enhance the susceptibility of the host to infectious complications [16].

The Mø is an extremely active metabolic cell which is located intricately within the multiple organs seen to fail during MOFS. The Mø is central to the regulation of the inflammatory process. Mø augments the inflammatory response locally to contain infectious foci and areas of tissue damage efficiently and effectively. However, when the inflammatory stimuli are able to escape local control and induce a disseminated activation of the tissue-fixed Mø, the inflammatory process is upregulated throughout the body with massive bystander injury leading to MOFS. Concomitantly, this excessive overresponse of inflammation leads to a subsequent consumption and downregulation or depression of the immune response leading to a enhanced susceptibility to subsequent infectious challenges. Our ability to identify and modulate the site and extent of the activation of the tissue-fixed Mø will allow us to ameliorate and hopefully prevent the ravages of the malignant systemic inflammation process and abrogate development of MOFS.

References

1. Carrico CJ, Meakins JL, Maier RV et al. (1986) Multiple-organ-failure syndrome. Arch Surg 121:196–208
2. Goris RJA, te Boekhorst TPA, Nuytinck JKS et al. (1985) Multiple organ failure: generalized autodestructive inflammation? Arch Surg 120:1109
3. Fry DE, Pearlstein L, Fulton, RL et al. (1980) Multiple system organ failure: the role of uncontrolled infection. Arch Surg 115:136–140
4. Maunder RJ (1985) Clinical prediction of the adult respiratory distress syndrome. Clin Chest Med 6:413–426
5. Henson PM, Larsen GL, Webster RO et al. (1982) Pulmonary microvascular alterations and injury induced by complement fragments: synergistic effect of complement activation, neutrophil sequestration, and prostaglandins. Ann NY Acad Sci 384:287–300
6. Takemura R, Werb Z (1984) Secretory products of macrophages and their physiological functions. Am J Physiol 246:C1–C9
7. Schraufstatter IU, Revak SD, Cochrane CG (1984) Proteases and oxidants in experimental pulmonary inflammatory injury. J Clin Invest 73:1175–1184
8. Bachofen M, Weibel ER (1977) Alterations of the gas exchange apparatus in adult respiratory insufficiency associated with septicemia. Am Rev Respir Dis 116:589–615
9. Baggiolini M, Walz A, Kunkel SL (1989) Neutrophil-activating peptide-1/interleukin-8, a novel cytokine that activates neutrophils. J Clin Invest 84:1045–1049
10. Martin TR, Aetman LC, Albert RK, Henderson WR (1984) Leukotriene B_4 production by the human alveolar macrophage: a potential mechanism for amplifying inflammation in the lung. Am Rev Respir Dis 129:106–111
11. Maier RV, Hahnel GB (1986) Is macrophage-induced microthrombosis during endotoxemia dependent on prostaglandin synthesis? J Surg Res 40:238–247
12. Dinarello CA (1984) Interleukin-1 and the pathogenesis of the acute-phase response. N Engl J Med 311:1413–1418
13. Tracey KJ, Beutler B, Lowry SF et al. (1986) Shock and tissue injury induced by recombinant human cachectin. Science 234:470–474
14. Fletcher JR, Disimone AG, Earnest MA (1990) Platelet activating factor receptor antagonist improves survival and attenuates eicosanoid release in severe endotoxemia. Ann Surg 211:312–316
15. Maier RV, Hahnel GB, Fletcher JR (1992) Platelet activating factor augments tumor necrosis factor and procoagulant activity. J Surg Res (in press)
16. Faist E, Mewes A, Strasser T et al. (1988) Aeteration of monocyte function following major injury. Arch Surg 123:287–292
17. Hershman MJ, Polk HC Jr, Pietsch JD et al. (1988) Modulation of infection by gamma interferon treatment following trauma. Infect Immun 56:2412–2416

Eicosanoids, Cytokines and Altered Metabolic Control in the Evolution of the Posttraumatic Host Defense Failure Syndromes: Adult Respiratory Distress Syndrome and Multiple Organ Failure Syndrome

J. H. Siegel

Host Defense Response After Trauma and Sepsis

Trauma of sufficient magnitude to induce a large volume of tissue injury and hypovolemic hemorrhagic shock results in a disparity between oxygen delivery and the oxygen consumption required to maintain cellular metabolic processes. As a result an oxygen debt is produced which forces the body cells into an anaerobic metabolic phase with increased production of lactic acid and a significant degree of metabolic acidemia [1]. The magnitude of this oxygen debt and the resultant metabolic acidemia have been shown to be quantitative predictors of mortality and the severity of the ischemic insult in experimental hemorrhagic shock [1] and also in blunt multiple trauma [2]. Initiation of hypovolemic, hemorrhagic shock has also been shown to induce bacterial translocation from the gut [3] and significant levels of circulating endotoxin have been demonstrated in humans following shock-producing traumatic injury [4]. Such shock patients have also been shown to have a higher incidence of postinjury sepsis and an increased frequency of development of the pulmonary failure syndrome known as adult respiratory distress syndrome (ARDS) or renal or hepatic failure, as well as a significant incidence of myocardial dysfunction. The various sequences of organ failures which occur have been characterized as the multiple organ failure syndrome (MOFS) [4].

Carefully analyzed with regard to physiologic, biochemical and clinical characteristics, the normal host-defense response to major trauma has been separated into two phases. The first of these has been characterized as the acute inflammatory phase and the second as the solid organ metabolic phase [5]. Although the aspects of the acute inflammatory phase can be demonstrated to be initiated immediately after injury or shock accompanied by severe metabolic acidosis and occur before the major features of the solid organ metabolic phase are recognizable, it is evident that very quickly both phases of the host-defense process occur together, and that there appears to be a powerful regulatory interaction between them.

Maryland Institute for Emergency Medical Services Systems 228 Greene Street, Baltimore, Maryland 21201-1595, USA

Host Defense Dysfunction
in Trauma, Shock and Sepsis
Eds. Faist/Meakins/Schildberg
© Springer-Verlag, Berlin Heidelberg 1993

Acute Inflammatory Response

This phase of the host-defense response can be characterized as involving a number of mediators released from the damaged tissue, the most prominent of which are the eicosanoids. These mediators result in the activation of the formed elements of blood, most notably the platelets and leukocytes (PMNs), with early aggregation, adherence to capillary membranes, and in the case of the PMNs subsequent respiratory burst activity. Some of the eicosanoids also cause initiation of macrophage and monocyte cytokine elaboration, which in turn results in stimulation of the endothelial cell to the synthesis of a leukocyte adherence protein (ELAM). The net result of all of these interactions is to produce an altered capillary membrane permeability at the nexus of PMN-endothelial cell interaction. Figure 1 summarizes the acute inflammatory phase of the host-defense response to be discussed below.

Eicosanoid Response

The posttrauma response in patients resuscitated from a shock-inducing episode following injury is associated with the release of large quantities of eicosanoids generated from the damaged cellular membranes of injured tissue and released from activated platelets and leukocytes [6, 7]. These eicosanoids are elaborated from the action of phospholipase A_2 on the phosphocholine portion of the damaged or altered cell membranes. This in turn induces the activation of the cyclooxygenase and lipoxygenase pathways of eicosanoid formation [8, 9].

Figure 2 shows the eicosanoid leukotriene B_4 (LTB_4) response over the first 8 days in a group of 31 posttrauma patients, 11 of whom had uncomplicated recoveries, 12 developed severe sepsis, and 7 early fulminant ARDS following their severe injury [7]. One of the most prominent features of the immediate eicosanoid response is the liberation of large quantities of the lipoxygenase derivative LTB_4, which has a powerful action on both PMN and macrophages, inducing respiratory burst activation, PMN aggregation, and PMN and macrophage adherence to capillary endothelium with leukosequestration. As demonstrated in Figs. 2 and 3, which shows the mean arterial base excess curves for these three trauma patient groups, the patients destined to be septic who were shown in Fig. 2 to have the highest postinjury LTB_4 plasma levels were also the group with the greatest base deficit on admission, reflecting a larger posthemorrhagic oxygen debt.

There is also an increased release of the cyclooxygenase derived eicosanoid prostaglandin E_2 (PGE_2), which has been defined as a universal immune suppressant [11, 12]. Concomitant with and also following the liberation of these two eicosanoids, it can be demonstrated that there is a subsequent rise in other cyclooxygenase eicosanoids, most notably $PGF_{1\alpha}$ and thromboxane A_2 (measured as thromboxane B_2) as well as PGF_2. These latter two mediators have been demonstrated to have a significant effect in promoting platelet

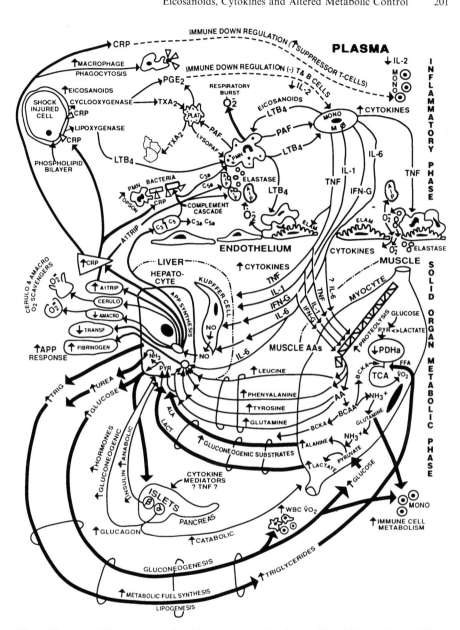

Fig. 1. The acute inflammatory and solid organ metabolic phases of host defense. (From [5])

aggregation and platelet endothelial adherence, and their rise is correlated with the initial thrombocytopenia seen immediately postinjury [6]. These data suggest that the magnitude of the posttraumatic ischemia is a critical factor in determining the quantitative release of the eicosanoid mediators. They also

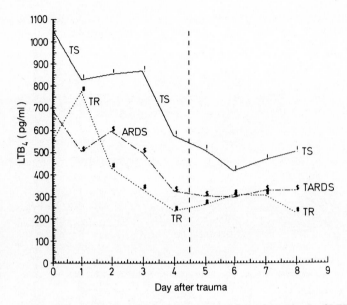

Fig. 2. LTB$_4$ elaboration after multiple trauma. Mean plasma levels of LTB$_4$ in patients with septic trauma (*TS*), Posttrauma ARDS (*TARDS*) and nonseptic non-ARDS trauma patients (*TR*). *Vertical dotted line*, approximate transition time between early preseptic and late clinically evident septic periods. (From [7])

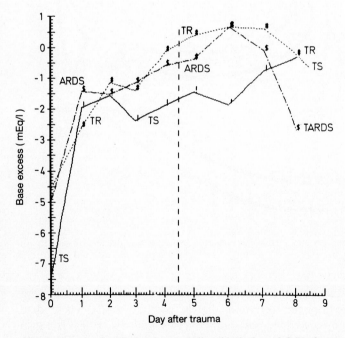

Fig. 3. Recovery from ischemic metabolic acidosis (base deficit) after trauma. (From [7]).

indicate that an excessive eicosanoid response over a period of several days immediately following injury is an early predictor of a subsequent host defense failure with evolution of invasive sepsis, prior to the laboratory or clinical delineation of a recognizable septic response [7].

A similar pattern of eicosanoid release has been demonstrated in trauma patients who develop the early fulminant posttraumatic ARDS [6]. However, the LTB$_4$ response and the subsequent interaction between the lipoxygenase, and cyclooxygenase-derived prostanoids has been demonstrated to be some-what more focused in time, and this focusing appears to be correlated with a pathophysiologically increased PMN respiratory burst activity occurring 8 –24 h later and correlated with evidence of impaired pulmonary gas exchange [6, 13].

Leukocyte Response

As shown in Fig. 4 for posttrauma patients who developed later sepsis, but also characteristic of all patients after major injury, there is an immediate postresuscitation leukopenia following the injury which has been demonstrated both clinically [6, 13] and experimentally [14, 15] to represent peripheral and pulmonary leukosequestration. This leukopenia response has been correlated experimentally with the leukotriene activation of leukocyte adherence proteins (CD18) which initiate the immediate adherence of PMNSs to the capillary

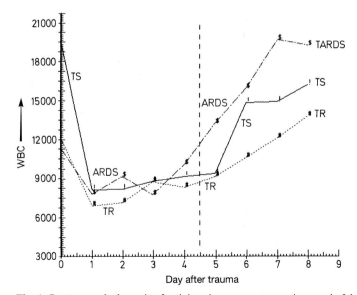

Fig. 4. Posttrauma leukopenia after injury in response to sepsis or early fulminant posttraumatic ARDS. (Legend, see Fig. 2; from [7])

endothelium [15, 16] The adherence response is also enhanced by the subsequent direct stimulation of endothelial cells to the production of ELAM proteins through the action of leukotrienes and of macrophage, and monocyte-generated tumor necrosis factor (TNF) [17–20].

As a result of the combined eicosanoid and cytokine interaction there is leukocyte aggregation, chemotaxis, and adherence to the capillary endothelium by PMNs which have been activated to increased respiratory burst activity with the release of superoxides and hydroxyl radicals [21, 22]. These activated leukocytes are also stimulated to adhere to and destroy damaged host tissues through the liberation of a variety of leukocyte-contained proteases (elastase and collagenase), and they are additionally activated to facilitate the opsonization and ingestion of bacteria whose membranes have been primed by the prior adherence of circulating C-reactive protein (CRP) and the complement cascade [23–28].

Another inflammatory mediator sequence initiator is thought to be effected through the medium of increased platelet-activating factor (PAF) and its precursor lyso-PAF [29]. There appears to be an important interaction between the activation of the platelets and that of the leukocytes through the medium of lyso-PAF liberated from platelet activation by tissue-released thrombin and collagen. Lyso-PAF appears to be converted to PAF in a cell–cell interaction between the platelet and the PMN to produce PAF. The generated PAF has the triple effect of inducing platelet activation, aggregation, and adherence to capillary endothelium, of initiating leukocyte and macrophage activation and macrophage cytokine releases and of inducing the elaboration of endothelial cell adherence proteins [29]. Thus PAF also plays a major role in bringing to culmination the total inflammatory response effect on the capillary membrane endothelium.

Monocyte-Macrophage Cytokine Responses

The final aspect of the formed element response to the inflammatory process initiated by the postinjury and/or endotoxin initiation of the eicosanoid response is the activation of the monocyte-macrophage population to the production of the cytokine mediators. In totality, these mediators affect nearly every aspect of the total immunologic and nonimmunologic host defense response.

The monocyte-macrophage activation to cytokine production elaborates immune mediators such as interleukin-2 (IL-2) which result in activation of T cells [30], interferon-gamma (INF-γ) which stimulates both the T and B cell populations [30] and IL-3 and the granulocyte and macrophage colony-stimulating factors (granulocyte CSF, CSF-1, granulocyte-macrophage CSF) which initiate the growth of the myeloid and lymphoid cell systems and thus have an amplifying role on monocyte-macrophage and leukocyte function [31]. In general, these aspects of immune function are unregulated by the leukotriene [18, 19, 32] and PAF effects [29] and to a large extent are down-regulated by PGE2 [11, 30].

However, with regard to the non immunologic component of the inflammatory phase of the host defense process there is clear evidence that the leukotriene and PAF response of the monocyte-macrophage population is to synthesize a series of monokines whose function is to enhance the increased permeability of the capillary endothelium by stimulating the endothelial cells to the production of ELAM and intercellular adhesion molecule (ICAM) proteins [14, 18, 19]. These in turn induce the adherence of PMN and macrophages with elaboration of leukocyte proteases and superoxide and hydroxyradicals which break the endothelial barrier [21, 22].

At the same time these cytokines, which include TNF, IL-1, IL-6, IFN-γ, as well as a variety of other interleukins whose function is not as well characterized, are permitted to leave the general circulation and enter the interstitium of organs remote from the primary site of traumatic injury or bacterial invasion. At these distant loci they can interact by binding to specialized receptors on the surface of the cells of the solid organs of the body which are involved in metabolic interorgan substrate-energy flux. These cytokine receptor interactions induce the mechanisms of skeletal muscle proteolysis, stimulate amino acid and lactate-mediated gluconeogenesis, and initiate the hepatic acute-phase protein (APP) synthesis response [34–43].

Finally, in addition to the previously noted TNF induction of endothelial cell elaborated leukocyte adherence molecules (ELAM, ICAM), there is evidence that fixed receptors on the endothelial cell are activated which induce the sequence of intravascular coagulation through activation of the intrinsic coagulation-kinin cascade based on Hageman factor dependent pathways. There is some evidence that there are fixed TNF-sensitive vascular receptor sites which include coagulation. These receptors may also be activated by bacterial endotoxins as well as by TNF, and under extreme circumstances endotoxin activation of these sites may induce the syndrome of disseminated intravascular coagulation.

Solid Organ Metabolic Phase of the Host Defense Response

The earliest findings that suggested a role for cytokines in the metabolic phase of host defense response were provided by the observation that cachetin, later shown to be identical with TNF, could induce a proteolytic response [35]. Other studies implied that a low molecular weight protein factor which was thought to be a breakdown product of IL-1 could also be responsible for the skeletal muscle proteolytic response [34]. Although recent in vitro studies have challenged the role of TNF in the induction of the proteolytic response [46], in vivo studies suggest that there is an interaction between the various cytokines released by a distant inflammatory process. This interaction enhances muscle proteolysis with release of muscle protein bound amino acids. This in turn induces the transamination of branched chain amino acid ammonia nitrogen, via glutamine synthesis, to the formation of alanine. As shown by Smith et al. [38], there is evidence that increasing circulating TNF in the presence of a distant sterile inflammatory process, which presumably results in the release of other cytokines as well, is correlated with increased levels of both alanine and skeletal muscle intracellular lactate. Other studies have suggested that IL-1 or IFN-γ can upgrade the number of cellular receptors to TNF [47], and vice versa, that this multiple cytokine interaction plays a potentiating role in inducing muscle proteolysis. Additional, as yet uncharacterized monokines have also been suggested as the mediators for muscle proteolysis [37]. Cytokines have also been implicated in the regulation of hepatic protein synthesis [39–43] and in pancreatic function [48]. Figure 1 summarizes the solid organ metabolic phase of the host defense response discussed below.

Cytokine Effects on Skeletal Muscle

The important aspect of this shift in the skeletal muscle equilibrium between muscle protein synthesis and breakdown is that the cytokine-mediated increased muscle formation of lactate, alanine, and glutamine (which can be later transaminated to alanine in gut) serves to produce the major substrates for hepatic and renal gluconeogenesis, when transported to these organs by the circulating blood. Of equal importance with regard to the formation of glutamine in skeletal muscle and its liberation into the circulation is the major role of this metabolic substrate for the oxidative metabolism of cells of the lymphoid system involved in the immunologic response. Thus, while monocyte-macrophage released IL-2 stimulates the immunologically active population of T and B cells to increased activity, the nonimmunologic cytokine mediator response induced by TNF, IFN-γ, and IL-1 also stimulates the solid organ metabolic phase to provide increased metabolic fuels to support the increased metabolism of the same T and B cells which are involved in an increased immunologic defense process.

Cytokine Effects on Liver Acute-Phase Protein Synthesis

The monocyte-synthesized cytokines which are allowed to leave the circulation to interact with the cell populations of the liver, as part of the solid organ metabolic phase of the host defense response, appear to induce their effect by a more complex set of cell–cell interactions. While there is evidence for a direct stimulating effect of at least one cytokine, IL-6, in the induction of hepatocyte APP synthesis in the formation of fibrinogen [41], the major effects of the cytokines in inducing or inhibiting hepatocyte protein synthesis appear to be through the medium of alteration of the Kupffer's cell–hepatocyte control mechanism [42, 43]. Evidence has been presented that cytokine interaction with receptors on the Kupffer's cells which are the fixed macrophages of the liver, are effected by a L-arginine mediated biochemical pathway in which the guanido nitrogen of L-arginine is oxidized to form the highly reactive molecule of nitric oxide which serves as the transmitter agent which actually stimulates the hepatocyte [43]

Studies have been carried out which suggest that IFN-γ, IL-1, or TNF can induce this pathway. More importantly, there is clear evidence of a potentiation of the effect of TNF, IL-1, and IL-6 on the Kupffer's cell production of nitric oxide in the presence of IFN-γ stimulation [41–43]. A similar effect was noted in the presence of bacterial endotoxin (lipopolysaccharide, (LPS) [43]. The exact nature of the hepatocyte response with regard to the synthesis and/or re-prioritization of hepatic APP appears to be a function of the interaction between these various cytokines and endotoxin, and the magnitude of the resulting nitric oxide response [42, 43]. While these relationships have not been explicitly defined, they suggest that the control of the hepatocyte APP synthesis and the nature and magnitude of the APP reprioritization which occurs in severe sepsis may be mediated by the interaction of circulating cytokines and LPS on the Kupffer's cell production of nitric oxide. As is discussed below, the ultimate hepatocyte APP response, which appears to be cytokine controlled, is of considerable importance in the septic modulation of the postinjury inflammatory component of the host defense response.

Cytokine Control of Hepatic Fuel Synthesis and Modulation
of the Pancreatic-Hepatic Endocrine Control Mechanisms

As noted earlier, a major aspect of the solid organ metabolic phase response is the increased synthesis of glucose by the liver from skeletal muscle-derived lactate and gluconeogenic amino acids. This process is in part driven by the increased quantity of gluconeogenic substrates liberated from muscle proteolysis and the resulting amino acid transamination process. However, the rate of gluconeogenesis is also controlled by the increased production of pancreatic glucagon which occurs in response to the host defense process, especially under septic conditions where both plasma glucagon and insulin may rise to extremely high levels. A direct hepatocellular-stimulating role of cytokines in mediating this process is not clear. However, there is suggestive evidence that either IL-1 or TNF may increase cytokine [48]. This has been demonstrated to result in increased pancreatic exocrine function and may be important in modulation of the pancreatic endocrine response (?) in the host defense process.

The second major area of hepatic fuel production in the solid organ metabolic phase of the host defense process is the increased magnitude of hepatic fatty acid and triglyceride synthesis with release of increased quantities of triglycerides into the circulation. The resulting hypertriglyceridemia is derived both from direct hepatic synthesis and from recycling of circulating fatty acids which enter the hepatocyte. This process is also driven in part by the increased gluconeogenic substrate presentation to the liver. There is evidence that in the presence of inflammation, and especially in the presence of sepsis, that some glucose-derived three-carbon fragments which enter the Krebs TCA cycle through the medium of acetyl-coenzyme A (CoA) are diverted from the mito-chondrial TCA cycle, at the level of citrate, into the formation of increased levels of cytosolic malonly-CoA, which is the mandatory precursor in fatty acid synthesis [50]. At the same time there is evidence of lipid recycling [51], which may represent malonyl-CoA inhibition of fatty acid oxidation and increased insulin-stimulated lipogenesis [50]. This is manifested by an increase in plasma triglycerides that may be enhanced by insulin, which is also increased in the plasma as part of the host defense response. The hyperinsulinemia may occur through the same mechanisms as are related to the glucagon increase since there is a rise in both plasma insulin and glucagon. However, the insulin-to-glucagon ratio may be altered, especially in the presence of sepsis. Whether the plasma insulin rise is also cytokine mediated, or whether it is a paracrine response to the hyperglycemia from increased gluconeogenesis remains to be demonstrated, but the net result is an enhanced lipogenesis and triglyceride formation. The increase in lipid substrates in the plasma alters the metabolic fuel substrates mix presented to the periphery and appears to be related to the increased body utilization of lipids and the fall in respiratory quotient seen in patients or animals with severe septic inflammatory processes [52].

Role of Hepatic Acute-Phase Proteins in Modulation of the Inflammatory Phase of the Host Defense Response

A critical aspect of the compensated host defense response is the modulation of the inflammatory phase by the hepatic synthesized APP. Under circumstances of nonseptic injury and in early sepsis this response may be seen as regulating the process by enhancing those aspects of the inflammatory process related to destruction of damaged cells and those facilitating opsonization and lysis of bacteria by PMNs and macrophages. At the same time, the APP response appears to reduce the potentially lethal effects of the activated PMN and macrophage on normal host tissues.

The hepatic production of CRP and the proteins of the complement sequence can be seen as enhancing the nonimmunologic defense responses. CRP has been demonstrated to bind to the exposed phospholipid membranes of damaged cells and is implicated in the activation of phospholipase A2 [26], with the initiation of the eicosanoid response, and the generation of chemotactic factors for leukocytes and monocyte-macrophages, which as noted earlier play a major role in mediating the inflammatory aspects of the host defense prospects [27, 28]. The complement sequence proteins which complex to bacterial mem-branes at the site of CRP binding release anaphylatoxins [53] and produce lethal lesions which induce bacterial destruction [54]. Complement proteins, as well as a variety of other hepatically synthesized protein factors, are associated with the coagulation cascade resulting in the generation of bradykinin and with the initiation of fibrinolysis [56]. The hepatic APP fibrinogen is also increased as part of the APP response and plays a major role in the coagulation process [24, 57].

A number of the hepatic APP are responsible for the binding of specific metal ions; these include hepatic metallothionein which binds zinc [58], ceruloplasmin which binds copper [24], as well as the iron-binding transport protein transferrin [24]. The later APP regulates extracellular free iron which participates in the conversion of hydrogen peroxide to hydroxyl ions as part of the superoxide response [59]. Iron binding to transferrin may also reduce the quantity of free iron available to bacteria, such as *Escherichia coli* whose lethality is a function of iron availability. In addition, the copper-binding APP ceruloplasmin plays a major role in dampening the inflammatory response by scavenging activated oxygen compounds such as the superoxides [60]. A similar role is played by α_2-macroglobulin which is also produced by lymphocytes and fiberblasts as well as by the liver [24]. The α_2-macroglobulin is also an antiprotease, as is α_1-antitrypsin, and these two APP play a role in reducing the leukocyte-liberated proteases which destroy both foreign and host proteins [21, 22, 61].

A considerable degree of study has involved the interrelationship between the superoxide radicals and the antiproteases, as modeled by α_1-antitrypsin, in regulating the capillary lesion induced when leukocytes and macrophages adhere to the ELAM-stimulated endothelial cells [21, 22]. Under ordinary circumstances the antiproteases inactivate the excess leukocyte elastase and collagenase liberated by contact stimulation of the PMN. However, the superoxide radicals have the capability of damaging the antiproteases to the point where they are inactivated and thus cannot antagonize the protease response. In the confines of the aggregated cells adherent to the capillary endothelial membrane it is speculated that the relative concentrations of superoxide and hydroxyl radicals may become extremely high, producing a complete inactivation of the antiproteases in the local setting. This would allow unregulated full activation of the protease molecules to alter the capillary basement membrane, thus permitting the normal degree of permeability change which occurs during inflammation to proceed to a pathophysiologic lesion. It has been suggested that when PMN superoxide generation is excessive, as it is the fulminant ARDS syndrome, it may thus mediate the extensive capillary permeability changes and the increased interstitial fluid occurring from the capillary leaks seen in this condition [6, 13].

Host Defense Failure Disease as a Manifestation of Hepatocellular Deregulation of the Inflammatory Response

In the normal response to traumatic injury, the acute inflammatory phase is accompanied by a solid organ metabolic phase with a cytokine-mediated Kupffer's cell–hepatocyte APP synthesis which results in a proportionate increase in both the facilitating and the inhibiting hepatic APP [62]. This early

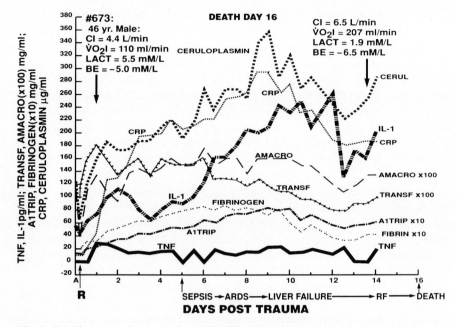

Fig. 5. Cytokine-acute phase protein relationships in posttraumatic sepsis and multiple organ failure: multiple bilateral rib fractures, bilateral hip fractures, right tibial fracture. Note reprioritization of APP beginning about day 7 with fall in transferrin followed by fibrinogen and α_2-macroglobulin as CRP and α_1-antitrypsin continue to rise.

inflammatory rise in APP is shown in Fig. 5 during the initial 5 days posttrauma prior to the onset of septic organ failure. In both nonseptic and early septic trauma these APP all rise, although there is a much larger percentage increase in CRP, α_1-antitrypsin, and fibrinogen. Ceruloplasmin also rises, but the levels of the other transport and the scavenging proteins such as transferrin and α_2-macroglobulin either rise slightly or remain relatively constant during the early postinjury inflammatory phase. In patients with nonseptic trauma who recover, all APP tend to fall toward baseline levels as the inflammatory response subsides.

However, as also shown in Fig. 5, when a posttrauma patients becomes septic and progresses into an early compensated septic phase (in this case from days 5 to 7), there is evidence of an initial alteration and reprioritization in the normal non-septic posttraumatic hepatic APP response. There is further enhancement of the plasma levels of the more rapid-turnover APP, such as CRP and α_1-antitrypsin. Generally, there is also an increased plasma level response in fibrinogen and sometimes in ceruloplasmin levels, but there is now evidence of no further increase or an initial down-regulation of the slow-turnover hepatic scavenger and transport proteins, α_2-macroglobulin, transferrin and albumin, and the circulating levels of these APP fall [62].

In severe sepsis especially in those patients who evolve septic MOFS, which always includes at least subtle hepatic dysfunction, there is evidence of marked

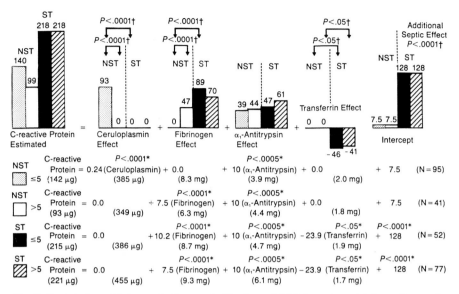

Fig. 6. Statistical model demonstrating reprioritization of APP in early and late posttraumatic sepsis, compared to nonseptic trauma patient values. *Height of bars*, relative change in each APP scaled in units of CRP equivalents. All differences significant, as indicated by Scheffé simultaneous comparison of all contrasts. (From [62] with permission)

reprioritization of the APP response [5, 62]. Under these circumstances (as seen in this case from day 9 until death at day 16) while there is some decrement in all APP, the rapid-turnover APP are still increased, and production of CRP α_1-antitrypsin and fibrinogen produce plasma levels which remain above normal control values. However, the carrier proteins such as transferrin and α_2-macroglobulin, as well as albumin, show evidence of a fall in plasma levels suggesting that a relative shift in protein synthesis has occurred with enhancement of some APP synthesis at the expense of others. The significance of these changes is shown in Fig. 6, which shows the changes in the various slower turnover APP relative to CRP, comparing nonseptic trauma to the early and late phases of septic trauma.

These human data are consistent with the in vitro hepatic coculture studies reported by Billiar et al. [63] in which increased levels of nitric oxide produced by activated Kupffer's cells in the presence of LPS or multiple cytokines cause inhibition of hepatocyte protein synthesis. In view of the evidence of an uncontrolled or run-away inflammatory response seen in these MOFS patients, many of whom also develop ARDS, it has been suggested that this reprioritization of APP synthesis results in a deregulation of the inflammatory response with an effective increase in the relative influence of the inflammatory enhancing APP such as CRP, in the coagulation APP fibrinogen, and in the antiproteases, while at the same time reducing the plasma concentrations of the superoxide scavengering and iron-binding APP [5]. Falls in the $\dot{O}_2^-$ scavenger APP are believed to increase the effectiveness of the superoxides in inactivating the antiproteases [21, 22], and the reduction in iron-binding APP may increase the rate of generation of hydroxyl radicals due to failure to control the Fentin reaction [59]. The accompanying multiple organ failure may be seen as a manifestation of deregulation of the host defense response.

Host Defense Failure Disease as the Cause of MOFS

In understanding the deregulation and loss of control of the inflammatory portion of the host defense response by the altered solid organ metabolic response, it is useful to contrast a normal posttraumatic host defense response with that which appears characteristic of the evolution of the multiple sequential organ failure syndrome characteristic of host defense failure disease (Fig. 1).

Normal Host Defense Response to Trauma

The initial host response to injury is characterized by an outpouring of eicosanoid mediators from the injured and ischemic tissues (Fig. 2) [6, 7]. The magnitude of this response is correlated in a general way with the severity of the metabolic shock characterized by the magnitude of the base deficit (Fig. 3) [7]. The initial rises in LTB_4 and PGE_2 are characterized by a contemporaneous leukopenia (Fig. 4) reflecting the early leukosequestration response mediated by the leukocyte adherence modules (CD18) [14, 15]. At the same time there appears to be the initiation of activation processes in the PMN that result in a progressive increase in PMN respiratory burst activation which becomes maximal between the 3rd and 4th days postinjury [6, 13], generally at a time when the leukosequestration persists and before the systemic leukemoid response is seen in severely injured patients or patients who become septic.

Immediately following the initial postresuscitation eicosanoid response there is evidence of stimulation of the synthesis of the rapid-turnover APP, CRP rises, followed closely or paralleled by the rise in α_1-antitrypsin and fibrinogen [62].

Systemic cytokine elaboration into the plasma is usually absent in relatively mild or intermediate-severity trauma [5], but in severe trauma especially that associated with transient profound ischemic shock there is often a burst of cytokine activity occurring between the 1st and 2nd days postinjury [5]. This is shown in Fig. 7. In general, TNF rises first, followed by IL-1, although these may be closely parallel in response. There may be be variable rise in IL-6 or IFN-γ, which appear to be related to the magnitude of the injury, since the former tends to rise in patients who develop the early posttraumatic ARDS and may be associated with a further rise in fibrinogen. However, in the normal host defense response, even to severe injury, cytokine elaboration into the plasma ceases as recovery progresses, and there is a reduction in the maximum levels of CRP toward normal as well as a fall in fibrinogen and α_1-antitrypsin [62]. In the normal recovery from nonseptic trauma the superoxide scavengering and

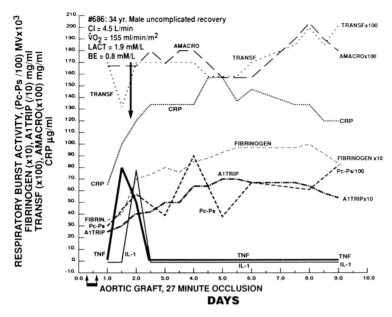

Fig. 7. Normal posttrauma cytokine and APP response after major trauma: aortic rupture with pseudoaneurysm, femoral, tibial, and radial fractures. (From [5])

transport proteins transferrin and α_2-macroglobulin and ceruloplasmin tend to maintain relatively steady labels or to rise slightly toward the end of the recovery period, and there is no evidence of reprioritization in these proteins.

The permeability changes which follow the initial leukopenia response and accompany the increased PMN respiratory burst activity occur within the first 24 h, generally become maximal at 72–96 h, and then slowly decay in patients who recover from the posttraumatic episode [13]. Leukopenia beyond the initial few hours appears to represent a combination of (a) LTB_4-activated leukocyte [18, 19] and (b) activated macrophage adherence to capillary membranes in response to the elaboration of the ELAM proteins in response to TNF [14, 64]. The capillary permeability response, which is generalized, results in a third space loss which may allow an increased cytokine access to the solid organs and appears to some degree to parallel in time the increase in muscle proteolysis and amino acid release with hyperalaninemia [65]. The concomitant hyperglycemic response following injury appears to reflect the combined effect of the cytokine mediators to increase the hepatofugal substrate flux of gluconeogenic amino acid substrates [35, 37, 38] as well as the enhanced skeletal muscle glycogenolytic and hepatic gluconeogenic enzymatic effects caused by the increased production of pancreatic glucagon [36, 48].

In contrast to the normal recovery sequence following trauma in the posttrauma organ failure syndromes, the initial ischemic response to injury is usually of greater magnitude, as reflected in the somewhat larger base deficit (Fig. 3), which reflects a greater oxygen debt. Those patients who develop sepsis within the first 4–6 days also appear to have a persistence of the elevated LTB_4 release response beyond the resuscitation period (Fig. 2) [7]. The post-trauma LTB_4 elaboration is paralleled by the release of PGE_2 and by a proportionate increase in the plasma levels of thromboxane and PGF_2, all of which have platelet-aggregating and vascoconstrictor properites [6].

However, the striking mediator differences in the septis patients who develop MOFS is the early and persistent elevation in plasma TNF, as evidence of a profound initial and continuing activation of the monocyte-macrophage population to the production of cytokines [5, 66]. In the severe, usually septic, cases the evolution of MOFS is paralleled by a rise or a continuing elevation in plasma IL-1 (Fig. 5) and by persistent or intermittent elevations of the other cytokines studied, most notably IL-6 and IFN-γ (not shown). These elevated plasma levels of multiple cytokines tend to persist throughout the period of evolving organ failure and often become even more exaggerated (Fig. 5) toward the end of the fulminant organ failure syndrome, just prior to the patient's death from multiple organ failures due to an uncontrolled solid organ metabolic response [5, 66].

As also shown in Fig. 5, one of the most characteristic biochemical features of this host defense failure process, as it evolves beyond the initial 4–5 days, is the significant reprioritization in the APP response (Fig. 6) [5, 62].

Clinically, the period of sustained cytokine mediator response is accompanied by persistent and excessive muscle wasting, marked by large increases in urinary 3-methylhistidine representing protein degradation, as well as by large increases in urinary urea nitrogen [65]. However, in contrast to the normal Ebb-phase proteolytic response in nonseptic trauma cases, in severe septic trauma associated with solid organ phase host defense dysfunction the urea nitrogen/3-methylhistidine ratio is increased, suggesting that a larger percentage of the amino acids released by the muscle proteolysis are irreversibly deaminated for gluconeogenesis or ketogenesis, rather then being made available for protein synthetic processes [65].

Another characteristic clinical biochemical feature of the septic MOFS solid organ host defense failure is the manifestation of a reprioritization of another family of hepatic synthetic processes. There is evidence of increased hepatic synthesis and increased hepatic reesterification of plasma free fatty acids with significant increases in plasma triglyceride levels, at the expense of cholesterol synthesis so that as triglycerides rise, cholesterol falls [48].

As host defense failure disease progresses, the clearances of most of the hepatically metabolized amino acids tend to be reduced [65, 68]. In specific tyrosine and phenylalanine clearances fall, so that the plasma levels of these aromatic amino acids rise, and there is generally a fall in the neutral amino acid clearances as well. Only the branched chain amino acids (whose utilization has been shown to be increased in skeletal muscle, heart, and liver) show increased clearances as the septic solid organ failure process progresses [68]. The essential branched chain amino acids are deaminated at a high rate to form their ketoacids, with a first NH_2^+ transamination via α-ketoglutarate to glutamine and a second NH_2^+ transamination with pyruvate to form the large quantities of alanine produced in septic MOFS. In this regard there is speculation from experimental evidence that in sepsis the relative synthetic rate of formation alanine may be disproportionately high so that the intracellular levels of glutamine as an intermediary in this process may fall [69, 70]. It has been suggested that this fall in intracellular glutamine may permit increased proteolysis or reduce the stimulus to protein synthesis thus enhancing the muscle wasting seen in this disease.

Discussion

A number of interesting speculations have been raised regarding the interactions of the various cytokines in including the hepatic APP reprioritization which is a characteristic feature of the process host defense failure [62]. Studies by Curran et al. [42] have shown that the inhibition of protein synthesis by the hepatocyte is a function of an increased production of nitric oxide caused by the synergistic action of multiple cytokines on the Kupffer's cell. It may be speculated that the nitric oxide inhibition is not uniform in degree with regard to all the proteins synthesized by he liver, but rather some proteins may escape this process or may even be enhanced in synthesis. Alternatively a differential effect of the cytokines on nitric oxide release by the Kupffer's cells may be the underlying phenomenon related to the hepatic protein reprioritization.

In a related investigation concerning the cytokine control of muscle proteolysis Smith et al. [38] have shown that in the presence of a remote sterile inflammatory abscess, administered circulating TNF produces a greater muscle proteolytic response than under circumstances where no remote inflammatory process exists. This suggests that even in the nonshock circumstance interaction between inflammatory mediators may be necessary to potentiate the muscle proteolytic process as well. This cytokine interaction, or up-regulation of cytokine receptors may account for the excessive muscle wasting seen in those MOFS individuals in whom multiple cytokines are persistently elevated in the plasma.

Finally, an interesting research question to be resolved by further studies is the role of glutamine and/or branched chain amino acids as glutamine precursors, in modulating the monocyte-macrophage cytokine response. Preliminary evidence by our group [71] suggests that severely ill septic patients given enriched branched chain amino acid total parenteral nutrition not only maintain somewhat higher levels of circulating glutamine but also appear to have marked decreases in the circulating levels of TNF, IL-1, and IL-6 compared to control septic patients managed with total parenteral nutrition having standard low branched chain amino acid content. These data, if confirmed, suggest that at least one of the factors involved in monocyte-macrophage cytokine production, after stimulation by the eicosanoid inflammatory mediators, may be the adequacy of nutritional support to the monocyte itself. Since approximately 35% of the oxidative metabolism in cells of the lymphoid system is related to glutamine, 40% to fatty acids, and only 10% to glucose [72], under septic conditions the production of increased quantities of these nonglucose fuels (glutamine by the muscle and fatty acids by the liver) may also serve as nutritional down-regulating factors to both support and control the monocyte generation of the cytokine mediators of the inflammatory and solid organ metabolic phases of the integrated host defense response.

Thus, the entire set of interrelations between the acute inflammatory phase and the solid organ metabolic phase of the host defense response can be seen as reinforcing and regulating each other through a variety of mechanisms. An excessive stimulation of production of the inflammatory mediators appears to cause a dysfunctional reprioritization of critical aspects of the solid organ metabolic response with a resultant deregulation of the total integrated host defense response. This deregulation leads to the overt clinical organ failures which we characterize as the ARDS and multiple or sequential organ failure syndromes.

Acknowledgements. The author would like to acknowledge the many colleagues whose work over the years has contributed to his conceptualization of this problem. In addition to those whose work is cited in the text or acknowledged in the figures, he would like to give recognition to those collaborators whose work, though cited, is still in progress or unpublished at the time of this manuscript: Diana Malcolm, Ph.D., C. Michael Dunham, M.D., Pietro Guadalupi, M.D., Charles E. Wiles, III, M.D., Tun Jen Ko, M.D., Edward E. Cornwell, III, M.D., Xi Hou Lin, M.D., Paolo Bruzzone, M.D., Michael Badellino, M.D., David Frankenfield, M.S., R.D., Joyce Smith, M.S., Joan C. Stoklosa, B.S., Kathleen Cotter, R.N., Chuka Jenkins, B.S., Steve Blevins, B.S., and Miklos Fabian, B.S.

References

1. Dunham CM, Siegel JH, Weireter L, Fabian M et al. (1991) Oxygen debt and metabolic acidemia as quantitative predictors of mortality and the severity of the ischemic insult in hemorrhagic shock. Crit Care Med 19:231–243
2. Siegel JH, Rivkind AI, Dalal S, Goodarzi S (1990) Early physiologic predictors of injury severity and death in blunt multiple trauma. Arch Surg 125:498–508
3. Baker JW, Dietch EA, Berg RD, Specian RD (1988) Hemorrhagic shock induces bacterial translocation from the gut. J Trauma 28:896–906
4. Baue AE (1975) Multiple progressive or sequential systems failures: a syndrome of the 1970's. Arch Surg 110:779–781
5. Siegel JH (1991) The liver as modulator of the host-defense response: host-defense failure disease as a manifestation of hepatic decompensation. In: Schlag G, Redl H, Siegel JH (eds) Second Wiggers-Bernard conference on shock, sepsis and organ failure. Springer, Berlin Heidelberg New York (in press)
6. Rivkind AI, Siegel JH, Guadalupi P, Littleton M (1989) Sequential patterns of eicosanoid, platelet, and neutrophil interactions in the evolution of the fulminant post-traumatic adult respiratory distress syndrome. Ann Surg 210:355–373
7. Guadalupi P, Siegel JH, Rivkind AI et al. (1991) Eicosanoid, physiological and inflammatory response relationships as early predictors of posttraumatic sepsis. Arch Surg (to be published)

8. Smith JB, Ingerman C, Kociss JJ, Silver MJ (1973) Formation of prostaglandins during aggregation of human blood platelets. J Clin Invest 52:965–969
9. Deby-Dupont G, Brawn M, Lamy M et al. (1987) Thromboxane and prostacyclin release in adult respiratory distress syndrome. Intensive care 13:167–174
10. Faist E, Storck M, Ertel W, Mewes A (1990) Posttraumatic immune suppression as initiator of organ failure. In: Schlag G, Redl H, Siegel J H (eds) First Wiggers-Bernard conference on shock, species and organ failure. Springer, Berlin Heidelberg New York, pp 307–328
11. Goodwin JS, Behrens T (1990) Humoral factors in immune suppression after injury. In: Schlag G, Redl H, Siegel JH (eds) First Wiggers-Bernard conference in shock, sepsis and organ failure. Springer, Berlin Heidelberg New York, pp 328–349
12. Rivkind AI, Siegel JH, Mamantov T, Littleton M (1991) Respiratory burst activation and the pattern of physiologic relationships in the evolution of the fulminant posttraumatic adult respiratory distress syndrome. Circ Shock 33:48–62
13. Goldman G, Welbourn R, Kobzek L et al. (1990) Tumor necrosis factor-α mediates acid aspiration induced systemic organ injury. Ann Surg 212:513–520
14. Vedder NB, Winn RK, Rice CL et al. (1988) A monoclonal antibody to adherence promoting leukocyte glycoprotien, CD_{18}, reduced organ injury and improves survival from hemorrhagic shock and resuscitation in rabbits. J Clin Invest 81:939–944
15. Harlan JM (1985) Leukocyte-endothelial interactions. Blood 65:513–525
16. Bevilacqua MP, Gimbrone MA (1987) Inducible endothelial function in inflammation and coagulation. Semin Thromb Hemost 13:425–433
17. McIntyre TM, Zimmerman GA, Prescott SM (1986) Leukotrienes C_4 and D_4 stimulate human endothelial cells to synthesize platelet-activating factor and bind neutrophils. Proc Natl Acad Sci USA 83:2204–2208
18. Hoover RL, Karnovsky MJ, Austen KF et al. (1984) Leukotriene B_4 action on endothelium mediates augmented neutrophil endothelial adhesions. Proc Natl Acad Sci USA 81:2191–2193
19. Meyer JD, Yurt RW, Duhaney R et al. (1988) Tumor necrosis factor enhanced leukotriene B_4 generation and chemotaxis in human neutrophils. Arch Surg 123:1454–1458
20. Babior BM (1983) Oxidants from phagocytes: agents of defense and destruction. Blood 64:959–966
21. Weiss SJ (1989) Tissue destruction by neutrophils. N Engl J Med 320:365–376
22. Kushner I, Kaplan MH (1961) Studies of acute phase protein I. An immunohistochemical method for localization of C-reactive protein in rabbits. Association with necrosis in local inflammatory lesions. J Exp Med 114:961–974
23. Koj A (1974) Acute phase reactants: their synthesis, turnover and biologic significance. In: Allison AC (ed) structure and function of plasma proteins vol 1. Plenum, New York, pp 73–131
24. Kushner I (1982) The phenemonon of the acute phase response. Ann NY Acad Sci 389:39–48
25. Volanakis JE (1982) Complement activation by C-reactive protein complexes. Ann NY Acad Sci 389:235–250
26. Mold C, DuClos TW, Nakayama S et al. (1982) C-reactive protein reactivity with complement and effects on phagocytosis Ann NY Acad Sci 389:251–262
27. Mortensen RF, Osmand AP, Lint TF, Gerwurz H (1976) Interaction of C-reactive protein with lymphocytes and monocytes. J Immunol 117:774–781
28. Braquet P, Touqui L, Shen TY, Vargafteg BB (1987) Perspectives in platelet-activating factor research. Pharmacolog Rev 39:97–145
29. Faist E, Ertel A, Mewes S et al. (1989) Trauma-induced alterations of the lymphokine cascade. In: Faist E, Ninneman J, Green D (eds) Immune consequences of trauma, shock, and sepsis. Springer, Berlin Heidelberg New York, pp 79–94
30. Guilbert LJ, Branch DR (1989) Regulation of hematopoiesis by growth factors: proliperation of the murine macrophage as a model for stimulatory and inhibitory effects. In: Faist, E Ninneman J, Green D. (eds) Immune consequences of trauma, shock and sepsis. Springer, Berlin Heidelberg New York, pp 35–44
31. Ninneman JL (1980) Prostaglandins and leukotrienes in monocyte T cell function in stress and trauma. In: Faist E, Ninneman, JL, Green D. (eds) Immune consequences of trauma, shock and sepsis. Springer, Berlin Heidelberg New York, pp 279–284
32. Yuo A, Kitagawa S, Suzuki I et al. (1989) Tumor necrosis factor as an activator of human granulocytes. Potentiation of the metabolisms triggered by the Ca^{2+} mobilizing agonists. J Immunol 142:1678–1684

33. Clowes GHA Jr, George BC, Villee CA Jr, Saravis CA (1981) Muscle proteolysis induced by a circulating peptide in patients with sepsis and trauma. N Engl J Med 305:545–552
34. Beutler B, Cerami A (1987) TNF: more than a tumor necrosis factor. N Engl J Med 316:378–385
35. Walters JM, Bessey PQ, Dinarello CA et al. (1986) Both inflammatory and endocrine mediators stimulate host responses to sepsis. Arch Surg 121:179–190
36. Goldberg AL, Kettelhut IC, Furono K et al. (1988) Activation of protein breakdown and prostaglandin E_2 production in rat skeletal muscle in fever is signaled by a macrophage product distinct from interleukin-1 or other known monokines. J Clin Invest 81:1378–1383
37. Smith JC, Siegel JH, Jawor D, Malcom D (1990) TNF enhances the skeletal muscle metabolic response to systemic inflammation. Circ shock 31(1):28 (abstract)
38. Dinarello CA (1984) Interleukin-1 and the pathogenesis of the acute phase response. N Engl J Med 311:1413–1418
39. Darlington GJ, Wilson DR, Lachman LB (1986) Monocyte-conditioned medium, interleukin-1 and tumor necrosis factor stimulate the acute phase response in human hepatoma cells in vitro. J Cell Biol 103:787–783
40. Baumann H, Onorato V, Gauldies J et al. (1987) Distinct sets of acute phase plasma proteins are stimulated by separate human hepatocyte-stimulating factors and monokines in rat hepatoma cells. J Biol Chem 262:9756–9768
41. Curran RD, Billiar TR, Stuehr DJ et al. (1990) Multiple cytokines are required to induce hepatocyte nitric oxide production and inhibit total protein synthesis. Ann Surg 212:462–471
42. West MA, Billiar TR, Mazuski JE et al. (1988) Endotoxin modulation of hepatocyte secretory and cellular protein synthesis is mediated by Kupffer cells. Arch Surg 123:1400–1405
43. Hasselgren PO, James JH, Benson DW et al. (1990) Is there a circulating proteolysis-inducing factor during sepsis? Arch Surg 125:510–514
44. Cybulsky MI, Chan MK, Movat HZ (1988) Acute inflammation and microthrombosis induced by endotoxin, interleukin-1 and tumor necrosis factor and their implication in gram negative infection. Lab Invest 58:365–378
45. Siegel JH, Cerra FB, Coleman B et al. (1979) Physiological and metabolic correlations in human sepsis. Surgery 86:163–193
46. Vary TC, Siegel JH, Nakatani T et al. (1986) A biochemical basis for depressed ketogenesis in sepsis. J Trauma 26:419–425
47. Wolfe RR, Herndon DN, Jahoor F et al. (1987) Effect of severe brain injury on substrate cycling by glucose and fatty acids. N Engl J Med 317:403–408
48. Nanni G, Siegel JH, Coleman B et al. (1984) Increased lipid fuel dependence in the critically ill septic patient. J Trauma 24:14–30
49. Hugli TE, Muller-Eberhard HJ (1975) Anaphylatoxins: C_3a and C_5a. Adv Immunol 26:1–53
50. Johnson RB, Stroud RM (1977) Complement and host defense against infection. J Pediatr 90:169–179
51. Mayer MM, Hammer CH, Michaels DW, Shin ML (1979) Immunologically mediated membrane damage: the mechanism of complement action and the similarity of lymphocyte-mediated cytotoxicity. Immunochemistry 15:813–831
52. Osmand AP, Mortensen RF, Siegel J, Gerwurz H Interactions of C-reactive protein with the complement system III. Complement-dependent passive hemolysis initiated by CRP. J Exp Med 142:1065–1077
53. Bernuau D, Rogier E, Feldman G (1983) Decreased albumin and increased fibrinogen secretion by single hepatocytes from rats with acute inflammatory reaction. Hepatology 3:29–33
54. Sobocinski PZ, Canterbury WJ Jr (1982) Hepatic metallothionein induction in inflammation. Ann NY Acad Sci 389:354–367
55. Goldstein S, Czapski G (1986) The role and mechanism of metal ions and their complexes in enhancing damage in biological systems or in protecting these systems from the toxicity of O_2. J Free Radic Biol Med 2:3–11
56. Goldstein IM, Kaplan HB, Edelson HS, Weissmann G (1979) A new function for ceruloplasmin as an acute phase reactant in inflammation: a scavenger of superoxide anion radicals. Trans Assoc Am physicians 92:360–369
57. Ohlsson K (1975) α-1 Antitrypsin and α-2-macroglobulin interactions with human neutrophil collagenase and elastase. Ann NY Acad Sci 256:409–419
58. Sganga G, Siegel JH, Brown G et al. (1985) Reprioritization of hepatic plasma protein release in trauma and sepsis. Arch Surg 120:187–199

59. Billiar TR, Curran RD, Stuehr DJ et al. (1989) Evidence that activation of Kupffer cells results in production of L-arginine metabolites that release cell associated iron and inhibit hepatocyte protein synthesis. Surgery 106:364–372

60. Rothlein R, Czajkowski M, O'Neill MM et al. (1988) Induction of intercellular adhesion molecule-1 on primary and continuous cell lines by pro-inflammatory cytokines: regulations by pharmacologic agents and neutralizing antibodies. J Immunol 141:1665–1669

61. Pittiruti M, Siegel JH, Sganga G et al. (1989) Determinants of urea production in sepsis: muscle catabolism, TPN, and hepatic clearance of amino acids. Arch Surg 124:362–372

62. Damas P, Reuter A, Gysen P et al. (1989) Tumor necrosis factor and interleukin-1 serum levels during severe sepsis in humans. Crit Care Med 17:975–978

63. Pittiruti M, Siegel JH, Sganga G et al. (1985) Increased dependence of leucine in posttraumatic sepsis: leucins/tyrosine clearance ratio as an indicator of hepatic impairment in septic multiple organ failure syndrome. Surgery 98:378–387

64. Vary TC, Siegel JH, Tall BD, Morris JG (1988) Pharmacologic reversal of abnormal glucose regulation, BCAA. utilization and muscle catabolism sepsis by dichloroacetate. J Trauma 28:1301–1311

65. Vary TC, Placko R, Siegel JH (1989) Pharmacologic modulation of increased release of gluconeogenic precursors from extrasplanchnic organs in sepsis. Circ Shock 29:59–76

66. Frankenfield D, Siegel JH, Badellino M et al. (1991) Nutritional modulation of cytokine production in human sepsis. (Work in progress.)

67. Newsholme EA, Newsholme P, Curi R et al. (1988) A role for muscle in the immune system and its importance in surgery, trauma, sepsis and burns. Nutrition 4:261–258

Diagnostic Role of New Mediators and Markers of Inflammation in Multiple Injured Patients

D. Nast-Kolb[1], C. Waydhas[1], M. Jochum[2], M. Spannagl[3], W. Machleidt[4], K.H. Duswald[1], and L. Schweiberer[1]

Introduction

The major cause of late death after severe blunt trauma is (multiple) organ failure (OF), which is a direct consequence of mediators released during primary tissue damage and circulatory shock. To further elucidate the role of inflammatory mediators in the development of OF we performed a prospective study in severely injured patients. In a second step we examined the early prognostic value of objective biochemical markers for death and the development of OF compared to the Injury Severity Score (ISS).

Patients and Methods

In the period 1986–1989, traumatized patients arriving at our emergency room were included in the prospective study if all of the following criteria were met: (a) severe injuries of at least two body regions (head/brain, thorax, abdomen, skeletal system) or three major fractures, (b) age between 16 and 70 years, and (c) less than 6 h between accident and admission to the emergency department. A total of 69 primary surviving patients entered the study. The mean ISS was 36 (range, 13–66). Between days 4 and 28, 11 patients died (median survival time, 19, days). Of survivors, 29 suffered from OF, and 29 had an event-free recovery. Three groups were formed: group 1, lethal OF ($n = 11$); group 2, reversible OF ($n = 29$); group 3, no OF ($n = 29$).

Laboratory testing and recording of clinical data was started within 30 min after arrival of the patient in the emergency department and continued on a 6-h basis. After 48 h the interval was extended to 24 h for a period of 14 days. After 2

---

[1] Chirurgische Klinik und Poliklinik, Klinikum Innenstadt der Universität München, Nußbaumstr. 20, 8000 Munich 2, FRG
[2] Abteilung für Klinische Chemie und Klinische Biochemie, Chirurgische Klinik und Poliklinik, Klinikum der Universität München, Nußbaumstr. 20, 8000 Munich 2, FRG
[3] Medizinische Klinik, Klinikum Innenstadt der Universität München, Nußbaumstr. 20, 8000 Munich 2, FRG
[4] Institut für Physiologische Chemie, Physikalische Biochemie und Zellbiologie der Universität München, Goethestr. 3, 8000 Munich 2, FRG

Host Defense Dysfunction
in Trauma, Shock and Sepsis
Eds. Faist/Meakins/Schildberg
© Springer-Verlag, Berlin Heidelberg 1993

weeks the clinical course was recorded until either transfer to a general ward or death. The biochemical markers studies are shown in the Fig. 1.

The following definitions were used:

Respiratory failure: need of mechanical ventilation and $pO_2/FiO_2 \leq 280$ or positive end-expiratory pressure ≥ 8 mmHg for at least 24 h

Renal failure: creatinine ≥ 177 μmol/l for at least 48 h

Liver failure: bilirubin ≥ 51 μmol/l for at least 48 h

Disseminated intravascular coagulation: (a) thrombocytes $\leq 100 \times 10^9/l$ or fall of $\geq 30\%$ in 24 n, (b) partial thromboplastin time ≥ 50 s for 24 h, (c) 22 reptilase time ≥ 22 s for 24 h

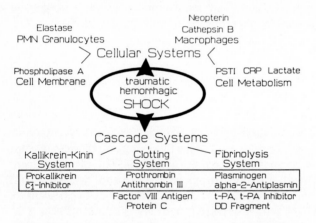

Fig. 1. Biochemical markers in traumatic hemorrhagic shock

Table 1. Complications ($n = 69$)

	Incidence (n)
Multiple organ failure	29
Sepsis	20
Respiratory Failure	42
Adult respiratory distress syndrome	17
Liver failure	42
Renal failure	17
Gastrointestinal failure	7
Disseminated intravascular coagulation	7
No complications	32

GI failure: endoscopically confirmed ulceration with bleeding, acalculous
          cholecystitis
MultipleOF: Failure of two or more organ systems at the same time

The complications of the 69 patients are shown in Table 1.

Statistical testing was done with the non parametric Wilcoxon test for two
samples. Differences were considered significant with *p* values below 0.05.

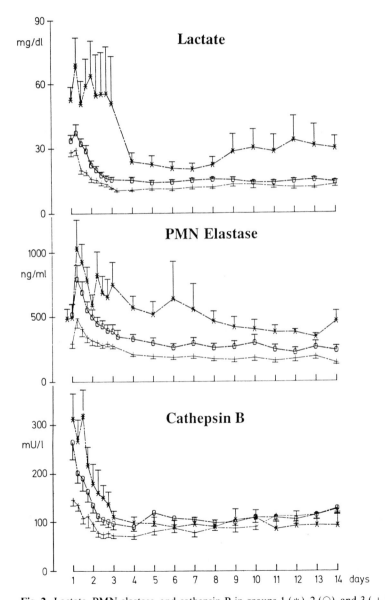

Fig. 2. Lactate, PMN elastase, and cathepsin B in groups 1 (∗), 2 (○), and 3 (+)

Results

The release of mediators and indicators of inflammatory reactions in the three outcome groups is displayed in Figs. 2–4 for those markers which showed clinical relevance. The following differences proved to be significant. A higher

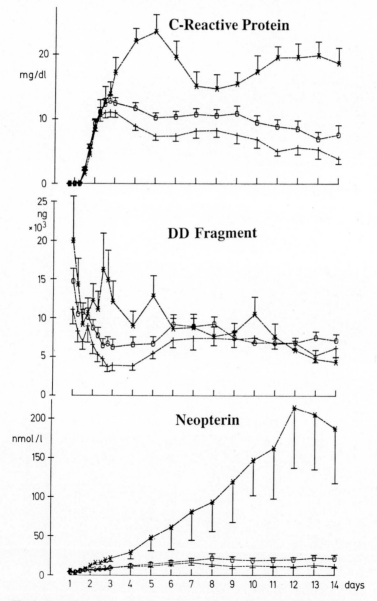

Fig. 3. C-reactive protein, DD fragment, and neopterin in groups 1 (∗), 2 (○), and 3 (+)

accumulation of lactate (Fig. 3) was observed in non survivors (group 1) compared to survivors with organ failure (group 2) throughout 14 days of observation. The level of polymorphonuclear leukocyte (PMN) elastase (Fig. 2) showed a highly significant difference in groups 1 and 2 versus group 3 throughout the whole observation period and in group 1 versus group 2 after the

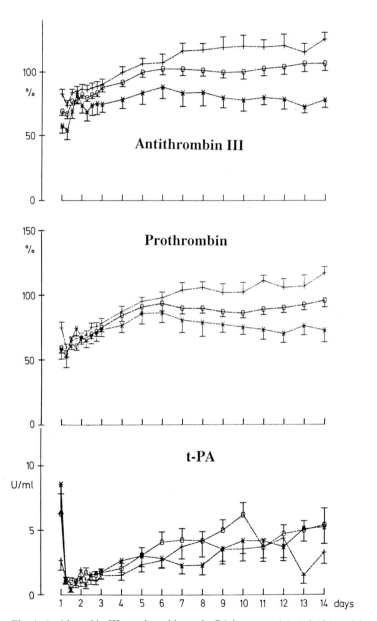

Fig. 4. Antithrombin III, prothrombin, and t-PA in groups 1 (∗), 2 (○), and 3 (+)

3rd day. Cathepsin B (Fig. 2) distinguished patients with OF (groups 1 and 2) from those with uneventful recovery (group 3) within the first 4 days. The production of C-reactive protein; (CRP; Fig 3) was different among all outcome groups starting on the 3rd day after trauma. The D-dimer fragment (Fig. 3) of group 3 differed from that of groups 1 and 2 at arrival, and the levels of all three groups differed between days 3 and 5. Neopterin (Fig. 3) was higher in group 1 (nonsurvivors) compared to survivors (groups 2 and 3) from the 2nd day onwards and between groups 2 versus 3 after the 4th posttraumatic day. Antithrombin III (Fig. 4) showed a lower inhibitory activity in groups 1 and 2 versus group 3 all the time and between groups 1 and 2 (nonsurvivors versus survivors with OF) after the 1st week. At arrival, prothrombin and tissue plasminogen activator (t-PA; Fig 4) distinguished between patients devoloping OF (groups 1 and 2) and those having an uneventful recovery (group 3). In the 2nd week prothrombin differed between survivors and nonsurvivors.

As OF often started on the 1 day, prediction of later OF was possible at hospital arrival, whereas a lethal outcome could be predicted within the first 3 days. The demonstrated mediators showed a reasonable accuracy in predicting OF and death with a higher validity than the ISS Table 2. The combination of the four factors with prognostic value for death (PMN elastase, CRP,

Table 2. Prognostic value for lethal outcome at hospital arrival[a] and at day 4

	ACC	Sens	Spec	PPV	NPV
Lactate[a] (> 45 mg/dl)	88%	60%	93%	60%	93%
Elastase (> 500 ng/ml)	90%	73%	93%	67%	95%
CRP (> 20 mg/dl)	88%	67%	98%	86%	95%
Neopterin (> nmol/l)	86%	75%	93%	67%	95%
ISS (> 50)	80%	36%	88%	36%	88%

ACC, Accuracy; Sens, sensitivity; Spec, specifity; PPV, positive, predicitive value; NPV, negative predictive value.
[a]Prognostic value at hospital arrival for lactate only.

Table 3. Prognostic value for organ failure at hospital arrival

	ACC	Sens	Spec	PPV	NPV
Cathepsin B (> 190 U/l)	90%	63%	86%	86%	62%
Elastase (> 200 ng/ml)	67%	84%	42%	68%	65%
Antithrombin III(< 80%)	66%	71%	58%	71%	58%
Prothrombin (< 70%)	61%	71%	60%	73%	58%
D-dimer fragment (> 12 000 ng/ml)	61%	62%	61%	70%	52%
t-PA (> 8 ng/ml)	57%	62%	54%	68%	48%
ISS (> 30)	61%	70%	48%	65%	54%

ACC, Accuracy; Sens, sensitivity; Spec, specifity; PPV, positive, predicitive value; NPV, negative predictive value,

Table 4. Prognostic value of the combination of four parameters for lethal outcome: elastase, CRP, neopterin, lactate

	(minimum of pathological factors)		
	3	2	1
Sensitivity	53%	73%	93%
Specifity	99%	87%	67%
PPV	89%	50%	34%
NPV	92%	95%	98%
Accuracy	92%	85%	61%

PPV, Positive predictive value; NPV, negative predicitve value.

neopterin, lactate) further improved the accuracy of prediction. More than three pathological results showed a very high risk of death; normal release of all mediators indicated survival (Table 3, 4).

Summary

Biochemical mediators showed a significant difference between traumatized patients with lethal, reversible, and no organ failure. These objective parameters of inflammation might give a more accurate description of injury severity and allow a better estimation of risk for OF than many trauma severity scores.

Intravascular Activation of Polymorphonuclear Neutrophils in Critically Ill Anergic Patients

J. M. Tellado[1] and N. V. Christou[2]

Introduction

Two major immune alterations are common among patients with multiple organ failure syndrome: a downregulation of the T-cell-mediated immunity and an aggressive neutrophil-endothelial interaction at the microvascular level. We intend to address the question whether in critical surgical illness the erosion of both arms of the immune system (specific and nonspecific) progress in parallel.

Material and Methods

Patient Selection. Critically ill surgical patients admitted to the Surgical intensive care unit (SICU) of the Royal Victoria Hospital (Montreal, Canada) with active infection and mounting a septic response were included in the present study after obtaining their informed consent. Patients receiving steroids, chemotherapy, radiotherapy, and massive blood transfusions (more then 5 units of blood) were excluded. Patients were classified as anergic or reactives according to their delayed-type hypersensitivity (DTH) skin test response.

Circulating and Exudative Neutrophil Isolation. Blood samples were drawn in preservative-free heparinized tubes and immediately processed. Aside from the initial red cell sedimentation in 10% dextran 70 at room temperature, the isolation on a Ficoll-Paque gradient (Pharmacia, Piskataway, New Jersey) was performed at 4 °C. After this step, polymorphonuclear neutrophils (PMN) were resuspended in HEPES buffer (HB) without Ca^{2+} (HEPES 30 mM, NaCl 110 mM, KCl 10 mM, MgCl$_2$ 1 mM, glucose 10 mM), washed twice, counted, and resuspended in HB at 4° until used.

PMN delivery was measured using the exudate skin window technique of Zimmerli et al. [1] as previously described [2]. Pooled human serum (75% in Hanks balanced salt solution with Ca^{2+} and Mg^{2+}) was used as an in vivo

[1] Cirugia General III, Hospital Gregorio Maranon, c/Dr. Esquerdo 46, 28007 Madrid, Spain
[2] Department of Surgery, McGill University, 687 Pine Avenue West, Montreal, Quebec, Canada H3A 1A1

Host Defense Dysfunction
in Trauma, Shock and Sepsis
Eds. Faist/Meakins/Schildberg
© Springer-Verlag, Berlin Heidelberg 1993

chemoattractant. Cells were harvested 18 h later. Non-specific esterase was used to count monocytes (less the 3% contamination) and trypan blue exclusion was used to assess cell viability, which was > 95%.

Plasma Lactoferrin.   Lactoferrin, a marker for secondary granules, was determined by an enzyme-linked immunosorbent assay (ELISA) technique [3]. Plates were read in an ELISA reader at 490 nm using buffers to blank the instrument. Optical densities were transformed to micrograms per milliliter according to a standard curve developed with purified human lactoferrin (Terochen, Ontario).

Equilibrium Binding of f-met-leu-phe-lys- and C5a Receptor.   PMN (10^5) were mixed either with f-met-leu-phe-lys (Fmlp)-fluorescein isothiocyanate (FITC) (10 nM) or C5a-FITC (50 nM, kindly provided by D. van Epps, Baxter Healthcare Corporation, Round Lake, Ill.) at equilibrium for 1 h. Nonspecific binding was determined in parallel, preincubating PMN with Fmlp and C5a in 100-fold excess. Fluorescence intensity was measured with a flow cytometer (FACSCAN, Becton and Dickinson) capturing > 10000 events/sample. Results are expressed as $\times 10^3$ receptors/cell (Fmlp) [4] or mean channel number (C5a).

Indirect PMN Immunostaining of Integrin Receptors.   Monoclonal antibodies CD11b/CR3, CD11c/CR4 and CDw29/Fn were incubated at 4° with PMN (10^7/ml) at saturating concentrations. The bound monoclonal antibody was stained with a FITC-labeled goat antimouse immunoglobulin G (IgG) and fixed with freshly diluted 1% paraformaldehyde. Analysis was performed using a flow cytometer and the peak fluorescence intensity transformed to binding sites $\times 10^3$/cell using microbeads (Flow Cytometry Standards, Research Triangle Park, NC).

Results

Plasma lactoferrin levels were higher in anergic than in reactive patients (Fig. 1), implying an intensive activation in the intravascular compartment. As a consequence of this, anergic patients showed an increased in the in vitro adhesion to nylon wool. This finding is in agreement with the surface expression of the adhesion receptors of the integrin superfamily showed in Table 1. There exists an increased gradient of adhesion receptors from controls to anergic patients, and this gradient prevails after PMN migration to inflammatory lesions.

We previously described an in vitro disorder of PMN chemotaxis in critically ill anergic patients [5]. We have now found that PMN cell delivery to inflammatory lesions is also lower in anergic than in reactive patients (Fig. 2). This is associated with anomalies in the number of chemotactic receptors both

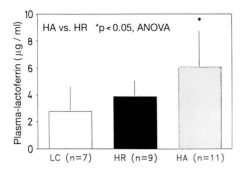

Fig. 1. Plasma lactoferrin concentration (μg/ml; mean $\pm$ SD) in critically ill surgical patients and laboratory controls (*LC*, controls; *HR*, reactive patients; *HA*, anergic patients). *$p < 0.05$ reactive vs anergic patients, ANOVA

Table 1. Adhesion receptors

	Controls ($n = 5$)	Reactives ($n = 6$)	Anergics ($n = 12$)
Circulating			
CR3	59 ± 12	67 ± 38**	123 ± 84**
CD11c	10 ± 2	13.8 ± 5.2*	20.6 ± 7.2*
FnR	21 ± 6	49 ± 27**	61 ± 27**
Exudate			
CR3	257 ± 65	270 ± 58	374 ± 189
CD11c	18 ± 3	25 ± 7	30 ± 15

$\times 10^3$ receptors/cell, mean $\pm$ SD.
*$p < 0.05$ A vs R; **$p < 0.01$ A vs R, ANOVA.

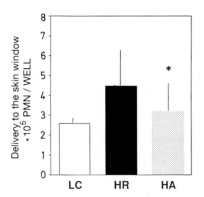

Fig. 2. PMN delivery to inflammatory lesions by means of the skin window technique. ** < 0.05 vs reactive patients or laboratory controls

in circulatins and exudate PMNs (Table 2). Intriguingly, Fmlp and C5a receptor expression follow the opposite pattern. The increased FMLP receptor number appears to correlate with the magnitude of the response observed after ligand challange [6]. The decreased C5a receptor number in anergic patients may be the result of receptor occupancy or lack of receptor recycling [7].

Table 2. Chemotactic receptors

	Controls (n = 5)	Reactives (n = 6)	Anergics (n = 8)
Circulating			
FmlpR	13.1 ± 3.1	20.9 ± 8.8	22.7 ± 9.1
C5a	347 ± 43	297 ± 135	220 ± 130
Exudate			
FmlpR	31.1 ± 2.4	46.8 ± 17.1	49.1 ± 15.8
C5a	255 ± 37	127 ± 42	122 ± 28

Mean ± SD.
FmlpR, $\times 10^3$ receptors/cell; C5a, mean channel number.

Discussion

The lack of response in the DTH skin test in critically ill patients is a step towards the multiple organ failure syndrome [8]. By contrast, this down-regulation of the specific T-cell-dependent immunity is associated with activation of nonspecific host defense mechanisms, e.g. neutrophils (as suggested by the increase in plasma lactoferrin and the production of superoxide in vitro). Our data fully support this hypothesis, suggesting in addition a cause–effect relationship between the intravascular activation of the PMN and the increased neutrophil-endothelial interaction (as indicated by the increased integrin receptors and the fall of cellular exudation to inflammatory lesions). The molecular mechanisms of this process are not fully understood, but better understanding may well provide insights into the differences between an acute physiological and a chronic uncontrolled inflammatory response.

Acknowledgements. This work was supported in part by the Medical Research council program grant PG-31. J.M.T. is recipient of the Lederle Fellowship on Surgical Infectious Diseases from the Canadian Surgical Research Fund. The technical skills of B. Giannias, B. Kapadia, and M. DeSantis are gratefully recognized.

References

1. Zimmerli W, Gallin JI (1987) Monocytes accumulate on rebuck skin window coverslips but not in skin chamber fluid. J Immunol Methods 96:11–17
2. Tellado JM, Giannias B, Kapadia B, Chartrand L, de Santis M, Christou NV (1990) Anergic patients before elective surgery have enhanced nonspecific host-defense capacity. Arch Surg 125:49–53
3. Rautenberg W, Neumann S, Gunzer G, Lang H, Jochum M, Fritz H (1986) Quantitation of human lactoferrin as an inflammation marker by an enzyme-linked immunoabsorbent assay (Elisa). Fresenius Z Anal Chem 324:364
4. Fay SP, Swann WN, Oades ZG, Sklar LA (1991) Direct, real-time analysis of ligand binding kinetics using a novel fluorescent peptides. (submitted)

5. Christou NV, Meakins J (1979) Neutrophil function in anergic surgical patients. Neutrophil adherence and chemotaxis. Ann Surg 190:557–564
6. Fletcher MP, Gallin JI (1980) Degranulation stimuli increase the availability of receptors in human neutrophils for the chemoattractant f-Met-Leu-Phe. J Immunol 124:1585–1588
7. Nelson RD, Hasslen SR, Ahrenholz DH, Solem LD (1987) Mechanisms of loss of human neutrophil chemotaxis following thermal injury. J Burn Care Rehabil 8:496–502
8. Marshall JC, Christou NV, Horn R, Meakins JL (1988) The microbiology of multiple organ failure. The proximal gastrointestinal tract as an occult reservoir of pathogens. Arch Surg 123:309–315

Mediators of Remote Lung Injury*

T. Lindsay[1], J. Hill[1], C. R. Valeri[2], D. Shepro[3], and H. B. Hechtman[1]

Introduction

Severe trauma and systemic sepsis are important precursors of life-threatening lung injury. Smaller injuries such as those occurring with brief periods of ischemia and reperfusion during abdominal aortic surgery result in transient lung dysfunction. The hallmark of injury is increased microvascular permeability, i.e., noncardiogenic pulmonary edema and hypoxia. This review will examine several models of remote organ injury that result in acute respiratory failure and will highlight the inflammatory mediators that appear to be responsible.

Two experimental preparations have been studied in detail, firstly, hindlimb ischemia and reperfusion and, secondly, acid aspiration. Early inflammatory mediators include the eicosanoids, thromboxane $(Tx)A_2$ and leukotriene $(LT)B_4$ [1]. These agents gain access to the circulation where they activate neutrophils, leading to the production of oxygen free radicals and degranulation occur, due largely to the production of cytokines leading to upregulation of the intercellular adhesion molecule (ICAM). Both neutrophil and endothelial cell cytoskeletal elements appear to play a role in adhesion and degranulation. Thus, the inflammatory response may lead to generalized lung injury in addition to the local hindlimb or acid-injured segment.

Thromboxane

Following release of a hindlimb tourniquet or infrarenal aortic crossclamp, the stable metabolite of TxA_2, TxB_2, appears in the plasma. The three- to fourfold rise in TxB_2 levels is rapid, and peaks within 10 min of reperfusion. Coincident with the rise in TxB_2 levels is a rapid rise in mean pulmonary artery pressure,

* Supported in part by the National Institutes of Health, grants GM 24891-11, GM 35141-03, HL 16714-13; the U. S. Navy Office of Naval Research, contract no. N00014-88-C-0118; the Brigham Surgical Group, Inc.; and the Trauma Research Foundation.
[1] Department of Surgery, Brigham and Women's Hospital, 75 Francis St., Boston, MA 02115, USA and Harvard Medical School, Cambridge, MA 02138, USA
[2] Naval Blood Research Laboratory, Boston, Massachusetts, USA
[3] Biological Science Center, Boston University, Boston, MA 02215, USA

which also rapidly returns towards control levels. Over the next several hours lung lymph flow and lung lymph protein clearance increase in the presence of an inflated left atrial balloon which assures a constant perfusion "bed". This documents an increase in lung microvascular permeability. Histological examination of the lungs has demonstrated foci of proteinaceous exudates in alveolar spaces as well as neutrophil sequestration in the alveolar capillaries. Thromboxane A_2 appears to be a key early mediator of these events. Pretreatment with a Tx synthetase inhibitor (OKY 046) will prevent the rise in plasma TxB_2, the transient increase in mean pulmonary artery pressure, neutrophil oxidative activity, and pulmonary leukosequestration, and the rise in lymph protein clearance. Using the Tx receptor antagonist SQ 29, 548, TxB_2 levels rise as expected. However, mean pulmonary artery pressure, neutrophil sequestration, and lung lymph protein clearance are unchanged from sham controls. One to two hours after ischemia, Tx produced by the lungs plays a key role in the pulmonary leukosequestration. The stimulus for pulmonary Tx synthesis is unknown, but its inhibition by bronchoalveolar lavage of an antagonist in a small lung segment will locally prevent neutrophil adhesion and permeability.

Leukotrienes

Leukotrienes also play a role in the lung injury following hindlimb ischemia. Both plasma LTB_4 and TxB_2 levels rose three- to fourfold at 2 min of reperfusion after 2 h of bilateral hindlimb ischemia in sheep. Treatment with the lipoxygenase inhibitor diethylcarbamazine (DEC) prevented lung neutrophil sequestration and lymph protein clearance remained at baseline levels. Plasma LTB_4 and TxB_2 levels did not rise in those animals treated with DEC. In other experimental settings DEC has been shown not to inhibit Tx synthesis. The results suggest that LTB_4 production is required for Tx synthesis. While this study emphasized the role of the chemoattractant/chemoactivating agent LTB_4, one cannot discount the indirect inhibition of TxA_2 production as a significant mechanism of action of DEC.

Neutrophils

The central role of the neutrophil following hindlimb ischemia was investigated in sheep made neutropenic either with hydroxyurea or nitrogen mustard administration. This prevented the rise in plasma TxB_2 levels, mean pulmonary artery pressure, and lymph protein clearance. While neutropenia experiments documented a role for neutrophils, more specific experiments have been carried out in rabbits using a monoclonal antibody (R 15.7) directed against the beta subunit of the CD11/CD18 neutrophil membrane glycoprotein complex. When

R 15.7 was given just prior to reperfusion it prevented the neutropenia usually observed within 10 min of reperfusion [2]. In addition, it prevented the increase in lung neutrophil sequestration, bronchoalveolar lavage protein, and lung wet to dry weight ratio that was observed in untreated animals. These data indicate that the CD18 complex is rapidly activated following reperfusion, probably by conformational changes, and implicate it as the key component of neutrophil adhesion and lung injury. Thus, neutrophil–endothelial cell adhesive interaction is a critical step in the cascade of events that follows hindlimb ischemia and leads to increased fluid and protein accumulation in the lungs.

Are these neutrophils activated prior to their adherence in the lung, and what stimulates their adhesion in the lung and not in other organs? Ten minutes of reperfusion following hindlimb ischemia has been shown to increase the intracellular production of H_2O_2 by the neutrophil. The same neutrophils when stimulated with phorbol myristate acetate (PMA) demonstrate enhanced H_2O_2 production. In animals treated with OKY 046 or SQ 29, 548, neutrophil H_2O_2 production was similar to those of sham controls. A direct relationship existed between plasma TxB_2 levels and the neutrophil production of H_2O_2. Thus, Tx stimulates the neutrophil's oxidative metabolism and enhances the oxidative response to PMA.

An in vitro study examined the adhesion of unstimulated neutrophils to pulmonary microvessel endothelial cells and aortic endothelial cells [3]. Unstimulated neutrophils were twofold more adherent to pulmonary microvessels than aortic endothelial cells. When neutrophils were stimulated with a Tx mimic, increased CD18-dependent adhesion to both types of endothelial cells was observed. These findings suggest that Tx stimulates both neutrophil oxidative metabolism and increased CD18-dependent adhesion following hindlimb ischemia reperfusion. Further, it indicates that the lung may be a preferential target organ secondary to the increased adhesiveness of neutrophils for the pulmonary microvessel endothelial cells. This does not negate the possibility that the low shear forces in the pulmonary circulation are important determinants of leukosequestration.

Reactive Oxygen Species

Oxygen free radicals are also thought to mediate organ injury following tissue ischemia [4]. Superoxide and H_2O_2 are believed to be the primary active oxygen metabolites produced by ischemic tissue upon reperfusion. The enzyme xanthine dehydrogenase can be converted during ischemia to the oxidase form, which with appropriate substrates will result in superoxide production once oxygen is reintroduced. A burst of oxygen free radical production is likely to occur during reperfusion and produce local damage. Remote injury may be secondary to free radicals produced by neutrophils. Treatment with superoxide dismutase and catalase coupled to polyethylene glycol (PEG SOD and PEG

CAT) or allopurinol reduced Tx production, the spike of mean pulmonary artery pressure, lung leukosequestration, and lung microvascular permeability. Since eicosanoid synthesis requires peroxy radicals it is possible that these intermediates were inhibited by PEG SOD and PEG CAT, and the true benefit of these agents may be the blocking of TxA_2 production. However, the inhibition of TxA_2 production by allopurinol was unexpected, unless one speculates that allopurinol is a free radical scavenger, or that oxygen free radicals from xanthine oxidase stimulate TxA_2 production. Nevertheless, Tx production in this model was inhibited by PEG SOD and PEG CAT or allopurinol administration and once again emphasizes the critical role of Tx in mediating the lung injury following hindlimb ischemia.

Cytokines

Infusion of the cytokine tumor necrosis factor-α (TNF-α) mimics endotoxemia and causes increased pulmonary permeability [5]. Secondly, TNF-α stimulates endothelium to upregulate ICAM-1 via de novo synthesis [6]. Also, TNF-α will stimulate neutrophils to produce and release superoxide and granular enzyme products. Thus, circulating TNF-α would seem to be a likely mediator of the remote lung injury that follows hindlimb ischemia. Using a 4-h period of hindlimb ischemia in rats, significant elevations in lung neutrophil sequestration, bronchoalveolar lavage (BAL) fluid protein content, and lung wet to dry weight ratio occurred after 4 h of reperfusion. The administration of TNF-α antiserum significantly reduced lung neutrophil sequestration, BAL fluid protein, and wet to dry ratio compared to rats receiving saline or control antiserum. However, lung neutrophil sequestration was not reduced to control levels. While LTB_4 and TxA_2 may stimulate early neutrophil activation and adhesion to basally expressed endothelial adhesion molecules, alone they do not induce endothelial adhesion proteins which are necessary for the later progressive neutrophil sequestration. These data suggest that TNF-α partially mediates the lung neutrophil sequestration, and the subsequent lung injury either by direct neutrophil activation or more likely by stimulation of increased pulmonary endothelial cell adhesive receptors.

   The role of cytokines in lung injury has also been investigated following liver and intestinal ischemia. Three cephelad lobes of the rat liver were made ischemic for 90 min and then reperfused [7]. Blood drawn during reperfusion from the suprahepatic vena cava demonstrated a rise in TNF-α levels at 30 min, followed by a decline to baseline over 4 h. Lung myeloperoxidase levels tripled 1 h following reperfusion and remained elevated for 12 h. Lung histology demonstrated significant alveolar flooding and hemorrhage at 12 h. The infusion of a polyclonal TNF-α antiserum before hepatic ischemia significantly reduced but did not abolish the increase in lung myeloperoxidase. Histologic sections revealed no alveolar flooding and reduced intraalveolar hemorrhage. Liver injury assessed by histology and transaminase release was also reduced. These results are similar to those quoted above regarding the hindlimb where the reduction in neutrophil sequestration was significant but not complete. Thus, it is possible that other cytokines may be involved in the upregulation of endothelial cell adhesion molecules, accounting for the incomplete suppression of neutrophil accumulation.

In a model of intestinal ischemia, TNF-α levels peaked 30 min following reperfusion [8]. Lung injury was assessed by the measurement of a permeability index using I^{125}-labeled albumen. Two hours after reperfusion the lung permeability index rose significantly, as did the lung myeloperoxidase content. TNF-α antiserum was able to reduce the lung permeability index but myeloperoxidase content was not reduced. Thus, this study is at variance with those mentioned above with respect to the effect of TNF-α in lung neutrophil sequestration. Despite this apparent difference, all three studies suggest that TNF-α is an important mediator of lung injury that follows remote ischemia. The role of other cytokines has yet to be delineated.

Acid Aspiration

Acid aspiration into one lung lobe causes both local neutrophil sequestration and systemic Tx synthesis. The aspirated lung demonstrates an increase in permeability and wet to dry weight ratio. Systemic neutrophil activation occurs, as demonstrated by a sevenfold increase in the intracellular production of H_2O_2. Injury to the nonaspirated lung is indicated by a significant rise in lung wet to dry weight ratio. Treatment with OKY 046 or SQ 29,548 prevented the neutrophil oxidative burst, minimized leukosequestration, and attenuated the increase in wet to dry weight ratio of the aspirated and nonaspirated lung. Thus, in this model of acid aspiration Tx also appears to be a key mediator of the local and remote injury.

Using the CD18 antibody R 15.7 just prior to acid aspiration, it was found that, 3 h following acid injury, the aspirated lung still sequestered polymorphonuclear leukocytes, while neutrophil sequestration in the nonaspirated lung was reduced to control levels. Reduction in permeability following R15.7 was only noted in the nonaspirated lung. Therefore, it appears that neutrophil adhesion on the aspirated side is CD18 independent.

Acid aspiration also leads to a multisystem organ injury. This is shown by increases in tissue myeloperoxidase levels and wet to dry weight ratios in heart and kidney. The systemic nature of the injury is similar to that produced by TNF-α infusion with systemic organ failure and associated leukosequestration.

A polyclonal TNF-α antiserum was administered 20 min following acid aspiration. Three hours later the groups treated with saline or control serum demonstrated significant leukosequestration in both lungs. Increases in BAL protein and lung wet to dry weight were observed, as were increases in heart and kidney myeloperoxidase content and wet to dry weight ratios. Treatment with TNF-α antiserum significantly reduced the leukosequestration and permeability in both lungs. Myeloperoxidase content in the heart and kindney as well as the organ wet to dry weight ratios were also reduced. Since de novo TNF-α synthesis is thought to be required for injury to occur, the protein synthesis inhibitor cyclohexamide was given 20 min following acid aspiration. Cyclohexamide was as effective as TNF-α antiserum in reducing the injury to both lungs. This experimental evidence supports the concept that TNF-α mediates a major component of the local and systemic injury and that this event is protein synthesis dependent. Although TNF-α was not detected in the plasma of many animals, this study still strongly supports TNF-α's role as a mediator in both local and systemic acid aspiration injury.

Cytoskeleton

One aspect of the inflammatory response is the alteration of the cytoskeleton of both neutrophils and endothelial cells. In assays of neutrophil diapedesis, cytoskeletal manipulation will modulate extravascular leukocyte accumulation in response to LTB_4, histamine, or zymosanactivated plasma. Phalloidin, a cyclic peptide from the *Amanita phalloides* mushroom, binds to F-actin and can reduce the macromolecular flux across endothelial cell monolayers. In rats, saline or phalloidin was used as a pretreatment 20 min prior to acid aspiration. Local treatment with phalloidin by lavage resulted in a reduction in local permeability but had no effect upon the nonaspirated lung. Neutrophil infiltration into the acid-aspirated lung was prevented while the rise in plasma TxB_2 and LTB_4 levels was unchanged by phalloidin administration.

Summary

Following ischemia and reperfusion or acid aspiration, the earliest inflammatory events occur within minutes and include tissue synthesis of Tx and LT. Entry of these eicosanoids into the circulation leads to rapid neutrophil activation manifested by H_2O_2 synthesis and conformational changes in the CD18 complex. The eicosanoids may also stimulate TNF-α synthesis by tissue monocytes and/or circulating leukocytes. Together with the eicosanoids TNF-α may act via positive feedback to promote local adhesion of neutrophils and a systemic inflammatory response by upregulation of remote endothelial adhesion proteins. Neutrophil–endothelial cell adhesion provides a microenvironment where released oxygen radicals and granular enzymes may disrupt the endothelial cytoskeleton and increase permeability. Differences exist between ischemic and aspiration injury in terms of mediators and the distribution of injury.

Regardless, a common group of agents are thought to be involved in both settings.

References

1. Klausner JM, Paterson IS, Mannick J, Valeri CR, Shepro D, Hechtman HB (1989) Reperfusion pulmonary edema. JAMA 261:1030–1035
2. Welbourn R, Goldman G, Lindsay T, Hill J, Shepro D, Hechtman HB (1991) Lung injury following hindlimb ischemia is mediated by neutrophil CD18 adherence receptors. FASEB J 5:6502 (Abstract)
3. Wiles M, Welbourn R, Goldman G, Hechtman HB, Shepro D (1991) Thromboxane-induced neutrophil adhesion to aortic and pulmonary microvesicular endothelium is regulated by CD18. Inflammation 15:181–199
4. Granger DN (1988) Role of xanthine oxidase and granulocytes in ischemia-reperfusion injury. Am J Physiol 255:H1269–1275
5. Tracey KJ, Beutler B, Lowry SF, Merryweather J, Wolpe S, Milsark IW, Hariri RJ, Fahey III, TJ, Zentella A, Albert JD, Shires GT, Cerami A (1986) Shock and tissue injury induced by recombinant human cachectin. Science 234:470–474
6. Bevilacqua MP, Prober JS, Mendrick DL, Cotran RS, Gimbrone MA (1987) Identification of an inducible endothelial-leukocyte adhesion molecule. Proc Natl Acad Sci USA 84:9238–9242
7. Colletti LM, Remick DG, Burtch GD, Kunkel SL, Stieter RM, Campbell DA (1990) Role of tumor necrosis factor in the pathophysiologic alterations after hepatic ischemia/reperfusion injury in rat. J Clin Invest 85:1936–1943
8. Caty MG, Guice KS, Oldham KT, Remick DG, Kunkel SI (1990). Evidence for a tumor necrosis factor induced pulmonary microvascular injury after intestine ischemia reperfusion injury. Ann Surg 212:694–700

3.3 Sepsis

Immunologic Dyshomeostasis in Multiple Organ Failure: The Gut–Liver Axis

J. C. Marshall

Introduction

Altered immunologic responsiveness is a cardinal feature of the syndrome of multiple organ failure (MOF). The mechanisms of immune dysfunction in MOF are largely unknown. Moreover, it is increasingly controversial whether the major clinical consequence of this dysfunction is *immunosuppression* resulting in enhanced susceptibility to infection and suggesting a need for therapies to stimulate the immune response [1, 2] or *overactivity* of the immune response with tissue injury the result of systemic activation of the inflammatory response, and a corresponding need for therapies to downregulate the endogenous response [3–5]. It is apparent, however, that alterations in normal immunologic homeostasis play a central role in the pathogenesis of the syndrome.

Interactions of the indigenous gastrointestinal flora with the gut-associated lymphoid tissues (GALT) and liver contribute to the normal maturation and regulation of systemic immunity [6, 7]. Changes in these interactions have been implicated in the sequelae of a variety of disease processes including trauma [8], radiation injury [9], cirrhosis [10], and certain autoimmune disorders [11]. It has been proposed that interactions between gut flora and host tissues are involved in the evolution of the clinical syndrome of MOF [12]. However, failure of the gut barrier with the entry of microorganisms and their products, and activation of local immunologic tissues in the gut and liver, are potential triggers for the state of immune dyshomeostasis which characterizes MOF.

Altered Gastrointestinal Flora in Critical Illness

The normal human gastrointestinal (GI) tract is a highly complex organ, consisting not only of host tissues but also of an indigenous microbial flora which exerts an important influence on physiologic and immunologic homeostasis. In health, the proximal GI tract is sterile or lightly populated with gram-positive organisms. Numbers of gram-negatives and anerobes increase

Toronto General Hospital, Eaton North 9-234, 200 Elizabeth Street, Toronto, Ontario, M5G 2C4, Canada

Host Defense Dysfunction
in Trauma, Shock and Sepsis
Eds. Faist/Meakins/Schildberg
© Springer-Verlag, Berlin Heidelberg 1993

Table 1. The most common microbial isolates from the upper GI tract of 34 critically ill surgical patients (from [17])

Organism	No. of patients[a]	Log CFU/ml	% Infected[b]	p[c]
Candida	15	4.4 ± 0.3	80	< 0.05
S. epidermidis	8	5.4 ± 0.6	75	< 0.05
Enterococcus	8	6.2 ± 0.5	50	NS
Pseudomonas	7	6.9 ± 0.4	86	< 0.005

[a] Number of patients colonized with organism.
[b] Percentage of colonized patients who had systemic infection with colonizing organism at any time during ICU stay
[c] Fisher's exact test comparing rates of infection with particular species in patients who were colonized with the organism versus those who were not.

progressively in the distal small bowel, reaching a density of 10^{11} organisms per gram of feces. More than 400 different bacterial species have been identified in the stool.

Studies of gut flora in the critically ill have demonstrated both qualitative and quantitative changes. Gastric, duodenal, and proximal jejunal colonization with gram negative aerobes and fungi is a prominent finding [13–16]. Upper gut colonization occurs early during the stay in the intensive care unit (ICU); bacterial concentrations approach those seen in the colon. We have investigated the relationship of proximal GI colonization to the development of ICU-acquired infection in a group of 34 surgical patients at high risk for the development of these infections [17]. The most common isolates from upper GI fluid were *Candida, Staphylococcus epidermidis, Pseudomonas,* and the enterococcus—the same organisms which predominate in all ICU-acquired infections [4, 18]. Upper gut colonization was significantly associated with the development of invasive infection (Table 1), not only pneumonia but also recurrent peritonitis, urinary tract infections, and bacteremias.

Similar findings of other descriptive studies support the conclusion that the upper GI/tract of the critically ill patient is an important reservoir of the organisms producing ICU-acquired infection [13, 16]. Moreover, rates of these infections can be reduced by measures designed to prevent upper gut colonization including selective decontamination of the digestive tract [19, 20] and the use of cytoprotective agents for stress ulcer prophylaxis [15]. Invasive infection of gut origin may arise as a consequence of the aspiration of contaminated gastric secretions or the translocation of viable microorganisms across the GI mucosa.

Gut Barrier Failure and Systemic Infection in Critical Illness

The normal gut harbors a volume of bacteria and bacterial products such as endotoxin which would be rapidly lethal were even a small portion of it introduced into the body. It is truly remarkable that an organ which has evolved biologically as a highly efficient absorptive site for nutrients should at the same time be so effective in preventing the entry of significant numbers of bacteria. The biologic barrier which prevents bacterial translocation is a complex one, consisting of the following anatomic, physiologic, microbiologic, and immunologic elements:

Anatomic
– Lower esophageal sphincter, pylorus, and ligament of Treitz—ensuring forward passage of luminal contents
– Tight junctions between mucosal epithelial cells
– Multilayered aggregations of lymphoid cells—intraepithelial lymphocytes, Peyer's patches, mesenteric lymph nodes

Physiologic
– Gastric acidity
– Normal GI motility
– Bile
– Mucus

Microbiologic
– Anerobic flora (colonization resistance)
– Competition for substrate
– Competition for mucosal binding sites
– Specific microbial factors

Immunologic
– GALT
– IgA secretion
– Immunologic priming by endogenous flora

Bacterial translocation can occur as a consequence of changes in the endogenous flora or impairment of normal barrier function.

Massive increases in the luminal concentrations alone are sufficient to cause the translocation of *Candida* in both experimental animals [21] and man [22]. Intestinal monoassociation with *Escherichia coli* induced by feeding antibiotic resistant organisms following suppression of the native flora similarly results in bacterial translocation to mesenteric lymph nodes [23]. Translocation in this latter model may result not so much from bacterial overgrowth as from the elimination of the normal anerobic flora; anerobes are recognized to be an important component of the gut barrier to translocation [24].

Under normal circumstances, the composition of the indigenous flora of a given individual is remarkably stable over time, both qualitatively and quantitatively. This stability is primarily a consequence of microbial interactions, through competition for nutritional substrate and binding sites and the production of factors regulating microbial growth. Van der Waaij demonstrated that the indigenous flora inhibits the proliferation of potential pathogens within the GI tract and termed this phenomenon "colonization resistance" [25]. Studies in which the normal flora is suppressed by orally administered antibiotics have shown that colonization resistance plays an important role in inhibiting the growth of both *Candida* [26] and *Pseudomonas* [27]. Anerobes are the predominant organisms which mediate colonization resistance [28]. In addition, it has been shown that a factor produced by *E. coli* can suppress gut proliferation of *Candida* in vivo [29]. Paradoxically then, one of the most important components of the gut barrier to bacterial translocation is the integrity of the indigenous flora.

Physiologic factors comprising the gut barrier function predominantly by regulating bacterial growth within the gut lumen. Bile duct obstruction, for example, results in both increases in cecal concentrations of gram-negative organisms and translocation of gram-negatives to mesenteric lymph nodes [30]. Maintenance of normal gastric acidity and of normal intestinal motility similarly minimizes microbial proliferation within the gut lumen. Translocation occurs in rats receiving intravenous total parenteral nutrition, and to a lesser extent in animals receiving such solution by mouth, but not in animals receiving normal chow [31]; the mechanism of the protective effect of enteral nutrition is not known.

Immunologic factors controlling the proliferation and translocation of gut organisms have not been well defined. Local production of IgA may regulate colonization by inhibition of bacterial adhesion, and it is known that jejunal colonization following surgical vagotomy occurs only in patients with isolated IgA deficiency [32]. IgA release in bile plays an important role in the regulation of luminal microbial ecology in rats [33] but is felt to be of less importance in humans. Impaired T cell immunity also appears to dispose to bacterial translocation [34].

The maintenance of stable patterns of microbial colonization by the mechanisms outlined above comprises a highly effective barrier to bacterial translocation across the gut wall. Low levels of translocation, however, probably occur on a regular basis, and studies of the mechanisms of translocation have revealed that organisms can pass into the host either directly through the gastrointestinal epithelium [35] or within macrophages circulating to regional lymph nodes [36]. Injury to the mucosa, however, results in greatly increased numbers of translocating organisms.

Experimental models of bacterial translocation mirror the spectrum of clinical disorders associated with MOF and its associated alterations in immune function, and include burns, endotoxemia, hemorrhage, and pancreatitis (reviewed in [37]). Reduced splanchnic blood flow occurs in all of these models, and experimental work demonstrating the importance of xanthine oxidase-generated oxygen intermediates in bacterial translocation [38] suggests a central role for reperfusion injury in the pathogenesis of translocation in models of critical illness.

Translocation of organisms from the gut into the body with resultant invasive infection provides a mechanism whereby gut flora can initiate the sequence of biologic events producing MOF. This process may, however, occur in the absence of invasive infection as a result of the activation of host mediator systems by absorbed endotoxin or as a consequence of microbial interactions with cells in the wall of the GI tract. Paneth's cells express messenger RNA for tumor necrosis factor [39], and immunologically activated colonic T cells have been shown to release both tumor necrosis factor and interferon gamma [40]. Thus gut flora may initiate the cytokine cascade leading to MOF by at least three separate mechanisms: (a) translocation of viable bacteria with systemic infection, (b) absorption of bacterial products with activation of mediator systems within the host, and (c) local interactions with the GALT resulting in local production and release of mediator substances. How important each of these processes is to the initiation and evolution of clinical MOF is unknown; however it is apparent that they can induce systemic immunologic alterations similar to those documented in MOF.

MOF as Dyshomeostasis: Infection, Sepsis, and Altered Immunity

The immunologic alterations of MOF and critical illness are extensive and complex, involving both nonspecific and specific effector mechanisms (reviewed in [41]). Suppression of T cell-mediated responses is striking—delayed type hypersensitivity (DTH) in vivo [42] and mitogen-stimulated lymphocyte proliferation in vitro [43]; certain B cell responses, on the other hand, may be normal or even augmented [44]. This pattern of immune dysregulation is identical to that which occurs in response to endotoxin [45] or macrophage activation [46] and therefore is better conceptualized as immune system activation rather than as immune system failure.

The syndrome of MOF is a dynamic process rather than a static event; its final expression reflects the interplay of a stimulus and the host response to that stimulus, producing a systemic state of disordered homeostasis or dyshomeostasis. Viewed from the perspective of immune homeostasis, the stimulus is infection, the response is the septic response, and the outcome is a spectrum of immunologic changes which both reflect systemic immunologic activation and predispose to further infectious complications. Increasing severity of organ dysfunction is associated with increasing susceptibility to ICU-acquired infection and increasing immune dysfunction reflected in impaired DTH (Fig. 1a, b), but also with an augmented rather than impaired host septic response reflected in greater elevations of clinical parameters such as temperature (Fig. 1c) and white cell count.

Gut Flora, the Liver, and Modulation of Systemic Immunity

The maturation and regulation of normal systemic immunity is profoundly influenced by the indigenous flora of the GI tract; conversely, alterations in that flora may induce systemic alterations in immunologic responsiveness.

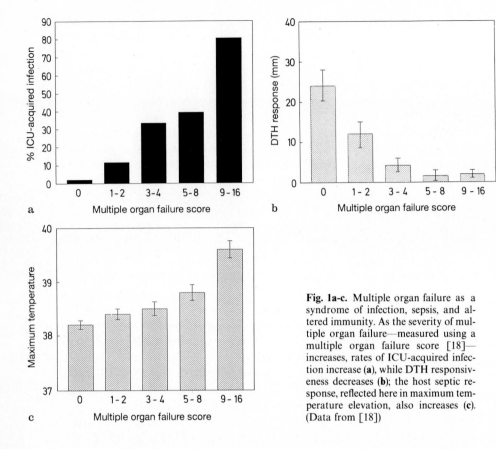

Fig. 1a-c. Multiple organ failure as a syndrome of infection, sepsis, and altered immunity. As the severity of multiple organ failure—measured using a multiple organ failure score [18]—increases, rates of ICU-acquired infection increase (**a**), while DTH responsiveness decreases (**b**); the host septic response, reflected here in maximum temperature elevation, also increases (**c**). (Data from [18])

Studies performed in germfree animals have helped to elucidate the role that the normal flora plays in the maturation of systemic immunity. Germfree mice fail to develop a primary DTH response following immunization with sheep red blood cells unless the GI tract is first colonized with gram-negative bacteria [47]. At the same time, this flora exerts a suppressive influence on the secondary antibody response of splenic lymphocytes, apparently as a result of the induction of suppressive activity in splenic macrophages [48]. Germfree animals are highly susceptible to lethal bacterial infection with *S. aureus* or *Klebsiella* but resistant to challenge with doses of endotoxin which would prove lethal to a conventional animal [49].

We studied the immunologic consequences of alterations in gut flora on the magnitude of the DTH response following recall challenge with the antigen keyhole limpet hemocyanin (KLH) in a rat model. Cecal ligation and puncture (CLP) resulted in both massive small bowel overgrowth with *E. coli* and suppression of DTH responsiveness. To investigate the relationship between these two phenomena, the endogenous flora was suppressed with oral antibiotics prior to CLP. Animals recolonized with antibiotic-resistant *E. coli* demonstrated significantly greater DTH suppression following CLP than did their saline controls; small bowel colonization alone was sufficient to induce this suppression [50]. Feeding killed *Candida* or *Pseudomonas* to normal animals over a 3-week period also induced DTH suppression; animals fed *S. epidermidis* or sheep red blood cells showed no such suppression. Although DTH reactivity was suppressed, the secondary antibody response to *Pseudomonas* was unaffected by prior feeding [51]. These data demonstrated that two organisms commonly isolated from the GI tract of the critically ill patient can, if present in high concentrations in the gut, induce the same systemic immune changes seen in critical illness, and that these changes are independent of bacterial viability.

Because macrophage activation by endotoxin induces suppression of DTH reactivity [52], and because hepatic Kupffer's cells account for fully 70% of the total population of macrophages in the body, we hypothesized that the activation of Kupffer's cells by endotoxin absorbed into the portal vein could produce systemic impairment of DTH reactivity. To test this hypothesis, live or killed bacteria were infused into either the portal vein or the systemic circulation via the inferior vena cava, and the effects on systemic immunity were assessed. Infusion of live *E. coli* or killed *Pseudomonas* into the portal vein resulted in significant DTH suppression when compared with either systemic infusion of these organisms of saline controls; suppression was not seen, however, when a gram positive organism—*S. fecalis*—was administered [53, 54]. The magnitude of DTH suppression correlated significantly with the calculated first-pass

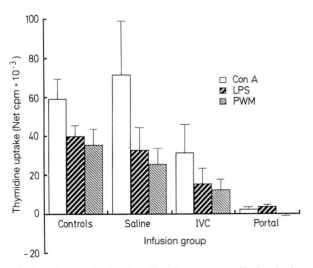

Fig. 2. Mitogen-stimulated proliferative responses of isolated splenocytes, 24 h following infusion of normal saline or 5×10^8 killed *Pseudomonas* into either the inferior vena cava (*IVC*) or portal vein. Splenocytes were stimulated with concanavalin A (*con A*), lipopolysaccharide (*LPS*), or pokeweed mitogen (*PWM*), and proliferation measured as the uptake of [^{3}H]thymidine. Suppression evident in cells from animals infused via the portal vein was found to be mediated by a soluble factor released by splenic adherent cells

extraction of the organism by the liver, and suppression could be ablated by portal infusion of the macrophage toxin carrageenan [53]. The ability of isolated splenic lymphocytes to proliferate in vitro in response to either a T cell (concanavalin A) or B cell (lipopolysaccharide) mitogen is also profoundly suppressed 24 h after portal but not systemic infusion of killed *Pseudomonas* (Fig. 2). Suppression is mediated by a soluble factor released by both splenic adherent cells and alveolar macrophages [55]; studies to identify the factor are in progress.

Summary: The Gut–Liver Axis in Multiple Organ Failure

It has become apparent that the conventional concept of MOF as the expression of uncontrolled infection [56] is inadequate to explain many features of the syndrome—its evolution in the absence of infection, its persistence despite the treatment of infection, and its variable and often unpredictable clinical expression. The concept of a gut–liver axis presented here provides a separate mechanism for the evolution of the syndrome. Briefly stated, the hypothesis suggests that changes in gut flora and barrier function occurring in the critically ill patient can set the stage for the immunologic dyshomeostasis which characterizes the syndrome. The gut serves as a reservoir of ICU-acquired infections, but perhaps more importantly the interaction of an altered gut flora with immune cells in the GALT and liver can initiate the mediator cascade which is seen clinically as sepsis and altered systemic immunity. The model is a reincarnation of concepts advanced by Fine and others more than 30 years ago [57], and before him by Metchnikoff at the turn of the century [58]. Tantalizing as the notion is to many of those involved in the care of the critically ill, there remains a wide gulf of speculation between the formulation of the hypothesis and its translation into therapies that can prevent or alter the course of MOF.

References

1. Meakins JL, Christou NV, Shizgal HM, MacLean LD (1979) Therapeutic approaches to anergy in surgical patients. Surgery and levamisole. Ann Surg 190:286–296
2. Polk HC Jr (1986) The enhancement of host defenses against infection—search for the holy grail? Surgery 99:1–6
3. Goris RJA, te Boekhorst TPA, Nuytinck JKS, Gimbrere JSF (1985) Multiple-organ failure. Generalized autodestructive inflammation? Arch Surg 120:1109–1115
4. Marshall JC, Sweeney D (1990) Microbial infection and the septic response in critical surgical illness. Sepsis, not infection, determines outcome. Arch Surg 125:17–23
5. Christou NV, Tellado JM (1989) In vitro polymorphonuclear neutrophil function in surgical patients does not correlate with anergy but 'activating' processes such as sepsis or trauma. Surgery 106:718–724
6. McGhee JR, Kiyono H, Alley CD (1984) Gut bacterial endotoxin: influence on gut-associated lymphoreticular tissue and host immune function. Surv Immunol Res 3:241–252

7. Dubos RJ, Schaedler RW (1960) The effect of the intestinal flora on the growth rate of mice and on their susceptibility to experimental infections. J Exp Med 111:407–417
8. Woodruff PWH, O'Carroll DI, Koizumi S, Fine J (1973) Role of the intestinal flora in major trauma. J Infect Dis 128 [Suppl]:S290–S294
9. Walker RI (1978) The contribution of intestinal endotoxin to mortality in hosts with compromised resistance: a review. Exp Hematol 6:172–184
10. Rutenburg AM, Sonnenblick E, Koven I, Aprahamian HA, Reiner L, Fine J (1957) The role of intestinal bacteria in the development of dietary cirrhosis in rats. J Exp Med 106:1–14
11. Penhale WJ, Young PR (1988) The influence of the normal microbial flora on the susceptibility of rats to experimental autoimmune thyroiditis. Clin Exp Immunol 72:288
12. Carrico CJ, Meakins JL, Marshall JC, Fry D, Maier RV (1986) Multiple-organ-failure syndrome. The gastrointestinal tract: the 'motor' of MOF. Arch Surg 121:196–208
13. Du Moulin GC, Hedley-White J, Paterson DG, Lisbon A (1982) Aspiration of gastric bacteria in antacid-treated patients: a frequent cause of postoperative colonisation of the airway. Lancet 1:242–244
14. Hillman KM, Riordan T, O'Farrell SM, Tabaqchali S (1982) Colonization of the gastric contents in critically ill patients. Crit Care Med 10:444–447
15. Driks MR, Craven DE, Celli BR et al. (1987) Nosocomial pneumonia in intubated patients given sucralfate as compared with antacids or histamine type 2 blockers. N Engl J Med 317:1376–1382
16. Gravey BM, McCambley JA, Tuxen DV (1989) Effects of gastric alkalization on bacterial colonization in critically ill patients. Crit Care Med 17:211–216
17. Marshall JC, Christou NV, de Santis M, Meakins JL (1987) Proximal gastrointestinal flora and systemic infection in the critically ill surgical patient. Surg Forum 38:89–91
18. Marshall JC, Christou NV, Horn R, Meakins JL (1988) The microbiology of multiple organ failure. The proximal GI tract as an occult reservoir of pathogens. Arch Surg 123:309–315
19. Stoutenbeek CP, van Saene HKF, Miranda DR, Zandstra DF (1984) The effect of selective decontamination of the digestive tract on colonisation and infection rates in multiple trauma patients. Intensive Care Med 10:185–192
20. Ledingham IMcA, Alcock SR, Eastaway AT, McDonaid JC, McKay IC, Ramsay G (1988) Triple regimen of selective decontamination of the digestive tract, systemic cefotaxime, and microbiological surveillance for prevention of acquired infection in intensive care. Lancet 1:785–790
21. Stone HH, Kolb LD, Currie CA, Geheber CE, Cuzzell JZ (1974) Candida sepsis: pathogenesis and principles of treatment. Ann Surg 179:697–711
22. Krause W, Matheis H, Wulf K (1969) Fuṅgaemia and funguria after oral administration of Candida albicans. Lancet 1:598–599
23. Berg RD, Owens WE (1979) Inhibition of translocation of viable Escherichia coli from the gastrointestinal tract of mice by bacterial antagonism. Infect Immun 25:820–827
24. Wells CL, Maddaus MA, Reynolds CM, Jechorek P, Simmons RL (1987) Role of the anaerobic flora in the translocation of aerobic and facultatively anaerobic intestinal bacteria. Infect Immun 55:2689–2694
25. Van der Waaij D, Berghuis de Vries JM, Lekkerkerk van der Wees JEC (1971) Colonization resistance of the digestive tract in conventional and antibiotic-treated mice. J Hyg 69:405–411
26. Kennedy MJ, Volz PA (1985) Ecology of Candida albicans gut colonization: inhibition of Candida adhesion, colonization, and dissemination from the gastrointestinal tract by bacterial antagonism. Infect Immun 49:654–663
27. Hentges DJ, Stein AJ, Casey SW, Que JU (1985) Protective role of intestinal flora against infection with Pseudomonas aeruginosa in mice: influence of antibiotics on colonizatioṅ resistance. Infect Immun 47:118–122
28. Wensinck F, Ruseler van Embden JGH (1971) The intestinal flora of colonization-resistant mice. J Hyg 69:413–421
29. Hummel RP, Ostreicher EJ, Maley MP, MacMillan BG (1973) Inhibition of Candida albicans by Escherichia coli in vitro and in the germfree mouse. J Surg Res 15:53–58
30. Deitch EA, Sittig K, Li M, Berg RD, Specian D (1990) Obstructive jaundice promotes bacterial translocation from the gut. Am J Surg 159:79–84
31. Alverdy JC, Aoys E, Moss GS (1988) Total parenteral nutrition promotes bacterial translocation from the gut. Surgery 104:185–190
32. McLoughlin GA, Hede JE, Temple JG, Bradley J, Chapman DM, McFarland J (1978) The role of IgA in the prevention of bacterial colonization of the jejunum in the vagotomized subject. Br J Surg 65:435–437

33. Alverdy JC, Chi HS, Sheldon GS (1985) The effect of parenteral nutrition on gastrointestinal immunity. The importance of enteral stimulation. Ann Surg 202:681–684
34. Owens WE, Berg RD (1980) Bacterial translocation from the gastrointestinal tract of athymic (nu/nu) mice. Infect Immun 27:461–467
35. Alexander JW, Boyce ST, Babcock GF, Gianotti L, Peck MD, Dunn DL et al. (1990) The process of microbial translocation. Ann Surg 212:496–512
36. Wells CL, Maddaus MA, Erlandsen SL, Simmons RL (1988) Evidence for the phagocytic transport of intestinal particles in dogs and rats. Infect Immun 56:278–282
37. Wells CL, Maddaus MA, Simmons RL (1988) Proposed mechanisms for the translocation of intestinal bacteria. Rev Infect Dis 10:958–979
38. Deitch EA, Ma L, Ma WJ, Grisham MB, Granger DN, Specian RD, Berg RD (1989) Inhibition of endotoxin-induced bacterial translocation in mice. J Clin Invest 84:36–42
39. Keshav S, Lawson L, Chung LP, Stein M, Perry VH, Gordon S (1990) Tumor necrosis factor mRNA localized T Paneth cells of normal murine intestinal epithelium by in situ hybridization. J Exp Med 171:327–332
40. Deem RL, Shanahan F, Targan SR (1991) Triggered human mucosal T cells release tumour necrosis factor-alpha and interferon-gamma which kill human colonic epithelial cells. Clin Exp Immunol 83:79–84
41. Abraham E (1989) Host defense abnormalities after hemorrhage, trauma, and burns. Crit Care Med 17:934–939
42. MacLean LD, Meakins JL, Taguchi K, Duignan JP, Dhillon KS, Gordon J (1975) Host resistance in sepsis and trauma. Ann Surg 182:207–217
43. Keane RM, Birmingham W, Shatney CM, Winchurch RA, Munster AM (1983) Prediction of sepsis in the multitraumatic patient by assays of lymphocyte responsiveness. Surg Gynecol Obstet 156:163–167
44. Nohr CW, Latter DA, Meakins JL, Christou NV (1986) In vivo and in vitro humoral immunity in surgical patients: antibody response to pneumococcal polysaccharide. Surgery 100:229–238
45. Morrison DC, Ulevitch RJ (1978) The effects of bacterial endotoxins on host mediation systems. Am J Pathol 93:527–617
46. Kirchner H, Holden HT, Herberman RB (1975) Splenic suppressor macrophages induced in mice by injection of Corynebacterium parvum. J Immunol 115:1212–1216
47. MacDonald TT, Carter PB (1979) Requirements for a bacterial flora before mice generate cells capable of mediating the delayed hypersensitivity reaction to sheep red blood cells. J Immunol 122:2624–2629
48. Mattingly JA, Eardley DD, Kemp JD, Gershon K (1979) Induction of suppressor cells in rat spleen: influence of intestinal stimulation. J Immunol 122:787–790
49. Dubos RJ, Schaedler RW (1960) The effect of the intestinal flora on the growth rate of mice and on their susceptibility to experimental infections. J Exp Med 111:407–417
50. Marshall JC, Christou NV, Meakins JL (1988) Small-bowel bacterial overgrowth and systemic immunosuppression in experimental peritonitis. Surgery 104:404–411
51. Marshall JC, Christou NV, Meakins JL (1988) Immunomodulation by altered gastrointestinal tract flora. The effects of orally administered, killed Staphylococcus epidermidis, Candida and Pseudomonas on systemic immune responses. Arch Med 123:1465–1469
52. Lagrange PH, Mackaness GB, Miller TE, Pardon P (1975) Effects of bacterial lipo-polysaccharide on the induction and expression of cell-mediated immunity. I. Depression of the afferent arc. J Immunol 114:442–446
53. Marshall JC, Lee C, Meakins JL, Michel RP, Christou NV (1987) Kupffer cell modulation of the systemic immune response. Arch Surg 122:191–196
54. Marshall JC, Rode H, Christou NV, Meakins JL (1988) In vivo activation of Kupffer cells by endotoxin causes suppression of nonspecific, but not specific, systemic immunity. Surg Forum 39:111–113
55. Marshall JC, Ribeiro MB, Chu PTY, Sheiner PA, Rotstein OD (1992) Portal endotoxemia stimulates the release of an immunosuppressive factor from alveolar and splenic macrophages. J Surg Res (in press)
56. Fry DE, Pearlstein L, Fulton RL, Polk HC (1980) Multiple system organ failure. The role of uncontrolled infection. Arch Surg 115:136–140
57. Fine J, Frank ED, Ravin HA, Rutenberg SH, Schweinburg FB (1959) The bacterial factor in traumatic shock. N Engl J Med 260:214–220
58. Metchnikoff E (1905) The nature of man. Studies in optimistic philosophy Putnam's, New York

Tumor Necrosis Factor and Other Cytokines as Mediators of Clinical Sepsis*

S. F. Lowry

Introduction

The clinical management of sepsis has benefited from breakthroughs in antimicrobial chemotherapy as well as other pharmacologic and technologic means of critical care support. Despite such advances, the course of patients suffering sepsis remains unpredictable and often protracted [1]. Disruptions of immunologic and metabolic homeostasis are well recognized sequelae of sepsis that contribute to the morbidity and mortality of chronic sepsis. In addition, variables related to the clinical status of patients prior to the onset of sepsis also appear to impact on the acute manifestations of sepsis.

Although the classical macroendocrine stress hormones contribute toward disruptions of normal immunologic [2] and metabolic [3] function attending sepsis, these macroendocrine mediator changes are not sufficient per se to reproduce the total spectrum of host responses to sepsis. Recent investigations have confirmed that other endogenously derived effector components contribute to altered immunologic and metabolic regulation during sepsis [4]. The cytokine class of mediators represents an important component of this alternative response pathway. The activities of individual cytokines demonstrable in vitro has generated significant interest in their potential contribution to sepsis, prompting efforts at detection of these proteins in septic and critically ill patients [5–7]. Unfortunately, the detection of increased cytokine levels in such patients has been sporadic and often lacking in specificity. This lack of in vivo human specificity precludes a precise definition for the role of cytokine mediators in clinical sepsis. As a consequence, the extent and importance of cytokine contributions during sepsis is currently inferred from in vitro work and animal experimentation.

The biological characteristics of cytokines and the data implicating them in clinical sepsis and injury have been reviewed [4, 8]. Despite extensive in vitro data referable to cytokine biology, extrapolation of such activity to the clinical setting remains fraught with caveats. Several aspects of cytokine biology render their evaluation in human systems exceedingly difficult. As these mediators are

* Supported in part by grants GM-34695, GM-40586, CA-52108, and P50 GM-26145 from the U. S. Public Health Service.
Laboratory of Surgical Metabolism, Cornell University Medical College, New York, NY, USA

produced by a diverse array of cell types, the study of cytokine regulation and tissue-specific activity may vary depending upon the cell population studied. This variability of tissue cytokine production and action is further complicated by the existence of polymorphic forms, not all of which are detectable as circulating species. The existence of biologically active cell-associated cytokines further complicates in vivo assessments of total cytokine activity. Additionally, complex in vivo regulatory systems serve to amplify or abrogate cytokine activity, often in synergy or antagonism with other cytokine or hormonal mediators. The complex and redundant nature of these endogenous regulatory systems requires a thorough assessment of cytokine and hormonal status both prior to and during the septic event. Unfortunately, little is currently understood regarding the potential beneficial influences exerted by cytokines in either the acute or chronic sepsis environment. It is likely that several cytokines, acting individually or synergistically, will prove to exert survival or reparative influences in the septic host. An obvious clinical corollary to this aspect of cytokine biology is that efforts to globally counteract cytokine activity may prove detrimental under certain circumstances.

Tumor Necrosis Factor and the Cytokine Cascade

The onset of sepsis initiates a complex cytokine cascade. Although a diverse system of such mediators are produced, tumor necrosis factor-α (TNF) is most widely identified as the cytokine exhibiting the potential for systemic and tissue specific injury. It is well documented that adverse cardiovascular and metabolic events similar to those of overwhelming sepsis may arise from excessive TNF activity [4, 8, 9]. These adverse events appear to be both species specific and dose dependent as evidenced by administration of large doses to animals [10] as well as lesser degrees of instability induced by infusion of TNF into humans [11]. Further, we have demonstrated that blockade of endogenously produced TNF utilizing monoclonal antibodies serves to confer survival benefit during overwhelming bacteremia [12]. Such a level of TNF activity also initiates the production of other proinflammatory cytokines in vivo [13], whereas a complex series of subsequent biochemical events are ultimately responsible for mediation of TNF-initiated tissue injury [14].

Despite the presumed role of TNF as a proximal mediator of many sequelae of sepsis, the detection of this cytokine in the circulation of infected experimental animals and humans remains problematic. Although TNF appearance is readily evident following the administration of large doses of either endotoxin or live bacteria in experimental models [13, 15], the incidence of detectable circulating TNF levels during chronic infectious conditions is less frequent [16, 17]. In clinical studies, prospective random sampling of infected patients often fails to detect TNF on a consistent basis [5–7]. This relatively infrequent detection of TNF precludes a consensus of opinion regarding the essential nature of TNF activity in the clinical sepsis syndrome. Several confounding variables are likely responsible for this sporadic detection of TNF. Principal among these is the intermittent nature of TNF production. Although circulating TNF is detected within 45–60 min after endotoxin challenge in experimental animals [15] as well as humans [18], even animals expiring from lethal gram-negative bacteremia exhibit only a monophasic appearance of TNF in the circulation [13]. Current evidence would suggest that chronic production of this cytokine may occur as the cell-associated form [16] or that production of the cell-associated and soluble species are highly compartmentalized. The extent of compartmentalized production of TNF and other cytokines is dependent upon both the site of TNF production as well as the intensity of the infectious stimulus [19]. Similar compartmentalized production of TNF has been demonstrated in man wherein the splanchnic organs appear to represent a significant proportion of the total body or necrosis factor production during endotoxinemic states [20]. It is also evident from our recent data that the opportunity to detect circulating forms of TNF is dependent upon the hormonal background antedating the onset of sepsis [21].

Evidence also suggests the likelihood of synergy between TNF and endotoxin or other humoral mediators during infection. Examples of this include the synergy between TNF and endotoxin in inducing hemorrhagic necrosis of tissues [22] as well as synergy between TNF and interleukin-1 (IL-1) for induction of altered substrate metabolism [23]. TNF as well as interferon-γ may also act synergistically toward the enhancement of leukocyte function [24], whereas TNF appears to participate with other cytokines and macroendocrine hormones in the redistribution of substrates between tissues [25].

TNF also precipitates the release of other immunologically important mediators both in vitro and in vivo, including the interleukins (IL-1, IL-2, IL-6, and IL-8) as well as more classical forms of neurohumoral peptides [4, 8]. Although detected with less frequency in the circulation of endotoxinemic or septic humans than is TNF, the IL-1 species are widely presumed to illicit significant immunologic and metabolic sequelae during sepsis. Recent studies evaluating a specific receptor antagonist to IL-1 have confirmed that modest alterations of hemodynamic function and some associated tissue injury are attributable to IL-1 activity during bacteremia or endotoxinemia [15]. While clearly not as potent as TNF with regard to initiating acute cardiovascular collapse and severe tissue injury, the pathologic tissue injury of IL-1 may prove to be exerted over a longer temporal sequence than that of TNF [17]. Thus, IL-1 and other TNF-inducible cytokines may serve as important mediators for the late sequelae of clinical sepsis [17].

Other proinflammatory cytokine mediators inducible by TNF appear to exert more specific tissue influences in the septic response. Among these, IL-6 currently appears to be a potential initiator of acute-phase synthesis. Although circulating levels of IL-6 are readily detectable during sepsis [26], studies defining its role as a shock-inducing agent are limited. Recent unconfirmed data suggests that blockade of the IL-6 response may be of benefit in terms of acute survival from experimental sepsis [27]. It is also evident that IL-6 or other sepsis-related cytokines such as IL-8 [28] exert highly specialized functions during chronic tissue injury and inflammatory states. These specialized functions render such cytokines less likely to be primary participants in the initiation of shock and other early systemic derangements of clinical sepsis.

Clinical Modifiers of Cytokine Appearance

As noted above, the ability to assess cytokine activity in the setting of clinical sepsis is limited by biologic variables related to their production, distribution, and postreceptor activities. Recent evidence documents that such variables may also be influenced by clinical and therapeutic conditions coexisting with or antedating the septic event. A consideration of these parameters permits additional insight into the regulation of cytokine activity during sepsis.

Prospective clinical studies have documented that nutritional state influences immune function [29] and the association of such disruptions in immune function also correlate with outcome from sepsis [30]. The spectrum of patients suffering septic events includes those whose antecedent nutritional state is adversely influenced by chronic disease as well as those who have suffered acute injury without overt malnutrition. This latter population nevertheless suffers from a significant incidence of sepsis during the course of hospitalization. Even though such patient populations have benefited from efforts to sustain nutritional status, recent data suggest that the route by which injured and critically ill patients receive nutrients may influence their susceptibility to infection and outcome from illness [31, 32].

The experimental and clinical data underlying the hypothesis that the route of nutrient provision influences regional and systemic cytokine activation have recently been reviewed [33] (Figs. 1, 2) We have sought to test this clinical hypothesis by utilizing the controlled in vivo model of endotoxinemia in man. To do so, healthy subjects were admitted to the hospital for a 1-week period of either oral feeding or total parenteral nutrition. At the completion of this dietary intervention phase, subjects were challenged with an intravenous bolus of endotoxin, and serial determinations of arterial counterregulatory hormones and cytokines as well as hepatic venous (splanchnic-derived) cytokine levels were performed [34]. Results supporting the hypothesis that antecedent alterations in the route of nutrient provision could significantly influence the regional and systemic appearance of TNF were obtained (Fig. 3). A differential magnitude of endotoxin-induced TNF appearance was evident, with parenterally fed subjects achieving greater levels of TNF within both hepatic venous and arterial blood in response to endotoxin. Additional observations suggested an association between the magnitude of circulating TNF levels and clinical responses, with parenterally fed subjects exhibiting a greater rise in core temperature, counter-regulatory hormone levels, and of acute phase (C-reactive)

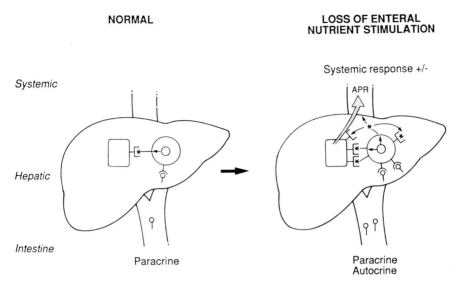

Fig. 1. A proposed mechanism for alterated hepatic Kupffer cell (*large circle*) and hepatocyte (*rectangle*) function during loss of enteral nutrient stimulation. Under normal conditions (*left*) there is minimal inciting antigen (♀). There is evidence of constitutive Kupffer cell cytokine production. This low level of activation likely produces a cell-associated form of cytokine (✳—) which interacts with specific receptors on the hepatocyte (↧). During conditions of liver exposure to loss of enteral nutrient stimulation (*right*), increased antigens of intestinal origin occurs. These antigens enhance production of cell-associated as well as soluble forms of cytokine (✳). These cytokines interact with hepatocytes to alter cellular function, including production of acute-phase proteins (*APR*). Soluble cytokine also serves to alter Kupffer cell capacity for further cytokine production by autocrine mechanisms. During such unstressed conditions, there may be no cytokine evident in the systemic circulation. (Adapted from [33])

protein production than their orally fed cohorts. These data are consistent with a significant nutritional influence in septic patients, particularly as such patients have often suffered from prolonged periods of inadequate enteral nutrient intake. The data are also consistent with our experimental data in animal models wherein a lack of enteral stimulation serves to prime hepatic Kupffer cells to chronically produce cell-associated forms of TNF [35].

In addition to the above clinical mechanism for regulation of cytokine production, recent data also suggests that the noncytokine hormonal milieu of septic patients also dramatically influences cytokine responses to sepsis. The existence of such regulatory pathways has been suggested by previous in vitro studies wherein components of the neurohumoral stress response system, such as glucocorticoids, transiently disrupt cellular production of TNF [36]. Although enhanced glucocorticoid appearance is evident following endotoxin administration in human models, this response is insufficient to abrogate either symptomatology or activation of the cytokine cascade [20, 37]. However, such models do not fully reproduce the hormonal environment encountered in injured and septic patients where sustained or intermittent periods of hyper-cortisolemia are frequently manifested.

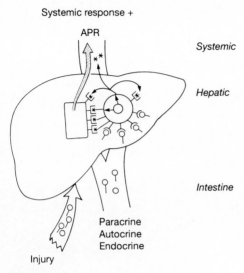

Systemic response +

APR

Systemic

Hepatic

Intestine

Paracrine
Autocrine
Endocrine

Injury

Fig. 2. A proposed mechanism for enhanced hepatic responses in patients experiencing loss of enteral nutrient stimulation and an associated or secondary infection. The predisposition to enhanced cytokine production by Kupffer cells is amplified by inciting antigen exposure from intestinal and injury sites. Increased hepatic injury responses, such as acute phase protein production, are now evident in the circulation. With this level of cytokine production, soluble mediator is detectable in the circulation and systemic responses consistent with cytokine appearance are observed. For symbols, see Fig. 1. (Adapted from [33])

Our recently completed studies have addressed the potential for hyper-cortisolemic conditions to serve as an endogenous mechanism for cytokine regulation. By utilizing the in vivo human model, we have sought to determine the influence of sustained elevations of circulating cortisol upon TNF appearance and clinical symptomatology. These studies have confirmed the capacity of exogenous glucocorticoid administration to acutely abrogate TNF responses to endotoxin in addition to confirming that clinical parameters such as increases in core temperature and symptoms are also alleviated by such treatment [19]. Nevertheless, more complex cytokine responses were obtained when such elevated cortisol levels were temporally removed from the period of endotoxin exposure. By contrast to the suppression of TNF responses observed by simultaneous administration of steroid and endotoxin, pretreatment with corti-costeroid followed by endotoxin administration 6–12 h later resulted in an exaggerated TNF and clinical response. These observations serve to emphasize the significance of both the antecedent and acute hormonal environment as determinants of clinical cytokine responses.

Clinical Management and the Scientific Interface

Experimental studies have demonstrated protection of the host against subsequent septic challenge by pretreatment with TNF. Conversely, abrogating

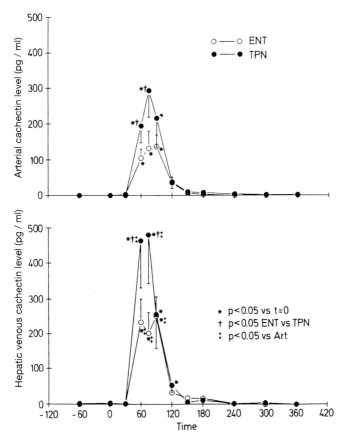

Fig. 3. Cachectin/TNF levels. TNF levels in the arterial (*Art*) and hepatic venous blood of volunteers before (*t* = 0) and after endotoxin injection. Subjects had received 7 prior days of either enteral feedings (*ENT*) or parenteral feedings (*TPN*). (Adapted from [34])

TNF activity using monoclonal antibodies may, under some circumstances, increase septic mortality. These observations underscore important, but often overlooked, components of cytokine activity, in that potential for exerting normal homeostatic regulation at low concentrations may subserve beneficial responses essential for survival of the septic host [38, 39]. Consideration of these influences are a necessary adjunct to efforts directed at global blockade of cytokine activity. Additional insights into this diversity of cytokine-related activity are necessary to permit future therapies directed at selective antagonism of adverse cytokine responses with simultaneous promotion of protective responses.

A complex array of clinical variables, including some outlined above, serve to complicate the interpretation of cytokine activity in humans. The existence of parallel in vivo systems for both cytokine amplification as well as for control of adverse consequences are increasingly evident. Given recent data suggesting that neutralization of inciting agents, such as endotoxin, can improve survival during septic conditions [40], efforts to expand these observations by direct antagonism of cytokine activity are currently underway. While it can be hoped that such therapy will prove of benefit in clinical management, such an outcome is by no means assured.

References

1. Cerra FB (1987) Hypermetabolism, organ failure, and metabolic support. Surgery 101:1–14
2. Calvano SE (1986) Hormonal mediation of immune dysfunction following thermal and traumatic injury. In: Davis JM, Shires GT (eds) Host defenses in trauma and surgery. Raven, New York, pp 111–142
3. Lowry SF (1986) Host metabolic response to injury. In: Davis JM, Shires GT (eds) Host defenses in trauma and surgery. Raven, New York, pp 169–190
4. Tracey KJ, Lowry SF (1989) The role of cytokines in septic shock. In: Tompkins RK (ed) Advances in surgery. Yearbook Medical Publishers, Chicago, pp 21–56
5. Marano MA, Fong Y, Moldawer LL, Wei H. Calvano SE, Tracey KJ, Barie PS, Manogue K, Cerami A, Shires GT, Lowry SF (1990) Serum cachectin/TNF in critically ill burn patients correlates with infection and mortality. Surg Gynecol Obstet 170(1):32–38
6. Debets JMH, Kampmeijer R, van der Linden MPMH, Buurman WA, van der Linden CJ (1989) Plasma tumor necrosis factor and mortality in critically ill septic patients. Crit Care Med 17(6):489–494
7. Damas P, Reuter A, Gysen P, Demonty J, Lamy M, Franchimont P (1989) Tumor necrosis factor and interleukin-1 serum levels during severe sepsis in humans. Crit Care Med 17(10):975–978
8. Fong Y, Moldawer LL, Shires GT, Lowry SF (1990) The biological characteristics of cytokines and their implication in surgical injury. Surg Gynecol Obstet 170(4):363–378
9. Tracey KJ, Beutler B, Lowry SF, Merryweather J, Wolpe S, Milsark IW, Hariri RJ, Fahey TJ, Zentella A, Albert JD, Shires GT, Cerami A (1986) Shock and tissue injury induced by recombinant human cachectin. Science 234:470–474
10. Tracey KJ, Lowry SF, Fahey TJ, Albert JD, Fong Y, Hesse D, Beutler B, Manogue K, Calvano SE, Wei H, Cerami A, Shires GT (1987) Cachectin/tumor necrosis factor induces lethal septic shock and stress hormone responses in the dog. Surg Gynecol Obstet 164;415–422
11. Starnes HF, Warren RS, Jeevanandam M, Gabrilove JL, Larchian W, Oettgen HF, Brennan MF (1988) Tumor necrosis factor and the acute metabolic response to tissue injury in man. J Clin Invest 82:1321–1325
12. Tracey KJ, Fong Y, Hesse DG, Manogue KR, Lee AT, Kuo GC, Lowry SF, cerami A (1987) Anti-cachectin/TNF monoclonal antibodies prevent septic shock during lethal bacteremia. Nature 330:662–664
13. Fong Y, Tracey KJ, Moldawer LL, Hesse DG. Manogue KR. Kenny J, Lee AT, Kuo GC, Allison A, Lowry SF, Cerami A (1989) Antibodies to cachectin/TNF reduce interleukin-1β and interleukin-6 appearance during lethal bacteremia. J Exp Med 170:1627–1633
14. Larrick JW, Wright SC (1990) Cytotoxic mechanism of tumor necrosis factor-α. FASEB J 4:3215–3223
15. Fischer E, Marano MA, Barber A, Hudson A, Lee K, Rock C, Hawes AE. Thompson RC, Hayes TJ, Anderson TD, Benjamin WR, Lowry SF, Moldawer LL (1991) Interleukin-1α administration can replicate the hemodynamic and metabolic responses to sublethal endotoxemia. AM J Physiol (in press)
16. Marano MA, Moldawer LL, Fong Y, Wei H, Minei J, Yurt R, Cerami A, Lowry SF (1988) Cachectin/tumor necrosis factor production in experimental burns and pseudomonas infection. Arch Surg 123:1383–1388
17. Gershenwald JE, Fong Y, Fahey TJ III, Calvano SE, Chizzonite R, Kilian PL, Lowry SF, Moldawer LL (1990) Interleukin-1 receptor blockade attenuates the host inflammatory response. Proc Natl Acad Sci USA 87:4966–4970

18. Hesse DG, Tracey KJ, Fong Y, Manogue KR, Palladino MA, Cerami A, Shires GT, Lowry SF (1988) Cytokine appearance in human endotoxemia and primate bacteremia. Surg Gynecol Obstet 166:147–153

19. Nelson S, Bagby GJ, Bainton BG, Wilson LA, Thompson JJ, Summer WR (1989) Compartmentalization of intraalveolar and systemic lipopolysaccharide-induced tumor necrosis factor and pulmonary inflammatory response. J Infect Dis 159:189–194

20. Fong Y, Marano MA, Moldawer LL, Wei H, Calvano SE, Kenney JS, Allison AC, Cerami A, Shires GT, Lowry SF (1990) The acute splanchnic and peripheral tissue metabolic response to endotoxin in man. J Clin Invest 85(6):1896–1904

21. Barber AE,Coyle SM, Fong Y, Fischer E, Marano MA, Calvano SE, Moldawer LL, Shires GT, Lowry SF (1990) Impact of hypercortisolemia on the metabolic and hormonal responses to endotoxin in man. Surg Forum 41:74–77

22. Rothstein JL, Schreiber H (1988) Synergy between tumor necrosis factor and bacterial products causes hemorrhagic necrosis and lethal shock in normal mice. Proc Natl Acad Sci USA 85:607–611

23. Tredget EE, Yu YM, Zhong S, Burini R, Okusawa S, Gelfand JA, Dinarello CA, Young VR, Burke JF (1988) Role of interleukin 1 and tumor necrosis factor on energy metabolism in rabbits. Am J Physiol 255:E760–E768

24. Djeu JY, Blanchard DK, Halkias D, Friedman H (1986) Growth inhibition of Candida albicans by human polymorphonuclear neutrophils: activation by interferon-g and tumor necrosis factor. J Immunol 137:2980–2984

25. Fong Y, Moldawer LL, Marano M, Manogue K, Tracey KJ, Wei H, Kuo G, Fischman DA, Cerami A, Lowry SF (1989) Cachectin/TNF or IL-1α induces cachexia with redistribution of body proteins. Am J Physiol 256(3):R659–R665

26. Guo Y, Dickerson C, Chrest FJ, Adler WH, Munster AM, Winchurch RA (1990) Increased levels of circulating interleukin 6 in burn patients. Clin Immunol Immunopathol 54:361–371

27. Starnes HF, Pearce MK, Tewari A, Yim JH, Zou J-C, Abrams JS (1990) Anti-IL-6 monoclonal antibodies protect against lethal escherichia coli infection and lethal tumor necrosis factor-α challenge in mice. J Immunol 145:4185–4191

28. VanZee KJ, DeForge LE, Fischer E, Marano MA, Kenney JS, Remick DG, Lowry SF, Moldawer LL (1991) Interleukin-8 circulates during septic shock, endotoxemia, and following interleukin-1 administration. J Immunol (in press)

29. Law DK, Dudrick SJ, Abdou NI (1973) Immunocompetence of patients with protein calorie malnutrition. Ann Intern Med 79:545

30. Poenaru D, Christou NV (1991) Clinical outcome of seriously ill surgical patients with intra abdominal infection depends on both physiologic (APACHE II score) and immunologic (DTH score) alterations. Ann Surg 213:130–136

31. Moore FA, Moore EE, Jones TN et al. (1989) TEN versus TPN following major abdominal trauma-reduced septic morbidity. J Trauma 29:916–923

32. McDonald WS, Sharp CW, Deitch EA (1991) Immediate enteral feeding in burn patients is safe and effective. Ann Surg 213:177–183

33. Lowry SF (1990) The route of feeding influences injury responses. J Trauma 30:510–515

34. Fong Y, Marano MA, Barber A, Wei H, Moldawer LL, Bushman ED, Coyle SM, Shires GT, Lowry SF (1989) Total parenteral nutrition and bowel rest modify the metabolic response to endotoxin in man. Ann Surg 210(4):449–457

35. Rock CS, Barber AE, Ng E, Jones WG, Roth MS, Moldawer LL, Lowry SF (1990) TPN vs. oral feeding: bacterial translocation, cytokine response and mortality following E. Coli LPS administration. Surg Forum 41:14–16

36. Beutler B, Krochin N, Milsark IW, Luedke C, Cerami A (1986) Control of cachectin (tumor necrosis factor) synthesis: mechanism of endotoxin resistance. Science 232:977–980

37. Richardson RP, Rhyne CD, Fong Y, Hesse DG, Tracey KJ, Marano MA, Lowry SF, Antonacci AC, Calvano SE, (1989) Peripheral blood leukocyte kinetics following in vivo lipopolysaccharide (LPS) administration to normal human subjects: Influence of elicited hormones and cytokines. Ann Surg 210(2):239–245

38. Echtenacher B. Falk W, Männel DN, Krammer PH (1990) Requirement of endogenous tumor necrosis factor/cachectin for recovery from experimental peritonitis. J Immunol 145:3762–3766

39. Sheppard BC, Fraker DL, Norton JA (1989) Prevention and treatment of endotoxin and sepsis lethality with recombinant human tumor necrosis factor. Surgery 106:156–162

40. Ziegler EJ, Fisher CJ, Sprung CL et al. (1991) Treatment of gram-negative bacteremia and septic shock with HA-1A human monoclonal antibody against endotoxin. N Engl J Med 324:429–436

The Protein C System in Septic Shock

F. B. Taylor

Summary Description of the Baboon Model of *Escherichia coli* Sepsis

Background

Septic shock can present a cruel paradox, for in spite of watchful care it occurs most often in the hospital. It occurs in a wide variety of patients ranging from premature neonates with necrotizing enterocolitis to the aged with burns limited to only 20%–30% of the body surface. It affects 30 000 out of one million admissions per year in the Veterans Administration (VA) system; approximately half of these are due to gram-positive and the other half to gram-negative organisms. Approximately 15 000 of this group of 30 000 patients die [1] in spite of diagnostic monitoring and treatment with appropriate antibiotics.

Sepsis due to gram-positive *Staphylococcus aureus* requires that the organisms be alive, breach the vascular wall, and multiply in the tissues, bringing the neutrophils after them. If uncontrolled, the live bacteria and neutrophils digest tissues, form abscesses, and in some unknown manner produce shock, multiple organ failure, and death.

Sepsis due to gram-negative *Escherichia coli*, on the other hand, does not require that the organisms be alive, nor that they gain access to the tissues. Instead, from their position in the cardiovascular reticuloendothelial system, they kill the host by turning the host's inflammatory and coagulant systems against the host.

In numerous in vitro and in vivo studies, investigators have focused on the effects of the endotoxin from these gram-negative organisms on the plasma and cellular components of the blood and blood vessels and on the inflammatory mediators released from these cells [2]. So much new information has been uncovered that it has become necessary to bring it into perspective by reexamining the natural history of *E. coli* sepsis in primates.

This review will therefore cover the following topics. First, the four stages of experimental *E. coli* shock as observed in the baboon will be described. Second, the effect of elevated levels of C4bBP and neutralization of the protein C/protein

---

Cardiovascular Biology Research Program, Oklahoma Medical Research Foundation, Oklahoma City, OK, USA

Host Defense Dysfunction
in Trauma, Shock and Sepsis
Eds. Faist/Meakins/Schildberg
© Springer-Verlag, Berlin Heidelberg 1993

S anticoagulant system on these four stages will be described. Third, the role of elevated levels of C4bBP in the development of this model of microvascular thrombosis (hemolytic uremic syndrome) will be discussed.

Description of the Baboon 2-h Infusion Model of *E. coli* Sepsis

Stage I (0–2 h). Figure 1 shows that as the concentration of *E. coli* organisms in plasma rises during the 2-h infusion of *E. coli*, the neutrophil concentration falls sharply. Coincident with this fall, at least some of the neutrophils adhere to the venous endothelium. This includes the veins and sinusoids of the major target organs, including the adrenals, liver, and kidney. This corresponds to what is seen in humans.

Stage II (2–6h). Figure 1 shows that this neutrophil response is followed by a sharp fall in the concentrations of *E. coli* organisms and fibrinogen. Coincidentally, and after these responses, blebs appear on the aortic endothelium and fibrin later appears on the surface of the intact endothelium of smaller vessels. This fibrin deposition is not extensive. Fibrin degradation products rise sharply

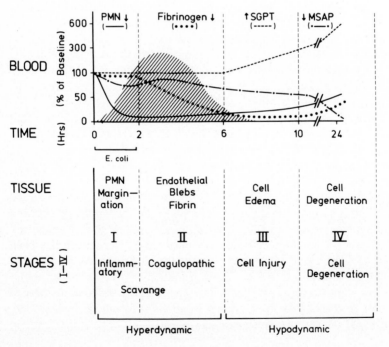

Fig. 1. The sequence of changes shown is divided into four stages: inflammatory (0–2 h), coagulopathic (2–6 h), cell injury (6–10 h), and cell degeneration (10 + h). The *hatched area* depicts concentration of *E. coli* organisms in blood; PMN, polymorphonuclear neutrophils; EM

and the platelet concentration falls gradually (not shown), while the white cell concentration remains low during this interval.

Stage III (6–10 h). Figure 1 shows that the fall in fibrinogen is followed by a rise in serum pyruvate transferase (SGPT) concentrations. Coincidentally, the endothelial fenestra of the adrenal and hepatic sinusoids are closed. Fluid accumulates in and between the parenchymal cells of the kidney and liver. The white cell concentration rises slightly. The fibrinogen concentration remains low. The vascular endothelium remains intact except in the adrenals, where there is focal extravasation of red blood corpuscles. During this interval, the platelet concentration and the mean blood pressure continue a slow, steady decline to approximately 50% of their baseline values.

Stage IV (10 + h). During this interval, death usually occurs at any time between 12 and 30 h. The white cell and fibrinogen concentrations rise to 50% of baseline values. The SGPT and other markers of cell injury continue to rise dramatically. At this point, there is irreversible degeneration of the organelles of hepatocytes and particularly of the epithelial cells of the proximal tubules of the kidney, findings similar to those reported in rats and monkeys. Finally, during this stage, the mean blood pressure and platelet concentration continue to fall until the time of death.

Figure 1 also illustrates the four divisions of the baboon response to *E. coli* infusion: inflammatory stage I, coagulopathic stage II, cell injury stage III, and cell degeneration stage IV; the more familiar cardiovascular hyperdynamic and hypodynamic stages are also shown in relation to these four stages.

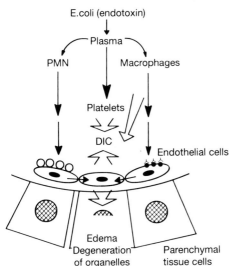

Fig. 2. Stages I–IV in relation to the hypothetical vascular endothelium and underlying parenchymal tissue. The inflammatory stage I involves neutrophils (*PMN*) and macrophages/monocytes which release mediators. These mediators perturb the vascular endothelium and initiate the coagulopathic stage II. The sum of platelet, macrophage, and endothelial procoagulant activity leads to a massive systemic disseminated intravascular coagulation response. Finally, in response to these explosive events occurring within the vasculature, the adjacent parenchymal tissue accumulates fluid (stage III) and ultimately undergoes degeneration (stage IV)

Figure 2 shows these four stages in relation to events in the blood vessels and tissues.

General Observations

First, *E. coli* organisms induce a massive intravascular inflammatory coagulant response which then affects the tissues (hypoxia, multiple organ failure). Unlike *S. aureus* organisms, which must remain alive and colonize tissues, the *E. coli* need not be alive nor colonize tissues in order to produce septic shock. Thus the principal field of battle in the case of *E. coli* is within the vasculature. Once within the baboon vasculature, there is a narrow range between the sublethal and lethal concentrations of *E. coli* (10^6 vs 10^7) organisms/ml plasma at 2 h. At some point within this narrow range, endotoxin appears in the plasma and the normally protective neutrophil and macrophage responses go out of control.

Second, the sequence of events leading up to the coagulopathic response suggests that it is caused by the preceding inflammatory response.

Third, during cell injury stage III and cell degeneration stage IV responses the vascular endothelium remains largely intact and the white cell and fibrinogen concentrations return toward their normal baseline values. This occurs in the face of cardiovascular collapse, a falling platelet count, and extensive injury and degeneration of the parenchymal tissue cells which underlie the intact endothelium.

Observations on the Protein C/Protein S System and the Role of C4bBP in Regulating the Baboon Response to *E. coli*.

Background

Protein S and protein C are two vitamin K-dependent plasma proteins involved in a natural anticoagulant pathway. Protein C is a precursor of the anticoagulant protease, activated protein C [3]. Protein C activation is catalyzed rapidly by a complex between thrombin and the endothelial cell surface protein, thrombomodulin [4]. Activated protein C functions as an anticoagulant through the selective inactivation of factors Va and VIIIa [5–7]. Protein S functions by enhancing the cell surface anticoagulant activity of activated protein C [8]. This appears to be accomplished both by increasing the affinity of the enzyme for the cell surface [9, 10] and by blocking the capacity of factor Xa to protect factor Va from inactivation by activated protein C [11]. In plasma, protein S circulates in at least two forms. Approximately 40% is free, and 60% is complexed to the complement regulatory protein C4bBP [12]. Only the free form retains protein S anticoagulant activity [13].

Deficiencies of either protein C or protein S are associated with an increased thrombotic tendency. For instance, homozygous protein C deficiency is responsible for purpura fulminans in some infants, which can lead to death if untreated [14–16]. Familial protein S deficiency can be divided into at least two separate classes. One results from decreased protein S antigen [17–20] and the other results from normal protein S antigen, but increased C4bBP-protein S complex with a concomitant decrease in free protein S [21]. In addition to the inherited deficiencies, several lines of evidence support the concept that the protein C anticoagulant pathway is downregulated in a variety of disease states, especially those associated with inflammation. For instance, exposure of endothelial cells to endotoxin [22], interleukin-1 [23], and tumor necrosis factor (TNF) [24–26] inhibits thrombomodulin activity on the surface of endothelial cells. In addition, protein C levels also decrease during disseminated intravascular coagulation (DIC) [27], further impairing the function of the anticoagulant pathway. Of particular interest to the present study, acquired deficiencies of protein S have been observed in inflammatory disease states such as systemic lupus erythematosus (SLE) [28] and DIC [29]. It has been proposed that the acquired deficiency of protein S in inflammation is due to increased plasma levels of the acute-phase protein C4bBP, and that this may contribute to coagulation abnormalities associated with inflammation by reducing the level of free protein S [28–31]. While there is an association between increased C4bBP levels and either thrombosis or DIC, no direct studies have demonstrated that elevation of C4bBP levels alone can contribute to a hypercoagulable state.

Previous studies have shown that inhibition of protein C activation rendered baboons considerably more hypercoagulable in response to sublethal *E. coli* infusion [32]. These studies suggest that protein C, and perhaps other components of the protein C anticoagulant pathway, play a role in a protective host response to *E. coli*. We have utilized this model to investigate the influence of increasing C4bBP levels, and hence decreasing free protein S levels, on the response to sublethal *E. coli*.

Observations

Before examining the influence of C4bBP on the response to *E. coli* in the baboon, it was important to demonstrate that C4bBP could inhibit protein S function in baboon plasma. Inhibition of protein S anticoagulant function would be manifested by a loss of the ability of activated protein C to function as a plasma anticoagulant. As anticipated, when the C4bBP concentration in baboon plasma was increased, the anticoagulant response to activated protein C was decreased (Fig. 3). C4bBP addition to plasma had no effect on the clotting time in the absence of added activated protein C.

In studying the effects of exogenous C4bBP on the response of the baboon to sublethal *E. coli*, we examined five groups of animals. They included animals infused with:sublethal *E. coli* (group 1); C4bBP alone (group 2); sublethal *E. coli*

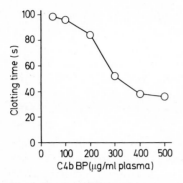

Fig. 3. Human C4bBP inhibits the ability of activated protein C to anticoagulate baboon plasma. The assay was performed in ten 75-mm glass test tubes at 37 °C. Sample addition was in the following order: 100 μl plasma, 100 μl, cephalin, 100 μl, 0.025 M calcium chloride, 50 μl buffer (see below), and 50 μl of a mixture of factor Xa and activated protein C. The concentrations of the factor Xa were adjusted to give a clotting time of 30 s in samples without activated protein C (approximately 2 ng/ml in the assay mixture) and the activated protein C concentration was adjusted to give a clotting time of 98 ± 8 s in this assay (at the same concentration of factor Xa). To examine the influence of C4bBP on the assay, 50 μl of 0.15 M NaCl, 0.02 M Tris-HCl, pH 7.5, or C4bBP in the same buffer were added to 100 μl baboon citrated plasma and incubated for 1 h at room temperature to allow the C4bBP–protein S complex to form. The C4bBP concentrations in the figure reflect the plasma concentrations and not the final concentration in the assay. The factor Xa and activated protein C were held constant and the only variable was the concentration of C4bBP present in the plasma

plus C4bBP (group 3); sublethal *E. coli* plus C4bBP saturated with protein S (group 4); and LD_{100} *E. coli* alone (group 5). Comparisons of the number of organisms infused and survival times of members of the five groups are presented in Table 1. All animals in the sublethal *E. coli* plus C4bBP and in the LD_{100} *E. coli* groups died in 27 h or less, while animals in the other three groups were permanent survivors (> 168 h). Thus, C4bBP supplementation exacerbates the response to sublethal *E. coli*. This deleterious effect, however, is largely prevented by supplementation with protein S.

The influence of C4bBP on fibrinogen consumption and TNF formation in response to sublethal *E. coli* is examined in Fig. 4. Figure 4a shows that infusions of sublethal *E. coli* alone and C4bBP alone induced no change in these parameters, whereas coinfusion of C4bBP with sublethal *E. coli* (Fig. 4b) was followed by a consumption of fibrinogen, appearance of TNF in plasma, and death (Table 1). In contrast, supplementation of the C4bBP with protein S largely prevented the fibrinogen consumption and TNF elaboration in response to sublethal *E. coli* (Fig. 4c). The supplementation also prevented death (Table 1). It should be noted that coinfusion of C4bBP with sublethal *E. coli* produced similar responses to those observed with LD_{100} *E. coli* with respect to fibrinogen consumption, plasma TNF levels, and survival (Fig. 4d, Table 1).

From these studies, the question arises as to whether the C4bBP functions solely by enhancing the coagulation response. To approach this problem, we utilized active site blocked factor Xa (DEGR-Xa). This protein has no clotting activity, but instead serves as an anticoagulant, presumably by complexing with

Table 1. Weight, sex, dose of *E. coli* and survival in control (sublethal *E. coli* alone, C4bBP alone, LD$_{100}$ *E. coli* alone) and experimental groups (sublethal *E. coli* plus C4bBP, sublethal *E. coli* plus C4bBP/protein S)

	Weight (kg)	Sex	Dose (10^{10} CFU/kg)	Survival (h)
Group 1	8.8	♀	0.45	> 168
(sublethal *E. coli* alone)	6.6	♂	0.37	> 168
	6.4	♂	0.43	> 168
	5.7	♂	0.45	> 168
Mean	7.27	–	0.43	–
SE	0.67	–	0.05	–
Group 2	4.6	♀	–	> 168
(C4bBP alone)	5.2	♂	–	> 168
	8.2	♀	–	> 168
Mean	6.0	–	–	–
SE	1.1	–	–	–
Group 3	3.9	♀	0.50	− 25
(sublethal *E. coli* + C4bBP)	2.7	♂	0.69	24
	2.3	♀	0.30	27
	5.2	♂	0.21	16
Mean	3.52	–	0.43	23
SE	0.65	–	0.11	1.21
Group 4	7.7	♀	1.83	> 168
(sublethal *E. coli* + C4bBP/PS)	10.0	♀	0.23	> 168
	3.2	♂	0.43	> 168
	7.3	♀	0.61	> 168
Mean	7.05	–	0.78	–
SE	1.41	–	0.36	–
Group 5	7.7	♂	6.60	12
(LD$_{100}$ *E. coli*)	7.3	♂	6.00	13
	6.9	♀	5.75	24
	7.1	♀	8.24	10
Mean	7.25	–	6.65	14.75
SE	0.09	–	0.28	1.57

CFU, colony-forming units; PS, protein S

factor Va and competing for the binding of activated factor X. As a result, it blocks prothrombin activation [33]. Figure 5 shows the effect of coinfusion of DEGR-Xa with LD$_{100}$ *E. coli* on the plasma levels of fibrinogen, TNF, and survival. It shows that while the coagulant response as monitored by fibrinogen consumption was completely inhibited by DEGR-Xa, the TNF response and lethal effects of LD$_{100}$ *E. coli* were not affected.

Table 2 compares changes in physiological responses to sublethal *E. coli* alone (group 1) with sublethal *E. coli* plus C4bBP (group 3). The fall in fibrinogen levels was accompanied by a reciprocal rise in fibrin degradation products (FDP) from time (T) + 120 to T + 360 min in the sublethal *E. coli* plus C4bBP group, whereas sublethal *E. coli* alone caused no significant changes in either of these parameters. The blood urea nitrogen and creatinine levels almost

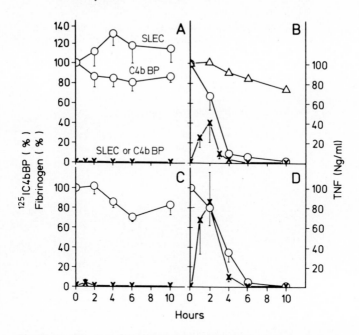

Fig. 4A–D. Elevation of C4bBP levels causes DIC and organ damage in response to sublethal *E. coli* (*SLEC*) infusion. Response of baboon plasma fibrinogen (O) and TNF (X) to infusion of C4bBP or sublethal *E. coli* (**A**); to infusion of sublethal *E. coli* (0.4×10^{10}CFU/kg) plus C4bBP (20 mg/kg) (**B**); to infusion of sublethal *E. coli* plus C4bBP saturated with an excess of protein S (20 mg/kg, 2.3 mg/kg respectively) (**C**); and to infusion of LD_{100} *E. coli* alone (4.0×10^{10}CFU/kg) (**D**). When either the C4bBP or C4bBP saturated with protein S were infused with *E. coli*, they were infused as a bolus at $T - 60$ min followed by infusion of *E. coli* beginning at 0 min and ending at $+ 120$ min. **B** also shows the relative (%) concentration of ^{125}I-labeled C4bBP during the response to coinfusion of C4bBP and sublethal *E. coli* (Δ). The half-life of C4bBP was 22 h $\pm$ 3 h

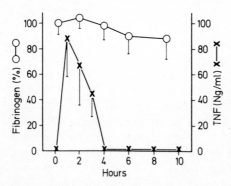

Fig. 5. DEGR-Xa inhibits the coagulant response to LD_{100} *E. coli*, but does not attenuate the inflammatory response or protect the animals. Response of baboon plasma fibrinogen (O) and TNF (X) to a bolus infusion of DEGR-Xa (1 mg/kg) at $T - 60$ min following by an infusion of LD_{100} *E. coli* (4.0×10^{10} CFU/kg) over a 2-h period beginning at T 0. The half-life of DEGR-Xa was 2 h. The data points indicate the mean response of four animals. All animals died within 30 h

doubled by 360 min in the sublethal *E. coli* plus C4bBP group, whereas in the sublethal *E. coli* alone group the changes in these two parameters were limited. The mean systemic arterial pressure (MSAP) remained stable except for a transient fall at $T + 120$ min in the sublethal *E. coli* plus C4bBP group. The

Table 2. Summary comparing the systemic arterial pressure, the sympathomimetic/inflammatory, the coagulant/fibrinolytic and cell injury responses to sublethal *E. coli* alone ($n = 4$) with those to sublethal *E. coli* plus C4bBP ($n = 4$)

	Time (min)					
	0	60	120	180	240	360
MSAP (mmHg)						
E. coli	105 ± 5.0	115 ± 6.0	97 ± 10.0	99 ± 8.6	96 ± 12.6	100 ± 4.2
E. coli + C4bBP	104 ± 3.3	89 ± 8.6	70 ± 6.8	89 ± 6.3	104 ± 3.2	102 ± 3.4
Heart rate (beats/min)						
E. coli	124 ± 8.8	154 ± 16.0	176 ± 21.1	182 ± 15.7	177 ± 17.2	175 ± 15.5
E. coli + C4bBP	147 ± 23.9	192 ± 10.3	220 ± 9.1	212 ± 16.0	212 ± 13.5	202 ± 11.8
Respiratory rate (/min)						
E. coli	33 ± 3.3	43 ± 8.8	41 ± 4.4	45 ± 5.0	43 ± 3.3	36 ± 3.3
E. coli + C4bBP	46 ± 9.9	58 ± 3.1	53 ± 3.8	65 ± 6.5 ($p \leq 0.05$)	62 ± 4.8 ($p \leq 0.03$)	62 ± 6.3 ($p \leq 0.02$)
Temperature (°C)						
E. coli	37.0 ± 0	36.5 ± 0.07	36.8 ± 0.43	37.2 ± 0.59	37.2 ± 0.71	37.7 ± 0.58
E. coli + C4bBP	36.8 ± 0.16	36.5 ± 0.20	37.0 ± 0.23	637.5 ± 0.26	38.0 ± 0.23	37.8 ± 0.27
WBC ($\times 10^3/100\,\mu l$)						
E. coli	7.7 ± 2.0	2.9 ± 0.81	2.0 ± 0.70	3.9 ± 2.0	4.1 ± 0.71	5.4 ± 2.1
E. coli + C4bBP	6.9 ± 0.78	3.0 ± 0.39	1.8 ± 0.14	1.7 ± 0.17	2.6 ± 0.62	3.1 ± 0.81
Fibrinogen (%)						
E. coli	100 ± 0	100 ± 0	84 ± 8.1	89 ± 7.2	87 ± 6.1	90 ± 4.5
E. coli + C4bBP	97 ± 2.8	93 ± 7.7	67 ± 14.7 ($p \leq 0.05$)	18 ± 14.2 ($p \leq 0.04$)	9 ± 8.3 ($p \leq 0.02$)	2 ± 1.3 ($p \leq 0.02$)
Platelets ($\times 10^3/\mu l$)						
E. coli	276 ± 37	264 ± 40	236 ± 41	212 ± 49	201 ± 45	184 ± 54
E. coli + C4bBP	173 ± 52	121 ± 20	117 ± 20	93 ± 26	112 ± 6 ($p \leq 0.05$)	39 ± 13 ($p \leq 0.03$)
FDP ($\mu g/dl$)						
E. coli	10 ± 0					10 ± 0
E. coli + C4bBP	10 ± 0		–	–	($p \leq 0.05$)	640 ± 0 ($p \leq 0.01$)
BUN (mg/dl)						
E. coli	15 ± 2					17 ± 2.3
E. coli + C4bBP	29	–	–	–	–	39 ± 6.6
CR (mg/dl)						
E. coli	0.46 ± 0.03					0.56 ± 0.06
E. coli + C4bBP	0.50	–	–	–	($p \leq 0.05$)	1.42 ± 0.43 ($p \leq 0.04$)

WBC, white blood cells; MSAP, mean systemic arterial pressure; FDP, fibrin degradation products; BUN, blood urea nitrogen; CR, cretinine

white cell and platelet counts fell in both groups. The white cells reached a nadir at 120 min followed by a return toward normal. The platelet response was different between the group 1 and 3 animals. Those given only sublethal *E. coli* exhibited a small but progressive decrease in platelets over the first 6 h, while those given both C4bBP and a sublethal *E. coli* infusion decreased their platelet number much more dramatically.

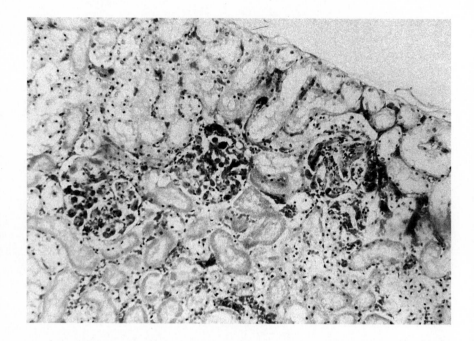

Fig. 6. Photomicrographs of kidney sections from animals receiving sublethal *E. coli* and C4bBP demonstrate necrosis and microvascular damage. A photomicroghaph magnified 10 times of an eosin-stained section of kidney from an animal (groups 3) that received sublethal *E. coli* and C4bBP and the tissues were processed immediately following death. Please note microvascular thrombosis involving the capillary loops of the renal glomeruli

Postmortem examinations were conducted on all baboons. Tissues were removed for analysis within minutes after death, thereby avoiding postmortem autolytic changes. Kidneys (Fig. 6) and adrenals removed from baboons receiving C4bBP plus sublethal *E. coli* (group 3) showed evidence of widespread microvascular thrombosis with extensive infarction and hemorrhage. Neither thrombosis nor hemorrhage was detected in these organs when the animals that received sublethal *E. coli* alone (group 1) or sublethal plus C4bBP saturated with protein S (group 4) were examined after 7 days.

Discussion of the Pathophysiologic and Clinical Implications of These Observations on the Role of C4bBP

Pathophysiologic Implications

Elevation of C4bBP levels in vivo converts a nonlethal phase response to a sublethal concentration of *E. coli* into a lethal shock response that includes DIC and organ damage. This demonstrates that increased levels of plasma C4bBP can influence the response to an inflammatory stimulus. The in vitro studies of the concentration-dependent effect of C4bBP on activated protein C anticoagulant activity are consistent with the concept that human C4bBP reduces the activity of free protein S in baboon plasma. The toxic contributions of elevated C4bBP to the response to *E. coli* appear to be mediated through its capacity to bind protein S since these toxic effects could be reversed by protein S addition. These studies raise the possibility that protein S might be of therapeutic value in some inflammatory disease states where C4bBP levels are elevated.

These observations extend the previous studies which demonstrated that activated protein C could protect animals from the lethal effects of *E. coli* [32]. In these studies, TNF appearance in plasma was usually suppressed [33], but this suppression has proven variable from animal to animal preventing definitive conclusions. In the studies reported here we observed that elevation of the C4bBP level is associated not only with DIC in response to sublethal *E. coli*, but also with lethality and the appearance of TNF in the plasma. This suggests that there is a link between protein S function and cytokine responses.

Clinical Implications

As seen in Fig. 6 the combined inflammatory coagulant response seen in association with *elevated* concentrations of C4bBP leads to a massive microvascular thrombosis. This is not seen following infusion of lethal *E. coli* in the absence of elevated levels of C4bBP. This might be characterized as a *delayed* response with death occurring after 30 h in which the inflammatory and coagulopathic responses are withstood, only to be followed by a massive microvascular thrombosis such as might be seen in hemolytic uremic syndrome (Table 3). This response might be viewed as delayed hyper-response of the coagulant system which, however, paradoxically occurs after the initial massive disseminated coagulopathy has resolved. This response might be viewed therefore as a second-generation coagulant response which, although more limited in intensity than the initial consumptive coagulopathy, is unaccompanied by a fibrinolytic response which otherwise would keep the microvasculature clear. The chief components of this delayed response include the acute-phase proteins, including C4bBP, which neutralizes protein S (cofactor for the anticoagulant, activated protein C). This is supported by the fact that this delayed lethal

Table 3. Microvascular thrombosis (days) (i.e., hemolytic uremic syndrome)

1. Blood pressure	→
2. Hematocrit (shistocytes)	↓
3. Pleural/peritoneal fluid	−
4. DIC	+
5. Microvascular thrombosis	+
6. Adrenal/renal infarction, hemorrhage	+

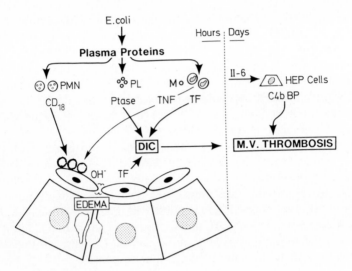

Fig. 7. Possible mechanism of the delayed response to *E. coli*. This is a two-step response in which the host is primed and then challenged by continuation of the inflammatory response. Priming involves an inflammatory stage I and coagulopathic stage II response which in this case is not sufficient to produce lethal shock or thrombosis. The host survives long enough to experience a rise in acute-phase proteins including C4bBP. The rise combined with continued inflammation or a second challenge stimulus is sufficient to produce widespread microvascular (*M.V.*) thrombosis such as that seen in hemolytic uremic syndrome. *HEP*, human epithelial cells; *Il-6*, interleukin-6; *M∅*, macrophages; *PL*, platelets; *Ptase*, prothrombinase; *TF*, tissue factors; *TNF*, tumor necrosis factor

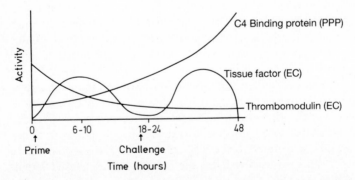

Fig. 8. The primary stimulus (TNF, LPS) upregulates the expression of the procoagulant receptor (tissue factor) and downregulates the expression of the anticoagulant receptor (thrombomodulin) by the endothelium. The increase of tissue factor expression is temporary and peaks at 6–10 h while the decrease of thrombomodulin expression is sustained. In addition, this primer stimulus induces a rise in the level of C4bBP and other acute-phase proteins which continue to rise over the 48-h period and beyond; C4bBP inhibits the protein S cofactor necessary for expression of anticoagulant activity by protein C (protein C is activated by the thrombin-thrombomodulin). Thus, at the time of the challenge stimulus conditions are set for an extensive microvascular thrombosis. That is, tissue factor expression is elevated for the second time under conditions where thrombomodulin expression is still depressed and where protein S function is inhibited by the high levels of C4bBP. This challenge stimulus could range from translocated *E. coli* organisms to virus particles

response with microvascular thrombosis can be reproduced by coinfusion of C4bBP with sublethal *E. coli.*

Figures 7 and 8 illustrate the principle which may be operative in the delayed (two-stage) response. There is a priming event which sets up conditions which favor development of microvascular thrombosis following a challenge or second stimulus. The conditions as hypothesized for this two-step model require that tissue factor expression by endothelium be upregulated and that thrombomodulin be downregulated at the time when the levels of acute-phase proteins in plasma including C4bBP are rising. The fact that this Schwartzman-like syndrome can be reproduced in one step by coinfusion of sublethal *E. coli* with C4bBP suggests that the elevated levels of the protein are the key factor in the triad (i.e., depressed thrombomodulin, elevated tissue factor, elevated acute-phase C4bBP) which produces microvascular thrombosis.

References

1. Hinshaw LB, Peduzzi P, Wilson M, et al. (1987) The veterans administration systemic sepsis cooperative study group: effect of high dose glucocorticoid therapy on mortality in patients with clinical signs of systemic sepsis. N Eng J Med 817:659
2. Taylor FB (1989) Baboon model of *E. coli* septic shock: staging and observations on the role of the vascular endothelium. In: Fuhrman BP, Shoemaker WC (eds) Critical care: state of the art, vol 10. Society of Critical Care Medicine, Fullerton, pp 251–284
3. Stenflo J (1988) The biochemistry of protein C. In: Bertina RM (ed) Protein C and related proteins. Churchill Livingstone, Edinburgh, p 21
4. Esmon, CT (1989) The roles of protein C and thrombomodulin in the regulation of blood coagulation. J Biol Chem 264:4743
5. Suzuki K, Stenflo J, Dahlback B, Teodorsson B (1983) Inactivation of human coagulation factor V by activated protein C. J Biol Chem 258:1914
6. Marlar RA, Kleiss AJ, Griffin JH (1982) Mechanism of action of human activated protein C, a thrombin-dependent anticoagulant enzyme. Blood 59:1067
7. Walker FJ, Chavin SI, Fay PJ (1987) Inactivation of Factor VIII by activated protein C and protein S. Arch Biochem Biophys 252:322
8. Harris KW, Esmon CT (1985) Protein S is required for bovine platelet suppression of activated protein C binding and activity. J Biol Chem 260:2007
9. Stern DM, Nawroth P, Harris KW, Esmon CT (1986) Cultured bovine aortic endothelial cells promote activated protein C-protein S-mediated factor Va inactivation. J Biol Chem 261:713
10. Walker F (1981) Regulation of activated protein C by protein S: the role of phospholipids in factor Va inactivation. J Biol Chem 256:11128
11. Solymoss S, Tucker MM, Tracy PB (1988) Kinetics of inactivation of membrane-bound factor Va by activated protein C. J Biol Chem 263:14884
12. Dahlback B (1983) Purification of human C4b-binding protein and formation of its complex with vitamin K-dependent protein S. Biochem J 209:847
13. Dahlback B (1986) Inhibition of protein Ca cofactor function of human and bovine protein S by C4b-binding protein. J Biol Chem 261:12022
14. Sills RH, Marlar RA, Montgomery RR, Deshpande GN, Humbert JR (1984) Severe homozygous protein C deficiency. J Pediatr 105:409
15. Seligsohn U, Berger A, Abend M, Rubin L, Attias D, Zivelin A, Rapaport SI (1984) Homozygous protein C deficiency manifested by massive venous thrombosis in the newborn. N Engl J Med 310:559
16. Griffin JH, Evatt B, Zimmerman TS, Kleiss AJ, Wideman C (1981) Deficiency of protein C in congenital thrombotic disease. J Clin Invest 68:1370

17. Schwartz HP, Fischer M, Hopmeier P, Batard MA, Griffin JH (1984) Plasma protein S deficiency in familial thrombotic disease. Blood 64:1297
18. Gladson CL, Scharrer I, Hach V, Beck KH, Griffin JH (1988) The frequency of type 1 heterozygous protein S and protein C deficiency in 141 unrelated young patients with venous thrombosis. Thromb Haemost 59:18
19. Schwartz HP, Heeb MJ, Lottenberg R, Roberts H, Griffin JH (1989) Familial protein S deficiency with a variant protein S molecule in plasma and platelets. Blood 74:213
20. Reitsma PH, Wouter ten Cate J, Bertina RM (1989) Partial protein S gene deletion in a family with hereditary thrombophilia. Blood 73:479
21. Comp PC, Doray D, Patton D, Esmon CT (1986) An abnormal plasma distribution of protein S occurs in functional protein S deficiency. Blood 67:504
22. Moore KL, Andreolia SP, Esmon NL, Esmon CT, Bang NU (1987) Endotoxin enhances tissue factor and suppresses thrombomodulin expression of human vascular endothelium *in vitro*. J Clin Invest 79:124
23. Nawroth PP, Handley DA, Esmon CT, Stern DM (1986) Interleukin-1 induces endothelial cell procoagulant while suppressing cell-surface anticoagulant activity. Proc Natl Acad Sci USA 83:3460
24. Nawroth PP, Stern DM (1986) Modulation of endothelial cell hemostatic properties by tumor necrosis factor. J Exp Med 163:740
25. Moore KL, Esmon CT, Esmon NL (1989) Tumor necrosis factor leads to the internalization and degradation of thrombomodulin from the surface of bovine aortic endothelial cells in culture. Blood 73:159
26. Conway EM, Rosenberg RD (1988) Tumor necrosis factor suppresses transcription thrombomodulin gene in endothelial cells. Mol Cell Biol 8:5588
27. Heeb MJ, Mosher D, Griffin JH (1989) Activation and complexation of protein C and cleavage and decrease of protein S in plasma of patients with intravascular coagulation. Blood 73:455
28. Comp PC, Vigano S, D'Angelo A, Thurnau G, Kaufman C, Esmon CT (1985) Acquired protein S deficiency occurs in pregnancy, the nephrotic syndrome and acute systemic lupus erythematosus (abstr). Blood 66:348a
29. D'Angelo A, Vigano-D'Angelo S, Esmon CT, Comp PC (1988) Acquired deficiencies of protein S: protein S activity during oral anticoagulatin, in liver disease, and in disseminated intravascular coagulation. J Clin Invest 81:1445
30. Boerger LM, Morris PC, Thurnau GR, Esmon CT, Comp PC (1987) Oral contraceptives and gender affect protein S status. Blood 69:692
31. D'Angelo SV, D'Angelo A, Kaufman C, Esmon CT, Comp PC (1987) Acquired functional protein S deficiency occurs in the nephrotic syndrome. Ann Intern Med 107:42
32. Taylor FB, Chang A, Esmon CT, D'Angelo A, Vigano-D'Angelo S, Blick K (1987) Protein C prevents the coagulopathic and lethal effects of *E. coli* infusion in the baboon. J Clin Invest 79:918
33. Taylor FB Jr, Stern DM, Nawroth PP, Esmon CT, Hinshaw LB, Blick KE (1986) Activated protein C prevents *E. coli* induced coagulopathy and shock in the primate (abstr). Circulation 74:64

Leukocyte-Endothelial Interactions in Trauma and Sepsis

H. Redl[1], G. Schlag[1], H. P. Dinges[2], R. Kneidinger[1], and J. Davies[3]

Polytrauma leads to the release of a multitude of mediators in the humoral and blood cell cascade systems. This mediator release among other reactions, results in interactions between endothelial cells (EC) and leukocyte, permeability changes, and organ dysfunction. This short review focuses on these EC-leukocyte interactions and compares the posttraumatic with the sepsis situation.

Leukostasis

Leukostasis is the most evident sign of EC-leukocyte interactions. We have previously demonstrated this event both in experimental [1] and in clinical [2] posttraumatic situations. Similar to the canine model, in our baboon model (originally based on Pretorius et al. [3]) leukostasis was found by measurement of myeloperoxidase content in lung and liver tissue. This technique was also used to study baboons after live *Escherichia coli* bacteremia in a hyperdynamic setting [4]. When these two model situations were compared, significantly more leukostasis was found in the sepsis situation (Table 1).

Leukostasis is the net effect of basically three different events (Fig. 1). (a) reduction in blood flow, (b) activation of leukocytes, and (c) changes in the endothelial surface. All three events lead to increased EC-leukocyte or leukocyte-leukocyte interaction and are generally related to an increased cell-to-cell adherence.

Flow Effects

The balance between polymorphonuclear granulocyte (PMN)/EC adhesive forces and hemodynamic dispersal forces is of major importance [5]. The shear forces are decreased in the postcapillary venules. Margination of leukocytes and

[1] Ludwig Boltzmann Institute for Experimental and Clinical Traumatology, Donaneschingenstr. 13, 1200 Wien, Vienna, Austria
[2] Institute of Pathology, University Graz, Graz, Austria
[3] Roodeplaat Research Laboratories, Pretoria, South Africa

Host Defense Dysfunction
in Trauma, Shock and Sepsis
Eds. Faist/Meakins/Schildberg
© Springer-Verlag, Berlin Heidelberg 1993

Table 1. Myeloperoxidase content of lung and liver tissue after either trauma or *E. coli* bacteremia in baboons (from [4])

	Myeloperoxidase lung	Wet weight mU/g liver
Polytrauma ($n = 6$)	188 (129–202)	463 (422–488)
Bacteremia ($n = 4$)	457[a] (354–476)	622[a] (468–716)

[a] $f < 0.05$.

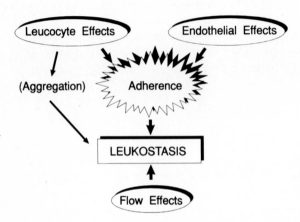

Fig. 1. Adherence as the central event, which leads to leukostasis, is based on changes in blood flow, leukocyte activation, and endothelial cell surface properties

their adhesion to the endothelium occurs almost exclusively in postcapillary venules [6]. House et al. [6] have provided experimental proof that adherence depends mainly on an increase in adhesive forces rather than on diminished shear stresses. Such diminished shear stress is found when blood flow is reduced, for example, due to hypovolemia, as in our polytrauma model, and a reduction of cardiac output down to one-third of normal values occurs. It must be noted that despite an increase in cardiac output with reinfusion and (over) normalization of blood flow leukostasis could not be significantly reduced [7], probably due to adhesion phenomena.

Leukocyte Effects

Among the various leukocyte populations PMN are the most fast-acting cells of the body's inflammatory response mechanism and are therefore the focus of EC-leukocyte interactions. Activation of PMN occurs via the action of humoral products (e.g., C5a), by bacterial products (e.g., chemotactic peptides; endotoxin—lipopolysaccharide, LPS) or cytokines (e.g., tumor necrosis factor, TNF; interleukin-8, IL-8).

Among the events caused by such mediators are respiratory burst, oxygen radical and enzyme release, together with upregulation of adherence molecules and increased adhesion (Fig. 2).

The increased adherence of PMN might result in aggregation, such as described by Craddock [8], which is caused by complement-derived ana-phylatoxins and is aggregated by platelets [9]. Aggregates formed in the peripheral circulation are then passively transported to the lung capillary bed and trapped (= leukostasis). Specific adhesion of PMN to the endothelial surface is provided via Fc, platelet-activation factor (PAF) receptors, and adhesion molecules [10], for example, the CDw18 complex. The CDw18 complex is part of the supergene integrin family and consists of glycoproteins arranged in one β-chain (CD18) and three different α-chains (CD11a, CD11b, CD11c) and can be influenced by several inflammatory mediators [11].

In addition to granulocytes, monocytes and lymphocytes also bind (e.g., to the endothelium [10, 12]) by means of these adhesive proteins. The relative contribution of each of these molecules to leukocyte/EC adhesion varies depending on the cell type and the stimulus used, as shown by Arnaout et al. [13].

It is difficult to monitor serially the increased adhesion of PMN as a result of PMN activation in vivo because only circulating (but not adherent) cells can be measured. Therefore the demonstration of PMN activation, of which PMN adhesion is one part, is performed more reliably by measurement of elastase release (plasma levels). Various groups have successfully used this method in the clinic [14]. We applied this method in the baboon (IMAC technique; Merck) [15] and found much higher elastase levels in severe septic than in traumatic baboons (Table 2).

Along with measurement of protease release, the oxygen radical release from PMN can be used as an activation parameter. In a study together with Inthorn et al. [16] we demonstrated PMN activation in postoperative and septic patients by whole blood chemiluminescence [17] as a measurement of oxygen radical formation during phagocytosis. The drawback of this method is that only circulating cells are quantified. In this study patients at the onset of sepsis had a higher PMN activity than in the postsurgical (trauma) state and thus corresponded to the higher activation state found in the septic as compared to

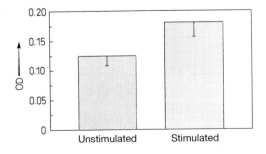

Fig. 2. Formyl-methionyl-leucyl-phenylalanine $(5 \times 10^{-7}\ mM)$ induced activation of human neutrophils (Percoll isolated) results in significantly increased adherence of the cells to a plastic cell culture disk—quantified by measurement of myeloperoxidase with 3, 3'-dimethoxybenzidine (O-dianisidine dihydrochloride) as substrate

Table 2. Plasma levels of PMN-specific elastase in baboon experiments with polytrauma or bacteremia (from [15])

Groups (h/animal)	Sepsis	Hypovolemic/ traumatic shock
0	6 ± 1.3	15 ± 2
2	270 ± 45.0	30 ± 6
4	262 ± 26.0[a]	62 ± 8
6	388 ± 31.0[a]	77 ± 15
8	304 ± 27.0	ND

[a] Sepsis statistically different from hypovoemic traumatic shock ($p < 0.05$) using Wilcoxon statistics.

the traumatic baboons. In the baboon model situation, one of the reasons for the higher activation state of leukocytes might be the *E. coli* related release of endotoxin into the plasma (up to 11 ng/ml), which was not seen in the trauma animals. Similarly most of the LPS inducible cytokines, except for IL-6, were found in the sepsis but seldom in the trauma situation [IL-6 trauma 11 (3–360) ng/ml, sepsis 4197 (1476–5468) ng/ml; in collaboration with U. Schade, Borstel, FRG].

The importance of PMN for tissue damage in general and of adhesion (molecule) upregulation during PMN activation is supported by numerous experimental studies with experimentally induced leukopenia which demonstrated that organ damage, for example in the lung, could be prevented [18–22]. Neutrophil depletion did not prevent edema formation in the lungs after endotoxin administration if depletion was performed with nitrogen mustard and not with hydroxyurea, in some but not in other studies [23]. In contrast, nitrogen mustard PMN depleted rabbits did not reveal lung injury induced by endotoxin and chemotactic peptide [24].

The importance of PMN-related adhesion is emphasized with the use of monoclonal antibodies (60.3, TS1/18, IB4) against the common CD-18 β-chain, since these antibodies possess a protective potential in hypovolemic shock [25] and against LPS-induced tissue injury [27, 28].

Endothelial Effects

One of the important tasks of EC is the communication between circulating blood cells and specific cells of the organs, with EC acting as "doorkeepers" in blood cell margination and extravasation. Along with this task, EC are important sites of synthesis of shock mediators and at the same time are target cells for many substances released during traumatic and septic shock [29].

The responses of EC to shock mediators differ according to the type of substance hitting the EC. In analogy to the local inflammatory scenario

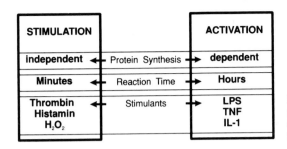

STIMULATION		ACTIVATION
independent ◀──	Protein Synthesis ──▶	dependent
Minutes ◀──	Reaction Time ──▶	Hours
Thrombin Histamin H_2O_2 ◀──	Stimulants ──▶	LPS TNF IL-1

Fig. 3. Probable time sequence of endothelial cell "stimulation" (e.g., by oxygen radicals, thrombin) and "activation" (e.g., by endotoxin or TNF)

acc. J.Pober

reviewed by Pober [30] we classify EC responses as *endothelial stimulation* (fast, protein synthesis independent response) or *endothelial activation* (slower, protein synthesis dependent response; Fig. 3).

EC stimulation occurs in response to agonists such as thrombin and histamine [31] or oxygen radicals [32]. Molecules involved in endothelial stimulation are primarily GMP-140 [31] and PAF [33] on the EC side as well as Lewis-X and PAF receptors as the PMN counterparts.

There has been recent in vivo data on this phenomena [34]. During gut ischemia and reperfusion PMN adherence in liver sinusoids was significantly diminished using PAF receptor antagonists (BN 52021), indicating the importance of this PAF/PAF receptor interaction. In the same setting antioxidant therapy was also partially successful (not synergistic with PAF antagonist) [35], thus indicating the possible involvement of oxygen radicals in this EC stimulation. Similar observations have been made in the splanchnic area [36].

A distinct series of events occur if EC are activated by LPS or cytokines. The in vitro inducible properties of the endothelium by LPS and cytokines include cytokine expression, procoagulant activity, immunologic functions, and increased adhesiveness for leukocytes due to expression of adherence molecules. These events are within the definition of endothelial activation. We can now demonstrate that such a (de novo) expression of adhesion molecules occurs in vivo under septic conditions in subprimate animal models [15]. This was shown using two different antibodies to the endothelial leukocyte adhesion molecule 1 (ELAM-1; Fig. 4). ELAM-1 serve to bind PMN via a sialyl-Lewis-X structure [37, 38]. ELAM-1 is not present on unstimulated EC in vitro and can be transiently induced (peak 4–6 h) by LPS, IL-1α, IL-1β, TNF, or LT [39, 40]. ELAM-1 together with intercellular adhesion molecule 1 (ICAM-1) is not only responsible for adherence, but also for neutrophil emigration [41]. We have previously shown massive cytokine release in the septic but not in the polytrauma situation in (baboon) models [42], which might also explain the differences in EC activation. Furthermore, circulating endotoxin in plasma is several log steps higher in sepsis than in trauma (S. Bahrami, unpublished results). Nevertheless, small amounts of endotoxin seen after polytrauma due to

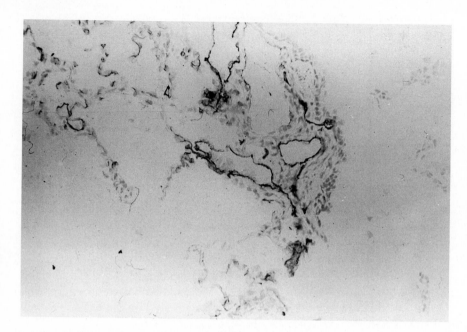

Fig. 4. ELAM-1 expression on the endothelial surface of vessels in lung specimen under septic conditions (Baboon live *E. coli* bacteremia model). (ELAM antibody ENA-1 was kindly supplied by Wim Buurman, Maastricht)

Table 3. Incidence of immunohistochemical identification (grades 0–3) of the adherence molecule ELAM-1 in baboon tissue from various organs after either polytrauma or sepsis (from [15])

	Septic shock		Traumatic shock	
	Number examined	Average score	Number examined	Average score
Lung	6	2.2 +	13	0.03 +
Liver	5	3.0 +	12	0.16 +
Kidney	3	2.7 +	9	0.8 +
Skin	2	3.0 +	2	0.5 +

bacterial translocation [43] might account for the few positive endothelial stainings in the trauma animals (Table 3).

ELAM-1 expression may serve as a marker for an "activated" EC state (as suggested by Pober [44]) and is one of the possible preconditions which lead to leukocyte-related EC damage, but of course we do not propose from our data that the ELAM-1 antigen expression causes leakiness. However, a recent study of immune complex induced alveolitis suggests that in vivo blocking of ELAM-1 with monoclonal antibodies has therapeutic effects [45].

Activated and EC-bound leukocytes may be responsible for the vascular leakiness which is associated with traumatic and septic shock. We observed in a series of animals such leakiness leading to edema formation in the lung, with a ratio of lung weights (medians) between the different protocols of 1:1.24:1.74 (sham:trauma:sepsis) [4].

In vitro findings on ELAM-1 are in contrast to those of ICAM-1 [46], which is present on unstimulated EC and is upregulated only by the same cytokines. We have now preliminary evidence (unpublished results) that the same holds true for septic shock conditions in vivo using our baboon model, but this upregulation is protracted as compared to ELAM-1, similar to the findings of Pober after local LPS injection.

The complementary adhesion molecules at the leukocyte surface (summarized in Fig. 5) are either constituitive (e.g., Lewis-X, LFA-1), are lost during PMN activation (e.g., LAM-1), or are upregulated, such as Mac-1 (CD11b/CD18).

All these EC-leukocyte interactions seem to be the prerequisite both for PMN extravasation and EC damage. Since EC changes (damage) lead to permeability changes and ultimately to edema formation, the EC-leukocyte interactions are of central importance in shock-induced organ damage. Adhering and activated PMN might be crucial in EC damage since a microenvironment is formed. In this environment mediators are released locally, and damage occurs because of insufficient neutralizing capacity (antiproteases, antioxidants). Such damage is attributed to oxygen radicals, proteases, or both.

From the current literature and our own in vivo studies in primates we conclude that leukostasis occurs both after trauma and sepsis but is more distinct in sepsis. There is clear evidence of PMN activation both in trauma and

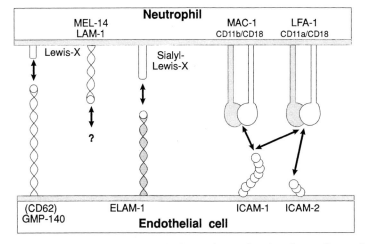

Fig. 5. Schematic diagram of EC-leukocyte interactions based on a figure of Springer [47] and further reports

sepsis, but again sepsis is a much stronger trigger mechanism. EC are probably involved in leukostasis, especially during sepsis when EC are "activated" with the de novo expression of adhesion molecules such as ELAM-1. This is hardly seen after trauma, when only low levels of LPS or cytokines are found. The importance of the adhesion phenomena can be derived from successful studies with specific blocking antibodies to the CD11/CD18–ICAM-1 interaction [25] and first results with anti ELAM-1 therapy [45].

Besides, neutralization of de novo expressed (or upregulated) adhesion molecules by antibodies, reducing PMN and EC activation should be considered as the primary therapeutic goal in the posttraumatic situation.

Acknowledgements. We thank E. Paul, A. Schießer, S. Mayer, and G. Leichtfried for invaluable technical assistance. The manuscript would not have been written without the help of E. Schwarz and G. Leichtfried. We thank all our many collaborators in these studies, D. Spragg for proof-reading, and the Lorenz Böhler Fonds for support.

References

1. Schlag G, Redl H (1980) Die Leukostase in der Lunge beim hypovolämisch-traumatischen Schock. Anaesthesist 29:606–612
2. Redl H, Dinges HP, Schlag G (1987) Quantitative estimation of leukostasis in the posttraumatic lung—canine and human autopsy data. Prog Clin Biol Res 236A:43–53
3. Pretorius JP, Schlag G, Redl H, Botha WS, Goosen DJ, Bosman H, van Eeden AF (1987) The 'lung in shock' as a result of hypovolemic-traumatic shock in baboons. J Trauma 27:1344–1353
4. Redl H, Schlag G, Dinges HP, Bahrami S, Buurman WA, Schade U, Ceska M (1991) Trauma and sepsis induced activation of granulocytes, monocytes/macrophages and endothelial cells in primates. In: Schlag G, Redl H, Siegel JH, Traber DL (eds) Shock, sepsis, and organ failure—second Wiggers Bernard conference. Springer, Berlin Heidelberg New York, pp 297–313
5. Mayrovitz H, Wiedeman M, Tuma R (1977) Factors influencing leukocyte adherence in microvessels. Thromb Haemost 38:823–830
6. House SD, Lipowsky HH (1987) Leukocyte-endothelium adhesion: microhemodynamics in mesentery of the cat. Microvasc Res 34:363–379
7. Redl H, Schlag G, Hammerschmidt DE (1984) Quantitative assessment of leukostasis in experimental hypovolemic-traumatic shock. Acta Chir Scand 150:113–117
8. Caddock PR, Hammerschmidt DE, White JG, Dalmasse AP, Jacob HS (1977) Complement (C5a) induced granulocyte aggregation in vitro. A possible mechanism of complement mediated leukostasis and leukopenia. J Clin Invest 60:260–264
9. Redl H, Hammerschmidt DE, Schlag G (1983) Augmentation by platelets of granulocyte aggregation in response to chemotaxins: studies utilizing an improved cell preparation technique. Blood 61:125–131
10. Wallis WJ, Hickstein DD, Schwartz BR, June CH, Ochs HD, Beatty PG, Klebanoff SJ, Harlan JM (1986) Monoclonal antibody defined functional epitopes on the adhesion promoting glycoprotein complex (CDw18) of human neutrophils. Blood 67:1007–1013
11. Tonnensen MG, Anderson DC, Springer TA, Knedler A, Avdi N, Henson PM (1989) Adherence of neutrophil to cultured human microvascular endothelial cells. Stimulation by chemotatic peptides and lipid mediators and dependence upon the Mac-1, LFA-1, p150,95 glycoprotein family. J Clin Invest 83:637–646
12. Bierer BE, Burakoff SJ (1988) T-cell adhesion molecules. FASEB J 2:2584–2590
13. Arnaout MA, Lanier LL, Faller DV (1988) Relative contribution of the leukocyte molecules Mol, LFA-1, and p150,95 (LeuM5) in adhesion of granulocytes and monocytes to vascular endothelium is tissue- and stimulus-specific. J Cell Physiol 137:305–309
14. Lang H, Jochum M, Fritz H, Redl H (1989) Validity of the elastase assay in intensive care medicine. Prog Clin Biol Res 308:701–706

15. Redl H, Dinges HP, Buurman WA, van der Linden CJ, Pober JS, Cotran RS, Schlag G (1991) Expression of endothelial leukocyte adhesion molecule-1 in septic but not traumatic/hypovolemic shock in the baboon. Am J Pathol 139: (in press)
16. Inthorn D, Szczeponik T, Mühlbayer D, Jochum M, Redl H (1987) Studies of granulocyte function (chemiluminescence response) in postoperative infection. Prog Clin Biol Res 236B:51–58
17. Redl H, Lamche H, Schlag G (1983) Red cell count dependence of whole blood granulocyte luminescence. Klin Wochenschr 61:163–164
18. Heflin Ac jr, Brigham KL (1981) Prevention by granulocyte depletion of increased vascular permeability of sheep lung following endotoxemia. J Clin Invest 68:1253–1260
19. Flick MR, Peral G, Staub NC (1981) Leukocytes are required for increased lung microvascular permeability after microemboli in sheep. Circ Res 48:344–351
20. Shasby DM, Fox RB, Haranda RN, Repine JE (1982) Reduction of the edema of acute hyperoxic lung injury by granulocyte depletion. J Appl Physiol 52:1237–1239
21. Johnson A, Malik AB (1980) Effect of granulocytopenia on extravascular lung water content after microembolization. Am Rev Respir Dis 122:561–566
22. Heath CA, Lai L, Bizios R, Malik AB (1986) Pulmonary hemodynamic effects of antisheep serum-induced leukopenia. J Leukoc Biol 3:385–392
23. Winn R, Maunder R, Chi E, Harlan J (1987) Neutrophil depletion does not prevent lung edema after endotoxin infusion in goats. J Appl Physiol 62:116–121
24. Worthen S, Haslett C, Rees AJ, Gumbay RS, Henson JE, Henson PM (1987). Neutrophil-mediated pulmonary vascular injury. Synergistic effect of trace amounts of lipopolysaccharide and neutrophil stimuli on vascular permeability and neutrophil sequestration in the lung. Am Rev Respir Dis 136:19–28
25. Vedder NB, Winn RK, Rice CL, Chi EY, Arfors KE, Harlan JM (1988) A monoclonal antibody to the adherence promoting leukocyte glycoprotein, CD18, reduces organ injury and improves survival from hemorrhagic shock and resuscitation in rabbits. J Clin Invest 81:939–944
26. Cooper JA, Neumann PH, Wright SD, Malik AB (1989) Pulmonary vascular sequestration of neutrophils in endotoxemia: role of CD18 leukocyte surface glycoprotein. Am Rev Respir Dis 139:A301
27. Kaslovsky RA, Horgan MJ, Lum H, McCandless BK, Gilboa N, Wright SD, Malik AB (1990) Pulmonary edema induced by phagocytosing neutrophils. Protective effect of monoclonal antibody against phagocyte CD18 integrin. Circ Res 67:795–802
28. Hernandez LA, Grisham MB, Twohig B, Arfors KE, Harlan JM, Granzer N (1987) Role of neutrophils in ischemia reperfusion induced microvascular injury. Am J Physiol 253:H699–H703
29. Schlag G, Redl H (1990) Endothelium as the interface between blood and organ in the evolution of organ failure. In: Schlag G, Redl H, Siegel JH (eds) Shock, sepsis, and organ failure—first Wiggers Bernard conference. Springer, Berlin Heidelberg New York, pp 210–271
30. Pober JS, Cotran RS (1990) The role of endothelial cells in inflammation. Transplantation 50:537–544
31. Geng JG, Bevilacqua MP, Moore KL, McIntyre TM, Prescott SM, Kim JM, Bliss GA, Zimmerman GA, McEver RP (1990) Rapid neutrophil adhesion to activated endothelium mediated by GMP 140. Nature 343:757–760
32. Patel KD, Zimmerman GA, Prescott SM, McEver RP, McIntyre TM (1991) Oxygen radicals induce human endothelial cells to express GMP-140 and bind neutrophils. J Cell Biol 112:749–759
33. Zimmerman GA, McIntyre TM, Mehra M, Prescott SM (1990) Endothelial cell associated platelet activating factor: a novel mechanism for signaling intercellular adhesion. J Cell Biol 110:529–540
34. Bühren V, Maier B, Hower R, Holzmann A, Redl H, Marzi I (1991) PAF-antagonist BN52021 reduces hepatic leukocyte adhesion following intestinal ischemia. Circ Shock 34:134–135
35. Marzi I, Bühren V, Schüttler A, Trentz O (1991) Recombinant human superoxide dismutase (rh-SOD) to reduce multiple organ failure after trauma—results of a prospective clinical trial. Circ Shock 34:145
36. Kubes P, Ibbotson G, Russell J, Wallace JL, Granger ND (1990) Role of platelet activating factor in ischemia reperfusion induced leukocyte adherence. Am J Physiol 259:G300–G305
37. Phillips ML, Nudelman E, Gaeta FCA, Perez M, Singhal AK, Hakomori SI, Paulson JC (1990) ELAM-1 mediates cell adhesion by recognition of a carbohydrate ligand sialyl le. Science 250:1130–1132

38. Walz G, Aruffo A, Kolanus W, Bevilacqua M, Seed B (1990) Recognition by ELAM-1 of the sialyl le determinant on myeloid and tumor cells. Science 250:1132–1135
39. Flynn WJ, Cryer HM, Garrison RN (1990) Angiotensin II arteriolar mediated constriction is not responsible for persistent intestinal hypoperfusion in rats resuscitated from hemorrhagic shock. Circ Shock 31:57
40. Leeuwenberg FM, Jeunhomme TMAA, Buurman WA (1989) Induction of an activation antigen on human endothelial cells in vitro. Eur J Immunol 19:715
41. Luscinskas FW, Cybulsky MI, Kiely JM, Peckins CS, Davis VM, Gomgrone MAjr (1991) Cytokine-activated human endothelial monolayers support enhanced neutrophil transmigration via a mechanism involving both endothelial-leukocyte adhesion molecule-1 and intercellular adhesion molecule-1. J Immunol 146:1617–1625
42. Redl H, Schlag G, Paul E, Davies J (1989) Monocyte/macrophage activation with cytokine release after polytrauma and sepsis in the baboon. Circ Shock 27:308
43. Schlag G, Redl H, Dinges HP, Davies J, Radmore K (1991) Bacterial translocation in a baboon model of hypovolemic-traumatic shock. In: Schlag G, Redl H, Siegel JH, Traber DL (eds) Shock, sepsis, and organ failure—second Wiggers Bernard conference. Springer, Berlin Heidelberg New York, pp 53–83
44. Pober JS (1988) Cytokine mediated activation of vascular endothelium. Physiology and pathology. Am J Pathol 133:426–433
45. Ward P (1991) Role of ELAM in inflammation in vivo. In: 2nd international congress on the immune consequences of trauma, shock and sepsis mechanisms and therapeutic approaches, Munich, abstract, p 22
46. Rothlein R, Dustin ML, Marlin SD, Springer TA (1986) A human intercellular adhesion molecule (ICAM-1) distinct from LFA-1. J Immunol 137:1270–1274
47. Springer TA (1990) Adhesion receptors of the immune system. Nature 346:425–434

Role of Oxygen Radicals in Multiple Organ Failure

H. P. Friedl[1], O. Trentz[1], G.O. Till[2], and P. A. Ward[2]

Introduction

Multiple organ failure (MOF) has become a recognized disease entity occurring in response to infection, vascular perfusion deficits, a persistent inflammatory focus, or a persistent focus of dead and/or injured tissue. At least four phases (shock, resuscitation, hypermetabolism and evidence of multiple organ failure) can be identified clinically. With MOF, the general pattern of the inflammatory response appears to be expressed both locally and systemically with the demonstrated changes of vascular permeability followed by exudation and the sequence of cell infiltrates characteristic of inflammation and, finally, the onset of repair mechanisms. A number of mechanisms appear to be associated with

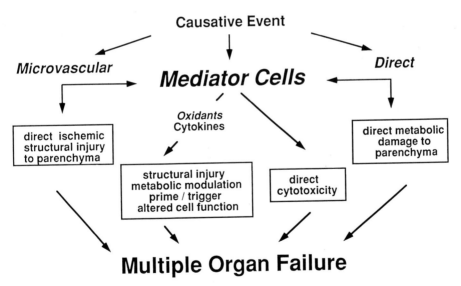

Fig. 1. Multiple organ failure: general mechanisms

[1] Departement Chirurgie, Klinik für Unfallchirurgie, Universitätsspital Zürich, CH-8091 Zürich, Switzterland
[2] Department of Pathology, University of Michigan Medical School, Ann Arbor, Michigan 48104-0602, USA

Host Defense Dysfunction
in Trauma, Shock and Sepsis
Eds. Faist/Meakins/Schildberg
© Springer-Verlag, Berlin Heidelberg 1993

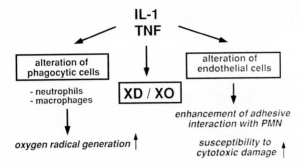

Fig. 2. Cytokines and oxygen-radical-mediated tissue injury

pathways leading to irreversible structural injury or metabolic disfuntion at the cell level (Fig. 1).

It appears that *xanthine oxidase, neutrophils*, and *endothelial cells* may play an important role in the initial phases of the MOF (Fig. 2), and that the *macrophage* assumes a dominant role through the secretion of cytokines and inflammatory mediators that induce, prime, or trigger oxidant pathways culminating in cell injury (Fig. 3).

Of the *cytokines* produced by macrophages, perhaps two of the most intensively studied and most relevant to the inflammatory process are interleukin-1β (IL-1β) and tumor necrosis factor-α (TNF-α). Both factors are proteins that are synthesized in macrophages and released after cell contact with any number of factors such as lipopolysaccharide (LPS) or immune complexes [1]. More often than not, both cytokines are produced simultaneously, although selective production of either IL-1 or TNF can occur.

Interactions of Cytokines With Xanthine Oxidase, Macrophages, and Neutrophils

Xanthine oxidase (XO) (EC 1.1.3.22) appears to play an important role in events related to ischemia–reperfusion injury in a variety of organs (reviewed in [2]). It has been demonstrated that this enzyme is derived by cleavage or by reversible oxidation of xanthine dehydrogenase (XD) (EC 1.1.1.204) [3, 4] and that the products of XO (superoxide anion and its conversion products, H_2O_2 and the hydroxyl radical) are either directly toxic to tissues or participate in generation of chemotactic lipids, which cause recruitment of neutrophils [2, 5, 6]. Inturn, oxygen products from activated neutrophils injure tissues [7]. XO has been found in endothelial cells from some species [8–10], and recently it has been shown that the interaction of activated neutrophils with endothelial cells results in conversion of XD to XO within endothelial cells [11]. This process appears to have biological implications, as the killing of endothelial cells by activated

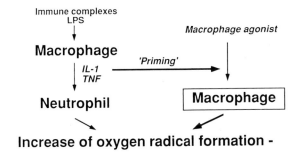

Fig. 3. Cytokines and oxygen-radical-mediated tissue injury

neutrophils can be attenuated if endothelial cells are pretreated with inhibitors of XO [11]. The ultimate killing of endothelial cells by activated neutrophils is related to H_2O_2 production by neutrophils [12].

In recent studies [13] we showed that peptide chemotactic mediators can interact directly with endothelial cells to bring about activation of XO (i.e., the conversion of XD to XO). Our data suggest that some inflammatory mediators (C5a, TNF-α, and N-formylmethionyl leucyl phenylalanine, fMLP; Table 1) have effects both on phagocytic cells as well as on potential targets such as endothelial cells, to bring about inimical consequences of the inflammatory response. Examples of the direct effect of these chemotactic peptides in endothelial cells are shown in Fig. 4. In these experiments, dose-response relations were determined, and the concentrations of peptide required to bring about 50% conversion of XD to XO (ED_{50}) were calculated. The results are shown in detail in Table 1.

C5a and TNF-α, which are products of complement activation and stimulated macrophages, respectively, can be generated at the interface of endothelial cells and blood leukocytes. In this manner, these products can lead to an amplification of the inflammatory response by engaging either effector (neutrophils) or target (endothelial) cells, or both. The nature of the process resulting in conversion of XD to XO is unknown except that this process is rapid and irreversible, as defined by the inability of XO to revert to XD in the presence of dithiothreitol (DTT). The fact that endothelial cells can respond to peptide mediators, which also stimulate phagocytic cells, underscores the complexity of events underlying how the inflammatory response brings about tissue injury and emphasizes the possibility that the generation of these peptide mediators in vivo may result in a multiplicity of events culminating in tissue injury.

With respect to the interactions of IL-1β or TNF-α with *phagocytic cells*, direct and indirect effects may alter the oxygen-radical-generating capacity of these cells (Fig. 5). Direct effects include the ability of IL-1β and TNF-α to stimulate *neutrophils*, with resultant production of oxygen radicals [14–17]. Dose ranges for IL-1 and TNF-α with respect to stimulation of human neutrophils are less than 5×10^{-9} M and 10^{-11}–10^{-8} M, respectively [14–17].

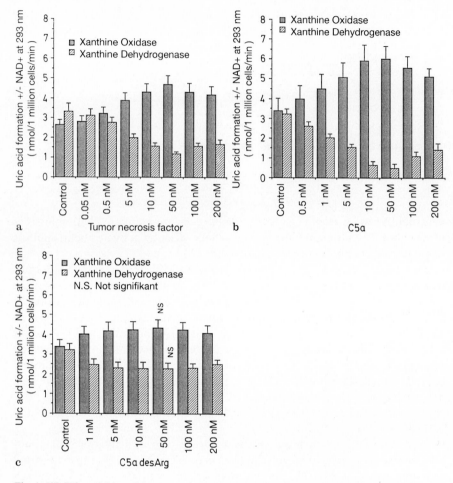

Fig. 4. XD/XO activities of lysates and supernatants of: **a** TNF-treated RPA endothelial cells. **b** C5a-treated RPA endothelial cells, and **c** C5a-desArg-treated RPA endothelial cells

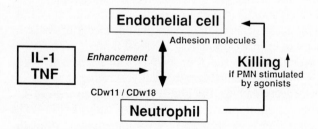

Fig. 5. Interactions of cytokines with endothelial cells

The oxygen-radical-generating responses under these conditions are of rather limited magnitude, rarely exceeding 25% of the total capacity of the neutrophil. Of equal interest regarding the mechanism of interaction of cytokines with phagocytic cells is the indirect effect of these mediators on macrophages. IL-1 and TNF have the ability to "prime" macrophages for accentuated oxygen responses when the cells come into contact with a macrophage agonist [18]. The "priming" phenomenon implies that the signal transduction pathway of the phagocytic cell is altered such that subsequent contact of the cell with an agonist results in a supernormal response.

Examples of the indirect (priming) effect of cytokines in phagocytic cells are shown in Fig. 6. Rat alveolar macrophages were incubated with increasing amounts of human recombinant TNF-α or IL-1, or with supernatant fluids from macrophages that were nonactivated or stimulated by contact with opsonized zymosan particles. Following these additions, the macrophages were placed in contact with immune complexes (containing rabbit immunoglobulin G, IgG) and the subsequent oxygen responses were measured.

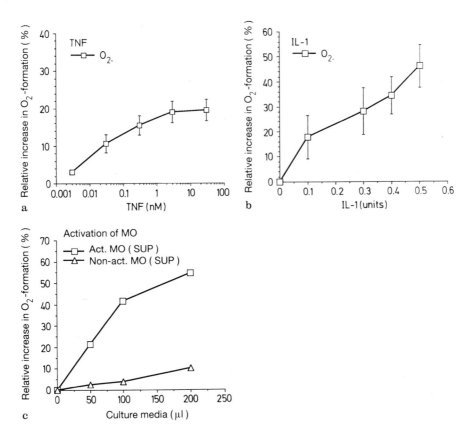

Fig. 6. Potentiated O_2^- response of alveolar macrophages: **a** TNF-α, **b** IL-1β, **c** activation of macrophages

As shown by Warren et al. [18], exposure to TNF caused a modest ($\sim 20\%$) but consistent increase in the oxygen radical response that had been triggered by the immune complexes. It is apparent that, by itself, TNF-α at the highest concentration did not directly cause an oxygen radical response in the absence of another agonist. Cell contact with IL-1 caused, in a dose-dependent manner, substantial enhancement (50% at the highest dose, 0.5 U) in the oxygen radical response of immune-complex-stimulated alveolar macrophages. Again, IL-1 in the absence of immune complexes caused virtually no increase in the baseline amount of oxygen radical production.

Macrophage contact with cytokine-rich supernatant fluids from activated alveolar macrophages (incubated with zymosan particles) resulted in enhanced (60%) oxygen radical responses of immune-complex-stimulated macrophages, while culture fluids from nonstimulated macrophages showed little or no evidence of an enhancement effect. In data not shown, supernatant fluids from activated macrophages in the absence of immune complexes did not cause an increase in the level of "background" oxygen radical production (< 1.5 nmol O_2^- in 20 min). Although the nature of the factor(s) in the supernatant fluids from activated macrophages is not known, it is reasonable to assume that the effects may be due to the presence of IL-1 or TNF-α, or both, in the supernatant fluids. The data stress that macrophage-generated cytokines can enhance substantially the oxygen radical responses of stimulated macrophages. In data not shown, the priming effect of IL-1, TNF, and supernatant fluids of activated macrophages has not been found in rat neutrophils, suggesting that the macrophage may be a more important target for indirect cytokine effects.

Interactions of Cytokines With Endothelial Cells

It has recently been reported [19, 20] that IL-1 and TNF-α alter endothelial cells (from human umbilical veins) in a manner that requires protein synthesis, such that adhesive interactions with neutrophils are greatly increased (Fig. 5). This phenomenon has been related to the appearance on the endothelial cell of a factor that interacts with the neutrophil. The most relevant adhesion promoting molecule on the endothelial cell appears to be ELAM-1. Adhesion promoting molecules on the neutrophil are next to the adhesion interaction molecule CD 11b/CD 18 heterodimer as well as the sial-Le^x molecule.

These observations have been extended by Varani et al. [12] with rat pulmonary artery endothelial cells and human neutrophils. For this experiment, endothelial cells were exposed to TNF-α (3 nM) for 5 or 18 h and then washed, after which nonstimulated human neutrophils were added and the adherence of neutrophils to the endothelial cells measured. Exposure of endothelial cells to TNF-α greatly enhanced the adhesiveness of the neutrophils to the altered endothelial cells. It should be pointed out that this adhesive interaction is noncytotoxic, provided a neutrophil agonist such as phorbol ester has not been added. The effects of the addition of such an agonist to the outcome of the neutrophil–endothelial cell interactions are prominent. In this study, endothelial cells were pretreated with 3 nM TNF for 18 h, washed, and then human neutrophils and phorbol ester were added. The data show a dramatic increase (104%) in the neutrophil-mediated cytotoxicity of endothelial cells that were altered by exposure to TNF-α. The TNF-α effects were abrogated by TNF-α antibody present during the 18-h period of exposure of endothelial cells to TNF. Similarly, the exposure of endothelial cells to IL-I before the addition of phorbol-ester-stimulated neutrophils also increased (by 48%) the cytotoxicity produced by activated neutrophils. These data indicate that cytokines may substantially alter the susceptibility of endothelial cells to the cytotoxic effects of activated neutrophils. The precise mechanisms by which endothelial cells are rendered more susceptible to injury is not currently known. The implication of these observations may be relevant to the well-known effects of TNF-α and IL-1 in causing multiorgan injury after experimental infusion of the cytokines into animals.

In Vivo Effects of Cytokines in Experimental Animals

Evidence is emerging that infusion of cytokines into experimental animals (and into humans) can, under certain conditions, result in inimical outcomes. In this respect, the most intensively studied cytokine has been TNF. Tissue damage follows LPS infusion and is targeted to specific organs including the small intestine [21], kidneys with resulting acute tubular necrosis, and lungs with respiratory failure [23].

In a study by Tracey et al. [23], tissue damage consisting of hemorrhagic necrosis and extensive acute inflammation was observed in the lungs after infusion of live gram-negative bacteria which induced TNF-α secretion. Tissue damage was also observed in the kidneys and adrenal glands. Pretreatment of animals with anti-TNF-α antibody completely blocked these histologic alterations. The direct infusion of human recombinant TNF-α into rats resulted in severe injury to the lungs, pancreas, kidneys, adrenals, and intestines [24]. Remick et al. [25] investigated the acute in vivo effects of human recombinant TNF-α given intravenously to mice. CBA/J mice which received 10 μg human recombinant TNF-α developed watery diarrhea, lethargy, piloerection, and tachypnea. At 2 h, analysis of peripheral blood showed the characteristic lymphopenia and neutrophilia [26]. Hemoconcentration was manifested by an increased hematocrit (46.6 $\pm$ 4 in TNF-α-treated animals vs 38.6 $\pm$ 0.5 in control animals). The small bowel was grossly distended with edema fluid. The major histologic alterations were confined to the small bowel in which villi were flattened and thinned with necrotic tips. Ultrastructural examination confirmed the light microscopic findings of necrotic epithelial cells. In addition, there was also damage to the blood vessels of the small intestine with gap formation and blebbing of the luminal surface of the endothelial cells. Within the interstitium of the lamina propria, extravasated neutrophils and red cells were present. In arterioles, neutrophils were marginated along the walls of the vessels. Vascular permeability studies using ^{125}I-labeled albumin provided quantitative assessment of fluid shifts and demonstrated a preferential fluid leak into the small intestine, even at the TNF-α dose of 100 µg. At higher doses, there is evidence of more generalized injuries. Preliminary laboratory data have suggested that at TNF-α doses of 10 µg, there is evidence of multiorgan injury, including significant pulmonary damage.

Finally, questions arise as to the exact role of cytokines in inflammatory reactions in vivo that have been triggered by a defined agonist. Answers to these questions should be forthcoming with the recent availability of antibodies to block endogenous cytokines in experimental animals. As noted above, IL-1, TNF-α, and supernatant fluids from activated macrophages can bring about enhanced oxygen responses in rat alveolar macrophages stimulated with IgG immune complexes. Preliminary evidence has demonstrated that in vitro incubation of rat alveolar macrophages or blood monocytes with IgG immune complexes causes 85% and 35% increases, respectively, in the content of IL-1 in the extracellular fluid, as compared to companion, nonstimulated phagocytic cells. Not surprisingly, these data indicate that rat tissue macrophages have a considerably greater capacity for cytokine formation than blood monocytes. In rats with acute lung damage induced by deposition of IgG immune complexes, the bronchoalveolar lavage fluids from these animals have revealed the presence of both IL-1 and TNF-α (10.8 and 26 U/ml, respectively), demonstrating that these cytokines are generated in the developing immune-complex-induced inflammatory reactions. The extent to which the presence of these cytokines contribute to the pathogenesis of the lung injury is currently under investigation.

Conclusion

There is abundant evidence that the cytokines IL-1 and TNF-α have important roles in the pathogenesis of tissue injury occurring during the initiation of the acute inflammatory reaction. The studies presented above indicate that IL-1 and TNF-α alter phagocytic cells in vitro, resulting in increased oxygen radical generation, and they can modify endothelial cells such that adhesive interactions with neutrophils are enhanced, as well as greatly increase the susceptibility of the endothelial cells to cytotoxic damage by activated neutrophils. In vivo, the infusion of TNF-α results in organ damage, with both epithelial and endothelial cell injury being especially evident. Finally, the detection of IL-1 and TNF-α in acute inflammatory reactions in the lung after deposition of immune complexes indicates that these cytokines are being generated in vivo; the data suggest that production of these cytokines may contribute to the outcome of organ injury.

References

1. Le J, Vilcek J (1987) Tumor necrosis factor and interleukin 1: cytokines with multiple overlapping biological activities. Lab Invest 56:234
2. Granger DM, Höllwarth ME, Parks DA (1986) Ischemia-reperfusion injury: role of oxygen derived free radicals. Acta Physiol Scand [Suppl] 548:47
3. Della Corte E, Stirpe F (1972) The regulation of rat liver xanthine oxidase. Involvement of thiol groups in the conversion of the enzyme activity from dehydrogenase (type D) into oxidase (type O) and purification of the enzyme. Biochem J 126:739
4. Batelli MG, Lorenzoni E, Stirpe F (1973) Milk xanthine oxidase type D (dehydrogenase) and type O (oxidase). Purification, interconversion and some properties. Biochem J 131:191
5. Perez HD, Weksler BB, Goldstein IA (1980) Generation of a chemotactic lipid from arachidonic acid by exposure to a superoxide-generating system. Inflammation 4:313
6. Petrone WF, English DK, Wong K, McCord JM (1980) Free radicals and inflammation: the superoxide dependent activation of a neutrophil chemotactic factor in plasma. Proc Natl Acad Sci USA 77:1159
7. Fantone JC, Ward PA (1982) Role of oxygen-derived free radicals and metabolites in leukocyte-dependent inflammatory reactions. Am J Pathol 107:395
8. Ratych RE, Chuknyiska RS, Bulkley GB (1987) The primary localization of free radical generation after anoxia/reoxygenation in isolated endothelial cells. Surgery 102:122
9. Jarasch ED, Grund C, Bruder G et al. (1981) Localization of xanthine oxidase in mammary gland epithelium and capillary endothelium. Cell 25:67
10. Rodell TC, Cheronis JC, Ohnemus CL et al. (1987) Xanthine oxidase mediates elastase-induced injury to isolated lungs and endothelium. J Appl Physiol 63:2159
11. Phan SH, Gannon DE, Varani J et al. (1989) Xanthine oxidase activity in rat pulmonary artery endothelial cells and its alteration by activated neutrophils. Am J Pathol (in press)
12. Varani J, Fligiel SEG, Till GO et al. (1985) Pulmonary endothelial cell killing by human neutrophils. Possible involvement of hydroxyl radical. Lab Invest 53:656
13. Friedl HP, Till GO, Ryan US et al. (1989) Mediator-induced activation of xanthine oxidase in endothelial cells. Faseb J 3(13):2512
14. Klempner MS, Dinarello CA, Gallin JI (1978) Human leukocyte pyrogen induces release of specific granule contents from human neutrophils. J Clin Invest 61:1330
15. Klempner MS, Dinarello CA, Henderson WR et al. (1979) Stimulation of neutrophil oxygen-dependent metabolism by human leukocytic pyrogen. J Clin Invest 64:996
16. Klebanoff SJ, Vades MA, Harlan JM et al. (1986) Stimulation of neutrophils by tumor necrosis factor. J Immunol 136:4220
17. Tsujimoto M, Tokota S, Vilcek J et al. (1986) Tumor necrosis factor provokes superoxide anion generation from neutrophils. Biochem Biophys Res Commun 137:1094
18. Warren JS, Kunkel SL, Cunningham TW et al. (1988) Macrophage-derived cytokines amplify immune complex-triggered oxygen responses by rat alveolar macrophages. Am J Pathol 130:489
19. Pober JS, Bevilacqua MP, Mendrick DL et al. (1986) Two distinct monokines, interleukin 1 and tumor necrosis factor, each independently induce biosynthesis and transient expression of the same antigen on the surface of cultured human vascular endothelial cells. J Immunol 137:1893
20. Pohlman TH, Staness KA, Beatty PG et al. (1986) An endothelial cell surface factor(s) induced in vitro by lipopolysaccharide, interleukin 1, and tumor necrosis factor-alpha increases neutrophil adherence by a CDw18 dependent mechanism. J Immunol 136:4548
21. Lillehei RC, Maclean LD (1958) The intestinal factor in irreversible endotoxin shock. Ann Surg 148:513
22. Morgan HR (1942) Pathologic changes produced in rabbits by a toxic somatic antigen derived from Eberthella typhosa. Am J Pathol 19:135
23. Tracey KJ, Fong Y, Hess DG et al. (1987) Anti-cachectin/TNF monoclonal antibodies prevent septic shock during lethal bacteraemia. Nature 330:662
24. Tracey KJ, Beutler B, Lowry SF et al. (1986) Shock and tissue injury induced by recombinant human cachectin. Science 234:470
25. Remick DG, Kunkel RG, Larrick JW et al. (1987) Acute in vivo effects of human recombinant tumor necrosis factor. Lab Invest 56:583
26. Remick DG, Larrick J, Kunkel SL (1986) Tumor necrosis factor-induced alterations in circulating leukocyte populations. Biochem Biophys Res Commun 141:818

Arachidonic Acid Metabolism in Endotoxemia and Sepsis: Therapeutic Approaches*

J. A. Cook[1], E. Li[1], and P. V. Halushka[2]

Arachidonic Acid Release and Metabolism

Administration of endotoxin to animals or stimulation of inflammatory cells with endotoxin has been shown to induce formation of lipids, peptides, and oxygen metabolites which are implicated as secondary mediators for endotoxin-induced shock sequelae [1]. One major class of mediators is the arachidonic acid metabolites.

Arachidonic acid, 5,8,11,14-eicosatetraenoic acid, is a component of cell membrane phospholipids. Four types of phospholipids, phosphatidylinositol, phosphatidylcholine, phosphatidylethanolamine, and phosphatidylserine serve as sources of arachidonic acid [2]. The release of arachidonic acid from phospholipids precedes its metabolism. Four different pathways may be involved in the release: (a) phospholipase A_2 cleaves arachidonic acid from the sn-2-acyl bond of the glycerol skeleton of phophatidylcholine and phosphatidylethanolamine; (b) phospholipase C converts phosphatidylinositol to inositol 1,4,5-triphosphate and diacylglycerol, which is further metabolized by diacylglycerol lipase to release arachidonic acid; (c) diacylglycerol kinase phosphorylates diacylglycerol to produce phosphatidic acid, which is subsequently metabolized by a phospholipase A_2 to produce free arachidonic acid; and (d) phospholipase D also metabolizes phospholipid into phosphatidic acid, which is subsequently metabolized to release arachidonic acid.

The free form of arachidonic acid is metabolized by the cyclooxygenase and lipoxygenase pathways (Fig. 1). Cyclooxygenase metabolizes arachidonic acid to prostaglandins PGG_2 and PGH_2, which are rapidly metabolized to thromboxane A_2 (TXA_2), prostacyclin (PGI_2), and other prostaglandins. TXA_2 and PGI_2 are unstable and rapidly undergo spontaneous hydrolysis to TXB_2 and 6-keto-$PGF_{1\alpha}$, respectively. The lipoxygenase pathways of arachidonic acid metabolism involve three species of lipoxygenase, the 5-lipoxygenase, the 12-lipoxygenase, and the 15-lipoxygenase [3]. The 5-lipoxygenase enzyme metabolizes arachidonic acid to 5-hydroperoxy-eicosatetraenoic acid (5-HPETE). The latter is further metabolized to 5-hydroxy eicosatetraenoic acid (5-HETE)

* This work was supported in part by NIHGM 27673.
[1] Department of Physiology, [2] Departments of Pharmacology and Medicine, Medical University of South Carolina, 171 Ashley Avenue, Charleston, SC 29425, USA

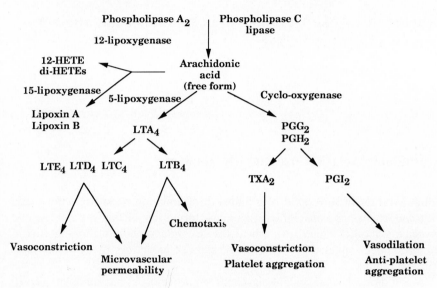

Fig. 1. Metabolic cascade of arachidonic acid and some pharmacological effects of eicosanoids

and leukotriene A_4 (LTA_4) is an unstable intermediate which is rapidly metabolized to di-HETEs, LTC_4 and LTB_4. LTC_4 is further metabolized to the sulfidopeptide leukotrienes LTD_4 and LTE_4.

The cyclooxygenase and 5-lipoxygenase products can pharmacologically mimic certain sequelae of endotoxic shock [4]. For example, TXA_2 induces vasoconstriction and platelet aggregation; PGI_2 and PGE_2 induce vasodilation, and PGI_2 induces inhibition of platelet aggregation. The leukotrienes C_4, D_4, and E_4 induce vasoconstriction and increases in microvascular permeability. LTB_4 induces chemotaxis of neutrophils, promotes degranulation of neutrophils, and increases microvascular permeability secondary to endothelial injury.

Increased Synthesis of Eicosanoids in Endotoxemia and Sepsis

Increased endogenous synthesis of eicosanoids in response to endotoxemia and sepsis can be shown in a variety of animal species and in man. In the rat with experimental endotoxemia and sepsis, increases in plasma levels of TXB_2 and 6-keto-$PGF_{1\alpha}$ have been demonstrated [4]. Similar profiles of TXB_2 and 6-keto-$PGF_{1\alpha}$ in plasma are observed in endotoxemic sheep [5, 6], pigs [7–10], horses [11, 12], and baboons [13, 14]. Increases in plasma levels of TXB_2 also parallel shock severity in patients dying of septic shock [15, 16]. Similarly, plasma levels of 6-keto-$PGF_{1\alpha}$ are increased in patients with severe sepsis [16, 17].

5-Lipoxygenase products are also increased in endotoxemic animals and patients with sepsis. In the endotoxemic rat, Hagmann et al. [18] reported increases in N-acetyl LTE_4, a stable metabolite of sulfidopeptide leukotrienes in bile. Chang et al. [19] measured increases in LTC_4 in the lung of rats with experimental endotoxemia. Increased plasma LTB_4 levels have been demonstrated in endotoxemic sheep [20]. Increased LTB_4 levels were also was measured in bronchoalveolar lavage fluid of endotoxemic pigs [21], and lung lymph in endotoxemic sheep [22]. Increases in sulfidopeptide leukotrienes and LTB_4 have been demonstrated in the bronchoalveolar lavage fluid of patients with adult respiratory distress syndrome (ARDS), complication associated with sepsis [23–25].

Effect of Eicosanoid Synthesis Inhibitors, Receptor Antagonists, and Essential Fatty Acid Deficiency

More direct evidence that eicosanoids mediate endotoxin-induced sequelae is provided by observations that inhibition of eicosanoid synthesis protects animals from endotoxic shock sequelae (Fig. 2). A reduction in eicosanoid synthesis can be induced by a dietary-induced deficiency in arachidonic acid substrate or by branch enzyme inhibitors. Essential fatty acid deficient (EFAD) rats produce decreased quantities of arachidonic acid metabolities and are resistant to endotoxin-induced mortality [26]. These rats are also more resistant to endotoxin-induced microvascular permeability changes [27]. Supplementation of arachidonic acid to EFAD rats reverses the resistance to endotoxin, indicating the importance of arachidonic acid in endotoxin-induced shock sequelae [28]. Pharmacological inhibition of eicosanoid synthesis or blockade of eicosanoid receptors have been used to elucidate their potential roles in shock sequelae (Fig. 2).

   Numerous nonsteroidal anti-inflammatory agents (NSAID) including indomethacin, acetylsalicyclic acid, flurbiprofen, and ibuprofen have been evaluated for potential therapeutic value in endotoxemia and sepsis in animal models [4]. These compounds when used in experimental sepsis or endotoxemia have generally been found to improve survival and/or survival time and reduce cardiopulmonary dysfunction and indices of tissue injury [4]. Among the most extensively studied of the NSAID is ibuprofen. In a variety of species with endotoxemia and sepsis, ibuprofen has been shown to improve systemic hypotension, pulmonary hypertension, protein and fluid extravasation, lung water flux, airway resistance, and oxygen delivery (Table 1). However, in some studies ibuprofen did not improve shock sequelae (Table 2). Ibuprofen also alters neutrophil (PMN) function including inhibition of PMN aggregation responses, organ influx, and adherence [29–32]. Some of these drug effects are dose-dependent. For example, low doses (3 mg/kg) of ibuprofen enhance endotoxin-induced alveolitis in rats, 10–20 mg/kg has no effect, and 30 mg/kg inhibits the alveolitis [33]. Certain beneficial effects therefore could be a result of pharmacological actions of ibuprofen other than inhibiting fatty acid cyclooxygenase.

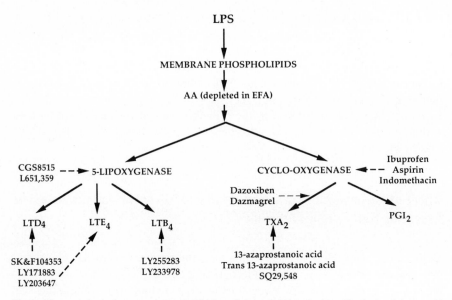

Fig. 2. Pharmacological approaches to inhibition of eicosanoid synthesis or blockade of eicosanoid receptors. Inhibition of synthesis or blockade of receptors are designated by the *dashed line*. The compounds listed at each step have been previously used to elucidate the potential involvement of arachidonic acid (*AA*) metabolites in septic and endotoxic shock

These include potential inhibition of LTB_4 production [34], superoxide anion production [32, 35], hydroxyl radicals [36], and burn-induced inhibition of fibrinolysis [37].

Pretreatment with TXA_2 synthase inhibitors or TXA_2 receptor antagonists improve survival time or attenuate certain shock sequelae in endotoxemic animals. The pathophysiological events ameliorated by these pharmacological agents include pulmonary hypertension [38, 39], reduction in cardiac output, hypotension [40, 41], decreased renal blood flow, decreased glomerular filtration rate [39, 41, 42], thrombocytopenia [38, 41–43], renal glomerular fibrin deposition [44], and renal glomerular microthrombi [41]. Most studies have shown that the beneficial effect of these drugs were not obtained if they were given after endotoxin. Other studies have failed to demonstrate improved outcome in sepsis and endotoxic shock [14, 45–48]. Presumably, in these experiments, mediators other than TXA_2 dominate to produce pathophysiological sequelae contributing to the development of shock and mortality.

TXA_2 receptor antagonists, unlike TXA_2 synthase inhibitors, do not alter plasma TXB_2 concentrations in response to endotoxin. Use of TXA_2 receptor antagonists in endotoxemia may have several advantages over use of TXA_2 synthase inhibitors. TXA_2 receptor antagonists block the effects of both PGH_2 and TXA_2 in activating TXA_2 receptors, do not produce shunting to PGI_2 production, and block the effects of TXA_2 already formed [38].

Table 1. Protective effects of ibuprofen in a variety of species in response to endotoxin and sepsis

Irritant	Species	Site	Inflammatory response prevented	Reference
Endotoxin	Rat	Systemic	Endotoxic shock	66
Endotoxin	Rat	Lung	Alveolitis (30 mg/kg)	33
Endotoxin/epinephrine	Rabbit	Ear lobe	Superoxide anion injury	67
Endotoxin	Dog	Aorta	PMN adherence	30
Endotoxin (Escherichia coli) i.v.	Dog	Lymph	Protein influx	68
Tumor necrosis factor	Dog	Systemic	Fever, hypotension	69
Endotoxin	Dog	Systemic	Hypodynamic	70
Endotoxin	Dog	Systemic	Hypotension	30
Endotoxin	Sheep, awake	Lung	Lung inflammation	71
Endotoxin	Sheep, awake	Heart, lung	Peroxidation (biphasic)	72
Endotoxin (Escherichia coli) i.v.	Sheep, awake	Heart, lung	Hyperdynamic, pulmonary hypertension	71
Endotoxin	Sheep	Heart	Contractility	73
Endotoxin (Escherichia coli)	Sheep, awake	Lung	Lipid peroxidation	74
Endotoxin	Sheep, awake	Lung	Airway, vascular resistance	75
Cecal ligation, perforation	Sheep	Lung	Lung water flux	76
Endotoxin	Pig	Organs	Decreases in organ blood flow	10
Endotoxin	Pig	Systemic	Hypotension	10
Endotoxin (Escherichia coli)	Pig	Mesenteric	Decreases in oxygen delivery	8
Endotoxin (Escherichia coli)	Pig	Systemic	Decreases in oxygen delivery	8
Pseudomonas aeruginosa	Pig	Lung	PMN emigration	31
Pseudomonas aeruginosa	Pig	Lung	Protein and fluid extravasation	77
Pseudomonas aeruginosa	Pig	Lung, BALF	Protein leakage	31

BALF, bronchoalveolar lavage fluid.

Table 2. Lack of a beneficial effect of ibuprofen on inflammatory responses to endotoxemia or sepsis in several animal models

Irritant	Species	Site	Unaffected responses	Reference
Endotoxin	Mice	Adrenalectomy	No effect on Mortality	78
Endotoxin	Rat	Lung	Alveolitis, no effect (10–20 mg/kg)	33
Endotoxin	Rat	Lung	Alveolitis, augmented (3 mg/kg)	33
Endotoxin	Rat	Heat	Decreases in contractility	79
B streptococcal shock	Rabbit	Systemic	Hemodynamic and hematology changes	80
Endotoxin	Dog	Blood	Hypoglycemia, hyperlactate, and glycerol fibrinolysis	81
Endotoxin	Dog	Lung	Pulmonary PMN stasis	30
Endotoxin	Sheep, awake	Lung	Permeability	72
P. aeruginosa	Pig	Alveolar macrophage	Down regulation of oxidant production	31
Pseudomonas ARDS	Pig	Lung	Albumin and fluid leak	82

The nonspecific 5-lipoxygenase inhibitor diethylcarbamazine improved survival of mice to endotoxic shock [18]. Using the 5-lipoxygenase inhibitor CGS8515, Matera et al. [49] demonstrated attenuation of endotoxin-induced hemoconcentration and hypotension in rats. Attenuation of endotoxin-induced neutropenia and concomitant oxygen radical synthesis by a 5-lipoxygenase inhibitor, AA-861, in the rat was also shown by Suematsu et al. [50]. In sheep, Coggeshall et al. [22] showed that a 5-lipoxygenase inhibitor, L-651, 392, blocked endotoxin-induced pulmonary hypertension, bronchoconstriction, and increased arterioalveolar oxygen difference and lung microvascular permeability.

Further evidence for the role of lipoxygenase products in endotoxin-induced shock sequelae is provided by studies using specific leukotriene receptor antagonists in experimental endotoxemia. Ahmed et al. [51] and Pacitti et al. [52] showed that the leukotriene receptor antagonist FPL 57231 attenuated endotoxin-induced bronchoconstriction and pulmonary hypertension in sheep and cats. In the rat, Smith et al. [53] showed that the LTD_4 receptor antagonist SKF104353 prevented endotoxin-induced hemoconcentration and thrombocytopenia and improved survival time. Cook et al. [54] also demonstrated a protective effect of LTD_4/E_4 receptor antagonist LY171883 on endotoxin-induced hypotension, hemoconcentration, and leukopenia in the rat. Both compounds were shown to prevent acute splanchnic permeability changes in the rat induced by endotoxin [55] and mesenteric ischemia in the pig [8]. More recently, the LTB_4 receptor antagonist LY255283 has been shown to attenuate endotoxin-induced leukopenia, hemoconcentration, and hypotension in the rat [56]. Another LTB_4 receptor antagonist LY255283, however, only transiently attenuated endotoxin-induced hypotension and hemoconcentration.

Therapeutic Approaches in Patients

The NSAID may have beneficial effects in the treatment of trauma or sepsis patients. Faist et al. [57] studied the effect of indomethacin in a randomized prospective study in 43 patients undergoing major surgical trauma. The cellular immune status was evaluated preoperatively and up to a week after surgery. In contrast to untreated patients, patients receiving indomethacin exhibited improved delayed-type hypersensitivity responses, mitogen-induced lymphocyte transformation, and a lower rate of opportunistic infections. The results suggest that NSAIDS, by preventing impairment of cell mediated immunity, may reduce susceptibility to postoperative surgery.

Short-course ibuprofen therapy in 30 patients with severe sepsis has been investigated in a randomized two-center study [58]. Ibuprofen (800 mg) or placebo (saline) was given as a rectal solution at the time of entry into the study and twice more at 4 h intervals. Vital signs and number of patients in shock at the time of entry into the study were similar. Seven of the eight patients in shock given ibuprofen reversed shock during the first 48 h compared to three out of eight in the placebo group. Because of the small number of patients, this was not of statistical significance ($p < 0.12$), but certain physiological measurements were significant (Table 3). Urinary levels of 2,3-dinor TXB_2 and 2,3-dinor 6-keto-$PGF_{1\alpha}$ were significantly reduced, along with febrile response, heart rate, and peak airway pressure responses. Importantly, there were no overt signs of renal toxicity. Similar beneficial actions of ibuprofen have been reported in human volunteers injected with endotoxin [59]. Ibuprofen pretreatment in these

Table 3. Effect of ibuprofen in the human sepsis syndrome

Physiological responses measured	Physiological responses improved by ibuprofen
Body temperature	$p < 0.02$
Mean arterial pressure	N.S.
Heart rate	$p < 0.01$
Systemic vascular resistance (6 placebo vs 9 ibuprofen)	N.S.
Minute ventilation	N.S.
Peak airway pressure	$p < 0.01$
PaO_2/PAO_2	N.S.
Serum creatinine	N.S.
Creatinine clearance	N.S.
Urinary 2,3-dinor TXB_2	$p < 0.05$
Urinary 2,3-dinor 6-keto-$PGF_{1\alpha}$	$p < 0.03$

Ibuprofen (800 mg) was given in sterile saline 20 ml rectally at time of entry into study and every four hour for a total of three doses (ibuprofen, $n = 16$; placebo, $n = 14$). Physiological responses were measured at 0, 4, 8, 12, 16, 24, 48 and 120 h upon entry into the study. Cardiac output was 12 ± 2 l/min in the ibuprofen group versus 18 ± 2 l/min in the placebo group at time of entry ($p < 0.05$). Other parameters were not significantly different at entry.

individuals reduced endotoxin-induced mylagia, trachycardia, fever, and plasma stress hormone responses [59].

These studies provide the impetus for more extensive studies of NSAID in trauma, sepsis, and ARDS. Combination therapy approaches with NSAID may also prove to be promising. Experimentally, combinations of drugs with NSAID have been more effective than single-drug treatments [60–65]. Of particular interest, in view of the demonstrated increases of lipoxygenase products in ARDS patients, will be the potential application of lipoxygenase inhibitors or LT receptor antagonists. Clinical studies with the latter compounds, however, must await the development of safe and selective compounds before such therapeutic approaches can be attempted.

References

1. Danner RL, Suffredini AF, Natanson C, Parilo JE (1989) Microbal toxins: role in the pathogenesis of septic shock and multiple organ failure. In: Bihari DJ, Cerra FB (eds) Multiple organ failure. Society of Critical Care Medicine, Fullerton, pp 151–192 (New Horizons, vol 3)
2. Lefkowith JB, Sprecher H, Needleman P (1986) The role and manipulation of eicosanoids in essential fatty acid deficiency. Prog Lipid Res 25:111–117
3. Handerson WR Jr (1989) Products of 12- and 15-lipoxygenase. In: Henson PM, Murphy RC (eds) Mediators of the inflammatory process. Elsevier, New York, pp 45–75
4. Cook JA, Halushka PV (1989) Arachidonic Acid Metabolism in Septic Shock. In:Bihari DJ, Cerra FB (eds) Multiple organ failure. Society of Critical Care Medicine, Fullerton, pp 101–124 (New Horizons, vol 3)
5. Morel DR, Huttemeier PC, Skoskiewicz MJ, Nguyenduy T, Melvin C, Robinson DR, Zapol WM (1987) Dose-dependent effects of a pyridoquinazoline thromboxane synthetase inhibitor on arachidonic acid metabolites and hemodynamics during E. coli endotoxemia in anesthetized sheep. Prostaglandins 33:879
6. Demling RH, Smith M, Gunther R, Flynn JT, Gee MH (1981) Pulmonary injury and prostaglandin production during endotoxemia in conscious sheep Am J Physiol 240:H348
7. Hardie EM, Olsen NC (1987) Prostaglandin and thromboxane levels during endotoxin-induced respiratory failure in pigs. Prostaglandins Leukotrienes Med 28:255
8. Fink MP, Rothschild HR, Deniz YF, Wang H, Lee PC, Cohn SM (1989) Systemic and mesenteric O_2 metabolism in endotoxic pigs: effect of ibuprofen and meclofenamate. J Appl Physiol 67:1950
9. Schrauwen E, Vandeplassche G, Laekman G, Houvenaghel A (1983) Endotoxin shock in the pig: release of prostaglandins and beneficial effects of flurbiprofen. Arch Int Pharmacodyn Ther 262:332
10. Nishijima MK, Breslow MJ, Miller CF and Traystam RJ (1988) Effect of naloxone and ibuprofen on organ blood flow during endotoxic shock in pig. Am J Physiol 225:H177
11. Bottoms GD, Templeton CB, Fessler JF, Johnson MA, Roesel OF, Ewert KM, Adams SB (1982) Thromboxane, prostacyclin and the hemodynamic changes in equine endotoxin shock. Am J Vet Res 43:999
12. Semrad SD, Moore JN (1987) Effects of multiple low doses of flunixin meglumine on reported endotoxin challenge in the horse. Prostaglandins Leukotrienes Med 27:169
13. Harris RH, Zmudka M, Maddox Y, Ramwell PW, Fletcher JR (1980) Relationships of TXB_2 and 6-keto-PGF1a to the hemodynamic changes during baboon endotoxic shock. In: Samuelsson B, Ramwell RW, Paoletti R (eds) Advances in prostaglandin and thromboxane research, vol 7. Raven, New York, pp 843
14. Casey LC, Fletcher JR, Zmudka MI, Ramwell PW (1987) Prevention of endotoxin-induced pulmonary hypertension in primates by the use of a selective thromboxane synthetase inhibitor, OKY 1581. J Pharmacol Exp Ther 222:441

15. Reines HD, Halushka PV, Cook JA, Wise WC, Rambo W (1982) Plasma thromboxane concentrations are raised in patients dying with septic shock. Lancet 24:174
16. Oettinger W, Berger D, Berger HG (1987) The clinical significance of prostaglandins and thromboxane as mediators of septic shock. Klin. Wochenschr 65:61
17. Halushka PV, Reines HD, Barrow SE, Blair IA, Dollery CT, Rambo W, Cook JA, Wise WC (1985) Elevated plasma 6-keto-prostaglandin F1a in patients in septic shock. Crit Care Med 13:451
18. Hagman W, Denzlinger C, Keppler D (1985) Production of peptide leukotrienes in endotoxin shock. FEBS Lett 180:309–313
19. Chang S-W, Westcott JY, Pickett WC, Murphy RC, Voelkel NF (1989) Endotoxin-induced lung injury in rats: role of eicosanoids. J Appl Physiol 66:2407–2418
20. Fujimoto K, Kobayashi T (1989) The role of leukotriene B_4 in endotoxin-induced lung injury in unanesthetized sheep. Respir Physiol 71:259–268
21. Olson NC, Dobrowsky RT, Fleisher LN (1988) Dexamethasone blocks increased leukotriene B_4 production during endotoxin-induced lung injury. J Appl Physiol 74:2100–2107
22. JW, Christman BW, Lefferts PL, Serafin WE, Blair IA, Butterfield MJ, Snapper JR (1988) Effect of inhibition of 5-lipoxygenase metabolism of arachidonic acid on response to endotoxemia in sheep. J Appl Physiol 65:1351–1359
23. Matthay MA, Eschenbacher WL, Goetzl EJ (1984) Elevated concentrations of leukotriene D_4 in pulmonary edema fluid of patients with adult respiratory distress syndrome. J Clin Immunol 4:479–483
24. Stephenson AH, Lonifro AJ, Hyers TM, Webster RO, Fowler AA (1988) Increased concentrations of leukotrienes in bronchoalveolar lavage fluid of patients with ARDS or at risk for ARDS. Am Rev Respir Dis 138:714–719
25. Antonelli A, Bufi M, De Blasi RA, Crimi G, Conti G, Mattia C, Vivino G, Lenti L, Lombardi D, Dotta A, Pontiere G, Gasparetto A (1989) Detection of leukotriene B_4, C_4 and of their isomers in arterial, mixed venous blood and bronchoalveolar lavage fluid from ARDS patients. Intensive Care Med 15:296–301
26. Cook JA, Wise WC, Callihan CS (1979) Resistance of essential fatty acid deficient rats to endotoxin shock. Circ Shock 6:333–342
27. Li EJ, Cook JA, Spicer KM, Tempel GE, Wise WC, Halushka PV (1990) Resistance of essential fatty acid-deficient rats to endotoxin-induced increases in vascular permeability. Circ Shock 28:249–255
28. Cook JA, Wise WC, Halushka PV (1981) Sensitization of essential fatty acid deficient rats to endotoxin by arachidonate pretreatment: role of thromboxane A_2. Circ Shock 8:69–76
29. Nielson VG, Webster RO (1987) Inhibition of human polymorphonuclear leukocyte functions by ibuprofen. Immunopharmacology 13:61–71
30. Balk RA, Jacobs RF, Tryka AF, Townsend JW, Walls RC, Bone RC (1988) Effects of ibuprofen on neutrophil function and acute lung injury in canine endotoxin shock. Crit Care Med 16: 1127–1131.
31. Jenkins JK, Carey PD, Byrne K, Sugerman HJ, Fowler AA III (1991) Sepsis-induced lung injury and the effects of ibuprofen pretreatment. Am Rev Respir Dis 143:155–161
32. Flynn PJ, Becker AK, Vercellotti GM, Weisdorf DJ, Craddock PR, Hammerchmidt DE, Lillehei RC, Jacob HS (1984) Ibuprofen inhibits granulocyte responses to inflammatory mediators, a proposed mechanism for reduction of experimental myocardial infarct size. Inflammation 8:33–44
33. Rinaldo JE, Pennock B (1986) Effects of ibuprofen on endotoxin-induced alveolitis: biphasic dose response and dissociation between inflammation and hypoxia. Am J Med Sci 29:29–38
34. Konstan MW, Vargo KM, Davis PB (1990) Ibuprofen attenuates the inflammatory response to Pseudomonas aeruginosa in a rat model of chronic pulmonary infection. Implications for anti-inflammatory therapy in cystic fibrosis. Am Rev Respir Dis 141:186–192
35. Schmeling DJ, Drongowski R, Coran AG (1989) The beneficial effects of ibuprofen on a lethal live E. coli septic model and the relationship of these effects to superoxide radical production. Prog Clin Biol Res 299:53–61
36. Hamburger SA, McCay PB (1990) Spin trapping of ibuprofen radicals—evidence that ibuprofen is a hydroxyl radical scavenger. Free Radic Res Commun 9:337–342
37. Rockwell WB, Ehrlich HP (1990) Ibuprofen in acute-care therapy. Ann Surg 211:78–83
38. Taneyama C, Sasao J, Senna S, Kimura M, Kiyono S, Goto H, Arakawa K (1989) Protective effects of ONO 3708, a new thromboxane A_2 receptor antagonist, during experimental endotoxin shock. Circ Shock 28:69

39. Cirino M, Morton H, MacDonald C, Hadden J, Ford-Hutchinson AW (1990) Thromboxane A_2 and prostaglandin endoperoxide analogue effects on porcine renal blood flow. Am J Physiol 258:F109

40. Svartholm E, Bergqvist D, Hedner U, Ljungberg J, Haglund U (1989) Thromboxane A_2-receptor blockade and prostacyclin in porcine *Escherichia coli* shock. Arch Surg 142:669

41. Fukumoto S, Tanaka K (1983) Protective effects of thromboxane A_2 synthetase inhibitors on endotoxin shock. Prostaglandins Leukotrines Med 11:179

42. Badr KF, Kelley VE, Rennke HG, Brenner BM (1986) Roles for thromboxane A_2 and leukotrienes in endotoxin-induced acute renal failure. Kidney Int 30:474

43. Olanoff LS, Cook JA, Eller T, Knapp DR, Halushka PV (1985) Protective effects of trans-13-APT, a thromboxane receptor antagonist, in endotoxemia. J. Cardiovasc Pharmacol 7:114

44. Westwick J, Fletcher MS, Kakkar VV (1983) Inhibition of thromboxane formation prevents endotoxin-induced renal fibrin deposition in jaundiced rats. Adv Prostaglandin Thromboxane Leukotriene Res 12:83

45. Butler RR, Wise WC, Halushka PV, Cook JA (1982) Thromboxane and prostacyclin production during septic shock. Adv Shock Res 7:133

46. Fletcher JR, Short BL, Casey LC Walker RI, Gardiner M, Ramwell PW (1983) Thromboxane inhibition in gram-negative sepsis fails to improve survival. Adv Prostaglandin Thromboxane Leukotriene Res 12:117

47. Furman BL, McKechnie K, Parratt JR (1984) Failure of drugs that selectively inhibit thromboxane synthesis to modify to endotoxin shock in conscious rats. Br J Pharmacol 82:289

48. Short BL, Miller MK, Stround CY, Fletcher JR (1983) Comparison of thromboxane inhibitors to cyclo-oxygenase inhibitors on survival in a newborn rat model for group B streptococcal sepsis. Adv Prostaglandin Thromboxane Leukotriene Res 12:113

49. Matera G, Cook JA, Hennigar RA, Tempel GE, Wise WC, Oglesby TD, Halushka PV (1988) Beneficial effects of a 5-lipoxygenase inhibitor in endotoxic shock. J Pharmacol Exp Ther 247:363–371

50. Suematsu M, Miura S, Suzuki M, Nagata H, Morishita T, Oshio C, Tsuchiya M (1988) 5-lipoxygenase inhibitor (AA-861) attenuates neutrophil-mediated oxidative stress on the venular endothelium in endotoxemia. J Clin Lab Immunol 25:41–45

51. Ahmed T, Wasserman MA, Muccitell R, Tucker S, Gazeroglu H, Marchette B (1986) Endotoxin-induced changes in pulmonary hemodynamic and respiratory mechanics. Role of lipoxygenase and cyclo-oxygenase products. Am Rev Respir Dis 134: 1149–1159

52. Pacitti N, Bryson SE, McKechnie K, Rodger IW, Parratt JR Jr (1987) Leukotriene antagonist FPL 57231 prevents the acute pulmonary effects of *Escherichia coli* endotoxin in cats. Circ Shock 21:155–168

53. Smith EF III, Kinter LB, Jagus M, Wasserman MA, Eckardt RD, Newton JF (1988) Beneficial effects of the peptidoleukotriene receptor antagonist SK&F 104353, on the responses to experimental endotoxemia in the conscious rat. Circ Shock 25:21–31

54. Cook JA, Wise WC, Halushka PV (1985) Protective effect of a leukotriene antagonist in endotoxic shock. J Pharmacol Exp Ther 235:470–474

55. Cook JA, Li EJ, Spicer KM, Wise WC, Halushka PV (1990) Effect of leukotriene receptor antagonists on vascular permeability during endotoxic shock. Circ Shock 32:209–218

56. Li EJ, Cook JA, Wise WC, Jackson WT, Halushka PV (1991) Effect of LTB_4 receptor antagonists in endotoxic shock in the rat. Circ Shock (in press)

57. Faist E, Ertel W, Cohnert T, Huber P, Inthorn D, Heberer G (1990) Immunoprotective effects of cyclo-oxygenase inhibition in patients with major surgical trauma. J Trauma 30:8–18

58. Bernard G, Reines HD, Metz CA, Halushka PV, Swindell SB, Higgins SB, Wright PE, Watts CA (1991) Effects of a short course of ibuprofen in patients with severe sepsis. Am Rev Respir Dis 144:1095–1101

59. Rivhaug A, Michie HR, Manson JM, Walters JM, Dinarello CA, Wolf S, Wilmore DW (1988) Inhibition of cyclo-oxygenase attenuates the metabolic response to endotoxin in humans. Arch Surg 123:162

60. Ogletree ML, Begley CJ, King GA, Brigham KL (1986) Influence of steroidal and nonsteroidal anti-inflammatory agents on the accumulation of arachidonic acid metabolites in plasma and lung lymph after endotoxemia in awake sheep. Measurements of prostacyclin and thromboxane metabolites and 12-HETE. Am Rev Respir Dis 133:55

61. Olson NC, Brown TT Jr, Anderson DL (1985) Dexamethasone and indomethacin modify endotoxin-induced respiratory failure in pigs J Appl Physiol 58:274

62. Sielaff TD, Harvey BS, Sugerman HJ, Tatum JL, Kellum JM, Blocher CR (1987) Treatment of porcine Pseudomonas ARDS with combination drug therapy. J Trauma 27:1313
63. Wise WC, Halushka PV, Knapp DR, Cook JA (1985) Ibuprofen methyprednisolone and gentamicin as conjoint therapy in septic shock. Circ Shock 17:59
64. Goto M, Zeller WP, Hurley RM (1990) Dexamethasone and indomethacin treatment during endotoxicosis in the suckling rat. Circ Shock 32:113
65. Butler RR, Wise WC, Halushka PV, Cook JA (1983) Gentamicin and indomethacin in the treatment of septic shock, effects on prostacyclin and thromboxane A_2 production. J Pharmacol Exp Ther 225:94–101
66. Wise WC, Cook JA, Halushka PV (1980) Ibuprofen improves survival from endotoxic shock in the rat. J Pharmacol Exp Ther 215:160–164
67. Ward PH, Maldonado M, Moreno M, Funther B, Vivaldi E (1990) Oxygen-derived free radicals mediate the cutaneous necrotizing vasculitis induced by epinephrine in endotoxin-primed rabbits. J Infect Dis 161:1020–1022
68. Hubbard JD, Janssen HF (1988) Increased microvascular permeability in canine endotoxic shock: protective effects of ibuprofen. Circ Shock 26:169–183
69. Evans A, Jacobs DO, Revhaug A, Wilmore DW (1989) Effects of tumor necrosis factor and their selective inhibition by ibuprofen. Ann Surg 209:312–321
70. Beck RR, Abel FL (1987) Effect of ibuprofen on the course of canine endotoxin shock. Circ Shock 23:59–70
71. Demling RH, Lalonde C, Goad MEP (1989) Effect of ibuprofen on the pulmonary and systemic response to repeated doses of endotoxin. Surgery 105:421–429
72. Demling RH, Lalonde C, Seekamp A, Fiore N (1988) Endotoxin causes hydrogen peroxide-induced lung lipid peroxidation and prostanoid production. Arch Surg 123:1337–1341
73. Huttemeier PC, Eliasen K, Ringsted C, Mongensen T, Jensen H, Nielsen SL (1989) Right and left ventricular performance during endotoxin-induced pulmonary hypertension in sheep. Clin Physiol 9:57–65.
74. Demling RH, Lalonde CC, Jin LJ, Ryan P, Fox R (1986) Endotoxemia causes increased lung tissue lipid peroxidation in unanesthetized sheep. J Appl Physiol 60:2094–2100.
75. Wright PE, Bernard GR (1989) Mechanisms of late hemodynamic and airway dynamic responses to endotoxin in awake sheep. Am Rev Respir Dis 140:672–678
76. Gnidec AG, Sibbard WJ, Cheung H, Metz CA (1988) Ibuprofen reduces the progression of permeability edema in an animal model of hyperdynamic sepsis. J Appl Physiol 65:1024–1032
77. Carey PD, Byrne K, Jenkins JK, Sielaff TD, Walsh CJ, Fowler AA Jr, Sugerman HJ (1990) Ibuprofen attenuates hypochlorous acid production from neutrophils in porcine acute lung injury. J Surg Res 49:262–270
78. Bertini R, Bianchi M, Ghezzi P (1988) Adrenalectomy sensitizes mice to the lethal effects of interleukin 1 and tumor necrosis factor. J Exp Med 167:1708–1712
79. Baum TD, Heard SO, Feldman HS, Latka CA, Fink MP (1990) Endotoxininduced myocardial depression in rats: effect of ibuprofen and SDZ 64-688, a platelet activating factor receptor antagonist. J Surg Res 48:629–634
80. Peevy KJ, Ronnlund RD, Chartrand SA, Boerth RC, Longenecker GL (1988) Ibuprofen in experimental group B streptococcal shock. Circ Shock 24:35–41
81. Jesmok GJ, Aono F, Simpson J, Borgia J (1987) Effect of ibuprofen on components of an actue systemic inflammatory response evoked by intravenous endotoxin administration in the conscious sheep. Prog Clin Biol Res 236A:333–346
82. Harvey CF, Sugerman HJ, Tatum JL, Sielaff TD, Lee EC, Blocher CR (1987) Ibuprofen and methylprednisolone in a pig Pseudomonas ARDS model. Circ Shock 231:175–178

Section 4

**Immune Mechanisms for the Control
of Infection Under Physiologic
and Stressful Conditions**

Biology and Function of Cytotoxic T-Cells

R. C. Bleackley

Introduction

Cytotoxic T lymphocytes (CTL) are major effectors in cell-mediated immune reactions. Once activated they search out and bind to cells that express inappropriate of "foreign" structures on their surfaces and, by a mechanism that remains unclear, program them to die. The CTL then move away to search for a new target, leaving the cell that has received the "Kiss of death" to literally explode. These cells are responsible for the rejection of transplanted organs and tissues, the eradication of virally infected cells, and probably the lysis of a variety of tumors. In addition, CTL may be involved in the destruction of normal cells and tissue in autoimmune disorders. Thus an understanding of the molecular basis of T-cell-mediated cytotoxicity is essential for the development of rational forms of immunotherapy.

Remarkable progress has been made in this area of research over the last few years [1]. This is due in large part to the availability of large quantities of interleukin-2. With this lymphokine, which is essential for the activation and growth of T lymphocytes, it has been possible to derive cloned functional cytotoxic T cell clones for biochemical and molecular genetic characterization.

The Search for Cytolytic Effector Molecules

Two approaches have been used to identify molecules involved in the cytolytic machinery. The first relied on the knowledge that, after maturation in the thymus, potential cytotoxic cells emerge in an inactive or precursor form (referred to as pCTL). Activation of pCTL occurs after interaction with cells that express "foreign" molecules and with regulatory cells that supply activation factors including interleukin-2. The activated CTL or T killer cells now possess the molecular machinery that enables them to bind to and destroy target cells. A search for molecules expressed specifically in activated CTL and not in a variety

Department of Biochemistry, University of Alberta, Edmonton, Alberta, Canada T6G 2H7

Host Defense Dysfunction
in Trauma, Shock and Sepsis
Eds. Faist/Meakins/Schildberg
© Springer-Verlag, Berlin Heidelberg 1993

of other cell types, including pCTL, was initiated using subtractive and differential screening of CTL cDNA libraries as it was believed that this group would include cytotoxicity-related molecules [2, 3, 4].

The second approach was prompted by the seminal experiments of Dourmaskin [5] who demonstrated ring-like lesions in the membranes of target cells that were being attacked by CTL. This observation suggested a similarity between CTL-mediated killing and complement-induced lysis (the lysis pathway of humoral immunity) and resulted in a search for the pore-forming proteins of CTL.

The Granule Exocytosis Model of Cytolysis

These experimental strategies recently converged when it was discovered that the molecules being characterized by both approaches were sequestered within cytoplasmic granules of CTL. Subsequently other molecules were purified from these intracellular packages (Table 1). The same organelles have previously been implicated in the killing mechanism following the observation that after target cell recognition the granules polarize to the contact surface between the two cells [13, 14]. It is believed that they contain the cytolytic effector molecules. Because of this packaging the CTL is protected from its own toxins that act on the target cell only after release from the granules by vectoral exocytosis (Fig. 1). A pore is formed within the target cell membrane through which other macromolecules can pass. Once inside the offending cell the CTL-derived molecules act on their substrates, thus setting off a chain of events that ultimately causes death of the target and fragmentation of its chromosomal contents.

Perforin and Proteases

The molecule responsible for pore-forming activity has been purified by a number of groups and named variously cytolysin, perforin, pore-forming protein, and C9-related protein [6, 7, 15]. It is a protein of molecular weight 66 K–75 K that polymerizes in the presence of calcium to yield a structure

Table 1. Molecules found in CTL/NK Granules

	Function
Perforin (Cytolysin)	Calcium-dependent pore-forming (like C9) [6, 7]
Proteases (granzymes)	Function unknown [3, 4, 8, 9]
Proteoglycans	Carrier molecule [10]
Leukolexin	TNF-like [11]
Arylsulphatase, Glucorinidase, Hexosaminidase	Lysosomal enzymes [12]

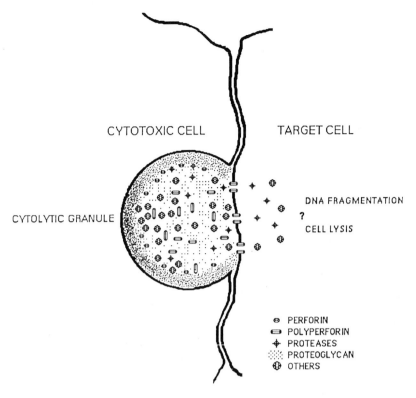

CYTOTOXIC CELL   TARGET CELL

CYTOLYTIC GRANULE

DNA FRAGMENTATION

?

CELL LYSIS

⊖ PERFORIN
⊟ POLYPERFORIN
✦ PROTEASES
∷ PROTEOGLYCAN
⊕ OTHERS

Fig. 1. The granule-exocytosis model of cell-mediated cytotoxicity. Upon binding of an activated cytotoxic T cell to its specific target the cytoplasmic granules polarize toward the contact surface between the two cells. As the granules fuse with the cytoplasmic membrane of the CTL their contents are exocytosed in high concentration close to the target cell. Released from the inhibitory environment of the granule, perforin polymerizes and inserts into the target cell membrane. This structure can act as a channel through which other granule-associated molecules can pass. The target cell DNA is fragmented and ultimately the whole cell explodes

capable of inserting into membranes and creating a channel through which other macromolecules can pass. When perforin was originally described it was believed to be the cytolytic effector. Indeed, in high concentrations purified perforin can cause lysis of cells. However, it is now clear that perforin-induced lysis occurs without DNA fragmentation in the target cell [16]. The relationship between DNA fragmentation and cell lysis is unclear but the degradation of target cell chromosomal DNA remains an important marker of the physiologically relevant event. Clearly perforin is a key member of the cytolytic machinery but is not the sole effector responsible for lysis.

The search for CTL-specific molecules led to the discovery of a novel family of serine proteases [3, 8, 17] that again suggested a degree of similarity with complement-mediated lysis. The role of the proteases in the killing mechanism remains unclear; however, their expression clearly correlates with the acquisition of cytotoxicity in killer cells [2, 4]. In addition, they have been shown, by both immunocytochemical techniques and protein purification methods, to be present within the cytotoxicity-related granules described earlier [9, 18].

Expression Correlates with Lytic Activity

In an in vivo model of transplant rejection in the mouse it has been demonstrated, by in situ hybridization, that there is a direct correlation between expression of these proteases and the progress of rejection [19]. This has led to an investigation of the value of using their expression as a marker of the rejection process in human organ transplant recipients. The preliminary evidence is that expression is clearly indicative of the early stages of rejection. It is hoped that they will also provide important clues concerning the molecule pathogenesis of autoimmune disorders and the basis of suppressed cell-mediated immune responses following trauma. There is already an early indication that the decline in cell-mediated immunity seen in the elderly correlates with a lower expression of the proteases.

It is tempting to speculate that correcting immune dysfunction could be achieved by specifically altering the levels of expression of the family of granule-associated genes. Thus increasing expression would be potentially useful in the treatment of viral infections or oncogenesis, and decreasing transcription could be therapeutic in autoimmune diseases or management of transplant recipients. Unfortunately the initial idea that all members would be controlled by the same regulatory system does not seem to be true. Indeed, in the case of the proteases, where work in this area has progressed somewhat further, each gene seems to be differentially regulated. Thus increasing cytotoxicity may be problematic, but decreasing it may be more realistic. Recently the specific expression of perforin mRNA using an antisense approach resulted in a significant decrease in cytotoxicity in vitro [20].

A Protease Substrate: Clinical Potential

The analysis of complex physiological responses at this level provides us with knowledge about the primary sequence of the molecules involved. Such detailed information can suggest novel therapeutic strategies involving rational drug design. In the case of one of the CTL-specific proteases (called cytotoxic cell protease 1 or CCP1), the primary amino acid sequence has been modeled using computer-assisted graphics to yield a predicted three-dimensional structure [21]. Careful analysis of the residues that line the binding pocket allow predictions to be made concerning the substrate specificity of the enzyme.

Serine proteases achieve their biological effect by cleaving a peptide bond at a specific amino acid sequence. For CCP1 it is believed that the peptide bond to be cleaved will be at an aspartic acid residue in the protein. This would make the substrate specificity of CCP1 unique among eukaryotic serine proteases. Most importantly for any potential clinical use, this fact suggests the possibility that CCP1 could be *specifically* inhibited while sparing other important related enzymes (e.g., blood clotting proteases). The first part of this prediction has now been validated and the specificity for aspartic acid in the substrate has been confirmed. The next challenge is to see if a selective inhibitor can be designed that would, if the proteases do play a key role in T-cell-mentioned cytotoxicity, lead to the development of a new class of immunosuppressive agents.

Other Molecules and Models

This brief review has focused on two classes of molecule that are believed to be involved in the granule-mediated killing mechanism of CTL. However, it should be noted that other granule-associated molecules have been described. Proteoglycans [10] are present that are believed to play an ancillary role in killing, possibly as binding sites and/or regulatory molecules for perforin and the proteases. Lymphotoxin is certainly involved in killing by some lymphocytes, and a recently described lymphotoxin-related molecule awaits further characterization [11]. Finally, granule-mediated cytotoxicity [22]. Undoubtedly other mechanisms do exist, and this makes eminent sense for the survival of the organism. The attraction of the mechanism described here is that it has moved beyond the purely phenomenological stage to where experiments can be designed to directly test it. Already the molecular knowledge gleaned from the studies described here can be used to study the molecular pathogenesis of disease progression and to suggest novel ways of gaining some therapeutic advantage.

Acknowledgements. The work described in this review was conducted by many laboratories throughout the world and, due to space constraints, is far from comprehensive. The author is an Alberta Heritage Foundation Medical Scientist and the research conducted in his laboratory was funded by the National Cancer Institute and Medical Research Council of Canada. Thanks to Mae Wylie for typing the manuscript and Michael Meier, MD, FRCP (C), for the initial rendering of Fig. 1.

References

1. Moller G (1988) Molecular mechanisms of T cell-mediated lysis. Immunol Rev 103:5–211
2. Lobe CG, Havele C, Bleackley RC (1986) Cloning of two genes that are specifically expressed in activated cytotoxic T lymphocytes. Proc Natl Acad Sci USA 83:1448–1452
3. Brunet JF, Dosseto M, Denizot F, Matter M-G, Clark WR, Haqqi TM, Ferrier P, Nabholz M, Schmitt- Verhulst A-M, Luciani M-F, Golstein P (1986) The inducible cytotoxic T-lymphocyte-

associated gene transcript CTLA-1 sequence and gene localization to mouse chromosome 14. Nature 322:268–271

4. Gershenfeld HK, Weissman IL (1986) Cloning of a cDNA for a T cell-specific serine protease from a cytotoxic T lymphocyte. Science 232:854–858

5. Dourmashkin RR, Deteix P, Simone CB, Henkart P (1980) Electron microscopic demonstration of lesions on target cell membranes associated with antibody-dependent cellular cytotoxicity. Clin Exp Immunol 43:554–560

6. Henkart PA, Millard PJ, Reynolds CJ, Henkart MP (1984) Cytolytic activity of purified cytoplasmic granules from cytotoxic rat large granular lymphocyte tumors. J Exp Med 160:75–93

7. Podack ER, Young JDE, Cohn ZA (1985) Isolation and biochemical and functional characterization of perforin 1 from cytolytic T-cell granules. Proc Natl Acad Sci USA 82:8629–8633

8. Lobe CG, Finlay BB, Paranchych W, Paetkau V, Bleackley RC (1986) Novel serine proteases encoded by two cytotoxic T lymphocyte-specific genes. Science 232:858–861

9. Masson D, Zamai M, Tschopp J (1986) Identification of granzyme A isolated from cytotoxic T lymphocyte granules as one of the proteases encoded by CTL-specific genes. FEBS Lett 208:84–88

10. Stevens RL, Kamada MN, Serafin WE (1989) Structure and function of the family of proteoglycans that reside in the secretory granules of natural killer cells and other effector cells of the immune response. Curr Top Microbiol Immunol 140:93–108

11. Liu CC, Steffen M, King F, Young JDE (1987) Identification, isolation, and characterization of novel cytotoxin in murine cytolytic lymphocytes. Cell 51:393–403

12. Millard PJ, Henkart MP, Reynolds CW, Henkart PA (1984) Purification and properties of cytoplasmic granules from cytotoxic rat LGL tumors. J Immunol 132:3197–3204

13. Zagury D, Bernard J, Thierness N, Feldman M, Berke G (1975) Isolation and characterization of individual functionally reactive cytotoxic T lymphocytes: conjugation, killing and recycling at the single cell level. Eur J Immunol 5:818–822

14. Yannelli JR, Sullivan JA, Mandell GL, Engelhard VH (1986) Reorientation and fusion of cytotoxic T lymphocyte granules after interaction with target cells as determined by high resolution cinemicrography. J Immunol 136:377–382

15. Tschopp J, Nabholz M (1990) Perforin-mediated target cell lysis by cytolytic T lymphocytes. Ann Rev Immunol 8:279–302

16. Duke RC, Persechini PM, Chang S, Liu CC, Cohen JJ, Young JDE (1989) Purified perforin induces target cell lysis but not DNA fragmentation. J Exp Med 170:1451–1456

17. Bleackley RC, Lobe CG, Duggan B, Ehrman N, Frégeau C, Meier M, Letellier M, Havele C, Shaw J, Paetkau V (1988) The isolation and characterization of a family of serine protease genes expressed in activated cytotoxic T lymphocytes. Immunol Rev 103:5–19

18. Redmond MJ, Letellier M, Parker JMR, Lobe CG, Havele C, Paetkau V, Bleackley RC (1987) A serine protease (CCP1) is sequestered in the cytoplasmic granules of cytotoxic T lymphocytes. J Immunol 139:3184–3188

19. Müeller C, Gershenfeld HK, Lobe CG, Okada CY, Bleackley RC, Weissman IL (1988) A high proportion of T lymphocytes that infiltrate H-2-incompatible heart allografts in vivo express genes encoding cytotoxic cell-specific serine proteases, but do not express the MEL 14-defined lymph node homing receptor. J Exp Med 167:1124–1136

20. Acha-Orbea H, Scarpellino L, Hertig S, Dupuis M, Tschopp J (1990) Inhibition of lymphocyte mediated cytotoxicity by perforin antisense oligonucleotides. EMBO J 9:3815–3819

21. Murphy MEP, Moult J, Bleackley RC, Gershenfeld H, Weissman IL, James MNG (1988) Comparative molecular model building of two serine proteinases from cytotoxic T lymphocytes. Proteins: structure, function, and genetics 4:190–204

22. Berke G (1988) Lymphocyte-mediated cytolysis. Effectors, lytic signals, and the mechanism whereby early membrane derangements result in target-cell death. Ann NY Acad Sci 532:314–335

Immune Response to Heat Shock Proteins

S. H. E. Kaufmann

Introduction

Species as diverse as bacteria and humans respond quite uniformly to environmental assaults: their cells produce a well-defined and highly conserved group of proteins, termed stress proteins or heat shock proteins (HSP). These hsp can be grouped into different families according to their apparent molecular weight, e.g., the hsp 60 family which is in the focus of this small treatise has an apparent molecular mass of 60 kDa [1]. Members of this family are extremely conserved and the bacterial and human cognates share about 60% sequence homology [2]. Although hsp levels are normally increased under stress, many hsp already perform important functions in the normal cell (see Fig. 1). Hsp 60 have a high peptide-binding activity which allows them to interact with other proteins in the cell [1]. In eukaryotes, hsp 60 is primarily localized in mitochondria where it facilitates unfolding and folding steps of protein translocation from the cytoplasmic into the mitochondrial compartment as well as the assembly of high molecular weight complexes [3]. The hsp 60 cognate of *Escherichia coli* has been termed GroEL. Together with another hsp, GroES, it facilitates protein folding and unfolding, protein translocation across membrane barriers, and protein secretion. Hsp 60 is an abundant bacterial polypeptide which makes up 1% –2% of the total protein content under normal conditions and increases up to Fivefold in certain stress situations.

Microbial Hsp and the Immune Response: Possible Role in Antibacterial Immunity

Until recently, heat shock was the most widely used assault used to induce hsp synthesis. More recently, however, several more physiologic stress conditions have been analyzed. Most importantly, increased hsp synthesis in *Salmonella typhimurium* organisms was observed after phagocytosis by murine macrophages [4]. This finding indicates that the professional phagocyte imposes

Department of Immunology, University of Ulm, Albert-Einstein-Allee 11, 7900 Ulm, FRG

Host Defense Dysfunction
in Trauma, Shock and Sepsis
Eds. Faist/Meakins/Schildberg
© Springer-Verlag, Berlin Heidelberg 1993

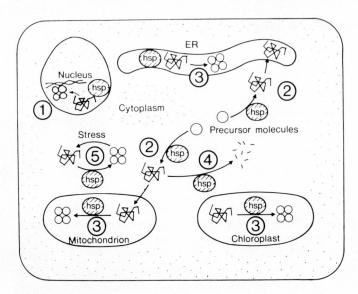

Fig. 1. Schematic illustration describing different functions of hsp in normal and stressed cells. *1*, Interference of hsp with steroid receptor binding to DNA; *2*, protein unfolding and translocation across intracellular membranes; *3*, protein folding and/or assembly of protein oligomers; *4*, protein degradation by hsp; *5*, interference with protein unfolding under heat or other assaults by hsp. *ER*, endoplasmic reticulum. For further details see [1]

strong stress stimuli upon intracellular parasites, which may increase their survival chance by elevating hsp synthesis.

Hsp 60 represents a dominant antigen of the cellular and hormonal immune response to many intracellular bacteria including the tubercle and leprosy bacilli. When mice have been immunized with *Mycobacterium tuberculosis*, about 20% of all T cells which respond to whole *M. tuberculosis* organisms are specific for hsp 60 (Fig. 2 [5]). Furthermore, in leprosy and tuberculosis patients strong T-cell responses to hsp 60 are observed [6]. Even in normal healthy individuals T cells with specificity to hsp 60 exist and both alpha/beta T cells and gamma/delta T cells recognize hsp 60 [7, 8]. Therefore, hsp 60-specific T cells are not indicative of clinical disease. It is assumed that hsp 60-specific T cells are activated and boosted by frequent contact with hsp from micro-organisms of low virulence. The abundant hsp production resulting from the stress bacteria being exposed to the inside of phagocytes, and the constant boosters by frequent contact with various microbes, could represent major reasons for the immunodominance of hsp. Although it is tempting to speculate that hsp 60-specific T cells provide a rapid first line of immune defense, their precise role in acquired resistance to intracellular bacteria needs to be further clarified.

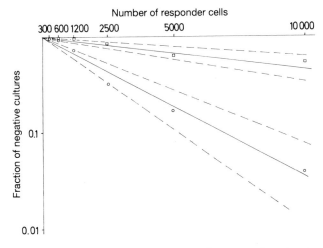

Fig. 2. Frequency analysis of T cells from *M. tuberculosis*-immune mice against whole *M. tuberculosis* organisms and hsp 60. Mice were immunized with killed *M. tuberculosis* and 10 days later lymph node cells collected. Purified T cells were stimulated with killed *M. tuberculosis* or hsp 60 or were left unstimulated. The linear regression line was calculated by the chi-square method and the frequency of antigen-reactive T cells was estimated by Poisson analysis. (Data reproduced with permission from [5])

Host Hsp and the Immune Response: Possible Role in Surveillance and Autoimmunity

Stress is not only imposed on the pathogen but also on the host cell. First, intracellular parasites compete for nutrients and other intracellular molecules and hence may stress their host cell. Second, parasitized host cells are under attack from immune effector mechanisms. Consistent with this assumption, evidence has been presented of increased hsp 60 levels in Schwann cells which had been infected with *Mycobacterium leprae* [9]. Furthermore, it has been found that Schwann cells infected with viable *M. leprae* become relatively resistant to destruction by non-specific killer cells [10]. Similarly resistance to killing was induced by more conventional assaults, such as heat shock. Thus, the production of hsp may provide a means for host cells to protect themselves against various assaults arising after they have become parasitized.

The remarkable conservation of hsp points to their potential role in surveillance and autoimmunity. Indeed, antibodies which recognize shared regions of mycobacterial and human hsp 60 have been described [9, 11]. Recently, we obtained evidence that one such antibody, ML30, which was originally raised against *M. leprae* and is specific for aminoacids 275–287 and 301–322 of mycobacterial and human hsp 60, respectively (17/22 amino acid identity), recognizes an epitope expressed on the surface of murine bone marrow-derived

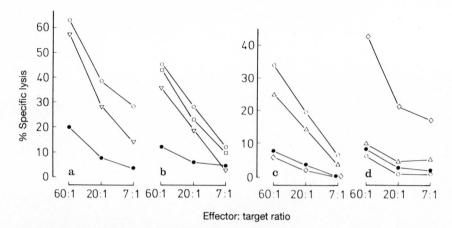

Fig. 3a–d. Lysis of peptide-pulsed macrophages or stressed macrophages by cytotoxic T lymphocytes (CTL) raised against mycobacterial *hsp 60*. **a–c** CTL were activated against tryptic digest of
mycobacterial hsp 60 or **d** ovalbumin and after wards their killer activity was tested on unstimulated
BMMØ (●); BMMØ pulsed with hsp 60 (○) BMMØ activated with interferon-γ (IFN-γ)-
containing T cell factors (▽); BMMØ activated with recombinant interferon-γ (r-IFN-γ) (△);
cytomegalovirus-infected *BMMØ* (□) and BMMØ pulsed with ovalbumin peptides (◇). (Data
reproduced with permission from [14])

macrophages [12]. Further studies are required to find out whether this surface
molecule is indeed an hsp cognate or whether it is of unrelated nature.

Peripheral blood leukocytes from normal healthy individuals comprise T
cells with specificity for epitopes shared by mycobacterial and human hsp 60.
This notion is based in our findings that synthetic peptides representing highly
conserved regions of hsp 60 are recognized by T cells after in vitro stimulation
with mycobacterial antigens [13]. These peptides are recognized in the context
of human leukocyte antigen (HLA) class II molecules.

In the murine system, it was found that T cells activated against tryptic
digest of mycobacterial hsp 60 specifically lyse stressed macrophages, leaving
unstressed macrophages virtually unaffected (Fig. 3 [14]). Stress was caused by
interferon-γ, heat, or viral infection. The relevant T cells express the CD8
phenotype, the alpha/beta T-cell receptor, and are class I restricted. Again, in
this case, the endogenous source of the peptides presented by stressed macrophages in the context of major histocompatibility complex (MHC) gene products remains unknown. However, it is tempting to speculate that it is hsp 60
itself. T cells and antibodies recognizing epitopes derived from host hsp should
be able to identify host cells suffering from various assaults such as infection,
inflammation, trauma, and transformation. Hence, they might perform an
important surveillance function. On the other hand, extensive tissue destruction
by hsp-reactive T cells might contribute to autoimmunity.

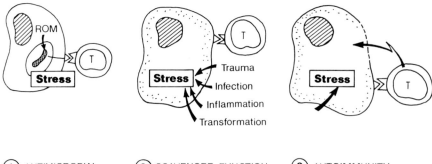

ANTIMICROBIAL
IMMUNITY

SCAVENGER FUNCTION

AUTOIMMUNITY

Fig. 4. Hypothetical scheme of the functional potential of T cells with specificity for hsp 60. *1*, Bacterial hsp are dominant antigens for atleast two reasons: first, abundant production by bacteria inside macrophages; second, constant boosters by hsp 60 epitopes shared by various microbes (*ROM*, reactive oxygen metabolites). *2*, T cells with specificity for hsp 60 could be involved in immune surveillance because they recognize and destroy stressed cells expressing hsp 60-derived epitopes. *3*, Recognition of stressed host cells by T cells with specificity for hsp 60 may, under certain conditions, lead to autoimmunity

Conclusion

This brief treatise focuses on the interesting liaison between hsp and the immune response. The broad distribution in the biosphere, the high conservation, and the abundant production under various stress conditions point to an important role of hsp 60 in antibacterial immunity, immune surveillance, and/or autoimmunity (Fig. 4).

Acknowledgements. The author is grateful to Mrs. R. Mahmoudi for typing the manuscript. Work from the author's laboratory received financial support from SFB 322, UNDP/World Bank/WHO Special Program for Research and Training in Tropical Diseases, German Leprosy Relief Association, EC India Science and Technology Cooperation Program, and the A. Krupp award for young professors.

References

1. Kaufmann SHE (1988) CD8$^+$ T lymphocytes in intracellular microbial infections. Immunol Today 9:168
2. Jindal S, Dudani AK, Singh B, Harley CB, Gupta RS (1989) Primary structure of a human mitochondrial protein homologous to the bacterial and plant chaperonins and to the 65-kiloDalton mycobacterial antigen. Mol Cell Biol 9:2279
3. Langer T, Neupert W (1991) Heat shock proteins hsp 60 and hsp 70: their roles in folding, assembly and membrane translocation of proteins. Curr Top Microbiol Immunol 167:3
4. Buchmeier NA, Heffron F (1990) Salmonella proteins induced following phagocytosis by macrophages are controlled by multiple regulons. Science 248:730

5. Kaufmann SHE, Vath U, Thole JER, v. Embden JDA, Emmrich F (1987) Enumeration of T cells reactive with *Mycobacterium tuberculosis* organisms and specific for the recombinant mycobacterial 64 kiloDalton protein. Eur J Immunol 17:351
6. Emmrich F, Thole J, van Embden J, Kaufmann SHE (1986) A recombinant 64 kiloDalton protein of *Mycobacterium bovis* BCG specifically stimulates human T4 clones reactive to mycobacterial antigens. J Exp Med 163:1024
7. Munk ME, Schoel B, Kaufmann SHE (1988) T cell responses of normal individuals towards recombinant protein antigens of *Mycobacterium tuberculosis*. Eur J Immunol 18:1835
8. Kabelitz D, Bender A, Schondelmaier S, Schoel B, Kaufmann SHE (1990) A large fraction of human peripheral blood $\gamma\delta^+$ T cells is activated by *Mycobacterium tuberculosis* but not by its 65 kD heat shock protein. J Exp Med 171:667
9. Kaufmann SHE, Schoel B, Koga T, Wand-Württenberger A, Munk ME, Steinhoff U (1991) Heat shock protein 60: implications for pathogenesis of and protection against bacterial infections. Immunol Rev (in press)
10. Steinhoff U, Wand-Württenberger A, Bremerich A, Kaufmann SHE (1991) *Mycobacterium leprae* renders Schwann cells and mononuclear phagocytes susceptible or resistant against killer cells. Infect Immun 59:684
11. Ivanyi J, Sinha S, Aston R, Cussell D, Keen M, Sengupta U (1983) Definition of species specific and cross-reactive antigenic determinants of *Mycobacterium leprae* using monoclonal antibodies. Clin Exp Immunol 52:528
12. Wang-Württenberger A, Schoel B, Ivanyi J, Kaufmann SHE (1991) Surface expression by mononuclear phagocytes of an epitope shared with mycobacterial heat shock protein 60. Eur J Immunol (in press)
13. Munk ME, Schoel B, Modrow S, Karr RW, Young RA, Kaufmann SHE (1989) Cytolytic T lymphocytes from healthy individuals with specificity to self epitopes shared by the mycobacterial and human 65 kDa heat shock protein. J Immunol 143:2844
14. Koga T, Wand-Württenberger A, DeBruyn J, Munk ME, Schoel B, Kaufmann SHE (1989) T cells against a bacterial heat shock protein recognize stressed macrophages. Science 245:1112

Prostaglandins Mediate the Expression of a 72-kDa Heat Shock Protein in Human Fibroblasts*

A. E. Heufelder[1,2], B. E. Wenzel[2], and R. S. Bahn[1]

Introduction

Highly conserved heat shock proteins (HSPs) function to maintain cellular homeostasis during stress [1]. At least in part, preservation by HSPs of cellular functions is achieved through protein refolding and degradation and export of damaged proteins [2] HSPs of different molecular weights are induced by various stimuli, including elevated temperatures, oxygen free radicals, tissue trauma caused by ischemia and reperfusion, inhibitors of energy metabolism, cytokines, and infectious microoganisms [1, 3]. Recently, immunological functions of HSPs in intracellular processing, membrane anchoring, and presentation of antigens have been suggested [4, 5]. Previous studies from this laboratory have focused on the induction of HSP expression in association with autoimmunity [6]. Prostaglandins and other inflammatory products are released locally by cells involved in immune reactions [7]. The purpose of this study was to determine whether prostaglandins may participate as mediators in the expression of a 72-kDa HSP (HSP 72) in cultured human fibroblasts.

Materials and Methods

Cell Cultures

Human pretibial fibroblasts were obtained from healthy individuals ($n = 3$) during surgery and cultured as described previously [8]. All culture strains were used between the third and sixth passage. Expression of HSPs was studied under baseline conditions (in the presence of 1% fetal bovine serum) and following a 3-h recovery from heat stress (43 °C for 90 min) or treatment with hydrogen peroxide (10^{-4} M H_2O_2 for 60 min) with or without a 48-h pretreatment with

* This work was supported in part by a postdoctoral grant from Deutsche Forschungsgeméinschaft (He 1485/2–1) and by the Mayo Clinic/Foundation

[1] Division of Endocrinology, Department of Internal Medicine, Mayo Clinic/Foundation, Rochester, MN 55905, USA

[2] Zell-und Immunbiologisches Labor, Klinik für Innere Medizin, Medizinische Universität Lübeck, 2400 Lübeck, FRG

indomethacin (10^{-6} M) or hydrocortisone (10^{-7} M). In some studies, prosta-glandin E_2 (PGE_2, 10^{-5}–10^{-9} M), indomethacin or hydrocortisone alone were added to the medium for 48 h. Throughout these studies, cell viability was found to be greater than 90% as assessed by trypan blue exclusion. Cells were harvested in 0.5% sodium dodecylsulfate using a rubber policeman. Protein concentrations were determined and cell lysates were either subjected immediately to gel electrophoresis or frozen at -70 °C until used.

Sodium Dodecylsulfate Polyacrylamide Gel Electrophoresis (SDS-PAGE) Immunoblotting and Quantitative Scanning Densitometry

Aliquots of cell lysates were mixed with standard sample buffer, heated, and applied to gels (4% acrylamide stacking gel, 10% acrylamide running gel) at a protein concentration of 70 µg/lane. Electrophoresis was performed with a standard buffer system at a constant current of 30 mA for 7 h. Following electrotransfer of proteins onto nitrocellulose (60 min at 1.0 A) membranes were presoaked in blocking buffer containing 5% non-fat dry milk for 2 h at 37 °C. The nitrocellulose was then incubated with anti-HSP 72 monoclonal antibody (Stress Gen Corp., Sidney, British Columbia, Canada) for 2 h at room temperature (1:1000 dilution in blocking buffer), washed four times and incubated with a 1:500 dilution of biotinylated anti-mouse immunoglobulin in blocking buffer for 1 h at room temperature. Following another four washes, blots were incubated with biotinylated streptavidin peroxidase performed complexes (1:400 dilution) for 30 min, washed again, and developed using a standard peroxidase substrate system with diaminobenzidine as the chromogen. Immunoblots were then air dried and subjected to scanning densitometry (550 nm) for quantitation of band intensity. Reactivity was measured and calculated as area under the curve (arbitrary units).

Indirect Immunofluorescence

Fibroblasts were plated directly on multichamber slides (Labtec No. 4808, Nunc Inc., Naperville, IL, USA) and grown to near confluence. Detection of HSP 72 was performed at baseline and following treatment with PGE_2 (10^{-7} M) for 48 h. Viable monolayers were washed with phosphate-buffered saline (PBS) containing 1% fetal bovine serum (FBS) and fixed for 10 min at -20 °C in 100% methanol. Airdried slides were rehydrated in PBS and preblocked with normal sheep serum (1:20 dilution) for 20 min at room temperature. Anti-HSP 72 mouse monoclonal antibody was applied for 1 h at room temperature (1:1000 dilution in PBS containing 1% bovine serum albumin, BSA). After several washes, cell monolayers were incubated with biotinylated anti-mouse immunoglobulin (1:100 dilution in PBS) for 1 h at room temperature, rinsed again, and incubated with fluorescein streptavidin (1:50 dilution in PBS) for 1 h at room temperature. Slides were washed, air dried, mounted, and visualized with a fluorescence microscope equipped with epiillumination ($\times$ 240). Parallel monolayers with the primary antibody replaced by unrelated monoclonal antibodies of the same isotype and by omitting each layer in turn were examined to assure specificity and to exclude cross-reactivities between the antibodies and conjugates employed.

Statistical Analysis

Samples of fibroblast culture extracts derived from three individuals and treated under identical conditions were run in duplicates. Intra- and interassay variabilities in our system have been determined previously [6]. Student's t test for the analysis of paired and unpaired data was used.

Results

No baseline expression of HSP 72 was detected in any fibroblast monolayer by either indirect immunofluorescence (Fig 1a) or sodium dodecylsulfate polyacrylamide gel electrophoresis (SDS-PAGE) and immunoblotting. Exposure to PGE_2 (10^{-7} M) strongly induced HSP 72 expression. This in vitro expression was primarily located in the perinuclear area of the cytoplasmic cellular compartment (Fig. 1b).

Both heat stress and treatment with hydrogen peroxide alone strongly induced HSP 72 expression (Fig. 2). Treatment of cell monolayers with indomethacin or hydrocortisone alone did not induce HSP 72 expression. Pretreatment of both heat-stressed and H_2O_2-treated cell monolayers with either indomethacin (10^{-6} M) or hydrocortisone (10^{-7} M) resulted in a similar and significant ($p < 0.005$) decrease in HSP 72 expression (Fig. 2).

Treatment of cell monolayers with increasing concentrations of PGE_2 (10^{-9})–10^{-5} M) enhanced the abundance of HSP 72 expression in a dose-dependent manner (Fig. 3). Pretreatment of monolayers with indomethacin (10^{-6} M) or dexamethasone (10^{-7} M) for 12 h prior to adding PGE_2 (10^{-7} M) did not result in a significant reduction of HSP 72 expression (Fig. 3).

Discussion

The expression of several HSPs, as well as serum antibodies against these HSPs, has been reported in a variety of infectious, inflammatory, and autoimmune conditions [3, 4, 9]. Oxygen free radicals, cytokines, and mediators of inflammation, generated or released at the site of tissue injury, have been implicated in the

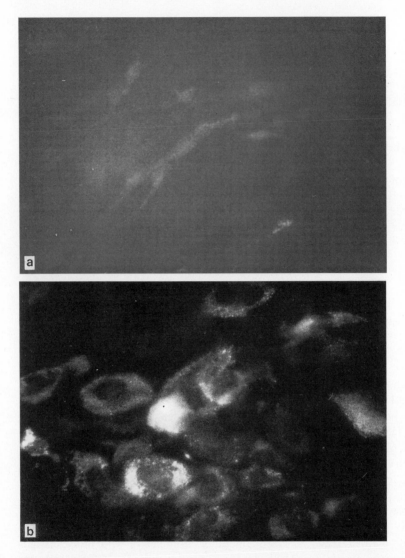

Fig. 1a,b. Detection by indirect immunofluorescence of HSP 72 expression in cultured fibroblasts **a** at baseline and **b** after a 48-h exposure to PGE_2 (10^{-7} M)

induction and modulation of HSPs [1, 4]. Prostaglandins are known a key mediators of inflammatory and immune reactions and can be detected locally at the site of tissue damage [10]. PGE_2 represents one of the major metabolites among the cyclooxygenase and lipoxygenase products generated by human fibroblasts [7, 10].

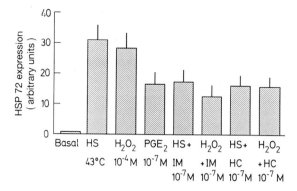

Fig. 2. Expression of HSP 72 in human fibroblasts at baseline and following recovery from heat stress (43 °C for 90 min) or treatment with H_2O_2 (10^{-4} M, 60 min). Where indicated, monolayers were pretreated with indomethacin (10^{-6} M) or hydrocortisone (10^{-7} M) prior to cellular stress. HSP reactivity was assessed by SDS-PAGE and immunoblotting and the resulting immunoblot bands were quantitated using scanning densitometry. Each *bar* represents the mean ± SD (given as arbitrary units) of duplicate samples derived from three individuals

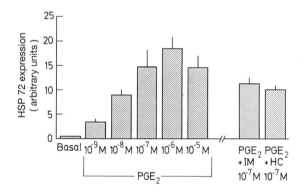

Fig. 3. Dose-response relationship between treatment (48 h) of fibroblast monolayers with increasing concentrations of PGE_2 and HSP 72 expression. HSP 72 expression was assessed by SDS-PAGE and immunoblotting and the resulting immunoblot bands were quantitated using scanning densitometry. Each *bar* represents the mean ± SD (given as arbitrary units) of duplicate samples derived from three individuals

In our culture system, a dose-dependent increase in HSP 72 expression was detected following the addition of increasing concentrations of PGE_2 to the medium, suggesting that this compound plays a role in the induction of HSP 72. As demonstrated by indirect immunofluorescence, HSP 72 was primarily located in the perinuclear area of the cytoplasmic compartment. When endogenous prostaglandin formation was blocked by pretreatment with indomethacin or hydrocortisone, HSP 72 expression following treatment with

PGE$_2$ was not significantly inhibited. In contrast, pretreatment of cell mono-layers with indomethacin or hydrocortisone prior to and during heat or chemical stress significantly ($p < 0.005$) reduced the abundance of stress-induc-ible HSP 72 expression. Thus, inhibition of prostaglandin formation prior to and during cellular stress reduced the abundance of detectable HSP 72 ex-pression. These results suggest a role for prostaglandins in mediating stress-induced HSP 72 expression in human fibroblasts and support results by other investigators demonstrating heat-induced synthesis of prostaglandins by fibrob-lasts [11]. In another study, induction of 68-kDa HSPs by cyclopentenone prostaglandins was closely associated with the G$_1$ block of cell cycle progression attributed to these prostaglandins [12]. Further, prostaglandins with antiproli-ferative activity have been found to induce synthesis of a member of the 70-kDa HSP family [13]. In our study, both a cyclooxygenase inhibitor, indomethacin, and an inhibitor of cyclooxygenase and lipoxygenase products, hydrocortisone, reduced HSP 72 expression to a similar degree. Therefore, among the arachi-donic acid metabolites, cyclooxygenase products may augment HSP 72 ex-pression to a greater extent than do lipoxygenase products.

In conclusion, various prostaglandin species are capable of inducing the expression of HSPs. We have demonstrated that cyclooxygenase products are potential second messengers in the process of stress-induced HSP 72 expression in human fibroblasts. This mechanism may play a role for conditions in infection, trauma, and autoimmunity, conditions in which inflammatory medi-ators contribute locally or systemically to tissue injury.

References

1. Lindquist S (1986) The heat-shock response. Annu Rev Biochem 55:1151–1191
2. Chiang HL, Terlecky SR, Plant CP, Dice JF (1989) A role for a 70-kilodalton heat shock protein in lysosomal degradation of intracellular proteins. Science 246:382–385
3. Winrow VR, Mc Lean L, Morris CJ, Blake DR (1990) The heat shock response and its role in inflammatory disease. Ann Rheum Dis 49:128–132
4. Kaufmann SHE (1990) Heat shock proteins and the immune response. Immunol Today 11:129–136
5. Vanbuskirk A, Crump BL, Margoliash E, Pierce SK (1989) A peptide binding protein having a role in antigen presentation is a member of the HSP70 heat shock family. J Exp Med 170:1799–1809
6. Heufelder AE, Wenzel BE, Gorman CA, Bahn RS (1991) Detection, cellular localization and modulation of heat shock proteins in cultured fibroblasts from patients with extrathyroidal manifestations of Graves' disease. J Clin Endocrinol Metab (submitted)
7. Plescia O, Racis S (1988) Prostaglandins as physiological immunoregulators. Prog Allergy 44:153–171
8. Bahn RS, Gorman CA, Woloschak GE, David CS, Johnson PM, Johnson CM (1987) Human retroocular fibroblasts in vitro: a model for the study of Graves' ophthalmopathy. J Clin Endocrinol Metab 65:665–670
9. Lamb JR, Bal V, Mendez-Samperio P et al. (1989) Stress proteins may provide a link between the immune response to infection and autoimmunity. Int Immunol 1:129–136
10. Mayer B, Rauter L, Zenzmaier E, Gleispach H, Esterbauer H (1984) Characterization of lipoxygenase metabolites of arachidonic acid in cultured human skin fibroblasts. Biochim Biophys Acta 795:151–161

11. Calderwood SK, Bornstein B, Farnum EK, Stevenson MA (1989) Heat shock stimulates the release of arachidonic acid and the synthesis of prostaglandins and leukotriene B_4 in mammalian cells. J Cell Physiol 141:325–333
12. Ohno K, Fukushima M, Fujiwara M, Narumiya S (1988) Induction of 68,000-dalton heat shock proteins by cyclopentenone prostaglandins. J Biol Chem 263:19764–19770
13. Santoro MG, Garaci E, Amici C (1989) Prostaglandins with antiproliferative activity induce the synthesis of a heat shock protein in human cells. Proc Natl Acad Sci USA 86:8407–8411

Glucocorticoid–Immune System Interactions in Injury and Sepsis*

S. E. Calvano

Introduction

Glucocorticoids have potent inhibitory effects on the immune system. Elevation of glucocorticoids causes a profound lymphopenia [1, 2] in the peripheral blood due to redistribution of lymphocytes to extravascular compartments [3, 4]. In addition to their role in modulating numbers of cells available to participate in and regulate immune responses, glucocorticoids also have direct suppressive effects on lymphocyte activity. T lymphocytes are much more strongly affected than are B lymphocytes. Inhibition of T-cell proliferation is the most commonly observed direct effect of elevated glucocorticoids [5, 6]. In turn, it has been established that inhibition of T-cell proliferation by glucocorticoids is due to suppression of interleukin-2 (IL-2) production which is obligatory for T-cell expansion [7, 8].

Elevation of endogenous glucocorticoids is observed during or after almost any stress including infection or injury [9]. Because immune dysfunction occurs during infection and/or after injury [10–12], a reasonable hypothesis to consider is that elevated glucocorticoids may play a role in mediating infection- or injury-induced immune disorders. To this end, the studies presented here evaluated plasma cortisol levels, and numerical, phenotypic, and proliferative changes in T lymphocytes following human burn injury and experimental endotoxemia in normal human volunteers. These hormonal, hematologic, and immunologic changes were then compared to those observed in normal human subjects subjected to a constant i.v. infusion of cortisol. It was postulated that if normal volunteers administered cortisol exhibited a pattern of T-lymphocyte modulation similar to those seen after burn or during experimental endotoxemia, this would support the hypothesis that glucocorticoid elevation after injury or during sepsis contributes to the immune dysfunction which occurs in these pathological conditions.

* Data condensed and reviewed in this paper have been previously published [12–14].
Department of Surgery, Cornell University Medical College, New York, New York, USA

Host Defense Dysfunction
in Trauma, Shock and Sepsis
Eds. Faist/Meakins/Schildberg
© Springer-Verlag, Berlin Heidelberg 1993

Materials and Methods

Burned Patients. Data presented are from three different groups of patients studied over a 4-year period. The number of patients in each group was 24, 30, and 26, respectively. The mean percentage of total body surface area (TBSA) burned varied from 30% to 44%. Blood samples were obtained at 24–48 h after injury. Controls were normal laboratory personnel (*n* = 50).

Experimental Endotoxemia. Twelve normal male volunteers were administered highly purified *Escherichia coli* lipopolysaccharide (LPS, 20 U/kg) by bolus i.v. injection, and blood was drawn hourly for the following 6 h. Control samples for each subject were those obtained prior to LPS injection.

Experimental Hypercortisolemia. Five normal male volunteers were administered hydrocortisone sodium succinate (3 μg/kg·min) by continuous i.v. infusion for 6 h. Blood was drawn at 4, 5, and 6 h during infusion. Control samples for each subject were those obtained prior to initiation of cortisol infusion.

Measurement of Plasma Cortisol. Plasma cortisol was quantified by a specific radioimmunoassay as previously described [13]. Three quality control samples containing low, medium, and high concentrations of cortisol were analyzed concurrently in each assay.

Lymphocyte Counts. Quantitative lymphocyte counts were performed on lysed whole blood by flow cytometric light scatter analysis [13, 14].

Lymphocyte Cell Surface Phenotyping. Analysis were performed on cells obtained either from lysed whole blood or by Ficoll-Hypaque gradient centrifugation. Lymphocytes were phenotyped by labeling with fluorescein isothiocynate (FITC)-conjugated monoclonal antibodies against CD3, CD4, and CD8 cell-surface markers followed by flow microfluorometry of light scatter-gated (forward × 90°) lymphocytes [12, 14].

Lymphocyte Blastogenesis. T-lymphocyte proliferation in the autologous or allogeneic mixed lymphocyte reactions, or in response to phytohemaglutinin (PHA) was performed as described previously [12, 13]. The dose of PHA employed was 0.1 μg/ml of a highly purified preparation from Wellcome Reagents.

Data Analysis. Data were analyzed either by Student's *t* test or by analysis of variance followed by Newman-Keuls' multiple range test.

Results

Plasma Cortisol

Table 1 presents plasma cortisol concentrations after burn injury or during experimental endotoxemia or hypercortisolemia. Relative to a group of 50 normal controls, cortisol was increased more than two fold to 48.4 μg/dl at 24–48 h after injury. During experimental endotoxemia, plasma cortisol increased to a peak of 33.7 μg/dl at 3 h after administration of LPS. Finally, during cortisol infusion, levels of this hormone reached a steady-state of 43–49 μg/dl by 4 h of infusion. Thus, burn patients at 24–48 h after postinjury and the experimental hypercortisolemic volunteers had virtually identical concentrations of cortisol while endotoxemic volunteers manifested peak levels that were about 10 μg/dl lower.

Lymphocyte Counts

Peripheral blood lymphocyte counts for the three groups are shown in Table 2. As the table demonstrates, data from burned patients is from 24–48 h postinjury, experimental endotoxemic subjects at 4 h after LPS administration (1 h after the peak in plasma cortisol concentrations, see paragraph immediately above), and experimental hypercortisolemic subjects after 6 h of cortisol infusion.

All three groups manifested significant ($p < 0.01$) lymphopenia that was correlated with elevated plasma cortisol. Although the lymphocyte counts for the burned patients at 24–48 h postinjury appeared to be somewhat higher ($725/mm^3$) compared to endotoxemic volunteers ($500/mm^3$) or cortisol infusion subjects ($534/mm^3$), control or baseline lymphocyte counts varied among the groups. Looking at difference scores for lymphocyte counts for the three groups, one obtains $1800 - 725 = 1075$ for the burned patients, $1625 - 500 = 1125$ for volunteers receiving LPS, and $1139 - 534 = 605$ for the hypercortisolemic subjects. Thus, the relative lymphopenia was similar for burned patients and experimental endotoxemic subjects but somewhat less for experimental hypercortisolemic volunteers.

Immunophenotype

Table 3 shows that the percentage of $CD3^+$ T cells declined significantly in all three groups. Further, this decline in the percentage of T cells could be accounted for almost entirely by a concomitant decrease in the percentage of $CD4^+$ helper/inducer T cells. There was little or no change in the percentage of $CD8^+$ suppressor/cytotoxic T cells. $CD8^+$ T cells did decline significantly in the

Table 1. Plasma cortisol concentrations after human burn injury or during experimental endotoxemia (LPS) or hypercortisolemia in normal human volunteers

Group								

Group	0ᵃ	1	2	3	4	5	6	24–48
			Time hours after burn or LPS/cortisol administration					
Burn	23.5 ± 1.2ᵇ	–	–	–	–	–	–	48.4 ± 4.5*
LPS	12.9 ± 2.1	19.7 ± 2.7	28.9 ± 2.7*	33.7 ± 3.2*	27.1 ± 2.6*	23.0 ± 2.3*	16.7 ± 2.0	–
Cortisol	9.3 ± 0.8	–	–	–	43.2 ± 3.1*	46.0 ± 3.4*	48.9 ± 5.7*	–

ᵃ Time 0 for the burn group is the mean of a separate group of normal controls.
ᵇ Mean ± SEM plasma cortisol in µg/dl.
* $p < 0.01$ vs time 0.

Table 2. Peripheral blood lymphocyte counts after human burn injury or during experimental endotoxemia (LPS) or hypercortisolemia in normal human volunteers

Group	Time hours after burn or LPS/cortisol administration			
	0[a]	4	6	24–48
Burn	1800 ± 250[b]	–	–	725 ± 112*
LPS	1625 ± 125	500 ± 68*	–	–
Cortisol	1139 ± 94	–	534 ± 76*	–

[a] Time 0 for the burn group is the mean of a separate group of normal controls.
[b] Mean $\pm$ SEM number of lymphocytes/mm^3.
* $p < 0.01$ vs time 0.

Table 3. T lymphocyte immunophenotype after human burn injury or during experimental endotoxemia (LPS) or hypercortisolemia in normal human volunteers

Group	T lymphocyte cell-surface marker expressed (time of assessment)					
	CD3		CD4		CD8	
	Before[a]	After[b]	Before	After	Before	After
Burn	71 ± 2[c]	41 ± 3**	47 ± 1	29 ± 3**	33 ± 1	32 ± 3
LPS	68 ± 2	55 ± 3**	47 ± 1	37 ± 2**	24 ± 1	21 ± 1**
Cortisol	68 ± 3	56 ± 4*	45 ± 2	31 ± 1**	24 ± 2	29 ± 2

[a] For the burn group, the mean of a separate group of normal controls; for the LPS and Cortisol groups, before administration of LPS and initiation of cortisol infusion, respectively.
[b] For the burn group, 24–48 h after injury; for the LPS group, 4 h after LPS administration; for the cortisol group, 6 h after the initiation of cortisol infusion.
[c] Mean $\pm$ SEM percent immunofluorescent-positive lymphocytes.
* $p < 0.05$, ** $p < 0.01$ vs "before".

experimental endotoxemia group, but the magnitude of this decline was only $24\% - 21\% = 3\%$. Statistical significance was achieved due to very low variability in the data. Thus, these data demonstrate a very similar pattern of change in immunophenotype after burn injury, after administration of LPS to normal volunteers, and during cortisol infusion to normal volunteers.

T-Cell Proliferation

At 24–48 h after burn injury, T-cell proliferation in the allogeneic mixed lymphocyte reaction (MLR) was not different from that of normal control subjects (Table 4). However, proliferative responses in the autologous MLR had significantly decreased after thermal injury especially for those patients with large burns. Four hours after administration of LPS to normal volunteers or after 6 h of cortisol infusion to normal subjects, proliferation to PHA was dramatically decreased (Table 5). The percentage inhibition of proliferation was

Table 4. T-lymphocyte proliferation in the allogeneic and autologous mixed lymphocyte responses after human burn injury

	Allogeneic MLR	Autologous MLR
Normal controls	21 000 ± 3800[a]	9 444 ± 1055
Burn (all)[b]	18 400 ± 3000	4 888 ± 1722*
Burn (> 60% TBSA)	–	1 411 ± 823**

[a] Mean ± SEM cpm [^{3}H] thymidine incorporation.
[b] Burn patients were studies 24–48 h after injury.
* $p < 0.05$, ** $p < 0.01$ vs normal controls.

Table 5. T-lymphocyte proliferation in response to PHA during experimental endotoxemia (LPS) or hypercortisolemia in normal human volunteers

	Before[a]	After[b]
LPS	47 803 ± 12 000[c]	13 012 ± 2000*
Cortisol	109 500 ± 19 500	3 500 ± 2500

[a] Before administration of LPS or initiation of cortisol infusion.
[b] 4 h after LPS administration or after 6 h or cortisol infusion.
[c] Mean ± SEM cpm [^{3}H] thymidine incorporation.
* $p < 0.01$ vs "before".

72% for the volunteers receiving LPS and 96% for the volunteers given cortisol infusions.

Conclusion

These studies have investigated hematologic and immunologic changes in three different human models where plasma cortisol concentrations are elevated to pathophysiologic levels. In all three situations, (1) human burn injury, (2) experimental endotoxemia in normal volunteers, and (3) experimental hypercortisolemia in normal volunteers, remarkably similar patterns of hematologic and immunologic change were observed. These included lymphopenia, a decrease in the percentage of CD3$^+$ T cells that could be accounted for by a concomitant decrease in the percentage of CD4$^+$ helper/inducer T cells, and defective T-cell proliferation in the autologous MLR or in response to PHA.

Of course, following burn injury or experimental endotoxemia, only a correlative relationship between elevated cortisol levels and immunologic defects could be discerned. The burn patients were studied in the early postinjury period (24–48 h), and it is obvious that these individuals had severe physiological derangements in addition to elevated glucocorticoids. Likewise, normal volunteers receiving LPS manifested fever, malaise, myalgia, hemodynamic changes, and elevations in tumor necrosis factor (TNF) and epinephrine [14–16], in addition to increased cortisol levels. Thus, in burned patients or experimental endotoxemic subjects, these other variables could be important mediators of immunologic change, and elevations in cortisol may simply have been correlative rather than causative in these situations.

However, the relationship between elevated cortisol and the observed changes in lymphocyte number, phenotype, and function is strengthened considerably by the cortisol infusions studies. In these experiments, plasma cortisol was specifically manipulated by a constant infusion which generated plasma levels of this hormone which were similar to those seen after burn injury or experimental endotoxemia (Table 1). Additionally, these normal subjects, unlike burned patients or normal subjects given LPS, were not distressed, did not have elevated epinephrine levels, and did not show changes in routine physiologic parameters. In spite of this, volunteers administered the cortisol infusions manifested hematologic and immunologic effects that were remarkably similar to those observed in burned patients or volunteers receiving LPS. It should be noted, however, that others [17, 18] have not observed a correlation between cortisol concentrations and defects in cell-mediated immunity after thermal injury.

If, by analogy to patients with acquired immunodeficiency syndrome (AIDS), a $CD4^+$ lymphocyte count of $< 500/mm^3$ is evidence of immunodeficiency, then the subjects in all three groups studied here were severely, albeit temporarily, immunocompromised. Combining data from Tables 2 and 3, the $CD4^+$ lymphocyte counts were: burned patients, $725 \times 0.29 = 210/mm^3$; experimental endotoxemic volunteers, $500 \times 0.37 = 185/mm^3$; and experimental hypercortisolemic volunteers, $534 \times 0.31 = 165/mm^3$.

Ilfeld et al. [19] demonstrated in vitro that the allogeneic MLR was relatively insensitive to inhibition by glucocorticoids. In contrast, proliferation in the autologous MLR was greatly depressed by the in vitro addition of physiological concentrations of cortisol. Thus, given that cortisol is elevated in burned patients, these results could explain why T-cell proliferation in the allogeneic MLR was unaffected by burn injury while proliferation in the autologous MLR was significantly depressed (Table 4). Others [20] have observed that mitogen-stimulated T-cell proliferation is sensitive to glucocorticoid-mediated inhibition in vivo.

References

1. Fauci AS, Dale DC (1974) The effect of in vivo hydrocortisone on subpopulations of human lymphocytes. J Clin Invest 53:240–246
2. Yu DTY, Clements PJ, Paulus HE, Peter JB, Levy J, Barnett EV (1974) Human lymphocyte subpopulations: effect of corticosteroids. J Clin Invest 53:565–571
3. Cohen JJ (1972) Thymus-derived lymphocytes sequestered in the bone marrow of hydrocortisone-treated mice. J Immunol 107:841–844

4. Levine MA, Claman HN (1970) Bone marrow and spleen: dissociation of immunologic properties by cortisone. Science 167:1515–1517
5. Blomgren H, Andersson B (1976) Steroid sensitivity of the PHA and PWM responses of fractionated human lymphocytes in vitro. Exp Cell Res 97:233–240
6. Neifeld JP, Tormey DC (1979) Effects of steroid hormones on phytohemagglutinin-stimulated human peripheral blood lymphocytes. Transplantation 27:309–314
7. Gillis S, Crabtree GR, Smith KA (1979) Glucocorticoid-induced inhibition of T-cell growth factor production. I. The effect on mitogen-induced lymphocyte proliferation. J Immunol 123:1624–1630
8. Larsson EL (1980) Cyclosporin A and dexamethasone suppress T cell responses by selectively acting at distinct sites of the triggering process. J Immunol 124:2828–2833
9. Liddle GW (1971) Regulation of adrenocortical function in man. In: Christy NP (ed) The human adrenal cortex Harper and Row, New York, pp 41–68
10. Miller CL, Baker CC (1979) Changes in lymphocyte activity after thermal injury. The role of suppressor cells. J Clin Invest 63:202–210
11. O'Mahony JB, Wood JJ, Rodrick ML, Mannick JA (1985) Changes in T-lymphocyte subsets following injury. Assessment by flow cytometry and relationship to sepsis. Ann Surg 202:580–586
12. Antonacci AC, Calvano SE, Reaves LE, Prajapati A, Bockman R, Welte K, Mertelsmann R, Gupta S, Good RA, Shires GT (1984) Autologous and allogeneic mixed-lymphocyte responses following thermal injury in man: the immunomodulatory effects of interleukin 1, interleukin 2, and a prostaglandin inhibitor, WY-18251. Clin Immunol Immunopathol 30:304–320
13. Calvano SE, Albert JD, Legaspi A, Organ BC, Tracey KJ, Lowry SF, Shires GT Antonacci AC (1987) Comparison of numerical and phenotypic leukocyte changes during constant hydrocortisone infusion in normal subjects with those in thermally injured patients at 24–48 hours following burn: hydrocortisone infusion mimics thermal injury with respect to changes in lymphocyte subset percentages. Surg Gynecol Obstet 164:509–520
14. Richardson RP, Rhyne CD, Fong Y, Hesse DG, Tracey KJ, Marano MA, Lowry SF, Antonacci AC, Calvano SE (1989) Peripheral blood leukocyte kinetics following in vivo lipopolysaccharide (LPS) administration to normal human subjects: influence of elicited hormones and cytokines. Ann Surg 210:113–119
15. Hesse DG, Tracey KJ, Fong Y, Manogue KR, Palladino MA Jr, Cerami A, Shires GT, Lowry SF (1988) Cytokine appearance in human endotoxemia and primate bacteremia. Surg Gynecol Obstet 166:147–153
16. Michie HR, Manogue KR, Spriggs DR, Revhaug A, O'Dwyer S, Dinarello CA, Cerami A, Wolff SM, Wilmore DW (1988) Detection of circulating tumor necrosis factor after endotoxin administration. N Engl J Med 318:1481–1486
17. Munster AM, Eurenius K, Katz RM, Canales L, Foley FD, Mortensen RF (1973) Cell-mediated immunity after thermal injury. Ann Surg 177:139–143
18. Wolfe JHN, Wu AVO, O'Connor NE, Saporoschetz I, Mannick JA (1982) Anergy, immunosuppressive serum, and impaired lymphocyte blastogenesis in burn patients. Arch Surg 117:1266–1271
19. Ilfeld DN, Krakauer RS, Blaese RM (1977) Suppression of the human autologous mixed lymphocyte reaction by physiologic concentrations of hydrocortisone. J Immunol 119:428–434
20. Webel Ml, Ritts RE Jr, Taswell HF, Donadio JV Jr, Woods JE (1974) Cellular immunity after intravenous administration of methyl-prednisolone. J Lab Clin Med 83:383–392

Hemorrhagic Shock Inhibits Myelopoiesis Independent of Bacterial Translocation*

D. H. Livingston, J. Hseih, T. Murphy, and B. F. Rush Jr.

Introduction

Hemorrhagic shock has been demonstrated to increase the susceptibility to bacterial infection [1–5]. Infection rates in patients who had sustained hemorrhagic shock complicating penetrating abdominal injury have been shown to be two to three times that for normotensive patients [4, 5]. Esrig demonstrated that a sublethal injection of endotoxin (lipopolysaccharide, LPS) resulted in significant mortality in rats following hemorrhagic shock [1]. This increased susceptibility to infection has been documented to persist for several days following shock in both rodent and murine models [2, 3]. Shock has also been demonstrated to result in numerous alterations in both cell-mediated and humoral immunity [3, 6, 7]. Among these is the failure of the bone marrow to mount a normal myelopoietic response to a challenge of intraperitoneal LPS following shock [8]. We have demonstrated that rats challenged with LPS after hemorrhagic shock resulted in a decline in the number of bone marrow granulocyte-macrophage colony-forming units (CFU-GM) compared with un-shocked rats [8]. Simultaneous with the loss of normal myelopoiesis is the appearance of serum factors inhibitory to CFU-GM growth.

Experimental data regarding translocation of bacteria and endotoxin from the gastrointestinal tract following hemorrhagic shock, thermal injury, and endotoxemia has been well described by Rush [9], Deitch [10], and others [11, 12]. Viable bacteria have been recovered from the mesenteric lymph nodes [13], lung [14], liver [14], and systemic blood [15] following experimental insult. Bacteria have also been recovered from the blood of trauma patients [16] and the mesenteric lymph nodes of patients undergoing celiotomy for intestinal obstruction [17]. Although translocation of bacteria and LPS has been demonstrated to occur, the clinical significance of these events remains uncertain. Selective decontamination of the gut in immunocompromised patients with hematologic malignancies has been demonstrated to reduce infection [18]. The impact of selective decontamination on intensive care unit (ICU) patients following trauma is less clear. Rush et al. have demonstrated that the germ-free

* Supported by NIH grants 2-RO1-GM37060 and 2-SO7-RRO5393 (Biomedical Research Support Grant).
Department of Surgery, UMD-New Jersey Medical School, Newark, NJ 07103, USA

state is associated with an improved survival following hemorrhagic shock [19]. Germ-free rats also contain less LPS in their gut than conventional animals although they should not be thought of as LPS deficient [19].

The purpose of these experiments were to define the contribution of bacterial translocation on the alteration of myelopoiesis following hemorrhagic shock. To achieve the goal we utilized the germ-free rat, which allowed us to compare the effects of hemorrhagic shock in animals with and without enteric bacteria. The impact of the severity of the shock model on myelopoiesis was also examined.

Materials and Methods

Animals

Adult male germ-free Sprague-Dawley rats weighing 350–400 g were purchased from Taconic Farms (Germantown, NY, USA) and shipped to our facility in sterile containers. Rats were transferred and housed in sterile isolators and maintained using standard gnotobiotic techniques [20]. Routine surveillance cultures taken from the isolators and from the cecum of these animals were consistently negative. Conventional rats were obtained from the same supplier and maintained in identical, but nonsterile, isolators. For the model of anesthetized hemorrhagic shock, adult female Sprague-Dawley rats weighing 200–225 g were purchased from Harlan Sprague-Dawley (Indianapolis, IN, USA). These animals were maintained under standard conditions in our animal facility. All animals were allowed food and water ad libitum and all experiments were reviewed and approved by the Animal Care and Use Committee of the New Jersey Medical School.

Hemorrhagic Shock

Several models of hemorrhagic shock were used in these studies. The model of unrestrained, awake hemorrhagic shock has been described [19]. Briefly, one day prior to shock rats were anesthetized with ketamine hydrochloride 100 mg/kg IP. An arterial catheter (PE-50) was inserted into the femoral artery and tunneled to exit the skin in the subscapular area. The catheter was connected to a swivel apparatus and the rat was allowed to waken from anesthesia. Twenty-four hours following catheterization the rats bled to a mean arterial pressure of 30 mmHg. This pressure was maintained until the animal required reinfusion of either 40% (30/40 shock) or 80% (30/80 shock) of the shed blood to maintain its blood pressure. The rats were then resuscitated with the remaining shed blood and approximately 1.5 volumes Ringer's lactate. Thereafter, animals were maintained on a constant infusion of Ringer's lactate and 20% glucose equal to twice the normal requirement. Control animals were treated identically but not subjected to shock.

The model of anesthetized hemorrhagic shock has also been previously described [2]. Briefly, rats were anesthetized with ketamine hydrochloride (50 mg/kg) and xylazine (15 mg/kg). The carotid artery was cannulated and the animals bled to a mean arterial pressure of 45 mmHg which was maintained for 45 min (45/45 shock). Animals were resuscitated to preshock blood pressure with the shed blood and 1.5 vol. normal saline. This preparation has a 15% mortality with all deaths occurring within the first 24 h following shock.

CFU-GM Assay

Both femurs were aseptically removed from a conventional rat and the bone marrow was obtained by flushing each femur with 10 ml of cold McCoy's medium supplemented with essential and non-essential amino acids, vitamins, pyruvate, serine, asparagine, glutamine, and penicillin/streptomycin (all reagents GIBCO, Grand Island, NY, USA) and passed twice through a 21-gauge needle to ensure cell separation. Bone marrow cells were centrifuged at 400 g and suspended in modified McCoy's medium at a concentration of 1×10^6 cells/ml. Bone marrow cells (1×10^5) were plated in triplicate on 35-mm tissue culture plates in 0.3% agar supplemented 10% volume per volume with heat-inactivated fetal calf serum (GIBCO, Grand Island, NY, USA) and either pokeweed mitogen spleen-conditioned medium (PWMSCM) or recombinant murine GM-CSF (a gift of Immunex, Seattle, WA, USA) as source of growth factors [21]. CFU-GM inhibitory activity of the serum was assayed by placing 100 µl of the serum sample (diluted to 20% serum in supplemented McCoy's medium) to be tested directly on the plate prior to the addition of the bone marrow/agar suspension. Plates were incubated for 7 days at 37 ° C in 5% CO_2 and scored for CFU-GM growth using an inverted microscope. CFU-GM colonies consisted of aggregates of more than 50 cells and clusters of between 5 and 50 cells.

Experimental Design

Rats were subjected to hemorrhagic shock as outlined and sacrificed either during shock or at various time-points following resuscitation for determination of plasma endotoxin and CFU-GM inhibitory capacity and blood cultures. Endotoxin was measured from plasma collected in dipyrogenated tubes and assayed by a quantitative colorimetric *Limulus* assay (QCL-1000, M.A. Bioproducts, Walkersville, MD, USA) as reported previously [15]. Pilot studies demonstrated that both plasma and serum was used depending on availability. Additional groups of rats were subjected to hemorrhagic shock for determination of survival.

342   D. H. Livingston et al.

Statistical analysis for survival data were determined using both chi-squared and life table analysis. Data for serum CFU-GM inhibitory activity was determined by comparing CFU-GM growth on plates containing shock serum with plates containing serum obtained from instrumented but unshocked rats (control) and results are reported as the percent of control. Statistical analysis of the percent inhibition was performed using the arcsin transformation on the percentage data followed by a two-tailed Student's t-test or a prior analysis of variance and least significant difference (LSD) test, where appropriate, on the transformed data. Significance was set a priori at the $p < 0.05$ level.

Results

The effect of the different models of hemorrhagic shock on survival are shown in Fig. 1. Germ-free rats had a significantly better survival at both 30/80 and 30/40 shock, than their germ-bearing counterparts. The differences were significant during shock and were maintained at all times following resuscitation ($p < 0.05$). There also were significant differences in survival between the two degrees of hemorrhagic shock (30/80 vs 30/40) in both the germ-free and conventional groups. The mortality of the anesthetized model of hemorrhagic shock (45/45) was 15% with all deaths occurring in the first 24 h.

Serum from rats subjected to hemorrhagic shock, regardless of the severity of the model or the germ-bearing status of the animal, significantly inhibited the growth of CFU-GM (Fig. 2). The inhibitory factors appeared in the serum during shock and were not effected by resuscitation. In germ-free rats, the inhibitory factors had been cleared from the serum by 24 h after shock. In contrast, serum from germ-bearing conventional rats still significantly inhibited myelopoiesis.

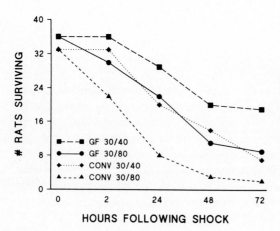

Fig. 1. Survival curves for both germ-free (*GF*) and conventional (*CONV*) rats subjected to 30/40 or 30/80 shock (see "Materials and Methods"). For both 30/40 and 30/80 models there are significant differences in survival at 24, 48, and 72 h between germ-free and conventional rats ($p < 0.05$). There was also an increase in mortality at all time-points ($p < 0.05$) in the 30/80 group vs those rats subjected to 30/40 hemorrhage

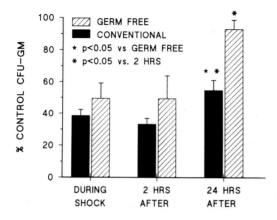

Fig. 2. Serum CFU-GM inhibitory activity from germ-free and conventional rats (pooled data from all models). Data (mean ± SEM) presented as a percentage of control (20% normal serum). Serum from conventional rats was significantly more inhibitory at 24 h than sera from germ-free animals. There is no difference between germ-free and control values ($n = 11$–17 rats per time-point)

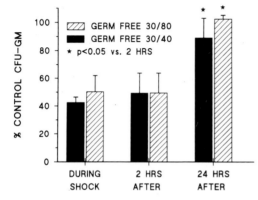

Fig. 3. There were no differences in CFU-GM inhibition between germ-free rats subjected to 30/40 or 30/80 hemorrhagic shock. Percentage growth at 24 h was not different from control ($n = 4$–8 rats per time-point)

The effect of the severity of the shock model was examined in both germ-free (Fig. 3) and conventional (Fig. 4) rats. In germ free animals there were no significant differences between the two models. Even at 30/80, a model with a 75% mortality at 72 h the inhibitory substances were cleared from the serum at 24 h. There were also no differences in CFU-GM inhibitory activity between the conventional rats. The data for conventional 30/80 rats were not different from the other two models. Two differences between the conventional models' shock are the presence of anesthesia and that rats subjected to 45/45 shock have not reached the decompensatory phase of shock. These factors had no impact on myelopoiesis. Serum CFU-GM inhibitory activity was unchanged immediately following resuscitation and it appears that reperfusion did not exacerbate the inhibition.

Serum from conventional rats continued to inhibit CFU-GM growth for up to 7 days following (Fig. 5). A dose-response curve was created using sera from conventional rats (Fig. 6) and demonstrates that as little as 5 μl of serum added to a 1-ml plate significantly inhibits CFU-GM growth.

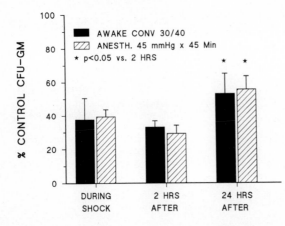

Fig. 4. There were no differences in CFU-GM inhibition between conventional (*CONV*) rats subjected to 30/40 or 45/45 hemorrhagic shock (*ANESTH.*) Percentage growth at 24 h remains significantly less than control (*n* = 4–7 rats per time-point)

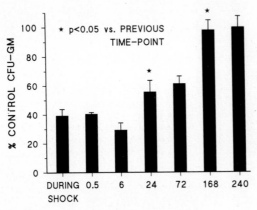

HOURS AFTER SHOCK

Fig. 5. Time course for the disappearance of CFU-GM inhibitory activity from the serum of conventional rats subjected to 45/45 hemorrhage. There is a significant increase in CFU-GM growth at 24 h compared with 6 h postshock. The decrease in growth from 0.5 to 6 h is not statistically significant. The inhibition does not disappear until 7 days following shock (*n* = 4–7 rats per time-point)

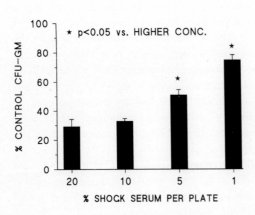

Fig. 6. Dose-response for CFU-GM inhibition from shocked sera obtained from conventional rats subjected to 45/45 shock. Significant differences are seen between 10%, 5%, and 1% shock serum per plate. (*n* = 7 rats)

Endotoxemia was present in approximately one-third of germ-free rats. There were no differences in the CFU-GM inhibition between germ-free animals who were positive for LPS and those who were negative. The rates of endotoxemia and bacteremia in germ-bearing conventional rats were 33%–50% and more than 70% respectively and also had no effect on CFU-GM growth.

Discussion

Hemorrhagic shock regardless of the model used resulted in a uniform inhibition of myelopoiesis. The inhibition was observed in both germ-free and conventional rats, at all levels of hemorrhagic shock, and whether or not anesthesia was used. There are numerous differences between the experimental models used in the laboratory and the severely injured patients on the trauma ward, and the search for comparable, relevant models continues. Older shock models which failed to include adequate resuscitation have been improved to make them more clinically relevant. All of the models described in the above experiments involved pure hemorrhagic shock without tissue injury and were measuring the shock component of injury alone. This is significantly different from what is seen in trauma patients since it has been shown that tissue trauma without shock results in a depression of immunity [22, 23]. All models also utilized low doses of heparin to maintain catheter patency. Chaudry et al. have recently developed a model of hemorrhagic shock without heparin [24] since this may improve blood flow during shock; our injured patients are never heparinized. While we recognize that several different models of shock were used in these experiments, all control animals also received identical treatment and CFU-GM inhibition was demonstrated in all animals subjected to shock.

The two models of shock used differed in two major respects: the presence of anesthesia, and whether or not the animal was allowed to reach the decompensatory phase of shock. In the awake models, all rats reach the decompensatory phase of shock where they require reinfusion of their shed blood to maintain the preselected mean pressure of 30 torr. The magnitude of the shock was controlled by selecting how much blood the animal would have to take back before being fully resuscitated. As was demonstrated, survival was significantly different for both germ-free and conventional 30/40 shock rats than for the rats made to take back 80% of their shed blood prior to resuscitation. In the timed model of shock, anesthetized rats were bled to a mean arterial pressure for 45 min. This time period is prior to the decompensatory phase of shock in almost all animals. The survival of this model is 85%, with almost all deaths occurring in the rats that begin to decompensate prior to 45 min. The data clearly demonstrate that it was not necessary to achieve a decompensatory phase of shock to result in the formation or release of serum inhibitors to myelopoiesis since conventional rats in both models demonstrated equivalent levels of inhibition. While germ-free rats were not subjected to a nondecompensatory model of hemorrhage, a significant number of these rats had not reached that point when they were sacrificed for the determination of intrashock CFU-GM inhibition.

Although the germ-bearing status of the rats had no impact on the release of the serum inhibitors, the recovery period was significantly longer in conventional rats. Serum from germ-free rats, at both degrees of shock, failed to inhibit CFU-GM 24 h after shock. In contrast, the serum from conventional rats continued to inhibit CFU-GM growth until 7 days following shock. The presence of the inhibitors to CFU-GM growth have also been associated with a failure of the animal to have the normal myelopoietic response to LPS. Prolonged recovery of other aspects of immune function have also been demonstrated in murine and rodent models of shock. Stephan et al. reported that IL-2 production [3] and macrophage antigen presentation [25] in mice were depressed for 3–4 days following shock. Livingston and coworkers have shown that rats have an increased susceptibility to bacterial infection for up to 5 days following shock [2]. The data presented in these experiments correlates well with those of other investigators.

One potential explanation for our findings would be that the immune response of the germ-free rat is diminished compared to conventional animals. Germ-free animals have been reported to be more resistant to the lethal effects of LPS than conventional littermates [26]. Rush has extended that observation to also include more resistant to hemorrhagic shock [19]. Kiyono et al. demonstrated however, that germ-free mice had greater in vitro immunogenic response to LPS than either germ-bearing or mono-associated mice [27]. A hyper-immune response to LPS has been associated with an increased mortality. Jurkovich and coworkers demonstrated a significant mortality to a sublethal dose of LPS in rabbits pretreated with interferon-gamma [28]. Although the entire immune response of the germ-free animals has not been elucidated, we feel that the presence of an intact immune system that is at least as reactive as that of conventional rats validates the use of gnotobiotic rats in these experiments.

In conclusion these experiments have demonstrated that hemorrhagic shock results in the creation or release of factors inhibitory to myelopoiesis independent of the severity of the shock model employed. Translocation of bacteria or endotoxin had no effect on the genesis of these factors, and we feel that ischemia alone probably accounts for their appearance. However, bacterial translocation did influence the disappearance of CFU-GM inhibitory activity from the serum of shocked animals and may play an important role in the persistent immune dysfunction and susceptibility to infection seen following shock and injury. The difficulty associated with quantifying small doses of LPS in the serum, and the markedly different LPS content of the gut between conventional and germ-free rats makes the contribution of endotoxemia independent of bacterial translocation CFU-GM inhibition difficult to interpret. Measurable LPS did not influence serum CFU-GM inhibitory activity and the future development of a endotoxin-depleted animal model in our laboratory may help to answer these questions.

References

1. Esrig BC, Frazee L, Stephenson SF et al. (1977) The predisposition to infection following hemorrhagic shock. Surg Gynecol Obstet 144:915–919
2. Livingston DH, Malangoni MA (1988) An experimental study of susceptibility to infection after hemorrhagic shock. Surg Gynecol Obstet 168:138–142
3. Stephan RN, Kupper TS, Geha AS, Baue AE, Chaudry IH (1987) Hemorrhage without tissue trauma produces immunosuppression and enhances susceptibility to sepsis. Arch Surg 122:62–67
4. Hofstetter SF, Pachter HL, Bailey AA, Coppa GF (1984) Prospective comparison of two regimens of prophylactic antibiotics in abdominal trauma: cefoxitin versus triple drug. J. Trauma 24:307–310
5. Jones RC, Thal ER, Johnson NA, Gollihar LN (1985) Evaluation of antibiotic therapy following penetrating abdominal trauma. Ann Surg 201:576–585
6. Fink MP, Gardiner M, MacVittie TJ (1985) Sublethal hemorrhage impairs the acute peritoneal inflammatory response in the rat. J Trauma 25:234–237
7. Abraham EH, Chang YH (1986) Cellular and humoral bases of hemorrhage-induced depression of lymphocyte function. Crit Care Med 14:81–86
8. Livingston DH, Gentile PS, Malangoni MA (1990) Bone marrow failure following hemorrhagic shock. Circ Shock 30:255–264
9. Sori AJ, Rush BF, Lysz TW et al. (1988) The gut as source of sepsis after hemorrhagic shock. Am J Surg 155:187–192
10. Deitch EA, Winterton J, Li M et al. (1987) The gut as portal of entry for bacteremia. Ann Surg 205:681–691
11. Wells CL, Maddus MA, Simmons RL (1988) Proposed mechanisms for the translocation of intestinal bacteria. Rev Infect Dis 10:958–979
12. Mora EM, Cardona MA, Simmons RL (1991) Enteric bacteria and ingested inert particles translocate to intraperitoneal prosthetic materials. Arch Surg 126:157–163
13. Deitch EA, Berg RD (1987) Endotoxin but not malnutrition promotes translocation of the gut flora in burned mice. J Trauma 27:161–165
14. Redan JA, Rush BF Jr, McCollough JN et al. (1990) Organ distribution of radiolabeled enteric *Escherichia coli* during and after hemorrhagic shock. Ann Surg 211:663–668
15. Rush BF, Jr, Sori AJ, Murphy TF et al. (1988) Endotoxemia and bacteremia during hemorrhagic shock. The link between trauma and sepsis? Ann Surg 207:549–554
16. Koziol JM, Rush BF Jr, Smith SM et al. (1988) Occurrence of bacteremia during and after hemorrhagic shock. J Trauma 28:10–16
17. Deitch EA (1989) Simple intestinal obstruction causes bacterial translocation in man. Arch Surg 124:699–701
18. Guiot HFL, et al. (1983) Selective antimicrobial modulation of the intestinal flora of patients with acute non-lymphocytic leukemia: a randomized double-blind placebo-controlled study. J Infect Dis 147:615–621
19. Rush BF Jr, Redan JA, Flanagan JJ et al. (1989) Does the bacteremia observed in hemorrhagic shock have clinical significance? A study in germ-free animals. Ann Surg 210:342–347
20. McLafferty MA, Goldmen P (1981) Germ free rats. In: □ Methods in enzymology. Academic, New York, pp 34–43
21. Metcalf D, Johnson GR, Mandel TF (1979) Colony formation in agar by multipotential hematopoietic cells. J Cell Physiol 98:401–411
22. Faist E, Mewes A, Strasser T et al. (1988) Alteration of monocyte function following major injury. Arch Surg 123:287–292
23. Polk HC Jr, George CD, Wellhausen SR et al. (1986) A systematic study of host defense processes in badly injured patients. Ann Surg 204:282–299
24. Wang P, Singh G, Rana MW, Ba ZF, Chaudry IH (1990) Preheparinization improves organ function after hemorrhage and resuscitation. Am J Physiol 244:R645–650
25. Stephan RN, Ayala A, Dean RE, Border JR, Chaudry IH (1989) Mechanism of immunosuppression following hemorrhagic shock: defective antigen presentation by macrophages. J Surg Res 46:553–556
26. Jensen SB, Mergenhagen SE, Fitzgerald RJ, Jordan HV (1963) Susceptibility of conventional and germ-free mice to the lethal effects of endotoxin. Proc Soc Exp Biol Med 113:710–717

27. Kiyono H, McGhee JR, Michalek SM (1980) Lipopolysaccharide regulation of the immune response: comparison of the responses to LPS in germ-free, *Escherichia coli*-monoassociated and conventional mice. Infect Immun 124:36–41
28. Jurkovich GL, Mileski WD, Maier RV et al. (1991) Interferon gamma increases sensitivity to endotoxin. J Surg Res 51:197–203

Monocyte HLA-DR Antigen Expression:
Its Reproducibility in Asymptomatic Volunteers
and Correlation with Clinical Infection*

W. G. Cheadle, M. J. Hershman, S. R. Wellhausen, and H. C. Polk Jr

Introduction

Trauma victims are an immunodepressed group of patients at high risk for infection because many facets of the immune response are depressed following severe injury [1–3]. These include delayed hypersensitivity [4], immunoglobulin production [5], and serum opsonic capacity [6], in addition to macrophage, lymphocyte, and neutrophil function [7, 8].

Failure of most (70%) peripheral blood monocytes to express the HLA-DR antigen by the 7th day after injury closely correlated with the development of infection and death in severely injured patients [9, 10]. In that study, incubation of patient monocytes with lipopolysaccharide (LPS) increased HLA-DR expression into the normal range in those who survived but not in those who died. Ertel et al. [11] and Ayala et al. [12] have correlated defective macrophage antigen presentation with decreased immune-associated expression following hemorrhage and infection.

Methods

Subject Age, Gender, Race, and Genetic Inheritance. Seventy-seven white volunteers (29 men and 48 women) had blood samples drawn to determine monocyte HLA-DR antigen expression [13]. The volunteers ranged in age from 20 to 91 years. To study the effect of race on monocyte HLA-DR antigen expression, blood samples were collected from an additional 20 black and 10 Asian volunteers who were in good health. Their monocyte HLA-DR antigen expression values were compared with values for the initial 77 subjects described above.

Determination of Monocyte HLA-DR Antigen Expression. The expression of HLA-DR antigen on monocytes was determined using fluorescent-labeled dual

* This work was supported by the John W. and Caroline Price Foundation, Price Institute of Surgical
Research, University of Louisville School of Medicine, Louisville, Kentucky.
Department of Surgery and Price Institute of Surgical Research, University of Louisville School of Medicine, Louisville, KY 40292, USA

monoclonal antibody staining and flow microfluorometric analysis as previously described [6]. In addition, paired aliquots of blood were incubated with LPS (10 µg/ml) for 2 h and then analyzed as described above.

Immunosuppressive Medication. Twenty-six patients who had undergone renal transplantation and who were on maintenance doses of immunosuppressive therapy had blood samples drawn for monocyte HLA-DR antigen determination. None had clinical or laboratory evidence of infection. The immunosuppressive regimens included prednisolone in four patients; cyclosporine and prednisolone in five; azathioprine and prednisolone in nine; and cyclosporine, azathioprine, and prednisolone in eight.

Elective Abdominal Operations. During the study period, 24 consecutive patients underwent elective laparotomy: ten for cholelithiasis, five for peptic ulcer, three for aortoiliac occlusive disease, three for colon carcinoma, two for diverticulosis, and one for aortic aneurysm. Blood samples to determine the monocyte HLA-DR antigen expression were drawn preoperatively and on postoperative days 1, 3, 5, 7, 10, 14, and 21.

Major Infection. Twenty-one patients who were randomly studied over a 6-month period included ten patients with bacteremia, nine with pneumonia, and two with necrotizing myofascitis. Nine of these patients died of their infection. One blood sample to determine monocyte HLA-DR antigen expression was drawn from each patient during the ongoing clinical episode of major infection.

Results

Effect of Subject Age, Gender, Race and Genetic Inheritance

The percentage of peripheral blood monocytes that expressed the HLA-DR antigen had a binomial distribution. The mean $\pm$ SEM was 85.0% $\pm$ 1.2%. After 2-h incubation with LPS, the mean percentage of monocytes expressing the antigen was increased to 94.0% $\pm$ 0.75%. Both the percentage of monocytes that expressed HLA-DR antigen and monocyte HLA-DR anitgen mean fluorescence intensity varied little with age. HLA-DR antigen expression in the 29 men was 86.4% $\pm$ 2.0%, which was similar to the mean of 84.1% $\pm$ 1.4% for the 48 women. There were no significant differences between the mean monocyte HLA-DR antigen expression of Asians (88.1% $\pm$ 2.6%), blacks, (78.0% $\pm$ 2.8%), or whites (85.0% $\pm$ 1.2%). There was also no significant difference in mean fluorescence intensity between subjects of different gender and race.

In determining the effect of delayed analysis on monocyte HLA-DR antigen expression, mean values decreased linearly from 86% at time 0 to 0% at 19 days.

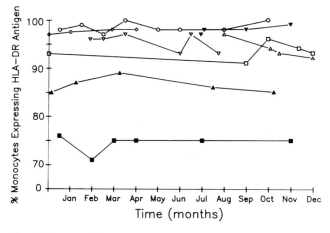

Fig. 1. Monocyte HLA-DR expression over long periods of time in eight subjects (each *symbol* denotes a different subject). (From [13])

Similarly, mean fluorescence intensity decreased from 156 to 0 in linear fashion over the same time period. Similarly, there was no apparent effect of cyclical variation on monocyte HLA-DR antigen expression (Fig. 1).

Effect of Immunosuppressive Therapy

The mean percentages of monocytes that expressed the antigen were similar: prednisolone alone 80.4% ± 6.0%; cyclosporine and prednisolone 82.1% ±9.2%; azathioprine and prednisolone 75.0% ± 5.9%; and azathioprine, prednisolone, and cyclosporine 81.4% ± 45%. Mean fluorescence intensity ranged from 161 to 229 and the mean was similar to the normal mean.

Effect of Abdominal Surgical Procedures and Wound Infection

Following general anesthesia and elective laparotomy, 19 of 24 patients recovered without infection. Five patients developed operative wound infection 5–7 days after operation, with pus discharging from the wound between 7 and 14 days postoperatively. The mean percentage of peripheral blood monocytes that expressed HLA-DR antigen in the 19 uninfected patients prior to operation was 85.6% ± 2.5% and the mean fluorescence intensity was 440 ± 92. The mean percentage of monocytes with HLA-DR antigen expression of these 19 patients was significantly reduced from the preoperative value on day 1 and 3 after surgery ($P < 0.01$), but rapidly returned towards preoperative values by postoperative day 5. Although preoperative values of the percentage of monocytes with HLA-DR antigen expression in the five patients who developed infection (80.0%

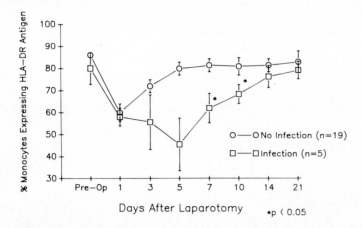

Fig. 2. Monocyte HLA-DR expression following general anesthesia and laparotomy and its relation to infection. *indicates difference ($P < 0.05$; Student's t test). (From [13])

$\pm 6.3\%$) were similar to the 19 uninfected patients, values were reduced compared with the uninfected group on postoperative days 3–10, achieving significance on the 7th and 10th postoperative days (Fig. 2). Mean fluorescence intensity, however, increased over the first 3 days postoperatively to 538 ± 75 in the uninfected patients before returning to preoperative levels at 1 week. In those patients who developed wound infections, mean fluorescence intensity was significantly less ($P < 0.05$) preoperatively (232 ± 91) than the group without infection and remained so for the first 7 days after surgery.

Effect of Major Infection

The mean value of $38.2\% \pm 2.0\%$ for monocyte HLA-DR antigen expression of the 21 patients with active major infection was significantly less than the mean of $85.0\% \pm 1.2\%$ for the normal distribution ($P < 0.01$). Although the mean monocyte HLA-DR antigen expression values of $32.4\% \pm 5.0\%$ for patients who died of sepsis was lower than the mean value of $43.7\% \pm 3.9\%$ for those who survived, there was no statistical significance (Fig. 3). However, the mean fluorescence intensity of the group that survived (95.1 ± 7.2) was significantly greater than that of those who died (73.9 ± 7.4; $P < 0.05$). After in vitro incubation with LPS, the 12 surviving infected patients had mean monocyte HLA-DR antigen expression values of $88\% \pm 3.3\%$, which was significantly greater ($P < 0.05$) than the mean value of $53\% \pm 6.5\%$ observed after LPS incubation in the nine patients who died (Fig. 3).

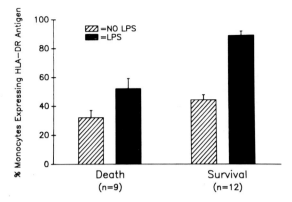

Fig. 3. Monocyte HLA-DR expression with and without LPS incubation and its relation to clinical outcome in 21 patients with severe infection. The difference between two LPS groups was significant (Student's *t* test). (From [13])

Discussion

Peripheral blood monocyte HLA-DR expression correlates significantly with patient outcome following major trauma, both in development and recovery from major infection and in death from such infection [9]. The present study of asymptomatic volunteers shows remarkable reproducibility. Little effect from age, race, or gender on the ability of the monocytes to express HLA-DR antigen or on mean fluorescence intensity was apparent. We found that HLA-DR expression decreased very quickly in stored blood, with no detectable surface antigen 19 days after collection. The assay of whole blood used in our laboratory avoids such cellular manipulation and induces minimal changes in HLA-DR antigen expression [14].

LPS is thought to induce migration of previously synthesized HLA-DR antigen within the cytoplasm to the cell surface [15]. The ability to express HLA-DR antigen after LPS incubation correlated with survival in the severely infected patients here as well as in a previous study of trauma patients [6]. Inability to express HLA-DR antigen, manifested by low percentages of monocytes that expressed this antigen after LPS incubation, was associated with a poor prognosis in these septic patients.

There was a lower mean percentage of monocytes that expressed HLA-DR antigen and lower mean fluorescence intensity in patients with postoperative infection and in those with severe sepsis. Of note was the group of 19 noninfected patients who had relatively high mean fluorescence intensity, compared with the overall volunteer group. There may be an increased expression in anticipation of major surgery in those destined to recover without infection; or, alternatively, this may have been a select group who had a relatively high normal mean fluorescence intensity value. The percentage of peripheral blood monocytes that express HLA-DR antigen appears to be an accurate marker of both the infection and diseases associated with immunodepression. However, immunosuppressive medication does not appear to reduce HLA-DR antigen expression either acutely or on a long-term basis. It seems likely that multiple mechanisms are in play that contribute to reduced HLA-DR expression, including influx of immature cells into peripheral blood that are low expressers, internalization of antigen, and increased antigen turnover. The data presented characterize such antigen expression as a valid correlate of major infection, which can also be used to identify the patient at high risk for such infection.

References

1. Faist E, Kupper TS, Baker CC, Chaudry IH, Dwyer J, Baue AE (1986) Depression of cellular immunity after major injury: its association with posttraumatic complications and its reversal with immunomodulation. Arch Surg 121:1000–1005
2. Ninnemann JL, Ozkan AN (1985) Definition of a burn injury-induced immunosuppressive serum component. J Trauma 25:113–117
3. O'Mahony JB, Palder SB, Wood JJ et al. (1984) Depression of cellular immunity after multiple trauma in the absence of sepsis. J Trauma 24:869–875
4. Meakins JL, Pietch JB, Bubenick O et al. (1977) Delayed hypersensitivity: indicator of acquired failure of host defenses in sepsis and trauma. Ann Surg 186:241–250
5. Hershman MJ, Cheadle WG, George CD et al. (1988) The response of immunoglobulins to infection after thermal and nonthermal injury. Am Surg 54:408–411
6. Polk HC Jr, George CD, Hershman MJ, Wellhausen SR, Cheadle WG (1988) The capacity of serum to support neutrophil phagocytosis is a vital host defense mechanism in severely injured patients. Ann Surg 207:686–692
7. Antonacci AC, Reaves LE, Calvano SE, Amand R, De Riesthal HF, Shires GT (1984) Flow cytometric analysis of lymphocyte subpopulations after thermal injury in human beings. Surg Gynecol Obstet 159:1–8
8. Christou NV, Meakins JL (1979) Neutrophil function in anergic surgical patients: neutrophil adherence and chemotaxis. Ann Surg 190:557–564
9. Hershman MJ, Cheadle WG, Kuftinec D, Polk HC Jr, George CD (1988) An outcome predictive score for sepsis and death following trauma. Injury 19:263–266
10. Polk HC Jr, George CD, Wellhausen SR et al. (1986) A systematic study of host defense processes in badly injured patients. Ann Surg 204:282–299
11. Ertel W, Meldrum DR, Morrison MH, Ayala A, Chaudry IH (1990) Immunoprotective effect of a calcium channel blocker on macrophage antigen presentation function, Ia expression and interleukin-1 synthesis following hemorrhage. Surgery 108:154–160
12. Ayala A, Perrin MM, Chaudry IH (1990) Defective macrophage antigen presentation following hemorrhage is associated with the loss of MHC class II (Ia) antigens. Immunology 70:33–39
13. Cheadle WG, Hershmann MJ, Wellhausen SR, Polk HC Jr (1991) HLA-DR antigen expression on peripheral blood monocytes correlates with surgical infection. Am J Surg 161:639–645
14. Appel SH, Wellhausen SR, Montgomery R, DeWeese RC, Polk HC Jr (1989) Experimental and clinical significance of endotoxin-dependent HLA-DR expression on monocytes. J Surg Res 47:39–44
15. McLeish KR, Wellhausen SR, Dean WL (1987) Biochemical basis of HLA-DR and CR3 modulation on human peripheral blood monocytes by lipopolysaccharide. Cell Immunol 108:242–248

Phenotypic and Functional Characteristics of Peripheral Blood Lymphocytes in a Defined Group of Polytrauma Patients

G. C. Spagnoli, M. Heberer, P. Vogelbach, R. Rosso, J. Jörgensen, and F. Harder

Introduction

A relevant percentage of polytrauma patients present severe impairments in immune status leading to an increased susceptibility to infections [1]. The nature and mechanisms underlying this defective immunoresponsiveness are poorly understood [2]. A number of studies have underlined the reduced in vitro proliferative capacity of peripheral blood lymphocytes from trauma patients upon stimulation with conventional mitogens, including phytohemagglutinin and concanavalin A [3].

Considering the pivotal role played by the T cell receptor complex (CD3-Ti) in the activation of T lymphocytes [4], the in vitro responsiveness of severely injured polytrauma patients to stimulation induced by mitogenic anti-CD3 monoclonal antibodies (MAb) was investigated in the current study. In parallel, phenotypic characteristics of the cell population under study were also analyzed.

Materials and Methods

Patients. Ten patients (six men, four women; mean age 32.9, range 16–66) were included in the study, presenting injury severity scores above or equal to 20 as defined by the American College of Surgeons [5]. Ten sex- and age-matched healthy donors were also studied.

Phenotypic studies. Heparinized whole blood samples (50 µl) were incubated for 15 min at room temperature in the presence of commercial, fluorochrome-labeled MAb (Becton Dickinson, Mountain View, CA, USA) at optimal dilution. Erythrocytes were then lysed by incubation (10 min, room temperature) in the presence of a commercial FACS lysing solution (Becton Dickinson). The cell suspension was repeatedly washed, and specific fluorescence was evaluated by FACScan cytofluorometer equipped with Simulset software, both from Becton Dickinson. Data are reported as percentage of the relevant cell population stained with the specific MAb.

Departments of Surgery and Research, Kantonspital, Spitalstr. 21, 4031 Basel, Basel, Switzerland.

Host Defense Dysfunction
in Trauma, Shock and Sepsis
Eds. Faist/Meakins/Schildberg
© Springer-Verlag, Berlin Heidelberg 1993

Functional Studies. Peripheral blood mononuclear cells (PBMNC) were isolated from heparinized blood samples by gradient centrifugation according to standard techniques [6]. Cells were then counted and resuspended in culture medium (RPMI additioned with 5% AB serum, glutamine, and antibiotics) at 10^6 cells/ml final concentration. T cell receptor complex specific activation [7] was provided by a mitogenic monoclonal antibody (CB3G, courtesy of Prof. Malavasi, Turin, Italy), used in ascitic form at a 1:10 000 final dilution. Cultures were established in 0.2-ml volumes in 96-well plates (Costar, Cambridge, MA, USA) and incubated for 72 h in humidified, 5% CO_2 atmosphere at 37 °C. Tritiated thymidine (0.5 μCi/well) was added for the last 6 h of culture. Cells were then harvested, and isotope incorporation was evaluated by beta counting according to standard procedures. Data were expressed as cpm ± standard deviation.

Results and Discussion

Initial phenotypic analysis performed on day 1 after trauma showed a significant increase in the percentage of mononuclear cells bearing classic monocyte markers such as CD14 and CD45 in the patient group as compared with healthy controls. On the other hand, no differences were detected in the percentages of $CD3^+$ cells in the two groups. It is of interest, however, that increased percentages of $CD8^+$ and decreased percentages of $CD4^+$ T lymphocytes were observed in patients as compared with healthy controls. In addition, no significant variations were observed as far as B and natural killer (NK) cells were concerned.

As transferrin receptor (TfR) represents an activation marker on lymphocytes, we also studied its expression in patients' cells. Again, only a nonsignificant decrease in the percentage of TfR^+ lymphocytes was detectable in the patient group (Table 1).

Table 1. Peripheral blood mononuclear cells subsets in healthy donors and polytrauma patients (day 1 after trauma)

	Healthy donors (n = 13)	Patients (n = 10)
Monocytes (CD14$^+$/CD45$^+$)[a]	18.2 ± 4	44.4 ± 10
T lymphocytes (CD3$^+$)[b]	73.6 ± 5	75.2 ± 8
CD4^{+b}	49.1 ± 5	37.5 ± 9
CD8^{+b}	35.1 ± 6	39.1 ± 7
B cells (CD12$^+$)[b]	11.9 ± 3	16.3 ± 6
NK cells (CD16$^+$/CD56$^+$)[b]	16.1 ± 5	9.6 ± 5
Transferrin-R^{+b}	23.4 ± 8	19.3 ± 7

[a] % of total MNC.
[b] % of gated lymphocytes.

At the same time, PBMNC from nine patients and controls were stimulated in vitro with anti-CD3 MAb in 3-day cultures. As reported in Table 2, lymphocyte proliferation, measured as [^{3}H] thymidine incorporation, was found to be significantly lower in the patient group compared with controls. These results prompted us to evaluate the proliferative capacity of anti-CD3 stimulated lymphocytes from eight polytrauma patients during their clinical course.

Our data, reported in Fig. 1, indicate that in four patients (L.W.,C. Z.,J.Z. and S.D.) a brisk, further decrease in anti-CD3 stimulated blastogenesis was observed within 2–4 days after the trauma followed by a recovery starting from days 4–10. In two other patients (J.W. and H.K.) an increase in responsiveness, although of different extent, was detected; no major variations were reported in the remaining two patients (B.G. and T.K.). It is of interest that during the

Table 2. Anti-CD3 induced proliferation in healthy donors and polytrauma patients (day 1 after trauma)

	Controls (n = 10)	Patients (n = 9)
Negative	271 ± 221	229 ± 176
αCD3	46.405 ± 18.347	25.084 ± 20561[a]

[a] AOV:$p = 0.0287$.

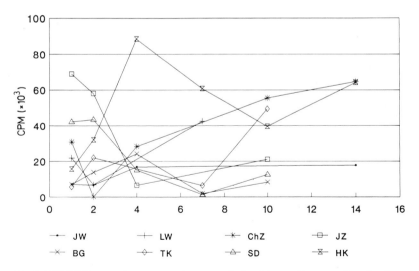

Fig. 1. PBMNC from polytrauma patients were isolated by gradient centrifugation from heparinized blood samples drawn on the indicated days. Cells were cultured in RPMI 5% AB serum in the presence of anti-CD3 MAb in ascitic form, at 1:10000 final dilution, for 3 days. Proliferation was measured by [^{3}H] thymidine incorporation and data expressed as cpm × 10^3. Symbols refer to data obtained from individual patients

observation period no significant variations of the percentages of $CD3^+$ cells were reported in patients PBMNC (data not shown).

Considering that anti-CD3 MAb activate lymphocytes by triggering the antigen receptor complex on T cells, thus mimicking the physiological interaction with HLA-bound antigenic peptides, our data underline that responsiveness to this stimulus could be markedly impaired in polytrauma patients, despite the presence of normal amounts of T cells. The mechanisms underlying this defective response warrants further investigations. At the present time, however, our data do not confirm a statistically significant correlation between in vitro anti-CD3 induced lymphoproliferation and the clinical course of the patients under study.

References

1. Delire M (1988) Immune disorders after severe injury. Ann Biol Clin 46:272–275
2. Richter M, Jodouin CA, Moher D, Barron P (1990) Immunologic defects following trauma: a delay in immunoglobulin synthesis by cultured B cells following traumatic accidents but not elective surgery. J Trauma 30:590–596
3. Howard RJ (1980) Cell-mediated immune defense against infection. Curr Probl Surg 17:267–316
4. Weiss A (1990) Structur and function of the T cell antigen receptor. J Clin Invest 86:1015–1022
5. Civil ID, Schwab CW (1988) The abbreviated Injury Scale, 1985 revision: a condensed chart for clinical use. J Trauma 28:87–90
6. Spagnoli GC, Ausiello CM, Cassone A, Casciani CU, Bellone G, Malavasi F (1987) Inhibitory effects of anti HLA-A-B-C heavy chain and anti beta 2 microglobulin monoclonal antibodies on alloantigen and microbial antigen induced immune responses in vitro. Scand J Immunol 25:555–565
7. Funaro A, Spagnoli GC, Ausiello CM, Alessio M, Roggero S, Delia D, Zaccolo M, Malavasi F (1990) Involvement of the multilineage CD38 molecule in a unique pathway of cell activation and proliferation. J Immunol 145:2390–2396.

Cell-Mediated Immunity During and After Cardiopulmonary Bypass

A. Paccagnella[1], S. De Angeli[2], M. Mordacchini[2], G. Caenaro[3], A. Nieri[2], P. Rosi[1], P. Michielon[1], M. Calò[1], G. Zanardo[1], L. Salvador[4], C. Furlan[5], and G. Simini[1]

Introduction

The effects of anesthesia and surgery on cellular immunological function has been extensively studied [1–4] but it has been shown that anesthesia in open heart surgery has only minor immunological effects [5]. In contrast, extracorporeal circulation (ECC) has been known to contribute to the morbidity and mortality of cardiac surgery because of a decrease in immunological function. This study has investigated the effects of ECC on cell-mediated immunity.

Patients and Methods

Twenty coronary patients admitted for open heart surgery were considered (mean age: 56.4 ± 8.4 years, number of coronary bypasses 3.3 ± 0.8, and duration of ECC: 103 ± 24 min). No immunological diseases were described and no immunosuppressive or immunostimulating therapies were carried out before surgery. The operations were performed under generalized hypothermia ($27\,°C$) as previously described [5]. No blood or plasma derivates were transfused during or after surgery. No complications occured and no high dose drugs were used in this group.

Blood samples were taken (a) before the induction of anesthesia, (b) before and, (c) after the ECC, (d) after surgery (at skin closure), (e) on postoperative day 1, and (f) on postoperative day 7. The following factors were examined: (a) activation of T lymphocytes (LY) by mitogens, (b) variation of LY subsets, and (c) study of white blood cells by scanning electronic microscopy (SEM). The mitogens were phytohemagglutinin (PHA) and concanavalin A (Con-A), used at 0.625, 1.25, 2.5, and $5\,\mu l\,ml^{-1}$ and 0.625, 1.25, 2.5, 5, and $10\,\mu l\,ml^{-1}$, respectively. The tests were performed according to Mottolesi [6]. LY subsets were obtained

[1] II Servizio Anestesia Rianimazione, Ospedale S. Maria de' Battuti, 31100 Treviso, Italy
[2] Centro di Immunoematologia-Trasfusionale, Ospedale S. Maria de' Battuti, 31100 Treviso, Italy
[3] Laboratorio Analisi Chimico-Fisiche, Ospedale S. Maria de' Battuti, 31100 Treviso, Italy
[4] Divisione Cardiochirurgica, Ospedale S. Maria de' Battuti, 31100 Treviso, Italy
[5] CUGAS Università di Padova, 35100 Padova, Italy

Host Defense Dysfunction
in Trauma, Shock and Sepsis
Eds. Faist/Meakins/Schildberg
© Springer-Verlag, Berlin Heidelberg 1993

using flow cytometry (FACScan Machine, Becton Dickinson Immunocytometry Systems, California) and quality controls were made according to Martini
[7]. SEM was performed using a StereoScan 2000 Microscope (Cambridge, UK)
[8]. Student's t test was used to compare the LY transformation and test of
variance was used to study the LY subsets variation. A p value of less than 0.05
was considered statistically significant and correlation test was used when
possible.

Results

The PHA and Con-A responses generally declined after anesthesia induction
and a further decrease was noted after the institution of ECC. A significant
variation was found for Con-A at 5 µl ml^{-1} in samples c, d, and e ($p < 0.01, 0.05$,
and 0.05 respectively) and at 1.2 µl ml^{-1} concentration in samples c, d, e, and f
($p < 0.05$). Analogous results were observed for PHA at 1.2 and 2.5 µl ml^{-1}
($p < 0.05$ vs baseline in samples c, d, and e). In the last sample a nonsignificant
depressed transformation was found for all Con-A concentrations (Fig. 1).

The analysis of LY subsets showed that ECC reduced the number of T and B
cells (Fig. 2) as follows: total B cells:$f = 3.56$, $p < 0.007$; percent B cells: 3.7,
$f = 3.7$, $p < 0.006$; total CD4: $f = 4.02$, $p < 0.004$.; percent CD4 $f = 1.2$, $p = $ n.s.;
total CD8:$f = 1.0$, $p = $ n.s.; percent-CD8:$f = 4.48$, $p < 0.002$; total CD57:
$f = 2.0, p = $ n.s.; percent CD57:$f = 1.1, p = $ n.s. Total white blood cells increased
significantly ($f = 1.2$, $p < 0.01$) mainly due to the rise in the number of granulocytes.

The SEM study performed before and after ECC showed a significant
decrease in LY membrane "villosity".

Discussion

In our previous study [5] the T lymphocyte reactivity showed a remarkable
decrease in cell activation starting in the early postoperative phase. The results
of the present study are consistent with these findings. The PHA and Con-A
responses that are a measure of T-cell function decrease in all patients even if the
maximal effects were observed after the ECC and on the first postoperative day.
These results also confirm previously studies performed in leukemic patients
[9, 10] and the Ryhaenen [11] and Salo [12] observations, who found depressed
LY transformation after the institution of ECC and surgery. In contrast with
Genetet [13], the T-cell-dependent lymphocyte responses are not completely
restored on the seventh postoperative day.

A significant reduction in total T-cells, T-helper cells, T-suppressor cells, and
B lymphocytes was noted after ECC and during postoperative time. These

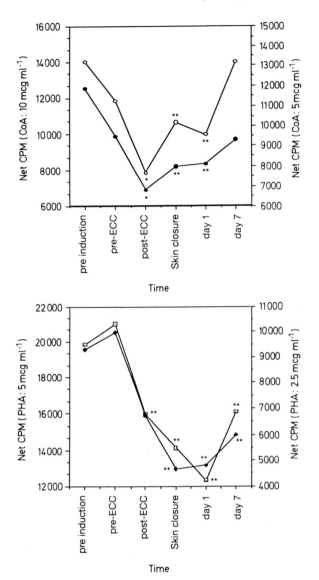

Fig. 1a – b. Activation of T lymphocytes by **a** PHA and **b** Con-A during and after cardiac surgery. *Open circles*, Con-A (10 µg ml⁻¹); *closed circles*, Con-A (5 µg ml⁻¹); *open boxes*, PHA (5 µg ml⁻¹); *closed boxes*, PHA (2.5 µg ml⁻¹). Statistical results versus baseline; $*p < 0.01$; $**p < 0.05$

findings confirm those in the report by Tønnesen [14], who observed a significant reduction in the number of T lymphocytes after cardiac surgery.

The villosity decrease in the white cell membrane observed in the present study seems to confirm a direct correlation between ECC and damage to the membrane structure. The absence of blocking factors suppressing the white

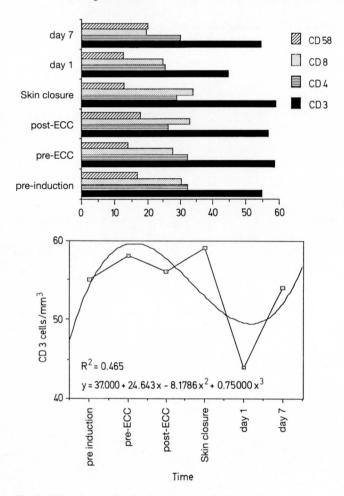

Fig. 2. T-lymphocyte distribution during and after cardiac surgery

blood cell reactivity in plasma samples obtained at the end of surgery [15] suggests that the impairment of LY function may be related either to the direct trauma or to the rapid plasma micro alterations due to the heart-lung machine, even though changes involving endocrine stress response or other variables could not be excluded. Although many studies have demonstrated that cardiac surgery and ECC cause a significant deterioration in cell-mediated immunological response, it is at present impossible to evaluate the real contribution of immunological impairment to postoperative septic complication rates. On the other hand, the immediate deterioration of skin test results following cardiac surgery [16] and the documented relationship existing between ECC time and

$$y = -0.93333 + 0.43280x + 0.30635x^2 - 4.0741e - 2x^3$$

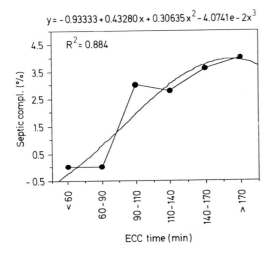

Fig. 3. Septic complications vs ECC time in 687 cardiac patients

septic complication (Fig. 3) seem to confirm the belief that prolonged open heart surgery may influence the outcome of ill patients.

References

1. Watkins J, Salo M (1982) Trauma, Stress and immunity in anesthesia and surgery. Butterworth, London
2. Tonnesen E, Mickley H, Grunnet N (1983) Natural killer cell activity during premedication, anesthesia and surgery. Acta Anesthesiol Scand 27:238–241
3. Hole A (1984) Pre- and postoperative monocyte and lymphocyte functions: effects of combined epidural and general anesthesia. Acta Anesthesiol Scand 28:367–371
4. Finlayson DC (1989) Immunologic changes in critically ill patients after anesthesia and surgery. Anesth Clin North Am 7:883–895
5. Paccagnella A, de Angeli S, Caenaro G et al. (1988) Variazioni della reattività T-linfocitaria in corso di bypass cardiopolmonare: indagine preliminare. Bypass 11:88–90
6. Mottolesi M, Apollony C, Carbone A (1978) Stimolazione linfocitaria in vitro: metodiche. In: Atti corso teorico-pratico di immunologia dei tumori, Roma
7. Martini, E, Dihautcourt JL, Brando B et al. (1989) First European quality control of cellular phenotyting by flow cytometry. Frison-Roche, Paris
8. Scala C, Pasquilli C (1987) Microscopia elettronica a scansione in biologia. CLEUB, Bologna
9. Paccagnella A, de Angeli S, Caenaro G et al. (1988) Cardiopulmonary bypass in leukemic patients. Ann Thorac Surg 45:588
10. Paccagnella A, Marconi L, de Angeli S et al. (1989) Alteration immunologique subordinnee au bypass cardiopulmonaire chez des malades leucemiques. CECEC 32:119–122
11. Ryhaenen P, Herva E, Hollmen A et al. (1979) Changes in peripheral blood leucocyte counts, lymphocytes subpopulations, and in vitro transformation after heart valve replacement. J Thorac Cardiovasc Surg 77:259–266
12. Salo M (1978) Effects of anesthesia and open heart surgery on lymphocyte responses to phytohaemagglutinin and concanavalin A. Acta Anesthesiol Scand 22:471–479
13. Genetet N, Sapene M, Genetet B et al. (1982) Modifications immunitaires après chirurgie cardiaque faite sous ciculation extra-corporelle. Nouv Press Med 6:433–437

14. Tønnesen E, Brinkløv MM, Christenen NJ et al. (1987) Natural killer cell activity and lymphocytes function during and after coronary artery bypass grafting in relation to the endocrine stress response. Anesthesiology 67:526–533
15. van Velzen-Blad H, Dijkstra YJ, Heijnen CJ et al. (1985) Cardiopulmonary bypass and host defence function in human being: II. Lymphocyte function. Ann Thorac Surg 39:212–217
16. Kress HG, Gehrsitz P, Elert O (1987) Predictive value of skin test in neutrophil migration, and C-reactive protein for postoperative infections in cardiopulmonary bypass patients. Acta Anesthesiol Scand 31:397–404

Alterations in Function and Phenotype of Monocytes from Patients with Septic Disease: Predictive Value and New Therapeutic Strategies

H. D. Volk[1], M. Thieme[1,2], U. Ruppe[1,2], S. Heym[1], W. D. Döcke[1], D. Manger[2], S. Zuckermann[2], A. Golosubow[3], B. Nieter[4], H. Klug[3], and R. van Baehr[1]

Introduction

Recently we described the usefulness of immune monitoring as a guide for immunosuppression in allograft recipients with septic complications [1]. From cytofluorometric analyses of mononuclear cells (MNC), the HLA-DR antigen expression on monocytes seems to be the most important diagnostic parameter for the clinical management of immunosuppressed patients with sepsis. A restitution of diminished HLA-DR antigen expression on monocytes after rapid decline of immunosuppression was associated with a favorable outcome of sepsis [1]. Further studies on surgical patients suffering from septic disease (peritonitis as septic focus) not receiving therapeutically induced immunosuppression confirmed the predictive value of HLA-DR antigen expression on monocytes for clinical outcome [2, 3]. Taking a proportion of HLA-DR+ monocytes lower than 20% as the threshold for predicting fatal outcome, we correctly classified survivors and nonsurvivors in all but one case ($n = 38$) between the 5th and 7th days after admission to the ICU.

Here we studied the expression of other markers on monocytes from septic patients with fatal outcome (and HLA-DR antigen expression < 20%). We then examined whether the phenotypic alterations in monocytes from such patients are associated with functional defects of these cells. We also analyzed whether T cell derived cytokines such as interferon-gamma (IFN-γ) or granulocyte-macrophage colony-stimulating factor (GM-CSF) can overcome the monocytic abnormalities in vitro. Based on these studies, we developed a new therapeutic strategy for patients with severe septic disease.

[1] Institute For Medical Immunology, Charité, Humboldt-Universität Berlin, Schumannstr. 20/21, 1040 Berlin, FRG
[2] Clinic For Surgery, Charité, Humboldt-Universität Berlin, Schumannstr. 20/21, 1040 Berlin, FRG
[3] Clinic For Intensive Care, Charité, Humboldt-Universität Berlin, Schumannstr. 20/21, 1040 Berlin, FRG
[4] Clinic For Internal Medicine, Charité, Humboldt-Universität Berlin, Schumannstr. 20/21, 1040 Berlin, FRG

Host Defense Dysfunction
in Trauma, Shock and Sepsis
Eds. Faist/Meakins/Schildberg
© Springer-Verlag, Berlin Heidelberg 1993

Patients and Methods

Included in this study were 38 septic patients admitted to a surgical intensive care unit (ICU). Septic disease was defined by bacteremia and typical clinical symptoms (fever, leukocytosis/leukopenia, altered differential blood film, splenomegaly, tachycardia, and in severe cases shock and multiple-organ failure). MNC were isolated from 20 ml citrated blood by standard procedure, stained with the appropriate monoclonal antibody (MAb), and analyzed cytofluorometrically as previously described [1, 4].

To test antigen-presenting activity, purified monocytes were pulsed for 2 h with tetanus toxoid (10 μg/ml) or anti-CD3 MAb (100 ng/ml) and cocultured with autologous or HLA-DR matched allogeneic purified lymphocytes for 3 or 7 days. [^{3}H] Thymidine incorporation was measured during the last 18 h. The spontaneous and PMA-induced (10 ng/ml) formation of reactive oxygen species by monocytes was measured cytofluorometrically using the method of Rothe et al. [5]. The spontaneous and endotoxin (lipopolysaccharide, LPS) induced secretion of tumor necrosis factor-alpha (TNF-α) and interleukin-6 (IL-6) were quantified by enzyme-linked immunosorbent assay (Quantikine, British-Biotechnology, UK) in supernatants of 4-h cultures of monocytes. To study the restitution of monocyte antigens in vitro, MNC were cultured for 2–4 days in RPMI-1640 supplemented with fetal calf serum (FCS), AB serum, or septic serum (20%) with or without IFN-γ (Roussel, France) or GM-CSF (Behring, FRG). Thereafter, cells were harvested and analyzed by cytofluorometry. Plasmapheresis was performed by exchanging 2.5 l plasma per session and volume restitution by fresh frozen plasma.

Results and Discussion

Phenotype of Monocytes. As described recently, septic patients with fatal outcome showed a persistently marked decrease both in proportion and absolute number of HLA-DR$^+$ monocytes. Between the 3rd and 5th days after admission to the ICU the threshold of 20% HLA-DR$^+$ monocytes allowed a correct prediction of the clinical outcome in more than 90% of cases. Patients with a low proportion of HLA-DR$^+$ monocytes also showed decreased expression of another HLA class II antigen, HLA-DQ (Table 1). However, the expression of HLA class I antigen on monocytes and lymphocytes was not disturbed, nor was the expression of HLA-class II antigens on B lymphocytes. The loss of HLA class II antigen expression was thus restricted to monocytes. Some other monocytic markers also showed abnormalities (Table 2) but were not consistently related to clinical outcome.

Functional assays. We examined whether the phenotypic changes of monocytes were associated with functional defects. As shown in Table 3, monocytes from

Table 1. Expression of HLA antigens on monocytes and lymphocytes from patients with fatal septic disease and healthy donors

HLA marker	Cells	Positive cells (%)		
		Patients[a] (n = 10)	Healthy donors (n = 20)	p Value
HLA-DR	Monocytes	12 ± 3	75 ± 3	< 0.01
	Lymphocytes	17 ± 4	14 ± 2	NS
HLA-DQ	Monocytes	1 ± 1	23 ± 4	< 0.01
	Lymphocytes	16 ± 3	14 ± 2	NS
HLA-A, B, C	Monocytes	96 ± 2	97 ± 1	NS
	Lymphocytes	98 ± 1	98 ± 1	NS
β_2-Microglobulin	Monocytes	97 ± 2	97 ± 1	NS
	Lymphocytes	97 ± 2	97 ± 1	NS

[a] Patients with HLA-DR antigen on monocytes less than 20% and fatal outcome were selected.

Table 2. Phenotypic changes of monocytes from patients with fatal septic disease

Normal expression	Decreased expression
HLA-A, B, C	HLA-DR
β_2-Microglobulin	HLA-DQ
CD11b	CD11c
CD15	KiM-2
CD18	4F2
CD68	CD14 (in the final phase)
CD71 (sometimes increased)	

Table 3. Loss of monocytic antigen-presenting activity

Cell source		Stimulatory Index[a]	
Monocytes (10%)	Lymphocytes (90%)	Tetanus toxoid (10 µg/ml)	CD3 MAb (0.1 µg/ml)
Healthy	Healthy	15 ± 5	25 ± 7
Patient[b]	Patient[b]	2 ± 2	6 ± 3
Patient[b]	Healthy	4 ± 3	7 ± 4
Healthy	Patient[b]	11 ± 5	19 ± 7

[a] Results expressed as mean ± SD (n = 5).
[b] Monocytes/lymphocytes from septic patients with immunoparalysis (HLA-DR[+] monocytes < 20%).

septic patients with fatal outcome (HLA-DR[+] monocytes < 20%) did not present tetanus toxoid or CD3 MAb to HLA-matched allogeneic lymphocytes from healthy subjects, while monocytes from septic patients with nearly normal HLA-DR antigen expression (> 50%; results not shown) presented both "antigens." Monocytes from former patients also showed a diminished capacity to form reactive oxygen species (ROS) in response to PMA as compared to healthy controls [132 $\pm$ 7 versus 96 $\pm$ 6 fluorescence channels (log scale); $p < 0.01$, Wilcoxon test]. The spontaneous formation of ROS did not significantly differ (62 $\pm$ 5 versus 64 $\pm$ 5). Furthermore, we tested the spontaneous and LPS-induced release of TNF-α and IL-6 by monocytes in short-term (4-h) cultures. Whereas the spontaneous release of TNF-α by monocytes from septic patients with fatal clinical outcome (HLA-DR antigen expression $< 20\%$) did not differ significantly from healthy subjects, monocytes from septic patients who survived (HLA-DR antigen expression $> 35\%$) spontaneously secreted five to ten times higher levels (Table 4). The LPS-induced secretion of TNF-α was comparable in all three groups. Similar results were observed for the spontaneous and LPS-induced IL-6 secretion (not shown). Based on these data, we termed the syndrome of phenotypic and functional abnormalities of monocytes with the leading parameter of diminished HLA-DR antigen expression ($< 20\%$) as "immunoparalysis."

Restitution of Monocytic Phenotype by Cytokines. It is well known that the HLA-class II antigen expression is regulated both negatively (endotoxin, products of phagocytosis; [6–8]) and positively (T cell-derived cytokines, such as IFN-γ and GM-CSF; [6, 7, 9, 10]). Therefore, we examined whether IFN-γ and GM-CSF are able to normalize in vitro the low HLA-DR antigen expression on monocytes derived from septic patients with immunoparalysis. As shown in Table 5, both cytokines were able to restore the diminished HLA-DR antigen expression, provided the cultures were supplemented with FCS or human AB serum. However, addition of serum from septic patients with immunoparalysis prevented the cytokine-mediated effects on HLA-DR antigen expression in six of eight cases. Remarkably, the normalization of other markers such as CD11c was not inhibited by serum factors (not shown). Neither protease inhibitors, anti-endotoxin MAb, anti-TNF MAb, nor scavenger of ROS did neutralize the inhibitory serum activity. The factor(s) was heat instable ($> 56\,°C$) and not dialyzable (m.w. > 6000 D).

Table 4. TNF-α secretion by monocytes

Cell source (patients)	n	TNF-α level (ng/ml)	
		Spontaneous release	LPS-induced release
Healthy subjects	8	105 $\pm$ 45	1025 $\pm$ 230
Nonsurvivors (HLA-DR $< 20\%$)	5	220 $\pm$ 90	1255 $\pm$ 310
Survivors (HLA-DR $> 35\%$)	8	1480 $\pm$ 230[a]	1520 $\pm$ 330

[a] $p < 0.01$, as compared to the other groups of patients.

Table 5. Effect of lymphokines on HLA-DR antigen expression on monocytes derived from septic patients with immunoparalysis

Lymphokine (100 U/ml)	Serum (20%)	HLA-DR$^+$ monocytes (%)
No	No	18 ± 5 ($n = 8$)
No	AB serum	17 ± 4 ($n = 8$)
IFN-γ	No	63 ± 12 ($n = 8$)
IFN-γ	AB serum	68 ± 10 ($n = 8$)
IFN-γ	Septic serum	31 ± 10 ($n = 8$)
GM-CSF	No	35 ± 7 ($n = 8$)
IFN-γ + GM-CSF	No	75 ± 12* ($n = 4$)
IFN-γ + GM-CSF	AB serum	78 ± 13* ($n = 4$)
IFN-γ + GM-CSF	Septic serum	52 ± 15* ($n = 4$)

MNC were cultured for 3 days in RPMI-1640 plus 5% FCS with or without cytokines and human serum supplements. Thereafter, the HLA-DR antigen expression on monocytes was determined by cytofluorometry.

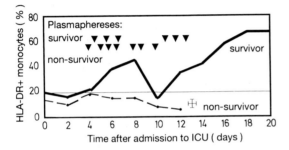

Fig. 1. Monitoring of HLA-DR$^+$ monocytes in septic patients. ———, Patient N. E., survivor; – – –, patient H. S., nonsurvivor

Plasmapheresis. To remove the inhibitory serum activity in vivo we initiated a clinical trial with plasmapheresis in septic patients with immunoparalysis. Only patients who showed repeatedly (days 1–2 and days 3–4) the signs of immuno-paralysis (HLA-DR$^+$ monocytes $< 20\%$) were included. Preliminary data demonstrate an improved survival rate in patients with immunoparalysis following repeated plasmapheresis. Whereas 22 of 24 patients died in the untreated control group, 8 of 14 patients in the plasmapheresis group survived (letality: 92% versus 43%; $p < 0.01$). Considering the course of monocytic markers, the number of plasmaphereses was three to ten for each patient. Two typical courses are shown in Fig. 1.

In summary, it was shown that the loss of HLA-class II antigen expression on monocytes from septic patients with fatal outcome was associated with other phenotypic changes as well as with functional defects such as diminished antigen presentation and formation of ROS. In contrast to monocytes from survivors, those from patients with fatal outcome and low HLA-DR antigen expression secreted low levels of TNF-α only. This observation was unexpected since TNF-α seems to be involved in the pathogenesis of septic shock [11]. However, TNF-α may also have some beneficial effects on the antimicrobial defense [11]. The functional and phenotypic alterations of septic monocytes suggest their diminished capacity for antimicrobiologic defense. Therefore we termed these functional breakdown immunoparalysis (principal parameter: HLA-DR$^+$ monocytes < 20%). Recovery from immunoparalysis within the 1st week after admission to the ICU as indicated by normalization of HLA-DR antigen expression on monocytes predicted a favorable clinical outcome [2, 3]. We observed similar findings in a part of immunosuppressed patients (allograft recipients) with septic complications [1]. In agreement with our results, Cheadle et al. [12] recently described the predictive value of the decrease in HLA-DR antigen expression on monocytes from patients following injury.

Preliminary data from the clinical trial on plasmapheresis support our concept of a new therapeutic strategy in septic disease based on selection of high-risk patients by immune monitoring and the use in these patients of the following therapeutic approaches in addition to the therapy commonly used: (a) plasmapheresis for removing suppressive serum factors, (b) immunostimulation by cytokines (IFN-γ and/or GM-CSF), and (c) inhibition of formation of suppressive factors by stimulated phagocytes (prostaglandin E synthesis inhibitors, scavengers of reactive oxygen species, surgical removal of septic focus and necrotizing tissue).

References

1. Volk HD, Reinke P, Falck P et al. (1989) Diagnostic value of an immune monitoring program for the clinical management of immunosuppressed patients with septic complications. Clin Transplant 3:246–252
2. Von Baehr R, Lohmann T, Heym S et al. (1990) Immunoparalysis in case of septicaemia. Z Klin Med 45:1133–1137
3. Volk HD, Lohmann T, Heym S et al. (1990) Decrease of proportion of HLA-DR$^+$ monocytes as prognostic parameter for the clinical outcome of septic disease. In: Masihi KN, Lange W (eds) Immunotherapeutic Springer, Berlin Heidelberg New York, pp 297–301
4. Falck P, Volk HD, Kiowski S et al. (1987) Characterization of mononuclear cells by means of monoclonal antibodies and cytofluorometry. Z Klin Med 42:2281–2284
5. Rothe G, Oser A, Valet G (1988) Dihydrorhodamine 123: a new flow cytometric indicator for respiratory burst activity in neutrophil granulocytes. Naturwissenschaften 75:354–355
6. Gruner S, Volk HD, Falck P, von Baehr R (1986) The influence of phagocytic stimuli on the expression of HLA-DR antigens: role of reactive oxygen intermediates. Eur J Immunol 16:212–215
7. Steeg PS, Johnson HM, Oppenheim JJ (1982) Regulation of murine macrophage Ia antigen expression by an immune IFN-like lymphokine: inhibitory effect of endotoxins. J Immunol 129:2402–2407
8. Heumann D, Vischer TL (1988) Immunomodulation by α_2-macroglobulin and α_2-macroglobulin-proteinase complexes: the effect on the human T lymphocyte response. Eur J Immunol 26:246–249
9. Janeway CA, Bottomly K, Babich J (1984) Quantitative variation in Ia antigen expression plays a central role in immune regulation. Immunol Today 5:99–105

10. Smith PD, Lamerson CL, Wong HL, Wahl LM, Wahl SM (1990) Granulocyte-macrophage colony-stimulating factor stimulates human monocyte accessory cell function. J Immunol 144:3829–3834
11. Beutler B, Cerami A (1989) The biology of cachectin/TNF — a primary mediator of the host response. Annu Rev Immunol 7:625–656
12. Cheadle WG, Hersman MJ, Wellhausen SR, Polk HC (1989) Role of monocyte HLA-DR expression following trauma in predicting clinical outcome. In: Faist E et al. (eds) Immune consequences of trauma, shock, and sepsis. Springer, Berlin Heidelberg New York, pp 119–122

Effects of Exercise on the Immune System with Special Reference to Natural Killer Cells

B. K. Pedersen

Introduction

Natural killer (NK) cells are defined as major histocompatibility complex (MHC)-independent cytotoxic lymphocytes that do not express the CD3 antigen. They commonly express certain cell surface markers such as CD16 (the NK cell Fc receptor) [1].

The biologic functions of NK cells have been claimed to be many. The most convincing results on the role of NK cells come from the virus era, showing that NK cells play a very important role in resistance against some (but not all) viruses, but definitely play a role against viruses from the herpes group [2]. Furthermore NK cells are believed to play a role in resistance against cancer [3].

NK cells are influenced by a number of other immunocompetent cells; their activity is enhanced by interferons (IFN) and interleukin-2 (IL-2) and down-regulated by certain prostaglandins. The NK cell response seems also remarkably variable and sensitive to a number of day-to-day stimuli, including smoking and alcoholism. Furthermore NK cells have been shown to be highly influenced by physical exercise and degree of training.

In the following a description of the NK cells in relation to acute physical exercise and long-term training will be given. As well as this, a short description of other parts of the immune system will be given and different aspects of importance for the understanding of the mechanisms behind the modulation of NK cell function will be dealt with. The focus will be on our own results with references to the work of others, but it is not the intention to give a full review.

Acute Physical Exercise and NK Cells

The effect of acute physical exercise on the NK cell function has been described with little or no controversy by several people [4–9].

Laboratory of Medical Immunology, TTA 754, Rigshospitalct University Hospital, Tagensvej 20 DU-2100 Copenhagen

Host Defense Dysfunction
in Trauma, Shock and Sepsis
Eds. Faist/Meakins/Schildberg
© Springer-Verlag, Berlin Heidelberg 1993

In our studies on the effect of exercise on the immune system, blood mononuclear cells (BMNC) were isolated before, during, and 2 and 24 h after bicycle exercise at 75% of $\dot{V}_{O_2max}$. Test persons were young, relatively untrained male students [7, 8].

During exercise the NK cell activity increased and the NK cell fraction (CD16+ cells) of BMNC increased in parallel. When BMNC were preincubated with IFN-α, IL-2, or the prostaglandin-inhibitor indomethacin, a significant increase in NK cell activity was registered at all times studied. During exercise the IL-2-enhanced NK cell activity increased significantly more than the IFN-α- and indomethacin-enhanced NK cell activity. These results strongly indicate that exercise induces an increase in the circulation of NK cells with an altered function. NK cells with a high IL-2 response capacity are recruited to the blood [7].

In another study by Targan et al. [9] it was shown that increased NK cell activity occurred during short moderate exercise for 5 min. Their results indicated that during moderate exercise a "new" population of active cells was derived probably from cells that could bind targets but were non-cytotoxic. The cytotoxic activity of these could be further augmented by in vitro boosting with IFN.

Two hours after maximal exercise the NK cell activity dropped to a low point. The decreased NK cell activity was probably not due to fluctuations among the NK cells as the proportion of CD16+ cells was normal. The fall in NK cell activity was probably due to inhibition by prostaglandins released by the elevated number of monocytes. In agreement with this, increased prosta- glandin production was found postexercise but the NK cell activity of mono- cyte-depleted mononuclear cells did not decrease postexercise. Furthermore, indomethacin in vitro and in vivo restored the suppressed NK cell activity post exercise.

We have examined the effect of 1 h of bicycle exercise at severe, moderate, and light exercise (75%, 50%, and 25% of $\dot{V}_{O_2max}$ in the same people with an interval of at least 1 week (Tvede and Pedersen, unpublished results). At all training intensities the percentage CD16+ cells increased to almost the same degree and returned to normal within 2 h. During severe, moderate, and light exercise the NK cell function increased, the suppression of NK cell function to below pre-exercise levels, which occurred 2 h after maximal exercise at 75% of $\dot{V}_{O_2max}$, did not occur during moderate and light exercise. Interestingly, while an increased concentration of monocytes was demonstrated 2 h postexercise at 75% of $\dot{V}_{O_2max}$, the monocyte concentration did not change following exercise at 50% or 25% of $\dot{V}_{O_2max}$. While light, moderate, as well as maximal physical exercise increase the NK cell activity, the post-exercise suppression of the NK cell function occurred following maximal exercise only. The finding that the monocyte concentration did not increase following submaximal exercise further supports the idea that the suppressed NK cell activity following severe exercise is due to the elevated concentration of monocytes releasing prostaglandins that down-regulate NK cell function.

Other Parts of the Immune System and Acute Physical Exercise

Leukocyte concentration increases during and after exercise. Neutrophil concentration increases during and a further three- to four- fold after exercise, while the lymphocyte concentration increases during and falls below prevalue post-exercise [10]

The percentage of CD3+ T cells (percentage of BMNC) falls due to a decrease in the CD4+ cell fraction, while the CD8+ cells do not alter. The percentage of CD19+ B cells does not change during or after exercise. The percentage of CD14+ monocytes does not change during, but increases two- to threefold after exercise [11].

The phytohematagglutinin (PHA)-induced lymphocyte proliferative response decreased during exercise and the IL-2-induced proliferative response increased, probably due to stimulation of T and NK cells, respectively [11, 12].

The B-cell function was suppressed during and especially following exercise. Tvede et al. [13] showed by estimating plaque-forming cells, decreased numbers of IgG-, IgM-, and IgA- secreting blood cells in relation to acute severe exercise.

Increased IL-1 and IL-6 production following exercise have been described, whereas the production of tumor necrosis factor alpha (TNF-α) IL-2, and IFN-γ did not fluctuate in relation to exercise [14].

We were unable to show any significant effect of heavy short-term exercise on the levels of erythrocyte, CR1, circulating immune complexes, and the complement C3 split products C3c and C3d [15].

Long-term Training and Cellular Immunity

NK cell activity and concentration of CD16+ cells were found to be elevated in elite cyclists when compared to sex- and age-matched controls [16].

BMNC subpopulations, lymphocyte proliferative response, and NK activity were measured under resting conditions in 29 highly trained male racing cyclists and in 15 untrained persons during a period of lowtraining intensity (winter). Fifteen of the trained and ten of the untrained persons were reexamined during a period of high training intensity (summer). Changes in any immune parameters from winter to summer did not differ significantly between the trained and untrained people. The NK cell activity was found to be highly significantly elevated in the trained vs the untrained subjects during low and during high training intensity, whereas the proliferative response and BMNC subsets did not differ between the two groups [17]. Evans et al. [18] and Thomsen et al. [15] showed elevated production of IL-1 in trained persons compared to untrained, whereas the production of IL-6 was only marginally elevated in trained persons [15]. The production of IL-2, TNF, and IFN did not differ between the two groups [15], neither did the CR1, immunocomplexes, or split products [15].

Tomasi et al. found lower levels of salivary IgA in skiers compared to controls [19].

To finally decide whether the immune status differs between trained and untrained persons during rest, longitudinal studies on the immune system in persons undergoing a regular training programme should be done.

Mechanisms of Action

Exercise induces an increase in a number of stress hormones, including catecholamines, growth hormone, β-endorphins, and cortisol. We have investigated the possibility that one or more of these hormones are responsible for the exercise-induced immunomodulation.

Epinephrine Selective administration of epinephrine to obtain plasma concentrations identical to those observed during bicycle exercise (75% of $\dot{V}_{O_2max}$, 1 h) showed that the modulation of BMNC subsets, NK activity, and lymphocyte function was closely mimicked by the administration of epinephrine [20]. However, epinephrine caused a minor increase in neutrophil concentration as compared to that induced by exercise.

Growth hormone Recently we have obtained results showing that in vivo injection of growth hormone in humans had no effect on BMNC subset, NK activity, or lymphocyte function, but induced a highly significant increase in neutrophil concentration (Kappel and Pedersen, unpublished observations).

β-Endorphins. When Fiatarone et al. [5] administered naloxone in vivo to young women who underwent a maximal bicycle test, the rise in NK cell activity was no longer significant. However, the rise in cells expressing the CD16 marker (NK cells) was not significantly different when compared to the group receiving placebo. We have preliminary results showing that when healthy young men were given an epidural analgesia that blocked the afferent impulses and inhibited an increase in β-endorphins and adrenocorticotropic hormone (ACTH) during exercise, this did not inhibit the exercise-induced increase in NK cell function or NK cell concentration. Based on these results we do not think that the β-endorphin response plays an important role in exercise-induced modulation of NK cells.

Cortisol. During bicycle exercise (75% of $\dot{V}_{O_2max}$, 1 h) only a minor increase in cortisol concentration is found (0.63 $\mu mol/l$ before exercise and 0.79 $\mu mol/l$ after) [7]. It cannot easily be predicted from the information how this minor increase in cortisol concentration can account for the exercise-induced immunomodulation, but cortisol might play a role in exercise training of longer duration.

In conclusion we find that epinephrine can account for the effect of physical exercise on NK activity, BMNC subsets, and proliferative responses, while epinephrine together with growth hormone might be responsible for the increase in neutrophil concentration following exercise.

References

1. Hercend T, Schmidt RE (1988) Characteristics and uses of natural killer cells. Immunol Today 9:291–293
2. Welsh RM (1986) Regulation of virus infections by natural killer cells. Nat Immun Cell Growth Regul 5:169–199
3. Burton RC (1988) Natural killer cells and cancer: a review. Aust NZJ Surg 58:761–765
4. Brahmi Z, Thomas JE, Park M, Dowdeswell IRG (1985) The effect of acute exercise on natural killer cell activity of trained and sedentary human subjects. J Clin Immunol 5:321–328
5. Fiatarone MA, Morley JE, Bloom ET, Donna M, Maskinodan T, Solomon GF (1988) Endogenous opioids and the exercise-induced augmentation of natural killer cell activity. J Lab Clin Med 112:544–552
6. MacKinnon LT, Chick TW, Tomasi TB (1987) The effect of exercise on secretory and natural immunity. Adv Exp Med Biol 216A:869–876
7. Pedersen BK, Tvede N et al. (1988) Modulation of natural killer cell activity in peripheral blood by physical exercise. Scand J Immunol 26:673–678
8. Pedersen BK, Tvede N et al. (1990) Indomethacin in vitro and in vivo abolishes post-exercise suppression of natural killer cell activity in peripheral blood. Int J Sports Med 11:127–131
9. Targan S, Britvan L, Dorey F (1981) Activation of human NKCF by moderate exercise increased frequency of NK cells with enhanced capability of effector-target cell lytic interactions. Clin Exp Immunol 45:352–360
10. Pedersen BK (1991) The influence of physical exercise on the cellular immune system— mechanisms of action. Int J Sports Med 12:523–529
11. Tvede N, Pedersen BK, Hansen FR, Bendix T, Christensen LD, Galbo H, Halkjær- Kristensen J (1989) Effect of physical exercise on blood mononuclear cell subpopulations and in vitro proliferative responses. Scand J Immunol 29:383–389
12. Tvede N, Pedersen BK, Hansen FR, Christensen LD, Galbo H, Andersen V, Halkjær-Kristensen J (1991) Exercise-induced changes in IL-2 proliferative response of peripheral blood mononuclear cells: Correlation to subpopulations and low-affinity IL-2 receptor expression (to be published)
13. Tvede N; Heilman C, Halkjær-Kristensen J, Pedersen BK (1989) Mechanisms of B-lymphocyte suppression induced by acute physical exercise. J Clin Lab Immunol 30:169–173
14. Haahr PM, Pedersen BK et al. (1991) Effect of physical exercise on the production of IL-1, IL-6, TNF, IL-2, and IFN. Int J Sports Med 12:223–227
15. Thomsen BS, Haahr PM, Rødgaard A, Tvede N, Hansen FR, Steensberg J, Halkjær-Kristensen J, Pedersen BK (1991) Complement receptor type one (CR1, CD35) on erythrocytes, circulating immune complexes, and complement C3 split products after short-term physical exercise and training Int J Sports Med (in press)
16. Pedersen BK, Tvede N, Christensen, Klarlund K, Kragbak S Halkjær-Kristensen J (1989) Natural killer cell activity in peripheral blood of highly trained and untrained persons. Int J Sports Med 10:120–131
17. Tvede N, Steensberg J, Baslund B, Halkjær-Kristensen J, Pedersen BK (1991) Cellular immunity in highly trained elite racing cyclists during periods of training with low and high intensity. Scand J Med Sci Sports 1:163–166
18. Evans WJ, Meredith CN, Cannon JG, Dinarello CA, Frontera WR, Hughes VA, Jones BA, Knuttgen HG (1986) Metabolic changes following eccentric exercise in trained and untrained men. J Appl Physiol 61:1864–1868

19. Tomasi TB, Trudeau FB, Czerwinsky D, Erredge S (1982) Immune parameters in athletes before and after strenuous exercise. J Clin Immunol 2:173–178
20. Kappel M, Tvede N, Galbo H, Haahr PM, Kjær M, Linstouw M, Klarlund K, Pedersen BK (1991) Epinephrine can account for the effect of physical exercise on natural killer cell activity. J Appl Physiol 70(6):2530–2534

Interaction of Immune, Interferon, and Opioid Systems in Professional Athletes

E. Gotovtseva[1], I. Surkina[1], P. Uchakin[1], M. Shchurin [2], S. Pschenichkin[2], N. Kost[2], A. Zozulya[2], and O. Ilyinsky[1]

Introduction

An integration of the immune system with the central nervous system and the endocrine system has been the subject of many recent studies in the field of "psychoneuroendocrine immunology".

Stress can significantly modulate the immune function via the nervous and endocrine system. It is well known that exercise stress can promote the release of pituitary hormones, particularly adrenocorticotropic hormone (ACTH) and β-endorphin [1, 3, 5]. Our previous studies showed that physical and psycho-emotional sport's stress in athletes resulted in immunodeficiency [2, 6].

It has therefore been suggested that opioid peptides (OP) and hormones play an important role in the development of stress-related immunological alterations. Our interest has focused upon the study of the relationship between immune, interferon, and opioid systems during physical and psychoemotional stress in athletes.

Subjects and Methods

Twenty-four professional skaters were examined during four different physical activities. (1) 2 weeks of moderate physical loadings, (2) 2 weeks of exhausting physical exercises, (3) acute extreme physical loading, and (4) the acute intensive psychoemotional stress of contest.

Peripheral blood mononuclear cells (PBMC) and plasma were collected 24 h after one day's rest following activities one and two above and 10 h and 8 h after activities three and four respectively.

To assess the immune, interferon, and opioid systems the following parameters were investigated: (a) the percentage and total number of active E and late E rosette-forming cells (Ea-RFC and E-RFC); (b) the ability of PBMC to

[1] Department of Neurohumoral Regulation, Central Research Institute for "Sport", Elizavetinsky pr. 10, Moscow, 107005, Russia
[2] Department of Clinical Immunology, National Center for Mental Health, Academy of Medical Science USSR, Zagorodnoe sh. 2, Moscow, 113152, Russia

Host Defense Dysfunction
in Trauma, Shock and Sepsis
Eds. Faist/Meakins/Schildberg
© Springer-Verlag, Berlin Heidelberg 1993

proliferate in response to phytohemagglutinin (PHA) and to produce interferon-gamma IFN-γ and interferon-alpha IFN-α in response to in vitro stimulation with PHA and with Newcastle disease virus (NDV) respectively, and (c) the level of activity of opioid-δ-receptor ligands (δ-ORL) in blood plasma.

Results

Moderate physical loadings in athletes did not change the percentage and total number of T lymphocytes or the proliferative activity of PBMC and its ability to produce IFN-α when compared with the results of the control group (non-athletes). The PBMC ability to synthesize IFN-γ was diminished, while the percentage of Ea-RFC and the level of δ-ORL activity in plasma were increased.

After 2 weeks of exhausting physical loadings, we observed a depressed PBMC responsiveness to PHA and a profoundly decreased production in IFN-γ 14 448 + 3156 cpm and 2.8 + 0.7 U/ml, respectively, compared with 55 000 + 2500 cpm and 52.5 + 0.3 U/ml in control). At the same time, the percentage of T lymphocytes, IFN-α production, and the level of δ-ORL activity in plasma were stable and corresponded to normal data.

The most pronounced changes in immune and opioid systems were registered after acute strenuous physical exercise and psychoemotional stress of competition. Alterations in the cellular immune response 10 h after acute physical loading included the depression of PBMC ability to proliferate in response to PHA (9333 + 2178 cpm) and to produce IFN-γ and IFN-α (2.5 + 0.5 U/ml and 14.5 + 2.5 U/ml, respectively). The percentage of T lymphocytes (47.0% + 5.8% in comparison to normal 75.0% + 8.4%) and Ea-RFC (23.8% + 4.8%) were also diminished. However, the level of δ-ORL activity in plasma did not change and was no different from the results obtained after long-term physical stress.

Eight hours after the psychoemotional stress of contest there was a significant decrease in the ability of PBMC to synthesize IFN-α (2.5 + 0.5 U/ml), IFN-γ (2.3 + 0.5 U/ml), and to proliferate in response to PHA (16 753 cpm). The percentage of Ea-RFC did not change and was comparative to baseline results obtained after exhausting physical loadings.

The most important finding was the diminished level of δ-ORL activity in plasma after extreme stress of competition (0.097 + 0.002 n mol equivalent in comparison to normal 0.13 + 0.001 nmol).

According to our data, professional athletes experience an increased risk of morbidity following long-term training and periods of competition.

Taking into consideration immunomodulating effects of OP, we carried out the pilot experiment to activate the opioid system by transcranial electro-stimulation (TES). Four volunteers, frequently suffering from respiratory diseases, took part in the study. TES was administered with the help of "Electronarcon-1" — anesthetic apparatus. Cutaneous electrodes were put on the frontal and occipital regions of the head. Combined direct and alternating currents with an intensity of 3–4 mA were used. The procedure was carried out once and continued for 30 min.

It was shown that TES enhanced the level of δ-ORL activity in plasma with the peak after 30 min (170% to normal data). The increased level of δ-ORL activity was still registered 6 h after TES was administered.

The released opioid peptides significantly modulated interferon response. In most cases we found a decrease in the ability of PBMC to synthesize IFN-α 6 h after TES; IFN-α production had recovered 24 h after TES. The OP-modulating effect on IFN-γ synthesis was just the same when its baseline level was normal. However, when the baseline level of IFN-γ production was low, we observed an increase in the ability of PBMC to produce IFN-γ 6 h after TES was administered and its decrease to baseline level after 24 h.

Conclusion

Our results are evidence that professional athletes experience some deficits in their immune function during exhausting physical and psychoemotional sport stress. Various alterations in immune status are closely connected with the dysregulation in the relationship between the immune and opioid systems. Our previous study showed that the stress-reaction of immune and opioid response occurs at different times. The peak of OP activity was registered immediately after exercise, while the immune and interferon systems reacted on exercise stress within 24 h (unpublished data).

Also, the increased level of δ-ORL activity in plasma is associated with the long-term stimulating effect of moderate physical loadings on the opioid system. It is necessary to mention that the results were obtained during 1 day's rest after moderate physical exercises. Our findings are in line with the data which testify the increase in the OP level in the blood of people going in for sport [4].

The results of OP activity, obtained 10 h and 8 h after acute physical and psychoemotional sport stress could be explained in another way, since these hours cover the recovery period of the opioid system after exercise stress. The delay in the recovery of OP activity 8 h after contest apparently testifies the profoundly depressed opioid response under acute psychoemotional stress of competition, but not the acute physical stress. TES of the opioid system modulates interferon functions. It is necessary to study TES as a method for obtaining further information on the adaptation process to stress.

References

1. Carr DB, Fishman SM (1985) Exercise and endogenous opioids. In: Fotherby K, Pal SB (eds) Exercise endocrinology, Vol 4. De Gruyter, Hawthorne, p. 155
2. Ershov F, Gotovtseva E (1989) Interferon status under stresses. Sov Med Rev E Virol 3:35

3. Farrell PA, Gates WK, Maksud MG, Morgan WP (1982) Increase in plasma β-endorphin/β-lipotropin immunoreactivity after treadmill running in humans. J Appl Physiol 52 (5):1245
4. Laatikainen T, Virtanen T, Apter D (1986) Plasma immunoreactive β-endorphin in exercise — associated amenorrhea. Am J Obstet Gynecol 154 (1):94
5. Rubinstein M, Stein S, Udenfriend S (1978) Characterization of pro-opiocortin, a precursor to opioid peptides and corticotropin. Proc Natl Acad Sci USA 75 (5):669
6. Surkina I, Gotovtseva E (1989) The immune state of female athletes and its correlation with menstrual function and conditions of sports acitivities. J Sports Train Med Rehabil 1:85

Section 5

**Inflammatory Mechanisms
in Traumatic and Septic Injury**

White Cells in Burn Patients

D.N. Herndon[1,2], T.C. Rutan[1], J.M. Mlakar[1], and D. Fleming[1]

Advances in the surgical treatment of burns have markedly decreased mortality over the last 10 years. In the United States, the advent of early massive excision and grafting of burns has increased the LD_{50} to 98% total body surface area (TBSA) burn in referral pediatric burn centers such as the Shriners Burns Institute—Galveston Unit. It is our prejudice that early excision of the burn wound within 24–72 h of the time of injury is absolutely essential in the very largest of third-degree burns, and the use of fresh cadaver skin as a temporary cover has become the standard of care. The physiologic and metabolic alterations following thermal injury continue despite these measures. We initially thought that if we excised and grafted the acute burn wound, the patients' immunologic and hypermetabolic responses would return to normal. Unfortunately, this has not been the case. Essentially, a burn patient is one whose outer defense, the skin, has been damaged and whose inner defense mechanism is totally befuddled.

The primary determinant of postburn immunosuppression appears to be the macrophage/monocyte which modulates helper-suppressor T-lymphocyte ratios and natural killer (NK) levels. The macrophage also synthesizes complement, generates plasminogen, and contributes to the microvascular clots that lead to the increased microvascular permeability near the burn wound and also in other organs. It may be particularly troublesome in the smoke-injured lung. The macrophage, activated in the burn wound and in the lungs, releases chemoattractants that cause neutrophil migration and margination, in turn causing increased vascular permeability. Production of vasoactive substances such as thromboxane (TxB) and leukotrienes is a recurrent theme following burn injury, and may augment the extent of the burn injury. The macrophage, in addition to recruiting leukocytes, also releases substances that modulate burn wound healing, alter immune function and upregulate metabolism. We believe that the hypermetabolic response to trauma and burns is primarily mediated by macrophages.

The hypermetabolic response to burn injury is the greatest of all such responses. Patients with multiple fractures, peritonitis, and cancer have shown an increase in metabolic rate, but the increase seen acutely postburn absolutely

[1] Shriners Burns Institute Galveston, Texas, USA
[2] University of Texas Medical Branch, Galveston, Texas, USA

Host Defense Dysfunction
in Trauma, Shock and Sepsis
Eds. Faist/Meakins/Schildberg
© Springer-Verlag, Berlin Heidelberg 1993

dwarfs the others [1, 2]. Metabolic expenditure can be twice normal in massive burns. Generally, if the patient is wrapped in bulky dressings and kept warm with external radiant heating devices, the metabolic rate is still 40%–60% above normal. The postburn response is characterized also by an increase in heart rate, with rates of 180–200 beats per minute (bpm) being common for children. A true temperature reset occurs between the 5th and 15th postburn day and remains up to 2 months in injuries of greater than 60% TBSA, regardless of the timing of burn wound closure. The temperature reset results in a core temperature that is around 38.6 °C [3, 4]. If we try to cool them to decrease their core temperatures, or give aspirin or acetaminophen, the patients produce more heat to compensate.

We maintain or increase body heat on a cellular level by cycling from glucose to phosphate and back, fructose to fructose-1-phosphate and back, and fatty acids and glycerol to triglycerides and back. These are all normal futile cycles that occur to produce energy and heat. Recent investigations have led us to understand that this is a catecholamine-influenced substrate cycling which maintains body temperature 2 °C above normal [5, 6]. The metabolic expenditure of burn injury can be decreased by warming the environment to about 32 °–34 °C. For the burned patient, thermal neutral is 33 °C, the temperature at which they are most comfortable. Whether elevated core temperature is good or bad is a philosophical point. We think temperature elevation and substrate cycling allow a more sensitive hormonal control on a cellular basis, so we hypothesize that increased temperature is appropriate in these patients. We do know that our current attempts to decrease temperature are counterproductive.

The afferent stimulus that causes this hypothalamic temperature reset, we believe, are monokines and prostanoids, specifically TxB, released from the inflammatory burn wound. The catecholamines are elevated sixfold and glucose flow is elevated three- to sixfold in burn patients relative to normals. Also increased are glucagon and cortisol. Insulin is near normal, but the ratio of the catabolic hormones (catecholamine and glucagon) to insulin is markedly elevated. Whether we feed burn patients or not, peripheral protein breaks down. Thus there is a net negative nitrogen balance.

Although we deliver a large amount of enteral calories which maintains total body weight, total body composition changes. Weight is distributed more to fat than to lean body mass. Patients catabolize protein; they become peripherally spindly and centrally fat. Their livers become grossly enlarged as the Kupffer cells become filled with fat. This all contributes to burn patients' eventual morbidity. A hormonal milieu is established by the macrophage and is not significantly altered either by early surgery or by aggressive feeding.

In the rat model, we have been able to decrease the hypermetabolism after burns by blockade of the adrenal network by adrenalectomy either with or without steroid support [4]. Thus the adrenal medulla or epinephrine is a primary mediator of the hypermetabolic response. In humans, one would expect that beta-adrenergic blockade could decrease the hypermetabolic response. We demonstrated that propranolol given intravenously (1 mg/kg every 6 h) effectively decreased heart rate in children with major burns to a more effective range for cardiac pumping activity [7]. The patients became relaxed, left ventricular stroke work index improved, and myocardial oxygen consumption decreased. However, propranolol did not affect resting energy expenditure. As we gave the beta-blocking agent, glucagon levels increased in a reciprocal fashion.

In burned humans, elevated catecholamines, glucagon and glucocorticoids operate to break down protein from skeletal muscle peripherally and recycle it to the liver where new glucose is made. We thought that new glucose in the form of total parenteral nutrition (TPN) would decrease morbidity and mortality in these patients. Actually, TPN given to a large number of patients [8, 9] starting at day 1 postinjury increased morbidity and had a greater negative impact on their immune system. We now recommend that TPN not be given routinely to burn patients. Almost all burn patients, even those over 80%–90% TBSA, can be supported with continuous enteral feedings of milk or similar substances to provide adequate calories.

In burns of 60% TBSA 10 days postinjury, leukocyte function is dramatically reduced [10]. Although the white cell counts are elevated at or above normal, leukocyte ability to phagocytize bacteria and to consume oxygen, an index of their ability to kill bacteria, is less than controls. This is not a plasma-mediated event; the cells themselves are exhausted. They are either immature or old and fatigued, and they function ineffectively. T-cell lymphocytic markers demonstrate similar debilitation and we think this is primarily due to these mediators. In a series of large burns with controls of the same age, the OKT3s are decreased significantly in burn patients relative to controls [11]. Again the helper-suppressor cell ratio is reversed from normal.

Why does the body respond this way? We believe that a massive burn injury produces tremendous amounts of antigens and that the macrophage is releasing messengers in an attempt to prevent an accidental autoimmune response as seen in certain other disease conditions. Not only are the T-cell helper-suppressor ratios reversed, but responses to phytohemagglutinin (PHA) are markedly depressed up to 14 days postinjury in rat burn models and up to 60–70 days postinjury in humans. The most disturbing cellular defect, and the one that has been predictive of mortality, has been a defect in NK cells [12].

NK cells have Fc receptors for IgG and they are functionally important in immunosurveillance against tumors and viral infection. Animal studies show that high NK activity causes an increased resistance to viral infections [13]. In our patient population, unfortunately, almost all convert to positivity for cytomegalovirus (CMV) and herpes simplex virus (HSV). NKs suppress both B and T cell responses in states such as Kawasaki syndrome, Crohn's disease, multiple sclerosis, chronic lymphocytic leukemia in children syndrome, and in major burn injury [14, 15]. NK cells are defective after major burn injury and demonstrate a more profound defect in burned patients who die than in those who live [12]. Of those that die, all die with viral manifestations.

In large burns, the percent NK activity in nonsurviving patients studied at the height of hypermetabolic response was quite low [12]. This defect in NK activity can be identified almost immediately postburn which allows some prediction of survival. It gradually returns to normal as the patient recovers.

The suppressive activity of burn serum can be expressed on normal NK cells [16]. Actually, this is a serum-dependent phenomenon in contrast to the leukocyte abnormality discussed above. In this circumstance, function of NK cells incubated with burn serum will be depressed. This depression is heat sensitive and not removed by dialysis.

We have tried some "magic bullets" to improve postburn immune response. Isoprinosine, a salt of paracetaminobenzene, enhanced blastogenic response of peripheral blood to PHA and concanavalin A (Con A) [17]. In high concentrations it inhibited introduction of suppressor cells by Con A and restored the antigen-presenting capabilities of autoimmune responses in mice. We saw a similar improvement in our animal model when we used interleukin-2 (IL-2) [18]. IL-2 is one of a few naturally occurring immunostimulators that also appears to decrease the hypermetabolic response. It appeared to work over a wide dosage range.

The condition most commonly associated with mortality following thermal injury is inhalation injury [19], and the leukocyte plays a major role. Of all burn deaths 20%–84% are associated with smoke inhalation injury [20]. In our experience, a large burn (> 50% TBSA) with significant inhalation injury is uniformly fatal in adult patients. Inhalation injury is a dramatic display of the immune response gone awry. We have found that white blood cells are primarily responsible for much of the pulmonary damage following inhalation injury. It is the leukocyte and its release of proteolytic enzymes and free oxygen radicals that is killing these patients.

As cells are destroyed and pulmonary alveolar macrophages are stimulated by the injury, chemotactic factors are released which bring leukocytes into the lung in large numbers. The injury is actually worsened due to the body's response to the injury. Polymorphonuclear leukocytes (PMNs) marginate in the pulmonary vasculature and migrate into the parenchyma [20], where they are activated and release proteolytic enzymes, free oxygen radicals, and eicosanoids. Enzymes and free radicals destroy mucosa and cause pulmonary vascular hyperpermeability. Eicosanoids, such as TxBs and prostacycline, alter blood flow and pulmonary vascular pressures. Interstitial pulmonary edema develops and is followed by fluid leaking into the tracheobronchial tree and alveoli. Intra-alveolar edema and hemorrhages occur along with damage to type I pneumocytes. Exposure of the alveolar basement membrane leads to hyaline membrane formation and further cast formation resulting in inadequate alveolar oxygen exchange. All of these factors (norcardiogenic pulmonary edema, decreased lung compliance, increased pulmonary transvascular protein flux, hyaline membrane formation, and shunting of blood in the pulmonary vasculature) contribute to the respiratory failure following inhalation injury. The damaged tracheobronchial epithelial surface and lung parenchyma are easy targets for opportunistic infections. Gut flora and pathogens from the infected burn wound (*Staphylococcus E. coli*, and *Pseudomonas*) are the most frequent organisms associated with the pneumonias developing after inhalation injury. If the patient does survive these insults, he is often left with significant lung disease from the fibrosis and loss of alveoli associated with the disease process and its treatment.

Animal studies have demonstrated that if white blood cells, specifically PMNs, are removed by nitrogen mustard or specific antibodies, most of the pulmonary damage following inhalation injury is prevented [21]. Extravascular lung water (EVLW) and measured lung lymph flow, both indicators of the amount of interstitial pulmonary edema, are decreased and eicosanoid release is attenuated. The animals do not develop irreversible pulmonary insufficiency and at autopsy their lungs do not show the histologic changes typical of inhalation injury [21]. Removing white cells from the circulation is effective, but impractical in humans who would succumb to sepsis in the absence of leukocytes to combat infection. We have since turned to the use of specific proteolytic inhibitors and free-radical scavengers to decrease pulmonary complications of inhalation injury. The problem again exists in that we must titrate these regimens to decrease the host response to reduce injury, but not to the extent that we render the patient incapable of responding to infectious insults.

Clearly a number of other cells and substances play a role in the modulation of the postburn leukocyte function. Histamines, serotonin, and kallikreins are important. The basal epithelial cell in the lung and in the burn wound may be an important source of TxB and other vasoactive mediators. Epithelial cells, damaged in the lung and in the skin, directly release chemotactic factors and activate the macrophage. The macrophage releases chemotactic factors which prime neutrophils and cause them to come to the site of injury where they marginate, migrate, and release oxygen radicals and proteolytic enzymes. This, in turn, causes the formation of the characteristic copious exudate on the burn wound and in the lung. It also causes bronchoconstriction and prostanoid activation which contribute to the hypermetabolic response protein degradation/bronchoconstriction in the lungs.

There is some mechanistic information to be gained from the use of all these agents. The early release of TxB causes pulmonary artery hypertension which can be reversed by the same antiprostanoids that decrease the metabolic derangements. In randomized controlled studies, we plan to use ibuprofen and other nonsteroidal anti-inflammatory agents in burn patients to block TxB production. Hopefully, we will suppress the ravages of the deranged host response but not depress the normal host immunocompetence. If we cannot titrate our antisuppression treatment appropriately, we will also decrease the hosts ability to kill bacteria, and we will increase damage.

References

1. Kinney JM, Long CL, Gump FE et al. (1968) Tissue composition of weight loss in surgical patients: I. Elective operations. Ann Surg 168:459

2. Long CL, Spencer JL, Kinney JM et al. (1971) Carbohydrate metabolism in man: effect of elective operations and major injury. J Appl Physiol 31:110
3. Wilmore DW, Long JM, Skreen RW et al. (1973) Studies of the effect of variations of temperature and humidity on energy demands of the burned soldier in a controlled metabolic room. Ft Sam Houston, US Army Institute of Surgical Research, Annual Report, Report Control Symbol MEDDH-288 (R1)
4. Herndon DN, Wilmore DW, Mason AD Jr et al. (1978) Development and analysis of a small animal model simulating the human postburn hypermetabolic response. J Surg Res 25:394
5. Goodall MC, Stone C, Haynes BW Jr (1957) Urinary output of adrenaline in severe thermal burns. Ann Surg 145:479
6. Wilmore DW, Long JM, Mason AD Jr et al. (1974) Catecholamines: mediator of the hypermetabolic response to thermal injury. Ann Surg 180:653
7. Herndon DN, Barrow RE, Rutan TC et al. (1988) Effect of propranolol administration on hemodynamic and metabolic responses of burned pediatric patients. Ann Surg 208:484
8. Herndon DN, Stein MD, Rutan TC et al. (1987) Failure of TPN supplementation to improve liver function, immunity, and mortality in thermally injured patients. J Trauma 27:195
9. Herndon DN, Barrow RE, Stein M (1989) Increased mortality with intravenous supplemental feeding in severely burned patients. J Burn Care Rehabil 10:309
10. Moran K, Munster AM (1987) Alterations of host defense mechanisms in burned patients. Surg Clin North Am 67:47
11. Bender BS, Winchurch RA, Thupari JN et al. (1988) Depressed natural killer cell function in thermally injured adults: successful in vivo and in vitro immunomodulation and the role of endotoxin. Clin Exp Immunol 71:120
12. Stein MD, Gamble DN, Klimpel KD et al. (1984) Natural killer cell defects resulting from thermal injury. Cell Immunol 86:551
13. Bancroft GJ, Shellam GR, Chalmer JE (1981) Genetic influences on the augmentation of natural killer cells during murine cytomegalovirus infection: correlation with patterns of resistance. J Immunol 126:988
14. Zieglar HW, Kay NE, Zarling JM (1980) Deficiency of natural killer cell activity in patients with chronic lymphocytic leukemia. Int J Cancer 27:321
15. Steinhauer EH, Doyle AT, Reed J et al. (1982) Defective natural cytotoxicity in patients with cancer: normal number of effector cells but decreased recycling capacity in patients with advance disease. J Immunol 129:2255
16. Stein MD, Herndon DN, Klimpel G (1985) Burn patient serum suppression of natural killer activity. Proc Am Burn Assoc 17:56
17. Singh H, Herndon DN (1989) Effect of isoprinosine on lymphocyte proliferation and natural killer cell activity following thermal injury. Immunopharmacol-Immunotoxico 11:631
18. Singh H, Herndon DN (1988) Augmentation of rat natural killer cell activity by interleukin-2 and interferon following thermal injury. Proc Am Burn Assoc 20:19
19. Silverstein P, Dressler DP (1970) Effect of current therapy on burn mortality. Ann Surg 171:124
20. Herndon DN, Thompson PB, Traber DL (1985) Pulmonary injury in burned patients. Crit Care Clin 1:79
21. Basadre JO, Sugi K, Traber DL et al. (1988) Effect of leukocyte depletion on smoke inhalation injury in sheep. Surgery 104:208

Fibronectin Degradation: An In Vitro Model of Neutrophil-Mediated Endothelial Cell Damage

K.D. Forsyth

Introduction

In this paper, a marker of surface damage to the endothelial cell induced by stimulated neutrophils, which is based on degradation of endothelial cell fibronectin is described. Details have been published previously [1]. The relevance of this observation to the in vitro assessment of vascular damage and the pathophysiological implications of fibronectin degradation on the surface of the endothelial cell are discussed.

Methods

Preparation of Endothelial Cells

Endothelial cells were cultured in the usual way and transferred to glass coverslips prior to analysis. Endothelial cells were studied either plain or treated with recombinant human interleukin-1 (rHIL-1). IL-1-treated endothelial cells were incubated at 37 °C for 4 h with 20 U/ml rHIL-1.

Preparation of Neutrophils

Neutrophils were prepared in the usual way, and reconstituted at 1×10^6 cells/ml in RPMI medium without phenol red containing 1% fetal calf serum (FCS) for the adhesion assay. For the assessment of fibronectin degradation, neutrophils at $2\text{-}3 \times 10^6$/ml in RPMI medium with 1% FCS were prepared and applied to endothelium on coverslips. For the production of neutrophil degranulation products by sonication, neutrophils at 5×10^6/ml in plain RPMI medium were sonicated until the neutrophils were totally disrupted as assessed histologically.

Department of Immunology, Princess Margaret Hospital, Perth, Western Australia

Host Defense Dysfunction
in Trauma, Shock and Sepsis
Eds. Faist/Meakins/Schildberg
© Springer-Verlag, Berlin Heidelberg 1993

Assay of Neutrophils on Cultured Endothelium

Do activated neutrophils or neutrophil release products alter cellular fibronectin morphology? The effect of neutrophils on endothelial cell fibronectin architecture was studied. Prepared neutrophils were committed to three different experimental procedures:

1. Unstimulated neutrophils (acting as control neutrophils) at 2×10^6/ml in RPMI medium with 1% FCS were applied to endothelium grown on coverslips at 37 °C for 120 min.
2. In parallel a second population of neutrophils (2×10^6/ml in RPMI with 1% FCS) were stimulated to degranulate on the endothelium by the addition of 1 μM formyl-methionyl-leucyl-phenylalanine (FMLP, Sigma). These activated neutrophils were applied to the endothelium for varying time periods up to 120 min.
3. A third population of neutrophils (5×10^6/ml in RPMI) were sonicated in protein-free buffer to release their intracellular contents, centrifuged, and the cell-free supernatant applied to endothelial cells on coverslips for varying time periods up to 120 min.

After incubation the neutrophils were gently washed off the endothelial cells, and the coverslips immunostained to assess cellular fibronectin morphology of the endothelium. Ten such experiments in each category were performed.

Neutrophil Degranulation

Neutrophils were stimulated to degranulate with 1 μM FMLP. Neutrophils were also sonicated in protein-free buffer to release their intracellular contents, the cells centrifuged, and the supernatants applied to endothelium grown on coverslips for assessment of fibronectin morphology.

Neutrophil Adhesion Assay

The adherence of neutrophils to purified plasma fibronectin applied to microtiter plates was studied. The surface of the wells were coated overnight in carbonate buffer pH 9.2 at 4 °C with 100 μl of a 1 mg/l fibronectin solution (Sigma). To produce degraded fibronectin in some of the wells, the supernatants from sonicated neutrophils were added to the wells for 60 min at 37 °C, followed by washing of the wells.

Identification of Fibronectin

Two immunoglobulin G(IgG) mouse monoclonal antibodies raised against human fibronectin were used (FN3 and FN4). One of these (FN3) is specific for cellular fibronectin, and does not cross-react with plasma fibronectin [2]. The epitope recognized by FN3 is lost from cellular fibronectin after limited proteolysis with α-chymotrypsin. The other (FN4) recognizes both cellular and plasma fibronectin [2]. In addition a rabbit polyclonal antibody for fibronectin (JMB1) was studied.

The endothelium that was assessed included resting endothelium, endothelium stimulated for 4 h with 20 U/ml r-IL-1, and endothelium pretreated with FMLP-stimulated neutrophils. Fibronectin morphology of the endothelial cells was assessed using the immunoperoxidase technique. The fibronectin antibodies were applied for 60 min at room temperature to endothelium grown on coverslips. After immunostaining with the antibodies, the coverslips were observed "blindly" by two observers, using the center portion of the coverslips. A scoring system was used to objectify the particular pattern seen. This scoring was as follows:

Normal	Fibrillar fibronectin (described in greater detail in "Results")
1 + degradation	Fibronectin strands which are noted to be uneven and "lumpy," indicating minor dissolution of the fibrillar structure
2 + degradation	Moderate dissolution of the fibrils, with patchy immunoreactive fibronectin present over the surface of the endothelial cells
3 + degradation	Total loss of recognizable fibronectin morphology, with diffuse immunoreactive material spread over the surface of the endothelium

Measurement of Fibronectin

In an attempt to assess whether fibronectin is released from endothelium as it becomes degraded and loses its normal architecture, two enzyme immunoassays (EIAs) were developed to measure cellular or total fibronectin. After incubation of stimulated neutrophils with endothelium for varying time periods, resulting supernatants were collected and assayed for fibronectin.

Total Fibronectin EIA. In order to achieve maximal accuracy, a competitive inhibition assay was used. Briefly, supernatant from the endothelial cultures was incubated overnight in a test tube with antihuman fibronectin antibody (Sigma). Also incubated overnight were a second series of microtiter plates which were coated with purified fibronectin (Sigma). The microtiter plates were then washed, blocked with bovine serum albumin (BSA), and the test tube mixture containing endothelial cell supernatant plus fibronectin antibody was added to the microtiter plates. The plates were incubated with antigoat peroxidase conjugated antibody, and the color developed with O-phenylenediamine/citrate buffer and read at 492 nm.

Cellular Fibronectin EIA. As purified cellular fibronectin is not available, and the FN3 antibody does not recognize plasma fibronectin, a competitive inhibition EIA as used for total fibronectin was not able to be used. Instead a capture EIA was developed. Briefly, microtiter plates were coated with a capture antibody–polyclonal goat antihuman fibronectin (Sigma). Plates were washed, blocked with BSA, and endothelial cell supernatant added. Plates were rewashed, FN3 antibody added, rewashed, and antimouse immunoglobulin conjugated to peroxidase (DAKO) added. This was then washed and developed as above.

Results

Identification of Endothelial Cell Fibronectin

1. Resting endothelium has fibronectin arranged in a characteristic fibrillar pattern on its surface.
2. The morphology of fibronectin on IL-1 stimulated endothelium was identical with that in resting endothelium.
3. Control (resting) neutrophils incubated with endothelium produced no change in fibronectin morphology. The incubation of neutrophils stimulated to degranulate with 1 µM FMLP on endothelium produced fragmentation and dissolution of the fibrillar pattern of fibronectin morphology in a time-dependent manner. After 30 min of incubation of activated neutrophils with endothelium, 1 + degradation had occurred. By 45 min this was 2 + , and by 60 min there was 3 + degradation (i.e., total dissolution) of the characteristic fibrillar architecture.

In the IL-1-pretreated endothelium incubated with activated neutrophils, the same sequence of fibronectin degradation occurred, but more rapidly. There was total (3 +) loss of fibronectin morphology by 30 min.

To further establish whether neutrophil release products were responsible for degrading the fibronectin, cell-free supernatants from neutrophils which were sonicated in protein-free buffer to release their intracellular contents induced 2 + degradation of fibronectin observed by 60 min.

Assessment of Fibronectin Release from Endothelium

Using a competitive inhibition EIA for fibronectin, release of fibronectin from the endothelial cells into the medium was measured. Assayed with JMB1 (recognizing both cellular and plasma fibronectin, and which detects fibronectin present in the FCS), no significant increase in fibronectin levels in the medium was detected in unstimulated endothelium following incubation with both resting and FMLP-stimulated neutrophils. However, in the IL-1-pretreated

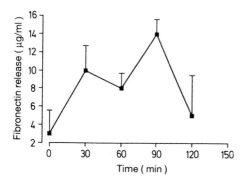

Fig. 1. Fibronectin release of IL-1-pretreated endothelium in 1% FCS. Endothelium was incubated with neutrophil supernatants for varying time periods up to 120 min and the fibronectin levels in the supernatant measured by EIA. Baseline levels of fibronectin in the medium were 3 μg/ml

endothelium, there was a progressive rise in measurable fibronectin, peaking between 60 and 90 min after incubation with neutrophil supernatants, followed by a return to baseline levels by 120 min (Fig. 1).

The maximal increase in fibronectin in the medium was 11 μg/ml. Since the FN3 epitope on cellular fibronectin is lost following proteolytic degradation, we would not expect to detect any cellular fibronectin in the endothelial supernatant with this antibody.

Using FN3 antibody as a capture in an EIA, this hypothesis was confirmed in that no cellular fibronectin was detected in the medium before or subsequent to neutrophil degranulation from both resting and IL-1-stimulated endothelium.

Neutrophil Adhesion to Degraded Fibronectin

Baseline adherence of neutrophils to plain plastic was 6% ± 1%, and to human plasma fibronectin 20 μg/ml on a plastic microtiter plate 5% ± 2% (Fig. 2). Neutrophils applied to the fibronectin-coated plate where the fibronectin was degraded showed 13% ± 4% adherence ($p < 0.005$), an increase of around 250%.

Discussion

The normal fibrillar architecture of the matrix glycoprotein fibronectin on the surface of the endothelial cell has been demonstrated in this study. The fibronectin has a distinct fibrillar pattern radiating over the surface of the endothelial cell. This architecture can be altered due to degradation of the fibronectin over 60 min by the addition to the endothelial cell of neutrophils which are activated by FMLP, or by neutrophil degranulation products. On IL-1-treated endothelium the same changes in fibronectin degradation are observed, but the changes are much more rapid, the mechanisms of which are

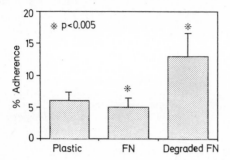

Fig. 2. Neutrophil adherence (as percentages) to uncoated plastic, to purified human fibronectin (*FN*; 20 μg/ml), or to fibronectin degraded by neutrophil release products (*degraded FN*). There is no increase in adhesion to purified fibronectin compared with uncoated plastic, but there is more than double adhesion to degraded fibronectin ($p < 0.005$), indicating that degraded fibronectin is stimulatory to neutrophils

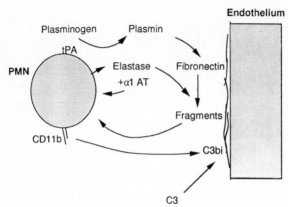

Fig. 3. Hypothetical schema of an amplification inflammatory loop involving fibronectin. Fibronectin degradation on endothelium is stimulatory for neutrophils, inducing further fibronectin degradation. *PMN*, neutrophil; *tPA*, tissue plasminogen activator present within the neutrophil, which converts plasminogen to plasmin; *α1 AT*, α_1-antitrypsin, which binds elastase

not understood. There is a concomitant increase in the number of neutrophils which adhere to degraded fibronectin.

These findings suggest an inflammatory mechanism acting at the luminal surface of the blood vessel—highly activated neutrophils may inappropriately release their intracellular contents as they adhere to the vessel wall. This degrades fibronectin. The degraded fibronectin augments further neutrophil adherence to the vessel wall. Hence degradation of endothelial cell fibronectin is likely to be of fundamental importance in amplifying inflammatory vascular damage. Hence the observation that activated neutrophils or their release products degrade fibronectin on the endothelial surface has important pathophysiological consequences, with the potential for inflammatory amplification loops to occur, augmenting endothelial cell damage (Fig. 3).

IL-1 caused a more rapid breakdown in the fibronectin on the endothelial cell following incubation with neutrophil degranulation products. IL-1 could be considered to have primed either the endothelial cell or surface fibronectin for breakdown, as IL-1 on its own had no detectable effect.

In situations where there is intravascular neutrophil degranulation such as may occur in severe sepsis, there are likely to be increased levels of IL-1 augmenting the breakdown and release of vascular fibronectin. This will amplify neutrophil-directed loss of vascular homeostasis and subsequent damage to the vessel wall.

References

1. Forsyth KD, Levinsky RJ (1990) Fibronectin degradation: an in-vitro model of neutrophil mediated endothelial cell damage. J Pathol 161:313–319
2. Keen J, Chang SE, Taylor-Papadimitrou J (1984) Monoclonal antibodies that distinguish between human cellular and plasma fibronectin. Mol Biol Med 2:15–27

Adenosine Inhibits Postischemic Leukocyte Adherence to the Endothelium of Postcapillary Venules via A_2 Receptor

D. Nolte, H. A. Lehr, and K. Messmer

Introduction

Ischemia and reperfusion lead to the activation of circulating leukocytes with ensuing accumulation, aggregation, and adhesion to the endothelium of post-capillary venules. Through the release of inflammatory mediators and cytotoxic enzymes and the formation of oxygen free radicals adherent leukocytes contribute to reperfusion injury [1, 2]. Therapeutic approaches such as leukocyte depletion by antineutrophil serum or blockage of leukocyte adhesion by monoclonal antibodies have been shown effectively to improve the outcome of reperfusion injury [3, 4]. Adenosine exerts several anti-inflammatory actions by the inhibition of oxygen free radical formation, release of inflammatory mediators, and leukocyte adherence to cultured endothelial cells [5-7]. These effects are mediated via interaction with the adenosine A_2 receptor [5].

The present study was performed to investigate the effects of adenosine on postischemic leukocyte/endothelium interaction in vivo and to determine the involved adenosine receptor.

Methods

For our study we used the dorsal skinfold chamber model in awake Syrian golden hamsters [8]. This preparation allows the investigation of the microcirculation of a striated skin muscle by intravital fluorescence microscopy. A 4-h ischemia was induced to the striated muscle by gently pressing the tissue against the cover slip with a silicone pad and an adjustable screw, just sufficient to empty the underlying vessels of blood. Leukocyte/endothelium interaction was assessed in four to six postcapillary venules (20–60 μm diameter) prior to ischemia and 30 min after reperfusion. For contrast enhancement leukocytes were stained with the in vivo fluorescent marker acridine orange (0.5 mg kg^{-1}

Dept. of Experimental Surgery, University of Heidelberg, Im Neuenheimer Feld 347, 6900 Heidelberg, FRG
Institute of Surgical Research, University of Munich, Clinic Großhadern, Marchioninistr. 15, 8000 Munich 70, FRG

Host Defense Dysfunction
in Trauma, Shock and Sepsis
Eds. Faist/Meakins/Schildberg
© Springer-Verlag, Berlin Heidelberg 1993

min^{-1} intravenously. Microscopic images were recorded on video tape and evaluated off-line using a computerized microcirculation analysis system [9]. Adherent leukocytes were expressed as cells per square millimeter of vessel surface. Red blood cell velocity was assessed using the two-window technique and a photometric analyzer (Velocity Tracker MOD 102 B, I.P.M., San Diego, CA, USA). Either saline (154 mM) or adenosine (10 mM; Sigma, Deisenhofen, FRG) or the adenosine A$_2$ receptor agonist CGS-21680 (10 μM; kindly provided by Dr. Jarvis, Ciba Geigy, NJ, USA) were infused via jugular vein at a constant rate of 3 μl/min, starting 15 min before release of ischemia and lasting until 30 min after reperfusion. At the given drug doses no changes in blood pressure or heart rate were observed.

Results

In control animals, ischemia-reperfusion elicited a dramatic increase of adherent leukocytes 30 min after reperfusion (Fig. 1). This enhancement was effectively reduced in animals treated with a continuous infusion of adenosine ($n = 6$ animals, $p < 0.01$ versus control, Wilcoxon test). Likewise, in animals treated with the adenosine A$_2$-receptor agonist CGS-21680 postischemic leukocyte/endothelium interaction was significantly reduced when compared to the saline-treated control animals ($p < 0.01$). Measurements of the microhemodynamic parameters of vessel diameter and red blood cell velocity showed no statistically significant differences between the three experimental groups.

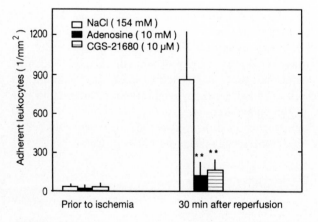

Fig. 1.

Discussion

These experiments demonstrate that intravenous infusion of adenosine inhibits postischemic leukocyte/endothelium interaction. Equipotent effects were obtained after intravenous infusion of the highly selective adenosine A_2 receptor agonist CGS-21680. Since no differences were observed between control and test animals regarding the parameters of vessel diameter and red blood cell velocity, the effects on leukocyte/endothelium interaction are not due to alterations of local microvascular blood flow.

Although other sites of adenosine action cannot be ruled out from this study, the present data suggest that the inhibition of postischemic leukocyte/endothelium interaction is mediated via adenosine A_2-receptor. Our results are in line with studies which have demonstrated that adenosine reduces leukocyte adherence to cultured endothelial cells via adenosine A_2 receptor [5].

The underlying molecular mechanism of adenosine action in postischemic leukocyte/endothelium interaction may be ascribed to the A_2 receptor mediated activation of adenylate cyclase [10]. Consequently, the rise in the intracellular cyclic AMP concentration may account for the decreased formation of oxygen free radicals and release of several inflammatory mediators [5, 7], as has been suggested by studies demonstrating that increased intracellular cyclic AMP concentration is associated with decreased leukocyte activation [11].

Recent studies indicate that adenosine alters the expression of immunocompetent receptors which is accompanied by changes of the intracellular cyclic AMP concentration [12]. It therefore remains to be investigated whether adenosine affects the expression of the leukocyte/endothelium interaction-mediating adhesion receptors [13].

The present study provides the first in vivo evidence of an adenosine A_2 receptor mediated inhibition of postischemic leukocyte/endothelium interaction and supports its role as a protective factor in postischemic reperfusion.

References

1. Granger DN, Benott JN, Suzuki M, Grisham MB (1989) Leukocyte adherence to venular endothelium during ischemia-reperfusion. Am J Physiol 257:G683
2. Mullane KM, Salmon JA, Kraemer R (1986) Leukocyte derived metabolites of arachidonic acid in ischemia-induced myocardial injury. Fed Proc 46:2422
3. Hernandez LA, Grisham MB, Twohig B, Arfors KE, Harlan JM, Granger DN (1987) Role of neutrophils in ischemia-reperfusion-induced microvascular injury. Am J Physiol 253:H699
4. Simpson PJ, Todd RF, Mickelson JK, Fantone JC et al (1990). Sustained limitation of myocardial reperfusion injury by a monoclonal antibody that alters leukocyte function. Circulation 81:226
5. Cronstein BN, Rosenstein ED, Kramer SB, Weissmann G, Hirschhorn R (1985) Adenosine: a physiologic modulator of superoxide anion generation by human neutrophils. Adenosine acts via an A_2-receptor on human neutrophils. J Immunol 136:1366
6. Cronstein BN, Levin RI, Belanoff J, Weissmann G, Hirschhorn G (1986) Adenosine: an endogenous inhibitor of neutrophil-mediated injury to endothelial cells. J Clin Invest 78:760

7. Peachell PT, Lichtenstein LM, Schleimer RP (1989) Inhibition by adenosine of histamine and leukotriene release from human basophils. Biochem Pharmacol 38:1717
8. Endrich B, Asaishi K, Götz A, Messmer K (1980) Technical report— a new chamber technique for microvascular studies in unanesthetized hamsters. Res Exp Med 177:125
9. Zeintl H, Sack F-U, Intaglietta M, Messmer K (1989) Computer assisted leukocyte velocity measurement in intravital microscopy. Int J Microcirc Clin Exp 8:293
10. Daly JW (1982) Adenosine receptors: targets for future drugs. J Med Chem 25:197
11. Omann GM, Allen RA, Bokoch GM, Painter RG, Traynor AE, Sklar LA (1987) Signal transduction and cytoskeletal activation in the neutrophil. Physiol Rev 67:285
12. Birch RE, Polmar SH (1986) Adenosine-induced immunosuppression: the role of the adenosine receptor-adenylate cyclase interaction in the alteration of T-lymphocyte surface phenotype and immunoregulatory function. Int J Immunopharmacol 8:329
13. Kuypers TW, Roos D. (1989) Leukocyte membrane adhesion proteins LFA-1, CR3 and p 150, 95: a review of functional and regulatory aspects. Res Immunol 140:461

Prostaglandin E$_1$ Inhibits the Stimulation of Neutrophils In Vitro and In Vivo and Improves Cardio-Respiratory Functions in Multiply Traumatized Patients at Risk of Adult Respiratory Distress Syndrome

A. Dwenger[1], M.L. Nerlich[2], E. Jonas[1], G. Schweitzer[1], J.A. Sturm[2], and H. Tscherne[2]

Introduction

The trauma-induced activation of granulocytes (PMN) and their functional alterations (increase in adherence, extracellular release of reactive oxygen derived agents and lysosomal enzymes) are believed to play a central role in the initiation and amplification of capillary endothelial cell (EC) damage and organ failure such as that in adult respiratory distress syndrome (ARDS) [1]. Prostaglandin E$_1$ (PGE$_1$) is known to inhibit several PMN functions involved in these processes. Because of this and its vasodilating actions, the immunomodulator PGE$_1$ seems a promising agent for the treatment of ARDS patients. Clinical trials were therefore started in recent years; however, the expected beneficial effects were not observed, presumably because of beginning the PGE$_1$ treatment only *after* the diagnosis of ARDS [2, 3]. Our study design called for treating patients at risk of ARDS *before* the onset of the disease to prevent or minimize very initial pathogenetic reactions of activated granulocytes by early PGE$_1$ infusion therapy. Additionally, the effects of PGE$_1$ on essential functions of granulocytes (adherence, oxygen radical production, enzyme release) and on EC/PMN interactions were investigated to enable a uniform and critical judgement about the proposed therapeutic approach and underlying pathomechanisms.

Methods

Inhibition by PGE$_1$ of Oxygen Radical Production and Enzyme Release from Isolated and Stimulated Human Granulocytes. From citrated venous blood of donors granulocytes were isolated by a two-step discontinuous Percoll gradient centrifugation [4], resuspended in Dulbecco's minimal essential medium (MEM; Boehringer-Mannheim, FRG) and preincubated with 0–1000 ng

[1] Abteilung für Klinische Biochemie, Medizinische Hochschule Hannover, Konstanty-Gutschow-Str. 8, 3000 Hanover 61, FRG
[2] Unfallchirurgische Klinik, Medizinische Hochschule Hannover, Konstanty-Gutschow-Str. 8, 3000 Hanover 61, FRG

Host Defense Dysfunction
in Trauma, Shock and Sepsis
Eds. Faist/Meakins/Schildberg
© Springer-Verlag, Berlin Heidelberg 1993

PGE$_1$/ml (Alprostadil, Schwarz Pharma, Monheim, FRG) for 10 min at 37 °C. This PMN suspension $(5-10 \times 10^6/ml)$ was used for the determination of (a) stimulus-induced oxygen radical production and of (b) stimulus-induced enzyme release. (c) Nylon fiber adherence and adherence-induced oxygen radical production were measured with diluted blood.

(a) The oxygen radical production was measured by luminol (0.4 mmol/l test) or lucigenin (0.23 mmol/l test; for lipopoly-saccharide, LPS, stimulation) enhanced chemiluminescence (CL) response in a Biolumat LB 9505 (Berthold, Wildbad, FRG) in the absence or presence of various stimuli of about 10^5 PMN/ml test volume in a total volume of 570 µl in 3.5 ml polystyrene vials. The stimuli were N-formyl-L-methionyl-L-leucyl-L-phenylalanine (FMLP; Sigma, Deisenhofen, FRG; 3.5×10^6 mol/l test), latex (Unisphere latex 22, 0.8 µm; Serva, Heidelberg, FRG; 2 µl/ml test), LPS (from *Escherichia coli* serotype no. 055:B5; Sigma; 20 ng/ml test), zymosan A (Sigma; 3.5 mg/ml test), and 4β-phorbol 12β-myristate 13α-acetate (PMA, Sigma; 5×10^{-6} mol/l test). The photon emission was recorded for 60 min; the specific CL response was calculated from the peak maximum values and referred to the specific CL response in the absence of PGE$_1$ as 100% for each stimulus. (b) The enzyme release was measured as follows. After PGE$_1$ preincubation the PMN suspension (about 5 $\times 10^6$ PMN/ml test) was supplemented with 100 µl pool plasma/ml test (to provide sufficient α_1-proteinase inhibitor for elastase complexation) and stimuli as described in (a). After 45 min of incubation at 37 °C and centrifugation β-N-acetylglucosaminidase (NAG; spectrofluorometry) and elastase (ELA; IMAC test, Merck-Darmstadt, FRG) were determined in the supernatant and cell pellet [4] and calculated as percentage of enzyme released. (c) For the determination of nylon fiber adherence and adherence-induced and lucigenin-enhanced CL production 100 µl citrated blood (preincubated with 0–1000 ng PGE$_1$/ml) plus 400 µl MEM and 10 µl lucigenin solution were incubated with (A) and without (B) 5 mg nylon fiber (Leuko Pak Leukocyte Filter, Code 4 C 2401, Fenwal Division, Travenol, Deerfield, USA) in 3.5-ml polystyrene vials. CL response was recorded for 30 min at 37 °C, the nylon fiber was removed, neutrophils were counted in A and B, and the adherence was calculated as a percentage.

Inhibition by PGE$_1$ of Oxygen Radical Production and Endothelial Cell Damage Caused by LPS-Primed Granulocytes. Cultered human umbilical cord vein endothelial cells were grown as a mono-layer and labeled with ^{111}In-oxine. The lucigenin-enhanced CL response during their interaction with LPS-primed granulocytes (isolated from blood after incubation with 20 ng LPS/ml for 20 min at 37 °C) was measured in dependency on the PGE$_1$ concentration as well as the concomitant ^{111}In release as a measure of EC damage [5].

PGE$_1$ Treatment of Patients at Risk of the ARDS. Subjects consisted of 19 multiply traumatized patients with ARDS predisposition (polytrauma scale, 42.3 ± 3.0). Nine patients were treated with 20 ng PGE$_1$/kg^{-1} min^{-1} immediately after admission to the ICU up to 6 days after trauma. Ten placebo patients served as a control group. Pulmonary and systemic hemodynamics and cardiorespiratory functions including cardiac index, compliance, Horovitz ratio, arterio-alveolar difference in oxygen tension, systemic and pulmonary vascular resistance, were monitored daily for up to 10 days after trauma. According to previously described methods [4, 6], we also measured the following biochemical parameters: plasma components such as elastase, CL inhibitory factor as microliters to reduce half-maximally the latex-induced stimulation of normal granulocytes ($\mu l_{11/2}$), total protein, albumin, lactate dehydrogenase, β-N-acetylglucosaminidase, cholinesterase, the elastase and myeloperoxidase content of blood granulocytes, CL response of blood, and isolated granulocytes.

Criteria for ARDS definition included PaO_2/FiO_2 of 150 mmHg, $PCWP \leq 18$ mmHg, compliance ≤ 50 ml/cmH$_2$O, diffuse bilateral infiltrations on chest roentgenogram, and extravascular lung water ≥ 9.5 ml/kg.

For statistical analysis the U test of Mann-Whitney was used. Differences between the patient groups were regarded as significant if p_6 or p_{10} < 0.05 (p_6/p_{10}, including data up to 6/10 days after trauma).

Results

The inhibition by PGE_1 of the oxygen radical production from isolated human granulocytes is shown in Fig. 1. The most effective inhibition was observed after stimulation with FMLP, followed by LPS, zymosan, latex, and PMA. NAG release was inhibited after stimulation with FMLP, latex, zymosan, and LPS but was not inhibited after PMA stimulation (Fig.2). Also, ELA release was inhibited after stimulation with FMLP, latex, zymosan, and LPS but not with PMA (Fig. 2). The nylon fiber adherence of granulocytes and the concomitantly observed oxygen radical production were inhibited by PGE_1 in a dose-dependent manner (Fig. 3). The correlation coefficient between adherence and CL

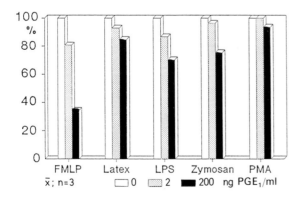

Fig. 1. Chemiluminescence response of isolated and PGE_1-pretreated human granulocytes after stimulation with FMLP, latex, LPS, zymosan, and PMA. CL response without PGE_1 = 100%

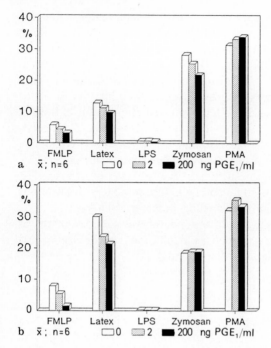

Fig. 2. β-N-Acetylglucosaminidase (**a**) and elastase (**b**) release (percentage of total granulocyte content) of isolated PGE_1-pretreated human granulocytes after stimulation for 45 min at 37 °C with FMLP, latex, LPS, zymosan, and PMA

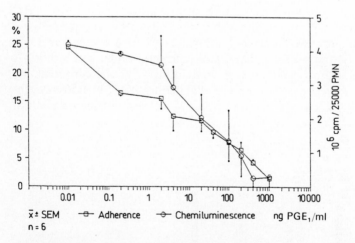

Fig. 3. Nylon fiber adherence (percentage) and CL response (10^6 cpm/25 000 PMN) of PGE_1-pretreated blood in relation to the PGE_1 concentration

response was $r = 0.945$. During the interaction of endothelial cells and LPS-primed granulocytes PGE_1 caused a dose-dependent reduction in oxygen radical production and EC damage (Fig. 4).

The results of the clinical study are presented in Table 1. From the cardio-respiratory parameters, an improvement by PGE_1 of cardiac functions (increase

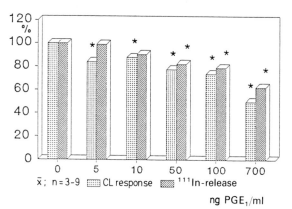

Fig. 4. Dose-dependent inhibition by PGE_1 of CL response and ^{111}In release during the interaction of LPS-treated human granulocytes and human endothelial cell monolayers. CL response and ^{111}In release without $PGE_1 = 100\%$. *, $p < 0.05$ (*U* test)

in cardiac index, decrease in systemic and pulmonary vascular resistance) and respiratory functions (increase in compliance and Horovitz ratio, decrease in $AaDO_2$) was observed. There was also a decrease in ARDS incidence from 4/10 in placebo patients to 2/9 in the PGE_1 group. Neutrophils were found to be protected by PGE_1 against in vivo stimulation (plasma elastase lower, CL inhibitory factor lower, elastase and myeloperoxidase in granulocytes higher, in vitro CL response of granulocytes higher) in comparison with placebo patients. Furthermore, there seemed to be a beneficial effect of PGE_1 on hepatocyte functions (plasma cholinesterase higher) and also a general cytoprotective effect (plasma lactate dehydrogenase and β-*N*-acetylglucosaminidase lower) as compared with placebo patients.

Summary and Conclusions

From in vitro experiments dose-dependent and significant inhibitory effects of PGE_1 were observed on oxygen radical production, enzyme release, nylon fiber adherence, and adherence-coupled oxygen radical production of isolated and stimulated human granulocytes. Also a dose-dependent inhibition by PGE_1 of oxygen radical production and endothelial cell damage was observed during the interaction of LPS- primed granulocytes and cultered human EC monolayers. Furthermore, the clinical study demonstrated that early PGE_1 infusion in patients at risk of the ARDS caused a significant increase in cardiac index and a significant decrease in systemic and pulmonary vascular resistance. Also, an essential improvement in compliance, Horovitz ratio, arterio-alveolar difference in oxygen tension and ARDS incidence was evident in this small series of patients. A larger study would be required to determine whether this improvement is statistically relevant. From the biochemical parameters the inhibition of neutrophil functions and neutrophil-mediated pathogenetic pathways as well as a general cyto-protection was demonstrated, confirming the pathogenetic mechanism of the neutrophil-mediated ARDS development and the validity of the therapeutic concept.

Table 1. Clinical and biochemical parameters of PGE_1-treated and placebo patients

Parameter	Group					
	PGE_1		Placebo		Significance	
	$\bar{X}_6$	$\bar{X}_{10}$	$\bar{X}_6$	$\bar{X}_{10}$	p_6	p_{10}
Cardiac index ($lm^{-2}\ min^{-1}$)	5.4	5.6	4.5	4.8	0.003	0.0008
Compliance (ml/cmH_2O)	39.9	38.8	35.8	34.0	0.148	0.085
Horovitz ratio (mmHg)	309.4	301.0	277.3	261.1	0.359	0.117
Arterio-alveolar difference in oxygen tension (mmHg)	155.3	152.0	169.5	178.9	0.419	0.328
Systemic vascular resistance ($dyn\ s^{-1}\ cm^{-5}$)	620	602	726	702	0.043	0.008
Pulmonary vascular resistance ($dyn\ s^{-1}\ cm^{-5}$)	149.6	145.6	189.3	187.6	0.008	0.001
Plasma elastase (µg/l)	88.4	75.9	112.5	110.8	0.12	0.005
Plasma CL inhibitory factor ($\mu l_{11/2}$)	35.2	33.8	30.4	29.9	0.008	0.009
Plasma total protein (g/l)	38.9	40.7	36.9	39.9	0.317	0.570
Plasma albumin (g/l)	20.3	19.7	18.6	19.2	0.113	0.898
Plasma lactate dehydrogenase (U/l)	287	303	366	380	0.019	0.004
Plasma β-N-acetylglucosaminidase (U/l)	9.7	10.2	10.4	10.9	0.337	0.362
Plasma cholinesterase (U/l)	2247	2070	1797	1754	0.0001	0.0001
Elastase in granulocytes ($U/10^9$ PMN)	94.6	82.7	85.8	77.5	0.012	0.074
Myeloperoxidase in granulocytes ($U/10^9$ PMN)	73.7	68.6	62.9	59.4	0.025	0.009
CL response of isolated granulocytes (10^6 cpm/25 000 PMN)	33.8	30.4	31.3	29.8	0.349	0.717
CL response of blood (10^6 cpm/200 000 PMN)	8.5	7.5	5.9	6.0	0.0005	0.011

$\bar{X}_6$, $\bar{X}_{10}$ = means of values over 6 or 10 days after trauma. p_6, p_{10} = p values for 6 or 10 days after trauma, calculated by the U test.

References

1. Tate RM, Repine JE (1983) Neutrophils and the adult respiratory distress syndrome. Am Rev Respir Dis 128:552–559
2. Holcroft JW, Vassar MJ, Weber CJ (1986) Prostaglandin E$_1$ and survival in patients with the adult respiratory distress syndrome: a prospective trial. Ann Surg 203:371–378
3. Bone RC, Slotman G, Maunder R, Silverman H, Hyers TM, Kerstein MD, Ursprung JJ, and the prostaglandin E$_1$ study group (1989) Randomized double-blind, multicenter study of prostaglandin E$_1$ in patients with the adult respiratory distress syndrome. Chest 96:114–119
4. Dwenger A, Schweitzer G, Regel G (1986) Bronchoalveolar lavage fluid and plasma proteins, chemiluminescence response and protein contents of polymorphonuclear leukocytes from blood and lavage fluid in traumatized patients. J Clin Chem Clin Biochem 24:73–88
5. Jonas E, Dwenger A, Funck M (1990) Effect of varying concentrations of prostaglandin E$_1$ on chemiluminescence response and endothelial cell damage during interaction between polymorphonuclear leukocytes and human endothelial cells. Fresenius Anal Chem 337:90–91
6. Dwenger A, Regel G, Schweitzer G, Funck M, Sturm JA, Tscherne H (1989) Cellular and humoral reactions of the nonspecific immune system of polytraumatized patients with and without the adult respiratory distress syndrome. In: Faist E, Ninnemann J, Green D (eds) Immune consequences of trauma, shock and sepsis. Springer, Berlin Heidelberg (New York), pp 241–246

Production and Characterization of Peptide-Specific Monoclonal Antibodies that Recognize a Neoepitope on Hog C5a

U. Höpken[1], A. Strüber[1], M. Oppermann[1], M. Mohr[2], K. H. Mücke[2], H. Burchardi[2], and O. Götze[1]

Introduction

Anaphylatoxins are generated from the serum proteins C3 and C5 during activation of either the classical or the alternative pathway of complement. Upon proteolytic cleavage by specific convertases the low molecular weight fragments C3a and C5a are released. Anaphylatoxins are under strict systemic control by the serum carboxypeptidase N which removes the COOH-terminal arginine, thus abrogating most of their biological functions. Besides their well-characterized effects (smooth-muscle contraction, vasodilatation, enhanced vascular permeability) the factors are assumed to contribute to numerous biological responses in vitro and in vivo. C5a is thought to be the most potent mediator of inflammatory reactions which involve the complement system. Experimental evidence showing that C5a promotes the synthesis of interleukin 1 and of tumor necrosis factor in human mononuclear cells in vitro has led some investigators to postulate a central role for C5a in the pathogenesis of septic shock and the adult respiratory distress syndrome [1, 2]. A number of animal studies have been performed to elucidate the role of complement in endotoxin-induced lung injury. Administration of gram-negative organisms or of purified lipopolysaccharide from gram-negative bacteria to experimental animals resulted in a variety of pathophysiologic alterations such as systemic hypotension, pulmonary hypertension, and a decrease in circulating leukocytes and platelets. The specific neutralization of proinflammatory components by the administration of blocking antibodies allows to directly assess the participation of mediators in complex in vivo situations. Beneficial effects of C5a-specific polyclonal IgG in animal models of sepsis have been described in the past [3-5]. These studies had been performed using antibodies which had not been fully characterized especially with respect to their reactivity with the native precursor protein C5. It can therefore not be excluded that the effects observed result from the inactivation of the precursor protein C5 and a subsequent block in the generation of C5b-9 complexes rather than from the neutralization of C5a. In addition, only C5a effects have been examined in these studies. The present study was designed to produce monoclonal antibodies (mAb) to porcine C3a and C5a.

Abteilung Immunologie and Zentrum Anästhesiologie, University of Göttingen, Kreuzbergring 57, 3400 Göttingen, FRG.

Host Defense Dysfunction
in Trauma, Shock and Sepsis
Eds. Faist/Meakins/Schildberg
© Springer-Verlag, Berlin Heidelberg 1993

Using a synthetic peptide as the immunogen, we obtained mAb that specifically react with C5a but not with C5, and which in addition block functional C5a activity.

Materials and Methods

Peptide Synthesis and Coupling to Bovine Serum Albumin. A 21 amino acid peptide C5a20C comprising the 20 amino acids of the C-terminus of the porcine C5a-fragment (YIANEVRAEQSHKNIELG) and an additional amino-terminal cysteine was synthesized in essence according to the solid-phase method of Merrifield. The peptide was purified by reversed-phase HPLC, and the fractions corresponding to the major peak were pooled and evaporated to dryness. The peptide was coupled to bovine serum albumin (BSA) through the amino-terminal cysteine using the hetereobifunctional reagent succinimidyl 4-(p-maleimidophenyl) butyrate [6].

Purification of Complement Proteins. The purification of porcine C5a and C3a was performed as described previously [7]. C5a was converted into the desArg form by incubating purified C5a at 1 mg/ml with carboxypeptidase B (Boehringer, Mannheim, FRG; final concentration 200 μg/ml) for 30 min at 37 °C.

Preparation of Peptide-Specific Monoclonal Antibodies. BALB/c-mice were immunized by repeated intraperitonea injection with C5a20C-BSA conjugate or purified C3a. The fusion was performed according to standard techniques using the myeloma cell line X63-Ag8.653. Culture supernatants were screened by a solid-phase enzyme-linked immunosorbent assay (ELISA) employing purified porcine C5a or C3a. Positive clones were detected using rabbit anti-mouse Ig peroxidase conjugates (Dako, Hamburg, FRG).

Enzyme-Linked Immunosorbent Assay Quantitation of C3a and C5a. Wells of microtiter plates were coated with a rabbit anti-mouse IgG fraction (Dako, Hamburg, FRG) in 50 mM carbonate buffer, pH 10.6 for 16 h at 4 °C. All further incubations were done at room temperature. After blocking of nonspecific binding sites with 1% gelatine, the neoepitope-specific anti-C5a mAb was administered (10 μg/ml) for 2 h. Purified C5a or plasma samples (diluted at least two-fold in phosphate-buffered solution, PBS, Tween 20 mM ethylenediamine tetraacetate, EDTA) were allowed to bind for 2 h and were detected by adding, in sequence, a biotinylated rabbit anti-C5a Ig fraction (5 μg/ml) and a 1000-fold dilution of streptavidin-peroxidase (Amersham, Braunschweig, FRG) in PBS-Tween. C5a determinations were carried out by the colorimetric analysis of peroxidase-mediated hydrolysis of 2 mM 2,2'-azino-di-(3-ethylbenzthiazoline sulfonate Boehringer, Mannheim, FRG) in the presence of 2.5 mM H_2O_2 using a microplate photometer (Dynatech MR 600; Dynatech, Denkendorf, FRG).

Calculations were performed by evaluating the absorbance at 630 nm. A microplate assay for the quantitation of porcine C3a/C3a(desArg) that relies on two different mAbs with specificities for epitopes on C3a was performed following the same protocol as described for the quantitation of C5a. To remove C3 from porcine plasma prior to the quantitation of C3a, wells of microtitration plates were filled sequentially with 1 part porcine EDTA plasma and 1 part precipitation medium. The precipitation medium contained 30 g polyethylene glycol (PEG) 6000 per 100 ml of 100 mM glycine HCl, pH 5.0 resulting in 15% PEG, pH 6.0 in the sample. After incubation (30 m in at room temperature) and centrifugation (20 min at 1000 g) the supernatant received 4 parts 0.2 M Tris-HCl, pH 7.8. Plasma was thus ten times diluted prior to the assay procedure [8].

C5a and C3a-Mediated ATP Release from Guinea Pig Platelets. A functional in vitro assay for the detection of biological C5a and C3a activities using the detection of ATP that was released from activated guinea pig platelets was performed as described previously [9].

Animal Experiments. Young pigs weighting 15–22 kg were used. Animals were anesthetized with midazolam and ketamine throughout the study and placed on a heating pad controlled by a rectal thermistor to keep the body temperature constant (37 °C). Tracheostomy was performed, and catheters were inserted into the left jugular vein and the left carotid artery for intravenous injections and blood pressure recordings. Sepsis was induced by the administration of *Escherichia coli* (0:2:H27; 10^9/kg body weight) during a period of 2 h. The control animal was given saline. The experiment was carried out for 4–6 h after completing the *E. coli* infusion.

Results and Discussion

The coupling efficiency of the C5a20C peptide to BSA and the specificity of the mAb was assessed by sodium dodecyl sulfate–polyacrylamide gel electrophoresis (SDS-PAGE) followed by immunoblotting. C5a20C-BSA and BSA were subjected to electrophoresis, transferred to nitrocellulose membranes, and stained with the neoepitope-specific mAb or with rabbit immunoglobulins to BSA. The mAb that were obtained after immunization with the peptide-BSA conjugate detected only C5a20C-BSA but not BSA (Fig. 1).

Ten murine mAb raised against the C5a20C peptide were found to be specific for a C5a neoepitope. These mAb reacted only with complement-activated porcine serum and failed to recognize hog C5 in normal plasma (Fig. 2). The detection limit of the C5a ELISA was 300 pg C5a/ml plasma. Two groups of murine mAb were generated, which recognized different epitopes of the C3a fragment. As the mAb against C3a reacted with both C3 and C3a, the removal of C3 from plasma prior to quantitation of C3a was essential. Only

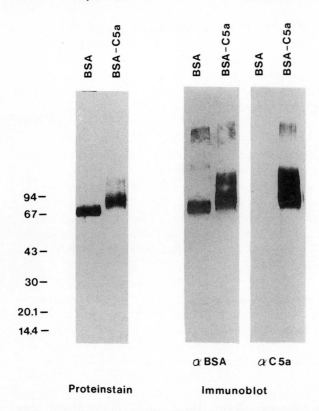

Fig. 1. Proteins were separated by SDS-PAGE and stained with Comassie-blue (*left*). Immunoblotting demonstrated the specificity for C5a of the obtained mAb. As expected, the C5a peptide BSA conjugate displayed higher molecular weight bands (*right*)

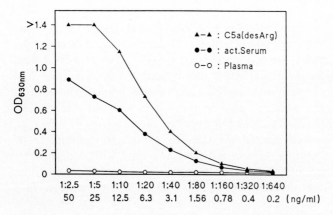

Fig. 2. C5a in zymosan-activated porcine serum but not C5 in EDTA plasma was detected by the neoepitope-specific mAb T13/9 using the established ELISA

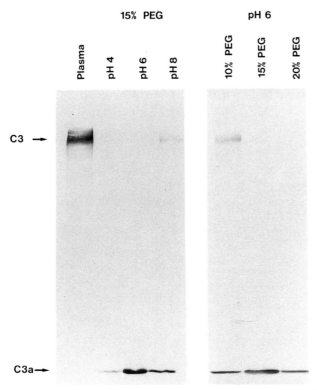

Fig. 3. Immunoblots of supernatants after precipitation of porcine plasma with acid PEG employing different PEG concentrations and pH values. C3/C3a from the supernatant of 1 ml plasma after precipitation was concentrated by anti-C3/C3a Sepharose beads and visualized by immunoblotting

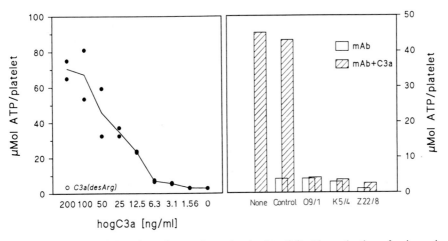

Fig. 4. C3a-induced ATP release from guinea pig platelets (*left*). The activation of guinea pig platelets by 50 ng C3a/ml is inhibited by the preincubation of C3a with a tenfold molar excess of C3a-specific mAb (*right*)

when plasma was precipitated with 15% PEG, pH 6.0, the supernatants contained no C3 as detected by SDS-PAGE followed by immunoblotting (Fig. 3). The detection limit of the C3a ELISA was 2 ng C3a/ml plasma.

Suboptimal concentrations of purified porcine C3a were preincubated with the tenfold molar excess of mAb for 16 h at 4 °C in the presence of 1 mM DL-mercaptomethyl-3-guanidinoethylthiopropanoicacid. C3a-induced ATP release

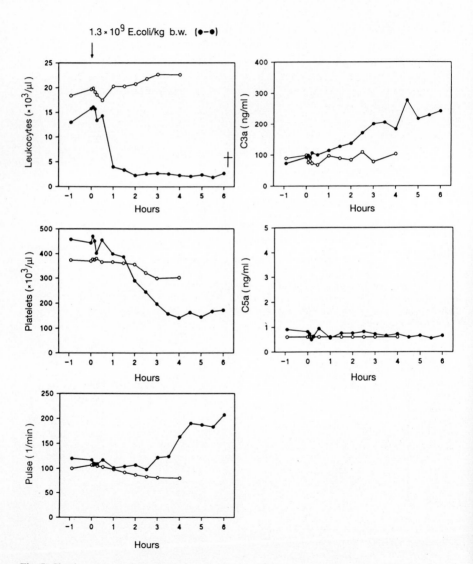

Fig. 5. Shock symptoms in a pig that received 1.3×10^9 *E. coli*/kg body weight (●-●) and in an untreated control (○-○). Whereas peripheral blood leukocyte and platelets counts and the pulse rate were significantly altered after *E.coli* infusion, plasma levels of the complement fragments remained unchanged

from guinea pig platelets was monitored (Fig. 4). All C3a-specific mAb totally inhibited porcine C3a activity in-vitro. Experiments on the C5a-mediated ATP release and inhibition of C5a activity by mAb are presently carried out.

Infusion of 1.3×10^9 *E.coli*/kg generated symptoms of shock as evidenced by hypotension, tachycardia, and decreased mean arterial blood pressure. The decrease in the number of circulating blood leukocytes was more pronounced than the reduction in platelets. None of the values returned to baseline levels during the observation time. No significant differences in the plasma levels of C5a were found among the untreated control and the experimental animal. A small increase in the plasma levels of C3a was observed (Fig. 5). The lack of a rise in C5a in this animal was interpreted as a sign for the rapid elimination of C5a from blood by its binding to specific receptors on granulocytes and monocytes. Further, the *E. coli* strain (0:2:H27) turned out to be capable of activating human but not porcine complement. These data suggest that apart from complement activation products various other immunological mediator systems may be involved in the pathogenesis of septic shock and adult respiratory distress syndrome. We are currently looking for other *E. coli* strains that activate the porcine complement system. Furthermore, C5a- and C3a-specific mAb will be employed in this animal model for both the specific quantitation of C5a/C3a generated in vivo and the prevention of the physiologic effects of these anaphylatoxins in this animal model.

Acknowledgements. This work was supported by the Deutsche Forschungsgemeinschaft (SFB 330, B11).

References

1. Okusawa S, Dinarello CA, Yancey KB, Endres S, Lawley TJ, Frank MM, Burke DF, Gelfand JA (1987) C5a induction of human interleukin 1: synergistic effect with endotoxin or interferon-gamma. J Immunol 139(8):2635–2640
2. Okusawa S, Yancey KB, van der Meer JW, Endres S, Lonnemann G, Hefter K, Frank MM, Burke JF, Dinarello CA, Gelfand JA (1988) C5a stimulates secretion of interleukin 1 beta and interleukin 1 alpha. J Exp Med 168(1):443–448
3. Smedegard G, Bui L, Hugli TE (1989) Endotoxin-induced shock in rat. Am J Pathol 135(3):489–497
4. Hangen DH, Stevens JH, Satoh PS, Hall EW, O'Hanley PT, Raffin TA (1987) Complement levels in septic primates treated with anti-C5a antibodies. J Surg Res 46:195–199
5. Stevens JH, O'Hanley P, Shaprio JM, Mihm FG, Satoh PS, Collins JA, Raffin TA (1986) Effects of anti-C5a antibodies on the adult respiratory distress syndrome in septic primates. J Clin Invest 77:1812–1816
6. Kitagawa T, Aikawa T (1976) Enzyme coupled immunoassay of insulin using a novel coupling reagent. J Biochem 79:233–236
7. Püschel GP, Oppermann M, Musehol W, Götze O, Jungermann K (1989) FEBS Lett 243:83–87
8. Schulze M, Götze O (1986) A sensitive ELISA for the quantitation of human C5a in blood plasma using a monoclonal antibody. Complement 3:25–39
9. Oppermann M, Schulze M, Götze O (1991) A sensitive enzyme immunoassay for the quantitation of human (C5a/C5a des Arg) anaphylatoxin using a monoclonal antibody with specificity for a neoepitope. Complement Inflamm 8:13–24

The Oxidative Burst Reaction of Neutrophils Is Reduced by the Acute Phase Serum Amyloid-A Protein

R. P. Linke, V. Bock, G. Valet, and G. Rothe

Introduction

The acute-phase reaction is considered to represent an adaptation of the organism toward meeting such life-threatening incidents as injury, necrosis, inflammation, sepsis, and tumor spread. The acute-phase reaction is induced by cytokines mainly from activated monocytes and macrophages and is characterized by changes in the concentration of definite plasma proteins, called acute-phase proteins. The concentration of such *positive* acute-phase proteins as α_1-proteinase inhibitor, complement factors, fibrinogen, haptoglobin, C-reactive protein, and serum amyloid-A protein (SAA) is increased, in contrast to a decrease seen in such *negative* acute-phase proteins as albumin or transthyretin [1].

SAA is the most sensitive acute-phase protein in man with a more than 1000-fold increase in concentration due to an increase in the hepatic level of SAA mRNA [2, 3]. SAA is a protein of 12 kDa, appearing in plasma at approximately 200 kDa [4] due to its association with high density [5] and other lipoproteins. It is composed of 104 amino acids [6] and is chemically heterogeneous [7]. SAA has been discovered to be the precursor of the protein thesaurosis amyloid-A (AA) amyloidosis, which is a sequela of recurrent acute-phase reactions in such prolonged inflammations as rheumatoid arthritis and familial Mediterranean fever. The AA protein, the hallmark of AA amyloidosis, is stored extracellularly in amyloid conformation and may result in severe disorders with a fatal outcome [8]. AA protein represents an N-terminal fragment of SAA (typically SAA 1-76). AA-fibrillar deposits can easily be diagnosed at the light and electron microscopic level using monoclonal antibodies [9, 10].

The function of SAA during the acute phase, however, is still unknown although B-cell suppression [11] and autocrine collagenase induction [12] has been described. Following our hypothesis that the humoral changes of the plasma proteins including SAA may influence the concomitantly changed cellular functions during the acute-phase reaction, we set out to examine (a) whether SAA binds to blood cells and (b) whether this binding alters cellular functions, in particular the oxidative burst response responsible for oxidative tissue destruction.

Max Planck Institute of Biochemistry, Am Klopferspitz 18a, D-8033 Martinsried/München, FRG

Host Defense Dysfunction
in Trauma, Shock and Sepsis
Eds. Faist/Meakins/Schildberg
© Springer-Verlag, Berlin Heidelberg 1993

Experimental Design and Results

Binding of SAA to Neutrophils. Highly purified SAA labeled with fluorescein isothiocyanate (FITC) was incubated with leukocytes isolated from heparinized blood of normal individuals by 1 g sedimentation on ficoll (Histopaque-1077, Sigma). After 1 h of exposure to SAA-FITC, the cells were washed in PBS, fixed in 1% paraformaldehyde, and examined by flow cytometry [13]. The cellular FITC fluorescence was measured simultaneously with side scatter (SSC). SSC permits the distinction of lymphocytes, monocytes, and neutrophils within a mixture of unseparated cells. Strong fluorescence was detected on neutrophils whereas lymphocytes revealed only low fluorescence, similar to the auto-fluorescence of cells not exposed to SAA-FITC [13].

The Inhibition of the Oxidative Burst of Neutrophils with SAA. To examine whether the binding of SAA was functionally effective, the oxidative burst reaction induced by the bacterial chemotactic peptide N-formyl-Meth-Leu-Phe (FMLP) was examined [13]. Indicator of the oxidative burst was the intracellular oxidation of dihydrorhodamine (DHR; Molecular Probes, Eugene, OR, USA) to the fluorescent product rhodamine 123 [14]. White blood cells were preincubated at $37\,^{\circ}$C for 15 min with 10 g/ml DHR, followed by cytochalasin B at 1 g/ml for another 15 min, before adding FMLP at 10^{-7} M for a further 15 min. The cells were then fixed (see above) and analyzed by flow cytometry.

The oxidative burst reaction of FMLP-stimulated neutrophils is characterized by a heterogeneous response with a strongly reactive subpopulation (Fig. 1b), in contrast to the basal homogeneous burst activity of unstimulated neutrophils (Fig. 1a). In the presence of SAA, however, the size of the FMLP-reactive neutrophil population is clearly reduced (Fig. 1c). Monocytes have a higher spontaneous burst activity than neutrophils. Yet, after stimulation with FMLP, the oxidative burst is not increased in monocytes, in contrast to that in neutrophils.

The inhibitory action of SAA on the oxidative burst of neutrophils was further confirmed in full acute-phase serum. To examine whether the inhibitory property of acute-phase serum was due to the presence of SAA, the monoclonal anti-AA/SAA antibody mc29 [9] was added to actue-phase serum before being used in the oxidative burst assay. The results revealed blocking of the inhibitory acute-phase serum function on the oxidative burst and proved SAA to be the principal inhibitory component of acute-phase serum.

This functional interference of a specific antibody could be used to localize the ligand by epitope analysis. Using synthetic peptides of the SAA molecule, the antigenic epitope of mc29 has been localized close to the conserved region of SAA [15]. This experiment therefore gives the first clue to the functional importance of the invariant SAA segment.

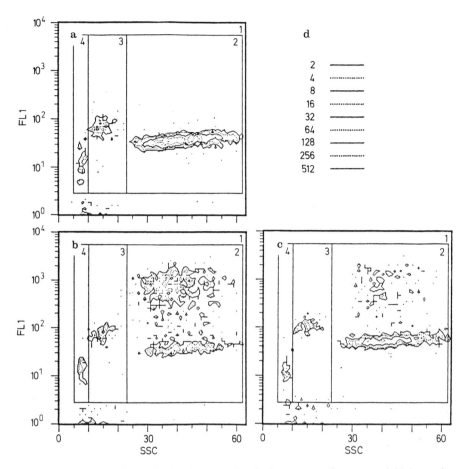

Fig. 1a–d. Reduction of the oxidative burst reaction in the presence of serum amyloid-A protein (SAA), as measured by dihydrorhodamine (DHR) oxidation and shown by flow cytometry. **a** Basal oxidative burst. **b** Oxidative burst reaction after stimulation with *N*-formyl-Meth-Leu-Phe (FMLP). **c** Reduction of the FMLP-induced oxidative burst reaction in the presence of SAA. **d** Conditions of evaluation: 2–512 density of events (contour levels). The position of neutrophils, monocytes and lymphocytes is indicated in *frames 2, 3* and *4,* respectively. FL, fluorescence, SSC, side scatter

Comment and Outlook

This data demonstrates that SAA binding to a specific binding site on neutrophils reduces the action of TNF-α and possibly that of other cytokines (IL-1β, IL-6) in a negative feedback regulatory loop. By way of successively increasing plasma levels, this leads to an increased oxidative burst response during sepsis [16]. In reducing the effect of these cytokines, SAA may reduce intravasal neutrophil activation and the ensuing self-destruction of the organism. The ligand domain of SAA for the interaction with a specific binding site on neutrophils was localized by the monoclonal antibody mc29. If this inhibitory principle can be utilized therapeutically, it could reduce the consequences of the overshooting neutrophil activation in inflammation, tissue injury, and sepsis.

References

1. Kushner I (1988) The acute phase response: an overview. Methods Enzymol 163:373–383
2. Lowell CA, Potter DA, Stearman RS, Morrow JF (1986) Transcriptional regulation of serum amyloid A gene expression. J Biol Chem 261:8453–8461
3. Selinger MJ, McAdam KPJ, Kaplan MM, Sipe JD, Vogel SN, Rosenstreich DL (1980) Monokine-induced synthesis of serum amyloid A protein by hepatocytes. Nature 285:498–500
4. Linke RP, Sipe JD, Pollock PS, Ignaczak TF, Glenner GG (1975) Isolation of a low-molecular weight serum component antigenically related to an amyloid fibril protein of unknown origin. Proc Natl Acad Sci USA 72:1473–1476
5. Benditt EP, Eriksen N (1977) Amyloid protein SAA is associated with high density lipoprotein from human serum. Proc Natl Acad Sci USA 74:4025–4028
6. Steinkasserer A, Weiss EH, Schwaeble W, Linke RP (1990) Heterogeneity of human serum amyloid A protein. Five different variants from one individual demonstrated by cDNA sequence analysis. Biochem J 268:187–193
7. Parmelee DC, Titani K, Ericsson LH, Eriksen N, Benditt EP, Walsh KA (1982) Amino acid sequence of amyloid-related apoprotein (apoSAA$_1$) from human high-density lipoprotein. Biochemistry 21:3298–3303
8. Glenner GG, (1980) Amyloid and amyloidosis. The β-fibrilloses. N Engl J Med 302:1283–1292, 1333–1343
9. Linke RP (1984) Monoclonal antibodies against amyloid fibril protein AA. Production, specificity and use of immunohistochemical localization and classification of AA-type amyloidosis. J Histochem Cytochem 32:322–328
10. Linke RP, Huhn D, Casanova S, Donini U (1977) Immunoelectron microscopic identification of human AA-type amyloid. Exploration of various monoclonal AA-antibodies, methods of fixation, embedding and other parameters for the protein-A gold method. Lab Invest 61:691–697
11. Benson MD, Aldo-Benson MA, Shirahama T, Borel Y, Cohen AS (1975) Suppression of in vitro antibody response by a serum factor (SAA) in experimentally induced amyloidosis. J Exp Med 142:236–241
12. Brinckerhoff CE, Mitchell TI, Karmilowicz MJ, Kluve-Beckerman B, Benson MD (1989) Autocrine induction of collagenase by serum amyloid-A-like and β_2-microglobulin-like proteins. Science 233:655–657
13. Linke RP, Bock V, Valet G, Rothe G (1991) Inhibition of the oxidative burst response of N-formyl peptide-stimulated neutrophils by serum amyloid-A protein. Biochem Biophys Res Commun 176:1100–1105
14. Rothe G, Oser A, Valet G (1988) Dihydrorhodamine 123: a new flow cytometric indicator for respiratory burst activity in neutrophil granulocytes. Naturwissenschaften 75:354–355
15. Frankenberger B, Modrow S, Linke RP (1991) Epitope mapping of amyloid-A protein using monoclonal antibodies. In: Natvig J, Natvig JB, Forre O, Husby B, Husebekk A, Skogen B, Sletten K, Westermark p (eds) Amyloid and amyloidosis. Kluwer, Dordrecht, pp 87–90
16. Fong Y, Tracey KJ, Moldawer LL, Hesse DG, Manogue KB, Kenney JS, Lee A, Kuo GC, Allison AC, Lowry SF, Cerami A (1989) Antibodies to cachectin/tumor necrosis factor reduce interleukin 1β and interleukin 6 appearance during lethal bacteremia. J Exp Med 170:1627–1633

Interaction of Pentoxifylline and Adenosine in the Inhibition of Superoxide Anion Production of Human Polymorphonuclear Leukocytes

M. Thiel, H. Bardenheuer, C. Madler, and K. Peter

Introduction

The nucleoside adenosine (ADO) has been shown to inhibit several leukocyte functions, such as the production of superoxide anions, degranulation, adherence, and cell-mediated cytotoxicity, and can enhance the chemotactic response of polymorphonuclear leukocytes (PMNL). These pharmacodynamic effects are also shared by pentoxifylline (PTX). ADO acts via specific receptors on the outer surface of the PMNL leading to the activation of the adenylate cyclase system. In contrast, the action of PTX has not yet been fully understood. In general, two modes of action might be considered in the inhibition of leukocyte functions. While the alkylxanthine PTX could act as an inhibitor of phosphodiesterases, it is also likely that PTX interferes with the specific ADO receptors thereby increasing intracellular cyclic adenosine monophosphate (cAMP). This latter possibility was supported by the findings that the specific ADO receptor antagonist BW A1433U was able to block PTX in restoring the chemotactic response of human PMNL after inhibition by tumor necrosis factor α (TNF-α) [12]. In order to elucidate these mechanisms, the influence of the combined action of PTX and ADO on the superoxide anion production was investigated in formyl-methionyl-leucyl-phenylalanine (FMLP)-stimulated PMNL. The pharmacological analysis [8] of the dose-response curves of ADO and PTX provide insight into the type of action of both substances. In addition, the effect of the ADO receptor antagonist 8-phenyltheophylline (8-PT) was compared with the ADO- and PTX-mediated inhibition.

Materials and Methods

Human PMNL were isolated from freshly drawn blood of healthy volunteers by Hypaque-Ficoll gradient and dextran sedimentation. Isolated cells were washed three times in Hanks buffered salt solution and kept in glass tubes at 4 °C after resuspension until use. Purity and viability of PMNL were more than 95% and superoxide anion production of PMNL was determined by lucigenin-enhanced

Department of Anesthesiology, University of Munich, 8000 Munich 70, FRG

Host Defense Dysfunction
in Trauma, Shock and Sepsis
Eds. Faist/Meakins/Schildberg
© Springer-Verlag, Berlin Heidelberg 1993

chemiluminescence [10]. The reaction mixture contained 10^5 PMNL and different agonists and was incubated in polystyrene cuvettes (10 min, 37 °C, final volume 500 µl) in the Biolumat counting chamber (Biolumat model 9505, Berthold, Wildbad, FRG). Thereafter, FMLP was injected the final concentrations of the components being as follows: FMLP 1×10^{-7} M, lucigenin 1×10^{-4} M, cytochalasin B 5×10^{-4} g/l, ADO 5×10^{-8}–1×10^{-3} M, PTX 10^{-6}–10^{-2} M, 8-PT 5×10^{-6} M. The specifity of lucigenin to detect superoxide anions was controlled in the presence of superoxide dismutase (SOD, EC 1.15.1.1, 5µg/ml), which abolished the chemiluminescence activity. Heat-inactivated SOD was without any effect on the chemiluminescence activity.

Results

Figure 1 shows the inhibition of the chemiluminescence activity of PMNL by increasing concentrations of ADO or PTX. As can be seen, the dose-response curve for ADO was sigmoid shaped, reaching a maximal value at 10^{-4} M and accounting for about 75% of the leukocyte's maximal activity under control conditions. In contrast, the inhibitory effect of PTX can be described by an exponential function. The chemiluminescence activity of PMNL was almost completely inhibited at 10^{-2} M. The half-maximal inhibition (IC_{50}) was about

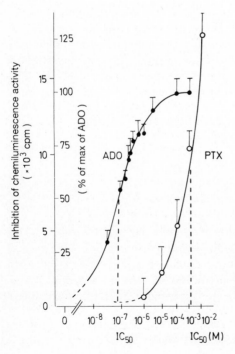

Fig. 1. Effect of ADO and PTX on FMLP-induced O_2^- production of human PMNL. PMNL (1×10^5) were stimulated with FMLP (1×10^{-7} M) in the presence of increasing concentraitons of ADO or PTX. Control chemiluminescence activity was $(19 \pm 1.2) \times 10^3$ cpm/10^5 PMNL (mean $\pm$ SE; n = 6–8)

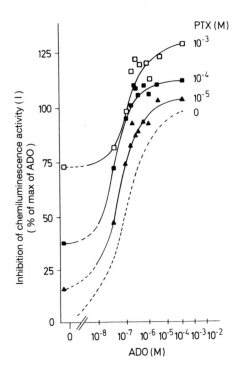

Fig. 2. Potentiation of the ADO-mediated inhibition by PTX. PMNL (1×10^5) were stimulated with FMLP (1×10^{-7} M) in the presence of increasing concentrations of ADO and different concentrations of PTX (mean $\pm$ SE; $n = 6-8$)

10^4 times lower for ADO than for PTX ($IC_{50} \approx 1 \times 10^{-7}$ M for ADO vs $Ic_{50} \approx 1 \times 10^{-4}$ M for PTX). When single concentrations of PTX were combined with ADO, PTX dose-dependently potentiated the inhibition mediated by ADO (Fig. 2). This potentiation was quantified by the determination of the dose factor of potentiation (DF) according to the method of PÖCH [8]. (Fig. 3). The DF is the factor by which a particular concentration of ADO has to be multiplied to obtain the same inhibition as in combination with PTX. This factor increased in proportion to the concentration of PTX in the range studied. In order to characterize the mechanism of potentiation the data were further analyzed by calculating the so-called corrected inhibition (CI) according to the following formula: $CI = (I - E)/(M - E)$ where I is the inhibition of any combination of ADO and PTX, E is the inhibitory effect of PTX alone, and M is the inhibition that is maximally reached with the combination of ADO and PTX [8] (Fig. 4). Because the values of the corrected inhibition were significantly higher for the drug combination than for ADO alone, the mechanism of drug potentiation was identified as a sequential synergism [8]. This type of potentiation could also be confirmed at a lower concentration of PTX (10^{-4} M; data not shown). Figure 5 shows the effect of the ADO receptor antagonist 8-PT on the chemiluminescence activity of PMNL in the presence of ADO or PTX. While the inhibitory influence of ADO on superoxide anion production was

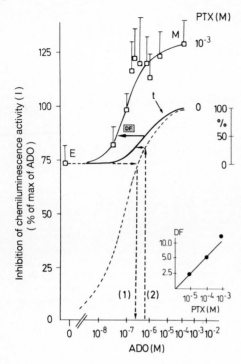

Fig. 3. Dose factor of potentiation (DF) of PTX for the ADO-mediated inhibition. DF is derived from a theoretical dose-response curve (*t*) according to the method of PÖCH [7]. The theoretical curve describes the effect of PTX and ADO assuming that PTX is equi-effective with the nucleoside. The theoretical curve is obtained as follows: (a) determination of the equi-effective dose of ADO and PTX (1) (b) obtaining the effects of the equi-effective dose of ADO (4×10^{-7} M) and any other concentration of ADO, as shown for the equi-effective dose of ADO itself (see ADO-response curve, 2). DF is the factor determined at half-maximal inhibition of the curve *t*, by which ADO's concentration has to be multiplied to obtain the same inhibition as in combination with PTX

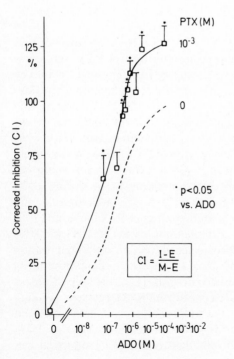

Fig. 4. Interaction between ADO and PTX in the inhibition of the chemiluminescence activity. The corrected inhibition was calculated by the formula shown. I, inhibition of any combination of ADO and PTX (see Fig. 3); E, inhibitory effect of PTX alone; M, maxmial inhibition of the combination of ADO and PTX. After correction (CI) the drug combination is significantly different from ADO alone. The inhibition of the chemiluminescence activity by ADO and PTX (mean $\pm$ SE; $n = 6$–8) is characterized by a sequential synergism (see [8])

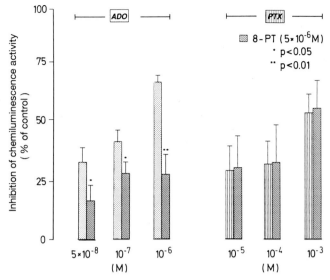

Fig. 5. Effect of the ADO receptor antagonist 8-PT on the ADO-and PTX-mediated inhibition of the chemiluminescence activity. PMNL (1×10^5) were stimulated with FMLP (1×10^{-7} M) in the presence of ADO or PTX and 8-PT (mean $\pm$ SE; $n = 6–8$)

significantly reduced by 8-PT, the ADO receptor antagonist was totally ineffective in the case of PTX.

Discussion

PTX has been proven to be an effective therapeutic tool in the prevention and therapy of experimentally induced multiple organ failure. In vitro studies demonstrated an inhibition of the release of cytotoxic agents from stimulated leukocytes and an increase in the cells' directed migration. PTX was effective even on those PMNL that had been primed before with cytokines [12]. Although a lot has been learned about the effects of PTX on particular cell functions, up to now only little was known about the biochemical pathways mediating these effects. Several studies demonstrated an increase of AMP associated with a decrease of intracellular calcium, suggesting interference of PTX with the formation of second messengers in PMNL [11, 12]. Interestingly, these pharmacodynamic effects are also shared by ADO, because the nucleoside can inhibit the production of reactive oxygen metabolites and can enhance chemotaxis. In addition, the close relationship between the increase in cAMP and the decrease in intracellular calcium was also demonstrated for ADO [6, 13]. It is therefore conceivable that both substances can effectively inhibit leuckocyte functions by the same mode of action. On the other hand, there is some evidence from our experimental studies that the inhibition of superoxide anion formation by ADO and PTX can be explained on the basis of different biochemical mechanisms. Interestingly, the dose-response curves relating both agents to the inhibition of radical formation exhibited a significant difference for PTX and ADO. In the case of ADO the curve demonstrated a sigmoid shape, reaching saturation at 10^{-4}–10^{-3} M. This result is in accordance with receptor-mediated processes. In contrast, the inhibition mediated by PTX increased exponentially, resulting in a total inhibition of the leukocyte activity. In addition the IC_{50} values were quite different for ADO and PTX. Assuming that both agents act via ADO receptors, PTX would be only a weak agonist at the receptor site compared to ADO. In this situation no potentiation of ADO by PTX is expected to occur, because the less effective "partial adenosine receptor agonist PTX" would antagonize the effect of the stronger agonist ADO [5]. However, when single concentrations of PTX were combined with ADO, PTX dose-dependently potentiated the effect of ADO. In addition, no effect was observed when the ADO receptor antagonist 8-PT [9] was used to reverse the inhibition mediated by PTX. Another conclusion that can be drawn from the dose-response curves is in support of the findings of Hand et al. [3]. This group reported that PTX is not acting as an uptake inhibitor of extracellularly released ADO. In this case a shift of the ADO dose-response curve to the left without any increase of the maximal inhibition would have been expected. These findings demonstrate that PTX neither acts via ADO-specific receptors nor does it block the uptake of extracellular ADO released by PMNL. Rather, they support a sequential synergism as the underlying mechanism of potentiation. This type of synergism was originally identified as the mode of potentiation in the case of the combination of an adenylate cyclase activator (orciprenalin) with a phospho-diesterase inhibitor (papaverin) in the relaxation of vascular smooth muscles [8]. Therefore the results of the present study most likely suggest the following interaction of ADO and PTX in the inhibition of the superoxide anion production of human PMNL: (1) ADO inhibits the production of superoxide anions by stimulating the adenylate cyclase via A2 receptors leading to an increase in intracellular cAMP [2, 6]; (2) PTX potentiates this effect by the inhibition of the enzyme phosphodiesterase, which degrades cAMP. However, it cannot be ruled out that PTX increases the efficacy of the ADO receptor system. For example, another alkylxanthine derivative (isobutylmethylxanthine) was shown to enhance the signal transduction mechanisms by its action on G proteins [7].

The drug potentiation reported here may be of clinical significance particu-larily in humans with septic shock. These patients are generally suffering from an imbalance in the oxygen supply-demand ratio. The oxygen deficit, however, is the driving force for the degradation of energy-rich adenine nucleotides, res-ulting in the enhanced formation of ADO. In agreement with this, Bardenheuer et al. [1] demonstrated fivefold higher plasma levels of ADO in patients with septic shock than in healthy volunteers. Therefore, PTX may exert its beneficial therapeutic effects in the septic state by the potentiation of endogenously formed ADO. This the more because the concentrations of PTX tested in our study were also achieved in man during oral administration of PTX at 3×400 mg/day, resulting in steady state plasma levels of PTX and its active main metabolite M1 of about 1×10^{-4} M [4].

References

1. Bardenheuer H, Forst H, Haller M, Peter K (1990) Influence of improved tissue oxygenation on plasma adenosine in septic patients. Intensive Care Med 16:S36
2. Cronstein Bn, Rosenstein ED, Kramer SB, Weissman G, Hirschhorn R (1985) Adenosine, a physiologic modulator of superoxide anion generation by human neutrophils. Adenosine acts via an A2 receptor on human neutrophils. J Immunol 135:1366–1371
3. Hand WL, Butera ML, King-Thompson NL, Hand DL (1989) Pentoxifylline modulation of plasma membrane functions in human polymorphonuclear leukocytes. Infect Immun 57:3520–3526
4. Herrmann R (1988) Pharmakokinetik des Pentoxifyllins. In: Senn E, Ernst E (eds) Pharmacological and physical therapy of peripheral vascular disease. Zuckerschwerdt, München, 91–97
5. Kenakin TP (1984) The classification of drugs and drug receptors in isolated tissue. Pharmacol Rev 36:165–209
6. Nielson CP, Crowley JJ, Morgan ME, Vestal RE (1988) Polymorphonuclear leukocyte inhibition by therapeutic concentrations of theophylline is mediated by cyclic-3′, 5′-adenosine monophosphate. Am Rev Respir Dis 137:25–30
7. Parsons WJ, Raukumar V, Stiles GL (1988) Isobutylmethylxanthine stimulates adenylate cyclase by blocking the inhibitory protein G_i. 34:37–41
8. Pöch G (1981) Quantitative Ermittlung potenzierender oder hemmender Kombinationswirkungen gleichsinnig wirkender Pharmaka. Drug Res 31:1135–1140
9. Smellie FW, Davis CW, Daly JW, Wells JN (1979) Alkylxanthines: inhibition of adenosine-elicited accumulation of cyclicAMP in brain slices and of brain phosphodiesterase activity. Life Sci 24:2475–2482
10. Stevens P, Hong D (1984) The role of myeloperoxidase and superoxide anoin in the luminol- and lucigenin-enhanced chemiluminescence of human neutrophils. Microchem J 30:135–146
11. Sullivan GW, Carper HT, Novik WJ, Mandell GL (1988) Inhibition of the inflammatory action of interleukin 1 and tumor necrosis factor (alpha) on neutrophil funciton by pentoxifylline. Infect Immun 56:1722–1729
12. Sullivan GW, Linden J, Hewlett EL, Carper HT, Hylton JB, Mandell GL (1990) Adenosine and related compounds conteract tumor necrosis factor-α inhibition of neutrophil migration: implication of a novel cAMP-independent action on the cell surface. J Immunol 145:1537–1544
13. Thiel M, Bardenheuer H (1989) Effect of adenosine on oxygen free radical production in human polymorphonuclear leukocytes. Ann Nutr Metab 33:228–229

Adhesive Interactions of Neutrophils with Endothelial Cells

C. W. Smith[1], O. Abbassi[2], S. B. Shappell[1], D. C. Anderson[1], L. V. McIntire[2], and T. K. Kishimoto[3]

The adhesion of neutrophils to endothelial cells appears to be necessary for their localization at sites of inflammation, and numerous studies show that the β_2 (CD18) integrins are involved in this process. For example, patients with CD18 deficiency have markedly reduced or absent β_2 integrins on their leukocytes, and biopsies of infected lesions reveal few if any neutrophils in extravascular tissues [1]. Additionally, it is now clear that anti-CD18 monoclonal antibodies (MAb) profoundly inhibit the extravasation of neutrophils at many different sites of inflammation in animal models [2]. Furthermore, a member of another family of adhesion molecules [3], LECAM-1 (also known as the MEL-14 antigen or peripheral lymph node homing receptor) was shown to participate in the extravasation of neutrophils in a murine peritonitis model [4]. LECAM-1 is a member of the LECAM family [3] and is constitutively expressed on the neutrophil surface.

In an effort to determine the relative contributions of the β_2 integrins and LECAM-1 to the interaction of neutrophils with endothelial cells, we used an in vitro model [5, 6] that assesses human neutrophil adhesion to monolayers of human umbilical vein endothelial cells (HUVEC) under conditions of flow intended to mimic the circumstances encountered by neutrophils in postcapillary venules. The experimental setup is shown in Fig. 1. As shown in Fig. 2, wall shear stresses between 0.5 and 3 dyn/cm^2 prevented the attachement of unstimulated neutrophils to unstimulated HUVEC. Since chemotactic stimulation is thought to induce neutrophil adhesion, fMet-Leu-Phe (FMLP) was added to the suspended neutrophils as they flowed over unstimulated HUVEC. Increases in adhesion were not seen until the wall shear stress was dropped to 0.5 dyn/cm^2. In contrast, stimulation of the endothelial cells with interleukin-1 (IL-1; 3 U/ml, 4 h) resulted in adhesion that withstood wall shear stresses of between 3 and 2 dyn/cm^2. The results suggested that different adhesive mechanisms resulted from the stimulation of each cell type.

Figure 3 indicates that the adhesion resulting from chemotactic stimulation was largely CD18 dependent since CD18-deficient cells failed to adhere at the low shear stress [7] and anti-CD18 MAb R15.7 blocked adhesion. In contrast,

[1] Section of Leukocyte Biology, Department of Pediatrics, Baylor College of Medicine, Houston, Texas, USA
[2] Biomedical Engineering Laboratory, Rice University, Houston, Texas, USA
[3] Boehringer Ingelheim Pharmaceuticals, Inc., Ridgefield, Connecticut, USA

Host Defense Dysfunction
in Trauma, Shock and Sepsis
Eds. Faist/Meakins/Schildberg
© Springer-Verlag, Berlin Heidelberg 1993

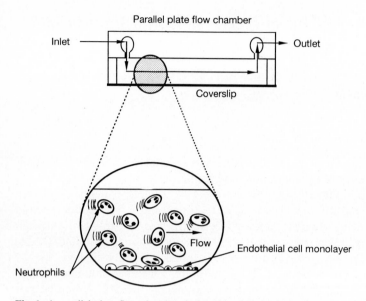

Fig. 1. A parallel plate flow chamber designed by L.V. McIntire (Rice University, USA) was used [6]. HUVEC were isolated as described [5] and cultured as a confluent monolayer on the lower coverglass as illustrated in the *enlarged view*. Neutrophil suspensions were passed through the chamber at a defined rate and neutrophil adhesion was recorded on videotape (10-min observation time) for subsequent computer assisted analysis.

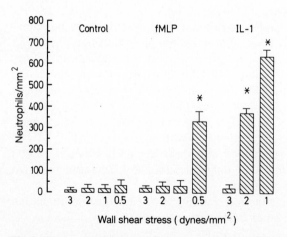

Fig. 2. Neutrophil adhesion to HUVEC monolayers under conditions of flow at the indicated wall shear stresses. The *control* condition was without stimulation of either neutrophils or HUVEC; the fMLP condition was the addition of fMLP (10^{-8} M) to the neutrophils immediately prior to passing them over unstimulated HUVEC; the IL-1 condition was with passage of unstimulated neutrophils over HUVEC that had been stimulated with IL-1 (3U/ml, 4 h). Results are expressed as the number of neutrophils adhering over a 10-min observation period per square millimeter of endothelial surface area $p < 0.01$, $n = 3$

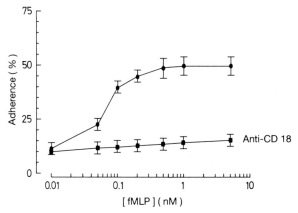

Fig. 3. Effects of anti-CD18 MAb R15.7 [5] on the increased adhesion caused by chemotactic (fMLP, concentrations indicated) stimulation. Antibody was present throughout the adhesion assay at 10 μg/ml. All points above 0.05 nM fMLP were significantly ($p < 0.01$) adherent and significantly ($p < 0.01$) inhibited by antibody ($n = 3$)

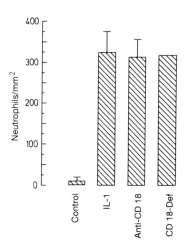

Fig. 4. Neutrophil-endothelial adhesion under conditions of flow at a wall shear stress of 2.00 dyn/cm^2. In this in vitro assay, evaluation involved four experimental conditions: control was the adhesion of unstimulated neutrophils to unstimulated endothelial cells; IL-1 was the level of adhesion of unstimulated neutrophils to IL-1-stimulated (4 U/ml, 4 h) HUVEC. The effect of anti-CD18 MAb on this condition and the adhesion of CD18-deficient (CD18-Def) neutrophils to IL-1 stimulated HUVEC were determined. Adhesion to IL-1 stimulated HUVEC was statistically significant, but anti-CD18 was without effect on this adhesion ($n = 5$)

as shown in Fig. 4, unstimulated CD18-deficient neutrophils adhered as well as normal cells to IL-1-stimulated HUVEC at higher shear stress and anti-CD18 MAbs were ineffective [6]. These results suggested qualitatively different adhesion mechanisms.

LECAM-1 was shown to participate in the adhesion to cytokine-stimulated HUVEC, as shown in Fig. 5, by two criteria. First, anti-LECAM-1 MAb DREG56 significantly reduced adhesion and, secondly, chemotactic stimulation reduced adhesion [5]. This latter result is logical in light of the finding by Kishimoto et al. [8] that chemotactic stimulation results in rapid and complete

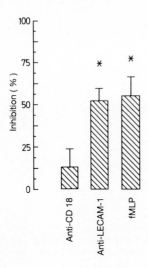

Fig. 5. Neutrophil-endothelial adhesion under conditions of flow at a wall shear stress of 1.85 dyn/cm²: effects of MAbs and chemotactic stimulation. The anti-CD18 MAb was R15.7 (10 μg/ml); anti-LECAM-1 was DREG56 (20 μg/ml); fMLP stimulation was 10^{-8} M, 30 min, 37 °C, prior to addition to the flow chamber. $*p < 0.01$; $n = 5$

shedding of LECAM-1 from the neutrophil's surface. That this is a plausible explanation for these present results is further supported by the lack of additive effects of anti-LECAM-1 and chemotactic stimulation.

The results thus far indicate that the β_2 (CD18) integrins play a minor role in neutrophil localization, yet patients with CD18 deficiency exhibit profound reduction in leuckocyte extravasation. We examined another step necessary for extravasation, transendothelial migration [7, 9, 10]. This event is promoted by stimulation of the HUVEC monolayers by cytokines such as IL-1 (3 U/ml for 4 h). Figure 6 illustrates the effects of the various MAbs on migration. Essentially opposite results were obtained from the studies of adhesion, i.e., anti-LECAM-1 failed to block migration but anti-CD18 completely inhibited it [7, 9, 10]. Both Mac-1 (CD11b/CD18) and LFA-1 (CD11a/CD18), two members of the β_2 integrin family, play partial and cooperative roles. CD18-deficient neutrophils fail to migrate under these conditions [9].

Nathan [11] documented an adherence-dependent enhancement of reactive oxygen production by neutrophils. This effect is entirely blocked by anti-CD18 MAbs and CD18-deficient neutrophils fail to show this oxidative burst [12, 13]. Figure 7 illustrates that this effect is dependent on one of the β_2 integrins, Mac-1 (CD11b/CD18) [13].

These results indicate that LECAM-1 and the β_2 integrins play distinct roles in the interaction of neutrophils with endothelial cells. LECAM-1 appears to contribute to margination under venous wall shear stresses and the β_2 integrins are responsible for transendothelial migration. Earlier studies in animal models indicate that both margination and transendothelial migration are necessary for extravasation since blocking either with MAbs is sufficient to markedly reduce inflammatory accumulation of neutrophils outside the vascular space. In addition, the oxidative burst, a mechanism of probable significance in neutrophil-

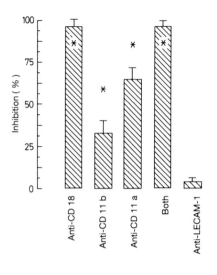

Fig. 6. Transendothelial migration of neutrophils through HUVEC monolayers that had been previously stimulated with IL-1 (3U/ml) for 3 h. A previously described technique was used. Neutrophils were incubated with MAbs for 5 min prior to contacting the monolayer. MAbs: R15.7 (anti-CD18), 904 (anti-CD11b), R3.1 (anti-CD11a), DREG56 (anti-LECAM-1). "*Both*" indicates combined use of 904 and R3.1. *$p < 0.01$ percent inhibition, $n = 5$

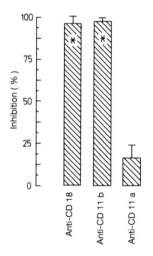

Fig. 7. Adherence-dependent H_2O_2 production: effects of MAbs. Neutrophils were incubated on plastic coated with keyhole limpet hemocyanin and stimulated with fMLP ($10^{-8}M$) as previously described [13]. See Fig. 6 for specific MAbs. *$p < 0.01$, $n = 5$

mediated tissue injury, is a CD18 (β_2 integrin) dependent phenomenon and may be therapeutically influenced by anti-Mac-1 (CD11b) antibodies.

References

1. Anderson DC, Springer TA (1987) Leukocyte adhesion deficiency: an inherted defect in the Mac-1, LFA-1, and p150,95 glycoproteins. Ann Rev Med 38:175–194
2. Carlos TM, Harlan JM (1990) Membrane proteins involved in phagocyte adherence to endothelium. Immunol Rev 114:5–28
3. Stoolman LM (1989) Adhesion molecules controlling lymphocyte migration. Cell 56:907–910

4. Jutila MA, Rott L, Berg EL, Butcher EC (1989) Function and regulation of the neutrophil MEL-14 antigen in vivo: comparison with LFA-1 and MAC-1. J Immunol 143:3318–3324
5. Smith CW, Kishimoto TK, Abbassi O, Hughes BJ, Rothlein R, McIntire LV, Butcher E, Anderson DC (1991) Chemotactic factors regulate lectin adhesion molecule 1 (LECAM-1)-dependent neutrophil adhesion to cytokine-stimulated endothelial cells in vitro. J Clin Invest 87:609–618
6. Lawrence MB, Smith CW, Eskin SG, McIntire LV (1990) Effect of venous shear stress on CD18-mediated neutrophil adhesion to cultured endothelium. Blood 75:227–237
7. Smith CW, Marlin SD, Rothlein R, Lawrence MB, McIntire LV, Anderson DC (1989) Role of ICAM-1 in the adherence of human neutrophils to human endothelial cells in vitro. In: Springer, TA, Anderson DC, Rosenthal AS, Rothlein R (eds) Leukocyte adhesion molecules: structure, function, and regulation. Springer Berlin Heidelberg New York, pp 170–189
8. Kishimoto TK, Jutila MA, Berg EL Butcher EC (1989) Neutrophil Mac-1 and MEL-14 adhesion proteins inversely regulated by chemotactic factors. Science 245:1238–1241
9. Smith CW, Marlin SD, Rothlein R, Toman C, Anderson DC (1989) Cooperative interactions of LFA-1 and Mac-1 with intercellular adhesion molecule-1 in facilitating adherence and trans-endothelial migration of human neutrophils in vitro. J Clin Invest 83:2008–2017
10. Smith CW, Rothlein R, Hughes BJ, Mariscalco MM, Schmalsteig FC, Anderson DC (1988) Recognition of an endothelial determinant for CD18-dependent human neutrophil adherence and transendothelial migration. J Clin Invest 82:1746–1756
11. Nathan CF (1987) Neutrophil activation on biological surfaces: massive secretion of hydrogen peroxide in response to products of macrophages and lymphocytes J Clin Invest 80:1550–1560
12. Nathan CF, Srimal S, Farber C, Sanchez E, Kabbash L, Asch A, Gailit J, Wright SD (1989) Cytokine-induced respiratory burst of human neutrophils: dependence on extracellular matrix proteins and CD11/CD18 integrins. Cell Biochem 109:1341–1349
13. Shappell SB, Toman C, Anderson DC, Taylor AA, Entman ML, Smith CW (1990) Mac-1 (CD11b/CD18) mediates adherence-dependent hydrogen peroxide production by human and canine neutrophils. J Immunol 144:2702–2711.

Endothelial Cell Stimulation by Anti-CD9 Antibodies

K. D. Forsyth

Introduction

The adhesion of neutrophils to endothelium is a fundamental early component of the inflammatory response. An understanding of adhesion events will enlarge our understanding of mechanisms involved in the inflammatory response.

The endothelial ligands that adhesion molecules of leucocytes bind to are relatively poorly defined. Three identified endothelial ligands are ICAM-1 (CD54, which binds LFA-1), ELAM-1 and GMP-140 (CD62). GMP-140 (also called platelet activation dependent granule to external membrane protein) is a glycoprotein heavily expressed by platelets after activation. This molecule has considerable homology to ELAM-1, is cytokine inducible, and induces neutrophil adhesion to endothelium [2]. Another 'platelet' antigen associated with adhesion is a 24-kDa protein (p24), identified by anti-CD9 antibodies [3]. Anti CD9 antibodies when added to platelets induce platelet aggregation, mediated at least in part by activation of a pertussis-toxin sensitive guanine nucleotide binding protein [4].

In this study we investigated further the role of CD9 and adhesion (for more details, see [1]). Specifically we investigated whether the CD9 antigen is expressed on endothelium, and if so whether anti-CD9 antibodies incubated with endothelium induce neutrophil-endothelial cell adhesion.

Methods

Preparation of Endothelial Cells. Endothelial cells were obtained from human umbilical cord veins and cultured in the usual way. Endothelial cells were used at the second to third passage. For immunoperoxidase analysis for endothelial antigen expression, the cells were transferred to 13-mm glass coverslips. For estimation of neutrophil adherence to endothelial cells, endothelium was transferred to Nunc (Denmark) 96-well tissue culture grade microtitre plates and allowed to grow to confluence—this generally occurred 2–3 days after seeding.

Department of Immunology, Children's Hospital Medical Centre, Box D184, GPO Perth 6001, Australia

Host Defense Dysfunction
in Trauma, Shock and Sepsis
Eds. Faist/Meakins/Schildberg
© Springer-Verlag, Berlin Heidelberg 1993

Cells were identified as endothelial cells by characteristic 'cobblestone' morphology when confluent, and by immunoperoxidase staining with a von Willebrand factor VIII antibody specific for endothelial cells.

Endothelial Antigen Expression. (a) The endothelial expression of CD9 was assessed using a conventional immunoperoxidase technique. Anti-CD9 culture supernatant monoclonal antibodies FMC56 [3] and 609-29 [5] were used. The control anti-MHC class I antibody was W6/32. The result of staining was assessed microscopically on a 0–3+ scale. Absence of staining was graded 0, with high intensity staining graded 3+. (b) Antigen expression by endothelium in culture exposed for varying time periods to the anti-CD9 antibodies. Anti-CD9 antibodies FMC56 and 609-29 were added to endothelium growing in culture on coverslips at 37 °C for varying time periods, ranging from 10 min to 2 h. At the end of the specified time period, the coverslips were removed from the wells, washed gently, fixed and immunoperoxidase stained with an anti-mouse IgG conjugated to peroxidase as above.

Neutrophil Antigen Expression. The suspension of purified neutrophils was prepared for flow cytometry in the usual way. The cells were incubated with the anti-CD9 antibodies on ice for 30 min, washed, followed by a 30-min incubation on ice with fluorescent conjugated anti-mouse antibody. After further washing fluorescent intensity of cell staining was estimated by a FACScan (Becton Dickenson) and Consort 30 software (Becton Dickenson).

Neutrophil Adhesion Assay. Neutrophils were reconstituted to 1.5×10^6 cells/ml in RPMI. Adherence to endothelium was quantitated with an alkaline phosphatase enzyme-linked immunosorbent assay.

Antibody Effect on Adhesion. (a) To assess whether anti-CD9 antibody or control antibody anti-MHC class I altered the neutrophil, inducing adhesion, these antibodies were incubated with neutrophils on ice for 30 min, followed by extensive washing. The neutrophils were then added to endothelium and adherence assessed. (b) To assess whether anti-CD9 antibodies altered the endothelial cell, inducing adhesion, anti-CD9 or anti-MHC class I antibodies were applied as tissue-culture supernatant to endothelium at 37 °C for varying time periods, followed by extensive washing of the endothelium with RPMI plus 1% fetal calf serum to remove free antibody. Neutrophils in RPMI were then added to the endothelium, and adherence was assessed.

Results

Endothelial Antigen Expression of CD 9. (a) By the immunoperoxidase technique human umbilical vein endothelium was found to stain heavily with both

Table 1. Co-incubation of anti-CD9 or control class I antibodies with endothelium in culture for varying time periods

Time (min) of antibody incubation	Class I expression	Fragmentation of Class I	CD9 expression	Fragmentation of CD9
10	2+	0	2+	0
20	3+	0	3+	0
40	3+	0	2+	1+
60	3+	0	0	3+
120	3+	0	1+	3+
240	3+	0	1+	3+

Endothelial expression by immunoperoxidase technique of class I and CD9 assessed on a 1+ (light staining) to 3+ (heavy staining) scale. Anti-CD9 induces a time-dependent loss of expression of CD9 antigen over 60 min not observed with the control class I antibody. There is in addition fragmentation of immunoreactive CD9/anti-CD9 material, it becoming spread in a disorganized way over the coverslip. This fragmentation of CD9 was not observed with the control class I antibody and suggests release of the CD9/anti-CD9 complex off the endothelium into the supernatant.

anti-CD9 antibodies (FMC 56 and 609–29). (b) Exposure of endothelium in culture to the anti-CD9 antibodies induced a time-dependent shedding of the antigen off the endothelial cell (Table 1). After 10–20 min of incubation of the antibodies with endothelium results were similar to those of antibody staining of fixed tissue (high antigen expression). However, with increasing time of coincubation, the density of staining of endothelial cells decreased, until at 60 min of incubation of antibody with endothelium there was not cellular expression of the CD9 antigen detected. Light endothelial cellular expression was noted at 120 min, consistent with new expression of the CD9 antigen. Scattered around the coverslip was disorganized, fragmented immunoreactive material. This disorganized material was first detectable at 30 min, reaching a maximum at 60 min, and remaining at a constant level for the remainder of the time studied (tabulated as fragmented CD9 in Table 1). The appearances would be consistent with shedding of the CD9/anti-CD9 complex off the endothelial cell. Throughout this time there was minimal change in class I expression, and no disorganized free immunoreactive material observed on the control class I coverslips.

Neutrophil Expression of CD9. Neutrophils do not express the CD9 antigen.

Effect of Anti-CD9 Antibody on adhesion. (a) Baseline levels of neutrophil adhesion to endothelium were 6%. Pre-incubation of neutrophils with anti-CD9 or control anti-MHC class I antibodies, followed by washing, had no effect on adhesion. (b) Pre-incubation of endothelium with anti-CD9 antibodies, followed by washing, produced a large increase in neutrophil adhesion; from baseline levels of 6% to 16%—an increase of 250%. This increase occurred rapidly in a time-dependent manner (Fig. 1), with maximal levels of augmented adhesion occurring by 15–20 min. To establish whether new protein synthesis was required for this increase, the adhesion assay was performed in the presence of

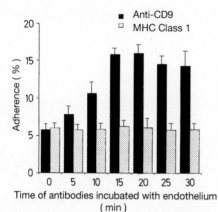

Fig. 1. Effect of anti-CD9 antibodies on neutrophil adhesion to endothelium. Endothelium was pretreated with anti-CD9 or control anti-class I antibody for varying time periods, and subsequent neutrophil adhesion to the endothelium was measured. Over a 15- to 20-min period of incubation of anti-CD9 antibody with endothelium, there is a 250% increase in the percentage of neutrophils adhering to the endothelium. Five experiments performed in each group, with $\pm$ 1 SD indicated

5 µg/ml cycloheximide. This augmentation of adherence occurred in the presence of cycloheximide.

Discussion

In this study we demonstrate that the classical 'platelet' antigen CD9 is expressed by human endothelial cells in culture. We also demonstrate that anti-CD9 antibodies incubated with endothelium rapidly stimulate a large increase in neutrophil adherence to endothelium. This increase in adherence is mediated by the endothelial cell, not the neutrophil, occurs rapidly, being maximal by 15–20 min, and is not dependent on new protein synthesis.

The increased adherence was mediated by the endothelium, not the neutrophil, as neutrophils were shown not to express the CD9 antigen, and prior incubation of anti-CD9 antibodies with neutrophils had no effect on adhesion. The increased adhesion occurred in the presence of a protein synthesis inhibitor, suggesting that binding of the anti-CD9 antibody to the CD9 antigen induces a change in the endothelial cell, perhaps through surface expression of a pre-formed adhesive element.

The majority of adhesion reactions involving the integrin superfamily occur through direct receptor-ligand interaction. It is an unusual observation that binding of an antibody to an antigen should elicit an alteration in adhesion. We consider it likely that anti-CD9 antibody binding to CD9 on the endothelial cell surface induces an activation change within the endothelial cell. Such an activation change is likely to result in expression of a new pre-formed adhesive ligand for the neutrophil, or an activation change to a constitutively expressed ligand to render it functional. Consistent with this is the observation that the binding of the CD9 ligand (anti-CD9 antibody) appears to induce shedding of the CD9/anti-CD9 complex off the endothelial cell, perhaps in a manner analogous to CD23. This shedding is maximal at the time of maximal augmentation of adhesion. This suggests that either the induced endothelial activation non-specifically leads to CD9 shedding, or the release products are stimulatory. The role of the release fragment of CD9, if any, remains to be determined.

References

1. Forsyth KD (1991) Anti-CD9 antibodies augment neutrophil adherence to endothelium. Immunology 72:292
2. Johnston GI, Cook RG, McEver RP (1989) Cloning of GMP-140, a granule membrane protein of platelets and endothelium: sequence similarity to proteins involved in cell adhesion and inflammation. Cell 56:1033
3. Zola H, Furness V, Barclay S, Zowtyj H, Smith M, Melo JV, Neoh SH, Bradley J (1989) The p24 leucocyte membrane antigen: modulation associated with lymphocyte activation and differentiation. Immunol Cell Biol 67:63
4. Jennings LK, Fox CF, Kouns WC, McKay CP, Ballou LR, Schultz HE, (1990) The activation of human platelets mediated by anti-human platelet p24/CD9 monoclonal antibodies. J Biol Chem 265:3815
5. Andrews PW, Knowles BB, Goodfellow PN (1981) A human cell surface antigen defined by a monoclonal antibody and controlled by a gene on chromosome 12. Somat Cell Genet 7:435

Decrease in Leukotriene Synthesis from Leukocytes Isolated in Septic Patients

H. Lessire[1], B. Miele[1], M. Pfisterer[1], T. N. Nguyen[1], E. Torwesten[1],
C. Puchstein[1], and B. M. Peskar[2]

Introduction

Many experimental and clinical investigations support the hypothesis that the leukotrienes are likely contributors to the nonhydrostatic edema associated with organ damage in sepsis [1–8]. In this study the capacity of leukocytes to synthesize leukotrienes was measured. The production of leukotriene C_4 (LTC_4) from leukocytes isolated in septic patients was compared to the values obtained in healthy volunteers.

Methods

Eight healthy volunteers and 14 septic patients were evaluated. Heparinized blood (20 U/ml) was withdrawn at 2- or 3-day intervals. After dextran sedimentation, the leukocytes were separated from contaminating erythrocytes by hypotonic lysis. The cells (1×10^6/ml) were suspended in a phosphate-buffered saline solution. Viability of the leukocyte preparation was assessed by the trypan blue dye exclusion test. After incubation for 20 min at 37 °C, leukocytes were stimulated by the addition of various Ca ionophore A23187 concentrations (0, 0.2, 1, 5, 10 μM) for 20 min at 37 °C. Once the reactions were stopped by rapid cooling on ice, the cell suspensions were centrifuged. The supernatants were collected and stored at − 20 °C for later analysis of LTC_4. Leukotriene concentrations were measured by radioimmunoassay [9]. For each blood collection a differential white blood cell count was performed after May-Grünwald-Giemsa staining, and a sepsis severity score [10] was calculated in the septic patients.

Statistical analysis of the data from healthy volunteers and septic patients was performed by the Mann-Whitney U test. A regression curve was plotted to correlate the sepsis severity score and the capacity of leukocytes to synthesize LTC_4. A p value of $\leqslant 0.05$ was considered statistically significant.

[1] Klinik für Anästhesiologie und operative Intensivmedizin, Marienhospital Herne 1, Ruhr-Universität Bochum, Hölkeskampring 40, 4690 Herne 1, FRG
[2] Abteilung für Experimentelle Klinische Medizin, Ruhruniversität Bochum 1, FRG
[3] Present address: Critical Case Unit, Clinique génésale Saint Jean, rue du marais, 104, 1000 Bruxelles, Belgium

Host Defense Dysfunction
in Trauma, Shock and Sepsis
Eds. Faist/Meakins/Schildberg
© Springer-Verlag, Berlin Heidelberg 1993

Results

The 14 septic patients had a sepsis syndrome caused by perinephretic abscess ($n = 1$), mediastinitis ($n = 2$), peritonitis ($n = 7$), or pneumonia ($n = 4$). Most of them showed one or more complications, such as septic shock, acute renal failure, noncardiogenic lung edema leading eventually to adult respiratory distress syndrome (ARDS), disseminated intravascular coagulation, or hyper-bilirubinemia. Their simplified acute physiologic score was 17.6 ± 3 [11]. Seven of the 14 patients (50%) died during hospitalization in the unit.

The leukocyte production of LTC_4 after Ca ionophore stimulation showed clear differences between the two study groups (Table 1). The concentrations of LTC_4 were significantly reduced in septic patients as compared to the control group ($p < 0.05$). All septic patients showed a shift to immature polymorpho-nuclear neutrophils (PMNs; mainly stab cells). In nonsurvivors the values of LTC_4 tended to remain low until death (Fig. 1a). In survivors LTC_4 production returned to normal values, even with enhancement during convalescence in certain of the patients (Fig. 1b).

Regression analysis showed a strong correlation between LTC_4 concentrations and sepsis severity score ($r = -.627$; $p < .001$; Fig. 2).

Discussion

The results showed a clear depression in leukocyte capacity to synthesize LTC_4 during sepsis. This decrease was directly related to the severity of sepsis. The exact causes of this reduced capacity are not yet established. Several metabolic and functional changes in the PMNs might explain this phenomenon. The leukocytes could have had a metabolic failure due to sepsis. A low energy charge due to inadequate production and utilization of energy-rich phosphates at the cell level could inhibit cell metabolism and LTC_4 production. Impaired cell metabolism accompanied by a decreased level of ATP was found in different tissues of patients with sepsis or after severe injury [12]. Similarly, Kopprasch et

Table 1. Concentrations of LTC_4 (pg/10^6 leukocytes) after stimulation with various concentrations of Ca ionophore A23187 in controls and septic patients.

	Ca ionophore (μM)			
	0.2	1	5	10
Control group ($n = 8$)	3858 ± 282	9184 ± 534	6786 ± 421	5381 ± 328
Septic patients ($n = 14$)	1031 ± 110^a	3216 ± 224^a	3835 ± 245^a	3520 ± 218^a

[a] $p < 0.05$

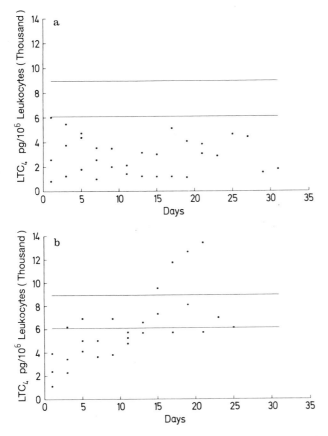

Fig. 1a,b. Concentration of LTC$_4$ in septic patients. **a** Nonsurvivors. **b** Survivors. The area between the two lines represents the mean value $\pm$ SEM obtained from leukocytes of healthy volunteers

al. [13] found a correlation between the severity of shock and the decrease in the energy state of rat liver cells. It therefore seems possible that a decreased capacity for biosynthetic reactions in leukocytes is the cellular expression of a catabolic state and even a generalized "sick cell syndrome." According to this hypothesis, many investigations in patients with ARDS showed alterations of several PMN functions, including adherence, chemotaxis, and chemiluminescence [14, 15]. Other studies, however, found increased immunological functions in similar experiments [16–18].

Another possible explanation for the decreased leukotriene generation is related to the appearance of many immature PMNs in the blood circulation. As seen in the differential white blood cell count, all spetic patients showed a marked shift to the left (mainly stab cells).

A decreased production of leukotrienes is not necessarily in opposition to the assumed role of leukotrienes in ARDS or in multiple system organ failure.

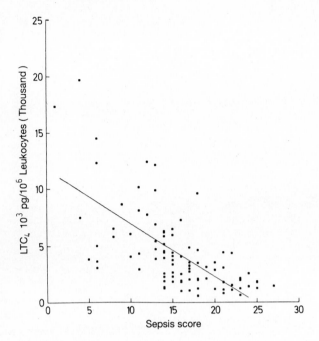

Fig. 2. Concentration of LTC$_4$ and sepsis severity score

The observed increase of LTC$_4$ concentration in the pulmonary edema fluid of patients with ARDS [1, 2, 5, 6] could be due to the local PMN increase in pulmonary capillaries. There are more PMNs in the bronchoalveolar lavage fluid from patients with ARDS than in controls by a factor of about 500–1000 [2, 19]. Such an accumulation could explain the increased amounts of LTC$_4$ in bronchoalveolar lavage fluid, although the synthesizing capacity of the leukocytes is reduced.

On the other hand, this in vitro depression could be due to in vivo hyperactivity; the cells isolated in septic patients could have been "exhausted" because of permanent stimulation. They could have developed a depletion of intracellular substrates serving the synthesis of leukotrienes. Köller [20] found that the synthesis of LTB$_4$ was depressed in severely burned patients. In one patient, however, addition of exogenous arachidonic acid led to a marked enhancement of LTB$_4$ synthesis. Davis [21] found the arachidonic acid levels of leukocyte membranes from patients with pulmonary failure to be significantly decreased.

During convalescence the enhancement of the LTC$_4$ synthesis could be attributed to a rebound effect once the cellular depression or the substrate depletion has resolved and/or to a frequently observed excess of eosinophils in the differential white blood cell count. In fact, eosinophils activated with the Ca ionophore A23187 are known to generate six- to tenfold more LTC$_4$ than PMNs [22].

In conclusion, further investigations of the possible mechanisms of the depressed capacity of leukotriene generation in septic patients are needed. Such investigations might have important therapeutic consequences, particularly as regards the use of drugs to inhibit the synthesis or activity of leukotrienes.

Acknowledgement. The authors thank Mrs. M. Krieger for her excellent technical assistance and Prof. E. A. Hopkins (Seminar für Sprachlehrforschung, Ruhr University of Bochum) for kindly reviewing this manuscript.

References

1. Mathay M, Eschenbacher W, Goetzel E (1984) Elevated concentration of leukotriene D_4 in pulmonary edema fluid of patients with the adult respiratory distress syndrome. J Clin Immunol 4:479–483
2. Stephenson A, Lonigro A, Hyers T (1988) Increased concentrations of leukotrienes in bronchoalveolar lavage fluid of patients with ARDS or at risk for ARDS. Am Rev Respir Dis 138:714–719
3. Coggeshall J, Christman B, Lefferts P et al. (1988) Effect of inhibition of 5-lipoxygenase metabolism of arachidonic acid on response to endotoxemia in sheep. J Appl Physiol 65:1351–1359
4. Brigham K, Sheller J (1989) Leukotrienes and ARDS Intensive Care Med 15:422–423
5. Antonelli M, Belufi M, De Blasi R et al. (1989) Detection of leukotriene B_4, C_4 and of isomers in arterial, mixed venous blood and bronchoalveolar lavage fluid from ARDS patients. Intensive Care Med 15:296–301
6. Antonelli M, Lenti L, De Blasi R et al. (1989) Differential evaluation of bronchoalveolar lavage cells and leukotrienes in unilateral lung injury and ARDS patients. Intensive Care Med 15:439–445
7. Sprague R, Stephenson A, Dahms T, Lonigro A (1989) Proposed role for leukotrienes in the pathophysiology of multiple system organ failure. Crit Care Clin 5/2:315–329
8. Gross D, Ben Dahan J, Landau E, Krausz M (1990) Effects of leukotriene inhibitor LY-171883 on the pulmonary response to *E. coli* endotoxemia. Crit Care Med 18:190–197
9. Aehringhaus U, Wölbling R, König W et al. (1982) Release of leukotriene C_4 from human polymorphonuclear leukocytes as determined by radioimmunoassay. FEBS Lett 146:111–114
10. Elebute E, Stoner H (1983) The grading of sepsis. Br J Surg 70:29–31
11. Le Gall JR, Loirat P, Alperovitch A et al. (1984) A simplified acute physiologic score for I.C.U. patients. Crit Care Med 12:975–977
12. Bergstrom J, Bostrom H, Fürst P (1976) Preliminary studies of energy-rich phosphagens in muscle from severely ill patients. Crit Care Med 4:197
13. Kopprash S, Hörkner U, Orlik H et al. (1989) Energy state, glycolytic intermediates and mitochondrial function in the liver during reversible and irreversible endotoxin shock. Biomed Biochim Acta 48:653–659
14. Venezio F, Westenfelder G, Phair J (1982) The adherence of polymorphonuclear leukocytes in patients with sepsis. J Infect Dis 140:351–352
15. Davis JM, Meyer JD, Philip SB et al. (1990) Elevated production of neutrophil leukotriene B4 precedes pulmonary failure in critically ill surgical patients. Surg Gynecol Obstet 170:495–500
16. Mac Gregor R (1977) Granulocytes adherence changes induced by hemodialysis, endotoxin, epinephrin and glucocorticoids. Ann Intern Med 86:35
17. Zimmerman G, Renzetti A, Hill H (1983) Functional and metabolic activity of granulocytes from patients with adult respiratory distress syndrome. Am Rev Respir Dis 127:290–300
18. Rossignon M, Khayat D, Royer C, Pouby J et al. (1990) Functional and metabolic activity of polymorphonuclear leukocytes from patients with adult respiratory distress syndrome: results of a randomized double-blind placebo-controlled study on the activity of prostaglandin E_1. Anesthesiology 72:276–281
19. Weiland J, Davis W, Holter J et al. (1986) Lung neutrophils in the adult respiratory distress syndrome. Am Rev Respir Dis 133:218–225

20. Köller M, König W, Brom J et al. (1989) Studies on the mechanisms of granulocyte dysfunctions in severely burned patients — evidence for altered leukotriene generation. J Trauma 29:435–445
21. Davis J, Yurt R, Barie P et al. (1989) Leukotriene B_4 generation in patients with established pulmonary failure. Arch Surg 124:1451–1455
22. Lewis R, Austen K (1984) The biologically active leukotrienes: biosynthesis, metabolism, receptors, functions and pharmacology. J Clin Invest 73:889–897

Aggravation of Ischemia-Reperfusion Injury in the Striated Muscle Microcirculation by Acute Endotoxemia

H. A. Lehr[1], K. Kawasaki[2], T. J. Galla[3], D. Nolte[1], and K. Messmer[1]

Introduction

Reperfusion injury after focal ischemia to organs and skeletal muscle has been implicated in the development of multi-organ failure (MOF) and death after primarily successful resuscitation from multiple injury and shock [1]. The gastrointestinal tract is particularly sensitive to underperfusion, and localized ischemia/reperfusion damage results in the breakdown of the intestinal mucosal barrier and facilitates the translocation of bacteria and endotoxin from the gut lumen into the liver and the systemic circulation, when the clearance capacity of the reticuloendothelial system is exhausted. Circulating endotoxin stimulates the synthesis and release of various proinflammatory mediators, including histamine, kinins, serotonin, platelet-activating factor, activated complement fragments, cytokines, and various metabolites of the arachidonic acid cascade. Through the release of these mediators, endotoxin contributes to the impairment of the microcirculation and finally the development of MOF [1].

The microcirculatory manifestations of ischemia/reperfusion injury are characterized by the activation and adhesion of circulating leukocytes to the endothelium of postcapillary venules, capillary plugging, and the breakdown of endothelial integrity. The present study was designed to investigate whether acute endotoxemia enhances the microcirculatory mainfestations of ischemia/reperfusion injury.

Methods

The study was performed using intravital fluorescence microscopy in the dorsal skinfold chamber model in Syrian golden hamsters [2]. This model permits the microscopic quantification of leukocyte/endothelium interaction in the microcirculation of the striated skin muscle. The techniques for chamber implantation

---

[1] Institut für Chirurgische Forschung, Klinikum Großhadern Univ. München Marchioninistr. 15,8000 München 70, FRG
[2] Dept. of Anesthesiology University of Kagoshima 1208-A Usuki-cho, Kagoshima 890 Japan
[3] Klinik für Verbrennungs- und Plastische Wiederherstellungschirurgie, Pauwelstr 5100 Aachen FRG

Host Defense Dysfunction
in Trauma, Shock and Sepsis
Eds. Faist/Meakins/Schildberg
© Springer-Verlag, Berlin Heidelberg 1993

and intravital microscopy have previously been described in detail [3]. A recovery period of 48–72 h between implantation of the observation chamber and the microscopic investigation was allowed to eliminate the effects of anesthesia and surgical trauma on the microvasculature. A 2 h ischemia was induced to the chamber tissue by gently pressing the skin muscle against the cover slip with a silicone pad and an adjustable screw, just sufficient to empty the blood vessels. Using acridine orange as in vivo leukocyte marker, adherent leukocytes were quantified in four to six postcapillary venules per chamber prior to ischemia and 2 h and 24 h after reperfusion. Adherent leukocytes were defined as cells that did not move or detach from the endothelial lining within the observation time of 1 min and are given as number of cells per square millimeter of endothelial surface as calculated from diameter and length of the vessel segment studied (200 μm). Endotoxin (*Salmonella abortus equi*, 0.1 μg/kg b.w.) was injected intravenously either 10 min prior to induction of ischemia (etox/ischemia; $n = 8$) or 10 min prior to reperfusion (etox/reperfusion; $n = 8$). Ischemia was likewise induced in control animals, receiving equivalent amounts of saline ($n = 8$). Endotoxin concentration in plasma was assessed at the time of reperfusion using a commercially available limulus amoebocyte lysate test (KabiVitrum, Munich, FRG).

Results

Under normal conditions, represented by the preischemic baseline situation, the majority of leukocytes did not interact with the endothelium of postcapillary venules, ranging in diameter from 10 to 60 μm (Fig. 1). In untreated control animals, ischemia/reperfusion elicited the adhesion of leukocytes to the endothelium of postcapillary venules with a maximum 2 h after reperfusion and a marked decline until 24 h thereafter. Leukocyte/endothelium interaction was significantly enhanced in endotoxin-treated animals. This effect was most

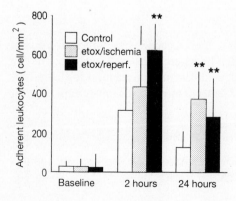

Fig. 1. Leukocyte adhesion to the endothelium of postcapillary venules prior to a 2-h ischemia and 2 h and 24 h after reperfusion. Adherent leukocytes are expressed as number of cells per square millimeter of endothelial surface. *Columns* represent measurements of 32–48 vessel segments in eight animals of each experimental group. Data are means ± SD. *Asterisks*, $p < 0.01$ as compared to corresponding values in saline-treated control animals

pronounced in animals in which endotoxin was administered only 10 min prior to reperfusion. This phenomenon can be ascribed to the considerably higher endotoxin plasma levels at the time of reperfusion in these animals (137 ± 119 versus 49 ± 23 pg/ml when endotoxin was injected 2 h earlier; $p < 0.05$, Wilcoxon test). In all endotoxin-treated animals postischemic leukocyte/endothelium interaction persisted at significantly higher levels as compared to control animals at 24 h after reperfusion, irrespective of whether endotoxin was administered prior to ischemia or reperfusion. As a response to ischemia/reperfusion, venular diameters increased and red cell velocities decreased to a comparable extent in all experimental animals (not shown), suggesting that the enhancement of postischemic leukocyte adhesion induced by endotoxin was not secondary to changes in microhemodynamic or wall shear force conditions.

Discussion

The principal observation of this study is that acute endotoxemia enhances and protracts leukocyte adhesion to the endothelium of postcapillary venules initiated by ischemia/reperfusion in striated muscle. The key role of leukocyte adhesion in the pathophysiologic sequelae of reperfusion injury has been inferred from experiments in which ischemia/reperfusion was significantly reduced by monoclonal antibodies directed toward leukocyte adhesion receptors CD11/CD18 or by neutrophil depletion [4]. These strategies also abrogate leukocyte adhesion [5] and tissue injury in response to acute endotoxemia [6], emphasizing the similarities between the two pathophysiologic conditions.

When endotoxin enters the circulation, it induces leukocyte/endothelium interaction through effects on both leukocytes and endothelium. Endotoxin enhances the expression of CD11/CD18 adherence receptors on the leukocyte surface [5], presumably through the action of leukotrienes, formed from arachidonic acid following endotoxin-mediated activation of complement and phospholipase A_2 [7]. On the other hand, endotoxin enhances the expression of endothelium-confined adherence receptors, either directly or through the action of interleukin-1 and tumor necrosis factor [8]. Finally, endotoxin stimulates the generation of cyclooxygenase products from arachidonic acid, oxygen free radicals [9], and the adhesion-promoting platelet-activating factor [10] and may thereby contribute to the extent of leukocyte/endothelium interaction.

The results of the present study suggest that the actions of acute endotoxemia and ischemia/reperfusion combine effectively to trigger the adhesion of leukocytes to the microvascular endothelium. In the clinical setting of trauma and shock, the combination of ischemia/reperfusion injury and acute endotoxemia may result in irreversible tissue damage and thereby promote the development of MOF. These considerations emphasize the importance of effective primary resuscitation, surgical interventions to remove ischemic tissue, and the elimination of endotoxin from the circulation [1].

References

1. Messmer K, Kreimeier U, Hammersen F (1988) Multiple organ failure: clinical implications to macro- and micro- circulation. In: Manabe H, Zweifach BZ, Messmer K (eds.) Microcirculation in clinical disorders. Springer, Berlin Heidelberg New York, p 147
2. Endrich B, Asaishi K, Goetz A, Messmer K (1980) Technical report—a new chamber technique for microvascular studies in unanesthetized hamsters. Res Exp Med 177:125
3. Lehr HA, Guhlmann A, Nolte D, Keppler D, Messmer K (1991) Leukotrienes as mediators in ischemia-reperfusion injury in a microcirculation model in the hamster. J Clin Invest (in press)
4. Hernandez LA, Grisham, MB Twohig B et al. (1987) Role of neutrophils in ischemia-reperfusion-induced microvascular injury. Am J Physiol 253:H699
5. Dal Nogare AR, Yarbrough WC Jr (1990) A comparison of the effects of intact and deacylated lipopolysaccharide on human polymorphonuclear leukocytes. J Immunol 144:1404
6. Heflin AC, Brigham KL (1981) Prevention by granulocyte depletion of increased vascular permeability of sheep lung following endotoxemia. J Clin Invest 68:1253
7. Brigham KL, Meyrick B (1986) Endotoxin and lung injury. State of the art. Am Rev Respi Dis 133:913
8. Pohlman TH, Stanness KA, Beatty PG, Ochs HD, Harlan JM (1986) An endothelial cell surface factor (s) induced in vitro by lipopolysaccharide, interleukin-1, and tumor necrosis factor-alpha increases neutropphil adherence by a CDw18-dependent mechanism. J Immunol 136:4548
9. Wilson ME (1985) Effects of bacterial endotoxins on neutrophil function. Rev Inf Dis 7:404
10. Chang SW, Feddersen CO, Henson PM, Voelkel NF (1987) Platelet-activiating factor mediates hemodynamic changes and lung injury in endotoxin-treated rats. J Clin Invest 79:1498

Selective Inhibition of Polymorphonuclear Leukocyte Oxidative Burst and CD11b/CD16 Expression by Prostaglandin E_2

J. A. Lieberman, J. M. Waldman, and J. K. Horn

Introduction

Following injury, prostaglandin E_2 (PGE_2) is released from stimulated mononuclear cells. Abnormally elevated levels of PGE_2 have been measured in supernatants of macrophages obtained from burned mice [1], and in post-traumatic patients PGE_2 suppresses interleukin-2 production by T lymphocytes [2]. Human polymorphonuclear leukocytes (PMN) contain on their surface an adhesion glycoprotein, identified as the receptor for C3bi (CR3) [3]. CR3 is a heterodimer composed of a 170-kDa α-chain (CD11b) and an invariant 95-kDa β-chain (CD18). Also contained on the PMN surface are several receptors for the Fc portion of immunoglobulins ($Fc_\gamma R$). In particular, the 50 to 70-kDa $Fc_\gamma R$ III is a low-affinity receptor that binds immune-complexed IgG and has been designated CD16 [4]. Together, these two surface proteins have been used to identify phenotypic subclasses of PMN [5].

Little is known regarding the effect of PGE_2 on the function of PMN. In this study, we examined the effects of 10^{-7} M PGE_2 upon normal human PMN. PMN function and phenotypic expression were assessed by measurements of basal and stimulated CD11b and CD16 antigen expression. Oxidative burst activity was measured with a sensitive assay for stimulated levels of intracellular H_2O_2.

Materials and Methods

Materials. Anti-CD16 (clone 3G8, fluorescein isothiocyanate conjugate) was obtained from AMAC (Westbrook ME) and anti CD11b (clone D12, phycoerythrin conjugate) from Becton Dickinson (San Jose CA). Phorbol myristate acetate (PMA), recombinant human C5a (rHC5a), and PGE_2 (Sigma, St. Louis MO) were prepared in working buffer to achieve a final concentration of 100 ng/ml, 10^{-8} M, and 10^{-7} M, respectively, when incubated with cells. 2',7'-Dichlorofluorescin diacetate (DCFH-DA) was obtained from Eastman Kodak (Rochester NY).

Departments of Surgery and Laboratory Medicine, University of California, San Francisco, CA 94143, USA

Host Defense Dysfunction
in Trauma, Shock and Sepsis
Eds. Faist/Meakins/Schildberg
© Springer-Verlag, Berlin Heidelberg 1993

Cell Preparation. PMN were obtained from ethylenediaminetetraacetate (EDTA) anticoagulated venous blood by lysis of red blood cells with buffered 0.89% ammonium chloride. Washed cells were then resuspended in 10 mM phosphate-buffered normal saline (PBS), pH 7.4, containing 0.1% gelatin, 5.0 mM glucose, 1.0 mM CaCl$_2$, and 0.6 mM MgCl$_2$ (PBSg^{2+}) for stimulation. Viability was determined with ethidium bromide and acridine orange [6].

CD11b/CD16 Expression. Cells (10^6 PMN/ml PBSg^{2+}) were exposed to buffer alone (control) or to soluble stimuli either alone or in sequence at 37 °C with agitation for the indicated time periods. Reactions were terminated by addition of an equal volume of cold (4 °C) PBSg containing 1% paraformaldehyde and 2.0 mM EDTA. Cells were stained with fluorescent-labeled monoclonal antibodies. For controls, monoclonal antibodies of the same immunoglobulin isotype directed against irrelevant antigens were used to characterize nonspecific binding.

Intracellular Hydrogen Peroxide Production. Measurement of intracellular H$_2$O$_2$ production was performed according to the method of Bass [7, 8]. Cells (10^6 PMN/ml PBSg^{2+}) were preincubated with 5.0 μM DCFH-DA, exposed to buffer alone (control) or to soluble stimuli either alone or in sequence, and incubated at 37 °C with agitation for the indicated time periods. Reactions were terminated by addition of 1.0 ml cold PBSg containing 5.0 mM sodium azide and 2.0 mM EDTA.

Flow Cytometric Analysis and Statistics. Cells were analyzed by quantitative flow cytometry using a Becton Dickinson FACScan. Forward angle light scatter and right angle light side scatter measurements were used to differentiate PMN. Logarithmic list mode data were collected for each sample on 10 000 events of interest. Single-parameter histograms were analyzed using Consort 30 software running on a Hewlett-Packard series 9000 computer. All data are expressed as mean $\pm$ SEM. Mean differences between experimental groups were compared by Student's paired t test, and differences with p values less than 0.05 were accepted as significant.

Results

Following isolation, the yield of white blood cells (WBC) ranged from 4.0 to 8.8 $\times$ 10^6 cells/ml whole blood. Viability for the cell mixtures ranged from 93% to 98%. PMN accounted for 46%–68% of the WBC mixtures.

The time course for CD11b expression by PMN is displayed in Fig. 1 and for CD16 in Fig. 2 as the percentage of baseline (37 °C) for the change in mean fluorescence. Incubation with PGE$_2$ did not produce any significant change in CD11b/CD16 expression. CD11b expression was augmented, however, by both

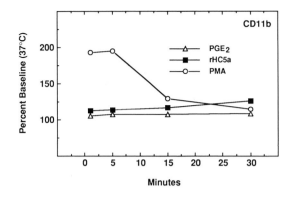

Fig. 1. Time course of CD11b expression by PMN. Data from three separate experiments is expressed as percentage of 37 °C baseline for mean fluorescence exhibited by PMN following exposure to various stimuli

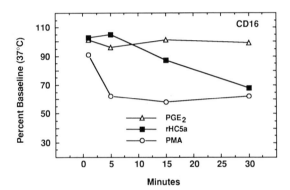

Fig. 2. Time course of CD16 expression by PMN. Data from three separate experiments is expressed as percentage of 37 °C baseline for mean fluorescence exhibited by PMN following exposure to various stimuli

rHC5a and PMA at 15 min. Loss of CD16 expression occurred with stimulation by either rHC5a or PMA. We examined the effect of preincubation of cells in the presence or absence of 10^{-7} M PGE$_2$ upon stimulated changes in CD11b/CD16 expression (Figs. 3, 4, respectively). PGE$_2$ markedly suppressed the increased expression of rHC5a-stimulated changes in CD11b/CD16 expression. In contrast, the PMA-stimulated changes in CD11b/CD16 expression were unaffected by PGE$_2$.

The time course for intracellular hydrogen peroxide production by PMN is displayed in Fig. 5. PGE$_2$ (10^{-7} M) did not alter the amount of H$_2$O$_2$ produced. In contrast, rHC5a was a mild stimulus for H$_2$O$_2$ production while PMA produced a profound increase in H$_2$O$_2$. To determine the effect of PGE$_2$ upon stimulated H$_2$O$_2$ production, we incubated PMN previously preloaded with 5.0 μM DCFH-DA with or without 10^{-7} M PGE$_2$ at 37 °C for 15 min and then exposed the cells to stimuli for an additional 15 min at 37 °C. Figure 6 shows that H$_2$O$_2$ production following exposure to rHC5a was suppressed to a significant degree by PGE$_2$. In contrast, H$_2$O$_2$ production stimulated by PMA was not affected.

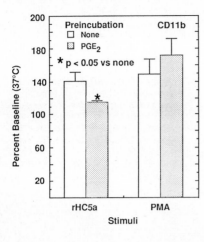

Fig. 3. Effects of PGE$_2$ upon the stimulated expression of CD11b by PMN. Data from six separate experiments are expressed as percentage of 37 °C baseline for mean ($\pm$ SEM) fluorescence exhibited by PMN following exposure to stimuli

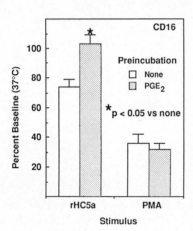

Fig. 4. Effect of PGE$_2$ upon the stimulated expression of CD16 by PMN. Data from six separate experiments are expressed as percentage of 37 °C baseline for mean ($\pm$ SEM) fluorescence exhibited by PMN following exposure to stimuli

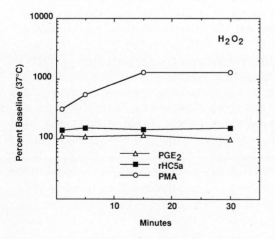

Fig. 5. Time course of intracellular hydrogen peroxide production by PMN. Data from three separate experiments is expressed as percentage of 37 °C baseline for mean fluorescence exhibited by PMN for intracellular levels of 2',7'-dichlorofluorescein following exposure to various stimuli

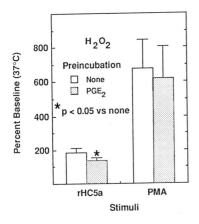

Fig. 6. Effect of PGE_2 upon the stimulated H_2O_2 by PMN. Data from six separate experiments are expressed as percentage of $37\,°C$ baseline for mean ($\pm$ SEM) fluorescence exhibited by PMN intracellular levels of $2',7'$-dichlorofluorescein following exposure to stimuli

Discussion

This study demonstrates that PGE_2 is capable of selectively suppressing some functional and phenotypic responses of human PMN. When exposed to the membrane receptor stimulus C5a, PMN produced less intracellular H_2O_2 when pretreated with $10^{-7}\ M\ PGE_2$. The same concentration of PGE_2 also interfered with C5a-induced changes in CD11b/CD16 expression. In contrast to the observations with C5a, PMA-induced intracellular H_2O_2 was not affected by PGE_2. Concomitantly, significant alterations of CD11b/CD16 expression were also not affected by pretreatment with PGE_2.

PMN respond to soluble stimuli by increasing the number of CR3 (CD11b) on their surface [9, 10], events that follow fusion of lysosomal membranes with the plasma membrane, thus mobilizing an internal store of CR3 to the PMN surface [11]. Following stimulation of PMN with formyl-methionyl-leucyl-phenylalanine the CD16 antigen is released from the surface of the PMN into the supernatant [12]. The clinical significance of this observation has not been determined.

To measure oxidative burst activity, we used a highly sensitive assay for intracellular production of H_2O_2 that detects changes in H_2O_2 within individual cells on the order of $10^{-18}\ M$ [7]. In this assay, both $2',7'$-dichlorofluorescin and $2',7'$-dichlorofluorescein are unable to leak out, and total cell fluorescence indirectly reflects intracellular hydrogen peroxide production. Our results indicate that membrane-stimulated oxidative burst activity was selectively inhibited by PGE_2, corroborating other reports that PMN taken from posttraumatic patients are less capable of generating oxidants [13].

An immunosuppressive role for PGE_2 has been reported in numerous in vitro studies [2, 14–16]. One study of in vivo effects of PGE_2 suggests that infusion of this agent failed to impair cell-mediated immunity [17]. This contrast between in vitro and in vivo effects has been resolved.

Ward et al. observed a suppressive effect of prostaglandins on superoxide production using rat PMN and soluble stimuli [18]. Other investigators have

J. A. Lieberman et al.: Selective Inhibition of Polymorphonuclear Leukocyte

demonstrated a direct inhibitory effect of PGE_2 on other PMN responses [19]. Our studies are consistent with these results in that intracellular hydrogen peroxide production stimulated by a chemotactic agent was suppressed by PGE_2, whereas PMA stimulation was unaffected. Further studies will be required to ascertain the mechanism for this selective inhibition of PMN by PGE_2.

References

1. Miller-Graziano CL, Fink M, Wu JY, Szabo G, Kodys K (1988) Mechanisms of altered monocyte prostaglandin E2 production in severely injured patients. Arch Surg 123:293–299
2. Faist E, Mewes A, Baker CC et al. (1987) Prostaglandin E2 (PGE2)-dependent suppression of interleukin 2 (IL-2) production in patients with major trauma. J Trauma 27:837–848
3. Fearon DT (1980) Identification of the membrane glycoprotein that is the C3b receptor of the human erythrocyte, polymorponuclear leukocyte, B lymphocyte, and monocyte. J Exp Med 152:20–30
4. Fleit HB, Wright SD, Unkeless JC (1984) Human neutrophil Fcγ receptor distribution and structure. Proc Natl Acad Sci USA 79:3275–3279
5. Babcock GF, Alexander JW, Warden GD (1990) Flow cytometric analysis of neutrophil subsets in thermally injured patients developing infection. Clin Immunol Immunopathol 54:117–125
6. Parks DR, Bryan VM, Oi VM, Oi VT, Herzenberg LA (1979) Antigen specific identification and cloning of hybridomas with a fluorescence activated cell sorter (FACS). Proc Natl Acad Sci USA 76:1962
7. Bass DA, Parce JW (1983) Flow cytometric studies of oxidative product formation by neutrophils: a graded response to membrane stimulation. J Immunol 130:1910–1917
8. Bass DA, Olbrantz P, Szejda P, Seeds MC, McCall CE (1986) Subpopulations of neutrophils with increased oxidative product formation in blood of patients with infections. J Immunol 136:860–866
9. Berger M, O'Shea J, Cross AS, Folks TM, Chused TM, Brown EJ, Frank MM (1984) Human neutrophils increase expression of C3bi as well as C3b receptors upon activation. J Clin Invest 74:1566
10. Kishimoto TK, Jutila MA, Berg EL, Butcher EC (1989) Neutrophil Mac-1 and MEL-14 adhesion proteins inversely regulated by chemotactic factors. Science 245:1238–1241
11. O'Shea J, Brown EJ, Seligmann BE, Metcalf JA, Frank MM, Gallin JI (1985) Evidence for distinct intracellular pools of receptors for C3b and C3bi in human neutrophils. J Immunol 134: 2580
12. Huizinga TW, van der Schoot CE, Jost C, Klaassen R, Kleijer M, von dem Borne AE, Roos D, Tetteroo PA (1988) The PI-linked receptor FcRIII is released on stimulation of neutrophils. Nature 333(6174):667–669
13. Davis JM, Dineen P, Gallin JI (1980) Neutrophil degranulation and abnormal chemotaxis after thermal injury. J Immunol 124:263–274
14. Freeman TR, Shelby J (1988) Effect of anti-PGE antibody on cell-mediated immune response in thermally injured mice. J Trauma 28:190–194
15. Snyder DA, Beller DI, Unanue ER (1982) Prostaglandins modulate macrophage Ia expression. Nature 299:263–265
16. Stephan RN, Conrad PJ, Saizawa M, Dean RE, Chaudry IH (1988) Prostaglandin E_2 depresses antigen-presenting cell function of peritoneal macrophages. J Surg Res 44:733–739
17. Waymack JP, Yurt RW (1988) Effect of prostaglandin E on immune function in multiple animal models. Arch Surg 123(11):1429–1432
18. Ward PA, Sulavik MC, Johnson KJ (1984) Rat neutrophil activation and effects of lipoxygenase and cyclooxygenase inhibitors. Am J Pathol 116(2):223–233
19. Styrt B, Klempner MS, Rocklin RE (1988) Comparison of prostaglandins E_2 and D_2 as inhibitors of respiratory burst in neutrophils from atopic and nonatopic subjects. Inflammation 12(3):213–221

The Role of Lysosomal Cysteine Proteinases as Markers of Macrophage Activation and as Nonspecific Mediators of Inflammation

W. Machleidt[1], I. Assfalg-Machleidt[1], A. Billing[2], D. Fröhlich[2], M. Jochum[3], T. Joka[4], and D. Nast-Kolb[5]

Introduction

A major portion of the lysosomal proteinases responsible for intracellular degradation of phagocytized proteins are cysteine proteinases, the "acid" cathepsins B, H, L, and S (see [1] for review). As we have shown previously [2, 3], increased cysteine proteinase activity is found in blood plasma of polytraumatized and septic patients as well as in local inflammatory secretions such as bronchoalveolar lavage fluid and peritonitis exudate. Most of this activity is due to cathepsin B, which is relatively stable at neutral pH (half-life about 30 min at pH 7.4) and is protected in the form of reversible complexes with its endogenous protein inhibitors (stefins, cystatins, and kininogens). Here we report some evidence for the role of cathepsin B as a marker of macrophage activation and of lysosomal cysteine proteinases as potential nonspecific mediators of inflammation.

Materials and Methods

Cysteine proteinase activity and complexed polymorphonuclear (PMN) elastase were determined by fluorometric assay and enzyme-linked immunosorbent assay as described [2, 3]. The organization of clinical studies and sampling protocols were reported in detail elsewhere [4, 5]. Proteolysis of fluorescein isothiocyanate IgG (Sigma) by human cathepsin B (Medor, Herrsching, FRG) and peritonitis exudate was performed as described [6].

[1] Institut für Physiologische Chemie, Physikalische Biochemie und Zellbiologie der Universität München, Geothestraße 33, 8000 Munich 2, FRG
[2] Chirurgische Klinik und Poliklinik der Universität München, Klinikum Großhadern,
[3] Abteilung für Klinische Chemie und Klinische Biochemie, Chirurgische Klinik Innenstadt der Universität München,
[4] Chirurgische Universitätskliniken, 4300 Essen, FRG
[5] Chirurgische Klinik Innenstadt der Universität München.

Host Defense Dysfunction
in Trauma, Shock and Sepsis
Eds. Faist/Meakins/Schildberg
© Springer-Verlag, Berlin Heidelberg 1993

Results and Discussion

Cathepsin B as Marker of Macrophage Activation. PMN granulocytes contain only minute amounts of cathepsin B (1.5 ng/10^6 cells), whereas high levels of cathepsin B, L, and H have been found in monocytes, macrophages, and other cells of the reticuloendothelial system [3, 7, 8]. Therefore cathepsin B may be considered as a marker for the activity of the monocyte/macrophage system. This hypothesis was supported by different patterns of release of cathepsin B and PMN elastase during inflammation in patients.

Cathepsin B of blood plasma after major trauma reaches its maximum at least 6 h earlier than complexed PMN elastase (Fig. 1). This early cathepsin B activity of blood plasma proved to be a sensitive and specific parameter for the prediction of subsequent multiple organ failure (Nast-Kolb et al., this volume). In all groups of patients, cathepsin B activity returned to only slightly elevated levels within 3 days after the trauma. Early cathepsin B activity does not discriminate between lethal and reversible organ failure. A nearly constant elastase/cathepsin B ratio around 300 was observed during the first 3 days in all patients, followed by a slow decrease in the groups with reversible organ failure and without organ complications. In patients developing lethal organ failure the elastase/cathepsin B ratio increased to 500–600 and remained high after the 3rd day (Fig. 2).

As determined with cell lysates, an elastase/cathepsin B ratio of 3000–6000 would be expected if both enzymes were released from PMN granulocytes [3].

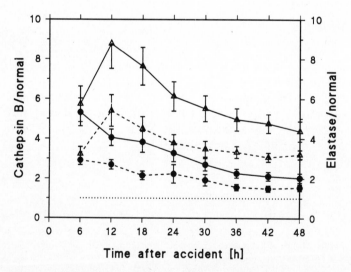

Fig. 1. Cathepsin B activity (●) and complexed PMN elastase (△) of blood plasma in the early phase after major trauma. Both enzymes were expressed as multiples of their normal values (50 mU/I for cathepsin B, 90 ng/ml for PMN elastase). Mean values ± SEM of 29 patients without organ complications (––––) and 29 patients with reversible multiple organ failure (———)

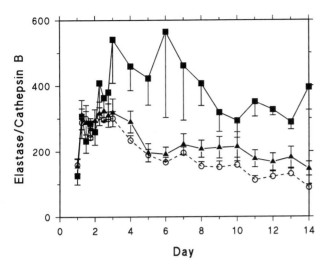

Fig. 2. Elastase/cathepsin B ratio in blood plasma of patients after severe multiple injury. Mean values ± SEM for 29 patients without organ complications (○), 29 patients with reversible multiple organ failure (▲), and 11 patients with lethal multiple organ failure (■)

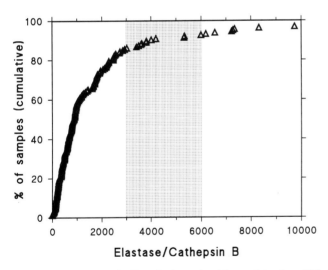

Fig. 3. Elastase/cathepsin B ratio in peritonitis exudates ($n = 166$). Cumulative percentage of samples as a function of increasing elastase/cathepsin B ratio. *Shaded area*, range of elastase/cathepsin B ratios found within lysates of PMN granulocytes from healthy persons

This ratio was indeed found in a few peritonitis exudates containing high numbers of neutrophils (Fig. 3). In the majority of samples, however, much lower elastase/cathepsin B ratios were observed, supporting the origin of cathepsin B from cells other than neutrophils. Elastase/cathepsin B ratios close

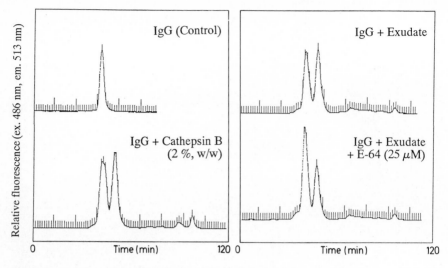

Fig. 4. Degradation of immunoglobulin G (IgG) by isolated human cathepsin B and by E-64 sensitive proteinase activity in peritonitis exudate. Fast gel chromatography of fluorescein isothiocyanate labeled IgG and its fragments on a Superose 12 column

to 1 were found in bronchoalveolar lavage fluid containing a large number of alveolar macrophages.

Cysteine Proteinases as Nonspecific Mediators of Inflammation. Direct evidence for a role of cysteine proteinases in proteolytic pathomechanisms of inflammation comes from studies with peritonitis exudates. Peritonitis exudates reveal strong proteolytic activity which is paralleled by deficient opsonic capacity and high levels of the lysosomal proteinases PMN elastase and cathepsin B [6]. Using fluorescence-labeled protein, degradation of IgG by cell-free supernatant of peritonitis exudate was demonstrated in vitro (Fig. 4). Part of this degradation can be prevented by addition of E-64, a specific inactivator of cysteine proteinases, indicating that lysosomal cysteine proteinases are involved. Catalytic amounts of isolated human cathepsin B (see Fig. 4) and L are able to proteolyse IgG in vitro effectively.

Conclusions

Cathepsin B seems to be a useful marker for the activity of phagocytes of the monocyte/macrophage system that can be followed easily in blood plasma and inflammatory secretions of patients. The observed very early release of cathepsin B after blunt major injury raises new questions about the role of macrophages in the reaction sequence of the inflammatory process.

Cysteine proteinases of monocytes/macrophages may play a role as non-specific mediators of inflammation comparable to that of the serine proteinases elastase and cathepsin G from PMN granulocytes.

Acknowledgements. We wish to thank Prof. Hans Fritz, Munich, for stimulating discussion and generous support. The expert technical assistance of Mrs. Gerda Behrens and Mrs. Rita Zauner is greatly appreciated. The investigations were supported by the Sonderforschungsbereich 207 of the University of Munich.

References

1. Barett AJ, Buttle DJ, Mason RW (1988) Lysosomal cysteine proteinases. In: ISI atlas of science: biochemistry. Institute for Scientific Information, Philadelphia, pp 256–260
2. Assfalg-Machleidt I, Jochum M, Klaubert W, Inthorn D, Machleidt W (1988) Enzymatically active cathepsin B dissociating from its inhibitor complexes is elevated in blood plasma of patients with septic shock and some malignant tumors. Biol Chem Hoppe Seyler 369 [Suppl]: 263–269
3. Assfalg-Machleidt I, Jochum M, Nast-Kolb D, Siebeck M, Billling A, Joka T. Rothe G, Valet G, Zauner R, Scheuber HP, Machleidt W (1990) Cathepsin B—indicator for the release of lysosomal cysteine proteinases in severe trauma and inflammation. Biol Chem Hoppe Seyler 371 [Suppl]: 211–222
4. Nast-Kolb D, Waydhas C, Jochum M, Spannagl M, Duswald KH, Schweiberer L (1990) Günstigster Operationszeitpunkt für die Versorgung von Femurschaftfrakturen bei Polytrauma. Chirurg 61:259–265
5. Billing A, Fröhlich D, Kortmann H, Jochum M (1989) Die Insuffizienz der intraabdominellen Infektabwehr bei eitrigen Peritonitis—Folge einer gestörten Fremdkörperopsonierung. Klin Wochenschr 67:349–356
6. Billing A, Fröhlich D, Assfalg-Machleidt I, Machleidt W, Jochum M (1991) Proteolysis of defensive proteins in peritonitis exudate: pathobiochemical aspects and therapeutical approach. Biomed Biochim Acta 50:399–402
7. Kominami E, Tsukahara T, Bando Y, Katunuma N (1985) Distribution of cathepsins B and H in rat tissues and peripheral blood cells. J Biochem 98:87–93
8. Howie AJ, Burnett D, Crocker J (1985) The distribution of cathepsin B in human tissues. J Pathol 145:307–314

Endothelin Mediates a Ca^{2+} Activation Signal in Human Monocytes

M. Huribal, D. S. Margolis, and M. A. McMillen

Introduction

Restoration of blood flow to ischemic organs after shock or vascular occlusion may result in further reperfusion damage. In animal models of reperfusion injury, the presence or absence of leukocytes significantly influences the severity of injury [1]. Some leukocyte factor(s) may be critical to the injury, and the aim of the current studies is to indentify those factors in underperfused vascular beds that might trigger the leukocyte component of this injury. Endothelin, a 21 amino acid peptide produced by the vascular endothelium, is a potent vasoconstrictor of vascular smooth muscle via a Ca^{2+}-dependent mechanism [2]. Endothelin may be a polyfunctional cytokine in that it also elicits intracellular ionized Ca^{2+} ($[Ca^{2+}]_i$) increase in anterior pituitary cells [3] and renal mesangial cells [4]. A series of studies were planned to evaluate whether endothelin mediates a Ca^{2+} activation signal in human peripheral blood mononuclear cells (H-PBMC), monocytes, or lymphocytes.

Materials and Methods

H-PBMC from 200 cm^3 heparinized blood of healthy donors were separated on Ficoll 1077 gradients and incubated overnight in tissue culture flasks at 37 °C in 5% CO_2 in RPMI 1640 (Sigma)/5% NuSera (Collaborative Research). Nonadherent cells were removed and subsequently treated with anti-CD8, anti-CD20, anti-OKM1 monoclonal antibodies (Ortho Laboratories), and magnetized heterologous goat anti-mouse antibodies (Advanced Magnetics) to obtain CD4(+) lymphocytes by negative selection. Cells were 90%–98% CD4(+) lymphocytes by flow cytometry performed on a Coulter Epics Flow Cytometer. Adherent cells were harvested with iced Ca^{2+}-free Hank's balanced salt solution and were 90%–95% monocytes by flow cytometry. H-PBMC, lymphocytes, and monocytes were loaded with Fura-2 AM (Molecular Probes), washed, and

Department of Surgery, Yale University and Yale Affiliate Regional Surgical Residency at Bridgeport, 950 Campbell Avenue, Westhaven CT 06515, USA

Host Defense Dysfunction
in Trauma, Shock and Sepsis
Eds. Faist/Meakins/Schildberg
© Springer-Verlag, Berlin Heidelberg 1993

8×10^6 cells placed inside a 2-ml cuvette inside a Perkin-Elmer LS5B spectro-fluorometer. Endothelin (Peninsula Laboratories) was added at 10^{-6}, 10^{-7}, 10^{-8}, 10^{-9}, 10^{-10} M. Phytohemagglutinin (PHA) lectin (Burroughs-Wellcome) was used as a control agonist. Fluorescence was measured on a Perkin-Elmer LS5B fluorescence spectrophotometer, and intracellular ionized Ca^{2+} was calculated on an IBM XT with Perkin-Elmer Fura-2 software [5].

Results

Endothelin increased $[Ca^{2+}]_i$ 110 ± 7 nM at 10^{-6} in Fura-2 loaded monocytes over a dosage range of 10^{-6}–10^{-10} (Fig. 1). This signal was different from other Ca^{2+} activation signals (Fig. 2) in monocytes/leukocytes (as represented by PHA) in that the endothelin-induced $[Ca^{2+}]_i$ increase was monophasic (Fig. 3) and did not extinguish with repeated doses of endothelin (Fig. 4). When Ca^{2+} was removed from the buffer, the Ca^{2+} signal was not affected (Fig. 5.)

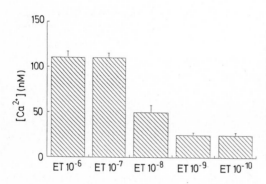

Fig. 1. Dose-response curve for endothelin-1 effect on intracellular ionized calcium. Endothelin-1 was added to FURA-2 loaded human monocytes at dosages of 10^{-6}, 10^{-7}, 10^{-8}, 10^{-9} and 10^{-10} M. Changes in intracellular calcium were measured as described in Materials and Methods. Intracellular calcium increase varied between 35 and 110 nM in a dose-response fashion when endothelin was added ($n = 6$, $p < 0.01$)

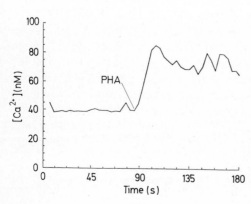

Fig. 2. Phytohemagglutinin-mediated biphasic increase in intracellular ionized calcium in 8×10^6 FURA-2 loaded monocytes (example of a single experiment)

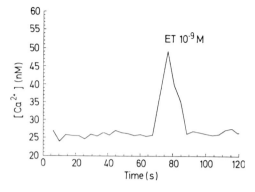

Fig. 3. Endothelin-mediated monophasic increase in intracellular ionized calcium in 8×10^6 FURA-2 loaded monocytes (example of a single experiment)

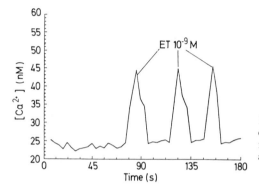

Fig. 4. Sequential addition of $10^{-9}\,M$ endothelin to FURA-2 loaded monocytes results in sequential calcium spikes (example of a single experiment)

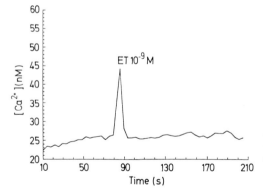

Fig. 5. Endothelin-mediated monophasic increase in intracellular ionized calcium in 8×10^6 FURA-2 loaded monocytes in calcium-free buffer. The magnitude and duration of the intracellular calcium increase is unaffected by removing extracellular calcium (example of a single experiment)

Discussion

Endothelin is a novel peptide of 21 amino acids originally isolated from cultured porcine aortic endothelial cells [6]. Three isoforms have been identified, and only endothelin-1 is of vascular endothelium origin [7]. The peptide is stored in a pre, pro form and is released when "endothelin-converting enzyme" is activated by thrombin, epinephrine, angiotensin II, arginine-vasopressin, transforming growth factor-β, phorbol ester (a protein kinase C, PKC, agonist) or Ca^{2+} ionophore A 23187 [8]. In human vascular smooth muscle cells 10^5 endothelin binding sites/cells have been observed in tissue culture [9]. Recent data suggest that endothelin may be a polyfunctional cytokine; it is a bronchoconstrictor and mediates a Ca^{2+} activation signal in cultured anterior pituitary cells and renal mesangial cells. Data in vascular smooth muscle cells suggest that endothelin transduces its intracellular message via phospholipase C cleavage of phosphatidylinositol biphosphate (PIP_2) into inositol trisphosphate (IP_3; which opens L-type Ca^{2+} channels as well as triggering the release of endoplasmic reticular Ca^{2+}) and diacylglycerol (DAG; which activates PKC). Endothelin has not been shown to effect intracellular cAMP [10].

PHA binds to several different surface receptors on lymphocytes (including CD3 and CD2) and monocytes and is a well-accepted control of a positive Ca^{2+} activation signal [11]. Lectins actually do not bind to receptors but rather to carbohydrates that glycosylate the receptor proteins. PHA binds to N-acetylgalactosamine. There are approximately 500 000 lectin binding sites per lymphocyte or monocyte, but most receptors are present in numbers between 5000 and 50 000. Therefore, it is likely that PHA controls in Ca^{2+} fluorescence studies represent the recruitment and activation of multiple and different receptors which utilize the $PIP_2 \rightarrow DAG + IP_3$ pathway. Competitive binding of PHA with a calcium agonist may suggest that agonist's receptor is normally glycosylated with N-acetylgalactosamine. However, other carbohydrates can also glycosylate receptors that utilize the $PIP_2 \rightarrow DAG + IP_3$ pathway. Pretreatment of monocytes with PHA does not block the endothelin signal, which suggests that the endothelin receptor is not glycosylated by N-acetylgalactosamine.

In these studies a $[Ca^{2+}]_i$ increment was observed in monocytes with a peak signal of $110 \pm 7\,\mathrm{n}M$ at 10^{-6} or $10^{-7}\,M$. This was compared to a signal of $240 \pm 20\,\mathrm{n}M$ observed with the lectin PHA. The endothelin signal was different from many other Ca^{2+} activation signals in lymphocytes and monocytes in that it was of short duration and was not sustained. It was therefore a monophasic signal. However, the endothelin-mediated Ca^{2+} signal was novel to monocytes. Studies with lymphocytes did not show any such signal. However, the Ca^{2+} signal observed was nevertheless well into the range known to produce biological activity.

Increases in monocyte $[Ca^{2+}]_i$ observed with Ca^{2+} ionophore or PHA have been shown to correlate with enhanced production of prostanoids [12] and superoxides and with secretion of interleukin-1, interleukin-6, and tumor necrosis factor [13], but no data yet exist describing the endothelin effect on these monocyte functions. Due to the peculiar morphology of the endothelin-induced Ca^{2+} activation signal, it is uncertain whether endothelin is the critical agonist for ischemic endothelial activation of monocytes in reperfusion injury, but studies are underway on the endothelin effect on the production of these mediators.

Summary

Endothelin increased $[Ca^{2+}]_i$ 110 nM in Fura-2 loaded human monocytes while the PHA control resulted in a 240 nM increase. Endothelin had no effect on lymphocytes or unseparated H-PBMC, although these populations increased $[Ca^{2+}]_i$ with PHA.

Conclusion

Endothelin mediates a novel $[Ca^{2+}]_i$ signal monocytes (but not lymphocytes) and may play a role in endothelium-leukocyte signaling which exacerbates reperfusion injury.

References

1. Entman ML, Michael L, Rosen RD, Dreyer WJ, Anderson DC, Taylor AA, Smith CW (1991) Inflammation in the course of early myocardial ischemia. FASEB J 5:2529–2537.
2. Yanagisawa M, Kurihara H, Kimura S, Tomobe Y, Kobayashi M, Mitsui Y, Yazaki Y, Goto K, Masaki T (1988) A novel potent vasoconstrictor peptide produced by vascular endothelial cells. Nature 332:411–415
3. Stojilkovic SS, Merelli F, Iida T, Krsmanovic LZ, Catt K (1990) Endothelin stimulation of cytosolic calcium and gonadotropin secretion in anterior pituitary cells. Science 248:1663–1666
4. Simonson MS, Dunn MJ (1990) Endothelin pathways of transmembrane signaling. Hypertention 15 [Suppl I]:I.5–I.12
5. Grynkiewicz G, Poenie M, Tsien R (1985) A new generation of Ca^{2+} indicators with greatly improved fluorescence properties. J Biol Chem 260:3440–3450
6. Yanagisawa H, Akihiro I, Ishikawa T, Kasuya Y, Kimura S, Kumagaye S, Nakajima K, Watamabe T, Sakakibara S, Goto K, Masaki T (1988) Primary structure, synthesis and biological activity of rat endothelin, and endothelium-derived vasoconstrictor peptide. Proc Natl Acad Sci USA 85:6064–6067
7. Inoue A, Yanagisawa M, Kimura S, Kasuya Y, Miyauchi T, Goto K, Masaki T (1989) The human endothelin family: three structurally and pharmacologically distinct isopeptides predicted by three separate genes. Proc Natl Acad Sci USA 86:2863–2867
8. Emori T, Hirata Y, Ohta K, Shichiri M, Marumo F (1989) Secretory mechanism of immunoreactive endothelin in cultured bovine endothelial cells. Biochem Biophys Res Commun 160:93–100
9. Clozel M, Fischli W, Guilly C (1989) Specific binding of endothelin on human vascular smooth muscle cell in culture. J Clin Invest 83:1758–1761
10. Simonson MS, Wann S, Mene P, Dubyak GR, Kester M, Nakazato Y, Sedor JR, Dunn MJ (1989) Endothelin stimulates phospholipase C, Na^+/H^+ exchange, c-*fos* expression, and mitogenesis in rat mesangial cells. J Clin Invest 83:708–712
11. Tsien RV, Pozzan T, Rink RJ (1982) Mechanism of disease: the calcium messenger system. J Cell Biol 94:325
12. Rasmussen H (1986) The calcium messenger system. N Engl J Med 314:1094–1100, 1164–1170
13. Ashman RF (1984) Lymphocyte activation. Fundamental immunology Ed. W. E. Paul, New York, pp 267–302

Nitric Oxide Synthesis in Sponge Matrix Allografts Coincides with the Initiation of the Allogeneic Response*

J. M. Langrehr, J. Stadler, T. R. Billiar, H. Schraut, R. L. Simmons, and R. A. Hoffman

Introduction

The investigation of the biological effects of nitric oxide ($\cdot N = O$) has been of increasing interest in the recent past. Nitric oxide is a product of oxidative L-arginine metabolism, in which L-arginine is metabolized to L-citrulline and $\cdot N = O$ by the yet not fully characterized enzyme $\cdot N = O$ synthase.

It has become evident through several reports that a constitutive enzyme system, which produces small amounts of $\cdot N = O$ constantly (e.g., in endothelial and cerebellar cells), exists as well as an inducible enzyme system, which is capable of producing large amounts of $\cdot N = O$ [1]. The latter enzyme system has been described primarily in macrophages, where $\cdot N = O$, produced by this system, has been shown to act microbiostatic [2–4]. Furthermore, $\cdot N = O$ produced in macrophage/tumor cell coculture systems has been shown to promote tumor cell cytostasis [5, 6]. These effects have been hypothesized to be due in part to the inhibition of aconitase (a rate-limiting enzyme of the citric acid circle) by $\cdot N = O$ [7]. Intracellular iron loss, inhibition of mitochondrial respiration, and inhibition of ribonucleotide reductase (a key enzyme in DNA synthesis) have also been shown to coincide with $\cdot N = O$ synthesis [6, 8, 9]. Reports from our laboratory indicated that Kupffer cell-mediated inhibition of hepatocyte protein synthesis is related to $\cdot N = O$ synthesis [10, 11].

Since many studies of $\cdot N = O$ production by macrophages utilized cytokines such as tumor necrosis factor alpha (TNF-γ), interleukin-1 (IL-1), and interferon gamma (IFN-γ), cytokines known to participate in cell-mediated immunity, we decided to determine if $\cdot N = O$ production played a role in the allograft response. Initially, we observed that nitrite/nitrate (NO_2^-/NO_3^-), the stable end products of oxidative L-arginine metabolism, accumulated in the supernatants of rat splenocyte mixed lymphocyte cultures. Subsequently, it was determined that proliferation and cytotoxic T-cell generation could only be detected in these cultures when N^G-monomethyl-L-arginine (NMA), a competitive inhibitor of $\cdot N = O$ production, was added to the cultures. Cytokines able to induce proliferation of the T-cell line, CTLL-2, were detected in the supernatants of cultures

---

* This work was supported by grants AI-16869 an GM-37753 from the National Institutes of Health, Bethesda, MD, USA. M. Langrehr and J. Stadler are supported by the German Research Council (La-621/2-2 and Sta-311/1-1, respectively).
Department of Surgery, University of Pittsburgh, USA

without NMA throughout the culture period. However, when NMA was present in the cultures, cytokines able to induce T-cell proliferation were observed early in the culture supernatants, but declined rapidly coincident with the onset of lymphocyte proliferation [12]. These findings lead us to investigate whether $\cdot N = O$ is produced in the in vivo allograft response. We utilized the previously described sponge matrix allograft model in the mouse [13–15] and adapted it for use in the rat.

Materials and Methods

In this model six polyurethane sponges, weighing 30 ± 2 mg, were implanted subcutaneously into Lewis (RTl^l) recipients and immediately injected with 10×10^6 syngeneic (Lewis) or allogeneic (ACI) splenocytes. On various days postgrafting, the sponges were harvested and tested for contamination and the sponge exudate fluid and the sponge graft infiltrating cells were recovered. Cytolytic activity of cells which had infiltrated an allogeneic graft became detectable on day 6, peaked on day 7 or 8, and rapidly waned by day 10 postgrafting (data not shown). This is different from the mouse sponge allograft model, where cytotoxicity appears later and lasts longer. The cytotoxicity of graft infiltrating cells was always donor specific and cytotoxicity by syngeneic graft infiltrating cells was never observed. To assess the $\cdot N = O$ production by graft infiltrating cells in vivo and in vitro, sponge fluid NO_2^-/NO_3^- and culture supernatant NO_2^- concentrations were determined using an automated procedure based on the Griess reaction [16]. All cultures were performed using standard cell culture techniques and Dulbecco's modified Eagle's medium (DMEM) or L-arginine-free DMEM (Gibco Inc., Grand Island, NY, USA) supplemented as previously described [12], with fetal calf serum (Gibco) as the serum source.

Results and Discussion

Our previous finding that $\cdot N = O$ production in mixed rat splenocyte mixed lymphocyte cultures inhibits proliferation and cytotoxic T-cell generation led us to assess the $\cdot N = O$ production in an in vivo allograft situation. When the sponge exudate fluid (the fluid which surrounds the graft infiltrating cells in vivo) was evaluated for the stable end products of $\cdot N = O$ synthesis, we observed that allogeneic sponge fluid consistently showed higher NO_2^-/NO_3^- levels than syngeneic sponge fluid (Table 1). This was statistically significantly different ($p \leq 0.05$) on day 6 postgrafting, when donor-specific cytotoxicity of graft infiltrating cells was first observed.

Since we have previously shown that small molecules such as NO_3^- rapidly disappear from the sponge fluid, and therefore the NO_2^-/NO_3^- concentration in

Table 1. Nitric oxide production in sponge allograft fluid

Day postgrafting	Sponge fluid NO_2^-/NO_3^- (μM)	
	Syngeneic	Allogeneic
4	19.3 ± 1.9	12.8 ± 3.4
6	17.8 ± 6.5	34.7 ± 7.0*
8	26.5 ± 4.6	30.3 ± 4.3

Sponges were implanted into Lewis recipients and immediately injected with 10×10^6 syngeneic (Lewis) or allogeneic (ACI) splenocytes. On various days postgrafting, the sponges were harvested, the sponge fluid was recovered and the NO_2^-/NO_3^- levels were determined. Results are expressed as mean ± SEM ($n = 3$).
*$p \leq 0.05$ by Student's t test

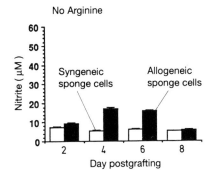
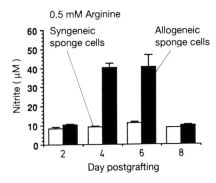

Fig. 1. The effect of L-arginine on ·N=O production by allograft infiltrating cells. Sponges were implanted into Lewis recipients and immediately injected with 10×10^6 syngeneic (Lewis) or allogeneic (ACI) splenocytes. On various days postgrafting, the graft infiltrating cells were recovered and the cells cultured for 2 days with or without L-arginine present in the media. Results are expressed as mean ± SD of replicates of six cultures. The ·N=O production by syngeneic cells was always significantly lower ($p \leq 0.01$ by Student's t test) than by allogeneic graft infiltrating cells

the sponge fluid represents the ongoing ·N=O production rather than the total ·N=O production, we recovered the graft infiltrating cells on various days postgrafting to determine their ability to synthesize ·N=O under defined conditions in vitro. We observed that allogeneic graft infiltrating cells produced significantly higher amount of ·N=O than syngeneic graft infiltrating cells when L-arginine was present in the culture medium (Fig. 1). Surprisingly, we observed that even when L-arginine was absent from the culture medium, allogeneic graft infiltrating cells harvested on days 4 and 6 postgrafting produced significantly higher amounts of ·N=O than cells recovered from a syngeneic graft on days 4 and 6 postgrafting. Further experiments showed that both syngeneic and allogeneic graft-infiltrating cells are capable of producing high amounts of

·N = O when stimulated with certain cytokines (such as IL-2 and IFN-γ, unpublished observations), whereas upon reexposure to the specific alloantigen only allograftinfiltrating cells demonstrated significant ·N = O production [17]. We therefore hypothesize that the cytokines produced in the in vivo allograft response are capable of stimulating graft infiltrating cells to produce ·N = O which, if acting as in vitro, might be able to temper the generation of an alloimmune response. Our findings confirm, to some extent, the recent study by Werner-Felmayer and co-workers. They speculated that cytokine-induced tetra-hydrobiopterin synthesis in murine fibroblasts is to provide the cells with the active cofactor for oxidative L-arginine metabolism [18]. Considering that the same group showed earlier that neopterin, an end product of the pteridine metabolism, is a marker of activation of the cellular immune system [19], it becomes obvious that further studies investigating the significance of ·N = O production in the allograft response are warranted.

References

1. Nathan CF, Stuehr DJ (1990) Does endothelium-derived nitric oxide have a role in cytokine-induced hypotension? J Nat Cancer Inst 82 (9):726–728
2. Granger DL, Hibbs JB Jr, Perfect JR, Durack DT (1988) Specific amino acid (L-arginine) requirement for the microbiostatic activity of murine macrophages. J Clin Invest 81:1129–1136
3. James SL, Glaven J (1989) Macrophage cytotoxicity against schistosomula of *Shistosoma masoni* involves arginine-dependent production of reactive nitrogen intermediates. J Immunol 143:4208–4212
4. Green SJ, Meltzer MS, Hibbs JB Jr, Nacy CA (1990) Activated macrophages destroy intracellular *Leishamania major* amastigotes by an L-arginine-dependent killing mechanism. J Immunol 144:278–283
5. Hibbs JB Jr, Read R, Taintor RR, Vavrin Z (1987) Macrophage cytotoxicity: role for L-arginine deiminase and amino nitrogen oxidation to nitrate. Science 235:473–476
6. Stuehr DJ, Nathan CF (1989) Nitric oxide. A macrophage product responsible for cytostasis and respiratory inhibition in tumor target cells. J. Exp. Med 169:1543–1555
7. Drapier JC, Hibbs JF Jr (1988) Differentiation of murine macrophages to express nonspecific cytotoxicity for tumor cells results in L-arginine dependent inhibition of mitochondrial iron-sulfur enzymes in the macrophage effector cells. J. Immunol 140:2829–2838
8. Wharton M, Granger DK, Durack DT (1988) Mitochondrial iron loss from leukemia cells injured by macrophages. A possible mechanism for electron transport chain defects. J. Immunol 141:1311–1317
9. Lepoivre M, Chenais B, Yapo A, Lemaire G, Thelauder L, Tenn JP (1990) Alterations of ribonucleotide reductase activity following induction of the nitrite-generating pathway in adenocarcinoma cells. J. Biol. Chem. 165:14143–14149
10. Billiar TR, Curran RD, Stuehr DJ, West MA, Bentz BG, Simmons RL (1989) An L-arginine-dependent mechanism mediates Kupffer cell inhibition of hepatocyte protein synthesis in vitro. J Exp Med 160:1467–1472
11. Curran RD, Billiar TR, Stuehr DJ, Hofmann K, Simmons RL (1989) Hepatocytes produce nitrogen oxides from L-arginine in response to inflammatory products of Kupffer cells. J Exp Med 170:1769–1774
12. Hoffman RA, Langrehr JM, Billiar TR, Curran RD, Simmons RL (1990) Alloantigen-induced activation of rat splenocytes is regulated by the oxidative metabolism of L-arginine. J Immunol 145:2220–2226
13. Roberts PJ, Hayry P (1976) Sponge matrix allografts: a model for analysis of killer cells infiltrating mouse allografts. Transplantation 21:437–445

14. Ascher NL, Chen S, Hoffman RA, Simmons RL (1983) Maturation of cytotoxic T cells within sponge matrix allografts. J Immunol 131:617–621
15. Bishop DK, Fergusen RM, Orosz CG (1990). Differential distribution of antigen-specific helper T cells and cytotoxic T cells after antigenic stimulation in vivo. A functional study using limiting delution analysis. J Immunol 144:1153–1160
16. Green LC, Wagner DA, Glogowski J, Skipper PL, Wishnok JS, Tannenbaum SR (1982). Analysis of nitrate, nitrite and (^{15}N)nitrate in biological fluids. Anal. Biochem 126:131–138
17. Langrehr JM, Hoffman RA, Billiar TR, Lee KKW, Schraut WH, Simmons RL. Nitric oxide synthesis in the in vivo allograft response: a possible regulatory mechanism. Surgery (in press).
18. Werner-Felmayer G, Werner ER, Fuchs D, Hausen A, Reibnegger G, Wachter H (1990). Tetrahydrobiopterin-dependent formation of nitrite and nitrate in murine fibroblasts. J. Exp. Med 172:1599–1605
19. Wachter H, Fuchs D, Hansen A, Reibnegger G, Werner ER (1989). Neopterin as marker for activation of cellular immunity: immunologic basis and clinical application. Adv. Clin. Chem 27:81

Neutrophil Elastase Induces Lung Injury Following Lower Limb Ischaemia

R. Welbourn[1], G. Goldman[2], D. Shepro[2] and B. Hechtman[1]

Introduction

Ischaemia-reperfusion injury in skeletal muscle is mediated in large part by adherent neutrophils [1]. If the mass of ischaemic tissue is large, reperfusion leads to acute lung injury, which is also dependent upon neutrophils. The injury mechanism is initiated by the generation of reactive oxygen species within the reperfused tissue [2, 3]. Inhibition of oxygen radical formation prevents the sequestration of neutrophils both within the reperfused tissue and also within the lungs. The effectiveness of oxygen radical inhibition in preventing reperfusion injury does not, therefore, document the mechanism by which the neutrophil induces injury in either setting [4, 5].

In vitro evidence implicates proteolytic enzymes, in particular elastase, as potent means by which stimulated adherent neutrophils may cause injury to endothelium [6, 7]. It seems likely that for neutrophils to injure endothelium in vivo, however, the secretion of oxygen radicals is also needed. This is because plasma contains regulatory proteins, principally α_1-proteinase inhibitor (α_1-PI), which prevent the destruction of normal tissues by elastase. Evidence suggests that neutrophil secretion of reactive oxygen species oxidizes α_1-PI sufficiently to allow unrestricted activity of free elastase [8, 9].

We studied how neutrophils cause lung injury in the setting of reperfusion following bilateral hindlimb tourniquet ischaemia in the rat. We found that elastase inhibition reduces the permeability without affecting neutrophil sequestration in the lung. Moreover, inhibition of oxygen radicals at a time when neutrophils had already sequestered in the lungs was as effective in preventing the injury, suggesting cooperative interaction between elastase and reactive oxygen species in determining injury.

Methods

Anaesthetized rats treated with saline ($n = 9$) or the specific neutrophil elastase inhibitor methoxysuccinyl-L-Ala-L-Ala-L-Pro—L-Val-chloromethylketone

---

[1] Department of Surgery, Brigham and Women's Hospital, Harvard Medical School, [2] Biological Science Center, Boston University, Boston, MA, USA

Host Defense Dysfunction
in Trauma, Shock and Sepsis
Eds. Faist/Meakins/Schildberg
© Springer-Verlag, Berlin Heidelberg 1993

(MAAPV, $n = 6$, 200 µg as a bolus, then 200 µg/h) underwent 4 h of bilateral hindlimb tourniquet ischaemia followed by 4 h of reperfusion. Sham procedures were undertaken in rats treated with saline ($n = 9$) or MAAPV ($n = 5$). After killing, the lungs were excised for estimation of myeloperoxidase activity, bronchoalveolar lavage was performed for protein leak and the wet to dry weight ratio was estimated. Seven other rats were subjected to ischaemia and were treated with polyethylene glycol (PEG) -conjugated superoxide dismutase (SOD, 1500 U/kg bolus) and PEG-catalase (CAT, 500 U/kg bolus) 2 h after the tourniquest were removed. Four sham rats were given SOD/CAT ($n = 4$).

Results and Discussion

Reperfusion led to neutrophil accumulation within the lungs (Fig. 1); there was permeability, indicated by bronchoalveolar lavage protein (Fig. 2), and also oedema, shown by an increase in the wet to dry weight ratio (Fig. 3). MAAPV reduced the injury without affecting neutrophil sequestration (Figs. 2, 3). Giving SOD and CAT 2 h after reperfusion did not affect neutrophil sequestration but was equally effective in reducing the lung injury (Figs. 2, 3). In sham animals neither MAAPV nor SOD/CAT induced neutrophil sequestration (23 ± 4 U/g and 16 ± 1 U/g respectively).

These results suggest that secretion of elastase, probably in conjunction with the generation of reactive oxygen species, is the mechanism by which sequestered neutrophils mediate lung permeability following bilateral hindlimb ischaemia and reperfusion [10]. In support of this hypothesis, we have found that the lung injury in this model can be prevented by selective depletion of circulating neutrophils or by preventing their microvascular adherence with an antibody directed against the CD18 glycoprotein [11, 12]. The observed reduction in injury therefore probably represents an effect of the elastase inhibitor and oxygen radical scavengers on neutrophil function. Indeed, we have

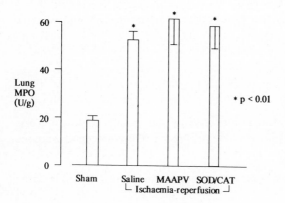

Fig. 1 Tourniquet release led to an increase in lung neutrophils, indicated by myeloperoxidase content, compared to shams. Neither MAAPV nor SOD/CAT prevented the rise in MPO content in reperfused animals. *$p < 0.01$ comparing all ischaemia/reperfusion groups to shams

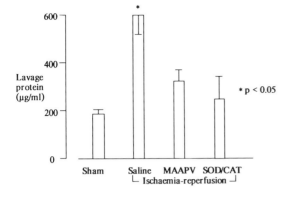

Fig. 2 Tourniquet release also led to an increase in protein concentration in bronchoalveolar lavage fluid. Both MAAPV and SOD/CAT reduced the rise in bronchoalvelar lavage fluid protein. *$p < 0.05$ compared to all other groups

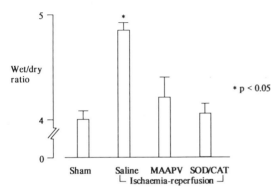

Fig. 3 The lung wet to dry weight ratio increased after tourniquet release. Both MAAPV and SOD/CAT reduced the rise in wet/dry ratio. *$p < 0.05$ compared to all other groups.

observed an increase in oxidative activity of circulating neutrophils following reperfusion in the same model [13].

It is unlikely that neutrophils can cause tissue injury solely by generation of oxygen metabolites, since oxygen radicals are very short-lived and are able to cause damage only over extremely short distances. An attractive hypothesis is that neutrophils use the system of elastase and oxygen metabolite secretion in a cooperative fashion to mediate cellular injury. Because close adhesion is required for neutrophils to injure endothelium, it is likely that this adhesive process creates a micro-environment in which α_1-PI is effectively inactivated by oxygen radicals so that secreted elastase might have unrestricted access to endothelium [7]. Present data provide evidence that this schema may be true in vivo.

References

1. Carden DL, Smith JK, Korthuis RJ (1990) Neutrophil-mediated microvascular dysfunction in postischemic canine skeletal muscle. Role of granulocyte adherence. Circ Res 66:1436–1444
2. McCord JM (1987) Oxygen-derived radicals: a link between reperfusion injury and inflammation. Fed Proc 46:2402–2406

3. Granger DN (1988) Role of xanthine oxidase and granulocytes in ischemia-reperfusion injury. Am J Physiol 255:H1269–H1275
4. Klausner JM, Paterson IS, Kobzik L, Valeri CR, Shepro D, Hechtman HB (1989) Oxygen free radicals mediate ischemia-induced lung injury. Surgery 104:192–299
5. Engler R (1987) Granulocytes and oxidative injury in myocardial ischemia and reperfusion. FASEB 46:2395–2396
6. Smedly LA, Tonnesen MG, Sandhaus RA et al. (1986) Neutrophil-mediated injury to endothelial cells. Enhancement by endotoxin and essential role of neutrophil elastase. J Clin Invest 77:1233–1243
7. Weiss SJ (1989) Tissue destruction by neutrophils. N Engl J Med 320:365–376
8. Carp H, Janoff A (1980) Potential mediator of inflammation. Phagocyte-derived oxidants suppress the elastase-inhibitory capacity of alpha$_1$-proteinase inhibitor in vitro. J Clin Invest 66:987–995
9. Ossanna PJ, Test ST, Matheson NR, Regiani S, Wiess SJ (1986) Oxidative regulation of neutrophil elastase-alpha-1 proteinase inhibitor interactions. J Clin Invest 77:1939–1951
10. Welbourn R, Goldman G, Paterson IS, Valeri CR, Shepro D, Hechtman HB (1991) Neutrophil elastase and oxygen radicals: synergism in lung injury following hindlimb ischemia. Am J Physiol (in press)
11. Klausner JM, Anner H, Paterson IS et al. (1988) Lower torso ischemia-induced lung injury is leukocyte dependent. Ann Surg 208:761–767
12. Welbourn R, Goldman G, Hill J, Lindsay T, Shepro D, Hechtman HB (1991) Lung injury following hindlimb ischemia is mediated via neutrophil CD 18 adherence receptors. FASEB (in press)
13. Paterson IS, Klausner JM, Goldman G et al. (1989) Thromboxane mediates the ischemia-induced neutrophil oxidative burst. Surgery 106:224–229

PMN Elastase in Local Infection

K. M. Peters[1], K. Koberg[1], H. Kehren[2], and K. W. Zilkens[1]

Polymorphonuclear (PMN) elastase, a proteolytic enzyme, is a biochemical marker for pathologic granulocyte stimulation [2, 4, 6]. In the presence of sepsis excessive neutrophil stimulation occurs, and significant amounts of PMN elastase are released into the plasma and serve as an indicator of the severity and prognosis of the disease [5, 7, 8]. Dittmer et al. found a positive correlation between the amount of liberated elastase and the severity of trauma [3]. In our current study we wanted to evaluate PMN elastase as a marker for the detection and follow-up of local infection of bone and joint.

Patients and Methods

In 62 patients with posttraumatic osteomyelitis and joint empyema the following markers of inflammation were tested preoperatively:
- PMN elastase
- C-reactive protein (CRP)
- Fibrinogen
- Erythrocyte sedimentation rate (ESR)
- Leukocyte count

In 21 patients with noninflammatory orthopedic diseases (nucleus prolapse, conservatively treated fractures) we evaluated a "diagnostic specificity" of these markers. In 33 patients with bone and joint infections these markers were also determined in the postoperative follow-up: the first determination was done 2–4 days postoperatively, the second 9–11 days, and the last 20–22 days.

PMN elastase was measured by an enzyme-linked immunoassay (IMAC-assay, F. Merck, Darmstadt, FRG), with a normal range of ≤ 40 µg/l. It was defined together with its antagonist (α-1-proteinase inhibitor) as the elastase α-1-proteinase inhibitor-complex. CRP was measured nephelometically by Na-Latex-CRP-reagent (Behring, Marburg, FRG), with a normal range ≤ 5 mg/l. The detection of fibrinogen was carried out as described by Clauss [1], with a normal range ≤ 4.5 g/l. ESR was measured according to Westergren (≤ 10

---

[1] Orthopedic Clinic, RWTH Aachen, 5100 Aachen, FRG
[2] Institute of Clinical Chemistry and Pathobiochemistry, RWTH Aachen, 5100 Aachen, FRG

Host Defense Dysfunction
in Trauma, Shock and Sepsis
Eds. Faist/Meakins/Schildberg
© Springer-Verlag, Berlin Heidelberg 1993

Westergren mm in 1 h) and leukocyte count was done automatically by Technicon H6000 (≤ 9 g/l). Neopterin was measured by a radioimmunoassay (IMMUtest Neopterin, Henning Berlin, FRG), with a normal range ≤ 10 nmol/l.

Results

In patients with posttraumatic osteomyelitis and joint empyema, PMN elastase had a sensitivity of 81% and was only exceeded by that of the very nonspecific ESR (sensitivity 90%). Sensitivity of other inflammation parameters was lower: CRP 71%, fibrinogen 54%, neopterin 37%, and leukocyte count 26% (see Fig. 1). Among the markers with high sensitivity (> 60%) PMN elastase had the highest specifity at 81% (see Fig. 2).

The results in the postoperative follow-up were similar: in the uncomplicated cases PMN elastase did not show a decisive postoperative rise and quickly returned to normal: after 2–4 days PMN elastase had normalized in 33% of cases and after 9–11 days in 63%. After 3 weeks 75% of the patients showed normal results. Normalization of CRP was slower: 13% after 2–4 days and 28% after 9–11 days. After 3 weeks CRP reached about the same level of normalization as PMN elastase (see Fig. 3). Even fibrinogen normalized faster than CRP in the postoperative follow-up. Determination of ESR was not useful in the postoperative follow-up of patients with bone and joint infections since after 3 weeks it had normalized in only 25% of cases.

Leukocytes did not react decisively. The initial postoperative leukocyte count was already within the normal range in more than 80% of cases. Neopterin was also not useful in the postoperative follow-up. However, elevated levels of leukocytes and neopterin were a decisive indication of severe postoperative inflammatory complications.

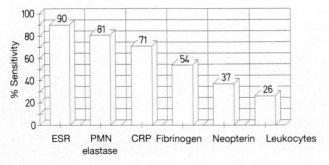

Fig. 1. Sensitivity of polymorphonuclear (PMN) elastase, C-reactive protein (CRP), erythrocyte sedimentation rate (ESR), fibrinogen, neopterin, and leukocyte count in preoperative management of patients with posttraumatic osteomyelitis and joint empyema ($n = 62$)

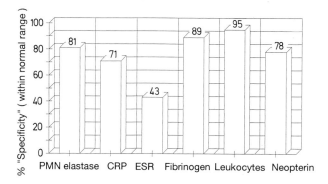

Fig. 2. "Diagnostic specificity" of PMN elastase, CRP, ESR, fibrinogen, neopterin, and leukocyte count in patients with non-inflammatory orthopedic diseases ($n = 21$)

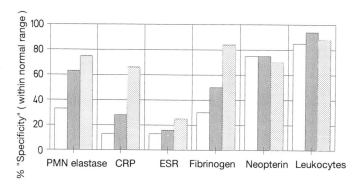

Fig. 3. Inflammation markers in postoperative follow-up of patients with posttraumatic osteomyelitis and joint empyema ($n = 33$). *Open bars*, 2–4 days surgery; *hatched bars*, 9–11 days after surgery; *stippled bars* 3 weeks after surgery

Discussion

Nowadays PMN elastase is a well-established marker for the diagnosis and prognosis of sepsis [2, 3, 5, 7, 8]. In our current study we were able to show that the detection of PMN elastase is not only important in severe general infection, but also in local infection of bones and joints.

In preoperative diagnositc management of patients with posttraumatic osteomyelitis and joint empyema, PMN elastase achieved a higher sensitivity than the classic inflammation markers. Diagnostic specifity was 81%. The high diagnostic validity of PMN elastase is especially helpful in the detection of bone inflammation, which even nowadays may be a diagnostic problem.

In the postoperative follow-up without any complications, PMN elastase normalized faster than CRP and ESR. Therefore, it is possible to distinguish earlier between septic and aseptic courses, which is decisive for postoperative treatment. Based on these findings we highly recommend PMN elastase for the preoperative detection and postoperative follow-up of bone and joint infection.

References

1. Clauss A (1957) Gerinnungsphysiologische Schnellmethode zur Bestimmung des Fibrinogens. Acta Haematol (Basel) 17:237
2. Dittmer H, Jochum M, Fritz H (1986) Freisetzung von granulozytärer Elastase und Plasmaproteinveränderungen nach traumatisch-hämorrhagischem Schock. Unfallchirurg 89:160
3. Dittmer H, Jochum M, Schmit-Neuerburg KP (1985) Der PMN-Elastase-Plasmaspiegel, ein biochemischer Parameter der Traumaschwere. Chirurg 56:723
4. Fritz H, Jochum M, Duswald KH, Dittmer H, Kortmann H (1984) Lysosomale Proteasen als Mediatoren der unspezifischen Proteolyse bei der Entzündung. In: Lang H, Greiling H (eds) Pathobiochemie der Entzündung. Springer, Berlin Heidelberg New York, p 75
5. Jochum M, Fritz H, Nast-Kolb D, Inthorn D (1990) Granulozyten-Elastase als prognostischer Marker. Dtsch Arztebl 87:1526
6. Kruse-Jarres JD, Kinzelmann T (1986) Pathobiochemistry and clinical role of granulocytes and their lysosomal proteinases in inflammatory processes. Arztl Laborat 32:185
7. Lang H, Jochum M, Fritz H, Redl H (1989) Validity of the elastase-assay in intensive care medicine. In: Schlag G, Redl H (eds) Second Vienna shock forum. Liss, New York, p 56
8. Redl H, Schlag G (1989) Möglichkeiten des biochemischen Monitoring bei Multiorganversagen. Intensivmedizin 26:345

Opioids from Immune Cells Interact with Receptors on Sensory Nerves to Inhibit Nociception in Inflammation

C. Stein[1], A. H. Hassan[2], R. Przewłocki[2], C. Epplen[2], C. Gramsch[2], K. Peter[1], and A. Herz[2]

Introduction

Recent evidence indicates that exogenous opioids can produce pronounced antinociceptive effects by interacting with local opioid receptors in peripheral inflamed tissue [1–4]. Activation of endogenous opioid systems by environmental stimuli, e.g., cold water swim (CWS), in rats with unilateral hindpaw inflammation similarly elicits localized opioid receptor-mediated antinociception in the inflamed paw [5]. The pituitary-adrenal axis, the classical source for circulating peripheral opioid peptides [6], is apparently not directly involved in producing this effect [7]. Another conceivable locus of origin for endogenous opioids in inflamed tissue is the immune system [8]. Immune cells have been shown to contain and release opioid peptides in vitro [9–11] and various types of such cells accumulate at sites of inflammation in vivo [12]. In the present study, we have examined tissue from normal and inflamed rat paws by radioimmunoassay (RIA) and immunocytochemistry for β-endorphin (β-EP), metenkephalin (ME), and dynorphin (DYN), the major representatives of the three endogenous opioid peptide families [13]. We report here the presence of significant amounts of immunoreactive β-EP and ME in inflamed tissue, apparently located in immunocytes. By the use of a monoclonal antiidiotypic antibody (anti-id-14) we demonstrate opioid receptors immunocytochemically on small diameter cutaneous nerves of the paw. Lastly, we show in vivo that antinociception induced by CWS in the inflamed paw is abolished by pretreatment with the immunosuppressive agent cyclosporin A (CsA) or by wholebody X-irradiation.

Materials and Methods

Subjects. Male Wistar rats (200 – 220 g) were housed individually in cages lined with sawdust. All testing was conducted in the light phase of a 12h/12h (8 A.M./8 P.M.) light–dark cycle.

[1] Department of Anesthesiology Ludwig-Maximilians University, Klinikum Grosshadern 8000 Munich 70, FRG
[2] Department of Neuropharmacology, Max Planck Institute of Psychiatry, 8033 Martinsried, FRG

Host Defense Dysfunction
in Trauma, Shock and Sepsis
Eds. Faist/Meakins/Schildberg
© Springer-Verlag, Berlin Heidelberg 1993

Induction of Inflammation. Rats received an intraplantar (i. pl) injection of 0.15 ml Freund's complete adjuvant (Calbiochem) into the right hind foot under brief ether anesthesia. The inflammation remained confined to the inoculated paw. All experiments were performed 4 days postinoculation.

Radioimmunoassays. Rats were decapitated, skin and adjacent subcutaneous tissue was dissected from the plantar surface of both hindpaws. The material was weighed and then incubated in 0.1 N HCl (six times the volume of the tissue) at 95 °C for 10 min. Following homogenization and centrifugation at 10 000 g for 20 min, supernatants were removed and filtered through YM 30 membranes (Amicon). Samples were then aliquoted, lyophilized, redissolved in RIA-buffer, and assayed for β-EP (1–31), ME, and DYN (1–17) as described previously [14].

Immunocytochemistry. Rats were anesthetized and perfused. The skin and adjacent subcutaneous tissue was dissected from both hindpaws, cut into small specimens, postfixed, and washed in phosphate buffered saline (PBS). The specimens were then dehydrated, cleared, and embedded in Paraplast Plus. Sections (5–7 µm) were cut, dewaxed, rehydrated, washed, and then immuno-stained using avidin-biotin peroxidase complex. Primary antisera used were: a monoclonal antibody against β-EP (3-E7) and polyclonal antibodies against β-EP, DYN, and ME. To demonstrate specificity of staining, the following controls were included: (1) preadsorption of primary antisera with excess of homologous antigen and (2) omission of either the primary antisera, the secondary antibody, or the avidin-biotin complex.

Visualization of opioid receptors was accomplished using the modified immunogold silver staining (IGSS) technique with Lugol's iodine and sodium thiosulfate pretreatment. Tissues from both inflamed and noninflamed paws were fixed and processed for Paraplast embedding as described above. The rehydrated sections were immersed in Lugol's iodine, treated with sodium thiosulfate, washed, and immersed in IGSS-buffer. Sections were then incubated for 20 min with neat goat serum, drained off, and directly overlayed with biotinylated anti-id-14, a mouse monoclonal antibody against opioid receptors. After washing, sections were covered with neat goat serum and incubated with AuroProbe LM streptavidin immunogold reagent. The following specificity controls were included: (1) preincubation of anti-id-14 with 3-E7 and (2) substitution of anti-id-14 with biotinylated normal mouse IgM or omission of the immunogold reagent. Further details are given in [14].

Algesiometry. Nociceptive thresholds were evaluated by use of a modified Randall-Sellito paw pressure test [4]. Animals (n = 5–6 per group) were gently restrained and incremental pressure was applied onto the hindpaw. The pressure required to elicit paw withdrawal, the paw pressure threshold (PPT), was determined. After baseline measurements, rats were subjected to CWS at 1 °–2 °C for 1 min as described previously [5] and PPTs were reevaluated repeatedly thereafter. Separate groups of rats received intraperitoneal CsA (0.75–3 mg per injection in 1 ml) or vehicle at 48, 24, and 4 h prior to testing. Four different groups were exposed to X-irradiation at a total dose of 0, 450, 900, and 1200 R, respectively, 48 h prior to testing.

Results

Significant amounts of immunoreactive β-EP (0.45 $\pm$ 0.05 pmol/g) and for ME (0.29 $\pm$ 0.05 pmol/g), but not of DYN, were found in inflamed tissue. Numerous inflammatory cells stained strongly with both the monoclonal and the polyclonal antibody to β-EP (Fig. 1B) and somewhat less intensely for ME (not shown). A small number of cells displayed a faint reaction to DYN (not shown). The intensity of immunoreactivity in the inflamed paw was most pronounced in the periphery of inflammatory foci within the plantar subcutaneous tissue. The opioid-containing cells had morphological appearances consistent with macrophages, mast cells, lymphocytes, and plasma cells (Fig. 1B). Opioid staining was almost entirely absent in noninflamed paws (Fig. 1A). Complete extinction of opioid like immunoreactivity was attained in the specificity control experiments (Fig. 1C). Further details are given in [14].

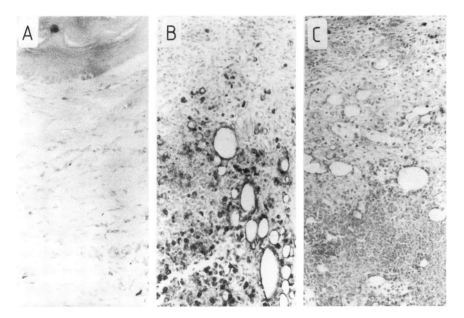

Fig. 1.A Opioid peptide staining in noninflamed paw. **B** Staining in inflamed paw. **C** Complete extinction of opiodlike immunoreactivity in the specificity control experiments

Intense staining of immunoreactive opioid receptors was detected on small diameter cutaneous nerves of both noninflamed and inflamed paws (Fig. 2A and B). In specificity control experiments this immunoreactivity was completely abolished (Fig. 2C).

Immediately following CWS the PPT increased significantly on the inflamed [$p < 0.01$, analysis of variance (ANOVA)] but not on the noninflamed paw [$p = 0.24$, ANOVA (Fig. 3A)]. This increase was dose dependently ($p < 0.001$, ANOVA) blocked by X-irradiation (Fig. 3B) and by CsA, but not by its vehicle (not shown).

Discussion

The first set of experiments demonstrate the presence of significant amounts of opioid peptides in immune cells of peripheral inflamed tissue. Immunoreactive opioid receptors were visualized on small diameter cutaneous nerves. Activation of such receptors by exogenous opioids can result in antinociception (1–4). Thus, it seemed likely that the endogenous opioid peptides seen in immune cells of the inflamed tissue could activate these receptors directly to exert a local inhibition of nociception. Indeed, immunosuppression by whole-body X-irradiation or

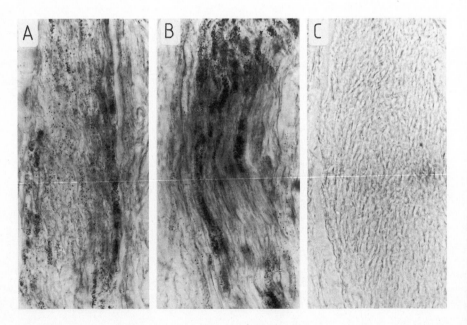

Fig. 2A-C. Opioid receptor staining on small diameter cutaneous nerves of **A** noninflamed and **B** inflamed paws. **C** Extinction control

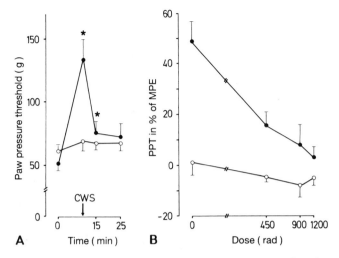

Fig. 3A. Paw pressure threshold (*PPT*) on inflamed and noninflamed rat paw following cold water swim (*CWS*). **B** The effect of X-irradiation and CsA on the increase in PPT. *Closed symbols,* inflamed paw; *open symbols,* noninflamed paw

CsA abolished the CWS-induced effect completely, thus demonstrating that immunocytes can be involved in intrinsic mechanisms of antinociception in inflammation.

Acknowledgements. We thank U. Bäuerle for artwork and J. T. and C. Epplen for continuous stimulating discussions. This work was supported by the Deutsche Forschungsgemeinschaft and International Anesthesia Research Society.

References

1. Ferreira SH, Nakamura M (1979) Prostaglandin hyperalgesia II: the peripheral analgesic activity of morphine, enkephalins and opioid antagonists. Prostaglandins 18:191–200
2. Joris JL, Dubner R, Hargreaves KM (1987) Opioid analgesia at peripheral sites: a target for opioids released during stress and inflammation. Anesth Analg 66:1277–1281
3. Stein C, Millan MJ, Shippenberg TS, Herz A (1988) Peripheral effect of fentanyl upon nociception in inflamed tissue of the rat. Neurosci Lett 84:225–228
4. Stein C, Millan MJ, Shippenberg TS, Peter K, Herz A (1989) Peripheral opioid receptors mediating antinociception in inflammation. Evidence for involvement of mu, delta and kappa receptors. J Pharmacol Exp Ther 248:1269–1275
5. Stein C, Gramsch C, Herz A (1990) Intrinsic mechanisms of antinociception in inflammation. Local opioid receptors and β-endorphin. J Neurosci 10:1292–1298
6. Guillemin RT, Vargo T, Rossier J, Minick S, Ling N, Rivier C, Vale W, Bloom FE (1977) β-Endorphin and adrenocorticotropin are secreted concomitantly by the pituitary gland. Science 197:1367–1369
7. Parsons CG, Członkowski A, Stein C, Herz A (1990) Peripheral opioid receptors mediating antinociception in inflammation. Activation by endogenous opioids and role of the pituitary-adrenal axis. Pain 41:81–93

8. Sibinga NES, Goldstein A (1988) Opioid peptides and opioid receptors in cells of the immune system. Ann Rev Immunol 6:219–249
9. Lolait SJ, Clements JA, Markwick AJ, Cheng C, McNally M, Smith AI, and Funder JW (1986) Pro-opiomelanocortin messenger ribonucleic acid and posttranslation processing of beta-endorphin in spleen macrophages. J Clin Invest 77:1776–1779.
10. Zurawski G, Benedik M, Kamp BJ, Abrams JS, Zurawski SM, and Lee FD (1986) Activation of mouse T-helper cells induces abundant preproenkephalin mRNA synthesis. Science 232:772–775.
11. Smith EM, Morril AC, Meyer WJ, Blalock JE (1986) Corticotropin releasing factor induction of leukocyte-derived immunoreactive ACTH and endorphins. Nature 321:881–882.
12. Male D, Champion B, Cooke A (1987) Inflammation In: Male D et al. (eds) Advanced Immunology. Lippincott, Philadelphia, pp 15.1–15.12
13. Höllt V (1986) Opioid peptide processing and receptor selectivity. Ann Rev Pharmacol Toxicol 26:59–77
14. Stein C, Hassan AHS, Przewłocki R, Gramsch C, Peter K, Herz A (1990) Opioids from immunocytes interact with receptors on sensory nerves to inhibit nociception in inflammation. Proc Natl Acad Sci USA 87:5935–5939

Section 6

Hepatocellular Injury in Ischemia, Trauma and Sepsis

An In Vitro Model of Hepatic Failure in Septic Shock

T. Hartung and A. Wendel

Introduction

Lipopolysaccharides (LPS) from gram-negative bacteria are known to be causally involved in the pathogenesis of septic shock and multiorgan failure, fulminant hepatic failure in patients with cirrhosis of the liver, and various other diseases [1]. In rodents sensitized, for example, by pretreatment with inhibitors of transcription [2] the administration of minute amounts of LPS causes acute hepatitis. Until now, this organotropic effect has not been successfully reproduced in a comparable in vitro model, i.e. in a system in which cytotoxicity toward isolated liver cells is caused by the presence of LPS. Neither LPS as such nor one of its known in vivo mediators including tumor necrosis factor (TNF), the cytotoxic monokine released following administration of LPS, showed significant hepatocytotoxicity in vitro [3].

We were interested in finding out what cellular or humoral components are required for an in vitro system of LPS-induced toxicity. The major aim was to establish similarities between in vitro findings and in vivo observations and to define possible dissimilarities compared to the available knowledge about the in vivo situation.

Materials and Methods

Substances. All substances used were purchased from commercial sources. The polyclonal sheep anti-mouse TNF-neutralizing serum (2.2×10^6 neutralizing units/ml) was from our laboratory. Murine recombinant TNF-α was a generous gift of Dr. Adolf, Boehringer Institut, Vienna, Austria.

Tissue Culture. Hepatocytes (PC) were prepared from male Fischer rats (F334, Charles River, body weight about 250–300 g, or Wistar chbb, Thomae) by the collagenase perfusion method according to Seglen [4]. Hepatocytes contained less than 1% Kupffer's, cells (KC) as judged by staining of unspecific esterase.

Biochemical Pharmacology, University of Konstanz POB 5560, 7750 Konstanz, FRG

Host Defense Dysfunction
in Trauma, Shock and Sepsis
Eds. Faist/Meakins/Schildberg
© Springer-Verlag, Berlin Heidelberg 1993

The proportion of nonparenchymal cells to parenchymal cells was enlarged by altering the centrifugation scheme (100 g instead of 50 g, as usual).

Cells were allowed to adhere for 2 h on collagen-coated six-well plates with 1.25×10^6 PC per ml. RPMI 1640 (Biochrom, Berlin) supplemented with penicillin/streptomycin (Sigma) and 10% calf serum (Serva, Heidelberg) was used as culture medium. Culture conditions were 37 °C, 40% oxygen, 55% nitrogen, and 5% carbon dioxide.

Assessment of In Vitro Hepatocytotoxicity. Incubations were started by replacing the supernatant with fresh medium. Putative effectors or inhibitors were added simultaneously. After a perincubation period of 30 min 1% of a stock solution of 1 mg/ml LPS in phosphate-buffered solution, i.e. 10 µg/ml LPS, was added. After 15.5 h of further incubation the supernatant was removed, and the remaining cells were lysed with 1 ml 0.1% Triton-X-100 (Serva, Heidelberg). Lactate dehydrogenase (LDH) release was taken as an indicator of cell death. The activity of LDH was determined separately in the medium and in the Triton lysate. Cytotoxicity was expressed as the proportion of LDH released into medium compared to the total amount of LDH present in the cells, i.e. the sum of both determinations.

TNF Assay. TNF was measured using a bioassay performed with the fibrosarcoma cell line WEHI 164 clone 13, according to Espevik and Nissen-Meyer [5].

Statistics. All in vitro experiments were performed in triplicate. Data are expressed as means ± SD; statistical analysis was performed using Student's *t* test.

Results and Discussion

With conventionally prepared hepatocytes from Fischer rats no significant LPS-induced cytotoxicity was observed (not shown). However, when the cells were prepared at higher centrifugation speed, a preparation was obtained which released significant activity of LDH in the presence of LPS (45%, basal 15%). This observation suggested that the preparation contained nonparenchymal cells of lower density which might be responsible for the phenomenon. In fact, using the esterase staining technique, the high-speed preparation contained 3% KC compared to less than 1% in the low-speed preparation. Figure 1 shows the time course of the enhancement of the LDH release from such a rat liver cell culture system in the presence and absence of LPS.

To check the specificity of this cytotoxic effect for LPS, 1 µg/ml polymyxin B as a known specific LPS binding agent was added. Under these conditions LDH

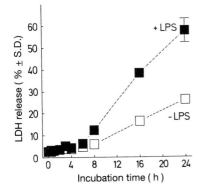

Fig. 1. Time course of LPS-induced cytotoxicity in liver cell cultures (10 µg/ml LPS)

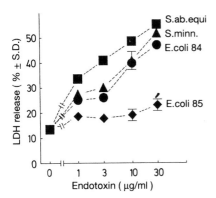

Fig. 2. Potency of different endotoxins to induce cytotoxicity in liver cells

release during the incubation period was identical to controls not exposed to LPS (data not shown).

Since a wide variety of endotoxins from different bacterial sources are known to be toxic in vivo, we studied various species of bacterial LPS in our system. The data presented in Fig. 2 demonstrate that any of the four endotoxins studied led to significant cytotoxicity in the incubation system, however, with different individual potency. To assess the contribution of nonparenchymal cells to the measured LPS-inducible LDH release, we performed several experiments in which KC function was impaired by various chemical or physical means. Inactivation of KC by either latex particles (0.5 µl/ml), gadolinium chloride (0.75 mg/ml), or methyl palmitate (1 mg/ml) led to significant reduction in the LPS-inducible LDH release from the cells by 33% ± 8%, 81% ± 5%, and 41% ± 12%, respectively. When the amount of KC was diminished by plastic adhesion (1 h) or centrifugal elutriation prior to plating, LPS-induced cytotoxicity was also inhibited by 52% ± 16% and 70% ± 13%, respectively. Upon elutriation and readditon of nonparenchymal cells, the LPS-induced cytotoxicity was partially restored (73% of the control).

Since evidence is available that in vivo TNF is one of the major pathogenic mediators of LPS, we considered whether TNF is detectable in the supernatant following stimulation of cells with LPS. The data in Fig. 3 demonstrate that TNF is produced under these conditions. Experiments shown in Fig. 4 demonstrate that in the KC/PC, i.e. the complete liver cell system, addition of sheep anti-mTNF antiserum significantly inhibited the LPS-induced cytotoxicity. On the other hand, when 0.1 µg/ml mTNF-α as such was added instead of LPS, no significant cytotoxicity resulted. However, when this amount of TNF was added in addition to 3 µg/ml LPS, LDH release after 16 h was 25% ± 10% higher than in control incubations containing only LPS. These findings are consistent with the view that LPS stimulates KC to release TNF, which in turn may exert deleterious effects on PC.

In vivo, mediation of LPS-induced hepatic injury by leukotriene D_4 (LTD_4) has been clearly demonstrated [6]. Data in Fig. 5 show that FPL 55.712, a known LTD_4 receptor antagonist, dose-dependently inhibits LPS-induced cytotoxicity after 0.5 h of preincubation. This result argues in favor of a analogous participation of LTD_4 in vitro. The aim of the final part of this study was to investigate the extent to which the in vitro model reflects the in vivo situation; in

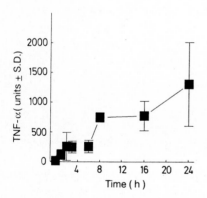

Fig. 3. Time course of LPS-induced production of TNF-α in liver cell cultures

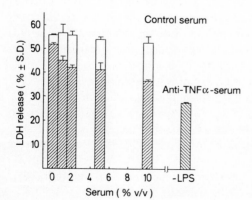

Fig. 4. Inhibition by anti-TNF-α antiserum of LPS-inducible cytotoxicity in culture

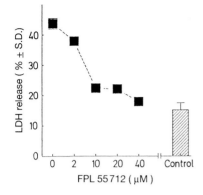

Fig. 5. Inhibition of LPS-inducible cytotoxicity in liver cells by FPL 55.712

other words, criteria as to the relevance of the model were collected. A comparison of the sensitivity of two different rat strains was made between the galactosamine/LPS model in vivo (300 mg/kg GalN plus 300 μg/kg LPS intraperitoneally; determination of serum transaminases after 16 h) and the responsiveness of cells prepared from these rat strains to LPS in vitro. Wistar rats were less sensitive to GalN/LPS-induced hepatitis than Fischer rats. When liver cells were prepared under identical conditions from both rat strains and then exposed to LPS, less then half of the LPS effect was found with the Wistar cells. These findings demonstrate a parallelism of the hepatic in vivo susceptibility and the in vitro responsiveness to LPS in these two animal strains. The findings summarized below indicate close similarity between the in vivo and the in vitro situation:

– Analogous sensitivity of different rat strains used.
– Concordant potencies of different LPS species; abrogation of LPS effect by polymyxin B.
– Attenuation by impairment of KC (latex, silica, gadolinium chloride, methyl palmitate).
– LPS tolerance after LPS administration in vivo or hepatectomy.
  Involvement of TNF-α:
  TNF-α is formed within cell cultures upon LPS stimulus.
  Partial protection by anti-rmu TNF-α serum.
  rmuTNF-α enhances LPS-induced cytotoxicity.
– Protection by pharmacological inhibitors/antagonists of LTD$_4$.

This coculture system provides a promising experimental approach to study potentially interesting compounds directed against endotoxins or some of their mediators in the course of primary drug screening.

Acknowledgements This project was supported by the Deutsche Forschungsgemeinschaft, SFB 156 "Mechanismen zellulärer Kommunikation", grant We686/12-1. The valuable contributions made by Dr. G. Tiegs as well as technical help by M. Klein and I. Görgen-Suckau are gratefully appreciated.

References

1. Bayston KF, Cohen J (1990) Bacterial endotoxin and current concepts in the diagnosis and treatment of endotoxemia. J Med Microbiol 31:73–83
2. Keppler D, Lesch R, Reutter W and Decker K (1968) Experimental hepatitis induced by D-galctosamine. Exp Mol Pathol 9:279–290
3. Rofe AM, Conyers RA, Bais R, Gamble JR, Vadas MA (1987) The effects of recombinant tumor necrosis factor (cachectin) on metabolism in isolated adipocyte, hepatocyte and muscle preparations. Biochem J 247:789–792
4. Seglen PO (1976) Preparation of isolated rat liver cells. Methods Cell Biol 13:29–83
5. Espevik T, Nissen-Meyer J (1986) A highly sensitive cell line, WEHI 164 clone 13, for measuring cytotoxic factor/tumor necrosis factor from human monocytes. J Immunol Methods 95:99–105
6. Tiegs G, Wendel A (1988) Leukotriene-mediated liver injury. Biochem Pharmacol 37:2569–2573

Ischemia-Reperfusion Injury of the Liver: Role of Neutrophils and Xanthine Oxidase

M. D. Menger[1], M. J. Müller[2], H. P. Friedl[3], O. Trentz[3], and K. Messmer[1]

Reperfusion of tissues after a period of ischemia is known to result in microvascular and endothelial injury. In this context activated neutrophils and xanthine oxidase have been suggested to play a major pathogenic role in a variety of inflammatory reactions associated with ischemia-reperfusion events [1]. Recent studies on ischemia-reperfusion have focused on the microcirculation, the primary target for leukocyte accumulation, leukocyte-endothelium interaction, and generation of oxygen-derived free radicals [2–4].

In addition to various organs, such as heart [5], striated muscle [6, 7], and skin [8], the microvasculature of the liver is known to be susceptible to ischemia-reperfusion injury [9, 10]. Within the hepatic microcirculation accumulation of leukocytes and the formation of oxygen radicals are thought to be a prominent feature during postischemic reperfusion. The purpose of our study was to evaluate the flow behavior of activated neutrophils within the hepatic microvasculature and to assess the formation of free oxygen radicals from xanthine oxidase in a rat model of warm ischemia-reperfusion of the liver, including small-bowel congestion.

Material and Methods

Sprague-Dawley rats (12 weeks old, 180–250 g body weight) were anesthetized with pentobarbital (50 mg/kg body weight; Abbott, North Chicago, IL), followed by tracheotomy and cannulation of the left carotid artery and jugular vein. A steady-state period of 15 min, including macrohemodynamic analysis (mean arterial blood pressure, heart rate) was followed by laparotomy and induction of complete liver ischemia and small-bowel congestion over 20 min by application of a microvascular clip to the hepatoduodenal ligament ($n = 8$). Thirty minutes after the onset of reperfusion the left liver lobe was exteriorized and placed on a plexiglass stage for intravital microscopy.

---

[1] Institute for Surgical Research, University of Munich, Chirurgische Forschung, LMU München, Marchioninistr. 15,8000 München 70, FRG
[2] Department of General Surgery, University of Saarland, Homburg/Saar, FRG
[3] Department of Trauma Surgery, University of Zurich, Switzerland

Host Defense Dysfunction
in Trauma, Shock and Sepsis
Eds. Faist/Meakins/Schildberg
© Springer-Verlag, Berlin Heidelberg 1993

Using intravital fluorescence microscopy and epi-illumination (100 W mercury lamp HBO, I_2 filterblock attached to a Ploemopak illuminator, excitation wavelength: 450–490 nm, emission wavelength: 515 nm; Leitz, Wetzlar, FRG the hepatic microvasculature was visualized after intravenous injection of acridine-orange (1 μM/kg body weight, Sigma Chemical, St. Louis, MO). Microvascular blood flow including the flow behavior of neutrophils was analyzed in sinusoids and postsinusoidal venules by videoframe recording of randomized lobular fields [11].

Blood samples were collected from the carotid artery and hepatic veins 40 min after declamping and analyzed spectrophotometrically [12] for xanthine oxidase activity (uric acid formation and superoxide anion generation), oxygen radical induced intravascular hemolysis, and liver enzyme activities (GOT, GPT, AP, GLDH) in plasma. Nonischemic (sham) animals ($n = 8$) served as controls.

Results

In two animals intravital microscopy revealed complete cessation of microvascular blood flow (no-reflow phenomenon) 30 min after declamping. The remaining six animals showed a reduction in microvascular blood flow during

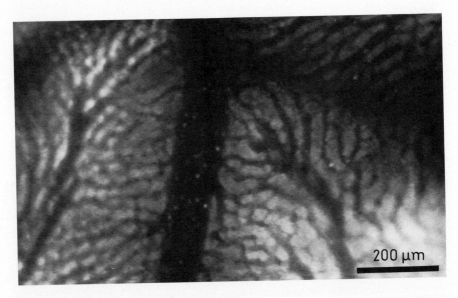

Fig. 1. Hepatic sinusoids and postsinusoidal venule of the rat liver following 20 min of liver ischemia and small-bowel congestion and 30 min of reperfusion. Note the distinct leukocyte accumulation and adherence within the postsinusoidal venule, while this phenomenon is less pronounced in the hepatic sinusoids. (Intravital fluorescence microscopy; *white dots*, leukocytes stained with acridine orange.

postischemic reperfusion. In particular, only 82.9% of the periportal sinusoids were perfused following ischemia-reperfusion as compared to 100% in controls. Concomitantly, activation of neutrophils was characterized by accumulation within the microvasculature and adherence to the microvascular endothelium. Within a complete sinusoidal segment (periportal, midzonal, pericentral) 25.6 ± 1.9 leukocytes were found adhesive as compared to control values of 2.4 ± 2.3 ($p < 0.05$, Mann-Whitney U test). However, leukocyte-endothelium interaction was even more pronounced in postsinusoidal venules (Fig. 1). Within these microvessels 402.8 ± 110.0 leukocytes/mm^2 endothelial surface were found adherent as compared to 2.5 ± 4.6 cells/mm^2 endothelial surface in nonischemic control livers ($p < 0.01$).

Leukocyte-endothelium interaction was accompanied by a significant increase of xanthine oxidase activity in the plasma of blood achieved from the hepatic veins (26.9 ± 4.7 versus control values of 6.8 ± 0.9 nmol uric acid formed ml^{-1} min^{-1}; $p < 0.05$). Assessment of oxygen radical induced intravascular hemolysis in the plasma effluent of the hepatic veins also revealed a significant difference between experimental (OD 0.066 ± 0.008) and sham animals (OD 0.004 ± 0.001; $p < 0.05$). In parallel GOT, GPT, AP, and GLDH were significantly increased with ischemic animals in comparison to non-ischemic controls.

Discussion

Microvascular ischemia-reperfusion in the rat liver is characterized by deterioration of microvascular blood flow in sinusoids, microvascular leukocyte accumulation, and leukocyte-endothelium interaction in sinusoids and, particularly, in postsinusoidal venules. These microvascular phenomena during ischemia-reperfusion were also demonstrated in vivo in other organs, including striated muscle [4, 6, 7, 13], mesenterium [2], and skin [8]. All of these studies emphasized that leukocyte-endothelium interaction occurs predominantly in postcapillary venules. While previous investigations on the hepatic microcirculation and leukocyte-endothelium interaction have considered only the hepatic sinusoids [14, 15], this is the first study, demonstrating in vivo that in the liver ischemia-reperfusion induced leukocyte-endothelium interaction is found most pronounced in postsinusoidal venules, as reported for striated muscle, mesenterium, and skin.

The accumulation of leukocytes within the microvasculature and their adherence to the endothelial surface is known to play a major role in the development of postischemic injury, since leukocyte depletion [16] as well as inhibition of leukocyte adherence [17, 18] attenuate vascular injury following ischemia-reperfusion.

In parallel with these microvascular phenomena, xanthine oxidase activity in plasma and oxygen radical induced intravascular hemolysis were found to be increased significantly during ischemia-reperfusion of the liver, indicating generation of oxygen derived free radicals. However, it should be taken into consideration that small-bowel congestion during clamping of the hepato-duodenal ligament may be in part responsible for the increase in xanthine oxidase activity during reperfusion (reoxygenation). In various studies Granger and coworkers demonstrated that ischemia-reperfusion in the small bowel is accompanied by xanthine oxidase mediated formation of oxygen radicals [1].

We conclude from our data that formation of oxygen radicals by xanthine oxidase might interact with the activation of neutrophils in situ and enhance leukocyte-endothelium interaction, probably triggered by a complement-dependent mechanism [12]. A recent study by Patel and coworkers [19] supports this hypothesis, demonstrating in vitro oxygen radical induced expression of granule membrane protein-140 (GMP-140), a membrane-associated glycoprotein which binds neutrophils to endothelial cells.

Acknowledgement. This work was supported by the Deutsche Forschungsgemeinschaft, Me 900/1-1 and Me 900/1-2.

References

1. Granger DN (1988) Role of xanthine oxidase and granulocytes in ischemia-reperfusion injury. Am J Physiol 255:H1269–H1275
2. Granger DN, Benoit JN, Suzuki M, Grisham MB (1989) Leukocyte adherence to venular endothelium during ischemia-reperfusion. Am J Physiol 257:G683–G688
3. Hernandez LA, Grisham MB, Twohig B, Arfors KE, Harlan JM, Granger DN (1987) Role of neutrophils in ischemia-reperfusion-induced microvascular injury. Am J Physiol 253:H699–H703
4. Lehr HA, Guhlmann A, Nolte D, Keppler D, Messmer (1991) Leukotrienes as mediators in ischemia-reperfusion injury in a microcirculation model in the hamster. J Clin Invest 87:2036–2042
5. Hearse DJ, Manning AS, Downey JM, Yellon DM (1986) Liver xanthine oxydase: a critical mediator of myocardial injury during ischemia and reperfusion. Acta Physiol Scand 548:65–78
6. Messina LM (1990) In vivo assessment of acute microvascular injury after reperfusion of ischemic tibialis anterior muscle of the hamster. J Surg Res 48:615–621
7. Suval WD, Duran WN, Boric MP, Hobson RW, Berendsen PB, Ritter AB (1987) Microvascular transport and endothelial cell alterations preceding skeletal muscle damage in ischemia and reperfusion injury. Am J Surg 154:211–218
8. Bartlett R, Funk W, Hammersen F, Arfors K-E, Messmer K, Nemir P (1986) Effect of superoxide dismutase on skin microcirculation after ischemia and reperfusion. Surg Forum 37:599–601
9. Parks DA, Granger DN (1988) Ischemia-reperfusion injury: a radical view. Hepatology 8:680–682
10. Jaeschke H, Farhood A, Smith CW (1990) Neutrophils contribute to ischemia/reperfusion injury in rat liver in vivo. FASEB J 4:3355–3359
11. Menger MD, Marzi I, Messmer K (1991) In vivo fluorescence microscopy for quantitative analysis of the hepatic microcirculation in hamsters and rats. Eur Surg Res 23:158–169
12. Friedl HP, Till GO, Trentz O, Ward PA (1989) Roles of histamine, complement, and xanthine oxidase in thermal injury of skin. Am J Physiol 135:203–217
13. Nolte D, Lehr HA, Messmer K (1991) Adenosine inhibits postischemic leukocyte-endothelium interaction in postcapillary venules of the hamster. Am J Physiol 261:H651–H655

14. Marzi I, Knee J, Bühren V, Menger MD, Trentz O (1991) Reduction of leukocyte-endothelial adherence following liver transplantation by superoxide dismutase. Surgery (in press)
15. Marzi I, Knee J, Bühren V, Menger MD, Harbauer G, Trentz O (1991) Hepatic microcirculatory disturbances due to portal vein clamping in the orthotopic rat liver transplantation model. Transplantation (in press)
16. Korthuis RJ, Grisham MB, Granger DN (1988) Leukocyte depletion attenuates vascular injury in postischemic skeletal muscle. Am J Physiol 254:H823–H827
17. Arfors K-E, Lundberg C, Lindbom L, Lundberg K, Beatty PG, Harlan JM (1987) A monoclonal antibody to the membrane glycoprotein complex CD18 inhibits polymorphonuclear leukocyte accumulation and plasma leakage in vivo. Blood 69:338–340
18. Vedder NB, Winn RK, Rice CL, Chi EY, Arfors K-E, Harlan JN (1990) Inhibition of leukocyte adherence by anti-CD18 monoclonal antibody attenuates reperfusion injury in the rabbit ear. Proc Natl Acad Sci USA 87:2643–2646
19. Patel KD, Zimmerman GA, Prescott SM, McEver RP, McIntyre TM (1991) Oxygen radicals induce human endothelial cells to express GMP-140 and bind neutrophils. J Cell Biol 112:749–760

Nitric Oxide Regulates Prostaglandin E$_2$ Release by Rat Kupffer Cells*

J. Stadler, B. G. Harbrecht, M. Di Silvio, R. D. Curran, M. L. Jordan, R. L. Simmons, and T. R. Billiar

Nitric oxide has recently been identified as an intermediate of mammalian nitrogen metabolism [1, 2]. This highly reactive radical is derived from the amino acid L-arginine and degrades within seconds into its stable end products nitrite and nitrate. Important biological functions of nitric oxide include regulation of vascular tone [1], inhibition of thrombocyte adherence and aggregation [3], as well as enhancement of macrophage cytotoxicity [4]. Macrophage nitric oxide biosynthesis is inducible, namely by inflammatory mediators such as lipopolysaccharide (LPS) [5]. Kupffer cells, the fixed macrophages of the liver, also produce nitric oxide in response to LPS [6]. In addition, LPS-stimulated Kupffer cells release cytokines, which induce nitric oxide synthesis in hepatocytes [7]. The role of nitric oxide in the septic liver is not very well understood. Experiments were undertaken to determine whether nitric oxide synthesis influences other functions of Kupffer cells, specifically the release of eicosanoids.

Material and Methods

Kupffer Cell Isolation and Culture Technique. Nonparenchymal liver cells were harvested from Sprague-Dawley rats (Harlan Sprague-Dawley, Madison, WI, USA) using a pronase perfusion technique as described by Emeis and Planque [8]. Kupffer cells were then separated from other nonparenchymal cells by centrifugal elutriation yielding 85%–95% Kupffer cells according to peroxidase staining. This cell preparation was cultured in Williams medium E (Gibco, Grand Island, NY, USA) as previously described [6] in 24-well plates at 5×10^5 cells/ml (1 ml/well). Following a preincubation period of 48 h LPS (*Escherichia coli* 0111:B4 from Sigma Chemical Co. St. Louis, MO, USA) and/or interferon-gamma (recombinant rat IFN-γ, Amgen Biologicals, Thousand Oaks, CA, USA) were added and culture supernatants harvested at various time points. At this time trypan blue exclusion of the cells was assessed.

* This work was supported by National Institutes of Health grants GM 44100 (T.R.B.) and GM 37753 (R.L.S.) J. S. was supported by a fellowship of the Deutsche Forschungs gemeinschaft, Bonn Germany (Sta 311/1-1).
Department of Surgery, University of Pittsburgh, Pittsburgh, PA, USA

Host Defense Dysfunction
in Trauma, Shock and Sepsis
Eds. Faist/Meakins/Schildberg
© Springer-Verlag, Berlin Heidelberg 1993

Determination of Prostaglandin E_2 Production. Prostaglandin E_2 (PGE_2) concentrations were measured in the culture supernatants using radioimmunoassay kits (Advanced Magnetic Inc., Cambridge, MA, USA) according to the manufacturer's instructions.

Determination of Nitrite and Enzyme Release. Nitrites (NO_2^-) were measured as stable endproducts of nitric oxide synthesis using a spectrophotometric assay based on the Greiss reaction [9]. Lactate dehydrogenase (LDH) levels were determined using a clinical chemistry analyzer.

Results and Discussion

As previously reported [6], exposure of Kupffer cells to LPS resulted in the induction of nitric oxide synthesis (Table 1). This effect was synergistically enhanced by the combination of LPS with IFN-γ, while IFN-γ alone did not induce significant nitric oxide production by Kupffer cells. This response of Kupffer cells to LPS and IFN-γ is similar to that of other macrophage-type cells [10]. Addition of the competitive inhibitor of nitric oxide synthesis N^G-monomethyl-L-arginine (NMA) in an equimolar concentration with L-arginine-suppressed nitric oxide synthesis almost completely.

   Similar to nitric oxide synthesis, PGE_2 production was also stimulated by a 24-h exposure to LPS (Fig. 1). Again, IFN-γ did not induce PGE_2 production by itself. In contrast to nitric oxide synthesis, IFN-γ had no significant effect on PGE_2 production when combined with LPS in the absence of NMA. However, inhibition of nitric oxide synthesis by the addition of NMA resulted in increased PGE_2 production stimulated by LPS alone and revealed a strong synergistic effect of IFN-γ in combination with LPS. This synergistic effect appears to be

Table 1. Nitric oxide synthesis by rat Kupffer cells in response to different stimulatory agents

Stimulatory agents		Nitrite release	
LPS (1.0 µg/ml)	IFN-γ(100 U/ml)	− NMA	+ NMA
−	−	2.4 ± 0.2	1.8 ± 0.2
−	+	4.4 ± 0.3	2.0 ± 0.2
+	−	$16.4 \pm 1.4^*$	3.9 ± 0.3
+	+	$39.3 \pm 2.6^*$	7.0 ± 0.4

$^*p < 0.001$ vs untreated Kupffer cells.
Kupffer cells were incubated under the conditions listed above for 24 h. Nitric oxide biosynthesis was inhibited by the addition of 0.2 mM NMA. Nitrites were measured in the culture supernatants as stable end products of nitric oxide synthesis. The results represent means $\pm$ SEM of four experiments.

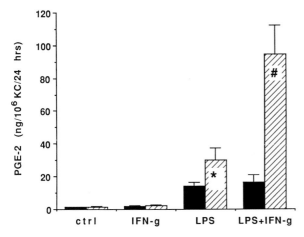

Fig. 1. PGE$_2$ production in response to different stimulatory agents. Kupffer cells were incubated in standard culture medium (*black columns*) or in the presence of 0.2 mM NMA (*hatched columns*) for 24 h 100 U/ml IFN-γ (*IFN-g*) and/or 1.0 μg/ml LPS were added as indicated. PGE$_2$ levels were determined using a radioimmunoassay. Data are presented as means ± SEM of four experiments. * $p < 0.05$ vs incubations without NMA; # $p < 0.005$ vs incubations without NMA

masked by the inhibitory effect of nitric oxide synthesis, which is simultaneously induced by the same mediators. When Kupffer cells were stimulated with LPS and IFN-γ, inhibition of nitric oxide synthesis with NMA led to a more than fivefold increase of PGE$_2$ production.

Several biological effects of nitric oxide may contribute to the inhibitory effect of PGE$_2$ production. Comparison of L-arginine-containing and L-arginine free culture media suggested that nitric oxide production may lead to decreased viability of macrophages [11]. In the present study neither stimulation nor inhibition of nitric oxide synthesis did affect cell viability (Table 2). This excludes the possibility that cell death is the cause of impaired PGE$_2$ production in the absence of NMA.

Table 2. Effect of nitric oxide synthesis on viability of Kupffer cells

Culture conditions				
LPS (1.0 μg/ml)	IFN (100 U/ml)	NMA (0.2 mM)	Trypan blue exclusion (%)	LDH Release (U/l)
−	−	−	87.3 ± 2.9	10.3 ± 3.5
−	−	+	83.5 ± 1.5	10.0 ± 3.2
+	+	−	85.1 ± 2.6	11.8 ± 2.4
+	+	+	82.7 ± 1.0	11.3 ± 2.5
Intentional lysis			0	152.3 ± 9.2

Kupffer cells were incubated for 24 h under the conditions listed above. The experiments represent the mean ± SE of three experiments

Well-established effects of nitric oxide include inhibition of protein synthesis [12] and inhibition of aerobic energy metabolism [5, 13]. Inhibition of cyclo-oxygenase production could explain the observed phenomenon, because continuous cyclooxygenase production is necessary to keep prostaglandin synthesis ongoing [14]. Inhibition of aerobic energy metabolism might not have such dramatic effects on the secretory capacity of macrophage-like cell types. In these cells mitochondrial respiration provides only a relatively small portion of the total energy pool [15]. A specific mechanism of alteration of enzyme activity may involve binding of nitric oxide to the heme-group in the catalytic center of the cyclooxygenase [16]. Nitric oxide binds vigorously to heme-groups [17] but a specific action on cyclooxygenase has not been demonstrated.

In conclusion, the presented results suggest that nitric oxide may play an essential role in the regulation of inflammatory processes in the liver and in other environments. In addition, studies on the interaction of nitric oxide and cyclooxygenase products may help to understand alterations in circulation, which are characteristic for sepsis.

References

1. Palmer RMJ, Ferrige AG, Moncada S (1987) Nitric oxide release accounts for the biological activity of endothelium-derived relaxing factor. Nature 327:524–526
2. Hibbs JB Jr, Taintor RR, Vavrin Z, Rachlin EM (1988) Nitric oxide: a cytotoxic activated macrophage effector molecule. Biochem Biophys Res Commun 157:87–94
3. Radomski MW, Palmer RMJ, Moncada S (1987) Endogenous nitric oxide inhibits human platelet adhesion to vascular endothelium. Lancet II:1057–1058
4. Stuehr DJ, Nathan CF (1989) Nitric oxide. A macrophage product responsible for cytostasis and respiratory inhibition in tumor target cells. J Exp Med 169:1543–1555
5. Stuehr DJ, Marletta MA (1985) Mammalian nitrate biosynthesis: mouse macrophages produce nitrite and nitrate in response to Escherichia coli lipopolysaccharide. Proc Natl Acad Sci USA 82:7738–7742
6. Billiar TR, Curran RD, Stuehr DJ, West MA, Bentz BG, Simmons RL (1989) An L-arginine-dependent mechanism mediates Kupffer cell inhibition of hepatocyte protein synthesis in vitro. J Exp Med 169:1467–1472
7. Curran RD, Billiar TR, Stuehr DJ, Hofmann K, Simmons RL (1989) Hepatocytes produce nitrogen oxides from L-arginine in response to inflammatory products of Kupffer cells. J Exp Med 170:1769–1774
8. Emeis JJ, Planque B (1976) Heterogeneity of cells isolated from rat liver by pronase digestion. J Reticuloendo Soc 20:11–29
9. Green LC, Wagner DA, Glogowski J, Skipper PL, Wishnok JS, Tannenbaum SR (1982) Analysis of nitrate, nitrite, and [^{15}N] nitrate in biological fluids. Anal Biochem 126:131–138
10. Ding AH, Nathan CF, Stuehr DJ (1988) Release of reactive nitrogen intermediates and reactive oxygen intermediates from mouse peritoneal macrophages. J Immunol 141:2407–2412
11. Albina JE, Mills CD, Henry WL Jr, Caldwell MD (1989) Regulation of macrophage physiology by L-arginine: role of the oxidative L-arginine deiminase pathway. J Immunol 143:3641–3646
12. Curran RD, Ferrari FK, Kispert PH, Stadler J, Stuehr DJ, Simmons RL, Billiar TR (1991) Nitric Oxide and nitric oxide-generating compounds inhibit hepatocyte protein synthesis. FASEB J 5:2085–2092
13. Stadler J, Billiar TR, Curran RD, Stuehr DJ, Ochoa JB, Simmons RL (1991) Effect of exogenous and endogenous nitric oxide on mitochondrial respiration of rat hepatocytes. Am J Physiol (in press)

14. Fu J-Y, Masferrer JL, Seibert K, Raz A, Needleman P (1990) The induction and suppression of prostaglandin H$_2$ synthase (cyclooxygenase) in human monocytes. J Biol Chem 265:16737–16740
15. Newsholme P, Gordon S, Newsholme EA (1987) Rates of utilization and fates of glucose, glutamine, pyruvate, fatty acids and ketone bodies by mouse macrophages. Biochem J 242:631–636
16. Hemler M, Lands WEM (1976) Purification of the cyclooxygenase that forms prostaglandins. Demonstration of two forms of iron in the holoenzyme. J Biol Chem 251:5575–5579
17. Ignarro LJ (1989) Endothelium-derived nitric oxide: actions and properties. FASEB J 3:31–36

C3a and C5a in Liver Transplantations During Bypass, Reperfusion, and the Postoperative Phase

M. Hartmann and L. Verner

Introduction

Activation of the complement cascade may be initiated either by the classical pathway—induced by antigen-antibody complexes—or by the alternative pathway [1] (Fig. 1). Triggers for the latter include proteinases, endotoxin, bacteria, and foreign surfaces. Activation of the alternative pathway results in amplification via feedback. This excessive reaction is considered to play an important etiological role in adult respiratory distress syndrome after trauma, operation, or sepsis [2–4].

We investigated the generation of anaphylatoxins, activated complement components with inflammatory activity. In patients undergoing liver transplantation plasma levels of the anaphylatoxins C3a and C5a were determined to evaluate (a) the effects of a veno-venous bypass which is used to harmonize hemodynamics during the anhepatic phase, and (b) whether C3a and C5a levels are suitable parameters for assessing graft function and rejection reaction.

Patients and Methods

In patients hepatocellular carcinomas and posthepatitic/cryptogenic cirrhoses ($n = 7$; patients A–G; Table 1) C3a and C5a were determined pre-, intra-, and early postoperatively. The timing of the 20 samples was as follows:
1: preoperatively
2: before anhepatic phase
3: beginning of anhepatic phase
4: 1 h anhepatic phase
5: end of bypass/declamping
6: 1 h after bypass/declamping
7: 2 h after bypass/declamping
8: 3 h after bypass/declamping
9: 1 h postoperatively
10–20: day 1; every other day

Department of Anesthesiology I, Hannover Medical School, Konstanty-Gutschow Str., 3000 Hannover 61, FRG

Host Defense Dysfunction
in Trauma, Shock and Sepsis
Eds. Faist/Meakins/Schildberg
© Springer-Verlag, Berlin Heidelberg 1993

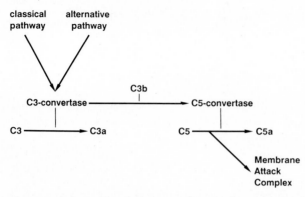

Fig. 1. The complement cascade

Table 1. Patient characteristics

Patient	Sex	Age (years)	Indication
A	M	50	CA (carcinoma)
B	F	45	PNC (post necrotic cirrhosis)
C	F	39	FULM (fulminant hepatic failure)
D	M	33	PNC
E	F	47	PNC
F	F	20	PNC
G	M	54	CA
H–L	4 M, 1 F	28–52	PNC

To avoid misinterpretation, additional investigations were made on the blood preparations transfused intraoperatively. Patients A–E were treated with a veno-venous bypass by means of the Bio-Medicus pump and TDMAC coated polyvinylchloride tubes (Argyle) with an average flow rate of 2000–4000 ml/min. Clamping of the large vessels was performed in patients F and G. In patients with posthepatitic cirrhoses ($n = 5$; H–L) blood samples for C3a and C5a were taken up to 3 weeks after the operation (see above).

The anaphylatoxins C3a and C5a were determined using an enzyme-linked immunosorbent assay as described by Klos and Bitter-Suermann [5]. In view of the large movements of fluid, hematocrit correction of all values obtained was performed according to the method described by Beaumont. Donor organ function was evaluated by liver-related blood chemistry, rejection by inflammatory parameters, histological, and cytological procedures. Hemodynamics, hemogram, and major clotting factors were measured at all times of sampling to investigate patient comparability.

Results

There was adequate substitution in all patients with respect to hemodynamics, hemogram, and major clotting factors. With one exception C3a was in the normal range in patients with and without bypass preoperatively and in the anhepatic phase. After termination of bypass or declamping, increased values were observed (normal range < 300 ng/ml; Fig. 2). With one exception (patient B) values were within or slightly exceeded the normal range of up to 5 ng/ml. After termination of the bypass or declamping, an increase was found in every patient. Values in patient B were influenced by the fact that all 6 U blood that he received intraoperatively showed markedly increased C5a levels (Fig. 3).

Averaging of the results of all seven patients shows that after reperfusion of the donor organ the generation of anaphylatoxins clearly exceeded normal values (Fig. 4). The postoperative investigations in patients H–L showed a rise over 3 weeks of up to twofold the normal range for C3a and up to fourfold the normal range for C5a, which, however, never reached those at the end of

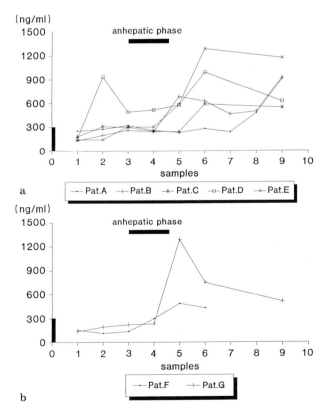

Fig. 2a, b. C3a plasma levels in orthotopic liver transplantation. **a** With bypass. **b** Without bypass

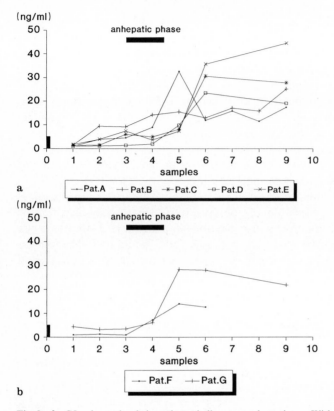

Fig. 3a, b. C5a plasma levels in orthotopic liver transplantation. **a** With bypass. **b** Without bypass

operation. No correlation was found with the initial nonfunction of the donor organ or acute rejection reaction. Anaphylatoxin levels showed no time dependency. Figure 5 presents the postoperative course of patient K, who developed a clinical episode of acute rejection.

Discussion

As a preliminary result in can be noted that with the reperfusion of the donor organ activated split products of the complement cascade are generated. This indicates that the analytical sensitivity of the enzyme-linked immunosorbent assay is sufficient, even for C5a. In contrast to the cardiopulmonary bypass, evidence seems to be provided that the foreign surface veno-venous bypass does not induce production of anaphylatoxins. This bypass-model may lead to a smaller extent of damage or to less regulator depletion [6]. On the other hand, a systemic error might have occurred by not measuring the parent molecules C3

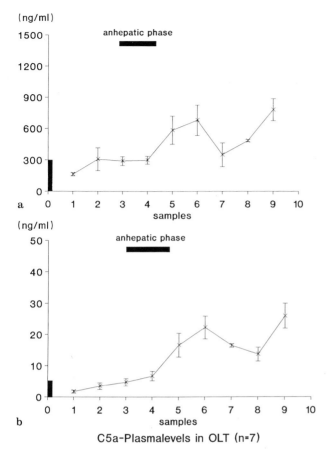

Fig. 4a, b. Mean plasma levels of anaphylatoxins in orthotopic liver transplantation ($n = 7$). **a** C3a. **b** C5a

and C5. Although the liver is known to be a site of synthesis, it is not fully understood to what extent this ability is compromised by certain diseases, or whether compensation is provided, for example, by macrophages [7, 8].

The marked complement activation after the graft is connected may be caused by several factors. Acidosis and anoxia following a release of proteinases or liver cell injury or impaired gall drainage may function as a trigger for the alternative pathway. Even with the liver's low immunological potential, classical activation is initiated through anti-idiotypic antibodies.

C3a and C5a levels dropped after the end of the operation but continued to exceed the normal range for at least 3 weeks. Further investigations are required to elucidate possible correlations with graft function and rejection reaction.

In conclusion, in patients undergoing liver transplantation reperfusion of the donor organ initiated activation of the complement cascade. Production of the

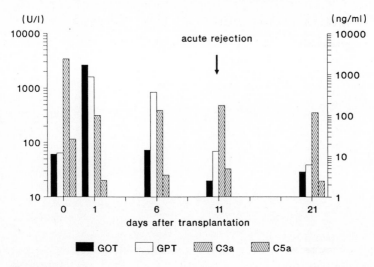

Fig. 5. Postoperative course of patient K. C3a, normal range (< 200 ng/ml); C5a, normal range (< 2 ng/ml)

anaphylatoxins C3a and C5a remained elevated during the first 3 weeks after transplantation. No correlation with organ dysfunction or rejection was found. The foreign surface bypass did not initiate activation of the alternative pathway.

References

1. Bitter-Suermann D (1983) Das Komplementsystem: physiologische Funktion und klinische Bedeutung. Dtsch Ärztebl 80:33
2. Heideman M, Hugli TE (1984) Anaphylatoxin generation in multisystem organ failure. J Trauma 24:1038
3. Hammerschmidt DE, Weaver LJ, Hudson LD, Craddock PR, Jacob HS (1980) Association of complement activation and elevated plasma-C5a with adult respiratory distress syndrome. Lancet 1:947
4. Westaby S (1983) Complement and the damaging effects of cardiopulmonary bypass. Thorax 38:321
5. Klos A, Ihring V, Messner M, Grabbe J, Bitter-Suermann D (1988) Detection of native human complement components C3 and C5 and their primary activation peptides C3a and C5a (anaphylatoxic peptides) by ELISA with monoclonal antibodies. J Immunol Med 111:241
6. Tamiya T, Yamasaki M, Maeo Y, Yamashiro T, Ogoshi S, Fujumato S (1988) Complement activation in cardiopulmonary bypass, with special reference to anaphylatoxin production in membrane and bubble oxygenators. Ann Thorac Surg 46:47
7. Alper CA, Johnson AM, Birtch AG, Moore FD (1969) Human C3: evidence for the liver as the primary site of synthesis. Science 163:286
8. Munoz LE, DeVilliers D, Markham D, Whaley K, Thomas HC (1982) Complement activation in chronic liver disease. Clin Exp Immunol 47:548

Effect of Superoxide Dismutase on Altered Hepatic Calcium Regulation During Gramnegative Sepsis

S. Rose[1], J. Dike[1], V. Bühren[1], O. Trentz[1], and M. M. Sayeed[2]

Introduction

Gram-negative infection after major surgery and abdominal trauma constitutes a serious complication with high mortality [5, 16]. Peritoneal abscess formation involves a variety of inflammatory cells and mediators which prevent the spread of a fulminant bacterial sepsis. Because of its prominent anatomical position and metabolic capabilities, the liver also plays a central role in supporting the septic host defense response during abdominal infection. Liver function derangements represent critical events in the sequence of multiple organ failure and the outcome of the septic syndrome.

Altered cellular Ca^{2+} regulation has been shown to occur in a variety of cell types. Cellular Ca^{2+} overload initiates a disturbance of cellular functions by activating cytolytic cascades and affecting hormonal and enzymatic pathways [9]. Preliminary studies in our laboratory demonstrated alterations in hepatocellular Ca^{2+} regulation during gram-negative intraabdominal infection. The Ca^{2+} channel blocker diltiazem not only prevented hepatocellular Ca^{2+} overload but also decreased oxygen free radical (OFR)-mediated membrane injury.

The purpose of the present study was to investigate a role of superoxide radical (SOR) in the alteration of hepatic Ca^{2+} homeostasis during gram-negative sepsis. Furthermore, we determined whether treatment of animals with the SOR-scavenging enzyme superoxide dismutase prevents OFR-mediated membrane injury.

Methods

In male Sprague-Dawley rats (250 g, $n = 7$ per group) intraabdominal gram-negative sepsis was induced by implantation of a fecal pellet (1 cm^3) impregnated with live *Escherichia coli* (100 colony forming unit, CFU) and *Bacillus fragilis* (10^4 CFU). In control rats either laparotomy was performed or a sterile pellet was implanted. Polyethylenglycol-bound superoxide dismutase (PEG-SOD, Sigma chemicals 5000 U/kg i.v.) with a half-life of about 35 h or its carrier

[1] Department of Trauma Surgery, Chirurgische Universitätsklinik, 6650 Homburg, FRG
[2] Department of Physiology, Loyola University School of Medicine, Maywood, IL, USA

Host Defense Dysfunction
in Trauma, Shock and Sepsis
Eds. Faist/Meakins/Schildberg
© Springer-Verlag, Berlin Heidelberg 1993

methoxy-polyethylenglycol (MG 5000, Sigma chemicals) was administered to the animals with implantation as a co-treatment. At 24 h post-implantation the rats were anesthetized with pentobarbital and hepatocytes were isolated. Briefly, after cannulation of the portal vein, livers were perfused for 7 min by a Ca^{2+}-free Krebs Ringer bicarbonate (KRB) solution. Additionally, the livers were perfused for 15 min with a KRB solution containing collagenase (Worthington, 14 mg/80 ml, 0.1 mM Ca^{2+}) [13].

Cytosolic Ca^{2+} concentrations, $[Ca^{2+}]_i$, were measured in hepatocytes (10 mg dry weight/ml) incubated for 30 min in Hank's solution (1 mM Ca^{2+}) containing the fluorescent calcium chelator indo-1/AM (final concentration: 10 μM) at 37 °C [6]. The hormone-stimulated response was the fluorescence signal (excitation: 332 nM, emmission: 400 nM) obtained 5 min after addition of vasopressin (100 nM). Maximum fluorescence (F_{max}) was determined using Ca^{2+}-agonist ionomycin (6.7 μM) and minimum fluorescence (F_{min}) was obtained by quenching with $MnCl_2$ (6 mM). Fluorescence signals were corrected for both the intrinsic fluorescence of non-loaded hepatocytes and leakage of indo-1 from loaded hepatocytes (40 mM $MnCl_2$). Cytosolic $[Ca^{2+}]_i$ was calculated using the equation $[Ca^{2+}]_i = K_d (F - F_{min})/(F_{max} - F)$, where K_d (250 nM) is the dissociation constant of the Ca^{2+}/indo-1 complex.

Cellular exchangeable Ca^{2+} was evaluated in hepatocytes (30 mg wet weight/ml) maximally loaded with $^{45}CaCl_2$ (0.05 MBq/ml) in Hank's medium at 37 °C [2]. When equilibrium was reached after 40 min, cells were washed and resuspended in non-radioactive medium to initiate Ca^{2+} washout. Cellular radioactivity was assessed using a scintillation counter after removing extracellular ^{45}Ca from loaded cells by a gradient [top, $LaCl_3$ (2.3 mM), 2.3 mM), pH 7.4; middle, silicone oil; bottom, $HClO_4$ (1.5 M)].

To determine lipid peroxidation products, conjugated dienes (CD) were extracted by chloroform/methanol (2:1 v/v) from lipids of lypholized liver tissue according to [4]. Aliquots of the chloroform phase were dried under nitrogen stream. The residue was dissolved in n-hexane and absorbance at 233 nm read against a n-hexane blank [12]. Total lipids were measured according to the method described by [3]. Thiobarbituric acid reactive substances (TBA-RS) were determined using the method of [11]. Sodium dodecyl sulfate (SDS)-acetic acid solution (pH 3.5) and aqueous solution of thiobarbituric acid were added to the tissue powder. After heating in an oil bath for 60 min at 95 °C the samples were cooled down and a mixture of n-butanol and pyridine (15:1, v/v) was added. After the addition of phosphotungstic acid and centrifugation, the absorbance of the organic layer was fluorometrically read at 532 nm. CD were expressed as: optical density (OD) units/mg total lipids and TBA-RS as: nmol/mg tissue. Statistical evaluations were made using an analysis of variance.

Results

Laparotomy or implantation of a sterile pellet had no effect on basal cytosolic free Ca^{2+} levels ($[Ca^{2+}]_i$) or cellular exchangeable Ca^{2+} as compared to

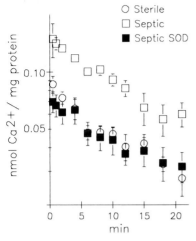

Fig. 1. Cellular exchangeable Ca^{2+} (nmol Ca^{2+}/mg protein) determined from isolated hepathocytes 24 h after the beginning of intraabdominal gram-negative sepsis. Values are expressed as x ± Standard error mean

healthy control animals. In contrast, $[Ca^{2+}]_i$ in septic animals was about five times higher than in sterile-implanted animals (738.3 ± 82 vs 147.7 ± 5 nmol/l). In septic animals treated with PEG-SOD, $[Ca^{2+}]_i$ was 157 ± 12 nmol/l. The vasopressin-induced magnitude of cytosolic $[Ca^{2+}]$ increase was attenuated in septic animals (175%) as compared to that in sterile-implanted animals (578%). PEG-SOD treatment of septic animals only slightly increased (237%) the amount of vasopressin-induced cellular $[Ca^{2+}]$.

As shown in Fig. 1, cellular exchangeable Ca^{2+} was significantly higher ($p < 0.001$) in septic animals compared to sterile-implanted animals (septic, 0.161 ± 0.02 nmol Ca^{2+}/mg protein; sterile, 0.077 ± 0.003 nmol Ca^{2+}/mg protein), but was significantly decreased ($p < 0.001$), when septic rats were treated with PEG-SOD (septic + PEG-SOD; 0.069 ± 0.002 nmol Ca^{2+}/mg protein). There was no effect of PEG-SOD administration on $[Ca^{2+}]_i$ and exchangeable Ca^{2+} in nonseptic, sterile-implanted animals.

Concentrations of CD and TBA-RS were significantly increased in liver homogenates of untreated septic animals when compared to untreated sterile-implanted animals ($p < 0.01$). A significant attenuation of hepatic lipid peroxidation ($p < 0.01$) was observed when septic animals were treated with PEG-SOD as indicated by a decrease in CD and TBA-RS to levels measured in control livers (Fig. 2)

Discussion

The present study demonstrated a protective effect of superoxide dismutase against alterations in hepatocellular Ca^{2+} regulation during gram-negative intraabdominal sepsis. Previous studies in our laboratory showed a disturbance in cellular Ca^{2+} regulation during endotoxic shock, which was prevented by the calcium channel blocker diltiazem [7, 13, 14]. The increased cytosolic $[Ca^{2+}]_i$

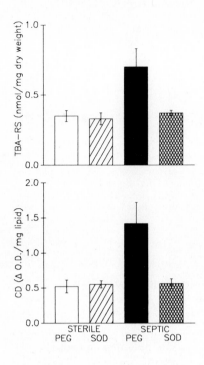

Fig. 2. Hepatic lipid peroxidation products during gram-negative sepsis: the effect of PEG superoxide dismutase (SOD) treatment. Values are expressed as x ± standard error of mean. *PEG*, methoxy-polyethylenglycol (MG 5000) as carrier of SOD; *SOD*, PEG-SOD, 5000 U/g

and cellular Ca^{2+} pool observed in septic animals was presumably due to an increase in cellular Ca^{2+} uptake and altered Ca^{2+} movements between the cytosolic and Ca^{2+} storing compartments, e.g., endoplasmic reticulum. Whereas treatment with PEG-SOD, at a time when sepsis was induced, did prevent cellular Ca^{2+} overload, it did not completely restore attenuated hormone response observed in septic animals.

A major source of oxygen free radical species during inflammation is the nicotinamide adenine dinucleotide phosphate, reduced (NADPH)-oxidase system of activated leukocytes, which is a potent generator of oxygen free radicals during bacterial killing [1]. Gram-negative infection and the release of endotoxin are also potent stimulators of macrophage release of cytokines like tumor necrosis factor (TNF) and interleukin-1 (IL-1) [8]. There is evidence that these inflammatory mediators stimulate the phagocytosis of polymorphonuclear leukocytes with secretion of proteases and oxygen free radicals, especially the highly reactive hydroxyl radical [16]. Since superoxide dismutase is known to catalyze the dismutation of superoxide radical to yield H_2O_2 and O_2 PEG-SOD could directly intercept the biochemical reactions leading to hydroxyl radical-mediated initiation of membrane lipid peroxidation. During the process of lipid peroxidation polyunsaturated fatty acids, phospholipids, and arachidonic acid are oxidatively degraded to a variety of lipid radicals. The initial step involves the abstraction of a hydrogen atom by the attack of a highly reactive hydroxyl radical yielding a lipid radical with CD structure. Further peroxidation results in the formation of lipid hydroperoxides and the final product,

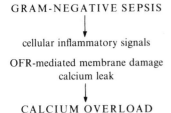

GRAM-NEGATIVE SEPSIS

cellular inflammatory signals

OFR-mediated membrane damage
calcium leak

CALCIUM OVERLOAD

calcium toxicity

altered cellular function

ORGAN FAILURE   **Fig. 3.** Free radical, calcium and hepatic injury

malondialdehyde. The increase in hepatic lipid peroxidation during gram-negative sepsis was attenuated by PEG-SOD treatment of the rats. Thus, PEG-SOD might have prevented changes in membrane integrity and ion permeability which could allow uncontrolled Ca^{2+} influx across hepatocyte plasma membrane, so-called "calcium leaks" [15] (Fig. 3). In vitro studies suggested that cellular Ca^{2+} overload caused irreversible cell injury by activation of cytolytic celular cascades like neutral proteases, endonucleases, and phospholipases [9]. Ca^{2+} toxicity with altered cellular functions might have deleterious consequences for host–defense mechansims in the septic organism and might finally result in organ failure.

Overall, prevention of sepsis-related cellular Ca^{2+} overload and tissue injury by PEG-SOD suggests oxygen free radical-mediated hepatic injury during gram-negative sepsis. This protective effect of PEG-SOD may be due either to a direct action of PEG-SOD against hepatocellular lipid peroxidation or to its modulation of signals from inflammatory cells.

References

1. Babior BM (1984) Oxidants from phagocytes: agents of defense and destruction. Blood 64:959–966
2. Barritt GJ, Parker JC, Wadsworth JC (1981) A kinetic analysis of the effects of adrenaline on calcium distribution in isolated rat liver parenchymal cells. J Physiol 312:29–55
3. Chiang SP, Gessert CF, Lowry OH (1957) Colorimetric determination of extracted lipids. Austin TX: Air Force University, School of Aviation Medicine, pp 56–63 (Res Rep 56–113)
4. Folch J, Lees M, Sloane-Stanley GH (1957) A simple method for the isolation and purification of total lipids from animal tissue. J Biol Chem 226:497–509
5. Goins WA, Rodriguez A, Joshi M, Jacobs D (1990) Intra-abdominal abscess after blunt abdominal trauma. Ann Surg 212:60–65
6. Grynkiewicz G, Poenie M, Tsien RY (1985) A new generation of Ca^{2+}-indicators with greatly improved fluorescence properties. J Biol Chem 260:3440–3450
7. Maitra SR, Sayeed MM (1987) Effect of diltiazem on intracellular Ca^{2+} mobilization in hepatocytes during endotoxic shock. Am J Physiol 253 (Regul Integr Comp Physiol 22): R545–R548

8. Movat ZH, Cybulsky MI, Colditz IG, Chan MKW, Dinarello CA (1987) Acute inflammation in gram-negative infection: endotoxin, interleukin-1, tumor necrosis factor, and neutrophils. Fed Proc 46:97–104
9. Nicotera P, Mc Conkey DJ, Dypbukt JM, Jones DP, Orrenius S (1989) Ca^{2+}-activated mechanisms in cell killing. Drug Metab Rev 20:193–201
10. Offenbart K, Bengmark S (1990) Intraabdominal infections and gut origin sepsis. World J Surg 14:145–203
11. Ohkawa O, Ohishi N, Yagi K (1979) Assay for lipid peroxides in animal tissues by thiolbarbituric acid reaction. Anal Biochem 95:351–358
12. Recknagel RO, Glende EA (1984) Spectrophotometric detection of lipid conjugated dienes. Methods Enzymol 105:331–337
13. Sayeed MM (1986) Alterations in cellular Ca^{2+} regulation in the liver in endotoxic shock. Am J Physiol 250 (Regul Integr Comp Physiol 19):R884–R891
14. Sayeed MM, Maitra SR (1987) Effect of diltiazem on altered cellular calcium regulation during endotoxic shock. Am J Physiol 253 (Regul Integr Comp Physiol 22):R549–R554
15. Siesjö BK (1989) Calcium and cell death. Magnesium 8:223–237
16. Ward PA, Jeffrey SW, Johnson KJ (1988) Oxygen radicals, inflammation, and tissue injury. Free Radic Biol Med 5:403–408

Role of Liver Macrophages (Kupffer Cells) in Bacterial Cell Wall-Induced Hepatic Inflammation*

T. Kossmann, C. Manthey, J. B. Allen, C. Morganti-Kossmann, K. Ohura, S. E. Mergenhagen, and S. M. Wahl

Introduction

Intraperitoneal injection of peptidoglycan-polysaccharide cell wall fragments from group A streptococci (SCW) results in the dissemination of the fragments primarily to the spleen, liver, bone marrow, and peripheral joints [1]. Early localization of SCW within Kupffer cells (KC) of the hepatic sinusoids is followed by acute hepatic edema and leukocyte infiltration. Although the acute inflammation resolves over the next 3–5 days, many KC remain laden with SCW antigens and granulomas develop over the next 2–3 weeks. The granulomas are composed primarily of macrophages, T lymphocytes, and less numerous neutrophils and mast cells [2]. Infiltrating fibroblasts encapsulate the granulomas and synthesize large amounts of collagen types I and III and other matrix proteins. In the final stage (12–24 weeks post injection) the chronic inflammatory reaction diminishes and the granulomas exhibit scar tissue. The role of KC in orchestrating the evolution of SCW-induced inflammation, granuloma formation, and fibrosis are not well elucidated.

In order to address the involvement of KC in the development of SCW-induced acute and chronic hepatic inflammation, KC were isolated from control and SCW-injected animals and examined for phenotypic and functional parameters relevant to their participation in granuloma formation.

Methods

KC from SCW-injected animals (1, 3, 14, and 21 days postinjection) were isolated following pronase digestion of liver using a modification of the protocol of Munthe Kaas [3]. After overnight culture, 90% of the adherent cells were KC, as determined by morphology and staining with a specific anti-KC receptor antibody (generous gift of Dr. Robert L. Hill, Duke University) using a sensitive

---

* T. K. was supported by a research fellowship from the Deutsche Forschungsgemeinschaft (K01078/1-1), Bonn, FRG
Cellular Immunology Section, Laboratory of Immunology, National Institute of Dental Research, National Institutes of Health, Bethesda, MD 20892, USA

immunoperoxidase technique (ABC Vectastain Kit, Vector Laboratories, Bur-lingham, CA, USA) [5]. KC supernatants were assayed for tumor necrosis factor (TNF), interleukin-1β (IL-1β), and transforming growth factor beta (TGF-β) bioactivity as described [2, 5]. Ribonucleic acid (RNA) was prepared from KC lysates using acid guanidinium thiocyanate phenol-chloroform extraction pro-cedure [6] and the resultant Northern blot was probed with labeled comple-mentary deoxyribonucleic acid (cDNA) inserts for human TNF-α [7], human IL-1β [8], and murine TGF-β1 [9]. Superoxide radical production was meas-ured by the reduction of ferricytochrome [10]. Chemotaxis was evaluated as described [11].

Results

The in vitro stimulation of adherent KC isolated from control animals with SCW at concentrations as low as 0.1 µg/ml resulted in the induction of TNF-α, IL-1β and TGF-β messenger (m)RNA (not shown) and the secretion of the peptides (Table 1). Although constitutive TGF-β1 mRNA levels were not augmented by SCW treatment, SCW did stimulate the secretion of latent TGF-β. Thus, SCW activation of KC in vitro induces these cells to synthesize cytokines which are important during the inflammatory process [12]. KC isolated from animals 1–21 days following SCW injection contained phago-cytized SCW as determined by immunolocalization. Moreover, these cells showed a biphasic elevation in chemotactic responses to C5a as compared to cells isolated from control animals (Table 2). No significant generation of superoxide radicals was observed by KC from either injected or noninjected animals when stimulated with phorbol myristate acetate (PMA) or with SCW in vitro (data not shown).

Table 1. SCW-induced KC cytokine production in vitro

Stimulus SCW (µg/ml)	Cytokine activity		
	TNF (U/ml)	IL-1β (U/ml)	TGF-β1 (pg/ml)
0	< 2	< 1	0
0.1	166	< 1	233
1.0	323	13	571
10	407	29	645

TNF-α activity was assayed by lysis of L929 fibroblasts, IL-1β by stimulation of thymocyte proliferation, and TGF-β by inhibition of thymocyte proliferation.

Table 2. Enhanced KC chemotaxis after SCW exposure in vivo

Days after SCW injection	Chemotactic activity (cells/field)	
	Control	C5a
0	4 ± 1	66 ± 4
1	26 ± 5	206 ± 9
7	12 ± 3	42 ± 2
21	23 ± 2	105 ± 5

Kupffer cells isolated from control (0) and SCW-injected animals (1–21 days after injection) were assayed for chemotactic activity to media (control) or C5a at 1×10^6 Kupffer cells/ml. Chemotactic activity is defined as the mean ($\pm$ SEM) number of Kupffer cells that migrated through the filter pores in three different fields in triplicate wells, for each condition.

Discussion

This study examined the functional effects of in vitro and in vivo exposure of rat KC to peptidoglycan-polysaccharide cell wall fragments. Isolated KC, exposed in vitro to SCW, were shown to express mRNA and secrete the peptides TNF-α, IL-1, and TGF-β. The multifunctional roles of TNF-α, IL-1 and TGF-β during inflammation suggest that these KC-derived mediators may promote leukocyte margination and extravascularization, activation of inflammatory cells, and increased availability of blood leukocytes necessary for granuloma formation. KC isolated from control and SCW-injected animals exhibited the ability to chemotax toward C5a, and migratory capacity was enhanced two- to threefold in cells 1 day after SCW injection. Thus KC have the capacity to migrate during the early phase of granuloma formation, which may facilitate the clearance of SCW, interactions of KC with other inflammatory cells, and the aggregation of SCW-containing cells to form the foci for granuloma formation.

KC from either control or SCW-injected animals did not generate substantial superoxide radicals after stimulation with PMA or with SCW. This is in contrast to other reports in which KC in the presence of phagocytizable material did produce superoxide radicals [13] and suggests that reactive oxygen intermediates may not play an important role in granuloma formation.

The rapid activation of KC by SCW in vitro and in vivo with the subsequent release of potent inflammatory cytokines implicates the participation of this population of cells, particularly in the initiation of SCW-induced liver inflammation. Moreover, the strategic location of these cells, with the potential release of inflammatory mediators into the circulation, may contribute to the systemic manifestations associated with these bacterial products.

References

1. Dalldorf FG, Cromartie WJ, Anderle SK, Clark RL, Schwab JH (1980) The relation of experimental arthritis to the distribution of streptococcal cell wall fragments. Am J Path 100:383–402
2. Wahl SM, Hunt DA, Allen JB, Wilder RL, Paglia L, Hand AR (1986) Bacterial cell wall induced hepatic granulomas. An in vitro model of T-cell-dependent fibrosis. J Exp Med 163:884–902
3. Munthe Kaas AC, Berg T, Seglen PO, Seljelid R (1975) Mass isolation and culture of rat Kupffer cells. J Exp Med 141:1–10
4. Allen JB, Malone DG, Wahl SW, Calandra GB, Wilder RL (1985) Role of the thymus in streptococcal cell wall-induced arthritis and hepatic granuloma formation. Comparative studies of pathology and cell distribution in athymic and euthmic rats. J Clin Invest 76:1042–1056
5. Dougherty S, Wahl SM (1990) Quantitation of transforming growth factor beta in conditioned media. In: Coligan JE, Kruisbeek AM, Margulies DH, Shevach EM, Strober W (eds) Current protocols in immunology, vol 1, 6.11.1–6.11.6. Greene and Wiley Interscience, New York
6. Chomezynski P, Sachi N (1987) Single step method of RNA isolation by acid guanidium thiocyanate-phenol-chloroform extraction. Anal Biochem. 162:156–159
7. Wang AM, Creasey AA, Ladner MB, Lin LS, Strickler J, Van Arsdell JN, Yamamoto R, Mark DF (1985) Molecular cloning of the complementary DNA for human tumor necrosis factor. Science 228:149–154
8. March CJ, Moseley B, Larsen A, Cerretti DP, Braedt G, Price V, Gillis S, Henney CS, Kronheim SR, Grabstein K, Conlon PJ, Hopp TP, Cosman D (1985) Cloning, sequence and expression of two distinct human interleukin-1 complementary DNAs. Nature 315:641–647
9. Derynck RJ, Jarret JA, Chen EY, Goeddel DV (1986) The murine-transforming growth factor-β precursor. J. Biol Chem. 261:4377–4379
10. Wahl SM, McCartney-Francis N, Hunt DA, Smith PD, Wahl LM, Katona IM (1987) Monocyte interleukin-2 receptor gene expression and interleukin-2 augmentation of microbicidal activity. J. Immunol 139:1342–1347
11. Allen JB, Manthey CL, Hand AR, Ohura K, Ellingsworth L, Wahl SM (1990) Rapid onset of synovial inflammation and hyperplasia induced by transforming growth factor β. J. Exp. Med 171:231–247
12. Wahl SM, McCartney-Francis N, Mergenhagen SE (1989) Inflammatory and immunomodulatory roles of TGF-β. Immunol. Today 10:258–260
13. Decker K (1990) Biologically active products of stimulated liver macrophages (Kupffer cells). Eur. J. Biochem. 192:245–261

Tumor Necrosis Factor Alpha Inhibits Hepatocyte Mitochondrial Respiration and Induces Release of Cytoplasmic Enzymes*

J. Stadler, B. G. Bentz, J. M. Langrehr, R. D. Curran, T. R. Billiar, B. G. Harbrecht, and R. L. Simmons

Tumor necrosis factor alpha (TNFα) has been identified as a major mediator of physiologic and pathophysiologic responses to infections and traumatic insults. While TNFα enhances tissue repair and host defense against microbials [1] at low concentrations, high concentrations lead to tissue damage and to a typical shock syndrome [2]. As endotoxin was shown to be one of the most important stimuli for TNFα release, it was subsequently demonstrated that many features of the septic shock syndrome are induced by TNFα [3]. In sepsis, Kupffer cells, the largest population of fixed macrophages in the body, are thought to be a major source of TNFα [4]. Due to their close relationship to Kupffer cells, hepatocytes are exposed to TNFα released from Kupffer cells in addition to TNFα coming from the intenstine into the portal bloodstream. Therefore, it may be relevant to investigate whether TNFα contributes to hepatocellular dysfunction, which is a serious problem in sepsis [5]. The mechanisms of TNFα-mediated cytotoxicity are not very well understood. One of the established effects of TNFα at the subcellular level is mitochondrial swelling [6] and a decrease of mitochondrial respiration in tumor cell lines [7]. Because endotoxemia also results in impaired mitochondrial function of hepatocytes [8] we undertook the following experiments to demonstrate whether this effect is also mediated by TNFα.

Material and Methods

Hepatocyte Isolation and Culture Technique. Hepatocytes were harvested from Sprague-Dawley rats (Harlan Sprague-Dawley, Inc., Indianapolis, IN, USA) using a collagenase perfusion technique as previously described [9]. Cell cultures were performed in Williams medium E (Gibco laboratories, Grand Island, NY, USA) supplemented with $10^{-6} M$ insulin, 2 mM L-glutamine, penicillin 10^5 U/l, streptomycin 100 mg/l, $10^{-8} M$ dexamethasone, and 10%

* This work was supported by National Institutes of Health grants MG 44100 (TRB) and GM 37753 (R.L.S). J. S. was supported by a fellowship of the Deutsche Forschungsgemeinschaft, Bonn, Germany (Sta 311/1-1). J. M. L. was supported by a fellowship of the Deutsche Forschungsgemeinschaft, Bonn Germany (La 621/2-2).
Department of Surgery, University of Pittsburgh, Pittsburgh, PA 15261, USA

Host Defense Dysfunction
in Trauma, Shock and Sepsis
Eds. Faist/Meakins/Schildberg
© Springer-Verlag, Berlin Heidelberg 1993

low endotoxin calf serum (HyClone Laboratories, Logan, UT, USA). Hepatocytes were placed in 75-cm^2 flasks at 12 ml/flask at a concentration of 1×10^6 hepatocytes/ml. Supernatants were harvested for determination of enzyme and nitrite release and the hepatocytes were detached from the flasks for respiration measurements using EDTA-trypsin.

Respiration Measurements. Respiration measurements were performed in a modification [10] of the method of Moreadith and Fiskum [11]. Briefly, hepatocytes were placed in respiration medium and permeabilized by the addition of 0.0075% digitonin. They were then washed and oxygen consumption measured using a Clark-type electrode. State 3 respiration, which is maximal respiratory activity under excess of all substrates and cofactors, was determined using specific substrates for the individual enzyme complexes of the mitochondrial respiratory chain. Complex I (NADH-ubiquinone oxidoreductase) was measured by addition of 5 mM malate/glutamate, complex II (succinate-ubiquinone oxidoreductase) by addition of 5 mM succinate, and complex IV (cytochrome oxidase) with 0.2 mM N,N,N',N'-tetramethyl-p-phenylenediamine (TMPD) in combination with 1 mM ascorbate.

Determination of Enzyme Release. Glutamate-oxalate transaminase (GOT) and glutamate-pyruvate transaminase (GPT) levels were measured in the culture supernatants using a clinical chemistry analyzer (Technicon RA-500, Technicon, Tarrytown, NY, USA).

Results and Discussion

To investigate whether mitochondrial respiration rates are influenced by lipopolysaccharide (LPS) or by TNFα hepatocytes were incubated either in regular culture medium or in the presence of LPS 10 μg/ml or TNFα 500 U/ml or 2000 U/ml. Oxygen consumption mediated by complex I, complex II, or complex IV was measured after an incubation period of 18 h. While exposure to LPS had no influence on mitochondrial respiratory activity, TNFα led to an inhibition of complex I and complex II activity in a concentration-dependent manner (Fig. 1). Complex I was most sensitive to the effect of TNFα and was reduced by the addition of TNFα 2000 U/ml to 67% of the activity of untreated cells. These results indicate that the inhibitory effect of endotoxemia [8] reflects the action of TNFα rather than the effect of LPS itself. The data also support our previous observation that supernatant from LPS-stimulated Kupffer cells inhibits the activity of the mitochondrial respiratory chain [9]. We have demonstrated that these supernatants contain up to TNFα 500 U/ml [12].

To determine whether the effect of TNFα on mitochondrial respiration is due to cell death or to specific inhibition of the mitochondrial enzyme complexes the release of intracellular enzymes was measured. Exposure to TNFα resulted

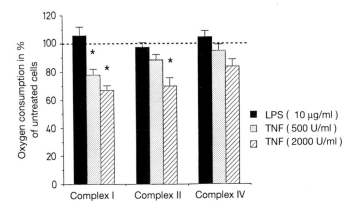

Fig. 1. Hepatocytes were incubated for 18 h in regular culture medium or with additions as indicated. Complex I activity was measured as malate/glutamate-dependent oxygen consumption, complex II as succinate-dependent respiration rate, and complex IV as TMPD/ascorbate-dependent respiration rate. The results represent means ± SEM of three experiments. *p < 0·01 vs untreated cells

Table 1. Effect of TNFα on the release of cytoplasmic enzymes by rat hepatocytes

Additions to culture medium	Enzyme release	
	GOT	GPT
– – – –	369 ± 23	61 ± 10
TNFα 500 U/ml	523 ± 97	57 ± 10
TNFα 2000 U/ml	540 ± 52*	87 ± 14
Intentional Lysis	5993 ± 296	398 ± 65

*p < 0.02 vs untreated hepatocytes.
Hepatocytes were incubated under the conditions listed above. Enzyme levels were determined in the culture supernatants. The results represent means ± SEM of eight experiments.

in the significant release of the cytosolic enzyme GOT (Table 1). However, the differences between untreated and TNFα-treated cells reached only 3% of the levels which were released by intentional lysis. The inhibition of 30% of mitochondrial respiratory capacity could therefore not be explained only by cell death.

In conclusion, our experiments show a direct inhibitory effect of TNFα on hepatocyte energy metabolism. The mechanisms by which TNFα leads to the inhibition of mitochondrial function remain to be elucidated. In vivo, this effect may be accompanied by the response from Kupffer cells which release oxygen radicals and other toxic agents when stimulated with TNFα [13]. This and the interaction with other inflammatory cytokines in sepsis may eventually enhance the effect of TNFα reported in the present study.

References

1. Old LJ (1990) Tumor necrosis factor. In: Bonavida B, Granger G (eds) *Tumor necrosis factor: structure, mechanism of action, role in disease and therapy.* Karger, Basel, pp 1–30
2. Beutler B, Cerami A (1990) Cachectin (tumor necrosis factor): an endogeneous mediator of shock and inflammatory response. In: Oppenheimer JJ, Shevach EM (eds) *Immunophysiology.* Oxford University press, New York, pp 226–237
3. Beutler B (1989) Orchestration of septic shock by cytokines: the role of cachectin (tumor necrosis factor). In: Roth BL, Nielsen TB, McKee AE (eds) *Molecular and cellular mechanisms of septic shock.* Liss, New York, pp 219–235
4. Decker K (1987) Biologically active products of stimulated liver macrophages (Kupffer cells). Eur J Biochem 192:245–261
5. Cerra FB (1987) Hypermetabolism, organ failure, and metabolic support. Surgery 101:1–14
6. Matthews N (1983) Anti-tumor cytotoxin produced by human monocytes: studies on its mode of action. Br J Cancer 48:405–410
7. Lancaster JR Jr, Laster SM, Gooding LR (1989) Inhibition of target cell mitochondrial electron transfer by tumor necrosis factor. FEBS Letts 248:169–174
8. Tavakoli H, Mela L (1982) Alterations of mitochondrial metabolism and protein concentrations in subacute septicemia. Infect Immun 38:536–541
9. Stadler J, Curran RD, Ochoa JB, Harbrecht BG, Hoffman RA, Simmons RL, Billiar TR (1991) Effect of endogeneous nitric oxide on mitochondrial respiration of rat hepatocytes in vitro and in vivo. Arch Surg 126:186–191
10. Stadler J, Billiar TR, Curran RD, Stuehr DJ, Ochoa JB, Simmons RL (1991) Effect of exogenous and endogenous nitric oxide on mitochondrial respiration of rat hepatocytes. Am J Physiol (in press)
11. Moreadith RW, Fiskum G (1984) Isolation of mitochondria from ascites tumor cells permeabilized with digitonin. Anal Biochem 137:360–367
12. Curran RD, Billiar TR, Stuehr DJ, Ochoa JB, Harbrecht BG, Flint SG, Simmons RL (1990) Multiple cytokines are required to induce hepatocyte nitric oxide production and inhibit total protein synthesis. Ann Surg 212:462–471
13. Matsuo S, Nakagawara A, Ikeda K, Mitsuyama M, Nomoto K (1985) Enhanced release of reactive oxygen intermediates by immunologically activated rat Kupffer cells. Clin Exp Immunol 59:203–220

Modulation of Hepatic Mitochondrial Fat Oxidation and Hepatic Gene Transcription by Tumor Necrosis Factor*

R. A. Barke[1], P. S. Brady[2], and L. J. Brady[2]

Introduction

Monocyte secretory mediators have been implicated in the regulation of metabolism following sepsis and trauma. Experimental evidence is increasing that cytokines are active in regulation of lipid metabolism at all levels. The regulation of hepatic fatty acid oxidation is dependent on the enzyme carnitine palmitoyltransferase (CPT), which has been described as the rate-limiting enzyme in hepatic mitochondrial β-oxidation of long-chain fatty acids. We hypothesized that tumor necrosis factor alpha (TNF-α) may modulate hepatic mitochondrial long-chain fatty acid oxidation and that this effect on fatty acid oxidation may be mediated by CPT gene transcriptional mechanisms. To investigate the effect of TNF-α on hepatic mitochondrial fatty acid oxidation and CPT gene expression, we studied TNF-α in vitro with respect to CPT gene transcription, CPT translation, and hepatic mitochondrial fatty acid oxidation to ketone bodies using either H4IIe rat hepatoma cell culture or rat hepatocytes in primary cell culture. Preliminary investigation suggested that TNF-α increased CPT mRNA in H4IIe rat hepatoma cell culture. To investigate the mechanism by which CPT gene expression is altered, we studied the role of protein kinase C or Ca^{2+} as mediators of the TNF-α effect on CPT gene transcription.

Materials and Methods

H4IIe Cell Culture

H4IIe cells (American Type Culture Collection, Rockville, MD, USA) were cultured in RPMI 1640 medium (Sigma Hybrimax) containing 2.5% (v/v) newborn calf serum and 2.5% fetal calf serum in equilibrium with 5% CO_2 in air at 37 °C. The cells were plated at 5×10^6 cells per 25-cm^2 flask and grown to confluence. Twelve hours prior to experimentation, the medium was replaced

* Supported in part by grants from the Research Core Center Grant NIH-DK34931, University of Minnesota, and the W.K. Kellogg Foundation.
Departments of [1]Surgery and [2]Food Science and Nutrition, University of Minnesota, Minneapolis, MN and the Minneapolis Veterans Administration Hospital, Minneapolis, MN 55417, USA

with serum-free medium. At the time of experimentation, the medium was replaced with either serum-free medium of the same composition (vehicle control) or serum-free medium with the assigned concentration of TNF-α. TNF-α was evaluated at 19.0-, 1.9-, and 0.19-nM concentrations. Each experimental set had three flasks assigned per treatment, time coupled with cells harvested at either 1, 2, 3, or 4 h. Each experimental set was repeated in triplicate. At the times indicated, the cells were harvested as described previously [1]. To exclude a toxic effect of TNF-α, cytotoxicity was evaluated in experimental protocols using trypan blue exclusion. Exposure of the H4IIe monolayers to either vehicle control or TNF-α plus vehicle control resulted in less than 20% cytotoxicity in experimental groups over the incubation period and no significant difference between groups as a function of time or TNF-α dose. Furthermore, microscopic examination of the flasks revealed no significant cellular alteration over the incubation period in any experimental group.

Primary Hepatocyte Cell Culture

Rat hepatocytes were harvested from male Sprague-Dawley rats maintained on Purina Lab Chow and water ad libitum by a modification of the methods of Reid and Jefferson [2] and Rojkind et al. [3] with final suspension in Williams E buffer. After final isolation, the cells were enumerated and viability determined by trypan blue exclusion (> 85% exclusion was considered acceptable). The cells were resuspended in RPMI 1640 buffer (Sigma Hybrimax), 5% (v/v) fetal bovine serum and 5% (v/v) newborn calf serum, dexamethasone (10 nM), and insulin (10 nM). Six to eight hours after the initial plating, the cells were checked for attachment and the medium changed to serum-free media. Twenty-four hours after isolation, the medium was replaced with either serum-free medium of the same composition (vehicle control) or serum-free medium with the assigned concentration of TNF-α (19.0 nM). The cells were harvested at 1, 2, 3, or 4 h using the identical experimental protocol as described above under "H4IIe Cell Culture" with cytotoxicity examined using trypan blue exclusion. Exposure of the rat hepatocytes to either vehicle control or TNF-α plus vehicle resulted in less than 20% cytotoxicity in all experimental groups over the incubation period and no significant difference between groups as a function of time. Furthermore, microscopic examination of the flasks revealed no significant cellular alteration over the incubation period in any experimental group.

Determination of CPT mRNA, Hepatic CPT Synthesis and Fat Oxidation

These methods are described briefly here and in detail by Brady et al. [4]. The full-length CPT cDNA clone (pBluescript$_{3A15.1.1.}$) was used as a probe [4]. Total RNA was formaldehyde denatured as described above and CPT mRNA quantified by northern and dot blotting. Samples with an A260/A280 ratio greater than 1.7 were considered acceptable. Similar sample loading per lane or per dot was confirmed spectrophotometrically based on A260. Ethidium bromide staining was used to verify that equal amounts of RNA were loaded per lane for northern blotting. The northern blots and dot blots were visualized by autoradiography and scanned densitometrically using Image v1.17 (National Technical Information Service, NTIS) on a Macintosh II computer. CPT protein synthesis was determined using [^{35}S]methionine incorporation as described by Culpepper and Liu [5] using rat hepatocytes in primary cell culture. Hepatocyte palmitate oxidation to ketone bodies was measured using [1-^{14}C]palmitate conversion to acid-soluble products in primary rat hepatocyte culture as described by Brady et al. [4].

Ethylene Glycol Tetra-acetic Acid and Acridine Orange Experiments

For experiments involving either ethylene glycol bis(beta amino-ethyl ether)N,N,N',N'-tetra-acetic acid (EGTA) or acridine orange, culture flasks were prepared with 5×10^6 rat hepatocytes per flask as outlined above. Experiments involving acridine orange or EGTA were divided into two groups: (1) the reference group (no pretreatment, (10 μM acridine orange pretreatment, or 3.0 mM EGTA pretreatment followed by sham vehicle control treatment); and (2) TNF-α group (no pretreatment, 10 μM acridine orange pretreatment, or 3.0 mM EGTA pretreatment followed by 19.0 nM TNF-α treatment). "Vehicle" refers to RPMI cell culture media. In either the reference group or the TNF-α group, rat hepatocytes were treated for 4 h with CPT mRNA, harvested, and analyzed as outlined above.

Statistics

Data were analyzed by analysis of variance (ANOVA) for a multifactor design using a general linear model with PC-SAS system (Statistical Analysis Systems, Cary, NC, USA). Statistical significance was accepted at $p < 0.05$.

Discussion

Figure 1 demonstrates the effect of TNF-α on CPT mRNA in H4IIe rat hepatoma cells and rat hepatocytes in primary culture. TNF-α (19.0 nM) significantly increased CPT mRNA in H4IIe cell culture. To confirm that the TNF-α-mediated effects on CPT transcription observed in H4IIe cells also occurs in rat hepatocytes, we demonstrated that TNF-α (19.0 nM) significantly increased CPT mRNA in rat hepatocyte primary cell culture. It should be recognized that the increase in CPT mRNA in response to TNF-α could also be

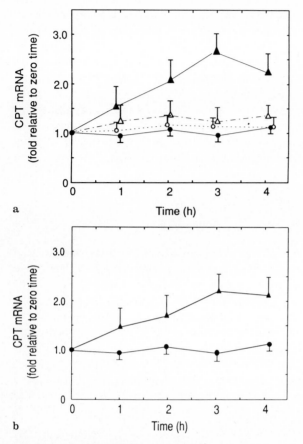

Fig. 1a, b. The effect of TNF-α on CPT gene transcription as measured by CPT mRNA in **a** H4IIe cell culture and **b** Primary hepatocyte cell culture. ●, Vehicle control; ○, TNF-α 0.19 nM; △, TNF-α 1.9 nM; ▲, TNF-α 19 nM; *bars*, SEM. TNF-α 19 nM > vehicle control, $p < 0.005$

the result of an increase in CPT mRNA half-life rather than increased transcription rate. Figure 2 shows the effect of TNF-α (19.0 nM) on CPT translation as measured by [^{35}S]methionine incorporation into CPT protein as a function of incubation time in rat hepatocytes. TNF-α significantly increased [^{35}S]-methionine incorporation into CPT protein, consistent with increased CPT protein translation. Similarly, the increase in [^{35}S]methionine incorporation into CPT protein in response to TNF-α also could be the result of an increase in CPT protein half-life rather than increased translation rate.

Figure 3 demonstrates the effect of TNF-α (19.0 nM) on hepatic mitochondrial [1-^{14}C]palmitate oxidation to acid soluble products as a function of incubation time in rat hepatocytes. TNF-α significantly increased [1-^{14}C]-palmitate oxidation to acid soluble products over the incubation period, consistent with increased TNF-α mediated ketogenesis. The increase in hepatic

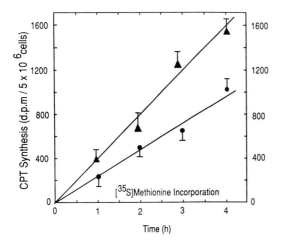

Fig. 2. The effect of TNF-α (19.0 nM; ▲) on CPT translation (CPT synthesis) as measured by [^{35}S]methionine incorporation into CPT protein. Linear regression: vehicle control (●), $y = 252x - 30$ ($r = 0.98$); TNF-α (▲), $y = 402x - 37$ ($r = 0.98$); $p < 0.01$

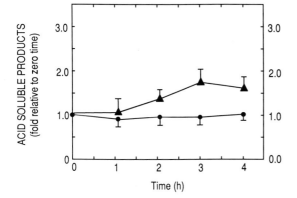

Fig. 3. The effect of TNF-α (19.0 nM) on the oxidation of [1-^{14}C]palmitate to ketone bodies as represented by acid soluble products. TNF-α (▲) > vehicle control (●), $p < 0.01$

mitochondrial long-chain fatty acid oxidation may be, in part, secondary to increased CPT gene transcription. The role of the TNF-α-induced increase in CPT gene expression on hepatic mitochondrial palmitate oxidation to acid soluble products is complicated by the fact that CPT activity is also controlled by allosteric (malonyl CoA inhibition) and covalent mechanisms (phosphorylation) [6, 7].

We must consider the relationship of this in vitro data to the known effects of sepsis in vivo on hepatic mitochondrial fatty acid oxidation and ketogenesis. Hepatic ketogenesis from long-chain fatty acids, in contrast to increased whole body fatty acid oxidation, has been shown to be depressed during sepsis [8, 9] both in vivo and in vitro using either perfused liver [8] or isolated hepatocytes from septic rats [9]. The present data suggest that TNF-α does not, at least directly, mediate the decrease in ketogenesis observed in sepsis using the rat model. This conclusion must be tentative and await in vivo confirmation since in vitro experiments are inherently limited secondary to cell culture effects (high

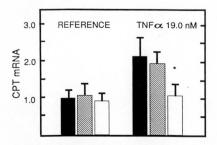

Fig. 4. In rat hepatocytes, pretreatment with EGTA (*white bar*), but not acridine orange (*hatched bar*), significantly inhibited the effect of TNF-α on CPT mRNA to baseline levels after a 4-h culture period. The *reference* group refers to the effect of sham treatment with vehicle alone on CPT mRNA. The *TNF-α 19.0 nM* group refers to the effect of treatment with TNF-α plus vehicle on CPT mRNA. *Black bar*, no pretreatment; *$p < 0.05$, TNF-α/no pretreatment > TNF-α/EGTA pretreatment. CPT mRNA calculated as change relative to zero time after 4-h incubation period.

prednisone, insulin, and media glucose concentrations) possibly altering the TNF-α-mediated effects on CPT and ketogenesis.

The Ca^{2+}-dependent phosphorylation of proteins has been recognized as a major regulatory mechanism of biological processes. We have previously demonstrated that phorbol myristate acetate (PMA, a diacylglycerol analogue) or calcium ionophore (A23187) resulted in increased CPT mRNA in rat hepatocytes, suggesting that protein kinase C or a Ca^{2+}-related mechanisms is involved in the transcriptional regulation of CPT [10]. We investigated whether these mechanisms of CPT gene induction are involved in the TNF-α-mediated increase in CPT mRNA. Figure 4 shows the inhibitory effect of pretreatment with EGTA (3 m*M*) on the TNF-α (19.0 n*M*) mediated increase in CPT mRNA measured after 4 h of incubation in rat hepatocytes. EGTA pretreatment but not acridine orange pretreatment resulted in significant inhibition of the TNF-α-stimulated increase in CPT mRNA to baseline levels.

The aminoacridines (acridine orange and related compounds) inhibit protein kinase C activity (Ca^{2+}/phospholipid-dependent enzyme) and the binding of diacylglycerol-like compounds such as PMA or phorbol dibutyrate [11]. The mechanism of protein kinase C inhibition by acridine orange involves both the catalytic and regulatory sites, with the predominant effect being inhibition of activation within the regulator domain of the enzyme [11]. In this study, acridine orange pretreatment had no effect on the TNF-α-mediated increase in CPT mRNA, suggesting that protein kinase C is not directly implicated in the signal transduction and the regulation of CPT gene expression. Release of Ca^{2+} from both extracellular and intracellular pools has been demonstrated to be involved in the cytoplasmic physiological response to TNF-α [12]. Calcium chelation with EGTA markedly decreased the CPT mRNA response following TNF-α, implicating an influx of extracellular Ca^{2+} in the control of CPT gene transcription. Thus, the present data suggest that TNF-α regulates the increase in CPT mRNA, in part, by a cytoplasmic Ca^{2+}-related mechanism but not diacylglycerol-induced activation of protein kinase C.

References

1. Wang L, Brady PS, Brady LJ (1989) Turnover of carnitine palmitoyltransferase mRNA and protein in H4IIE cells. Effect of cyclic AMP and insulin. Biochem J 263:903–908
2. Reid TM, Jefferson DM (1984) Culturing hepatocytes and other differentiated cells. Hepatology 4(3):548–559
3. Rojkind M, Gatmaitan Z, Mackensen S, Giambrone MA, Ponce P, Reid LM (1980) Connective tissue biomatrix: its isolation and utilization for long-term cultures of normal rat hepatocytes. J Cell Biol 87(1):255–263
4. Brady PS, Feng YX, Brady LJ (1988) Transcriptional regulation of carnitine palmitoyltransferase synthesis in riboflavin deficiency in rats. J Nutr 118:1128–1136
5. Culpepper JA, Liu AYC (1983) Pretranslational control of tyrosine aminotransferase synthesis by 8-bromo-cyclic AMP in H-4 rat hepatoma cells. J Biol Chem 258(22):13812–13819
6. Harano Y, Kashiwagi A, Kojima H, Suzuki M, Hashimoto T (1985) Phosphorylation of carnitine palmitoyltransferase and activation by glucagon in isolated rat hepatocytes. FEBS Lett. 188(2):267–272.
7. McGarry JD, Foster DW (1980) Regulation of hepatic fatty acid oxidation and ketone body production. Annu Rev Biochem 49:395–420.
8. Wannemacher RW, Pace JG, Beall FA, Dinterman RE, Petrella VJ, Neufeld HA (1979) Role of the liver in regulation of ketone body production during sepsis. J Clin Invest 64:1565–1572.
9. Neufeld HA, Pace JE, Kaminski MV, George DT, Jahrling PB, Wannemacher RW, Beisel WR (1980) A probable endocrine basis for the depression of ketone bodies during infectious or inflammatory state in rats. Endocrinology 107:596–601.
10. Barke RA, Brady PS, Brady LJ (1991) The Ca^{2+} second messenger system and IL-1α modulation of hepatic gene transcription and mitochondrial fat oxidation. Surgery (accepted for publication)
11. Hannum YA, Bell RM (1988) Aminoacridines, potent inhibitors of protein kinase C. J Biol Chem 263(11):5124–5131
12. Sugama K, Kuwano K, Furukawa M, Himeno Y, Satoh T, Arai S (1990) Mycoplasmas induce transcription and production of tumor necrosis factor in a monocytic cell line, THP-1, by protein kinase C-independent pathway. Infect Immun 58(11):3564–3567

Increased Leukocyte Adhesion in Liver Sinusoids Following Superior Mesenteric Artery Occlusion in the Rat

V. Bühren, B. Maier, R. Hower, M. D. Menger, and I. Marzi

Introduction

Endotoxemia and bacterial translocation due to an injured mucosal barrier may occur following shock or vascular occlusion due to an intestinal ischemia/reperfusion injury [1, 2]. It has been suggested that this sequence of events contributes to the development of multiple organ failure after shock and trauma [3–5]. The importance of gut-derived toxins (e.g., endotoxin) in inducing the release of cytokines such as TNF-α or other inflammatory mediators is well known [6, 7]. However, the precise sequence of pathophysiological events taking place in the liver due to intestinal reperfusion injury has not been completely elucidated.

The aim of our study was to assess leukocyte–endothelial adhesion in liver sinusoids after intestinal ischemia and reperfusion induced by clamping of the superior mesenteric artery (SMA shock). Therefore, we applied in vivo fluorescence video microscopy to rat livers as described recently [8]. Because the importance of oxygen free radicals in the mechanism of ischemia/reperfusion injury of the gut is well accepted [9, 10], we evaluated the effect of recombinant human superoxide dismutase (rh-SOD) during reperfusion of the ischemic gut.

Methods

In pentobarbital anesthesia (50 mg/kg i.p.), one carotid artery and jugular vein were cannulated in female Sprague-Dawley rats (250 g; $n = 5$-6/group). After laparotomy and during steady-state conditions, baseline hemodynamic and metabolic parameters were registrated. Then, the superior mesenteric artery (SMA) was clamped for 60 min in all but control animals. After declamping and a 30 or 60 min reperfusion period, respectively, the livers were exposed under an intravital microscope (Lietz, Wetzlar, FRG, Fluotar 10x, 545 nm filter). Using the leukocyte marker acridine orange (1 µmol/kg; Sigma, Deisenhofen, FRG) leukocyte–endothelial interactions were observed in 5 liver lobules/rat for 30 s. Sublobular adhesion characteristics were determined off line by frame-

Department of Trauma Surgery, University of Saarland, D-6650 Homburg/Saar, FRG

Host Defense Dysfunction
in Trauma, Shock and Sepsis
Eds. Faist/Meakins/Schildberg
© Springer-Verlag, Berlin Heidelberg 1993

Table 1. Leukocyte adhesion in rat liver sinusoids after superior mesenteric artery occlusion: Experimental groups, treatment, hematocrit, pH, and base excess values

	Group				
	Control	30 min reperfusion		60 min reperfusion	
		Shock	Shock/SOD	Shock	Shock/SOD
Treatment	NaCl 0.9%	NaCl 0.9%	40 mg/kg rhSOD	NaCl 0.9%	40 mg/kg rhSOD
Hematocrit					
Baseline	44.75 ± 1.48	45.5 ± 2.6	44.3 ± 2.6	46.58 ± 1.6	41.4 ± 5.0
Shock	47.0 ± 2.8	49.4 ± 3.3	48.4 ± 3.9	46.46 ± 2.4	44.4 ± 7.0
Reperfusion	48.0 ± 1.7	39.7 ± 4.0	47.6 ± 3.2	53.0 ± 0.84	52.4 ± 7.0
pH					
pH baseline	7.48 ± 0.04	7.32 ± 0.06	7.35 ± 0.07	7.28 ± 0.02	7.29 ± 0.02
pH shock	7.32 ± 0.03	7.34 ± 0.07	7.35 ± 0.02	7.31 ± 0.02	7.29 ± 0.04
pH reperfusion	7.33 ± 0.02	7.35 ± 0.04	7.35 ± 0.02	7.28 ± 0.04	7.36 ± 0.07
Base excess (mol/l)					
Baseline	− 4.15 ± 2.5	− 3.1 ± 2.5	− 3.0 ± 1.6	− 1.63 ± 1.7	− 0.14 ± 2.8
Shock	− 3.4 ± 2.0	− 5.1 ± 2.6	− 5.2 ± 2.4	− 3.21 ± 1.9	− 3.95 ± 2.7
Reperfusion	− 4.6 ± 4.5	− 9.5 ± 3.7	− 5.7 ± 1.7	− 9.47 ± 2.4	− 8.42 ± 6.8

Data are expressed as means ± SD.

by-frame analysis of videotaped images. To reduce intestinal reperfusion injury, (rh-SOD (40 mg/kg body weight; Grünenthal, Aachen, FRG) was injected i.v. in a blinded fashion during the first 30 min of reperfusion in the SOD groups and compared to NaCl-treated shock groups and sham-operated controls. Microcirculation characteristics were assessed either 30 or 60 min after declamping as indicated in Table 1.

Results

Substantial changes of hematocrit, pH, and base excess were not observed due to the rh-SOD therapy after 30 and 60 min of reperfusion after SMA shock (Table 1). The mean arterial blood pressure (MABP) dropped slightly after laparotomy (Fig. 1). Following declamping the MABP dropped again and remained at a lower comparable level in shock and shock/SOD groups.

Leukocyte adhesion, which was distinguished between permanently (> 20 s) and temporarily (≤ 20 s) adhesion, rose during reperfusion period after superior mesenteric artery occlusion. The percentage of permanent leukocyte adhesion was not increased after 30 min of reperfusion. However after 60 min of reperfusion, permanant adherence of leukocytes to the sinusoidal wall rose from 3.3% ± 0.7% in controls to 10.7% ± 5.2% in the periportal area (Table 2). In contrast, the percentage of temporarily adherent leukocytes were elevated as early as after 30 min of reperfusion in periportal and midzonal areas (Table 3). After 60 min of reperfusion, 22.8% ± 5.6% of temporarily adherent leukocytes were found periportally (Table 3). Attenuation of temporary and permanent leukocyte adhesion was noted particularly after 60 min when rh-SOD was given (periportally 6.4% ± 1.2% and 3.4% ± 1.2%, respectively, $p < 0.05$, Tables 2, 3).

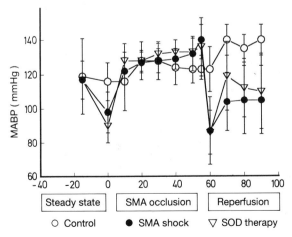

Fig. 1. Mean arterial blood pressure (MABP) before, during, and after superior mesenteric artery occlusion in the rat. Data are expressed as means ± SEM

Table 2. Permanent leukocyte adhesion and effect of rhSOD after superior mesenteric artery occlusion

Group	Treatment	Reperfusion	Periportal (%)	Midzonal (%)	Pericentral (%)
Control	NaCl 0.9%	No	3.3 ± 0.7	3.1 ± 1.1	1.3 ± 0.8
Shock	NaCl 0.9%	30 min	4.7 ± 2.7	3.6 ± 1.6	2.4 ± 2.0
Shock	rhSOD	30 min	3.1 ± 1.6	4.7 ± 4.7	1.1 ± 1.1
Shock	NaCl 0.9%	60 min	10.7 ± 5.2	5.5 ± 3.0	2.3 ± 1.6
Shock	rhSOD	60 min	3.4 ± 1.2*	3.1 ± 0.3	0.3 ± 0.4*

Percentage of leukocytes adherent longer than 20 s of the hepatic sinusoidal wall. All observed leukocytes, circulating or adherent during the 30 s observation period per microscopic field represent 100%. Mean ± SD.
*, $p < 0.05$ vs rhSOD-treated group vs sodium chloride-treated group.

Table 3. Temporarily adherent leukocytes and effect of rhSOD after superior mesenteric artery occlusion

Group	Treatment	Reperfusion	Periportal (%)	Midzonal (%)	Pericentral (%)
Control	NaCl 0.9%	No	4.2 ± 3.1	6.0 ± 1.4	3.5 ± 1.5
Shock	NaCl 0.9%	30 min	10.6 ± 5.6	9.5 ± 4.2	5.3 ± 2.6
Shock	rhSOD	30 min	8.7 ± 4.4	5.9 ± 2.7	2.6 ± 0.9*
Shock	NaCl 0.9%	60 min	22.8 ± 5.6	22.8 ± 5.8	6.9 ± 1.6
Shock	rhSOD	60 min	6.4 ± 1.2*	4.8 ± 1.2*	1.2 ± 0.5*

Percentage of leukocytes adherent between 0.2 s and 20 s to the hepatic sinusoidal is given. All observed leukocytes, circulating or adherent during the 30 s observation period per microscopic field represent 100%. Mean ± SD.
*, $p < 0.05$ vs rhSOD-treated groups vs sodium chloride-treated groups ($n = 6$ per group).

Discussion

In the immediate follow-up period after SMA shock, no relevant beneficial effects of rh-SOD on metabolic parameters were observed. Similarly, the MABP did not show significant improvements, which is consistent with the results reported by others [11]. While no effect on the macrohemodynamical parameters were found, a significant effect of rh-SOD on leukocyte adhesion in the liver microvasculature was registrated 60 min after reperfusion. The fact that after 30 min of reperfusion no increase of permanent adherent leukocytes and only a minor increase of temporary adherent leukocytes was observed indicates a time-dependent process inducing leukocyte adhesion in the liver. This may be due to the manifestation of the intestinal reperfusion injury leading to an injured mucosal barrier, thus allowing an influx of endotoxin in the portal circulation [12]. However, it was shown recently that as early as 5 min after declamping of the occluded superior mesenteric artery, pathologic endotoxin levels in the portal vein were detected in the baboon [1]. Therefore, it seems likely that endotoxemia does not directly influence the leukocyte adhesion to the hepatic sinusoidal wall. As a consequence, the generation of secondary messengers probably requiring protein synthesis may be involved. It is well known that TNF-α or interleukin synthesis are time-dependent processes and this fits with the effects and time course of our study [6, 13, 14]. These events may cause the upregulation of adhesion sites either on endothelial cell surfaces such as ELAM-1 or ICAM-1, or on leukocytes such as Mac-1, gmp 140 [6, 15, 16]. Taken together, prevention of free radical-mediated reperfusion injury of the gut by superoxide dismutase indicates that the complex sequence of events contributing to the pathological adhesion of leukocytes to liver sinusoids may be attenuated at an early step.

Acknowledgements. This study was supported in part by the Deutsche Forschungsgemeinschaft (Ma 1119/2−1).

References

1. Gathiram P, Wells MT, Raidoo D, Borck–Utne JG, Gaffin SL (1989) Changes in lipopolysaccharide concentrations in hepatic portal and systemic arterial plasma during intestinal ischemia in monkeys. Circ shock 27:103–109
2. Deitch EA, Bridges W, Baker J, Ma J–W, Ma L, Grisham B, Granger N, Specian RD, Berg R (1988) Hemorrhagic shock-induced bacterial translocation is reduced by xanthine oxidase inhibition or inactivation. Surgery 104:191–198
3. Carrico CJ, Meakins JL, Marshall JC, Fry D, Maier RV (1986) Multiple-organ-failure syndrome. Arch Surg 121:196–208
4. Bounous G (1990) The intestinal factor in multiple organ failure and shock. Surgery 107:118–119.
5. Mallik AA, Ishizaka A, Stephens KE, Hatherill JR, Tazelaar HD, Raffin TA (1989) Multiple organ damage caused by tumor necrosis factor and prevented by prior neutrophil depletion. Chest 95:1114–1120.
6. Pober JS, Cotran RS (1990) Cytokines and endothelial cell biology. Physiol Rev 70:427–452
7. Michie HR, Manogue KR, Spriggs DR, Revhaug A, O'Dwyer S, Dinarello CA, Cerami A, Wolff SM, Wilmore DW (1988) Detection of circulating tumor necrosis factor after endotoxin administration. N Engl J Med 318:1481–1486.
8. Marzi I, Takei Y, Knee J, Menger MD, Gores GJ, Bühern V, Trentz O, Lemasters JJ, Thurman RG (1990) Assessment of reperfusion injury by intravital fluorescence microscopy following liver transplantation in the rat. Transplant Proc 22:2004–2005.
9. McCord JM (1985) Oxygen-derived free radicals in postischemic tissue injury. N Engl J Med 312:159–163.
10. Granger DN, Höllwarth ME, Parks DA (1986) Ischemia-reperfusion injury: role of oxygen-derived free radicals. Acta Physiol Scand Suppl 548:47–63.
11. Wang J, Chen H, Wang T, Diao Y, Tian K (1990) Oxygen-derived free radicals induced cellular injury in superior mesentric artery occlusion shock: protective effect of superoxide dismutase. Circ Shock 32:31–41.
12. Tamakuma S, Rojas-Corona R, Cuevas P, Fine J (1971) Demonstration of a lethal endotoxemia of intestinal origin in refractory non-septic shock. Ann Surg 173:219–224.
13. Colletti LM, Burtch GD, Remick DG, Kunkel SL, Strieter RM, Guice KS, Oldham KT, Campbell DA Jr (1990) The production of tumor necrosis factor alpha and the development of a pulmonary capillary injury following hepatic ischemia/reperfusion. Transplantation 49:268–272.
14. Cybulsky MI, McComb DJ, Movat HZ (1989) Protein synthesis dependent and independent mechanisms of neutrophil emigration: different mechanisms of inflammation in rabbits induced

by interleukin-1, tumor necrosis factor alpha or endotoxin versus leukocyte chemoattractants. Am J Pathol 135:227–237.

15. Jutila MA, Berg EL, Kishimoto TK, Picker LJ, Bargatze RF, Bishop DK, Orosz CG, Wu NW, Butcher EC (1989) Inflammation-induced endothelial cell adhesion to lymphocytes, neutrophils, and monocytes. Role of homing receptors and other adhesion molecules. Transplantation 48:727–731.

16. Kishimoto TK, Jutila MA, Berg EL, Butcher EC (1989) Neutrophil Mac-1 and MEL-14 adhesion proteins inversely regulated by chemotactic factors. Science 245:1238–1241.

Section 7

**Cytokines and Modulation of
Cytokine Action**

Gene Knockout:
New Approach to the Physiology of Cytokines

F. F. Csaikl[1,2], U. N. Csaikl[1], and S. K. Durum[1]

Introduction

Advances in the last decade in both molecular biology and mammalian embryology make it possible to study gene structure–function relationships in new ways. Cloning techniques have become routine and the body of genomically cloned genes is increasing daily. With reliable DNA transfection methods like DNA microinjection or electroporation it is possible to transfer altered genes into established cell lines, where they can stably integrate into chromosomes [1–4]. For studies of gene function in vivo, genetic material can be introduced into mice and other species; such transgenics are in wide use for studying overexpression of gene products [5] and promoter function [6] or for expression of inhibitory molecules [7].

While transgenic animals can give much useful information, the real physiological function of a gene would best be determined by deleting it, then studying the physiological consequences. For example, in the study of interleukin-1 (IL-1), one could overexpress the gene in transgenics. However, overexpression of IL-1 under a major histocompatibility (MHC) class I promoter has so far been lethal (Young, personal communication), and even if it were tolerated, such an approach would be most useful in understanding the pathologies induced by IL-1, not its physiological roles.

Deleting the IL-1 gene would, on the other hand, give us understanding of its physiological roles, i.e., Is IL-1 really required for inflammation and immune processes? Is it involved in keratinocyte growth or brain function? Is it good or bad in trauma, sepsis and burn models? It is now possible to study such questions by creating mice with specific gene deletions, and a few laboratories have succeded in producing mice with genetic deletions. This has been achieved through first producing genetic deletions in pluripotent embryonic stem (ES) cells in vitro, then using these ES cells to create mice with genetic deletions. In this article we will briefly outline these new methods for deleting specific genes in mice, cite a few successful examples, and discuss design of vectors to delete the IL-1β gene.

[1] National Cancer Institute, Laboratory of Molecular Immunoregulation, Biological Response Modifiers Program, Bldg 560, Rm 31-45, Frederick, MD 21702–1202, USA
[2] National Cancer Institute, BCDP, Program Resources Inc., Dyn Corp, Frederick, MD, USA

Host Defense Dysfunction
in Trauma, Shock and Sepsis
Eds. Faist/Meakins/Schildberg
© Springer-Verlag, Berlin Heidelberg 1993

Gene Knockout: What It Can Be Used For

DNA molecules introduced into a mammalian cell can integrate into the genome, and this occurs mainly at random sites in the genome. But occasionally, the introduced DNA finds its homologous sequence in the genome and displaces it. This rare event, in which an introduced gene replaces the endogenous gene, is termed "homologous recombination." The process of homologous recombination can be used to introduce genetic alterations into the genome, and these alterations can be limited to the gene under study while other genes remain untouched.

Homologous recombination opens the way for two different applications: the first is to correct naturally occuring mutations in a particular gene; the second is to introduce mutations with the aim of blocking the gene. The latter is termed gene "targeting" or "knockout" and allows creation of cell lines or whole organisms with artificially altered genetic information or even animals entirely depleted of certain gene functions.

From ES Cells to a Mouse

ES cells are derived from the inner cell mass of the blastocyst. They are propagated in vitro under stringent conditions and retain the ability to differentiate into all tissue types if placed back into a blastocyst. It is critical to maintain the pluripotency of the ES cell line, which stays in this pluripotent phase only for a restricted number of cell passages.

To create mice with targeted genes, ES cells are first manipulated in vitro so as to produce the desired genetic alteration in one allele of the gene. ES cells are then injected into a mouse blastocyst, which is placed into the uterus of a foster mother; normal development leads to the birth of a mouse. The mouse is chimeric, consisting of a mixture of cells, those derived from the genetically manipulated ES cell and those from the normal blastocyst.

If the gonads of the chimera are derived from the ES cell, then the altered genome can be propagated through breeding to a normal mouse. The progeny will be heterozygous mice with one targeted allele and one normal allele. To produce mice that are homozygous for the targeted allele, heterozygous brothers and sisters are mated. Some of these offspring will be completely depleted of the particular gene.

The effects of such a knockout experiment can be variable and often surprising, and in Table 1 are listed several possible outcomes. The most difficult outcome to analyze would be one effecting very early events in development. If, for example, heterozygotes are never successfully produced, this could be because both normal alleles of the gene in question are required for viability of ES cells, embryos, or gametes. Similarly, homozygotes may not survive beyond early stages of development.

Table 1. Possible effects of gene targeting

Effect	Gene	Reference
No detectable effect		(not reported)
Defect in function of adults or juveniles	$\beta_2 m$	[12]
Defect in development (deformation or variation in size)	IGF-2	[8]
Lethal Effect, Postnatal	Wnt-1 (int-1)	[10]
Lethal effect, prenatal	int-1	[9]
Lethal in early stage; no implantation of the embryo		(not reported)

Since this technology is very new, only a few successful gene targeting experiments have been reported, some of which are indicated in Table 1. Chimeric animals with a disruption of one allele of an insulin-like growth factor II gene were found to be fertile but smaller than their wild type litter mates [8]. This outcome verifies the importance of insulin-like growth factor as a secondary mediator of the action of the pituitary growth hormone.

A more deleterious effect is described for the targeted disruption of the murine int-1 protooncogene [9, 10]. While mice heterozygous for the int-1 null allele are normal and fertile, homozygotes show severe abnormalities in midbrain and cerebellar development, or even may die before birth. This implies an important role for int-1 in brain development.

Mice carrying a null mutation for both alleles of the c-src protooncogene suggest an essential role for src in bone formation. These mutants were deficient in bone remodeling and developed osteopetrosis, leading to death within the first few weeks of birth [11].

Inactivation of the β_2-microglobulin ($\beta_2 m$) gene resulted in homozygous mice with immunological abnormalities [12]. Without $\beta_2 m$, there is no surface expression of class I MHC products. These mice fail to develop CD4$^-$CD8$^+$ T-cells in the thymus, verifying the importance of MHC on thymic epithelium in the development of this T-cell subset. $\beta_2 m$-less mice were otherwise normal and fertile, which is somewhat surprising, since class I MHC products are abundantly expressed on most cells of the body.

Homologous Recombination: Nature Works for You

The basic underlying mechanism for knockout experiments is homologous recombination. Although the molecular mechanisms of this process are far from being understood it is a basic method for yeast geneticists [13, 14]. It is frequently used to correct mutations or to verify cloned genes by introducing them into a mutant yeast strain deficient in this gene [15]. By using specific yeast strains with a defined genetic background these experiments are comparatively easy to monitor.

Whereas in mammalian cells, integration is usually at random sites and rarely by homologous recombination, in yeasts integration events seem to be

Table 2. Comparison of gene targeting in yeast and mammalian cells

	Mammals[a]	Yeast[b]
Cells/experiment	10^6–10^8	10^7–10^8
DNA amount/experiment (µg)	20	15
Total integrations	10^3–10^4	1–10
Homologous integrants	1–10	1–10

[a] compiled from [8–10, 19, 21–23].
[b] Calculated from [15] and unpublished data (Csaikl and Csaikl).

restricted to homologous regions and random insertions were found to be rather infrequent. In mammalian cells, detecting the rare cell with a homologously recombined gene is very laborious because of the high rate of random integrants. If calculations for the rate of homologous integration are based on the amount of cells used for transfections, homologous recombination events are similar in yeast and mammalian cells (Table 2). Thus the difference between yeast and mammalian cells is not that the latter undergo less homologous recombination, but that they have much more random integration.

In contrast to the aforementioned yeast strains which carry genetic markers enabling the investigator to screen for a certain phenotype, most mammalian genes would not be selectable in this way. Thus, to knock out the IL-1β gene in ES cells, it is not possible to screen at the phenotypic level, that is for production of IL-1β. Thus different types of drug selection procedures are used to help distinguish homologous from random integrants (discussed below). The polymerase chain reaction is a fast and (in theory) easy way to help identify clones with homologous recombinations [16]. However, spurious polymerase chain reactions are so common that in many laboratories, the more laborious genomic Southern blot has been used to screen hundreds of clones for a homologous integration event.

Gene Technology: Creating Targeting Vectors

Another crucial step in the whole experiment is the design of the targeting vector. The constructs generally contain at least three parts: a region homologous to the target gene (this directs the DNA to its target), a drug selection gene, and a simple vector backbone. As shown in Fig. 1, two types of vectors can be used, replacement vectors and insertion vectors.

In replacement vectors, gene knockout occurs by replacing a part of the coding sequence with foreign DNA sequences (neomycin resistance gene can be used both to disrupt the targeted gene, as well as a selectable marker gene). In insertion vectors, none of the host genetic material is actually lost, but the exon/intron structure is interrupted by introduced sequences. Mutations and/or stop codons contained in the introduced sequence can also be used to interrupt

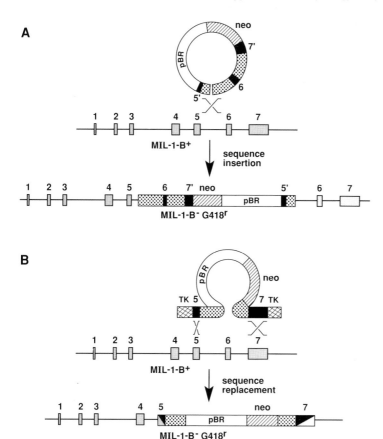

Fig. 1A, B. Gene knockout vectors: two approaches for disrupting mouse IL-1β by gene targeting. **A** Sequence insertion targeting vector. **B** Sequence replacement targeting vector

the targeted allele. Frequencies that lead to a successful targeting event are similar using either replacement or insertion vectors [17].

Because of the comparatively high background of random integration events an enrichment procedure is necessary. One approach is to use a drug resistance gene, such as *neo*, which has been depleted of its own promoter. The promoterless *neo*, integrating at most random sites, would not be transcribed and cells would be neomycin sensitive. However, after homologous recombination, for example into the IL-1β gene, the promoterless *neo* would be activated by the chromosomal IL-1β promoter, turning on transcription of *neo*, resulting in neomycin resistance.

Addition of a poly-A tail at the end of *neo* should terminate transcription, so transcription of the 3′ regions of the targeted gene is not resumed. A synthetic translation initiation site should help to get a functional resistance gene protein.

Linearization within the region of homology increases the recombination frequency.

For replacement vectors, an elegant enrichment procedure termed "positive-negative" selection was described [18]. This procedure takes advantage of the finding that random integration events primarily happen via the ends of the transfected DNA sequence. This is different from homologous recombination, where the break points occur internally, within the region of homology. To exploit this, a drug sensitivity gene is placed distal to the homologous region of the targeting plasmid. If this construct is integrated randomly into the chromosome, the drug sensitivity gene is retained, and such cells would be killed by the drug. Cells with homologous recombination were found to lose such distal nonhomologous sequences, and would thus not be killed by the drug.

The drug sensitivity gene used in positive-negative selection has been the herpes simplex virus thymidine kinase (HSV-tk). Thus, HSV-tk converts the antiviral drugs acyclovir or gancyclovir into toxic nucleotide analogs. By adding this gene to the targeting cassette, cells retaining this randomly integrated "negative" selection gene are eliminated by gancyclovir. The drawback of this enrichment procedure is that the use of a nucleoside analog like gancyclovir has the potential of causing random mutations. An additional drawback is that not only homologous recombinants lose the HSV-tk gene, but so do a number of random integrants; hence the procedure is leaky, with many false positives.

Although both replacement and insertion targeting vector approaches were used successfully in the past, it is not clear yet which one is superior.

Problems: Obstacles Between ES Cells and Transgenic Mice

During the screening process embryonic stem cells must be kept in culture in order to identify the recombinants, during which it is important to maintain the pluripotency of the ES cells. As long as ES cells are cocultured on a feeder layer of primary embryonic fibroblasts they retain their embryonic phenotype; however, after removal from the feeder cells they differentiate spontaneously. Another way to inhibit the differentiation of ES cells is by use of murine leukemia inhibitory factor (LIF) or the homologous human cytokine (termed human interleukin differentiation activity or HILDA). Recombinant LIF is produced in bacteria [19] and recombinant HILDA is expressed from yeast or cos cells [17]. It is especially important to maintain ES cells in the un-differentiated state since undifferentiated ES cells injected into blastocysts efficiently participate in germline chimera production [19]. In gene targeting experiments the germline colonization of the mutated ES cells was found to be a critical step.

Different ES cell clones in different laboratories appear, from the published results, to differ widely in their ability to reconstitute mice, despite the fact that many laboratories work with ES cell lines originating from the same source.

Perhaps there are real differences in ES cells, or on the other hand prolonged culture or simple lab-to-lab variability in tissue culture conditions may account for this variability.

The number of normal cells of the inner cell mass remaining in the blastocyst after injection of ES cells may also be crucial: a certain amount of damage of this cell mass appears to be necessary for colonization by ES cells, whereas too much damage impairs the blastocyst.

Germline transmission of targeted genes has been difficult to achieve. This is partly due to difficulties for ES cell lines to produce germ cells, but also because many experiments have focused on genes with possible impacts on development and differentiation. Thus, targeted cytokine genes, which we believe to be primarily involved in inflammation and immunity, may find better success in being transmitted through the germline, because they may not be needed in early development and differentiation.

Conclusions and Implications for Cytokine Research

By targeting genes, we will have the opportunity to explore the role of single gene products in the enormously complex milieu of the body. This new technology will have a major impact on research using whole animals. Thus, studies of immune suppression following trauma, sepsis, burns, and shock will certainly use mice with targeted cytokine genes in the next few years.

The old technology allowed study of cytokines in vivo by blocking their actions with antibodies or inhibitors, but these agents are imperfect, have many side effects, and cannot be used for sustained periods. To illustrate the impact on research of a mouse with a single mutation in a cytokine, consider the natural mutations in mice of the kit ligand and its receptor [24]. The *steel* locus encodes kit ligand and the *white spotting* locus encodes the receptor (kit). Mutations in these genes have been studied extensively over 30 years (only recently were the genes precisely identified). Mutations in either kit ligand or kit genes produce similar phenotypes. These phenotypes have been studied in much detail and include defects in producing melanocytes, gametes, erythrocytes, and mast cells. Because of these natural mutations, the kit ligand is the only cytokine today whose in vivo physiology is reasonably well understood. Gene targeting will allow study of all the cytokines.

We will also be able to study multigene effects. For example, to analyze the combined roles of IL-1 and tumor necrosis factor (TNF), we can produce mice with double deletions simply by breeding IL-1-less mice with TNF-less mice.

Gene knockout is not a routine procedure. It takes considerable expertise at multiple levels of biology and several years of intensive effort, and there is no assurance that the gene of interest can be successfully targeted. But the technology has progressed rapidly, and we anticipate advances in the basic methodologies of gene targeting as more laboratories become involved.

Acknowledgements. We thank Drs. J.J. Oppenheim, R. Fenton and D. Longo for critical review of the manuscript.

References

1. Capecchi MR (1987) High efficiency transformation by direct microinjection of DNA into cultured mammalian cells. Cell 51:503–512
2. Zimmer A, Gruss P (1989) Production of chimeric mice containing embryonic stem (ES) cells carrying a homoeobox Hox 1.1 allele mutated by homologous recombination. Nature 338:150–153
3. Boggs SS, Gregg RG (1986) Efficient transformation and frequent single-site, single-copy insertion of DNA can be obtained in mouse erythroleukemia cells transformed by electroporation. Exp Haematol 14:988–994
4. Thomas KR, Capecchi MR (1987) Site-directed mutagenesis by gene targeting in mouse embryo-derived stem cells. Cell 51:503–512
5. Robey EA, Fowlkes BJ, Gordon JW, Kioussis D, von Boehmer H, Ramsdell R, Axel R (1991) Thymic selection in CD8 transgenic mice supports an instructive model for commitment to a CD4 or CD8 lineage. Cell 64:99–107
6. Young, HA, Komschlies KL, Ciccarone V, Beckwith M, Rosenberg M, Jenkins NA, Copeland NG, Durum SK (1989) Expression of human IFNγ genomic DNA in transgenic mice. J Immunol 143:2389
7. Chaffin KE, Beals CR, Wilkie TM, Forbush KA, Simon MI, Perlmutter RM (1990) Dissection of thymocyte signaling pathways by in vivo expression of pertussis toxin ADP-ribosyltransferase. EMBO J 9:3821–3829
8. DeChiara TM, Efstratiadis A, Robertson EJ (1990) A growth-deficiency phenotype in heterozygous mice carrying an insulin-like growth factor II gene disrupted by targeting. Nature 345:78–80
9. Thomas KR, Capecchi MR (1990) Targeted disruption of the murine int-1 proto-oncogene resulting in severe abnormalities in midbrain and cerebellar development. Nature 346:847–850
10. McMahon AP, Bradley A (1990) The Wnt-1 (int-1) proto-oncogene is required for development of a large region of the mouse brain. Cell 62:1073–1085
11. Soriano P, Montgomery C, Geske R, Bradley A (1991) Targeted disruption of the c-src proto-oncogene leads to osteopetrosis in mice. Cell 64:693–702
12. Koller BH, Marrack P, Kappler JW, Smithies O (1990) Normal development of mice deficient in β_2M, MHC class I proteins, and CD8$^+$ T cells. Science 248:1227–1230
13. Hinnen A, Hicks JB, Fink GR (1978) Transformation of yeast. Proc Natl Acad Sci USA 75:1929–1933
14. Orr-Weaver TL, Szostak JW, Rothstein RJ (1981) Yeast transformation: a model system for the study of recombination. Proc Natl Acad Sci USA 78:6354–6358
15. Csaikl U, Csaikl F (1986) Molecular cloning and characterization of the MET6 gene of Saccharomyces cerevisiae. Gene 46:207–214
16. Saiki RK, Gelfand DH, Stoffel S, Scharf SF, Higuchi R, Horn RT, Mullis KB, Erlich HA (1988) Primer-directed enzymatic amplification of DNA with a thermostable DNA polymerase. Science 239:487–491
17. Baribault H, Kemler R (1989) Embryonic stem cell culture and gene targeting in transgenic mice. Mol Biol Med 6:481–492
18. Mansour SL, Thomas KR, Capecchi MR (1988) Disruption of the proto-oncogene int-2 in mouse embryo-derived stem cells: a general strategy for targeting mutations ot non-selectable genes. Nature 336:348–352
19. Pease S, Williams RL (1990) Formation of germ-line chimeras from embryonic stem cells maintained with recombinant leukemia inhibitory factor. Exp Cell Res 190:209–211
20. Bradley A, Evans M, Kaufman MH, Robertson E (1984) Formation of germ line chimeras from embryo derived teratocarcinoma cell lines. Nature 309:255–256
21. Johnson RS, Sheng M, Greenberg ME, Kolodner RD, Papaioannou VE, Spiegelman BM (1989) Targeting of nonexpressed genes in embryonic stem cells via homologous recombination. Science 245:1234–1236

22. Stanton BR, Reid SW, Parada LF (1990) Germ line transmission of an inactive N-myc allele generated by homologous recombination in mouse embryonic stem cells. Mol Cell Biol 10:6755–6758
23. Thomas KR, Folger KR, Capecchi MR (1986) High frequency targeting of genes to specific sites in the mammalian genome. Cell 44:419–428
24. Flanagan JG, Chan DC, Leder P (1991) Transmembrane form of the *kit* ligand growth factor is determined by alternative splicing and is missing in the SI^d mutant. Cell 64:1025–1035

The Role of Interleukin-1 and Other Macrophage-Derived Cytokines in Macrophage–T-Cell Interactions

L. S. Davis and P. E. Lipsky

Introduction

Interleukin-1 (IL-1) is produced by a wide variety of cells, including monocytes, lymphocytes, endothelial cells, microglial cells, keratinocytes, and chondrocytes [1–8]. IL-1 appears to play a variety of roles in maintaining normal physiologic responses ranging from inducing slow wave sleep to increasing brain blood flow [9, 10]. However, IL-1 also plays a major role in host defense by inducing fever and contributing to the inflammatory response [11, 12]. As a potent immunologic mediator, IL-1 has been implicated as a major contributor to acute states such as shock, burns, and acute arithritides as well as chronic disease states such as diabetes, rheumatoid arthritis, kidney diseases, and a variety of other conditions [13–21].

One mechanism whereby IL-1 promotes both acute and chronic inflammation is the induction of T-cell-derived cytokines [11, 13]. Once activated, T cells can produce a number of cytokines such as IL-2, interferon-γ (γ-IFN), and tumor necrosis factor-α (TNF-α) that induce further IL-1 production [22–24]. Although many cell types can produce IL-1-like substances, monocytes and macrophages are thought to be the major cell type producing IL-1 at sites of inflammation [13, 25]. IL-1 has two biochemically distinct forms derived from two distinct genes. Both are produced by activated macrophages [26, 27]. Although IL-1α and IL-1β share less than 50% homology at the nucleic acid level, they appear to bind to the same receptors and share similar activities [24, 28]. IL-1β is secreted whereas IL-1α is thought to remain largely in a membrane-bound form [24]. IL-1β is the predominant species in humans, accounting for 90% of the total IL-1 mRNA produced by monocytes [24]. However, recent studies have suggested that IL-1α, and in some circumstances IL-1β, can also be produced by T cells. IL-1α is produced by murine T cell clones, human T cell clones, and freshly isolated human CD4$^+$ T cells activated with a combination of anti-CD2 and anti-CD28 monoclonal antibodies (mAb) [29–31]. Unlike monocyte production of IL-1, which occurs during the first 24 h after stimulation, small amounts of IL-1α mRNA were detectable 48–96 h after initial stimulation of freshly isolated T cells [30]. Therefore, IL-1α produced by

Harold C. Simmons Arthritis Research Center, Department of Internal Medicine, University of Texas Southwestern Medical Center, 5323 Harry Hines Boulevard, Dallas, TX 75235-8884, USA

Host Defense Dysfunction
in Trauma, Shock and Sepsis
Eds. Faist/Meakins/Schildberg
© Springer-Verlag, Berlin Heidelberg 1993

T cells probably does not effect early activation events but may promote ongoing responsiveness during T-T interactions.

IL-1 has been shown to play an important role in T cell proliferation and differentiation [13, 24, 25]. Moreover, exogenous IL-1 is required for IL-2 production and responsiveness in some long-term cultured T cell lines and certain single cell cultures, supporting the notion that IL-1 produced by other cells can be critical for the responses of some T cell subpopulations [32–34]. Although much of the enhanced T cell response produced by macrophage-secreted factors is the result of IL-1 activity, IL-6 and TNF-α can also play a role in facilitating T cell activation [22, 35, 36]. Moreover, T cell proliferation and cytokine release can occur in the complete absence of IL-1 [37]. The costimulatory role of IL-1 appears to be especially important when the stimulus or presence of other costimulatory cytokines is limiting or when stimulation of poorly responsive T cell subsets is examined. It has become clear that several features are critical in determining the role of IL-1 and other monocyte cytokines in T cell activation. The first is the nature and intensity of the stimulus. The second is the nature of the responding T cell. CD4$^+$ and CD8$^+$ cells contain subsets of memory (CD45RO$^+$) and naive (CD45RA$^+$) cells that have distinct patterns of responsiveness to various cytokines as well as stimuli. The third consideration is the nature and presence of other costimulatory cytokines. And finally, the nature of the T cell response assayed (i.e., proliferation versus cytokine production or cytotoxicity) determines the requirement for costimulation by IL-1.

The Effects of IL-1 on T Cell Activation and Responsiveness Vary with the Stimulus

Several conflicting experiments have been reported on the ability of IL-1 to support mitogen-induced responses. Some studies have suggested that IL-1 can completely replace the requirement for accessory cells in mitogen-induced T cell proliferative responses [38, 39]. This work was contradicted by the observation that resting guinea pig T cells had an absolute requirement for accessory cells in order to respond to phytohemagglutinin (PHA) [40, 41]. IL-1 was shown to enhance responses in these cultures but it could not completely replace accessory cells. Similar results were observed for human T cells stimulated with the mitogens PHA, concanavalin A (Con A) and anti-CD3 mAb bound to sepharose beads [42, 43]. Accessory cell independent responses were obtained when T cells were cultured with phorbol myristate acetate (PMA) and IL-1. It was postulated that PMA was capable of replacing monocyte contact in promoting T cell cycle progression whereas IL-1 induced IL-2 synthesis. Other studies indicated that the role of the accessory cell was to engage the mitogen, allowing prolonged contact between the T cell receptor and the stimulus [44, 45]. These studies were supported by the observation that anti-CD3 mAbs

immobilized to the bottom of a microtiter well were capable of inducing purified
T cells to proliferate and produce IL-2 in the complete absence of accessory cells
or IL-1 [37]. The density of the anti-CD3 mAb was critical since other studies
demonstrated that the same anti-CD3 mAb immobilized on a bead was not able
to induce a T cell response even in the presence of IL-1 [42, 43]. By contrast,
others observed that anti-CD3 bound to a bead was sufficient to generate T cell
activation in the presence of IL-1 [39]. The differences in these reports are likely
to relate to the density of the T cells, the number of residual contaminating
accessory cells in the T cell populations, or the density of anti-CD3 bound onto
the beads.

Experiments using highly purified Ia-negative T lymphocytes containing less
than 0.1% macrophages were used to dissect the effects of IL-1 on human T cell
activation and IL-2 production and proliferation [22]. The ability of IL-1 to
promote T cell responses was studied using a variety of stimuli. In bulk cultures,
where limiting numbers of macrophages were present, optimal concentrations of
PHA induced T cell proliferative responses that were not enhanced by the
addition of exogenous IL-1. In the complete absence of accessory cells, the
potent anti-CD3 mAb 64.1 also induced maximal responses that were not
enhanced by exogenous cytokines including IL-1. When suboptimal concentrations of these stimuli were employed, T cell responses were enhanced by IL-1 or
TNF-α (Fig. 1). IL-1 and/or TNF-α enhanced the number of T cells that entered
the cell cycle from a resting state and the percent of cells expressing IL-2
receptors. IL-1β but not TNF-α also increased the amount of IL-2 detectable in
culture supernatants and steady state levels of IL-2 mRNA, resulting in enhanced DNA synthesis (Fig. 2). Both IL-1 and TNF-α were most effective when
added at the initiation of culture and were required at least 24 h before the
termination of culture in order to observe an increase in DNA synthesis. The
lack of effect of cytokine addition late in culture may be explained by the fact
that late in culture T cells are capable of producing TNF-α and IL-1α [29–31,
46, 47]. Thus, these studies indicated that IL-1 and TNF-α could enhance

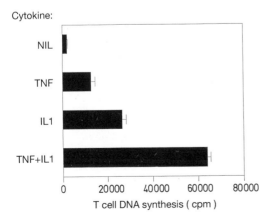

Fig. 1. IL-1β and TNF-α augment mitogen-stimulated T cell DNA synthesis.
T cells (1×10^5) were stimulated with
anti-CD3 mAb (64.1; 20 ng/well) alone
or in the presence of IL-1β (150 pM) or
TNF-α (12 nM) or both and assayed
for [^{3}H]thymidine incorporation at
96 h. Values are expressed as mean
cpm $\pm$ SEM

PHA Cytokine:

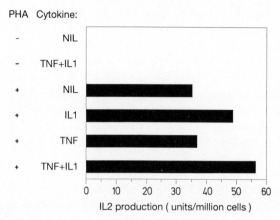

Fig. 2. IL-2 production induced by IL-1β and TNF-α. T cells (2.5 × 10^5/ml) were stimulated with immobilized anti-CD3 (64.1; 200 ng/well) in the presence or absence of IL-1β (150 pM) and/or TNF-α (12 nM) for 16 h. The supernatants were harvested and assayed for IL-2 in a standard CTLL assay. CTLL were cultured with varying supernatant dilutions and [^{3}H]thymidine incorporation was determined after a 28-h culture. Values are expressed as U/10^6 cells.

responses when strong stimuli were used in suboptimal concentrations. IL-1 exerted an effect on both IL-2 production and IL-2 receptor expression whereas TNF-α did not increase IL-2 production but did enhance IL-2 receptor expression, indicating that macrophage factors can independently influence T cell growth and cytokine production.

Different results were observed when limiting numbers of CD4$^+$ T cells were used and the frequency of responding cells was analyzed for cell growth and cytokine production [33, 34]. In the absence of exogenous cytokines or accessory cells, optimal concentrations of PHA or 64.1 in soluble or immobilized form could not induce colony formation in cultures containing one T cell per well. However, these stimuli could induce IL-2 responsiveness since in the presence of IL-2 about one-fourth of the cultures stimulated with immobilized PHA or 64.1 could generate colonies. In contrast, growth was not observed when cells were stimulated with immobilized PHA in combination with IL-1β, TNF-α, or the anti-CD28 mAb 9.3. Moreover, no growth was observed after stimulation with immobilized 64.1 in combination with IL-1β, TNF-α, or IL-6 alone. However, the cytokines and co-stimulatory antibody did enhance IL-2-supported responses, suggesting that they could each induce IL-2 responsiveness, but in the absence of cell-cell contact could not generate sufficient IL-2 production to support colony growth. The only cytokine that could support T cell growth in the absence of IL-2 was the T cell growth factor IL-4, which alone induced a small percentage of T cells to grow. The combination of IL-2 and IL-4 did not enhance responses above what was seen with IL-2 alone. When the T cells were cocultured with Epstein-Barr virus- (EBV)-transformed B cells as accessory cells immobilized anti-CD3- or PHA-induced minimal growth in the absence of IL-2, but growth in the presence of IL-2 was markedly enhanced. These results suggested that, in the absence of cell contact, IL-2 but not other cytokines was required to support most T cell growth. Moreover, some subpopulations of T cells required monocyte-derived cytokines to become IL-2 responsive. Finally, the studies also suggested that immobilization of the stimulus could replace accessory cell signals required for some T cells to become activated.

Limiting dilution cultures were also used to assess the requirements for individual CD4$^+$ T cells to produce IL-2 [33, 34]. When soluble or immobilized PHA was used as the stimulus, no IL-2 production was detected even when IL-1β or anti-CD28 mAb was added to the cultures. However, when accessory cells were present, IL-2 could be detected in over 10% of the cultures in some experiments. A very potent immobilized anti-CD3 mAb (64.1) could induce about 1.4 in 1000 T cells to produce IL-2 in the absence of accessory cells or cytokines. The addition of IL-4 or TNF-α did not increase the frequency of IL-2 producing cells in these cultures. However, paraformaldehyde-fixed accessory cells or IL-1β did induce a small increase in the frequency of IL-2-producing cells, and untreated accessory cells induced about 10% of the cells to produce IL-2. These experiments, therefore, again show that there are distinct patterns of cytokine involvement in the induction of IL-2 responsiveness versus IL-2 production. Whereas all of the monocyte cytokines tested could enhance the number of IL-2-responsive cells in these cultures, only IL-1β in the presence of the most potent immobilized anti-CD3 mAb, 64.1, enhanced the frequency of IL-2-producing cells. None of the cytokines could compare with intact viable accessory cells in the number of IL-2 producers generated with either stimulus. Therefore these studies suggest that each of the monocyte cytokines can upregulate T cell IL-2 responsiveness, whereas only IL-1 enhances IL-2 production, but only when the stimulus is sufficient to generate a series of primary signaling events that are required for T cell activation.

In bulk T cell cultures, some stimuli induced a weak or partial activation of T cells in the complete absence of accessory cells that could be costimulated by IL-1. However, responses to these mitogens in the presence of exogenous cytokines were never as great as that observed in the presence of accessory cells. For example, the anti-CD3 mAb OKT3 when immobilized onto the bottom of a microtiter well was a relatively weak stimulus in the absence of accessory cells [48, 49]. Enhancement of OKT3-induced responses by IL-1 was observed even when optimal concentrations of the mAb were employed. Soluble anti-CD2 mAbs also were weak stimulators of CD4$^+$ T cell activation in the complete absence of accessory cells, and these responses were enhanced by IL-4 alone or in combination with IL-1 and IL-6 [48, 49]. The finding that much greater responses to OKT3 or anti-CD2 mAb were always observed when intact accessory cells were present than was seen with any combination of exogenous cytokines suggested that only a subset of T cells was directly responsive to cytokines after stimulation with these mitogens as opposed to PHA or 64.1, which appeared to induce a majority of T cells to become cytokine responsive in bulk cultures [37, 43]. As previously mentioned, PMA induces partial T cell activation as indicated by IL-2 receptor expression without concomitant IL-2 production. In the absence of a costimulus or accessory cells, the combination of IL-1 and PMA induced IL-2 gene transcription and T cell proliferation in highly purified human T cells. Thus, PMA was an effective mitogen in the presence of IL-1.

These results indicate that several factors determine whether IL-1 could enhance T cell responses. Some stimuli, such as PHA and presumably Con A, were accessory cell dependent regardless of whether they were presented to the T cells in soluble or immobilized form [33]. IL-1 enhanced proliferative responses when accessory cells were present but either the numbers were suboptimal or, when the accessory cell numbers were optimal, the mitogen concentrations were suboptimal. Other stimuli, such as anti-CD3 mAb were accessory cell dependent in soluble form and accessory cell independent when immobilized [37, 43, 48]. The ability of IL-1 to promote anti-CD3-induced responses was determined by the form of the antibody (soluble vs immobilized) or the density of the antibody [37]. PMA and anti-CD2-induced T cell proliferation was enhanced by IL-1 after monocyte depletion. Thus, T cells are heterogeneous in their response to mitogens and mitogens have varying requirements for costimulatory signals. When primary activation events induced by mitogen stimulation are sufficient, monocyte cytokines, such as IL-1, can promote IL-2 production and T cell proliferation. However, the data suggest that monocyte cytokines are limited in their capacity to transduce activation signals and therefore cannot completely replace costimulatory signals provided by intact accessory cells that are required for some mitogens.

The Effect of IL-1 and other Cytokines on T Cell Subsets

The biochemical pathway of IL-1 signal transduction has not been delineated in T cells. Evidence has been presented that suggests that IL-1 effects cells by activating either an A or C kinase [50–52]. IL-1 has been shown to stimulate diacylglycerol production and/or a transient rise in cyclic adenosine monophosphate (cAMP) that could be mimicked by a brief exposure to cAMP elevating agents such as forskolin [50–54]. IL-1 also has been reported to costimulate expression of the DNA binding proteins c-Jun and NF-kappa B [52, 55]. Whether the biochemical signals generated vary with the subset of T cells studied is unknown. However, recent experiments suggest that different patterns of responses to IL-1 can be seen when the human naive and memory $CD4^+$ T cell subsets are analyzed. These differences in responsiveness appear to reflect the differential ability of various stimuli to induce IL-1 responsiveness rather than resulting from a total lack of responsiveness to IL-1 by a specific subset of T cells, as observed in the murine system [56]. For example, memory T cells, but not naive T cells, demonstrated enhanced responses when stimulated with immobilized OKT3 and IL-1 compared to responses obtained with OKT3 alone (Fig. 3). By contrast, naive cells responded vigorously to the combination of PMA and IL-1, whereas much less of an IL-1 effect was observed with PMA-stimulated memory cells. Interestingly, IL-6 had virtually no effect on either

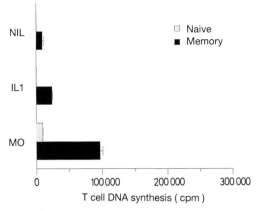

Fig. 3. The effect of IL-1β on OKT3-stimulated memory and naive T cell proliferation. CD4⁺ T cells purified by negative selection panning were further separated into naive (CD45RA⁺) and memory (CD45RA⁻) cells by panning using an anti-CD45RA mAb (2H4). T cells (5 × 10⁴/well) were cultured in wells containing immobilized OKT3 (200 ng/well) in the presence or absence of recombinant IL-1β (10 U/ml) or monocytes (5 × 10⁴/well). T cell DNA synthesis was assessed by [³H]thymidine incorporation after a 72-h incubation. Values are expressed as mean cpm ± SEM

subset after PMA stimulation, again emphasizing the differences in the costimulatory effects of monocyte-derived cytokines.

When bulk cultures of naive (CD45RA⁺) and memory (CD45RA⁻) CD4⁺ T cells were cultured with immobilized anti-CD3 mAbs, cytokine effects varied depending on the particular stimulus. Optimal concentrations of immobilized 64.1 induced maximal proliferative responses by memory cells that were not effected or only slightly augmented by the addition of IL-1β, IL-2, IL-4, and IL-6 alone or in combination (Fig. 4). Naive cells responded equally well to

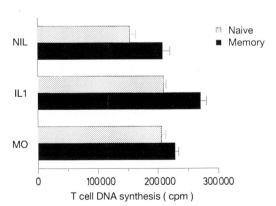

Fig. 4. Immobilized anti-CD3 mAb (64.1) induces maximal stimulation of naive and memory T cells. CD4⁺T cells were separated into naive and memory cells and cultured as described in Fig. 3

immobilized 64.1 and responses were augmented by IL-2, IL-4, and IL-6, alone or in combination with IL-1. However, IL-1 alone had no effect on the responses generated by either subset. Optimal concentrations of immobilized OKT3 induced proliferative reponses in cultures of memory cells but responses of naive cells were minimum. IL-1β and IL-2, but not IL-6, enhanced memory cell responses to immobilized OKT3. Whereas IL-2 and IL-4 appeared to augment naive cell responses slightly, IL-1β and IL-6 had no effect. With optimal stimulation using another anti-CD3 mAb, Rw24, Wasik and Morimoto [57] reported that mitogen-stimulated naive CD4$^+$ T cells proliferated preferentially to IL-4 and IL-1 synergized with IL-4. IL-6, but not IL-1, synergized with IL-2, and this effect was also more marked in the naive subset. The memory subset was more responsive than the naive subset when anti-CD3 concentrations were suboptimal. Under these conditions memory cell responses were augmented by both IL-1 and IL-6. Therefore, these subsets appeared to display complex patterns of cytokine responsiveness that varied with the concentration and particular anti-CD3 mAb used for the primary stimulation.

The role of cytokines in anti-CD2-stimulated proliferative responses has also been investigated. Neither naive or memory CD4$^+$ T cells responded to high concentrations of soluble anti-CD2 mAbs T11$_2$ and T11$_3$ in the complete absence of accessory cells (Fig. 5). Naive T cells had a nominal response to anti-CD2 at various concentrations in the presence of monocytes. The response approached that of memory T cells when the cultures were supplemented with IL-2. In the absence of accessory cells naive T cells responded to IL-6, and this response was also enhanced by IL-2, whereas IL-1 and IL-4 had much less of an

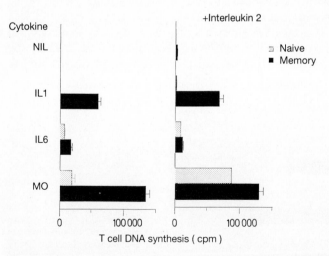

Fig. 5. Effect of monocyte cytokines on anti-CD2 mAb-stimulated T cell responses. Memory or naive cells were purified as described in Fig. 3 and cultured with soluble anti-CD2 mAb (T11$_2$ and T11$_3$; 1:500 ascites dilution) in the presence or absence of IL-1β (10 U/ml), IL-6 (10 U/ml), or monocytes (5 × 10^4/well), with or without IL-2 (5 U/ml). T cell DNA synthesis was assessed after a 72-h incubation.

effect in the presence or absence of IL-2. None of the responses obtained with cytokines equaled responses obtained in the presence of intact accessory cells. In the presence of accessory cells, memory T cells stimulated with optimal concentrations of anti-CD2 exhibited maximal responses that could not be augmented by cytokines. Small responses were obtained without accessory cells in the presence of IL-6 or IL-4 alone or in combination with IL-2. On the other hand, IL-1 greatly augmented anti-CD2 responses and they were further enhanced by IL-2. Thus, in the absence of accessory cells IL-6 was most effective at enhancing naive T cell responses whereas IL-1 enhanced memory responses stimulated by anti-CD2 mAb.

A previous report has suggested that memory cells can respond directly to anti-CD2 mAb in the absence of accessory cells because they have the capacity to secrete IL-6 after stimulation, whereas naive cells cannot produce IL-6 unless stimulated with the potent combination of PHA and PMA [58]. IL-6 could completely reconstitute accessory cell function and induce low levels of IL-2 production in cultures of naive T cells in these experiments. Horgan et al. [59] also reported that soluble anti-CD2 responses could be reconstituted with cytokines. In these studies, anti-CD2 mAbs (9.1 and 95-5-49) induced small proliferative responses in memory cell but not naive cell cultures in the absence of costimulatory signals. Both subsets responded vigorously to anti-CD2 in combination with anti-CD28, anti-CD44, or IL-1 and IL-6. Memory cells, but not naive cells, proliferated optimally in the presence of monocytes. The differences in the results in these studies may be explained by the differences in anti-CD2 mAbs, the methods of purifying naive and memory cells, or the number of contaminating cells that could perform some accessory cell function. Regardless of the differences, these studies indicate that naive and memory cells have distinct requirements for accessory cell signals. Whereas memory cells responded optimally to accessory cells and were far more responsive to monocyte-derived cytokines, especially IL-1, naive T cells responded less well to anti-CD2 in the presence of accessory cells and IL-6 appeared to be the most effective cytokine at reconstituting naive T cell responses. One interpretation of the data is that anti-CD2 is a much more effective stimulus for memory cells than for naive cells. Therefore, as stated previously, when the primary activation signal is sufficient cytokines can augment the response. The lack of a costimulatory effect of cytokines in some cultures with naive cells may be explained by the lack of this primary activation signal. Finally, the results again document that the nature of the activating stimulus as well as the intrinsic responsiveness of the T cell subset determines the capacity of different monocyte-derived cytokines to deliver costimulatory signals.

Because of the complex nature of the results obtained using a variety of stimuli and naive or memory cells, experiments using these same stimuli were carried out in the presence of cyclosporin A (CYA) to attempt to dissect the effects of the cytokines in the absence of endogenous cytokine production. In the presence of CYA, immobilized 64.1 responses were almost completely abolished and the addition of any combination of cytokines was only able to recover about one-third of the response of each subset. When immobilized OKT3 was used, only IL-2 reconstituted memory cell responses, and this response was further augmented by IL-1 or IL-6. Cytokine responsiveness was left mostly intact when T cells were stimulated with PMA in the presence of CYA. Under these conditions naive cells responded vigorously to IL-1 and IL-4 alone or in combination, but less well to IL-2 or IL-6. By contrast, memory cells responded best to the combination of IL-1 and IL-2 and less to IL-1 and IL-4. IL-2, IL-4, and IL-6 all had minimal costimulatory effects.

Since the T cells were responding to IL-1 in the absence of exogenous IL-2 it was to interest to explore the effects of IL-1 on IL-2 production by memory and naive T cells in the presence of CYA. For these studies, high concentrations of immobilized 64.1 were used to generate maximum IL-2 production from both subsets. IL-2 production was assessed after a 24-h culture. In the presence of CYA 50–100 ng/ml almost no IL-2 was detected in 64.1-stimulated memory or naive CD4$^+$ T cell cultures (Fig. 6). Memory cell IL-2 production was restored by the addition of IL-1, whereas IL-4 had no effect. The combination of IL-1 and IL-4 did not further enhance IL-2 production. However, when naive cells were analyzed IL-1 alone partially restored IL-2 production, whereas the combination of IL-1 and IL-4 synergized to enhance IL-2 production markedly in these cultures. IL-4 alone also had no effect on naive cell IL-2 production. Therefore, these studies suggest that IL-1 induces IL-2 production in these cultures by a cyclosporin-resistant pathway. Moreover, memory T cells appeared to be much

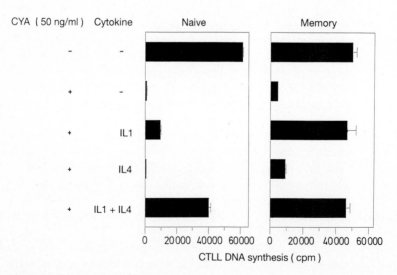

Fig. 6. IL-1β costimulates IL-2 production via a cyclosporin A-resistant pathway. Memory and naive T cells were purified as described in Fig. 3. T cells (1×10^5/well) stimulated with immobilized 64.1 (200 ng/well) were cultured with or without cyclosporin A in the presence or absence of IL-1β (10 U/ml), IL-4 (10 U/ml), or both, and IL-2 production was assessed by CTLL-induced DNA synthesis.

more responsive to the direct effects of IL-1 than naive T cells under these culture conditions.

Summary

Mononuclear phagocytes and their secreted cytokines play an important role in amplifying the responses of T lymphocytes. These cells and the cytokines not only provide signals that amplify T cell cytokine release, but they also facilitate T cell responsiveness to other cytokines, such as IL-2 or IL-4. The macrophage-derived cytokine IL-1 accounts for much of the enhancement of T cell responses by macrophage-secreted factors, although other macrophage-derived cytokines, including IL-6 and TNF-α can also facilitate various aspects of T cell activation. The data indicate a number of features of IL-1 activity in facilitating T cell responses. First, for many T cells, activation, proliferation, and cytokine release can occur in the complete absence of signals provided by IL-1, although a distinct subset of T cells growing in single cell cultures clearly requires IL-1 to respond to maximal stimulation through the CD3 complex even in the face of superoptimal concentrations of IL-2. Additional features of the role of IL-1 in promoting T cell activation have become apparent by dissecting the cellular responses in detail. At least four features are critical determinants of the role of IL-1 in facilitating T cell responsiveness. The first is the nature or intensity of the stimulus. The second is the nature of the responding T cells. Especially critical in this regard is whether the responding T cells are memory (CD45RO$^+$) or naive (CD45RA$^+$) subsets. The third feature is the nature and presence of costimulatory cytokines. The fourth is the nature of the response analyzed, with cytokine production and responsiveness exhibiting different degrees of stimulation. Although IL-1 and other macrophage-derived cytokines can exert a variety of effects on T cell responsiveness, these specific aspects of the response play a critical role in determining their impact.

References

1. Chao P, Francis L, Atkins EF (1977) The release of an endogenous pyrogen from guinea pig leukocytes in vitro. J Exp Med 145:1288
2. Gery I, Lepe-Zuniga JL (1983) Interleukin 1: uniqueness of its production and spectrum of activities. In: Pick E (ed) Lymphokines, Vol 9. Academic, New York, pp 109–126
3. Matsushima K, Procopio A, Abe H, Scala G, Ortaldo JR, Oppenheim JJ (1985) Production of IL 1 activity by normal human peripheral blood B lymphocytes. J Immunol 135:1132
4. Stern DM, Bank I, Nawroth PP, Cussimeris J, Kisiel W, Fenton JW II, Dinarello CA, Chess L, Jaffe EA (1985) Self-regulation of proccoagulant events on the endothelial cell surface. J Exp Med 162:1223
5. Giulian D, Baker TJ, Young DG, Shih L-CN, Brown DC, Lachman LB (1985) Interleukin 1 as a mediator of brain growth. In: Kluger MJ, Oppenheim JJ, Powanda MC (eds) The physiologic, metabolic, and immunologic actions of interleukin 1. Liss, New York, pp 133–142

6. Sauder DN, Carter CS, Katz SI, Oppenheim JJ (1982) Epidermal cell production of thymocyte activating factor (ETAF). J Invest Dermatol 79:34

7. Ollivierre F, Gubler U, Towle CA, Laurencin C, Treadwell BV (1986) Expression of IL-1 genes in human and bovine chondrocytes: a mechanism for autocrine control of cartilage matrix degradation. Biochem Biophys Res Commun 141:904

8. Iribe H, Koga T, Kotani S (1983) Stimulating effect of MDP and its adjuvant-active analogue on guinea pig fibroblasts for the production of myelocyte-activating factor. J Exp Med 157:2190

9. Tobler I, Borbely AA, Schwyzer M, Fontana A (1984) Interleukin-1 derived from astrocytes enhances slow wave activity in sleep EEG of the rat. Eur J Pharmacol 104:191

10. Dascombe MJ, Rothwell NJ, Sagay BO, Stock MJ (1989) Pyrogenic and thermogenic effects of interleukin 1 beta in the rat. Am J Physiol 256:E7

11. Dinarello CA (1984) Interleukin-1. Rev Infect Dis 6:51

12. Beeson PB (1948) Temperature-elevating effect of a substance obtained from polymorphonuclear leukocytes. J Clin Invest 27:524

13. Lipsky PE, Davis LS, Cush JJ, Oppenheimer-Marks N (1989) The role of cytokines in the pathogenesis of rheumatoid arthritis. Springer Semin Immunopathol 11:123

14. Okusawa S, Gelfand JA, Ikejima T, Connolly RJ, Dinarello CA (1988) Interleukin 1 induces a shock-like state in rabbits. Synergism with tumor necrosis factor and the effect of cyclooxygenase inhibition. J Clin Invest 81:1162

15. Clowes GHA Jr, George BC, Villee CA Jr, Saravis CA (1983) Muscle proteolysis induced by a circulating peptide in patients with sepsis or trauma. N Engl J Med 308:545

16. Kupper TS, Deitch EA, Baker CC, Wong WC (1986) The human burn wound as a primary source of interleukin-1 activity. Surgery 100:409

17. Baracos V, Rodemann HP, Dinarello CA, Goldbert AL (1983) Stimulation of muscle protein degradation and prostaglandin E_2 release by leukocytic pyrogen (interleukin-1) N Engl J Med 308:553

18. Malawista SE, Duff GW, Atkins E, Cheung HS, McCarty DJ (1985) Crystal-induced endogenous pyrogen production. A further look at gouty inflammation. Arthritis Rheum 28:1039

19. Di Giovine FS, Duff GW (1990) Interleukin 1: the first interleukin. Immunol Today 11:13

20. Werber HI, Emancipator SN, Tykocinski ML, Sedor JR (1987) The interleukin 1 gene is expressed by rat glomerular mesangial cells and is augmented in immune complex glomerulonephritis. J Immunol 138:3207

21. Bendtzon K, Mandrup-Poulsen T, Nerup J, Nielsen JH, Dinarello CA, Sevenson M (1986) Cytotoxicity of human pI 7 interleukin-1 for pancreatic islets of Langerhans. Science 232:1545

22. Hackett RJ, Davis LS, Lipsky PE (1988) Comparative effects of tumor necrosis factor-α and IL-1β on mitogen-induced T cell activation. J Immunol 140:2639

23. Fischer H, Helund G, Kalland T, Sjogren HO, Dohlsten M (1990) Independent regulation of IFN-gamma and tumor necrosis factor by IL-1 in human helper T cells. J Immunol 145:3767

24. Dinarello CA (1989) Interleukin-1 and its biologically related cytokines. Adv Immunol 44:153

25. Oppenheim JJ, Kovaks EJ, Matsushima K, Durum SK (1986) There is more than one interleukin 1. Immunol. Today 7:45

26. Dinarello CA (1986) Multiple biological properties of recombinant human interleukin 1 (beta). Immunobiology 172:301

27. March CJ, Mosley B, Larson A, Cerretti DP, Braedt G, Price V, Gillis S, Henney CS, Kronheim SR, Grabstein K, Conlon PJ, Hopp TP, Cosman D (1985) Cloning and sequence expression of two distinct human interleukin-1 complementary DNAs. Nature 315:641

28. Dower SK, Kronheim SR, Hopp TP, Cantrell M, Deeley M, Gillis S, Henney CS, Urdal DL (1986) The cell surface receptors for interleukin 1α and interleukin 1β are identical. Nature 324:266

29. Acres RB, Larsen A, Conlon PJ (1987) IL 1 expression in a clone of human T cells. J Immunol 138:2132

30. Cerdan C, Martin Y, Brailly H, Courcoul M, Flavetta S, Costello R, Mawas C, Birg F, Olive D (1991) IL-1α is produced by T lymphocytes activated via the CD2 plus CD28 pathway. J Immunol 146:560

31. Tartakovsky B, Kovacs EJ, Takacs L, Durham SK (1986) T cell clone producing an IL-1-like activity after stimulation with antigen-presenting B cells. J Immunol 137:160

32. Zlotnik A, Daine B (1986) Activation of IL1-dependent and IL1-independent T cell lines by calcium ionophore and phorbol ester. J Immunol 136:1033

33. Vine JB, Geppert TD, Lipsky PE (1988) T4 cell activation by immobilized phytohemagglutinin:

differential capacity to induce IL-2 responsiveness and IL-2 production. J Immunol 141:2593–2600

34. Vine JB, Geppert TD, Lipsky PE (1989) Precursor frequency of human T4 cells responding to stimulation through the CD3 molecular complex: role of various cytokines in promoting growth and IL2 production. Cell Immunol 124:212–226

35. Houssiau FA, Coulie PG, Olive D, van Snick J (1988) Synergistic activation of human T cells by interleukin 1 and interleukin 6. Eur J Immunol 18:653

36. Ceuppens JL, Baroja ML, Lorre K, van Damme J, Billiau A (1988) Human T cell activation with PHA: the function of IL-6 as an accessory signal. J Immunol 141:3866·

37. Geppert TD, Lipsky PE (1987) Accessory cell independent proliferation of human T4 cells stimulated by immobilized monoclonal antibodies to CD3. J Immunol 138:1660

38. Dinarello CA, Canon JG, Mier JW, Bernheim HA, Lapresete G, Lynn DL, Love RN, Webb AC, Auron PE, Reuben RC, Rich A, Wolfe SM, Putney SD (1986) Multiple biological activities of human recombinant interleukin 1. J Clin Invest 77:1734

39. Williams JM, Deloria D, Hansen JA, Dinarello CA, Lortscher R, Shapiro HM, Strom TB (1985) The events of primary T cell activation can be staged by use of sepharose-bound anti-T3 (64.1) monoclonal antibody and purified interleukin 1. J Immunol 135:2249

40. Davis L, Lipsky PE (1985) Signals involved in T cell activation. I. Phorbol esters enhance responsiveness but cannot replace intact accessory cells in the induction of mitogen-stimulated T cell proliferation. J Immunol 135:2946–2952

41. Davis L, Lipsky PE (1986) Signals involved in T cell activation. II. Distinct roles of intact accessory cells, phorbol esters, and interleukin 1 in activation and cell cycle progression of resting T lymphocytes. J Immunol 136:3588–3596

42. Chatila TA, Schwartz DH, Miller R, Geha RS (1987) Requirement for mitogen, T cell-accessory cells contact, and interleukin 1 in the induction of resting T-cell proliferation. Clin Immunol Immunopathol 44:235–247

43. Davis L, Vida R, Lipsky PE (1986) Regulation of human T lymphocyte mitogenesis by antibodies to CD3. J Immunol 137:3758

44. Davis LS, Lipsky PE (1989) T cell activation induced by anti-CD3 antibodies requires prolonged stimulation of protein kinase C. Cell Immunol 118:208

45. Weiss A, Manger B, Imboden J (1986) Synergy between the T3/antigen receptor complex and Tp44 in the activation of human T cells. J Immunol 137:819

46. Cuturi MC, Murphy M, Costa-Giomi MP, Weinmann R, Perussia B, Trinchieri G (1987) Independent regulation of tumor necrosis factor and lymphotoxin production by human peripheral blood lymphocytes. J Exp Med 165:1581

47. Christmas SE, Meager A, Moore M (1987) Production of interferon and tumour necrosis factor by cloned human natural cytotoxic lymphocytes and T cells. Clin Exp Immunol 69:441

48. Mitchell LC, Davis LS, Lipsky PE (1989) Promotion of human T lymphocyte proliferation by IL-4. J Immunol 142:1548–1557

49. Lorre K, van Damme J, Ceuppens JL (1990) A bidirectional regulatory network involving IL2 and IL4 in the alternative CD2 pathway of T cell activation. Eur J Immunol 20:1569

50. O'Neill LAJ, Bird TA, Sakalatvala J (1990) Interleukin 1 signal transduction. Immunol. Today 11:392

51. Munoz E, Beutner U, Zubiaga AM, Huber BT (1990) IL-1 activates two separate signal transduction pathways in T helper type II cells. J Immunol 146:136

52. Mizel SB, Shirakawa F, Chedid M (1990) Signal transduction pathway for interleukin-1 In: Cambier JC (ed) Ligands, receptors, and signal transduction in regulation of lymphocyte function. American Society for Microbiology, Washington, pp 297–320

53. Rosoff PM, Savage N, Dinarello CA (1988) Interleukin-1 stimulates diacylglycerol production in T lymphocytes by a novel mechanism. Cell 54:73

54. Shirakawa F, Yamashita U, Chedid M, Mizel SB (1988) Cyclic AMP-an intracellular second messenger for interleukin-1. Proc Natl Acad Sci USA 85:8201

55. Muegge K, Williams TM, Kant J, Karin M, Chiu R, Schmidt A, Siebenlist U, Young HA, Duram SK (1989) Interleukin-1 costimulatory activity on the interleukin-2 promoter via AP-1. Science 246:249

56. Greenbaum LA, Horowitz JB, Woods A, Pasqualini T, Reich EP, Bottomly K (1988) Autocrine growth of CD4$^+$ T cells. Differential effects of IL-1 on helper and inflammatory T cells. J Immunol 140:1555

57. Wasik MA, Morimoto C (1990) Differential effects of cytokines on proliferative response of

human CD4$^+$ T lymphocyte subsets stimulated via T cell receptor-CD3 complex. J Immunol 144:3334
58. Kasahara Y, Miyawaki T, Kato K, Kanegane H, Yachie A, Yokoi T, Taniguchi N (1990) Role of interleukin 6 for differential responsiveness of naive and memory CD4$^+$ T cells in CD2-mediated activation. J Exp Med 172:1419
59. Horgan KJ, van Seventer GA, Shimizu Y, Shaw S (1990) Hyporesponsiveness of "naive" (CD45RA$^+$) human T cells to multiple receptor-mediated stimuli but augmentation of responses by co-stimuli. Eur J Immunol 20:1111

Interleukin-1-Induced Hypotension and the Effect of an Interleukin-1 Receptor Antagonist *

C. A. Dinarello

Vascular Effects of Interleukin-1 and Tumor Necrosis Factor

The systemic effects of high doses (> 1µg/kg) of intravenously administered interleukin (IL-1) in animals include hypotension, decreased systemic vascular resistance, depressed myocardial function, lactic acidosis, leukopenia, thrombocytopenia, vascular leak, pulmonary congestion, and tissue neutrophilic infiltration with necrosis [1, 2]. The hypotensive effects of intravenously administered IL-1 in humans have been observed at doses below 1 µg/kg, and hypotension is the major clinical response limiting the maximal dose tolerated to 300 ng/kg [3]. The hypotensive effect of IL-1 may occur via various mechanisms. One mechanism appears to be due to cyclooxygenase products, and IL-1 and tumor necrosis factor (TNF) act synergistically in increasing prostaglandin E (PGE) in a variety of cells. The hypotension following an IL-1/TNF injection in rabbits is blocked by cyclooxygenase inhibitors [1]. Arterial perfusion with IL-1 increases prostanoid synthesis, which lowers the pain threshold to bradykinin [4]. TNF potentiates these effects of IL-1. IL-1 inhibits vascular smooth muscle contraction, but this is independent of prostaglandin synthesis. The inhibition of smooth muscle contraction by IL-1 appears to be due to an L-arginine-dependent increase in nitric oxide production, which leads to increased guanylate cyclase activity [5, 6].

Cultured endothelial cells exposed to IL-1 increase the expression of adhesion molecules, which leads to the adherence of leukocytes to endothelial surfaces. The mechanism for tissue neutrophil infiltration is primarily dependent on the induction of the adhesion molecules rather than on activation of neutrophil itself. For example, tissue damage due to endotoxin can be reduced by passive immunization with antibodies which block the adhesion molecules.

IL-1-treated endothelial cells also increase procoagulant activity, tissue factor, PGE_2, PGI_2, platelet activating factor (PAF), plasminogen activator inhibitor production [7], enhancement of thrombin-induced von Willebrand's factor, and the synthesis of other cytokines including IL-1 itself.

* These studies are supported by NIH grant AI 15614.
Department of Medicine, Tufts University and New England Medical Center, Boston, MA 02111, USA

IL-1 Production During Sepsis

In humans with infections, endotoxemia, trauma, burns, or acute bouts of rheumatoid arthritis, or undergoing organ transplant rejection, levels of IL-1β are elevated [8, 9]. In patients with sepsis, the levels of TNF in the circulation increase proportionally with the severity of hypotension and organ failure [8]. However, circulating levels of IL-1β tend to decrease with increasing severity. IL-1 may be only transiently elevated and hence a single measurement may not reflect the amount of production of these cytokines. On the other hand, IL-6 levels are also elevated in these patients and correlate with the disease severity. Measurement of IL-6 concentrations in the circulation can be a better indicator of the amount of IL-1 produced than measurement of the actual levels of IL-1. In some experimental models, the amount of IL-6 appears to be under the control of IL-1 [10].

In animal models of shock and gram-negative sepsis, TNF levels rise rapidly after the injection of bacteria or endotoxin, reach peak levels at 60–90 min, and then decrease; IL-1 levels rise slowly and reach peak elevation at 180 min. Similar kinetics have been observed in human subjects injected with endotoxin [8, 9]. In rabbits, the amount of IL-1 and TNF which circulates correlates with the degree of hypotension [11]. Furthermore, complement activation, induction of IL-1 and TNF, shock, and organ damage take place in the absence to endotoxemia [11]. In fact, IL-1 and TNF are produced during gram-positive sepsis, and correlate with the degree of hypotension even in the absence of staphylococcal exotoxins. These experiments support the concept that the production of IL-1 and TNF is the common denominator to the development of shock, rather than the presence of lipopolysaccharide endotoxins or various exotoxins.

Naturally Occurring Inhibitors of IL-1 Activity

Polypeptides which *specifically* inhibit IL-1 have been detected in the serum of humans injected with bacterial endotoxin [12], the urine of febrile patients [13], supernatants of human monocytes adhering to immunoglobulin G- (IgG)-coated surfaces [14], and the urine of patients with monocytic leukemia [15]. IL-1-specific inhibitory molecules of 52–66 kDa secreted from a human myelomonocytic cell line [16] have also been reported. The IL-1 receptor antagonist (IL-1ra) was originally called the "IL-1 inhibitor" [15, 17]; it was a 23- to 25-kDa protein purified from the urine of patients with monocytic leukemia [15, 17, 18]. Natural IL-1 inhibitor blocked the ability of IL-1 to stimulate synovial cell PGE$_2$ production and thymocyte proliferation [15, 17, 19]. It is unclear whether similar IL-1-specific inhibitory activities found in the serum during endotoxemia [12], in the urine of patients with fever [13], or secreted from myelomonocytic cell lines [16] share identity with the IL-1ra. The

IL-1 inhibitor blocked the binding of IL-1 to receptors on T-cells and fibroblasts but did not affect the binding of TNF or IL-2 to their receptors [17, 19].

Using the IL-1 inhibitor purified from adherent monocytes [14, 20], the molecule was cloned [21]. The cDNA sequence codes for a polypeptide of approximately 17 kDa with a 26% amino acid homology to IL-1β and a 19% homology to IL-1α. Conserved amino acids revealed a 41% homology of the IL-1ra to IL-1β and 30% to IL-1α.

Similar to the naturally occurring IL-1 urinary inhibitor [17], the recombinant IL-1 inhibitor competes with the binding of IL-1 to its cell surface receptors. Because of its sequence homology and mode of activity, the IL-1 inhibitor was renamed the IL-1 receptor antagonist (IL-1ra). The IL-1ra blocks IL-1 activity in vitro and in vivo. In vitro, the IL-1ra appears to occupy the IL-1RtI on T-cells and fibroblasts with nearly the same affinity as bone fide IL-1 but without demonstrable agonist activity [20]. The human IL-1ra also blocks the binding of IL-1 to human cells bearing the IL-1RtII such as neutrophils and B-cells [22] as well as human peripheral myelomonocytic leukemia cells [23]. Using murine T-cells (IL-1RtI), the human IL-1ra blocks the binding of IL-1 at nearly equimolar concentration; however, a 10–50-fold molar excess of the IL-1ra is required to block the binding of human IL-1 to human type II receptor-bearing cells [22].

Effect of IL-1ra on Septic Shock

The administration of the IL-1ra prevents death in rabbits due to lipopolysaccharide [24]. The intravenous injection of *Escherichia coli* in rabbits produces several parameters of the septic shock syndrome, namely, hypotension, decreased systemic vascular resistance, leukopenia, thrombocytopenia, and tissue damage. When rabbits were pretreated with the IL-1ra, only a transient and mild hypotensive episode was observed, whereas severe and sustained hypotension with a 50% mortality was observed in control rabbits [25]. There were also reduced numbers of tissue infiltrating neutrophils. In these studies the circulating levels of TNF and IL-1β were unchanged. These results suggest that TNF may be responsible for the initial fall in blood pressure but that IL-1 is playing an essential role in the progression of the shock state. The human IL-1ra also prevents lethal *Klebsiella pneumonae* sepsis in newborn rats [26] and *Escherichial. coli*-induced hypotension in baboons (Moldawer, personal communication).

Other Effects of the IL-1ra Data support a role for IL-1 in the pathogenesis of colitis; rabbits injected with soluble immune complexes develop tissue inflammatory cell infiltration, edema, and necrosis of the lower colon. However, when treated with the IL-1ra, a marked decrease was observed [27]. An autocrine role for IL-1 has been proposed in leukemia in which IL-1 production by leukemic blasts is uncontrolled and results in production of colony-stimulating factors (CSFs). Recent studies have shown that the IL-1ra blocked the spontaneous proliferation as well as spontaneous production of granulocyte–macrophage CSF, IL-1, and TL-6 in peripheral blood or bone marrow-derived acute myelogenous leukemia cells from over 25 patients [23]. When IL-1ra was removed after a 48-h exposure, the leukemic cells showed evidence of death during a subsequent 72-h incubation.

Acknowledgement. The author thanks Drs. Sheldon M. Wolff and Jeffery A. Gelfand for their contributions to this review.

References

1. Okusawa S, Gelfand JA, Ikejima T, Connolly RJ, Dinarello CA (1988) Interleukin 1 induces a shock-like state in rabbits. Synergism with tumor necrosis factor and the effect of cyclooxygenase inhibition. J Clin Invest 81:1162–1172
2. Tredget EE, Yu YM, Zhong S, Burini R, Okusawa S, Gelfand JA, Dinarello CA, Young VR, Burke JF (1988) Role of interleukin 1 and tumor necrosis factor on energy metabolism in rabbits. Am J Physiol 255:E760–E768
3. Smith J, Urba W, Steis R, Janik J, Fenton B, Sharfman W, Conlon K, Sznol M, Creekmore S, Wells N, Elwood L, Keller J, Hestdal K, Ewel C, Rossio J, Kopp W, Shimuzut M, Oppenheim J, Longo D (1990) Interleukin-1 alpha: results of a phase I toxicity and immunomodulatory trial. Am Soc Clin Oncol 9:717
4. Schweizer A, Feige U, Fontana A, Muller K, Dinarello CA (1988) Interleukin-1 enhances pain reflexes. Mediation through increased prostaglandin E2 levels. Agents Actions 25:246–251
5. Beasley D, Schwartz JH, Brenner BM (1991) Interleukin-1 induces prolonged L-arginine-dependent cyclic guanosine monophosphate and nitrite production in rat vascular smooth muscle cells. J Clin Invest (in press)
6. Beasley D (1990) Interleukin 1 and endotoxin activate soluble guanylate cyclase in vascular smooth muscle. Am J Physiol □
7. Dejana E, Breviario F, Erroi A, Bussolino F, Mussoni L, Gramse M, Pintucci G, Casali B, Dinarello CA, van Damme J, Mantovani A (1987) Modulation of endothelial cell functions by different molecular species of interleukin 1. Blood 69:695–699
8. Cannon JG, Tompkins RG, Gelfand JA, Michie HR, Stanford GG, van der Meer JWM, Endres S, Lonnemann G, Corsetti J, Chernow B, Wilmore DW, Wolff SM, Dinarello CA (1990) Circulating interleukin-1 and tumor necrosis factor in septic shock and experimental endotoxin fever. J Infect Dis 161:79–84
9. Michie HR, Manogue KR, Spriggs DR, Revhaug A, O'Dwyer S, Dinarello CA, Cerami A, Wolff SM, Wilmore DW (1988) Detection of circulating tumor necrosis factor after endotoxin administration. N Engl J Med 318:1481–1486
10. Gershenwald JE, Fong YM, Fahey TJ3, Calvano SE, Chizzonite R, Kilian PL, Lowry SF, Moldawer LL (1990) Interleukin 1 receptor blockade attenuates the host inflammatory response. Proc Natl Acad Sci USA 87:4966–4970
11. Wakabayashi G, Gelfand JA, Jung WK, Connolly RJ, Burke JF, Dinarello CA, (1991) *Staphylococcus epidermidis* induces complement activatio, TNF, IL-1, a shock-like state and tissue injury in rabbits without endotoxemia: comparison to *Escherichia coli.* J Clin Invest (in press)
12. Dinarello CA, Rosenwasser LJ, Wolff SM (1981) Demonstration of a circulating suppressor factor of thymocyte proliferation during endotoxin fever in humans. J Immunol 127:2517–2519
13. Liao Z, Grimshaw RS, Rosenstreich DL (1984) Identification of a specific interleukin-1 inhibitor in the urine of febrile patients. J Exp Med 159:125–136
14. Arend WP, Joslin FG, Thompson RC, Hannum CH (1989) An IL-1 inhibitor from human monocytes. Production and characterization of biologic properties. J Immunol 143:1851–1858
15. Seckinger P, Dayer JM (1987) Interleukin-1 inhibitors. Ann Inst Pasteur Immunol 138:461–516

16. Barak V, Treves AJ, Yanai P, Halperin M, Wasserman D, Biran S, Braun S (1986) Interleukin-1 inhibitory activity secreted by a human myelomonocytic cell line (M20). Eur J Immunol 16:1449–1452
17. Seckinger P, Lowenthal JW, Williamson K, Dayer JM, MacDonald HR (1987) A urine inhibitor of interleukin-1 activity that blocks ligand binding. J Immunol 139:1546–1549
18. Mazzei GJ, Seckinger PL, Dayer JM, Shaw AR (1990) Purification and characterization of a 26-kDa competitive inhibitor of interleukin 1. Eur J Immunol 20:683–689
19. De Balavoine JF RB, Williamson K, Seckinger P, Cruchaud A, Dayer JM (1986) Prostaglandin E2 and collagenase production by fibroblasts and synovial cells is regulated by urine-derived human interleukin 1 and inhibitor(s). J Clin Invest 78:1120–1124
20. Hannum CH, Wilcox CJ, Arend WP, Joslin FG, Dripps DJ, Heimdal PL, Armes LG, Sommer A, Eisenberg SP, Thompson RC (1990) Interleukin-1 receptor antagonist activity of a human interleukin-1 inhibitor. Nature 343:336–340
21. Eisenberg SP, Evans RJ, Arend WP, Verderber E, Brewer MT, Hannum CH, Thompson RC (1990) Primary structure and functional expression from complementary DNA of a human interleukin-1 receptor antagonist. Nature 343:341–346
22. Granowitz EV, Mancilla BD, Clark BD, Dinarello CA (1991) The IL-1 receptor antagonist blocks IL-1 binding to the IL-1RtII on human neutrophils and B-cells. Clin Res (in press)
23. Rambaldi A, Torcia M, Bettoni S, Barbui T, Vannier E, Dinarello CA, Cozzolino F (1990) Modulation of cell proliferation and cytokine production in acute myeloblastic leukemia by interleukin-1 receptor antagonist and lack of its expression by leukemic cells. Blood 76:114a
24. Ohlsson K, Bjork P, Bergenfeldt M, Hageman R, Thompson RC (1990) Interleukin-1 receptor antagonist reduces mortality from endotoxin shock. Nature 348:550–552
25. Wakabayashi G, Gelfand JA, Burke JF, Thompson RC, Dinarello CA (1991) A specific receptor antagonist for interleukin-1 prevents E. coli-induced shock. FASEB J (in press)
26. Mancilla J, Garcia P, Dinarello CA (1991) Either interleukin-1 or the interleukin-1 receptor antagonist prevent lethal sepsis in newborn rats. Clin Res (in press)
27. Cominelli F, Nast CC, Clark BD, Schindler R, Llerena R, Eysselein VE, Thompson RC, Dinarello CA (1990) Interleukin-1 gene expression, synthesis and effect of specific IL-1 receptor blockade in rabbit immune complex colitis. J Clin Invest 86:972–980

Interleukin-8 (Neutrophil-Activating Peptide-1) and Related Chemotactic Cytokines

M. Baggiolini

Introduction

Neutrophils are recruited into inflamed or infected tissues by a variety of chemotactic agonists that differ in chemical structure and mode and site of formation, and act via separate receptors. They include the anaphylatoxin C5a formed upon complement activation via the classical or the alternative pathway, fMet-Leu-Phe and other bacterial N-formylmethionyl peptides, and two lipids, the arachidonic acid oxygenation product leukotriene B_4(LTB_4) and the alkyl phospholipid derivative platelet activating factor (PAF) [1].

These agonists activate neutrophils and some other blood phagocytes, inducing chemotaxis and the release of microbicidal and digestive products. The mechanism of signal transduction involved is only partly understood. Two elements are believed to be essential, a rise of the cytosolic free calcium concentration ($[Ca^{2+}]_i$) and the activation of protein kinase C. The need for enhanced $[Ca^{2+}]_i$ is suggested by the fact that depletion of the intracellular storage pool Ca^{2+} prevents exocytosis and the respiratory burst [2]. On the other hand, protein kinase C appears to be necessary for the respiratory burst, since this response is induced by phorbol esters or permeant diacylglycerols which act directly on the kinase [3], and is prevented by staurosporine and other kinase inhibitors [4]. Other important elements are guanosine triphosphate (GTP)-binding proteins, which control all receptor-mediated responses of neutrophils as indicated by inhibition with B. pertussis toxin [5].

Neutrophil-activating Peptides

Interleukin-8 (IL-8) was originally identified in the culture supernatants of human blood mononuclear phagocytes stimulated with endotoxin [see 6]. From the cDNA coding for IL-8, which was cloned a few months before the protein was isolated and identified as a neutrophil activator [7], it was deduced that the peptide is generated as a precursor of 99 amino acids. The mature form

Theodor-Kocher Institute, University of Bern, P.O. Box 99, CH-3000 Bern 9, Switzerland

Host Defense Dysfunction
in Trauma, Shock and Sepsis
Eds. Faist/Meakins/Schildberg
© Springer-Verlag, Berlin Heidelberg 1993

consists of 79 residues. Several variants resulting from amino-terminal processing are found in biological fluids, and the most abundant ones are those consisting of 72 and 77 amino acids [8].

IL-8 has considerable sequence homology with peptides from platelet α-granules, i.e., platelet basic protein (PBP), connective tissue-activating peptide III (CTAP-III) and platelet factor 4 (PF-4), and with other human peptides, γ-interferon-inducible protein (γ-IP-10) and gro melanoma growth stimulatory activity (gro/MGSA), the product of the gro gene [6]. All these peptides have four cysteines in virtually identical positions, which form disulfide bridges that are essential for the biological activity [9].

Biological Properties of IL-8

The biological profile of IL-8 is very similar to that of two well-established chemotactic peptides, C5a and fMet-Leu-Phe. IL-8 activates the motile apparatus of the cell, leading to shape change and migration, and induces the expression of complement receptors (CR1, CR3), the release of enzymes from the granules and other storage organelles, and the respiratory burst [6, 10]. The mechanism of signal transduction involved in these responses is also similar. All IL-8-mediated responses depend on GTP-binding proteins that are blocked by B. pertussis toxin. Other inhibitory treatments are Ca^{2+} depletion or wortmannin, which both prevent exocytosis and the respiratory burst without affecting the shape changes [11, 12], and staurosporine, a protein kinase inhibitor, which inhibits the respiratory burst, but not exocytosis [4]. Human neutrophils have selective receptors for IL-8 which are comparable in numbers and affinity to those for C5a or fMet-Leu-Phe [13, 14]. We have recently obtained evidence for the presence of two IL-8 receptors which also bind neutrophil-activating peptide 2 (NAP-2) and gro/MGSA [15].

IL-8 appears to be more selective for neutrophils than other chemotactic agonists. It has low activities on monocytes, [16] eosinophils [17], and basophils, which respond significantly only upon pretreatment with IL-3 or granulocyte-macrophage colony-stimulating factor (GM-CSF) [18]. IL-8 was reported to be chemotactic for lymphocytes [19]. After injection into the human skin, however, no lymphocyte infiltration was observed [20].

Effects In Vivo

IL-8 is effective in several animal species and its effects were studied in rodents. Intradermal injection in rabbits induces plasma exudation and a massive neutrophil accumulation. The infiltration is long-lasting and apparently exclusive to neutrophils [21, 22]. Neutrophil infiltration is also induced by E. coli lipopolysaccharide (LPS). In this case, however, the effect is indirect and depends on the induction of a secondary mediator, possibly IL-8 itself. Massive neutrophil infiltration is also observed upon intradermal injection of IL-8 in rats, mice, and guinea pigs. The long duration of action is probably due to the remarkable resistance of IL-8 to enzymatic inactivation and denaturation [9].

IL-8 Is Produced by Many Cells

IL-8 was originally identified in the culture supernatants of blood monocytes exposed to LPS. It was then discovered that it is produced by a wide variety of cells upon stimulation. IL-8 mRNA is expressed in fibroblasts, macrophages, endothelial cells, lung epithelial cells [6], and, as found more recently, in retinal pigment cells [23] and hepatoma cells [24] after stimulation with IL-1 or tumor necrosis factor (TNF). These observations were fundamental to the understanding of the potential role of IL-8 in pathology. IL-8 qualifies as a neutrophil chemotaxin of tissue origin, whose production appears to be controlled by two classical inflammatory cytokines, IL-1 and TNF. In this respect, IL-8 clearly differs from other chemotaxins like C5a, fMet-Leu-Phe, LTB_4 and PAF, which are not induction-dependent and which derive from cells and proteins that enter inflamed tissues, rather than from the tissues themselves.

Neutrophil-Activating Peptide-2 and *gro*/MGSA, Two IL-8 Analogues

Neutrophil-activating peptide 2 (NAP-2) was originally identified in the culture supernatants of stimulated human blood mononuclear cells [25]. It corresponds to the 70 carboxy-terminal amino acids of PBP and has some structural homology with PF-4, like PBP a component of the α-granules. NAP-2 is not stored in platelets or other cells present in the cultures. It is formed by proteolytic cleavage of PBP and/or CTAP-III, which are released upon platelet activation [26]. It has the typical properties of chemotactic receptor agonists and induces $[Ca^{2+}]_i$ changes, chemotaxis, and exocytosis at similar concentrations to IL-8. By contrast, the precursors PBP and CTAP-III, and the homolog PF-4, are virtually inactive at 100–10000 times higher concentrations [27].

   gro/MGSA (melanoma growth-stimulatory activity) was orginally described as a growth factor for a human melanoma cell line [28] with a sequence corresponding to that derived from the *gro* cDNA described by Anisowicz et al. [29]. *gro*/MGSA, which has marked sequence homology to IL-8, was chemically synthesized and tested for neutrophil-stimulating properties. Like IL-8 and NAP-2, *gro*/MGSA induced a rapid and transient $[Ca^{2+}]_i$ rise, the exocytosis of elastase and chemotaxis in human neutrophils. Upon intradermal injection in rats, it elicited a massive and long-lasting neutrophil infiltration [30]. This profile of activity indicates that *gro*/MGSA is biologically related to the neutrophil-activating peptides and shares with them potent proinflammatory effects.

Pathophysiological Considerations

The involvement of IL-8 in inflammatory disease is suggested by its occurrence in the scales of psoriatic patients [31]. Such lesions contain, in addition, high levels of IL-1 which could function locally as one of the inducers of IL-8 production. In this disease, IL-8 could be the mediator of the massive accumulation of neutrophils in the microabscesses that are characteristic of the lesions [6]. IL-8 is also believed to be a major cause of neutrophil invasion into the synovial fluid in inflammatory joint diseases since it is produced by IL-1-stimulated synovial cells [32]. We have recently observed that mononuclear cells from the blood or synovial fluid of patients with rheumatoid arthritis, in contrast to cells of healthy individuals, release IL-8 spontaneously, and can be triggered to produce much higher levels by stimulation which IL-1, TNF, and immune complexes [33]. Neutrophil accumulation is prominent in certain lung diseases like idiopathic pulmonary fibrosis and asbestosis. Because of their high contents of neutral proteinases [34], neutrophils are generally considered to be the main effectors of parenchymal cell injury and breakdown of interstitial structures. A comparable situation is encountered in the adult respiratory distress syndrome, where elastase and other neutral proteases, in concert with respiratory burst-derived radicals, are implicated in the irreversible damage of the lung [35, 36]. The presence of neutrophil attractants differing from C5a in the bronchoalveolar lavage fluid of patients with inflammatory lung diseases has been repeatedly reported in the past (see [6, 9] for references).

The information thus far available suggests that the activity and tissue distribution of *gro*/MGSA is similar to that of IL-8, since it was found to be expressed in endothelial cells and fibroblasts upon stimulation with IL-1 [30]. The mode of formation and biodistribution of NAP-2, by contrast, is completely different as it depends on the release of precursors from activated platelets and their processing by phagocyte proteases [26]. In contrast to IL-8 and *gro*/MGSA, NAP-2 is assumed to form almost exclusively within the vascular bed, where it could play a role in attracting neutrophils into thrombotic deposits.

References

1. Sha'afi RI, Molski TFP (1988) Activation of the neutrophil. Prog Allergy 42:1
2. Grzeskowiak M, della Bianca V, Cassatella MA, Rossi F (1986) Complete dissociation between

the activation of phosphoinositide turnover and of NADPH oxidase by formyl-methionyl-leucyl-phenylalanine in human nuetrophils depleted of Ca2$^+$ and primed by subthreshold doses of phorbol 12, myristate 13, acetate, Biochem Biophys Res Commun 135:785

3. Dewald B, Payne TG, Baggiolini M (1984) Activation of NADPH oxidase of human neutrophils. Potentiation of chemotactic peptide by a diacylglycerol. Biochem Biophys Res Commun 125:367

4. Dewald B, Thelen M, Wymann MP, Baggiolini M (1989) Staurosporine inhibits the respiratory burst and induces exocytosis in human neutrophils. Biochem J 264:879

5. Okajima F, Katada T, Ui M (1985) Coupling of the guanine nucleotide regulatory protein to chemotactic peptide receptors in neutrophil membranes and its uncoupling by islet-activating protein, pertussis toxin. A possible role of the toxin substrate in Ca2$^+$-mobilizing receptor-mediated signal transduction. J Biol Chem 260:6761

6. Baggiolini M, Walz A, Kunkel SL (1989) Neutrophil-activating peptide-1/interleukin 8, a novel cytokine that activates neutrophils. J Clin Invest 84:1045

7. Schmid J, Weissmann C (1987) Induction of mRNA for a serine protease and a beta-thromboglobulin-like protein in mitogen-stimulated human leukocytes. J Immunol 139:250

8. Lindley I, Aschauer H, Seifert JM, Lam C, Brunowsky W, Kownatzki E, Thelen M, Peveri P, Dewald B, von Tscharner V, Walz A, Baggiolini M (1988) Synthesis and expression in *Escherichia coli* of the gene encoding monocyte-derived neutrophil-activating factor: biological equivalence between natural and recombinant neutrophil-activating factor. Proc Natl Acad Sci USA 85:9199

9. Peveri P, Walz A, Dewald B, Baggiolini M (1988) A novel neutrophil-activating factor produced by human mononuclear phagocytes. J Exp Med 167:1547

10. Thelen M, Peveri P, Kernen P, von Tscharner V, Walz A, Baggiolini M (1988) Mechanism of neutrophil activation by NAF, a novel monocyte-derived peptide agonist. FASEB J 2:2702

11. Wymann MP, Kernen P, Deranleau DA, Baggiolini M (1989) Respiratory burst oscillations in human neutrophils and their correlation with fluctuations in apparent cell shape. J Biol Chem 264:15829

12. Dewald B, Thelen M, Baggiolini M (1988) Two transduction sequences are necessary for neutrophil activation by receptor agonists. J Biol Chem 263:16179

13. Samanta AK, Oppenheim JJ, Matsushima K (1989) Identification and characterization of specific receptors for monocyte-derived neutrophil chemotactic factor (MDNCF) on human neutrophils. J Exp Med 169:1185

14. Besemer J, Hujber A, Kuhn B (1989) Specific binding, internalization, and degradation of human neutrophil-activating factor by human polymorphonuclear leukocytes. J Biol Chem 264:17409

15. Moser B, Schumacher C, von Tscharner V, Clark-Lewis I, Baggiolini M (1991) Neutrophil-activating peptide 2 and gro/melanoma growth-stimulatory activity interact with neutrophil-activating peptide 1/interleukin 8 receptors on human neutrophils. J Biol Chem. 266:10666

16. Walz A, Meloni F, Clark-Lewis I, von Tscharner V, Baggiolini M (1991) [Ca^{2+}]$_i$ changes and respiratory burst in human neutrophils and monocytes induced by NAP-1/interleukin-8, NAP-2 and gro/MGSA. J Leukocyte Biol 50:279

17. Kernen P. Wymann MP, von Tscharner V, Deranleau DA, Tai PC, Spry CJ, Dahinden CA, Baggiolini M (1991) Shape changes, exocytosis and cytosolic free calcium changes in stimulated human eosinophils. J Clin Invest 87:2012

18. Dahinden CA, Kurimoto Y, de Weck AL, Lindley I, Dewald B, Baggiolini M (1989) The neutrophil-activating peptide NAF/NAP-1 induces histamine and leukotriene release by interleukin 3-primed basophils. J Exp Med 170:1787

19. Larsen CG, Anderson AO, Oppenheim JJ, Matsushima K (1989) Production of interleukin-8 by human dermal fibroblasts and keratinocytes in response to interleukin-1 or tumour necrosis factor. Immunology 68:31

20. Leonard EJ, Yoshimura T (1990) Neutrophil attractant/activation protein-1 (NAP-1 (interleukin-8)). Am J Respir Cell Mol Biol 2:479

21. Colditz I, Zwahlen R, Dewald B, Baggiolini M (1989) In vivo inflammatory activity of neutrophil-activating factor, a novel chemotactic peptide derived from human monocytes. Am J Pathol 134:755

22. Colditz IG, Zwahlen RD, Baggiolini M (1990) Neutrophil accumulation and plasma leakage induced in·vivo by neutrophil-activating peptide-1. J Leukocyte Biol 48:129

23. Elner VM, Strieter RM, Elner SG, Baggiolini M, Lindley I, Kunkel SL (1990) Neutrophil chemotactic factor (IL-8) gene expression by cytokine-treated retinal pigment epithelial cells. Am J Pathol 136:745

24. Thornton AJ, Strieter RM, Lindley I, Baggiolini M, Kunkel SL (1990) Cytokine-induced gene expression of a neutrophil chemotatic factor/IL-8 in human hepatocytes. J Immunol 144:2609
25. Walz A, Baggiolini M (1989) A novel cleavage product of beta-thromboglobulin formed in cultures of stimulated mononuclear cells activates human neutrophils. Biochem Biophys Res Commun 159:969
26. Walz A, Baggiolini M (1990) Generation of the neutrophil-activating peptide NAP-2 from platelet basic protein or connective tissue-activating peptide III through monocyte proteases. J Exp Med 171:449
27. Walz A, Dewald B, von Tscharner V, Baggiolini M (1989) Effects of the neutrophil-activating peptide NAP-2, platelet basic protein, connective tissue-activating peptide III and platelet factor 4 on human neutrophils. J Exp Med 170:1745
28. Richmond A, Balentien B, Thomas HG, Flaggs G, Barton DE, Spiess J, Bordoni R, Francke U, Derynck R (1988) Molecular characterization and chromosomal mapping of melanoma growth stimulatory activity, a growth factor structurally related to beta-thromboglobulin. EMBO J 7:2025
29. Anisowicz A, Bardwell L, Sager R (1987) Constitutive overexpression of a growth-regulated gene in transformed Chinese hamster and human cells. Proc Natl Acad Sci USA 84:7188
30. Moser B, Clark-Lewis I, Zwahlen R, Baggiolini M (1990) Neutrophil-activating properties of the melanoma growth-stimulatory activity. J Exp Med 171:1797
31. Schroder JM, Christophers E (1986) Identification of C5ades arg and an anionic neutrophil-activating peptide (ANAP) in psoriatic scales. Pulmonary and systemic immunoregulatory changes during the development of experimentally asbestos-induced lung inflammation. Role of local macrophage-derived chemotactic factors in accumulation of neutrophils in the lungs. J Invest Dermatol 87:53
32. Watson ML, Westwick J, Fincham NJ, Camp RD (1988) Elevation of PMN cytosolic free calcium and locomotion stimulated by novel peptides from IL-1-treated human synovial cell cultures. Biochem Biophys Res Commun 155:1154
33. Seitz M, Dewald B, Gerber N, Baggiolini M (1991) Enhanced production of neutrophil-activating peptide-1/interleukin-8 in rheumatoid arthritis. J Clin Invest 87:463
34. Baggiolini M, Schnyder J, Bretz U, Dewald B, Ruch W (1980) Cellular mechanisms of proteinase release from inflammatory cells and the degradation of extracellular proteins. Ciba Found Symp 75:105
35. Hunninghake GW, Gadek JE, Lawley TJ, Crystal RG (1981) Mechanisms of neutrophil accumulation in the lungs of patients with idiopathic pulmonary fibrosis. J Clin Invest 68:259
36. McGuire WW, Spragg RG, Cohen AB, Cochrane CG (1982) Studies on the pathogenesis of the adult respiratory distress syndrome. J Clin Invest 69:543

Cellular and Molecular Mechanisms that Regulate the Production of Interleukin-8: The Potential Role of Chemotactic Cytokines in Acute Respiratory Distress Syndrome and Multiple Organ Failure

S. L. Kunkel[1], S. W. Chensue[1], T. J. Standiford[2], and R. M. Strieter[2]

Introduction

In order for functional inflammatory cells to arrive at sites of reactivity, a complex cascade of events must be set in motion. These events are characterized by cell-to-cell interactions that involve either intimate cell contact or contact established by soluble mediators. A strict requirement for successful cell movement appears to be the regulated order in which the above interactions occur. The elicitation of leukocytes from the vasculature to an area of interstitial inflammation is maintained via a series of specific, regulated steps. For example, very early during an inflammatory reaction physical and structural changes within the small venules may dictate early leukocyte responses. These proximal events may include alterations in physical properties, such as pH, oxygenation, and viscosity, as well as changes in blood flow and vessel tone (vasoconstriction-/dilation). These early changes can occur locally within minutes and appear to "prime" the inflammatory region for subsequent events.

These subsequent events are likely dependent upon the expression of early response cytokines from leukocytes within the vessel lumen. Interestingly, preliminary studies have identified the induction of specific cytokines that appear to be under the influence of oxygen concentration. Proximal mediators such as interleukin-1 (IL-1) and tumor necrosis factor-alpha (TNF-α) are important soluble signals that are involved in the initiation of leukocyte movement [1, 2]. These cytokines are instrumental in inducing the expression of adherence proteins from the endothelium (ICAM-1, ELAM, VCAM), as well as causing the expression of the CD11/CD18 family of adherence proteins by phagocytic leukocytes. In the confines of a vessel with reduced blood flow, the expression of adherence proteins allows for intimate cell contact between leukocytes and the endothelium. This adherence event is one of the first well-characterized cellular interactions that can be histologically observed during inflammation. The binding phenomenon between leukocytes and endothelial cells can be observed at the ultrastructural level, as can be seen from the electron micrograph in Fig. 1, which clearly demonstrates cell-to-cell contact. The initial interactions that lead to the adherence of leukocytes to the vascular wall must be

[1] Department of Pathology and [2] Division of Pulmonary Medicine, Department of Internal Medicine, University of Michigan Medical School, Ann Arbor, MI 48109-0602, USA

Host Defense Dysfunction
in Trauma, Shock and Sepsis
Eds. Faist/Meakins/Schildberg
© Springer-Verlag, Berlin Heidelberg 1993

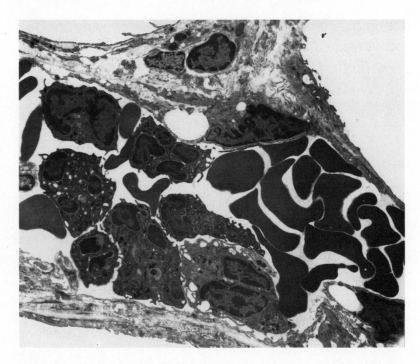

Fig. 1. Electron microscopic assessment of the movement of leukocytes from the lumen of a vessel through the endothelial cell barrier

a conserved response, as this histological picture is observed in a number of inflammatory reactions independent of the initiating agent or organ location. One of the interesting aspects regarding the adherence reaction is its reversibility. In order to have successful recruitment of leukocytes from the vessel to an area of inflammation, the cells must bind and then move from the vascular lumen/wall into the interstitium. The transient adherence of these cells and the mechanism(s) which govern this event are one of many enigmas that surround in vivo chemotaxis.

While adherence is an important proximal event, necessary for cell recruitment, other distal events are likely to be important in maintaining this reaction. These include the ability of cells to clear the basement membrane barrier and follow a signal gradient into an area of inflammation. The importance of the elicitation of leukocytes into an area of inflammation is clearly underscored by the redundancy of chemotactic factors which have been previously found. These chemotaxins include peptides, polypeptides, and lipid mediators (Table 1). Most of these factors are structurally unrelated and exert their effects via specific receptors. Although these inflammatory mediators possess potent activity, their specificity for individual cell populations is limited. An interesting physical/chemical attribute of these factors is the short half-life found in vivo. It is

Table 1. A number of redundant peptide, polypeptide, and lipid mediators comprise the various chemotactic factors with potential biologic activity

Bacterial-derived fMLP	Fibronectin
Complement-derived C5a	Collagen fragments
Transforming growth factor	Platelet-derived growth factor
Leukotriene B	Platelet-activating factor
Interleukin-8	Monocyte chemotactic protein

Table 2. Partial listing of the members of the supergene family of chemotactic cytokines that possess a high degree of structural homology

Interleukin-8	Platelet factor 4
Platelet basic protein	Macrophage inflammatory protein
Growth-related onogene (GRO)	Neutrophil-activating peptide 2
Connective tissue-activating protein III	β-thromboglobulin

apparent that many of the mediators found in Table 1 possess limited activity over a prolong time span. This is particularly true of the bacteria-derived f-methionyl-leucyl-phenylalanine (fMLP), the split product of the fifth component of complement (C5a), and the lipid metabolites leukotriene B_4 (LTB_4) and platelet-activating factor (PAF).

Numerous investigations have identified the importance of the above chemotactic factors during inflammation, but recent studies have identified other chemotaxins as being important in maintaining a successful recruitment response [2–5]. These additional chemoattractants belong to a family of related polypeptides that are expressed by both immune and nonimmune cells [6–10]. The identification of these proteins has generated increased excitement in the research area of chemotactic factors, as they possess relatively specific activity for neutrophils, monocytes, and lymphocytes [2, 11]. These chemotactic cytokines share a high degree of homology with a number of other inflammatory proteins (Table 2). The chemotactic cytokines are identified according to the position of the four cysteine residues found in their amino acid structures. One of these factors has been identified as a neutrophil chemotactic factor/activating factor, also known as interleukin-8 (IL-8). IL-8 is an 8000-dalton peptide that is synthesized as a 99-amino-acid precursor with a leader sequence of 22 amino acids [12, 13]. Interestingly, IL-8 is processed at the amino terminus, resulting in the expression of mature IL-8 protein possessing either 69, 72, or 77 amino acids. This chemotactic cytokine is an active chemoattractant and activating polypeptide for neutrophils in the range of 1–100 ng/ml. In addition, IL-8 has been shown to possess chemotactic activity for lymphocytes at pg/ml concentrations. As identified in Table 2, IL-8 belongs to a novel supergene family including murine macrophage inflammatory peptide 2 (MIP-2), platelet factor 4 (PF-4), chicken v-*src*-inducible protein (9E3), interferon-γ inducible protein (IP-10), growth-related oncogene/melanoma growth and stimulatory activity

(GRO/MGSA), platelet basic protein (PBP), and its cleavage products: β-thromboglobulin (β-TG), connective tissue activating protein III (CTAP III), and neutrophil activating peptide 2 (NAP-2). A number of cell types produce IL-8. The most prominent cellular source of IL-8 appears to be mononuclear phagocytes, such as monocytes and alveolar macrophages. In addition, endothelial cells, fibroblasts, epithelial cells, and smooth muscle cells have also been identified as important sources of IL-8. This chemotactic cytokine has been shown to be relatively resistant to pH changes, alterations in temperature, and mild proteolytic degradation [14]. The stability of IL-8 suggests that this factor may have prolonged activity during inflammation and in vivo may serve as an important leukocyte chemoattractant.

The Establishment of Cytokine Networks

Kupffer Cell–Hepatocyte Interactions

It is becoming increasing apparent that cell-to-cell communication circuits between mononuclear phagocytes and surrounding nonimmune parenchymal cells that characterize a given tissue are important events in establishing an inflammatory response, e.g., we have shown that pulmonary epithelial cells [15] and hepatocytes [8] can possess important effector cell activity during inflammation via IL-1 or TNF-dependent IL-8 production. We have studied this network interaction between proximal and distal cytokines. As shown in Fig. 1, human hepatoma cells challenged with IL-1 demonstrated a time- and dose-dependent increase in the expression of steady state IL-8 messenger ribonucleic acid (mRNA). Concentrations of IL-1 in the pg/ml range proved to be effective in the induction of IL-8 mRNA. In addition, a kinetic analysis of IL-8 mRNA expression demonstrated the presence of steady state IL-8 by 1 h after stimulation and this expression lasted in excess of 24 h. Interestingly, hepatocytes treated with lipopolysaccharide (LPS), a major immune-activating agent released from gram-negative bacteria, did not induce an increase in the expression of IL-8 mRNA. These findings suggest that in order for the hepatocyte to synthesize a chemotactic factor important in LPS-initiated inflammation, this cell must first come into contact with a host-derived cytokine such as IL-1 or TNF.

To further explore the necessity for soluble mediators to dictate cell-to-cell interactions, we conducted studies to assess the communication circuits between LPS-treated Kupffer cells and hepatocyte-derived IL-8 expression. In these investigations, conditioned medium from LPS-stimulated human Kupffer cells was overlaid on cultured human hepatocytes. At specific time points, steady state levels of hepatocyte IL-8 mRNA were assessed by Northern blot analysis. As shown in Fig. 2, the conditioned medium from the LPS-challenged Kupffer cells was active in causing an increase in the expression of hepatocyte IL-8

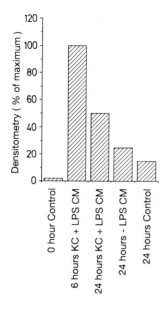

Fig. 2. Laser densitometry of autoradiographs of Northern blot analyses for hepatocyte IL-8 mRNA expression induced by conditioned media (*CM*) derived from LPS-treated human Kupffer cells (*KC*)

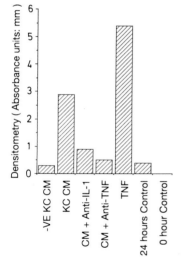

Fig. 3. Laser densitometry of Northern blot analyses of hepatocyte IL-8 mRNA by LPS-treated Kupffer cell (*KC*) conditioned media (*CM*) treated with neutralizing antibodies to IL-1 or TNF

mRNA. The addition of Kupffer cell condition media to hepatocytes induced significant levels of hepatocyte-derived IL-8 mRNA during 6- and 24-h study periods. To determine if IL-1 or TNF could be influencing the expression of hepatocyte IL-8 mRNA levels, the conditioned medium from LPS-treated Kupffer cells was first treated with neutralizing antibody to either human IL-1 or TNF. Treatment with anti-IL-1 or anti-TNF suppressed the ability of Kupffer cell conditioned media to cause hepatocyte IL-8 mRNA by approximately 70% and 80%, respectively (Fig. 3). Preimmune serum had no suppressive effect in this system. These studies are important, as they describe the ability of a resident noninflammatory cell to play an important effector role, via the generation of a hepatocyte-derived neutrophil chemotactic factor, during an inflammatory response in the liver.

Alveolar Macrophage-Pulmonary Epithelial Cell Interactions

In addition to the above interactions of Kupffer cells and hepatocytes there are other examples of cell-to-cell interactions that may result in the noninflammatory cell constituents of tissue acquiring effector cell activity. Our recent studies have shown that LPS-treated alveolar macrophages from nondisease, nonsmoking volunteers can network with type II-like pulmonary epithelial cells and/or pulmonary fibroblasts [15]. This interaction sequentially leads to the production of important cytokines from the resident lung cells. As shown in Fig. 4, human type II-like pulmonary epithelial cells treated with IL-1 or TNF could synthesize a neutrophil chemotactic factor in a time-dependent manner. Furthermore, this activity could be suppressed by the addition of specific neutralizing antibody to IL-8. While the cytokines IL-1 and TNF were found to be effective in increasing the production of IL-8 by a resident cell population from the lungs, LPS was not nearly as effective. Although the addition of LPS to cultured type II-like cells did induce the expression of an activity that promoted neutrophil chemotaxis (Fig. 4), an assessment of the culture supernatant by enzyme-linked immunosorbent assay (ELISA) demonstrated that the LPS-treated cells were not producing IL-8 (Fig. 5). Thus, LPS does not appear to stimulate the production of IL-8 by the pulmonary type II-like cells. This identical stimulus specificity, as demonstrated by human hepatocytes and type II-like epithelial cells, has also been identified in human dermal and pulmonary fibroblasts. Since previous studies in our laboratory and others have identified

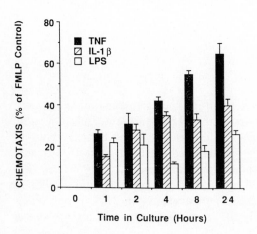

Fig. 4. Kinetics of the production of a neutrophil chemotactic factor (IL-8) by human type II-like pulmonary epithelial cells treated with either IL-1 or TNF

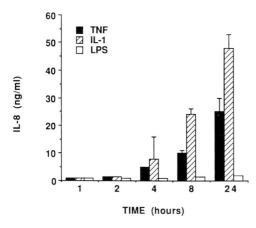

Fig. 5. Induction of IL-8 antigenic activity (by ELISA) by IL-1 and TNF, but not LPS, stimulated human type II-like pulmonary epithelial cells

the production of IL-1 and TNF by LPS-stimulated human alveolar macrophages, we were interested in establishing the role of cytokine networks in the lung via alveolar macrophage–epithelial cell interactions. Cell-free conditioned media from human alveolar macrophages was incubated with the type II-like epithelial cells in the presence or absence of specific neutralizing antibody to IL-1 or TNF. At specific time points, the epithelial cells were assessed for the expression of IL-8 mRNA. Using laser densitometry to assess IL-8 level from the Northern blots of the epithelial cells, we observed that antibodies to IL-1 or TNF, individually or in combination, resulted in a 44%, 28%, and 83% reduction in steady state IL-8 mRNA levels. This cell-to-cell interaction that is mediated by soluble polypeptides is a typical example of cytokine networking and is likely to be a major mechanism whereby normal resident cells in any given organ can play an important role as an immunologic effector cell.

Role of Cytokine Networks in Sepsis and Acute Respiratory Distress Syndrome

There is growing evidence that the pathophysiologic manifestation of many disease states is due to the production of a variety of protein mediators produced via cytokine networks. While the major sources of proximal cytokines appear to be mononuclear cells of the immune system, other resident tissue cells can synthesize distal cytokines. When these cytokines are produced in excess or are aberrantly regulated, they can exert pathologic consequences. There is strong evidence to support this contention, as the clinical manifestation of septic shock may be due in part to the exaggerated production of IL-1 and TNF [16–19]. Postulated sources of these cytokines have been either sessile, fixed tissue macrophages or peripheral blood monocytes. Recently, we have examined the production of TNF, IL-1α and IL-1β and IL-6 in vivo in an animal model of endotoxemia [20]. These studies have provided several lines of interesting experimental data: specifically, after administration of LPS to mice, both IL-1 and TNF were demonstrated by immunohistochemistry within the hepatic sinusoidal macrophages (Kupffer cells). This information lends evidence to the idea that fixed tissue macrophages are important sources of cytokines during endotoxemia. The staining patterns for IL-1 and TNF in vivo were identical to those found in in vitro studies. Interestingly, the antigenic expression of IL-6 by Kupffer cells was not detected, although IL-6 bioactivity could be identified in the serum of the LPS-challenged animals. In the serum TNF bioactivity was detected first, followed by IL-6 and IL-1. These data are in support of other investigations which demonstrated similar kinetics of cytokine expression using a baboon challenged with *Escherichia coli* [18] or rabbit challenged with meningococcus [17]. As compared to the in vitro production of cytokines by cultured macrophages, our studies suggest that synthetic events are accelerated and under complex regulation in vivo. The cascade of cytokine production reflects a highly refined level of gene expression and regulation. The sequential synthesis of specific cytokines is undoubtedly the key to the subsequent pathologic events that are observed during endotoxemia and/or sepsis. For example, the rapid onset of hypotension and other physiologic parameters that are associated with shock are likely due to the acute expression of TNF and potentially IL-1. The delayed or prolonged synthesis of IL-6 and IL-1 may be involved in mediating distal events such as the pyrogenic response, acute phase response, and the cortisol response.

Much of our data provide support for the role of cytokine networking during pathologic states: specifically, the key role of proximal mediators such as TNF in initiating the cascade-like induction of other polypeptide mediators. Furthermore, it is possible that the network phenomenon may extend beyond cytokine-cytokine interactions and may include an intimate relationship between humoral mediators and cytokines. Recent studies have shown that C5a, the split product of the fifth component of complement, can induce both IL-1 and TNF expression by human monocytes [21]. Since it is well established that endotoxemia can lead to significant complement activation, a situation exists that could network cytokines with other humoral mediators. Thus, the life-threating consequences of disease, such as sepsis and multiple organ failure, may be mechanistically mediated via the exaggerated involvement of many inflammatory systems acting in concert with each other. The potential end result is an accelerated and synergistic action of the host resulting in a clinical picture of septic shock.

Conclusion

There is little doubt that the analysis of cytokine networks both in vitro and in vivo are crucial to our understanding of the role of cytokines in the pathology of diseases. In order to design more effective/selective therapies for such enigmatic states as sepsis and the devastating consequence of multiple organ failure, increased understanding of the source, kinetics of synthesis, synergistic activities, and regulation at the cellular and molecular levels must be secured. Further studies addressing the above issues will likely result in novel pharmacologic and biotechnological interventions, such as the use of a cocktail of anticytokine antibodies, cytokine receptor antagonists, antioxidants, and next-generation antibiotics. Continued basic and clinical research into the mechanisms driving the pathologic consequences of these disorders offers hope for the development of effective interventions.

Acknowledgements. The authors wish to thank Robin Kunkel for expert graphics. This work was supported in part by National Institutes of Health grants HL 02401, HL 31237, HL 31963, and HL 35276. Dr. Strieter is a RJR Research Scholar.

References

1. Pohlman TH, Stanness KA, Beatty PG, Ochs HD, Harlan JM (1986) An endothelial cell surface factor(s) induced in vitro by LPS, IL-1, and TNF increases neutrophil adherences by a CDW 18-dependent mechanism. J Immunol 136:4548–4557
2. Matsushima K, Oppenheim JJ (1989) Interleukin-8 and MCAF: novel inflammatory cytokine inducible by IL-1 and TNF. Cytokine 1:2–13
3. Anisowicz A, Bardwell L, Sager R (1987) Constitutive overexpression of a growth-related gene in transformed Chinese hamster and human cells. Proc Natl Acad Sci USA 84:7188–7192
4. Baggiolini M, Walz A, Kunkel SL (1989) Neutrophil-activating peptide-1/Interleukin-8, a novel cytokine that activates neutrophils. J Clin Invest 84:1045–1049
5. Brown KD, Zurawski SM, Mosmann TR, Zurawski G (1989) A family of small inducible proteins secreted by leukocytes are members of a new super family that includes leukocytes and fibroblast-derived inflammatory agents, growth-factors, and indicators of various activation processes. J Immunol 142:679–687
6. Strieter RM, Kunkel SL, Showell HJ, Remick DG, Phan SH, Ward PA, Marks RM (1989) Endothelial cell gene expression of a neutrophil chemotactic factor by TNF, LPS, and IL-1. Science 243:1467–1469
7. Strieter RM, Phan SH, Showell HJ, Remick DJ, Marks RM, Kunkel SL (1989) Monokine-induced neutrophil chemotactic factor gene expression in human fibroblasts. J Biol Chem 264:10621–10626
8. Thornton AJ, Strieter RM, Lindley I, Baggiolini M, Kunkel SL (1990) Cytokine-induced gene expression of a neutrophil chemotactic factor/IL-8 in human hepatocytes. J Immunol 144:2609–2613
9. Strieter RM, Chensue SW, Basha MA, Standiford TJ, Lynch JP, Baggiolini M, Kunkel SL (1990) Human alveolar macrophage gene expression of interleukin-8 by tumor necrosis factor, lipopolysaccharide, and interleukin-1. Am J Respir Cell Mol Biol 2:321–326
10. Elner VM, Strieter RM, Elner SG, Baggiolini M, Lindley I, Kunkel SL (1990) Neutrophil chemotactic factor (IL-8) gene expression by cytokine treated retinal pigment epithelial cells. Am J Pathol 136:745–750
11. Larsen CG, Anderson AO, Appella E, Oppenheim JJ, Matsushima K (1989) Neutrophil-activating protein (NAP-1) is also chemotactic for lymphocytes. Science 243:1464–1469
12. Yoshimura T, Matsushima K, Oppenheim JJ, Leonard FJ (1987) Neutrophil chemotactic factor produced by lipopolysaccharide stimulate human blood mononuclear leukocytes: partial characterization and separation from interleukin-1. J Immunol 139:788–793
13. Matsushima K, Morishita K, Yoshimura T, Lavu S, Kobayashi Y, Lew W, Appella E, Leonard EJ, Oppenheim JJ (1988) Molecular cloning of a human monocyte-derived neutrophil chemo-

tactic factor (MDNCF) and the induction of MDNCF mRNA by interleukin-1 and tumor necrosis factor. J Exp Med 167:1883–1893

14. Thelen M, Peverri P, Kernen P, von Tscharner V, Walz A, Baggiolini M (1988) Mechanism of neutrophil activation by NAF, a novel monocyte-derived peptide agonist. FASEB J 2:2702–2706

15. Standiford TJ, Kunkel SL, Basha MA, Chensue SW, Lynch JP, Toews GB, Westwick J, Strieter RM (1990) Interleukin-8 gene expression by a pulmonary epithelial cell line: a model for cytokine networks in the lung. J Clin Invest 86:1945–1953

16. Fong Y, Tracy KJ, Lowry SF, Cerami A (1989) Biology of cachectin. In: Sorg C (ed) Cytokines: macrophage-derived cell regulatory factors, vol 1. Karger, Basel, pp 74–88

17. Waage A, Brandtzaeg P, Halstensen A, Kierulf P, Espevik T (1987) The complex pattern of cytokines in serum from patients with meningococcal septic shock. Association between interleukin-1, interleukin-6, and fatal outcome. J Exp Med 169:333–338

18. Tracey KJ, Fong Y, Hesse DG, Manogue KR, Lee AT, Lowry SF, Cerami A (1987) Anti-cachectin/TNF monoclonal antibodies prevent septic shock during lethal bacterial. Nature 330:662–664

19. Remick DG, Strieter RM, Eskandari MK, Nguyen DT, Genord MA, Kunkel SL (1990) Role of tumor necrosis factor in lipopolysaccharide-induced pathologic alterations. Am J Pathol 136:49–60

20. Chensue SW, Terebuh PD, Remick DG, Scales WE, Kunkel SL (1991) In vivo biologic and immunohistochemical analysis of interleukin-1 alpha, beta, and tumor necrosis factor during experimental endotoxemia. Am J Pathol 138:395–402

21. Okusawa S, Yancey KB, van der Meer JWM, Endres S, Dinarello CA, Gelfand JA (1988) C5a stimulates secretion of tumor necrosis factor from human mononuclear cells in vitro. Comparison with secretion of interleukin-1 beta. J Exp Med 168:443–448

Generation and Properties of Neutrophil-Activating Peptide 2 (NAP-2)

A. Walz[1], F. Meloni[1], R. Zwahlen[2], I. Clark-Lewis[3], and B. Car

Introduction

Neutrophil-activating peptide 2(NAP-2) is a peptide which was first isolated from the culture supernatants of stimulated human blood mononuclear cells [1]. Sequence analysis and carboxy-terminus determination showed that it consists of 70 amino acids and results from the truncation of platelet basic protein (PBP) [2] and connective tissue activating peptide III (CTAP-III) [3], both of which are released from alpha granules following platelet stimulation. NAP-2 has considerable sequence homology with neutrophil-activating peptide 1/interleukin-8 (NAP-1/IL-8) [1], melanoma growth-stimulatory activity (gro/MGSA) [4, 5], platelet factor 4 (PF-4) [6], and γ-IP10, a γ-interferon inducible cytokine [7] (Fig. 1).

We have compared the effects of highly purified NAP-2, NAP-1/IL-8, gro/MGSA-α, PBP, CTAP-III, PF-4, and γ-IP10 on human neutrophils. NAP-1/IL-8, gro/MGSA-α, and NAP-2 are similar in their potency to induce chemotaxis and cytosolic free calcium rise, but vary in their ability to induce exocytosis and the respiratory burst response. The other peptides tested were essentially inactive [8]. The in vivo effect of human NAP-2, NAP-1/IL-8, and gro/MGSA-α was tested in rabbits and rats by intradermal injection.

Formation of NAP-2

NAP-2 was first detected in supernatants of human blood mononuclear cells stimulated with lipopolysaccharide (LPS) or lectins [9]. Subsequently, it was demonstrated that the formation of NAP-2 depends on the presence of platelets in the monocyte cultures [10]. Neither platelets nor monocytes alone are able to produce NAP-2. Monocytes cultured in the presence of LPS produced NAP-1/IL-8 in addition, with no marked increase in NAP-2 formation. But, under these conditions, three amino-terminal NAP-2 variants, consisting of 73,

---

[1] Theodor Kocher Institute, University of Bern, Switzerland
[2] Institute of Veterinary Pathology, University of Bern, Switzerland
[3] Biomedical Research Centre, University of British Columbia, Vancouver, Canada

Host Defense Dysfunction
in Trauma, Shock and Sepsis
Eds. Faist/Meakins/Schildberg
© Springer-Verlag, Berlin Heidelberg 1993

```
                              * *                    *              *
NAP-1/IL-8              SAKELRCQCIKTYSKPFHPKFIKELRVIESGPHCANTEIIVKLSD-GRELCLDPKENWVQRVVEKFLKRAENS


NAP-2                  AELRCMCIKTTS-GIHPKNIQSLEVIGKGTHCNQVEVIATLKD-GRKICLDPDAPRIKKIVQKKLAGDESAD

CTAP-III       NLAKGKEESLDSDLYAELRCMC·····-·································_·································

PBP       SSTKGQTKRNLAKGKEESLDSDLYAELRCMC·····-································_·································


gro/MGSA-α             ASVATELRCQCLQTLQ-GIHPKNIQSVNVKSPGPHCAQTEVIATLKN-GRKACLNPASPIVKKIIEKMLNSDKSN

gro/MGSA-β             ·PL··············-···L······K···················-·Q········M·········KNG···

gro/MGSA-γ             ···V·············-···L········R··················-·K········M·Q·····I··KGST·


PF4                    EAEEDGDLQCLCVKTTS-QVRPRHITSLEVIKAGPHCPTAQLIATLKN-GRKICLDLQAPLYKKIIKKLLES


γ-IP10                 VPLSRTVRCTCISINQ-PVNPRSLEKLEIIPASQFCPRVEIIATMKKKGEKRCLNPESKAIKNLLKAVSKEMSKRSP
```

Fig. 1. Alignment of the amino acid sequences of neutrophil-activating peptide 1/interleukin-8 (NAP-1/IL-8), neutrophil-activating peptide 2 (NAP-2), its precursor peptides platelet basic protein (PBP) and connective tissue activating peptide III (CTAP-III), three members of melanoma growth stimulatory activity (gro/MGSA), platelet factor 4 (PF4), and γ-interferon inducible peptide 10 (γ-IP10). The sequences are aligned according to their four characteristic cysteine residues (*)

74, and 75 residues, were also found [10]. No NAP-1/IL-8 or NAP-2 was detected when lymphocytes were substituted for monocytes.

The formation of active and stable NAP-2 from purified CTAP-III can be observed under cell-free conditions with monocyte supernatants or by the addition of chymotrypsin and leukocyte cathepsin G [10, 11]. Neutrophil elastase and a number of other proteases, on the other hand, rapidly degrade CTAP-III without the formation of an active intermediate [11].

Biological Activities In Vitro

NAP-2 was found to be a powerful activator of human neutrophils in vitro, inducing cytosolic free calcium changes, chemotaxis, and exocytosis at concentrations between 0.3 and 10 nM [8]. By contrast, its precursors PBP and CTAP-III had little, if any, activity at concentrations up to 100 nM [8]. Highly purified PF-4, previously reported to be chemotactic for neutrophils, monocytes, and fibroblasts and to induce neutrophil granule release [12], was found to be at least 1000-fold less effective than NAP-2 on neutrophil stimulation. NAP-2 was equipotent with NAP-1/IL-8 and gro/MGSA-α as a stimulus of cytosolic free calcium changes and chemotaxis, but weaker than these as a stimulus of exocytosis (Table 1) [8, 13]. NAP-2 and gro/MGSA-α are inducers of the respiratory burst in human neutrophils. Their efficacy, however, is low compared to that of NAP-1/IL-8 or other agonists such as f-Met-Leu-Phe or C5a

Table 1. Neutrophil responses to NAP-1/IL-8, PBP, CTAP-III, NAP-2, and *gro*/MGSA-α

	NAP-1/IL-8	PBP/CTAP-III	NAP-2	*gro*/MGSA-α
Ca²⁺ rise	+ + +	–	+ + +	+ + +
Chemotaxis	+ + +	–	+ + +	+ + +
Exocytosis	+ + +	–	+ +	+ +
Respiratory burst	+ +	n.d.	+	+
PMN infiltration (rabbit)	+ + +	n.d.	+ + +	+ + +
PMN infiltration (rat)	+ + +	n.d.	+	+ + +

[14, 15]. In contrast to chemotaxis and induction of cytosolic calcium, the respiratory burst response measured in human neutrophils shows considerable variation between individuals. This suggests that the signal transduction pathway for this cellular response differs. The specific enhancement of this signal transduction pathway can be achieved through concanavalin A priming, which results in a massive enhancement of the rate and duration of the respiratory burst induced by NAP-1/IL-8, NAP-2, and gro/MGSA-α [15].

N-amino-terminal variants of NAP-2 with 3, 4, and 5 additional amino acids were found to induce cytosolic free calcium changes and exocytosis, but biological activity was about 10 times lower than that of NAP-2 [10].

In Vivo Activity

The in vivo activity of NAP-2 was tested in rats and rabbits by the intradermal injection of 10^{-9}–10^{-12} mol/site. Similar concentrations of NAP-1/IL-8 was used for comparison. In the rat skin gro/MGSA-α was tested in addition to the two other peptides. Neutrophil infiltrates within the skin were scored in the lower and upper dermis 4 h after injection. Total scores for the skin samples

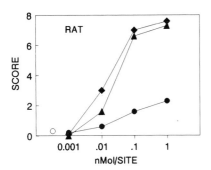
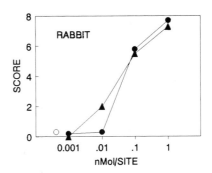

Fig. 2. Neutrophil accumulation in rat and rabbit skin 4 h after injection of NAP-1/IL-8 (▲), NAP-2 (●), gro/MGSA-α (◆), and phosphate-buffered saline (○). Each *point* represents score values from six injection sites (two sites per animal). Scores were determined from neutrophil counts in the upper dermis and in the lower dermis (range 0–8)

were obtained by adding both counts. In the rabbit skin the scores for NAP-1/IL-8 and NAP-2 were essentially identical at all four concentrations tested (Fig. 2). A gradual decrease of neutrophil scores was recorded with diminishing concentrations of chemoattractants, reaching background levels at $10^{-11} - 10^{-12}$ mol/site. At $10^{-9}-10^{-10}$ mol/site a massive neutrophil migration from venules into the surrounding tissue was observed. In the rat skin, however, NAP-2 is approximately three fold less effective than either NAP-1/IL-8 or gro/MGSA-α. It is not known whether this discrepancy is due to an indirect effect, such as proteolytic degradation, or to poor chemotactic potency of human NAP-2 for rat neutrophils.

Possible Role for NAP-2 in Pathophysiology

Whereas the biological effects on neutrophils vary only slightly for NAP-1/IL-8, NAP-2, and gro/MGSA-α, their mode of formation and cellular origin are strikingly different, implying different in vivo roles, under normal and pathological conditions. NAP-1/IL-8 is produced and secreted by mononuclear phagocytes and a variety of tissue cells in response to stimulation with LPS, IL-1 or TNF (for review see [1, 16]). NAP-2, on the other hand, is produced by the proteolytic processing of inactive precursors released from platelet alpha granules. Normal plasma levels of platelet release products such as PBP and CTAP-III are probably too low to serve as a precursor pool for NAP-2 formation. However, one might expect much higher local concentrations of such peptides under conditions where thrombi are formed and blood flow is reduced, thus facilitating the development of focal intravascular inflammatory sites.

NAP-2 could conceivably play a role in thrombolysis. The presence of neutrophils in platelet aggregates suggests the presence of chemoattractants. Furthermore, it was recently demonstrated that activated platelets translocate GMP-140 to the surface, where it may serve to anchor neutrophils [17]. In addition, NAP-1/IL-8 (and possibly also NAP-2) upregulates the leukocyte adhesion receptor CD11b/CD18 (CR3) on human neutrophils [18]. This receptor not only recognizes ligands on endothelial cells but also binds to fibrinogen [19], thus providing another potential anchor of the neutrophil to the thrombus. Neutrophils can degrade thrombi by the release of proteases such as urokinase plasminogen activator and elastase, and thus facilitate the recanalization of an obstructed vessel.

NAP-2 may also contribute to neutrophil activation and subsequent tissue damage caused by neutrophil elastase and reactive oxygen species. Significant NAP-2 formation might occur under conditions of increased platelet activation. High levels of "β-thromboglobulin" and PF-4 have been observed in the serum of patients with hemostatic failure after cardiopulmonary bypass surgery [20, 21] and in bronchoalveolar lavage fluids of patients with the adult respiratory distress syndrome (ARDS) [22, 23]. In both cases the levels of

β-thromboglobulin correlated with the severity of the tissue damage attributed to neutrophil activation.

Since the two prerequisites for NAP-2 formation, activated neutrophils and platelets, frequently occur together, the potential exists for the involvement of NAP-2 in a wide variety of pathophysiological conditions, ranging from wound healing to atherosclerosis.

References

1. Baggiolini M, Walz A, Kunkel SL (1989) Neutrophil-activating peptide-1/interleukin 8, a novel cytokine that activates neutrophils. J Clin Invest 84:1045–1049
2. Holt JC, Harris ME, Holt AM, Lange E, Henschen A, Niewiarowski S (1986) Characterization of human platelet basic protein, a precursor form of low-affinity platelet factor 4 and beta-thromboglobulin. Biochemistry 25:1988–1996
3. Castor CW, Miller JW, Walz DA (1983) Structural and biological characteristics of connective tissue activating peptide (CTAP-III), a major human platelet derived growth factor. Proc Natl Acad Sci USA 80:765–769
4. Anisowicz A, Bardwell L, Sager R (1987) Constitutive overexpression of a growth-regulated gene in transformed Chinese hamster and human cells. Proc Natl Acad Sci USA 84:7188–7192
5. Haskill S, Peace A, Morris J, Sporn SA, Anisowicz A, Lee SW, Smith T, Martin G, Ralph P, Sager R (1990) Identification of three related human GRO genes encoding cytokine functions. Proc Natl Acad Sci USA 87:7732–7736
6. Deuel TF, Keim PS, Farmer M, Heinrikson RL (1977) Amino acid sequence of human platelet factor 4. Proc Natl Acad Sci USA 74:2256–2258
7. Luster AD, Ravetch JV (1987) Biochemical characterization of a gamma interferon-inducible cytokine (IP-10). J Exp Med 166:1084–1097
8. Walz A, Dewald B, von Tscharner V, Baggiolini M (1989) Effects of the neutrophil-activating peptide NAP-2, platelet basic protein, connective tissue activating peptide III and platelet factor 4 on human neutrophils. J Exp Med 170:1745–1750
9. Walz A, Baggiolini M (1989) A novel cleavage product of beta-thromboglobulin formed in cultures of stimulated mononuclear cells activates human neutrophils. Biochem Biophys Res Commun 159:969–975
10. Walz A, Baggiolini M (1990) Generation of the neutrophil-activating peptide NAP-2 from platelet basic protein or connective tissue-activating peptide III through monocyte proteases. J Exp Med 171:449–454
11. Car BD, Baggiolini M, Walz A (1991) Formation of neutrophil-activating peptide 2 from connective tissue-activating peptide III by different proteases. Biochem J (in press)
12. Deuel TF, Senior RM, Chang D, Griffin GL, Heinrikson RL, Kaiser ET (1981) Platelet factor 4 is chemotactic for neutrophils and monocytes. Proc Natl Acad Sci USA 78:4584–4587
13. Moser B, Clark-Lewis I, Zwahlen R, Baggiolini M (1990) Neutrophil-activating properties of the melanoma growth-stimulatory activity. J Exp Med 171:1797–1802
14. Dewald B, Payne TG, Baggiolini M (1984) Activation of NADPH oxidase of human neutrophils. Potentiation of chemotactic peptide by a diacylglycerol. Biochem Biophys Res Commun 125:367–373
15. Walz A, Meloni F, Clark-Lewis I, von Tscharner V, Baggiolini M (1991) [Ca^{2+}]$_i$ changes and respiratory burst in human neutrophils and monocytes induced by NAP-1/IL-8, NAP-2 and gro/MGSA. J Leukocyte Biol (in press)
16. Matsushima K, Oppenheim JJ (1989) Interleukin 8 and MCAF: novel inflammatory cytokines inducible by IL 1 and TNF. Cytokine 1:2–13
17. Hamburger SA, McEver RP (1990) Gmp-140 mediates adhesion of stimulated platelets to neutrophils. Blood 75 (3):550–554
18. Detmers PA, Olsen-Egbert E, Peveri P, Walz A, Baggiolini M, Cohn ZA (1989) Neutrophil activating factor (NAF) enhances the binding activity of CD11b/CD18. FASEB J 3:A1087–A1087

19. Wright SD, Weitz JI, Huang AJ, Levin SM, Silverstein SC, Loike JD (1988) Complement receptor type three (CD11b/CD18) of human polymorphonuclear leukocytes recognizes fibrinogen. J Exp Med 171:1155–1162
20. Wachtfogel YT, Kucich U, Greenplate J, Gluszko P, Abrams W, Weinbaum G, Wenger RK, Rucinski B, Niewiarowski S, Edmunds LH Jr et al. (1987) Human neutrophil degranulation during extracorporeal circulation. Increased anticoagulation during cardiopulmonary bypass by aprotinin. Blood 69:324–330
21. Van Oeveren W, Kazatchkine MD, Descamps Latscha B, Maillet F, Fischer E, Carpentier A, Wildevuur CR (1985) Deleterious effects of cardiopulmonary bypass a prospective study of bubble versus membrane oxygenation. J Thorac Cardiovasc Surg 89:888–899
22. Idell S, Maunder R, Fein AM, Switalska HI, Tuszynski GP, McLarty J. Niewiarowski S (1989) Platelet-specific alpha-granule proteins and thrombospondin in bronchoalveolar lavage in the adult respiratory distress syndrome. Chest 96:1125–1132
23. Idell S, Kucich U, Fein A, Kueppers F, James HL, Walsh PN Weinbaum G, Colman RW, Cohen AB (1985) Neutrophil elastase-releasing factors in bronchoalveolar lavage from patients with adult respiratory distress syndrome. Am Rev Respir Dis 132:1098–1105

Soluble and Cell Surface Receptors for Tumor Necrosis Factor

H. Engelmann[1], D. Aderka[2], Y. Nophar[1], O. Kemper[1], C. Brakebusch[1], H. Holtmann[3], and D. Wallach[1]

Introduction

Tumor necrosis factor (TNF) represents a remarkable example for the dichotomic nature which characterizes some molecules classified as cytokines. No other cytokine combines such enormous beneficial and detrimental potential. Discovered initially as a serum factor with dramatic antitumor effects [1], TNF eventually emerged as the mediator with a wide spectrum of activities. Activation of neutrophils and vascular endothelium, induction of major histocompatibility complex (MHC) antigens, supresion of lipogenesis, increased procoagulatory activity and bone erosion, stimulation of fibroblast growth and increased production of proinflammatory compounds like prostaglandins are just some of TNF's multiple effects [2]. In vivo this plethora of TNF effects combines to give the multi-facetted picture of inflammation resulting in increased host resistance against various pathogens [3–5] or the destruction of tumors. However, TNF appears also to be a molecule with exceptional capacity for harm. It seems to play a key role in the pathogenesis of endotoxin shock [6], fatal bacterial meningitis [7], graft versus host disease [8], and cerebral malaria [9]. The tissue damage caused by this cytokine may even cause the death of the host.

The paradox that a molecule meant for the elimination of pathogens mediates even more damage to the host has raised enormous interest in finding approaches to influence the action of TNF. Aiming at rational and effective ways of manipulating TNF's effects, we tried to gain detailed knowledge of the mechanisms by which the organism controls the function of TNF. Our studies indicate that the two TNF receptors play a central role in the natural regulation of TNF function. Both receptors exist in a soluble and a membrane-associated form. This dual mode of molecular existence opens many interesting possibilities by which the TNF receptors may contribute to producing the exceptionally large spectrum of in vivo and in vitro responses to TNF. Some of these possibilities are addressed experimentally and discussed in this study.

---

[1] Department of Molecular Genetics and Virology, Weizmann Institute of Science, Rehovot, Israel
[2] Department of Medicine T, Ichilov Hospital, Tel-Aviv, Israel
[3] School of Medicine, Hanover, FRG

Host Defense Dysfunction
in Trauma, Shock and Sepsis
Eds. Faist/Meakins/Schildberg
© Springer-Verlag, Berlin Heidelberg 1993

Results and Discussion

Soluble TNF Receptors as TNF Antagonists

As central molecules in the pathways initiating the cellular responses to TNF, the cell surface receptors for TNF (TNF-Rs) were a preferred target of cytokine research. Yet the low abundance of the TNF-Rs precluded their detailed analysis. The isolation and characterization of the TNF-Rs resulted eventually from research efforts aiming at a different goal. The simultaneous search of three groups for naturally occuring TNF antagonists led to the discovery of two previously unknown proteins which inhibited the cytotoxicity of TNF in vitro (see Fig. 1) [10–13]. These proteins, which are found in minute amounts in human urine, exerted their effect by high-affinity binding to TNF. Accordingly, they were called TNF binding proteins (TBP I and TBP II).

First experimental evidence that the two TNF binding proteins found in human urine were actually soluble forms of two cell surface TNF-Rs came from studies demonstrating their immunological relationship [13]. Rabbit antisera against the TBPs inhibited the binding of TNF to its cell surface receptors. Furthermore, the antisera immunoprecipitated the TNF-Rs extracted from HeLa or U937 cells; each antiserum recognized one of the two receptors (see Fig. 2).

Molecular cloning of the two cDNAs encoding the type I and type II TNF-Rs with the help of nucleotide probes deduced from amino acid sequence data of the TBPs finally reconfirmed that the TNF binding proteins were soluble forms of the TNF-Rs [14–16].

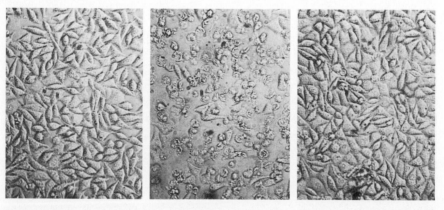

Fig. 1. Inhibition of TNF cytotoxicity by soluble TNF-R *Left*, control A9 cells treated for 14 h with cycloheximide only (CHI, 50 µg/ml). *Middle*, dead cells after treatment with recombinant TNF-α (5 U/ml) + CHI. *Right*, cells treated with TNF + CHI in the presence of urine-derived soluble TNF-Rs [12].

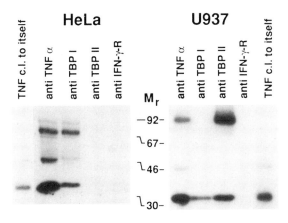

Fig. 2. Immunoprecipitation of the TNF-Rs using antisera against two urinary TNF binding proteins. ^{125}I-TNF was crosslinked with bis(sulfosuccinimidyl) suberate (BS^3) to the cell surface receptors of HeLa or U937 cells. Detergent extracts (1% Triton X 100) of the cells were incubated with rabbit antiserum to TBP I, TBP II, TNF, or the interferor-γ receptor, all at dilutions of 1:100, followed by precipitation of the immunecomplexes with protein A beads. The precipitated proteins were analyzed by sodium dodecylsulfate polyacrylamide gel electrophoresis (SDS PAGE) on a 7.5% acrylamide gel. For comparison, BS^3-treated TNF was analyzed in the same way [34]

Structural Features of the TNF-Rs

Cloning of the cDNAs encoding for the two TNF-Rs, achieved by several groups in parallel [14, 15, 17, 18], permitted a detailed structural analysis of the two TNF-Rs. Both receptors are glycoproteins with predicted molecular sizes of 58 kDa (type I TNF-R) and 75 kDa (type II TNF-R). Both receptors show molecular partition into extracellular, hydrophobic transmembrane, and intracellular domains. Neither the intracellular nor the transmembrane domains of the two receptors appear to be related. However, their extracellular domains share common molecular architecture. Computer-aided sequence analysis demonstrated that the extracellular domains of both receptors consist of four repeating segments in which the cystein residues are found in highly conserved positions (Fig. 3a). No conclusion about the signal transduction mechanisms of either TNF-R could be drawn from the structural characteristics of the intracellular domains. Sequence motifs like Gly-x-Gly-x-x-Gly, known to characterize protein kinases and various nucleotide binding proteins [19], are not present in the intracellular domains of the TNF-Rs. This suggested that the TNF-Rs transduce their signals either via a presently unknown pathway or that both receptors require additional associated proteins which couple them to known second messenger systems.

Both membrane TNF-Rs exist in corresponding soluble forms (Fig. 3a). Amino acid sequence comparison of the urine-derived soluble TNF-Rs with

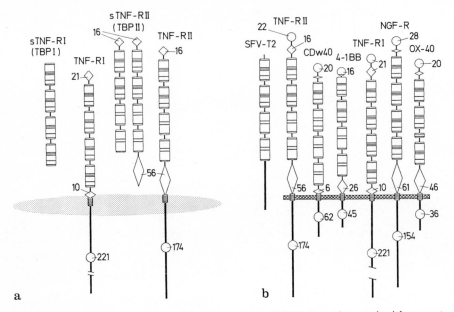

Fig. 3a. Schematic presentation of soluble and cell surface TNF-R. Repeating cystein-rich segments in the extracellular domains are *boxed*. Cysteins are symbolized by *horizontal lines*. *Circles* symbolize leader sequences, *diamonds* other non homologous parts. Inserted *numbers* indicate the size in amino acid residues. **b** The TNF-NGF receptor family

their cell surface form show identity between the soluble TNF-Rs and large parts of the extracellular domains of the cell surface TNF-Rs [15]. Thus the soluble TNF-R I matches exactly the four cystein-rich repeats characterizing the extracellular domain of this receptor (unpublished data, Fig. 3a). The soluble TNF-R II seems to exist in two molecular forms. The 30-kDa form present in human urine appears identical to the four cystein-rich repeats of the type II TNF-R. A recently discovered 40-kDa form of the type II TNF-R [16] apparently corresponds to the complete extracellular domain of this receptor.

The unique architecture of the extracellular domain of the two TNF-Rs classifies them as members of a new family of proteins (Fig. 3b). One member of particular interest is the nerve growth factor (NGF) receptor [20]. Other molecules sharing the structural characteristics of this family are three receptors with yet unknown ligands: CDw40 [21], a B cell antigen, and two proteins which are expressed on activated T lymphocytes, 4-1 BB [22] and OX-40 [23]. An unusual relative of the TNF-Rs is the T2 protein in the shope fibroma virus (SFV) genome [24]. Besides having remarkable homology with the TNF-R II, this protein was reported to bind TNF with high affinity [25]. Whether or not this protein is part of a specific escape mechanism of SFV-infected cells from TNF-mediated destruction is as yet unclear.

Mechanism of Production of Soluble (TNF-Rs)

The suggested regulatory role of the soluble TNF-Rs as TNF antagonists gives central importance to the mechanism of soluble TNF-R formation and the regulation of this process. Three possible modes of production for the soluble forms of the TNF-Rs can be considered: (1) Soluble and cell surface form may be encoded by two different genes. (2) The two receptor forms may be translated from two different mRNAs produced from one gene by alternative splicing, as suggested for the soluble interleukin-4 (IL-4) and IL-7 receptors [26, 27]. (3) Proteolytic cleavage of the cell surface TNF-Rs may occur. Our studies indicate, at least for the soluble TNF-R I, that the last mechanism is the most likely one [15]. Northern blot analysis did not reveal transcripts smaller than the full size of the TNF-R I cDNA in any of the cells examined. Even in HT-29 cells which constitutively produce the soluble TNF-R I no additional mRNA could be detected. Furthermore, CHO cells transfected with the cDNA for the complete TNF-R I in a suitable expression vector express not only the membranous but also the soluble TNF-R, meaning that the full-length transcript encodes both forms.

The information on the regulation of the production of the soluble TNF-Rs is limited. A recent study indicates that the formation of the soluble TNF-Rs can be subject to effective enhancement by specific stimuli [28]. Stimulation of human neutrophils with N-formyl-Met-Leu-Phe was found to result within minutes in an extensive decrease of the cell surface expressed TNF-R and an accompanying release of soluble TNF-Rs. Protein phosphorylation may play a role in the activation of TNF-R shedding since phorbol esters also trigger this process. A study examining the regulation of cell surface expression of the colony stimulating factor receptor (CSF-R) also indicates that receptor shedding may be controlled by the activity of certain kinases [29].

Possible Role of the soluble TNF-Rs as Regulators of TNF Function in vivo

Although there is still little evidence that receptor shedding is indeed a specific mechanism serving in vivo for the control of the respective ligand, it seems unlikely that the soluble TNF-Rs are just waste products without biological function. To gain further information on the physiological role of the soluble TNF-Rs we examined human serum for their presence. Using immunoasays (ELISA) for both TNF-Rs we found, for 40 healthy control individuals, mean serum levels of 0.8 ± 0.2 ng/ml for soluble TNF-R I and 3.2 ± 0.6 ng/ml for soluble TNF-R II. Significant increases of 10- to 100-fold were found in the serum of patients with various inflammatory and noninflammatory disorders, surprisingly also in patients with different malignancies (Table 1) [30] ([30] and Aderka et al., unpublished data). Elevated TNF-R serum levels correlated with the TNF neutralizing capacity of the respective serum, suggesting that the

Table 1. Disorders with elevated serum levels of soluble TNF-R I and TNF-R II

Infectious inflammatory disorders	Autoimmune diseases	Malignancies
Sepsis/septic shock Malaria	Systemic lupus erythematosus (30)	Solid tumors (e.g., colon carcinoma [31] -Leukemia (e.g., CLL)

soluble TNF-Rs antagonize TNF also in vivo [30]. Studies of the extent of correlation between soluble TNF-R serum levels and disease severity are currently in progress. An as yet unresolved question is also the source of the soluble TNF-Rs in the examined disease states.

Neutralization of ligand effects is not the only possible regulatory function of a soluble receptor. As demonstrated by the soluble IL-6 receptors, soluble receptors may as well enhance ligand activities [31]. More importantly, the interaction between the ligand and its soluble receptor most likely changes the pharmacological behavior of the ligand. Decreased biological clearance rate of the receptor-ligand complex or altered availability of the receptor-bound ligand to degradation processes may also be part of the biological function of the soluble receptor. Enhancement of TNF effects by soluble TNF-Rs is observed for effects which require continuous presence of TNF for longer periods, like the acceleration of fibroblast growth (D. Aderka, unpublished observations). Apparently, the soluble TNF-Rs protect the biologically active TNF trimer from decomposition.

Receptor shedding represents a powerful alternative to receptor internalization as a mechanism of receptor downregulation. The receptorless state would result in inability of the target cell to respond to the respective ligand. Assuming that the shed soluble receptors neutralize the ligand, one may postulate a supplementary function of the soluble TNF-Rs in the induction of the TNF-refractory state. Studies on the autoregulatory role of TNF demonstrate that TNF itself, as well as IL-1, may induce irresponsiveness to the toxic effects of TNF in vivo and in vitro [32]. TNF inhibition by soluble TNF-Rs could contribute to these phenomena.

The TNF-Rs as Signal Transducing Elements

The absolute requirement for TNF-Rs for the induction of TNF effects has been a matter of controversy. One suggestion was that TNF itself triggered the intracellular events which initiate the response to TNF, assigning the TNF-Rs the role of shuttle molecules transporting TNF into the cell's interior [33]. However, studies with ligand mimetic antibodies to the type I TNF-R demonstrated clearly that the initiation of TNF responses is a function of the TNF-Rs [34]. Several effects characteristic of TNF could be mimicked with antibodies directed against the TNF-R I. The antibodies were cytotoxic to TNF-sensitive cells, induced the production of prostaglandin E_2, stimulated the growth of normal fibroblasts, and inhibited the growth of chlamydiae. The capability of anti-TNF-R I antibodies to induce TNF-like effects correlated with their ability to cause aggregation of the TNF-Rs. Thus, monovalent F(ab) fragments of the mimetic antibodies as well as several monoclonal antibodies against the TNF-R I failed to induce TNF-like effects. However, when the F(ab) fragments

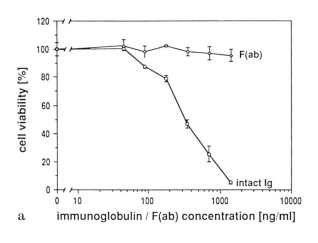

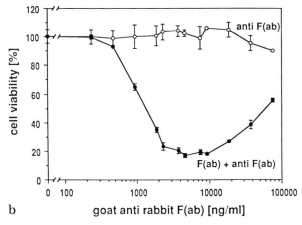

Fig. 4a, b. TNF-like effects of anti-TNF-R I antibodies depend on receptor aggregation. SV80 cells were pretreated at 4 °C with rabbit anti-TNF-R I immunoglobulin or the monovalent F(ab) fragments thereof and then incubated for 16 h at 37 °C, either in the presence or absence of anti-rabbit immunoglobulin antibodies with 50 μg/ml CHI. Viability of the cells was determined by the neutral red uptake method. **a.** □ Anti-TNF-R I + CHI; ○ F(ab) + CHI. **b** ● F(ab) + CHI and anti-Ig; ○ medium + CHI and anti-Ig or the monoclonal antibodies were cross-linked with anti-immunoglobulin antibodies they regained their biological activity (see Fig. 4). This suggested that induced receptor aggregation is a basic molecular mechanism for the initiation of TNF responses. In view of the trimeric structure of TNF one might even speculate that TNF itself triggers its effects by receptor aggregation. Studies showing that monomeric TNF is biologically less active support such a hypothesis [35].

Summary

The identification of two naturally occuring TNF inhibitors as soluble TNF-Rs enabled the isolation and molecular characterization of the receptors for TNF. Biologically, the two TNF-Rs seem to play an essential role in the regulation of TNF function. In their cell surface form, the TNF-Rs are a prerequisite for the initiation of TNF responses. The soluble TNF-Rs in turn may act as TNF antagonists. Complex changes in the pharmacological behavior of TNF are an expected consequence of the interaction between TNF and the soluble TNF-Rs. Substantial changes in TNF responsiveness may also result from the process of soluble TNF-R production itself: Effective downregulation of the TNF-Rs leads eventually to target cell refractoriness. Depending on the situation, the TNF-Rs may thus trigger or prevent, enhance or antagonize TNF function. These findings outline the TNF-Rs as molecules of central importance for the regulation of TNF function and predestine them as targets for therapeutic manipulations.

References

1. Carswell EA, Old LJ, Fiore N et al. (1975) An endotoxin-induced serum factor that causes necrosis of tumors. Proc Natl Acad Sci USA 72:3666–3670
2. Beutler B, Cerami A (1989) The biology of cachectin/TNF-A primary mediator of host response. Ann Rev Immunol 7:625–655
3. Parant MA, Parant FJ, Chedid LA (1980) Enhancement of resistance to infection by endotoxin induced serum factor from *Mycobacterium bovis* BCG-infected mice. Infect Immunol 28:654–659
4. Taverne J, Matthews N, Depledge P et al. (1984) Malarial parasites and tumor cells are killed by the same component of tumor necrosis serum. Clin Exp Immunol 57:293–300
5. Blanchard DK, Djeu JY, Klein TW et al. (1988) Protective effects of tumor necrosis factor in experimental *Legionella pneumophila* infections in mice via activation of PMN function. J Leukocyte Biol 43:429–435
6. Tracey KJ, Beutler B, Lowry SF et al. (1986) Shock and tissue injury induced by recombinant human cachectin. Science 234:470–474
7. Waage A, Halstensen A, Espevik T (1987) Association between tumor necrosis factor and fatal outcome in patients with meningococcal disease. Lancet 1:355–357
8. Piguet PF, Grau G, Allet B et al. (1987) Tumor necrosis factor (TNF) is an effector of skin and gut lesions of the acute phase of graft-vs. -host disease. J Exp Med 166:1280–1289
9. Grau GE, Fajardo LF, Piguet P-F et al. (1987) Tumor necrosis factor (cachectin) as an essential mediator in murine cerebral malaria. Science 237:1210–1212

10. Olsson I, Lantz M, Nilsson E et al. (1989) Isolation and characterization of a tumor necrosis factor binding protein from urine. Eur J Haematol 42:270–275

11. Seckinger P, Isaaz S, Dayer J-M (1989) Purification and biologic characterization of a specific tumor necrosis factor α inhibitor. J Biol Chem 264:11966–11973

12. Engelmann H, Aderka D, Rubinstein M et al. (1989) A tumor necrosis factor-binding protein purified to homogeneity from human urine protects cells from tumor necrosis factor cytotoxicity. J Biol Chem 264:11974–11980

13. Engelmann H, Novick D, Wallach D (1990) Two tumor necrosis factor-binding proteins purified from human urine. Evidence for immunological cross-reactivity with the cell surface tumor necrosis factor receptors. J Biol Chem 265:1531–1536

14. Schall TJ, Lewis M, Koller KJ et al. (1990) Molecular cloning and expression of a receptor for human tumor necrosis factor. Cell 61:361–370

15. Nophar Y, Kemper O, Brakebusch C et al. (1990) Soluble forms of tumor necrosis factor receptors (TNF-Rs). The cDNA for the type I TNF-R cloned using amino acid data of its soluble form, encodes for both the cell surface and a soluble form of the receptor. EMBO J 9:3269–3278

16. Kohno T, Brewer MT, Baker SL et al. (1990) a Second tumor necrosis factor receptor gene product can shed a naturally occurring tumor necrosis factor inhibitor. Proc Natl Acad Sci USA 87:8331–8335

17. Loetscher H, Pan Y-CE, Lahm H-W et al. (1990) Molecular cloning and expression of the human 55 kd tumor necrosis factor receptor. Cell 61:351–359

18. Smith CA, Davis T, Anderson D et al. (1990) A receptor for tumor necrosis factor defines an unusual family of cellular and viral proteins. Science 248:1019–1023

19. Kamps MP, Taylor SS, Seflon BM (1984) Direct evidence that oncogenic tyrosine kinases and cyclic AMP-dependent protein kinases have homologous ATP-binding sites. Nature 310:589–591

20. Johnson D, Lanahan A, Buck CR et al. (1986) Expression and structure of the human NGF receptor. Cell 47:545–554

21. Stamenkovic I, Clark EA, Seed B (1989) A B-lymphocyte activation molecule related to the nerve growth factor receptor and induced by cytokines in carcinomas. EMBO J 8:1403–1410

22. Kwon BS, Weissman SM (1989) cDNA sequences of two inducible T-cell genes. Proc Natl Acad Sci USA 86:1963–1967

23. Mallet S, Fossum S, Barcley AN (1990) Characterization of the MRC OX40 antigen of activated CD4 positive T lymphocytes—a molecule related to nerve growth factor receptor. EMBO J 9:1063–1068

24. McFadden G (1988) in: Darai G (ed) Viral diseases in laboratory and captive animals. Nijhoff, Boston, pp 37–62

25. Smith CA, Davis T, Wignal J et al. (1990) T2 open reading frame from shope fibroma virus (SFV) encodes a soluble form of the human type I TNF receptor. Lymphokine Res 9:584

26. Mosley B, Beckmann MP, March CJ et al. (1989) The murine interleukin-4 receptor: molecular cloning and characterization of secreted and membrane bound forms. Cell 59:335–348

27. Goodwin RG, Friend D, Ziegler SF et al. (1990) Cloning of the human and murine interleukin-7 receptors: demonstration of a soluble form and homology to a new receptor superfamily. Cell 60:941–951

28. Porteu F, Nathan C (1990) Shedding of tumor necrosis factor receptors by activated human neutrophils. J Exp Med 17:599–607

29. Downing JR, Roussel MF, Sherr CJ (1989) Ligand and protein kinase C downmodulate the colony-stimulating-factor 1 receptor by independent mechanisms. Mol Cell Biol 9:2890–2896

30. Aderka D, Engelmann H, Hornik V et al. (1991) Increased serum levels of soluble receptors for tumor necrosis factor in cancer patients. Cancer Res (in press)

31. Taga T, Hibi M, Hirata Y et al. (1989) Interleukin-6 triggers the association of its receptor with a possible signal transducer, gp130. Cell 58:573–581

32. Wallach D, Holtmann H, Engelmann H et al. (1988) Sensitization and desensitization to lethal effects of tumor necrosis factor and IL-1. J Immunol 140:2994–2999

33. Smith MR, Munger WE, Kung H-F et al. (1990) Direct evidence for an intracellular role for tumor necrosis factor-α. J Immunol 144:162–169

34. Engelmann H, Holtmann, H, Brakebusch C et al. (1990) Antibodies to a soluble form of a tumor necrosis factor receptor have TNF-like activity. J Biol Chem 265:14497–14504

35. Smith RA, Baglioni C (1987) The active form of tumor necrosis factor is a trimer. J Biol Chem 262:6951–6954

Regulation of Cytokine Synthesis Through Cyclic Nucleotides*

S. Endres, H. J. Fülle, B. Sinha, D. Stoll, and R. Gerzer

Recent studies have shown that the addition of phosphodiesterase inhibitors to mouse macrophages can suppress tumor necrosis factor (TNF) production [1, 2] putatively by raising the intracellular concentration of cyclic 3',5'-adenosine monophosphate cAMP [3]. Our current studies addressed three questions: First, is there a suppressive effect of phosphodiesterase inhibitors on TNF production by monocytes of human origin? Second, is this effect specific for TNF or does it also affect the synthesis of other cytokines such as interleukin-1β (IL-1β)? And third, is the effect of phosphodiesterase inhibitors on cytokine production mediated by accumulation of cAMP levels alone or also of cyclic 3',5'-guanosine monophosphate (cGMP) levels?

Human peripheral blood mononuclear cells (MNC) were stimulated by the addition of lipopolysaccharide (LPS; *E. coli* 055:B5, Sigma, Munich Fig. 1). Within 1 min after LPS, various agents were added, such as theophylline or pentoxifylline (Albert-Roussel, Wiesbaden, FRG), prostaglandin E$_2$ (PGE$_2$, Sigma) or 3-morpholinosydnonimine (SIN 1, Cassella-Riedel AG, Frankfurt Main, FRG). Incubation of one of the duplicate tubes was terminated after 1 h for determination of cGMP and cAMP; incubation of the other tube was terminated after 20 h for determination of TNF and IL-1β.

TNF [3] and IL-1β[4] were determined by specific radioimmunoassays (RIA) as previously described. cAMP and cGMP were measured by RIA after ethanol extraction as previously described [5]. Theophylline exhibited a dose-dependent suppression of TNF production induced by LPS 100 ng/ml in human MNC [6]. TNF synthesis was suppressed to 50% of control by about 200 μM and was maximally suppressed by 1000 μM theophylline (Fig. 2). By contrast, synthesis of IL-1β was unaffected by theophylline doses as high as 1000 μM. Pentoxifylline, another phosphodiesterase inhibitor, was effective at even lower concentrations, reaching half-maximal suppression at about 80 μM. Addition of PGE$_2$ 1000 ng/ml to MNC stimulated with LPS 1000 ng/ml also suppressed TNF production by 85% with production of IL-1β not significantly affected.

Cyclic nucleotide levels were unchanged after incubation with LPS alone. Addition of pentoxifylline led to a dose-dependent rise in total cAMP. In

* Supported by a grant from the Deutsche Forschungsgemeinschaft (En 169/2-2). H. J. Fülle was a scholar of the Boehringer-Ingelheim Fond.
Medizinische Klinik, Klinikum Innenstadt der Universität München, Ziemssenstr.1, 8000 Munich 2, FRG

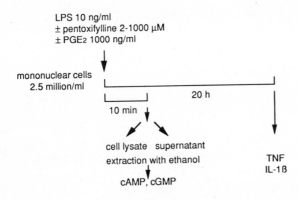

Fig. 1. Experimental protocol for the simultaneous measurement of cyclic nucleotides and cytokines formed in LPS-stimulated MNC

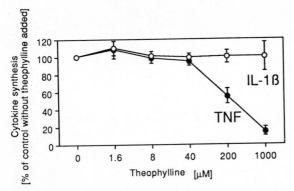

Fig. 2. Suppression of LPS-induced synthesis of TNF but not of IL-1β by theophylline

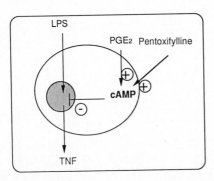

Fig. 3. Probable mechanisms of suppression of TNF synthesis by pentoxifylline or PGE_2

contrast, the concentration of cGMP changed only marginally, independent of considering intracellular, extracellular, or total cGMP. Also, the PGE_2-induced suppression of TNF production was accompained by a marked increase of total cAMP.

Thus, the observed effect of phosphodiesterase inhibitors appears to be mediated by an increase of intracellular cAMP concentration (Fig. 3) since (a) addition of phosphodiesterase inhibitors leads to a marked increase of cAMP,

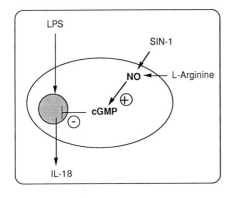

Fig. 4. Possible mechanism of suppression of IL-1β synthesis via No. No is added exogenously by addition of the NO donar SIN 1 or formed endogenously after addition of L-arginine

while cGMP is only marginally elevated; (b) raising cAMP by induction with PGE$_2$ leads to the same suppression of TNF production; and (c) raising cGMP with SIN 1 does not inhibit TNF synthesis (see below).

A suppressive effect of phosphodiesterase inhibitors on TNF production by mouse macrophages has been reported in previous studies. Renz et al. [1] found that TNF production was decreased by 90% using 1000 µM theophylline. Strieter et al.[2] compared the effect of different phosphodiesterase inhibitors on TNF production and identified pentoxifylline as the most potent agent.

As a tool for studying the effect of cGMP on cytokine synthesis we used the compound 3-morpholino-sydnonimine (SIN 1). SIN 1 is the active metabolite of the clinically used drug molsidomine. SIN 1 spontaneously releases nitric oxide (NO), which stimulates soluble guanylate cyclase and increases cGMP formation.

Addition of SIN 1 (100 µM) to LPS-stimulated MNC indeed increased the levels of cGMP. This resulted in a decreased production of IL-1β, while synthesis of TNF was unaffected. The suppression was detectable at all concentrations of LPS studied [7]. To further elucidate this phenomenon we also investigated whether endogenously formed NO (from L-arginine) would exert the same effect on IL-1β synthesis. We found that addition of L-arginine to L-arginine-free medium reduced the amount of LPS-induced IL-1β in MNC [8]. In summary, it appears that cGMP acts as a negative signal in the induction of IL-1β synthesis (Fig. 4).

Acknowledgements. The authors thank Dr. S. E. Graber (Nashville, TN, USA) for providing antibodies to cAMP and cGMP and Dr. Charles A. Dinarello for providing antiserum to IL-1β and TNF.

References

1. Renz H, Gong JH, Schmidt A, Nain N, Gemsa D (1988) Release of tumor necrosis factor-α from macrophages. Enhancement and suppression are dose-dependently regulated by prostaglandin E$_2$ and cyclic nucleotides. J Immunol 141:2388–2393

2. Strieter RM, Remick DG, Ward PA, Spengler RN, Lynch III JP, Larrick J, Kunkel SL (1988) Cellular and molecular regulation of tumor necrosis factor-alpha production by pentoxifylline. Biochem Biophys Res Comm 155:1230–1236

3. van der Meer JWM, Endres S, Lonnemann G, Cannon JG, Ikejima T, Okusawa S, Gelfand JA, Dinarello CA (1988) Concentrations of immunoreactive human tumor necrosis factor alpha produced by human mononuclear cells in vitro. J Leukocyte Biol 43:216–223

4. Endres S, Ghorbani R, Lonnemann G, van der Meer JWM, Dinarello CA(1988) Measurement of immunoreactive interleukin-1β from human mononuclear cells: optimization of recovery, intra-subject consistency and comparison with interleukin-1α and tumor necrosis factor. Clin Immunol Immunopathol 49:424–438

5. Heim JM, Gottmann K, Weil J, Haufe MC, Gerzer (1988) Is cyclic GMP a clinically useful marker for ANF action? Z Kardiol 77 [Suppl 2]:41–46

6. Endres S, Fülle HJ, Sinha B, Stoll D, Dinarello CA, Gerzer R, Weber PC (1991) Cyclic nucleotides differentially regulate the synthesis of tumor necrosis factor-α and interleukin-1β in human mononuclear cells. Immunology 72:56–60

7. Fülle HJ, Endres S, Sinha B, Stoll D, Weber PC, Gerzer R (1991) Effects of SIN-1 on cytokine synthesis in human mononuclear cells. J Cardiovasc Pharmacol 17 (Suppl. 3):in press

8. Fülle HJ, Harings R, Stoll D, Sinha B, Endres S, Gerzer R (1991) L-arginine stereo specifically modulates production of interleukin-1β and tumor necrosis factor-α in human mononuclear cells (abstract) FASEB J in press

Removal of Circulating Cytokines by Hemodialysis Membranes In Vitro

G. Lonnemann[1], R. Schindler[1], C. A. Dinarello[2], and K. M. Koch[1]

Introduction

The cytokines interleukin-1 (IL-1α and IL-1β) and tumor necrosis factor alpha (TNFα) produced by activated mononuclear leukocytes are important mediators of the host response to infection and injury [1]. As IL-1β and TNFα act synergistically in the induction of a shock-like state after intravenous injection into laboratory animals [2], these cytokines are likely to be involved in the pathogenesis of septic shock. During experimental fever induced by intravenous injection of endotoxin into humans, serum levels of TNFα [3] and IL-1β [4] are elevated. Recent publications reported elevated circulating concentrations of IL-1β and TNFα in children with severe infectious purpura [5] and in patients with meningococcal infection [6] or septic shock [4]. The latter studies also describe a correlation between plasma TNFα concentrations and severity of disease. As the highest levels of TNFα were found in patients who died these studies suggest that the reduction in circulating cytokines could be beneficial to critically ill patients.

We have previously demonstrated that hemodialysis membranes, depending on their physical and chemical compositions, are able to bind and clear human monocyte-derived IL-1 and iodinated IL-1α added to protein-free tissue culture medium which was recirculated in a closed loop in vitro dialysis system [7]. We have now extended these studies using a modification of the previously described dialysis model [7] in order to better simulate the in vivo situation. Instead of using protein-free media, the blood compartment (Fig. 1) contained heparinized donor blood. In the first set of experiments, iodinated recombinant IL-1α or TNFα was added to the blood and the time-dependent distribution of these cytokines was studied in the closed loop dialysis system, in which diffusion is the predominant transport mechanism across the dialyzer membrane. In the second part, whole blood was prestimulated with endotoxin for 12 h and recirculated in the blood compartment; plasma concentrations of natural, immunoreactive IL-1β and TNFα were measured during in vitro hemodialysis.

[1] Department of Nephrology, Hanover School of Medicine, 3000 Hanover 61, FRG
[2] Department of Medicine, New England Medical Center Hospital and Tufts University School of Medicine, Boston, MA 02111, USA

Host Defense Dysfunction
in Trauma, Shock and Sepsis
Eds. Faist/Meakins/Schildberg
© Springer-Verlag, Berlin Heidelberg 1993

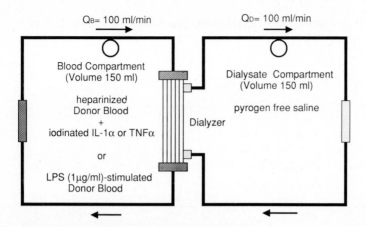

Fig. 1. The in vitro hemodialysis system. The *arrows* indicate the direction of flow in the two compartments. Q_B, blood flow; Q_D, dialysate flow.

Materials and Methods

Iodination of Human Recombinant IL-1α and TNFα

Recombinant human IL-1α (kindly supplied by Dr. Peter Lomedico, Hoffmann La Roche, Nutley, NJ, USA) and TNFα (kindly supplied by Dr. Alan Shaw, Glaxo, Geneva, Switzerland) were iodinated following the same protocol. Five microgram of protein was labeled with 0.5 mCi ^{125}I (New England Nuclear, Boston, MA, USA) using 10 µg chloramin T (Sigma) in 0.25 M phosphate buffer, pH = 7.4. Following a reaction time of approximately 20 s, 100 µg sodium metabisulfite (Sigma) was added to stop the reaction. ^{125}I-IL-1α and ^{125}I-TNFα were purified by gel chromatography on two Sephadex G50 columns equilibrated with phosphate-buffered saline containing 0.25% bovine serum albumin. Fractions were collected and two peaks of ^{125}I activity were detected in both fractionations. The first peak contained labeled protein (^{125}I-IL-1α or ^{125}I-TNFα) which was biologically active as determined by standard bioassays (lymphocyte activating factor assay for IL-1α, fibroblast cytotoxicity assay on L929 cells for TNFα). The specific activity of the labeled cytokines was approximately 60 µCi/µg for ^{125}I-IL-1α and 35 µCi/µg for ^{125}I-TNFα. Sodium dodecyl sulfate–polyacrylamide gel electrophoresis and fluorography confirmed the purity of the labeled cytokines.

In vitro Hemodialysis Experiments

We used a closed loop in vitro hemodialysis system as described in Fig. 1. Hollow fiber dialyzers with three different membranes were studied: Cuprammonium (Clirans, Terumo Corp., Tokyo, Japan), AN 69 (Filtral, Hospal Medical Corp., Nuremberg, FRG) and polysulfon (Hemoflow, Fresenius AG, Bad Homburg, FRG). All three dialyzers had a surface area of approximately 1.2 m². Pyrogen-free standard blood tubing sets were aseptically attached to the dialyzers and the blood compartment as well as the dialysate compartment were rinsed with 2 l pyrogen-free saline each. Following the rinsing procedure, the dialysate compartment was filled with pyrogen-free saline (total volume 150 ml) and recirculated with a flow rate of $Q_D = 100$ ml/min. The saline in the blood compartment was replaced by 150 ml freshly drawn, heparinized (10 U/ml) human donor blood which was recirculated with a flow rate of $Q_B = 100$ ml/min. During in vitro hemodialysis for 2 h the dialyzer was kept at 37 °C.

In order to study the ability of the three different dialyzers to remove iodinated cytokines, 20 000 cpm/ml of ^{125}I-IL-1α or ^{125}I-TNFα (equivalent to approximately 500 pg/ml for both cytokines) was added to donor blood circulating in the blood compartment of the closed loop system and the kinetics of distribution of these labeled cytokines were studied during 2 h of in vitro hemodialysis.

The amounts of iodinated IL-1α or TNFα added to the blood compartment at time zero were assigned a value of 100%. The total amount of radioactive IL-1α or TNFα recovered from the blood compartment and the dialysate compartment was calculated by the product of the radioactivity in 1-ml samples and the volume of the fluid in the two compartments. The amount of cytokines was expressed as a percentage of the radioactivity added to the blood at time zero, corrected for sampling loss and volume gain or loss due to ultrafiltration. At each time of measurement (2, 5, 15, 30, 60, and 120 min of in vitro hemodialysis), the total amount of radioactivity recovered from the blood and the dialysate was added and the difference between this sum and 100% (the mass balance error) was assumed to be due to adsorption of IL-1α or TNFα to the dialyzer membrane.

The percentage of adsorbed cytokines at each time of measurement was calculated as follows:

$$\% \text{ membrane bound} = [1 - (BC_t + DC_t)/BC_0] \times 100$$

where BC_t was the total amount of labeled cytokine recovered from the fluid phase of the blood compartment at time t, DC_t the amount of labeled cytokine in the fluid phase of the dialysate compartment at time t, and BC_0 the amount of labeled cytokine added to the blood compartment at time zero.

In the second part of these studies, we stimulated heparinized donor blood with lipopolysaccharide (LPS) from *Escherichia coli* (055:B5; Sigma, 1 μg/ml) for 12 h at 37 °C. Previous studies have demonstrated that after 12 h of whole blood stimulation plasma concentrations of immunoreactive IL-1β and TNFα have reached maximal levels and do not increase further with prolonged incubation time (R. Schindler, unpublished observation). The LPS-stimulated blood was filled into the blood compartment and the time-dependent distribution of immunoreactive cytokines was measured in plasma samples using radioimmunoassays (RIA) for IL-1β [8] and TNFα [9]. For IL-1β determinations plasma samples were extracted by the chloroform method in order to remove plasma components interferring with the RIA [10]. The total amounts of immunoreactive cytokines present in the blood compartment and the dialysate during recirculation as well as the amounts lost by adsorption to the dialyzer were calculated as described previously for iodinated cytokines.

Results

Removal of Iodinated IL-1α and TNFα from Blood During In Vitro Hemodialysis

The distribution of ^{125}I-IL-1α (total amount = 75 ng) in the closed loop system during in vitro hemodialysis with cuprammonium, AN 69, and polysulfon

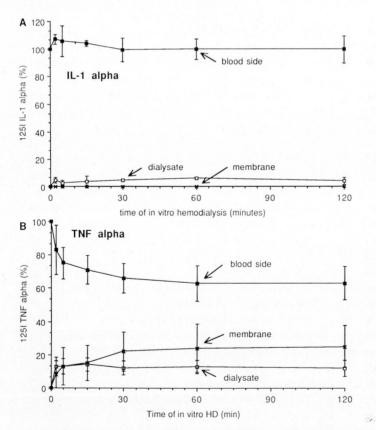

Fig. 2A, B. Time-dependent distribution of **A** ^{125}I-IL-1α and **B** ^{125}I TNFα during 2 h of in vitro hemodialysis (*Hb*) with cuprammonium dialyzers (*n* = 3, mean ± SD). Results are expressed in percent of total TCA-precipitable radioactivity added to the blood compartment at time zero

dialyzers is shown in Figs. 2 and 3 ($n = 3$ for each membrane). When cuprammonium dialyzers were used, there was no loss of radioactivity from the blood compartment and no activity appeared in the dialysate, and therefore no ^{125}I-IL-1α was assumed to be adsorbed to cuprammonium (Fig. 2a). With AN 69 (Fig. 3a), the total amount of ^{125}I-IL-1α in the blood compartment dropped to 25% within 30 min, 25% was detected in the dialysate, and the amount of adsorbed ^{125}I-IL-1α reached 50% within this time. Testing polysulfon (Fig. 3b), the total amount of ^{125}I-IL-1α in the blood compartment dropped to 40%, and 60% of the total was recovered from the dialysate. Since the sum of radioactivity recovered from both compartments was 100%, we assume that no ^{125}I-IL-1α was adsorbed to polysulfon.

In the AN 69 and polysulfon experiments, approximately 95% of the radioactivities recovered from the dialysate compartments, like the activities added to the blood compartments, were precipitable with trichloroacetic acid (TCA). Therefore, the activity recovered from the dialysate was predominantly the intact ^{125}I-IL-1α peptide rather than free iodine.

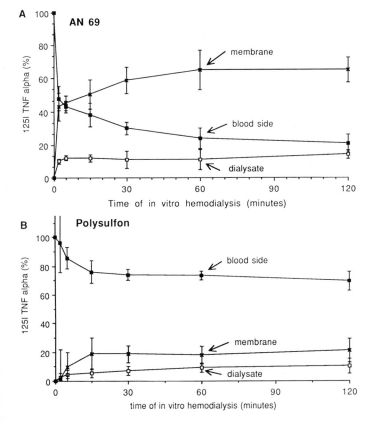

Fig. 3A, B. Time dependent distribution of ^{125}I-IL-1α during 2 h of in vitro hemodialysis with **A** AN 69 and **B** polysulfon dialyzers ($n = 3$, mean $\pm$ SD). Results are expressed in per cent of total TCA-precipitable ^{125}I-IL-1α activity added to the blood compartment at time zero

The distribution curves for ^{125}I-TNFα (total amount = 75 ng) in the closed loop system were slightly different. With cuprammonium dialyzers (Fig. 2b) the amount of ^{125}I-TNFα in the blood compartment dropped to 63% within 60 min of in vitro hemodialysis, 13% of the radioactivity was recovered from the dialysate, and the mass balance error was 24% at this time. During in vitro hemodialysis with AN 69 (Fig. 4a), ^{125}I-TNFα in the blood compartment, like ^{125}I-IL-1α, dropped to 25% within 60 min. However, only 11% of ^{125}I-TNFα (compared to 25% for ^{125}I-IL-1α) was recovered from the dialysate, and so the amount of adsorbed ^{125}I-TNFα was approximately 64%. With polysulfon (Fig. 4b), ^{125}I-TNFα was less effectively removed from the blood than ^{125}I-IL-1α. The amount ^{125}I-TNFα in the blood compartment dropped to 75%, and only very small amounts (8% of total compared to 60% of total ^{125}I-IL-1α) were recovered from the dialysate. The mass balance error and therefore the adsorbed amount of 5[125]I-TNFα was approximately 17%.

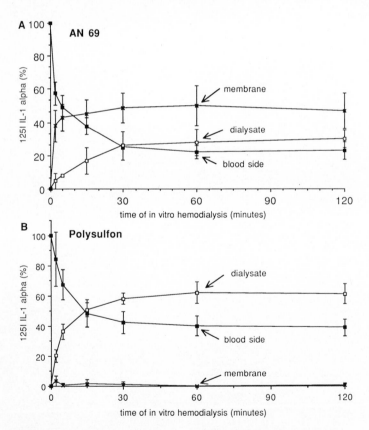

Fig. 4A, B. Time-dependent distribution of ^{125}I-TNFα during 2 h of in vitro hemodialysis with **A** AN 69 and **B** polysulfon dialyzers (*n* = 3, mean ± SD). Results are expressed in percent of total TCA-precipitable ^{125}I-TNFα activity added to the blood compartment at time zero

After in vitro hemodialysis with all three membranes, samples taken from both compartments were subjected to TCA precipitation. Of the ^{125}I-TNFα added to the blood compartments, 85% was TCA precipitable. In contrast, only 15% of the radioactivity detected in the dialysate compartment of AN 69 and polysulfon dialyzers was precipitable by TCA. Counts recovered from the dialysate side of cuprammonium dialyzers were not precipitable. These results indicate that less than 15% of the radioactive substances detected in the dialysate compartments were intact ^{125}I-TNFα.

Removal of LPS-Induced Immunoreactive IL-1β and TNFα from Blood during In Vitro Hemodialysis

The distribution of immunoreactive IL-1β (total amount 1.5 µg) in the closed loop system during in vitro hemodialysis with AN 69 and polysulfon dialyzers is shown in Fig. 5 (the data represent one out of two similar experiments.). With

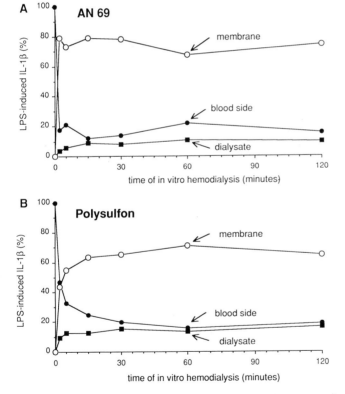

Fig. 5A, B. Time-dependent distribution of LPS-induced immunoreactive IL-1β during 2 h of in vitro hemodialysis with **A** AN 69 and **B** polysulfon dialyzers ($n = 1$). Results are expressed in percent of total IL-1β measured in the blood before start of the recirculation

AN 69 (Fig. 5a), the amount of IL-1β in the blood compartment dropped to 15% within 30 min, 10% was detected in the dialysate, and the amount of adsorbed IL-1β reached 75% within this time. Testing polysulfon (Fig. 6b), the amount of IL-1β in the blood compartment dropped to 20%, and 15% of the total was recovered from the dialysate; consequently, 65% was assumed to be adsorbed to the polysulfon membrane.

The distribution curves for immunoreactive TNFα in the closed loop system were slightly different. During in vitro hemodialysis with AN 69 (Fig. 6a), TNFα in the blood compartment dropped to 12% within 60 min. However, no TNFα (compared to 10% for IL-1β) was recovered from the dialysate, so the amount of adsorbed TNFα was approximately 88%. With polysulfon (Fig. 6b), TNFα was less effectively removed from the blood than IL-1β. The total amount of TNFα in the blood compartment dropped to 40%, and only very small amounts (3% of total compared to 15% of total IL-1β) were recovered from the dialysate. The mass balance error and therefore the amount of TNFα adsorbed to polysulfon was approximately 57%.

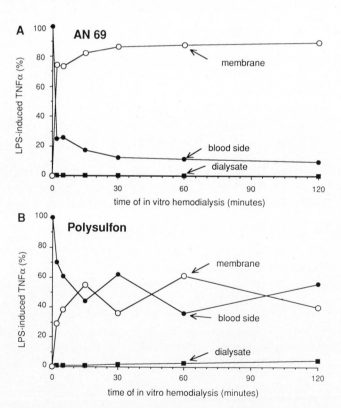

Fig. 6A, B. Time-dependent distribution of LPS-induced immunoreactive TNFα during 2 h of in vitro hemodialysis with **A** AN 69 and **B** polysulfon dialyzers ($n = 1$). Results are expressed in percent of total TNFα measured in the blood before start of the recirculation

Discussion

The results demonstrate that circulating cytokines can be removed from whole blood during hemodialysis. The amount of cytokines removed from the blood compartment depends on the type of dialyzer membrane used in the circuit. With cuprammonium dialyzers only negligible amounts of TNFα or IL-1α were removed. Using dialyzers with highly permeable membranes such as AN 69 and polysulfon which are known to clear substances with a molecular weight of up to 40 000, removal of TNFα, IL-1α, and IL-1β (molecular weights approximately 17 000) during hemodialysis could be expected. However, with the exception of polysulfon, which cleared ^{125}I-IL-1α by diffusion into the dialysate, significant amounts of cytokines disappeared from the blood compartment but were not detectable in the dialysate compartment. Although we did not measure the amount of cytokines bound to the dialyzer and tubings, the only plausible explanation for the observed mass balance error in the closed loop system is adsorption of cytokines to the dialyzer membrane. In particular, the experiments investigating the removal of LPS-induced cytokines suggest that adsorption to highly permeable membranes is the most effective mechanism removing circulating IL-1 and TNFα during hemodialysis. Adsorption to the tubings alone as well as to the cuprammonium membrane seems to be negligible as experiments with cuprammonium dialyzers in the vitro system did not remove any ^{125}I-IL-1α and very little ^{125}I-TNFα from the blood.

In addition to the different membrane effects, cytokine-dependent differences were demonstrated. Although IL-1α, IL-1β, and TNFα are peptides with similar molecular weights, they are handled differently by the two high-flux membranes (polysulfon and AN 69) tested in this study. Both IL-1α and IL-1β penetrate the AN 69 and the polysulfon membranes in significant amounts whereas TNFα does not. Therefore, diffusive clearance in addition to adsorption plays a role during hemodialysis only for IL-1. The mechanism to remove TNFα is almost exclusively adsorption. Because of the higher binding capacity of AN 69 compared to polysulfon under the conditions of closed loop circulation, AN 69 removes more TNFα than polysulfon in our model.

The ability of synthetic dialyzer membranes to adsorb both cytokines is unique but not specific since similar effects have been described for cytochrome C, complement components [11], and β_2-microglobulin [12]. It remains unclear why IL-1, but not TNFα, penetrates these highly permeable membranes. However, differences in the three-dimensional structure of IL-1 and TNFα may be important. IL-1 is an all beta-folded molecule [13] which might facilitate the passage of this molecule through the membrane, whereas the tertiary structure of TNFα is a mixture of beta-sheets and alpha helixes [14]. In addition, it was found that the biologically active form of TNFα is most likely a trimer [15] with an estimated molecular weight of 51 000. Such a large trimeric molecule is likely to be rejected by molecular size exclusion even when highly permeable membranes are used.

The maximal amount of circulating cytokines removable by adsorption to synthetic dialyzer membranes is difficult to estimate using the results of the present study because the adsorptive capacity of both membranes was not saturated. When the total amounts of circulating cytokines were increased from 75 ng (Figs 3, 4) to 1.5 µg (Figs 5, 6) the percentage of cytokines adsorbed (60%–80%) did not decrease as one would expect reaching saturation. Therefore, 1.5 µg (10 ng/ml) TNFα or IL-1β was not sufficient to saturate the adsorptive capacity of AN 69 and polysulfon. On the other hand, with lower amounts of circulating cytokines (75 ng = 0.5 ng/ml) adsorption did not reach 100%. These data suggest that over a wide range of cytokine levels in blood (0.5–10 ng/ml), adsorbed cytokines are equilibrated with circulating levels with a constant percentage of 60%–80% being removed by adsorption.

With regard to the in vivo situation in treating patients with severe sepsis, who have been reported to have plasma TNFα and IL-1β levels of up to 500 pg/ml [4], one could speculate that hemodialysis with cytokine-adsorbing dialyzers could reduce these levels to 100–200 pg/ml, which is still above normal (≤ 50–70 pg/ml) [4]. Further reduction of circulating cytokines to normal levels would require replacement of the cytokine-adsorbing dialyzer in the extracorporal blood circuit, because equilibration between adsorbed and circulating cytokines is complete within 15 min of blood contact to the membrane. These speculations are based on constant circulating cytokine concentrations, which cannot be assumed during ongoing sepsis. Therefore, in vivo evaluations are required to prove or disprove a beneficial effect of hemodialysis with cytokine-adsorbing dialyzers in the treatment of septic shock.

Acknowledgments. The authors thank Dr. Peter Lomedico (Hoffmann La Roche) and Dr. Alan Shaw (Glaxo) for providing human recombinant IL-1α and human recombinant TNFα. We are indebted to Dr. Stefan Endres, Dr. Jos van der Meer, Dr. Joseph Cannon, Scott Orencole, Herle Lindemann, and Marion Knollmann for their help and technical assistance.

References

1. Dinarello CA (1989) Adv Immunol 44:153–205
2. Okusawa S, Gelfand JA, Ikejima T, Connolly RJ, Dinarello CA (1988) J Clin Invest 81:1162–1172
3. Michie HR, Manogue KR, Spriggs DR, Revhaug A, O'Dwyer S, Dinarello CA, Cerami A, Wolff SM, Wilmore DW (1988) N Engl J Med 318:1481–1486
4. Cannon JG, Tompkins RG, Gelfand JA, Michie HR, Stanford GG, van der Meer JWM, Endres S, Lonnemann G, Corsetti J, Chernow B, Wilmore DW, Wolff SM, Burke JF, Dinarello CA (1990) J Infect Dis 161:79–84
5. Girardin E, Grau GE, Dayer JM, Roux-Lombard P, the J5 Study Group, Lambert PH (1988) N Engl J Med 319:397–400
6. Waage A, Halstensen A, Espevik T (1987) Lancet 1:355–357
7. Lonnemann G, Koch KM, Shaldon S, Dinarello CA (1988) J Lab Clin Med 112:76–86
8. Endres S, Ghorbani R, Lonnemann G, van der Meer JWM, Dinarello CA (1988) Clin Immunol Immunopathol 49:424–438
9. Van der Meer JWM, Endres S, Lonnemann G, Cannon JG, Ikejima T, Okusawa S, Gelfand JA, Dinarello CA (1988) J Leukocyte Biol 43:216–223

10. Cannon JG, van der Meer JWM, Kwiatkowski D, Endres S, Lonnemann G, Burke JF, Dinarello CA (1988) Lymphokine Res 7:457–467
11. Cheung AK, Chenoweth DE, Otsuka D, Henderson LW (1986) Kidney Int 30:74–80
12. Floege J, Wilks M, Shaldon S, Koch KM, Smeby LC (1988) Nephrol Dial Transplant 3:784–789
13. Cohen FE, Dinarello CA (1987) J Leukocyte Biol 42:548
14. Jones EY, Stuart DI, Walker NPC (1989) Nature 338:225–228
15. Smith RA, Baglioni C (1987) J Biol Chem 262:6951–6957

Modulation of Monokine Production In Vitro by Human Intravenous Immunoglobulin

J. P. Andersson[1], S. Nagy[2], and U. G. Andersson[2]

Introduction

The mechanisms by which intravenous Ig acts in modulation of inflammatory diseases are unclear. One postulated effect operates by affecting cytokine production, interfering with ligand binding to interleukin (IL) receptors, or stimulating monocytes to IL-1 receptor antagonist release. In this study the attempt was made to elucidate whether the anti-pyretic effect of intravenous Ig in inflammatory conditions is caused by a direct suppression of monokine production. Mononuclear cells were isolated from healthy blood donors and stimulated with lipopolysaccharide (LPS) or *Borrelia burgdorferi* spirochetes (Bb) for induction of tumor necrosis factor-alpha (TNF-α), IL-1, and IL-6 in the absence or presence of intravenous Ig. The cytokine production was studied at a single cell level.

Materials and Methods

Individual peripheral blood monocytes obtained from healthy blood donors which produced IL-1 (-α and -β), IL-6, and TNF-α after in vitro stimulation were identified by cytokine specific monoclonal antibodies and indirect immuno-fluorescence technique [1]. LPS or Bb were used to induce TNF-α, IL-1α, and -β, and IL-6 production in cultures. Peak synthesis occurred 2.0 h after initiation of the cultures for TNF-α, at 6.0 h for IL-6, and at 8.0 h for IL-1α and -β (Fig. 1) in the majority of the monocytes [2]. The monocytes were identified by two-color staining using a monocyte-specific monoclonal antibody.

Results

IL-6 was produced by 64% $\pm$ 8% or 71% $\pm$ 9% (mean $\pm$ SD) of the monocytes not exposed to intravenous Ig after LPS or Bb stimulation, respectively ($n = 12$).

[1] Department of Infectious Diseases, Karolinska Institute, Karolinska Hospital, Box 60 500, 104 05 Stockholm, Sweden
[2] Department of Immunology, Arrhenius Laboratories for Natural Sciences, Stockholm University, 10691 Stockholm, Sweden

Host Defense Dysfunction
in Trauma, Shock and Sepsis
Eds. Faist/Meakins/Schildberg
© Springer-Verlag, Berlin Heidelberg 1993

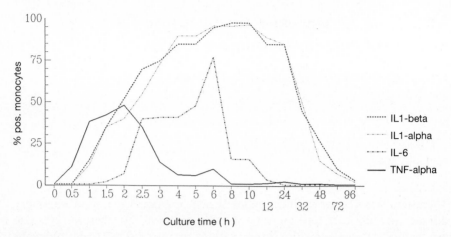

Fig. 1. The kinetics of TNFα, IL-1α, IL-1β and IL-6 production in monocytes after LPS (10ng/ml) stimulation. The incidence is given as the percentage of cytokine producing cells per total number of monocytes. The frequency of monocytes varied between 15–22% in all experiments. The figure represent one of four experiments with similar results.

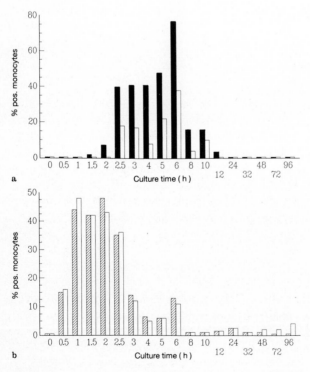

Fig. 2a, b.

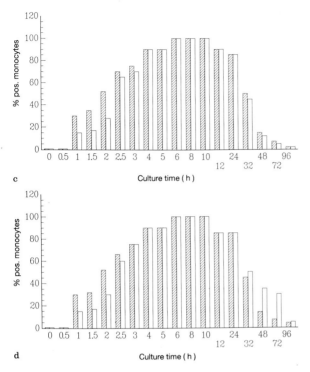

c

d

Fig. 2a–d. The kinetics of a)TNFα, b) IL-1α, c) IL-1β and d) IL-6 production after LPS (10ng/ml) stimulation in the presence or absence of IVIg (6mg/ml). Cells were harvested at indicated intervals and the incidence of cytokine producing monocytes is given as the percentage per total number of Mac 387 positive monocytes, as assessed by two-color immunofluorescence staining. A significant inhibition of IL-6 production was noticed in the IVIg supplemented cultures ($p < .001$)

A dose-dependent and significant reduction in the number of IL-6 producing cells was noted in the intravenous Ig supplemented cultures ($p < .003$). In these cultures 24% ± 12% or 29% ± 12% of the monocytes made IL-6 in response to LPS or Bb. Kinetic studies indicated a sustained significant inhibition of IL-6 production during 24 h of culture ($p < .001$; Fig. 2a). In contrast, TNF-α, IL-1α and -β synthesis was not inhibited by intravenous Ig at a dose of 6 mg/ml. LPS or Bb stimulation resulted in 47% ± 18% or 69% ± 7% TNF-α producing cells versus 48% ± 9% or 59% ± 8% in intravenous Ig supplemented cultures (Fig. 2b). LPS stimulation induced IL-1α and -β production in 100% of the monocytes at 8 h. No inhibition was evident for IL-1α or -β by intravenous Ig addition) (Fig. 2c,d).

These results indicate downregulation of IL-6 but not TNF-α or IL-1α and -β production by intravenous Ig. A direct antigen neutralization is an unlikely explanation for divergent effects observed on monokine production after intravenous addition.

References

1. Sander B, Andersson J, Andersson U (1991) Assessment of cytokines by immunoflourescence and the paraformaldehyde-saponin procedure. Immunol Rev 119:65–93
2. Andersson J, Andersson U (1990) Human intravenous immunoglobulin modulates monokine production in vitro. Immunology 71:372–376

Transforming Growth Factor β1 Upregulates the Interleukin-2 Receptor α Promoter

C. S. Cocanour, F. M. Orson, D. Thomas, and S. Rich

Introduction

The transforming growth factor β (TGF-β) are multifunctional cytokines intimately involved in development, maintenance, and repair. In the immune system, TGF-β are known to have potent growth inhibitory properties [1, 2] as well as influencing immunoglobulin subclass expression [3] and major histocompatibility complex (MHC) antigen expression [4, 5]. In order to examine the complex effect of TGF-β1 on T cell regulation we determined the effect of TGF-β1 on the interleukin-2 receptor α (IL2Rα) promoter using a Jurkat T cell line stably transfected with the IL2Rα promoter fused to the reporter gene for chloramphenicol acetyl transferase (CAT).

Materials and Methods

Cell Lines. The human leukemia T cell line, Jurkat, was transfected with a plasmid containing the -471 to $+109$ region of the IL2Rα promoter fused to the CAT gene using electroporation. A second plasmid (pHEBO) containing the hygromycin resistance gene was cotransfected as a selection marker. Stable transfectants were identified and assayed for CAT production. Transfectant 1.4 was used throughout the course of these experiments.

CAT Assay. Following cell culture, the cells were washed and cell extracts prepared. CAT activity was detected by a scintillation method in which chloramphenicol is acetylated with ^{3}H-labeled acetyl-CoA, permitting its partitioning into the organic scintillant. Counts per minute were normalized per 10^6 viable cells.

Experimental Design. The lectin PHA (4 μg/ml) and the phorbol ester PDB (4 ng/ml) were used alone or in combination with increasing concentrations of TGF-β1 for stimulation of the IL2Rα/CAT-transfected cell line 1.4. Cells were cultured for 48 h, then cell extracts prepared for CAT enzyme measurement.

University of Texas Medical School at Houston, and Baylor College of Medicine, Houston, TX 77030, USA

Host Defense Dysfunction
in Trauma, Shock and Sepsis
Eds. Faist/Meakins/Schildberg
© Springer-Verlag, Berlin Heidelberg 1993

Results

Transfected cells stimulated with PHA/PDB and TGF-β1 at concentrations greater than 0.1 ng/ml showed a 1.5- to 2-fold increase in CAT activity when compared to cells stimulated with PHA/PDB alone (see Fig. 1). TGF-β1 alone, at concentrations greater than 10 ng/ml, increased CAT activity 3- to 4-fold above non-mitogen-stimulated cells. At picomolar concentrations of TGF-β1, CAT activity decreased to baseline non-mitogen-stimulated levels. Although not statistically significant, this decrease was seen again on repeat experiments with an increased range of TGF-β1 concentrations (see Fig. 2).

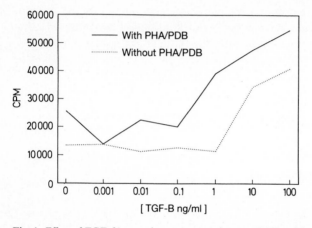

Fig. 1. Effect of TGF-β1 at various concentrations on CAT activity in transfected cell line 1.4

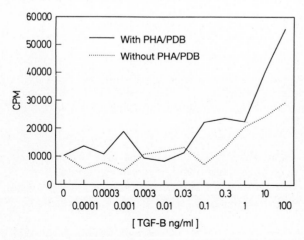

Fig. 2. Effect of TGF-β1 over an expanded concentration range

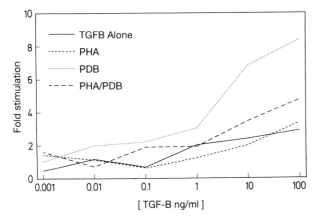

Fig. 3. Effect of TGF-β1 alone and in combination with PHA, PDB, and PHA + PDB

When PHA and PDB stimulation were examined separately in association with TGF-β1, picomolar concentrations of TGF-β1 augmented PDB stimulation of CAT activity more than PHA. At higher concentrations of TGF-β1, the augmentation of PDB stimulation is significantly greater than that of PHA (Fig. 3).

Discussion

Nearly all cells possess functional TGF-β receptors and almost all cells are capable of making at least one of the five known isoforms [6, 7]. In the immune system, macrophages [8], T cells [1], B cells [2], and lymphokine-activated killer cell precursors [9] have all been reported to secrete TGF-β following activation. The effect of TGF-β on the T cell response is complex. Normal T lymphocytes regulate their own proliferative responses by secretion of several growth factors: IL-2, IL-4, IL-6, and TGF-[1, 10, 11, 12, 13]. Activated T lymphocytes secrete IL-2 and form IL-2 membrane receptors within 4–8 h after activation. IL-2 secretion and IL-2 receptor expression reach peaks at 48–72 h [14, 15]. These events are accompanied by DNA synthesis, and proliferation and expansion of the T cell population.

TGF-β messenger (m)RNA can be identified in as little as 2 h following T cell activation, but secretion of TGF-β does not occur until 24 h and does not reach a maximum until 72–96 h after stimulation [1]. This time course suggests that TGF-β may play a role in downregulating IL-2 secretion or inducing the synthesis of other factors abrogating T cell proliferation. This is supported by reports that TGF-β can inhibit proliferation of T cells induced by either lectins [1, 16] or anti-CD3 antibody [17]. TGF-β decreases the expression of the IL-1 receptor as well as blocking IL-1-induced IL-2-production and proliferation

[18]. TGF-β has been found to inhibit IL-2-induced proliferation [1, 19, 20, 21, 22], in addition to inhibiting IL-2 mRNA production [23], and IL-2 protein production ([18, 20]; J. Lin and S. Rich, unpublished).

The IL-2 receptor (TAC, CD25) has been shown to be important in T cell growth. TGF-β has been shown to inhibit IL2R expression in activated human T cells and in a murine T helper cell line [1, 20], while having no effect on IL2R expression in a murine cytolytic T cell line [18]. In an immature, CD8$^-$, weakly CD4$^+$ T cell line (EL4), TGF-β has been shown to induce IL2R (TAC) expression (J. Lin and S. Rich, unpublished).

Our data suggest that TGF-β1 may upregulate IL2Rα expression at the promoter level in Jurkat. Higher concentrations of TGF-β1 appear to be able to increase activity of the IL2Rα promoter without additional mitogen stimulation. TGF-β1 augments PDB stimulation more than that of PHA, suggesting that TGF-β1 may affect these cells through the same pathways used by PHA.

These data also suggests that TGF-β1's down regulation of IL-2-responsive cells may be through a mechanism similar to that of glucocorticoids. TGF-β1 upregulates the receptor, which binds more IL-2, thus clearing the system of IL-2 and down regulating the response. Further studies will be necessary to confirm this action.

References

1. Kehrl JG, Wakefield LM, Roberts AB, Jakowlew S, Alvarerz-Mon M, Derynck R, Sporn MB, Fauci AS (1986) Production of transforming growth factor β by human T lymphocytes and its potential role in the regulation of T cell growth. J Immunol 163:1037–1050
2. Kehrl JH, Roberts AB, Wakefield LM, Jakowlew S, Sporn MB, Fauci AS (1986) Transforming growth factor β is an important immunomodulatory protein for human B lymphocytes. J Immunol 137:3855
3. Lebman DA, Lee FD, Coffman RL (1990) Mechanism for transforming growth factor B and IL-2 enhancement of IgA expression in lipopolysaccharide-stimulated B cell cultures. J Immunol 144:952–959
4. Schluesener HJ (1990) Transforming growth factors type β1 and β2 suppress rat astrocyte autoantigen presentation and antagonize hyperinduction of class II major histocompatibility complex antigen expression by interferon-γ and tumor necrosis factor-α. J Neuroimmunol 27:41–47
5. Zuber P, Kuppner MC, Tribolet MD (1988) Transforming growth factor-down-regulates HLA-DR antigen expression on human malignant glioma cells. Eur J Immunol 19:1623–1626
6. Cheifetz S, Weatherbee JA, Tsang MLS et al. (1987) The transforming growth factor-B system, a complex pattern of cross-reactive ligands and receptors. Cell. 48:409–415
7. Ellingsworth L, Nakayama D, Dasch J et al. (1989) Transforming growth factor beta 1 (TGFB1) receptor expression on resting and mitogen-activated T cells. J Cell Biochem 39:489–500
8. Assoian RK, Fleurdelys BE et al. (1987) Expression and secretion of type B transforming growth factor by activated human macrophages. Proc Natl Acad Sci USA 84(17):6020–6024
9. Kasid A, Bell GI, Director EP(1988) Effects of transforming growth factor Bon human lymphokine-activated killer cell precursors. Autocrine inhibition of cellular proliferation and differentiation to immune killer cells. J Immunol 141:690
10. Morgan DA, Ruscetti FW, Gallo RC (1976) Selective in vitro growth of T-lymphoctyes from normal human bone marrow Science. 193:1007–1008
11. Smith KA (1980) T-cell growth factor. Immunol Rev 51:337–357

12. Fernandez-Botran R, Sanders VM, Oliver KG, Chen YW, Krammer PH, Uhr JW, Vitetta ES (1986) Interleukin 4 mediates autocrine growth of helper T cells after antifenic stimulation. Proc Natl Acad Sci USA 83:9689
13. Uyttenhove C, Coulie PG, VanSnick J (1988) T cell growth and differentiation induced by interleukin-4P1/IL-6, the murine hybridoma/plasmacytoma growth factor. J Exp Med 167:1417–1427
14. Depper JM, Keonard WJ, Kronke M et al. (1984) Regulation of interleukin-2 receptor gene expression: effects of phorbol diester, phospholipase C, and reexposure to lectin or antigen 14. J Immunol 133:3054–3061
15. Greene WC, Leonard WJ, Depper JM et al. (1986) The human interleukin-2 receptor: normal and abnormal expression in T cells and in leukemias induced by the human T-lymphotropic retroviruses. Ann Intern Med 105:560–572
16. Ellingsworth LR, Nakayama D, Segarini P et al. (1988) Transforming growth factor-Bs are equipotent growth inhibits of interleukin-1 induced thymocyte proliferation. Cell Immunol 114:41–54
17. Stoeck MH, Sommermeyer H, Miescher S et al. (1989) Transforming growth factor beta 1 and beta 2 as well as milk growth factor decrease anti-CD3-induced proliferation of human lymphocytes without inhibiting the anti-CD32-mediated increase of CA2-i and the activation of protein kinase C. FEBS Lett 249:289
18. Dubois CM, Ruscetti FW, Palaszynski EW, Falk LA, Ossenheim JJ, Keller JR (1990) Transforming growth factor β is a potent inhibitor of interleukin 1 (IL-1) receptor expression: proposed mechanism of inhibition of IL-1 action. J Exp Med 172:737–744
19. Newcom SR, Kadin ME, Ansari AA (1988) Production of transforming growth factor-beta activity by Ki-1 positive lymphoma cells and analysis of its role in the regulation of Ki-1 positive lymphoma growth. Am J Pathol 131:569
20. Ruegemer JJ, Ho SN, Augustine JA, Schlager JW, Bell MP, McKean DJ, Abraham RT (1990) Regulatory effects of transforming growth factor-β on IL-2- and IL-4-dependent T cell-cycle progression. J Immunol 144:1767–1776
21. Stoeck M, Miescher S, MacDonald HR, von Fliedner V (1990) J Cell Physiol 141:65–73
22. Espevik T, Waage A, Faxvaag A, Shalaby MR (1990) Regulation of interleukin-2 and interleukin-6 production from T-cells: involvement of interleukin-1 β and transforming growth factor-β. Cell Immunol 126:47–56
23. Schluesener HJ, Lider O (1989) Transforming growth factors β1 and β2: cytokines with identical immunosuppressive effects and a potential role in the regulation of autoimmune T cell function. J Neuroimmunol 24:249–258

Section 8

**Cytokines in Acute Phase
States and Trauma**

Interactions of Immunopathological Mediators (Tumor Necrosis Factor-α, TGF-β, Prostaglandin E₂) in Traumatized Individuals

C. L. Miller-Graziano, G. Szabo, K. Kodys, and B. Mehta

Introduction

Characterization of monokine action in septic shock is complicated by the interactive nature of the cytokines and the unusual activation status of the posttrauma macrophage-monocytes (MØ). The response of preseptic trauma patients' MØ to bacterial stimuli is exaggerated when compared to normals' MØ [1, 2]. MØ from trauma patients not only produce elevated tumor necrosis factor-α (TNF-α) levels, but the TNF-α which patients' MØ produce is primarily cell-associated rather than secreted TNF-α as produced by normals' MØ [1, 3, 4]. The trauma patients' MØ TNF-α is often resistant to prostaglandin E₂ (PGE₂) downregulation [3]. One hypothesis explaining this posttrauma aberrant monokine function is that the microenvironment around trauma patients' MØ consists of high concentrations of secondary inducers of monokines (for example, substance P, immunoglobulin monomers, and complement split products), as well as elevated cytokines. It is the concomitant presence of these trauma-induced mediators during subsequent MØ induction that results in deranged monocyte responses, such as exaggerated production of some monokines and depression of both MØ antigen-presenting function and MØ plasminogen-activator production. Some examples of altered cytokine response capacities of trauma patients' MØ versus normals' MØ are given in this section, and the implication for prophylactic therapy is discussed. The effects of FcRI cross-linking, cyclo-oxygenase inhibitors, lipoxygenase products, transforming growth factor-β, (TGF-β) and interleukin (IL) 4 on trauma patients' MØ are compared and contrasted with those same mediators' effects on normals' MØ.

FcγRI Cross-Linking Activation

Trauma patients' peripheral blood monocytes exhibit increased numbers of cells with high densities of the 72-KDa FcγRI receptor for IgG [1, 2, 5]. These high-density FcγRI expressing MØ can be stimulated by the circulating nonspecific

Department of Surgery, University of Massachusetts Medical School, 55 Lake Avenue North, Worcester, MA 01655, USA

Host Defense Dysfunction
in Trauma, Shock and Sepsis
Eds. Faist/Meakins/Schildberg
© Springer-Verlag, Berlin Heidelberg 1993

immunoglobulins which are characteristically elevated in trauma patients [1, 5, 6]. Stimulation of MØ by cross-linking their FcγRI produces increased PGE$_2$ activity and increased TNF-α levels, as well as increased IL-6 production [2, 7–9]. All of these mediators (IL-6, TNF-α and PGE$_2$) are excessively elevated in trauma patients [1, 4, 10, 11]. In our experiments, we simultaneously cross-link/activate the FcγRI and selectively enrich for this cross-linked MØ population by rosetting the MØ with anti-Rh coated human erythrocytes. In the absence of an interferon-gamma (IFN-γ) prime, the stimulation of normals' MØ through their FcγRI receptor and enrichment in this manner leads to a predominantly cell-associated rather than secreted TNF-α response (Fig. 1).

By cross-linking normals' MØ FcγRI, we are able to induce normals' MØ to mimic the TNF-α response pattern of immunoaberrant trauma patients' MØ. This predominance of MØ cell-associated versus secreted TNF-α is not only typical of the trauma patient but may be also a major contributor to their septic shock syndrome. Cell-associated TNF-α is proposed as being more efficient in delivery of cytotoxic activity than secreted TNF-α [12, 13]. We have previously demonstrated that patients' MØ concomitantly produce large amounts of cell-associated TNF-α and PGE$_2$ [1, 3]. In vitro induction of even greater PGE$_2$ production still did not result in decreased TNF-α levels [3]. These data suggested that patients' MØ were uniquely in vivo primed so that their TNF-α

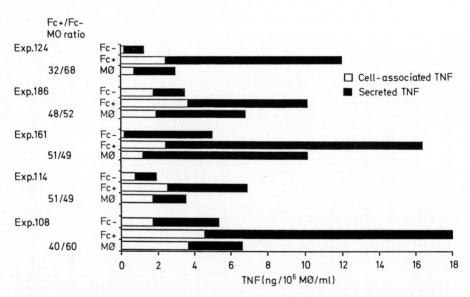

Fig. 1. FcγRI stimulation augments cell-associated MØ TNF-α. MØ were stimulated by FcRI receptor cross-linking with anti-Rh erythrocyte rosetting. Fc^+, the rosetting population of MØ; Fc^-, the nonrosetting MØ. MØ are the nonstimulated whole population. TNF-α was measured in MØ lysates (cell-associated) and supernates (secreted) using the LM bioassay. Data are presented as nanograms per 10^6 recovered MØ per milliliter. The ratios of the FcγRI$^+$ and FcγRI$^-$ MØ subsets (Fc$^+$/Fc$^-$ MØ Ratio) within the unseparated MØ population (MØ) are shown for each experiment. There was a different individual blood donor for each experiment

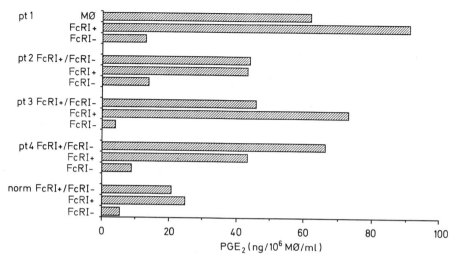

Fig. 2. Stimulation by cross-linking FcRI induces greater PGE_2 levels in patients' versus normals' MØ. Supernates from 16-h cultures of equal numbers of $Fc\gamma RI^+$ cross-linked (anti-Rh erythrocyte rosetted), non-cross-linked $Fc\gamma RI^-$ (nonrosetting), remixed populations $Fc\gamma RI^+/Fc\gamma RI^-$ (MØ separated by anti-Rh erythrocyte rosetting and then combined at the proper ratio so that the whole population is also stimulated by FcRI cross-linking), and MØ (whole population before rosetting) were assessed for PGE_2 levels during enzyme-linked immunosorbent assay (ELISA). Results from four separate patients are shown, and the normal control is the mean of the corresponding normal controls. Data are presented as nanograms per 10^6 recovered MØ per milliliter

messenger RNA production was not affected by the elevated cyclic AMP levels resulting from elevated PGE_2 levels. Such insensitivity of MØ TNF-α production to PGE_2 downregulation has been previously reported for normals' MØ under unusual stimulation conditions [14–16].

Another demonstration of the unique preactivated state of trauma patients' MØ can be seen in their response to $Fc\gamma RI$ cross-linking. Although $Fc\gamma RI$ cross-linking induces elevated PGE_2 levels in normals' monocytes, this stimulation induces even greater PGE_2 levels in the patients' MØ (Fig. 2). Patients' MØ are already activated for PGE_2 production, and their freshly isolated MØ population are often already maximally stimulated to produce PGE_2 even before in vitro $Fc\gamma RI$ cross-linking. It is our contention that in this case these patients' MØ have already been $Fc\gamma RI$ cross-link/activated in vivo.

Activation by Cyclo-oxygenase and Lipoxygenase Products

The posttrauma activation state of the trauma patients' MØ alters profoundly the way in which trauma patients' MØ respond to subsequent stimuli. As is illustrated in Fig. 3, addition of the cyclo-oxygenase inhibitor indomethacin, in the absence of an IFN-γ prime, to freshly isolate normals' MØ, only minimally

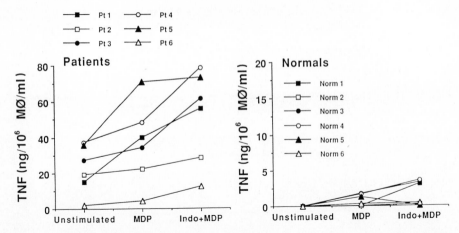

Fig. 3. Indomethacin augments TNF-α levels in patients' activated MØ. Equal numbers of MØ were cultured either unstimulated (media only), MDP (20 μg/ml) stimulated, or indomethacin (*Indo*; 10^{-6} *M*) plus MDP (20 μg/ml) stimulated. After 16 h of culture, the TNF-α level was measured using the LM bioassay. The data are reported as total TNF-α in nanograms per 10^6 recovered MØ per milliliter

increases their TNF-α production in response to the synthetic gram-positive bacterial cell wall analogue muramyl dipeptide (MDP). In contrast, MØ freshly isolated from patients 8–10 days after major injury (injury severity score > 25), show significant TNF-α production in response to MDP. These patients' TNF-α production is even more exaggerated in the presence of indomethacin (Fig. 3). Since these trauma patients' MØ production of TNF-α is independent of PGE_2 downregulation [1, 3], the indomethacin effect must be explained by some mechanism other than a cyclo-oxygenase decrease of PGE_2 levels.

One well-described effect of blocking the cyclo-oxygenase pathway is to increase lipoxygenase product production [17, 18]. Previous investigators have described a small but significant augmentary effect of leukotriene B_4 (LTB_4) on normal MØ production of TNF-α [19, 20]. We examined the TNF-α augmenting effect of adding 10^{-7} *M* exogenous LTB_4 to normals' MØ stimulated with 100 U IFN-γ plus 20 μg/ml MDP. Since we assay TNF-α in the LM bioassay, we can simultaneously assess both the TNF-α levels in MØ culture supernates and in the MØ cell lysates [21]. All TNF-α measured is completely neutralizable with anti-TNF-α antibody. We found that LTB_4 does augment MØ TNF-α production, and that in some individuals, an enhancement of cell-associated as well as secreted TNF-α levels is observed (Fig. 4). This is particularly interesting because the indomethacin-enhancing effect of patients' MØ occurs primarily in the cell-associated component of TNF-α activity (Fig. 5). In fact, if normal MØ are FcγRI cross-link/activated and enriched, the subsequent augmenting effects of LTB_4 on their TNF-α production are greatly increased (Fig. 6). As previously shown, FcγRI cross-linking increases the induction of cell-associated TNF-α in

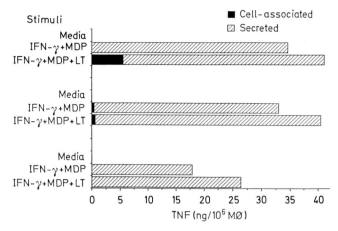

Fig. 4. LTB$_4$ increases IFN-γ plus MDP stimulated MØ TNF-α. Equal numbers of either patients' or normals' MØ were cultured for 16 h in media only, IFN-γ (100 U/ml) plus MDp (20 µg/ml) or IFN-γ (100 U/ml) plus LTB$_4$ (*LT*; 10^{-7} M) plus MDP (20 µg/ml). Both secreted and cell-associated TNF-α was measured (as in Fig. 1) using the LM bioassay. Data are presented as nanograms per 10^6 recovered MØ per milliliter

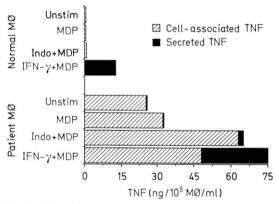

Fig. 5. Indomethacin primarily increases patients' cell-associated TNF-α. Equal numbers of either patients' or normals' MØ were cultured for 16 h without stimuli (media only), with MDP (20 µg/ml) with indomethacin (*Indo*; 10^{-6} M) plus MDP (20 µg/ml), or with IFN-γ (10 U/ml) plus MDP (20 µg/ml). Cell-associated and secreted TNF was measured using the LM bioassay. Data are presented as nanograms per 10^6 recovered MØ per milliliter

normals' MØ. Addition of LTB$_4$ to these FcγRI activated normal MØ has a much more pronounced enhancing effect on TNF-α levels than LTB$_4$ addition to the same MØ without FcγRI preactivation. These data again demonstrate that the activation state of the patients' MØ alter their subsequent response to other mediators or to mediator therapy.

The augmenting effect of LTB$_4$ on MØ TNF-α production is also independent of any PGE$_2$ effect (Fig. 6). LTB$_4$ does not enhance all MØ mediator

642   C. L. Miller-Graziano et al.

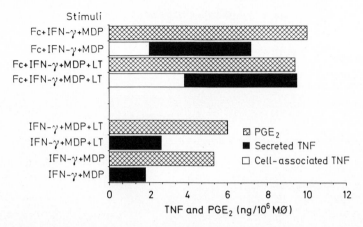

Fig. 6. LTB_4 stimulates increased cell-associated and secreted TNF-α levels in FcγRI cross-linked normal MØ independently of PGE_2 levels. Equal numbers of MØ either FcRI cross-linked (anti-Rh erythrocyte rosetting) or whole MØ population (nonrosetted) were cultured with IFN-γ (100 U/ml) plus MDP (20 μg/ml) or IFN-γ (10 U/ml) plus MDP (20 μg/ml) plus LTB_4 (LT; 10^{-7} M). MØ supernates were assayed for PGE_2 using the ELISA described in Fig. 2 and for secreted TNF-α in the LM bioassay. Cell lysates were also assayed for cell-associated TNF-α. Both TNF-α and PGE_2 are reported in nanograms per 10^6 recovered MØ per milliliter

production equally. In those in vivo activated trauma patients with elevated MØ PGE_2 and TNF-α, LTB_4 further enhances TNF-α and IL-6 levels, but has no effect on IL-1 or PGE_2 stimulation. Normal MØ, which have been FcγRI cross-link/activated, also show enhanced IL-6 and TNF-α production when additionally stimulated with LTB_4, but the levels of cytokines produced are still significantly below those seen in the FcγRI activated trauma patients' MØ (Fig. 7).

These data suggest the following: first, LTB_4 significantly augments MØ TNF-α induction primarily in unusually activated MØ (i.e., trauma patients or FcγRI$^+$ normals); second, LTB_4 enhancement of TNF-α, like the indomethacin effect, primarily affects cell-associated TNF-α; third, MØ PGE_2 levels are not affected by LTB_4 so that reduction in PGE_2 activity cannot account for the LTB_4 enhancing effect on TNF-α; and fourth, LTB_4 enhances patient FcγRI cross-linked MØ more than normal FcγRI cross-linked MØ. All of these data are consistent with the hypothesis that the TNF-α enhancing effect of cyclo-oxygenase blockade seen in trauma victims might result from lipoxygenase shunting and increased LTB_4 levels.

The final experiment in this series examined the effect of adding both a cyclo-oxygenase and lipoxygenase inhibitor to FcγRI$^+$ activated normals' or trauma patients' MØ. If the indomethacin-enhancing effect was the result of lipoxygen-ase shunting, then simultaneous addition of a lipoxygenase inhibitor should abrogate this enhanced response. In four experiments, the lipoxygenase in-hibitor nordihydroguaiaretic acid (NDGA) was added at 40 μM to normals' or monokine aberrant trauma patients' MØ. When indomethacin at 10^{-7} M was

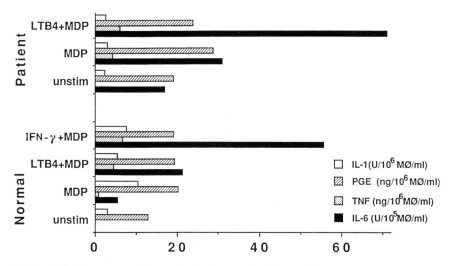

Fig. 7. LTB_4 effect on monokine production in $Fc\gamma RI^+$ MØ. $Fc\gamma RI^+$ MØ were selected by rosetting with anti-Rh coated erythrocytes. Equal numbers of $Fc\gamma RI^+$ MØ from either patients' or normals' were cultured for 16 h unstimulated (media only), with MDP (20 µg/ml) or, with LTB_4 (10^{-7} M) plus MDP (20 µg/ml). IL-1 was measured in the MØ supernates using the D10.G4.1 cell bioassay and reported as units per 10^6 recovered MØ per milliliter. PGE_2 was assayed in the supernates by ELISA and reported as nanograms per 10^6 recovered MØ per milliliter. TNF-α was measured using the LM bioassay and presented as nanograms per 10^6 recovered MØ per milliliter. The MØ supernates were also assayed for IL-6 using the B9 cell bioassay and reported as units per 10^5 recovered MØ per milliliter

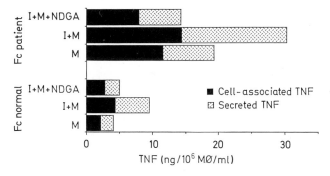

Fig. 8. Lipoxygenase inhibitor decreases indomethacin enhanced TNF-α levels. Both normal and patient MØ were FcRI cross-linked (anti-Rh erythrocyte rosetted) and cultured with either MDP alone (M; 20 µg/ml) indomethacin (10^{-6} M) plus MDP (I + M; 20 µg/ml), or indomethacin (I; 10^{-6} M) plus MDP (20 µg/ml) plus the lipoxygenase inhibitor nordihydroguaiaretic acid (I + M + NDGA; 40 µM). After 16 h of culture, both secreted and cell-associated TNF-α were measured using the LM cell bioassay. TNF-α is presented as nanograms per 10^6 recovered MØ per milliliter

added along with MDP (bacterial cell wall analogue) to $Fc\gamma RI^+$ activated normals' or patients' MØ, enhanced production of TNF-α was observed. Simultaneous addition of NDGA to these cultures completely abrogated the indomethacin-enhancing effects (Fig. 8). These data indicate that the enhancing effect of indomethacin addition on MØ TNF-α production is due to the indomethacin augmentation of the lipoxygenase pathway and not to its inhibition of cyclo-oxygenase production. The data also illustrate again the greatly elevated TNF-α response of trauma patients' MØ and that subsequent stimulation of patients' intensely activated MØ leads to exaggerated responses.

TGF-β Activation

This laboratory has previously published that trauma patients' MØ which are producing aberrant TNF-α levels are also producing greatly enhanced levels of TGF-β [21]. TGF-β is a 27-kDa homodimer with immunosuppressive activity for both T cell and B cell proliferation [22]. Besides its effect in depressing T cell production of IL-2, IL-4, and IFN-γ, TGF-β also can profoundly alter MØ function [22, 23]. TGF-β has been reported to both increase and decrease biologically active TNF-α levels depending on the TGF-β dose and the activation state of the MØ when TGF-β is added [22, 23].

In a number of experiments, we added 2.4 ng/ml exogenous TGF-β to both normals' MØ and immunoaberrant trauma patients' MØ. TGF-β addition had little or no effect on the PGE_2 levels produced by normals' MØ. However, addition of exogenous TGF-β to patients' MØ resulted in increased PGE_2 production particularly in those patients whose PGE_2 levels were already

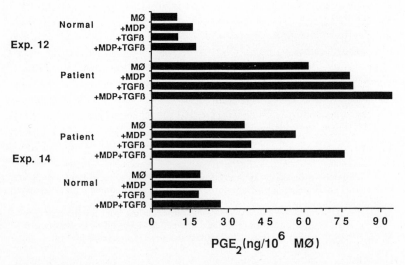

Fig. 9. TGF-β increases patients' MØ PGE_2 levels more than normals'. Equal numbers of both patients' and normals' MØ were cultured for 16 h. MØ alone (media only), with MDP (20 μg/ml), TGF-β (2.4 ng/ml), or with MDP (20 μg/ml) plus TGF-β (2.4 ng/ml) were assessed for PGE_2 levels. PGE_2 was measured in the supernates by ELISA and presented as nanograms per 10^6 recovered MØ per milliliter

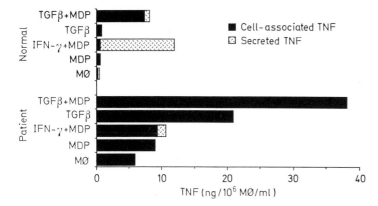

Fig. 10. Effect of TGF-β on MØ TNF-α production. Equal numbers of normals' or patients' MØ were cultured for 16 h unstimulated (media only), with MDP (20 µg/ml), IFN-γ (10 U/ml) plus MDP (20 µg/ml), TGF-β (2.4 ng/ml), or with TGF-β (2.4 mg/ml) plus MDP (20 µg/ml). Secreted and cell-associated TNF-α was measured using the LM cell bioassay and reported as nanograms per 10^6 recovered MØ per milliliter

elevated (Fig. 9). When TGF-β was added to normal MØ in the presence of MDP, small amounts of cell-associated TNF-α were induced, but little or no secreted TNF-α (Fig. 10). Addition of TGF-β alone had no effect on normal MØ. However, addition of 2.4 ng/ml exogenous TGF-β to patients' MØ who already had in vivo activated TNF-α production, resulted in a significant increase in MØ cell-associated TNF-α levels. Costimulation of patient MØ with TGF-β and MDP produced an even greater augmentation of MØ cell-associated TNF-α levels (Fig. 10). MØ secreted TNF-α levels induced by IFN-γ plus MDP were actually reduced by TGF-β addition. This dichotomy may explain the conflicting results reported on TGF-β effects on TNF-α production.

These data imply that TGF-β can decrease IFN-γ plus MDP induced TNF-α secretion in normals' MØ. However TGF-β can augment TNF-α levels in trauma patients' MØ activated by trauma induced mediators. The implication of this dichotomy for trauma patients is as follows. Trauma patients' MØ are producing elevated TGF-β levels [24]. The trauma patient's MØ TGF-β is directly suppressive to T cell proliferation, B cell proliferation, and T cell lymphokine production [22, 23, 25]. This suppressive activity of TGF-β contributes to the immunosuppressed state of the trauma victim. In addition, these elevated posttrauma TGF-β concentrations are present when the patients' MØ are stimulated by other trauma mediators and by bacterial products. The presence of TGF-β during MØ activation alters the subsequent response of patients' MØ to other stimuli. In the presence of TGF-β, MØ PGE_2 responses are increased, and MØ TNF-α responses are predisposed toward greatly elevated levels of cell-associated TNF-α. The trauma patients' MØ also seem more sensitive to these TGF-β effects. TGF-β has been shown to stimulate upregulation of its own receptor [23, 26]. We are currently examining trauma patients' MØ to determine whether increased presence of TGF-β receptors accounts for their increased sensitivity to TGF-β mediated effects on PGE$_2$ and TNF-α. The presence of elevated TGF-β levels in the posttrauma microenvironment contributes to the trauma patients' MØ aberrant monokine responses.

TGF-β does not equally augment all monokine production in the trauma patients. IL-6 production does not seem to be increased in the trauma patients' MØ by exogenous TGF-β when TNF-α levels are increased. This again may reflect the MØ activation state (Fig. 11). At other postinjury periods when TNF-α is not predominant we have observed some TGF-β mediated increase in IL-6. As with TNF-α, TGF-β has been reported to both increase and decrease IL-6 levels [22, 23]. The increased sensitivity of immunoaberrant trauma patients'

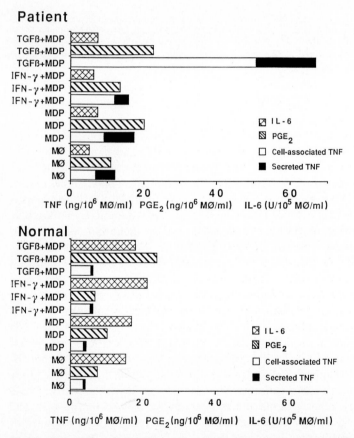

Fig. 11. TGF-β effect of monokine production. Both normals' and patients' MØ were cultured for 16 h either alone (media only), with MDP (20 µg/ml), IFN-γ (10 U/ml) plus MDP (20 µg/ml) or, with TGF-β (2.4 ng/ml) plus MDP (20 µg/ml). IL-6 was measured in the supernates using the B9 cell bioassay and reported as units per 10^5 recovered MØ per milliliter. The supernates were assayed for PGE$_2$ using an ELISA and reported as nanograms per 10^6 recovered MØ per milliliter. Both cell-associated and secreted TNF-α were measured using the LM cell bioassay and presented as nanograms per 10^6 recovered MØ per milliliter

MØ to TGF-β and the presence of elevated levels of TGF-β alter the patients' in vivo response to immunotherapeutic modalities administered. For example, treatment of the patients' MØ with IFN-γ altered the effect of TGF-β on TNF-α production, reducing TGF-β's augmenting effect. Since TGF-β is produced in a latent form, the ability of the MØ to activate TGF-β is dependent on their activation state [27]. Some of the TGF-β produced by trauma patients is already activated in the culture supernates [24]. These data indicate that the trauma patients' MØ are also producing proteolytic enzymes to activate the latent TGF-β which they themselves or other cell types produce [27]. The availability of activated TGF-β in the microenvironment of trauma patients' MØ is another cause of their altered TGF-β responses. Taken together, the data presented in this section strongly suggest that the results of administering prophylactic mediators to trauma patients can be quite different than the administration of these mediators in an *Escherichia coli* induced septic shock model. The trauma induced microenvironment is quite varied from the uncomplicated bacteria induced septic shock microenvironment in that many unique mediators are present.

Interleukin-4 Immunomodulation

Examining the in vitro ability of different mediators to affect trauma patients' MØ function provides an approximation of the patients' in vivo response to prophylactic mediators. Our laboratory has examined the ability of the T cell lymphokine IL-4 to moderate trauma patients' excessive monokine activity [28]. IL-4, an activator of T helper lymphocytes type II is also a potent inducer of B cell proliferation [29]. IL-4 downregulates some human monocyte functions while potentiating others [30–34]. The human IL-4 activity of human MØ appears quite different than the murine IL-4 activity on murine macrophage [26, 31]. IL-4 has been shown to downregulate human MØ production of IL-1, TNF-α, IL-6, and PGE$_2$ in response to LPS stimulation [31, 34].

We examined the ability of exogenously added IL-4 to downregulate aberrant mediator production by patients' MØ. Patients' or normals' MØ stimulated with MDP have increased PGE$_2$ activity. As can be seen in Fig. 12, patients' MØ were in vivo preactivated and produced immunosuppressive levels of PGE$_2$ (> 35 ng/10^6 MØ). Stimulation with MDP further elevated the MØ PGE$_2$ activity. Addition of IL-4 over a concentration range of 0.5–25 ng/ml downregulated the patients' MØ PGE$_2$ levels in a dose-dependent fashion. Addition of 5–25 ng/ml IL-4 decreased PGE$_2$ levels to the non-immunosuppressive normal range (< 35 ng/10^6 MØ). Simultaneously assessed normal MØ PGE$_2$ levels were also reduced by IL-4 addition (Fig. 12). Interestingly, addition of IL-4 to patients' MØ in the same concentration range (5–25 ng/ml) reduced their TNF-α production but did not return it to normal levels. (Fig. 13). As can be seen in Fig. 13, patients' MØ were producing considerable cell-associated TNF-α due solely to their in vivo stimulation.

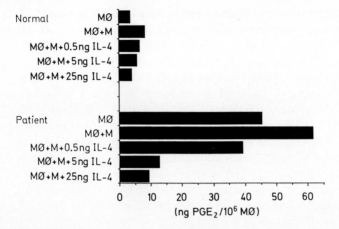

Fig. 12. IL-4 downregulates elevated MØ PGE$_2$ levels in trauma patients. Equal numbers of both patients' and normals' MØ were cultured either without stimuli (media only), with MDP (20 µg/ml), or with IL-4 (at concentrations of 0.5 ng/ml, 5 ng/ml, and 25 ng/ml) in combination with MDP (20 µg/ml). PGE$_2$ was assayed using an ELISA and reported as nanograms per 10^6 recovered MØ per milliliter

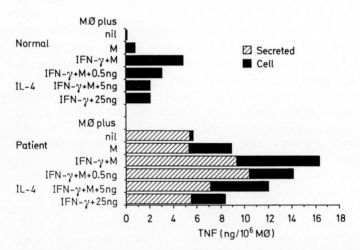

Fig. 13. IL-4 downregulates elevated TNF-α production by trauma patients' MØ. Equal numbers of normals' and patients' MØ were cultured for 16 h with either media only, MDP (20 µg/ml), IFN-γ (10 U/ml) plus MDP (20 µg/ml), or IFN-γ (10 U/ml) plus MDP (20 µg/ml) plus IL-4 (0.5 ng/ml, 5 ng/ml, or 25 ng/ml). Both secreted and cell-associated TNF-α was measured using the LM cell bioassay. Data is presented as nanograms per 10^6 per milliliter

Further stimulation of patients' MØ with MDP-induced production of additional secreted TNF-α. MDP does not induce significant secreted TNF-α in normals' MØ if an IFN-γ prime is not copresent. Addition of a suboptimal prime with IFN-γ (10 U/ml) induced a significant secreted TNF-α response in both the patients' and normals' MØ. The patients' MØ also increased their cell-associated TNF-α production while normals' MØ produced no cell-associated TNF-α (Fig. 13). Addition of 5ng/ml IL-4 downregulated the normals' IFN-γ plus MDP induced TNF-α response by more than 65%. In contrast, 25 ng/ml IL-4 was only able to downregulate patients' secreted TNF-α by 50% and their cell-associated TNF-α by 50%. Patients' MØ TNF-α levels were still abnormally elevated even in the presence of 25 ng/ml IL-4. These data imply that IL-4 can down modulate patients' aberrant monokine responses, but that the effective dose required for control of TNF-α induced septic shock might be unrealistic for a clinical situation. A combinational therapy of IL-4 plus other immune modulators might be more effective in controlling the aberrant cytokine levels of significantly immunoaberrant trauma patients.

Summary

In summary, MØ from immunoaberrant trauma patients produce abnormally elevated levels of IL-6, PGE$_2$ and TGF-β, as well as TNF-α. These patients' MØ TNF-α is insensitive to PGE$_2$ downregulation and largely consists of cell-associated TNF-α. The in vivo activated MØ from these patients are aberrant in their response to the cyclo-oxygenase inhibitor indomethacin in that their TNF-α levels are abnormally augmented by indomethacin. These patients' abnormal increase in MØ TNF-α levels in response to indomethacin appears to be a result of increased sensitivity to stimulation by lipoxygenase products, particularly LTB$_4$. The patients' trauma-activated MØ are not just more sensitive to LTB$_4$ but also to other trauma-induced mediators in the microenvironment.

Cross-linking the patients' MØ FcγRI, as would occur in vivo by excessive circulating immunoglobulin, results in exaggerated production of TNF-α, IL-6, and PGE$_2$ by patients' MØ. As shown in this chapter immunoaberrant patients' MØ also have increased sensitivity to TGF-β. Excessive MØ-produced TGF-β is available in the posttrauma microenvironment [24]. This TGF-β is activated from its latent form by MØ-produced proteolytic enzymes [27]. The posttrauma MØ is now autocrine stimulated by its own TGF-β. The posttrauma activated MØ produces both greater PGE$_2$ activity and augmented levels of cell-associated TNF-α in response to the activated TGF-β in its microenvironment. The normal unactivated MØ is unaffected or even depressed by exogenous TGF-β. The PGE$_2$ and TNF-α responses of normal MØ that have been preactivated by FcγRI cross-linking and then exposed to TGF-β parallels the patients' MØ responses in kind but not quantity.

The response of trauma-activated patients' MØ to TGF-β is different from normals' and leads to questions about the actual response of patients' MØ to in vivo therapy. The T cell lymphokine IL-4, which has previously been demonstrated to have regulatory effects on MØ responses, was examined. IL-4 was effective in downregulating patients' elevated MØ PGE$_2$ activity, but was less effective in correcting the patients' MØ aberrant TNF-α responses. The unusual activation of trauma patients' MØ by trauma-generated mediators such as complement split products, circulating immunoglobulin, and fibrin degradation products results in a preactivated monocyte. The subsequent response of this in vivo activated MØ to bacterial stimuli or other trauma-generated mediators varies greatly from that of normals' monocytes. These altered MØ response potentials can be predicted by assessing the trauma patients' MØ in vitro for their response to potential mediators or immunotherapeutic modalities.

Acknowledgements. This study was supported by Grants GM 36214 from the United States Public Health Service and DAMD 17-86-C-6097. The muramyl dipeptide was a gift from the Ciba-Geigy Co., Basel, Switzerland. The human recombinant IL-4 was a generous gift from Dr. S. Gillis (Immunex) and IL-6 was a generous gift of D. S. Clark (Genetics Institute).

References

1. Miller-Graziano CL et al. (1990) J Trauma 30:S86
2. Szabo G et al. (1991) J Clin Immunol 11:326
3. Takayama T et al. (1990) Arch Surg 125:29
4. Munoz C et al. (1991) Eur J Immunol 21:2177
5. Miller-Graziano CL et al. (1988) Arch Surg 123:293
6. Ertel W et al. (1989) Arch Surg 124:1437
7. Debets JMH et al. (1988) J Immunol 141:1197
8. Krutmann J et al. (1990) J Immunol 145:1337
9. Debets JMH et al. (1990) J Immunol 144:1304
10. Pullicino EA et al. (1990) Lymphokine Res 9:231
11. Ayala A et al. (1991) Am J Physiol 210:R167
12. Patek PQ et al. (1989) Immunol 67:509
13. Liu C-C et al. (1989) Proc Natl Acad Sci USA 86:3286
14. Kunkel SL et al. (1988) Methods Achiev Exp Pathol 13:240
15. Renz H et al. (1988) J Immunol 141:2388
16. Pace JL et al. (1984) Mol Immunol 21:249
17. Goodwin J et al. (1988) In: Biology of the leukotrienes. NY Acad Sci, p 201
18. Schade U et al. (1989) Lymphokine Res 8:245
19. Lee J et al. (1989) Agents Actions 27:277
20. Rola-Pleszczynski M et al. (1988) In: Biology of the Leukotrienes NY Acad Sci, p 218
21. Szabo G et al. (1990) J Leukoc Biol 47:206
22. Palladino MA et al. (1990) Transforming growth factor-βs. Ann NY Acad Sci 593:181
23. Wahl SM et al. (1990) Transforming growth factors-βs Ann Acad Sci 593:188
24. Miller-Grazino CL et al. (1991) J Clin Immunol 11:95
25. Kehrl JH et al. (1991) J Immunol 146:4016
26. Wong HL et al. (1991) J Immunol 147:1843
27. Twardzik DR et al. (1990) Transforming growth factors-βs. Ann NY Acad Sci 593:276
28. Szabo G et al. (1991) J Clin Immunol 11:336
29. Paul WE et al. (1987) Annu Rev Immunol 5:429
30. Zlotkik A et al. (1987) J Immunol 138:4275
31. Essner R et al. (1989) J Immunol 142:3857
32. Donnelly RP et al. (1990) J Immunol 145:569
33. Hart PH et al. (1989) Proc Natl Acad Sci USA 86:3803
34. Lee JD et al. (1990) J Leukoc Biol 47:475

In Vitro Production and Secretion of Interleukin-1 by Human Monocytes After Surgical Trauma

M. L. Vuotto[1], E. Bresciano[1], D. Mancino[1], M. T. Ielpo[1], M. R. Mosti[1], G. De Martino[2], and A. Barbarisi[2]

Introduction

Interleukin-1 (IL-1) is a cytokine produced by different cells, the principal ones being mononuclear phagocytes. This cytokine functions as a key mediator in the organism's response to various stimuli principally modulating target cell growth and differentiation. IL-1 is part of a complex of soluble mediators forming the biological and molecular cornerstone of the lymphomonokine network that, in turn, links the immune system to other systems [2].

Under physiological conditions IL-1 blood levels are very low since normally the cells do not secrete it. Any alteration, of inflammatory, immunitary, or traumatic origin, may trigger the gene transcription with a rapid rise in blood IL-1 [3, 5, 7, 11, 13]. Elective surgery is a good model of programmed trauma. Therefore, we evaluated in vitro both spontaneous and lipopolysaccharide (LPS)-stimulated synthesis and release of IL-1 by monocytes from patients that had undergone this procedure.

Materials and Methods

Population. Thirty patients (18 males and 12 females) were included in the study. The mean age was 42 years. All those with immune disease, recent blood transfusions, and those who had regularly taken immune-modulating drugs or narcotics in the 6 months preceeding the study were excluded, as were subjects with jaundice, excised spleen, recurrent or local infection, nutritional deficiency, metabolic disease, neoplasia, and liver or renal disease. The sera of all subjects were screened for anti-HIV antibodies.

After evaluation of operative risk, using the classification of the American Society of Anesthesiologists (with no one exceeding class I), patients underwent elective surgery which was either clean or clean-contaminated [10]. None of the operations lasted more than 120 min. Each was performed under standardized

[1] Institute of General Pathology and Oncology, First School of Medicine and Surgery, University of Naples, Naples, Italy
[2] Institute of Surgery and Surgical Therapy, First School of Medicine and Surgery, University of Naples, Naples, Italy

Host Defense Dysfunction
in Trauma, Shock and Sepsis
Eds. Faist/Meakins/Schildberg
© Springer-Verlag, Berlin Heidelberg 1993

general anesthesia (thiopentone + N_2O + fentanyl) by the same surgical team. None of the patients received a blood transfusion, during or after surgery. Antibiotic prophylaxis was carried out with second-generation cephalosporins. Samples of blood were drawn prior to surgery (PSD), and on the second and seventh postoperative days (POD).

Monocyte Cultures. Mononuclear cells were taken from samples of peripheral blood by Ficoll-Paque fractioning, (Pharmacia, Uppsala, Sweden). These were washed three times with phosphate-buffered solution and resuspended in the same medium at a concentration of $2 \times 10^6/ml$. The percentage of monocytes was evaluated by a cytofluorimeter using a anti-CD14 MAb (Leu-M3; Becton Dickinson, Mountain View, CA, USA). Suspensions of cells were performed to obtain the same number of monocytes in all cultures. Cells were finally suspended in RPMI 1640 (Flow Laboratories, Irvine, Scotland), containing 2.5% heat-inactivated fetal calf serum (FCS), 2 mM L-glutamine and antibiotics (complete RPMI). Aliquots of 1 ml cell suspensions were distributed onto 24 sterile well dishes (Falcon Oxnard, USA); after 2 h incubation at 37 °C in 5% CO_2 in air, the nonadherent cells were removed by RPMI 1640 washing. Approximately 90% of the adherent cells (AC) were esterase positive and, after staining with Giemsa, revealed the typical monocyte morphology. The cells were more than 95% viable as assessed by the trypan blue exclusion test.

IL-1 Production. The AC from each well were incubated at 37 °C in 5% CO_2 in air for 24 h in 1 ml of complete RPMI 1640 containing 1 μg/ml indomethacin (final concentration) in the absence or in the pesence of 20 μg/ml LPS (*Escherichia coli*, 055:B55; Difco Laboratories, Detroit, MI USA). After incubation the supernatants were collected and centrifuged at 250 g for 10 min, sterilized on 450 μm Millipore filters and stored at − 80 °C until used. To determine cell-associated IL-1 activity the AC were washed three times with Hank's balanced salt solution (Flow Laboratories). One ml of Eagle's medium (Flow Laboratories) containing 5% FCS was added to each well and the cells lysed by three freeze-thaw cycles. The lysates were filtered and stored at − 80 °C until used [1, 6, 9].

IL-1 Assay. Using a costimulatory assay, murine thymocytes were assayed for IL-1 activity [5, 9]. Briefly, thymocyte suspension in RPMI 1640 was obtained from 5 to 8-week-old female C3H/HeJ mice. The cells were washed with the same culture medium and resuspended ($10^7/ml$) in complete RPMI 1640, to which 2-mercaptoethanol had been added (2.5×10^{-5} M). Aliquots of 100 μl of the cell suspension were incubated, in triplicate, for 72 h in 96 flat-bottomed well dishes (Falcon), at 37 °C in 5% CO_2 in air. Phytohemagglutinin 50 μl; 1 μg/ml; Wellcome, Beckenham, England) and 50 μl of serial dilution from the samples were added to each well. Recombinant IL-1 α (20 U/ml; Boehringer Mannheim, FRG) was used for the positive control. Twenty-four hours before the end of incubation 0.5 μCi of [^{3}H] thymidine (2 Ci/mmol; Amersham, Buckinghamshire, England) were added to the culture. Microcultures were sacrificed with a semiautomatic cell harvester (Skatron, Lier, Norway) and the radioactivity determined by liquid scintillation counter (LKB-Wallac, Turku, Finland). Results were evaluated by the Student's t-test.

Results

Supernatants of cultures incubated in the absence of LPS show a slight increase in IL-1 activity only on the second POD. LPS-stimulated AC show a marked IL-1 release that significantly increased on second POD and returned to the basal level on the seventh POD (Fig. 1).

Cell-associated IL-1 activity also appears to be significantly increased on the second POD. both in unstimulated and in LPS-stimulated AC. On the seventh POD however, this activity decreases in unstimulated AC, although this is still higher than that on the PSD, while in LPS-stimulated AC the levels are very near to those on the second POD (Fig. 1).

Conclusions

Our study shows an overall postoperative activation of AC that is expressed with an increase of both spontaneous and LPS-stimulated synthesis and release of IL-1. This result is principally evident on the second POD and tends to return to the basal values on the seventh POD.

The changes in IL-1 production and secretion postoperatively are not due to the secretion of PGE_2 by cultured monocytes since we have added indomethacin, a well-known cyclooxygenase inhibitor, to the culture medium [4, 9]

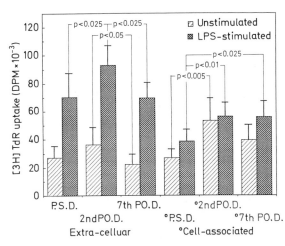

Fig. 1. Pre and postoperative IL-1 activity from mononuclear adherent cells, unstimualted (□) and stimulated with lipopolysaccharide (□), in the presence of 1 μg/ml indomethacin. Results are expressed as mean ± S.D. of [³H] thymidine uptake in triplicate cultures of C3H/HeJ mouse in a costimulatory assay. P. S. D., prior to surgery; P. O. D., postoperative day

Studies are in progress to determine the amount of α-or β-forms occurring in extra and intracellular IL-1.

References

1. Bacle F, Haeffner-Cavaillon N, Laude M, Couturier C, Kazatchkine MD (1990) Induction of IL-1 release through stimulation of the C3b/C4b complement receptor type one (CR1, CD35) on human monocytes. J immunol 144:147–152
2. Dinarello CA, Savage N (1989) Interleukin-1 and its receptor. Crit Rev Immunol 9 (1):1–20
3. Faist E, Ertel W, Mewes A, Alkan S, Walz A, Strasser T (1989) Trauma-induced alterations of the lymphokine cascade. In: Faist E, Ninnemann J, Green DR (eds) Immune consequences of trauma, shock, and sepsis. Springer, Berlin Heidelberg New York, pp 79–94
4. Faist E, Mewes A, Backer CC, Strasser Th, Alkan SS, Rieber P, Heberer G, (1987) Prostaglandin E₂ (PGE)₂-dependent suppression of interleukin-2 (IL-2) production in patients with major trauma. J Trauma 27:837–848
5. Faist E, Mewes A, Strasser T, Walz A, Alkan S, Baker C, Ertel W, Heberer G (1988) Alteration of monocyte function following major injury. Arch Surg 123:287–292
6. Gery l, Schimdt IA (1985) Human interleukin 1. In: Di Sabato G, Langone JJ, Van Vunakis H (eds) Methods in enzymology, vol 116. Academic, New York, pp 456–467
7. Green DR, Faist E (1988) Trauma and the immune response. Immunol Today 9:253–254
8. Meakins JL (1988) Host defense mechanisms in surgical patients: effect of surgery and trauma. Acta Chir Scand Suppl 550:43–53
9. Mizel SB (1981) Production and quantitation of lymphocyte-activating factor (interleukin-1). In: Herskowitz HB, Holden HT, Bellanti JA, Ghaffar A (eds) Manual of macrophage methodology. Dekker, New York, pp 407–416
10. National Academy of Sciences-National Research Council, Division of Medical Sciences; ad hoc Committee on trauma NAS-NRC (1964) Post-operative wound infections: the influence of ultraviolet irradiation of the operating room and various other factors. Ann Surg: 160 (Suppl 2)
11. Ninnemann JL (1989) The immune consequences of trauma: an overview. In: Faist E, Ninnemann JL, Green DR (eds) Immune consequences of trauma, shock, and sepsis. Springer, Berlin Heidelberg New York, pp 3–8
12. Rodrick ML, Wood JJ, Gribc JT, O'Mabony JB, Davis CF, Moss NK, Blazar BA, Demcing RH, Mannick JA (1986) Defective IL-2 production in patients with severe burns and sepsis. Lymphokine Res 5:75–80
13. Wood JJ, Rodrick ML, O'Mahony JB, Palder SB, Saporoschetz I, D'Eon P, Mannick JA (1984) Inadequate interleukin-2 production. A fundamental immunological deficiency in patients with major burns. Ann Surg: 311–320

The Biological Characteristics of Cytokines and Their Interactions with Prostaglandins Following Hemorrhagic Shock

W. Ertel[1], E. Faist[1], and I. H. Chaudry[2]

Trauma, burn, and surgical injury as well as shock and sepsis stimulate the production and the release of a variety of endogenous mediators. These mediators, in turn, initiate immunological, circulatory, hematologic, metabolic, and histological alterations that are integral to the response of the host to injury or bacteremia. The role of classic endocrine hormones such as catecholamines, cortisol, thyroxine, or adrenocorticotropic hormone (ACTH) have been extensively studied in the past [1–3]. Recently, however, attention was directed from these classic hormones to a new class of proteins, collectively termed cytokines, as important endogenous mediators of the inflammatory response. These proteins differ from classic hormones in that cytokines are bioactive at very low concentrations, are produced by a wide array of different cell types at multiple sites within the body, are differentially synthesized in various concentrations dependent on the challenge and/or the nature of the initiating stimulus or the location, and have important autocrine and paracrine as well as endocrine functions.

Cytokines have beneficial or detrimental properties, depending upon the amount and the type of the released cytokine. At low concentrations, the cytokines stimulate antimicrobial functions and the healing of the wound. They also mobilize substrate stores and activate the humoral and cellular immune system. At high concentrations cytokines produce hypotension, metabolic alterations, and a shocklike status with severe tissue damage. With such diverse influences on biological functions, it is not surprising that an exaggerated or prolonged secretion of these proteins may be detrimental for the host. Specifically, aberrant secretion of cytokines is thought to be responsible, at least in part, for the changes in the host during and following severe infection or septic shock.

The most widely studied and essential cytokines are tumor necrosis factor-alpha (TNF-α)/cachectin, interleukin-1 (IL-1), and interleukin-6 (IL-6). Cachectin/TNF-α is produced by blood monocytes [4], alveolar macrophages [5], hepatic Kupffer cells [6], peritoneal macrophages [7], and endothelial and natural killer cells [8]. TNF-α has been found to play a central role during and after infection causing hypotension [9], adult respiratory distress syndrome

---

[1] Chirurgische Klinik und Poliklinik der Ludwig-Maximilians-Universität München, Klinikum Großhadern, 8000 Munich 70, FRG
[2] Department of Surgery, Michigan State University, East Lansing, MI, 48824, USA

Host Defense Dysfunction
in Trauma, Shock and Sepsis
Eds. Faist/Meakins/Schildberg
© Springer-Verlag, Berlin Heidelberg 1993

(ARDS) [10], severe metabolic changes [11, 12], and tissue damage [13] leading to multiple organ failure and death. The marked elevation of serum levels during meningococcal sepsis in patients correlated with the fatal outcome [14]. IL-1, released by blood monocytes, tissue macrophages, endothelial cells, blood neutrophils, and B lymphocytes [15] was initially described as a comitogen for T-lymphocyte proliferation [16] and has been found to promote myelopoiesis [17, 18], but also causes fever [19], increases permeability of endothelial cells [20], and stimulates procoagulant activity [21]. IL-6 is released by fibroblasts, monocytes, macrophages, keratinocytes, and endothelial cells [22]. Besides the activation and stimulation of B-cell functions [23], IL-6 enhances the synthesis of hepatic proteins during injury [24, 25]. Furthermore, IL-6 represents an endogenous pyrogen that acts by inducing the production of prostaglandins [26]. In addition, the levels of IL-6 appear to correlate with the acute phase response in patients with burns [27].

A large number of in vitro and in vivo studies demonstrated a close relationship between these three cytokines. TNF seems to be the first mediator released following trauma or sepsis [28], thus upregulating the synthesis and release of IL-1 [29], IL-6 [30, 31], and arachidonic acid metabolites such as prostaglandin E_2 (PGE_2) [32]. IL-6 on the other hand, down-regulates the synthesis of TNF and IL-1 by blood monocytes [4]. The expression of cachectin/TNF-α is tightly controlled, both on the transcriptional and the translational level. Kunkel et al. [33] showed that PGE_2 plays a pivotal role in the regulation of TNF synthesis via a negative feedback mechanism. In parallel to TNF, IL-1 induces the release of PGE_2 [34], while PGE_2 down-regulates the activation of IL-1 on a posttranscriptional level [35]. Cachectin/TNF-α also elicits the release of the counterregulatory hormones glucagon, cortisol, and epinephrine in vivo [36]. In a primate model of bacteremia, the release of these hormones and the cytokines IL-1β and IL-6 could be blocked by the administration of antibodies specific for cachectin/TNF-α [37, 38]. IL-1 acts on the neuroendocrine axis, stimulating the release of pituitary neurohormones, including the ACTH, thyroid-stimulating hormone, and somatostatin [39–41]. IL-1 also directly elicits adrenal corticoid release and pancreatic release of both insulin and glucagon [42, 43]. IL-6 can enhance the production of IL-2 in vitro [44] and IL-2 can increase the translation of cachectin/TNF-α messenger ribonucleic acid (mRNA) and protein [45, 46]. Cytokine mediators also exhibit synergy among themselves in addition to the interactions with other mediators. For example, Kindler et al. [47] demonstrated that TNF-α is able to up-regulate its own gene expression, translation, and secretion. The synergistic interaction of cachectin/TNF-α and IL-1 in many types of tissue including pituitary cells, bone, vascular endothelial cells, skin fibroblasts, and islets of Langerhans, are well described [48]. Cachectin/TNF-α is synergistic with interferon-gamma (IFN-γ) in their antiproliferative effects on certain human and murine cell lines [49] and in their enhancement of fungus killing by polymorphonuclear cells [50]. The combined systemic infusion of cachectin/TNF-α and IL-1 into conscious rabbits produce hemodynamic instability, alterations in expenditure of energy and hypertriglyceridemia, whereas infusions of each cytokine alone at comparable doses yield only minimal effects [51].

In patients with thermal injury, severe soft tissue trauma, or after prolonged surgical procedures, a broad spectrum of alterations with regard to cytokine and prostanoid synthesis and release occurs. There is evidence that the release of TNF-α, IL-6, and PGE_2 by macrophages is dramatically increased, while IL-1 secretion is significantly depressed after surgery [52]. These alterations in cytokine and prostaglandin release are of great biological significance, since these mediators predominantly regulate the immune system of the host [53]. With regard to the elevated release of immunosuppressive mediators, the host is rendered to an increased susceptibility to infection and sepsis. This is documented by the fact that sepsis is the major nonneurological cause of death associated with trauma, thermal injury, and major surgery and carries an overall mortality rate of 60% [54]. Although a large number of investigations have examined and continue to examine the effects of various forms of trauma on the cytokine cascade, the immune system and their interactions, very few studies are being carried out to precisely study the interactions of cytokines and prostaglandins in a well-defined model of simple hemorrhage or trauma. Trauma consists of various components such as severe blood loss, soft tissue trauma, the release of toxic peptides, the migration of bacteria, emergency operations, and prolonged anesthesia. The complexity of this issue made it very difficult in previous studies to clearly elucidate the alterations in cytokine and prostaglandin cascade following trauma and sepsis. Thus, there was a need to separate the complex alterations which occur during and after trauma. Since hemorrhage is a prevalent complication in trauma victims arising from soft tissue and bone injury, as well as frequently being encountered during complex surgical procedures, a simple murine model of hemorrhage and resuscitation was developed [55]. The model was a nonlethal, fixed blood pressure model which allowed us to precisely study the alterations in cytokine production and release as well as the interactions among these mediators and PGE_2.

Although serum/plasma levels of cytokines and prostaglandins, respectively, do not necessarily reflect mediator concentrations in the tissue, it was important to define the alterations in circulating cytokine levels which occur following hemorrhage. As little as 30 min into hemorrhage significant levels of circulating TNF-α are detectable [56]. The enhancement of TNF in serum revealed its peak levels after 2 h with a tendency towards baseline values after 24 h [56, 57]. TNF-α could not be detected in significant amounts in either sham controls, normal, stressed, or in the shed blood samples [56]. Although IL-6 had not increased after 30 min, circulating IL-6 was found to be significantly elevated after 2 h, which persisted slightly but not significantly, for up to 24 h after the induction of hemorrhagic shock [57]. In contrast to TNF-α, small amounts of IL-6 were, however, detected in serum harvested from stressed animals and in the shed blood of animals subjected to hemorrhage [56]. Since endotoxin represents a potent mediator of the release of both TNF and IL-6, and since it has been suggested that endotoxin might be released via bacterial translocation during hemorrhage [58], circulating endotoxin levels were determined during and after hemorrhagic shock and correlated with the alterations in cytokine profiles. While minimal levels of endotoxin could be detected under all conditions, no marked increase in systemic endotoxin was seen in hemorrhaged animals that could be attributed to hemorrhage per se [56]. However, it cannot be excluded that following hemorrhagic shock, some bacteria and/or endotoxin are released due to translocation from the gut. However, the amounts are so small that they are cleared through the reticuloendothelial system of the liver, (i.e., Kupffer cells), thus resulting in no significant elevation of endotoxin in plasma. This hypothesis is confirmed by the fact that Kupffer cells, and not the other macrophage populations, produce up to tenfold higher amounts of TNF-α, IL-6, and IL-1 2 h following hemorrhage [57, 58]. This activation can be, in part, due to hypoxia. However, transient endotoxemia may also stimulate Kupffer cells to synthesize and release these inflammatory mediators in high amounts. Thus, the Kupffer cells, because of their location and largest macrophage pool in the whole body, may predominantly influence serum/plasma levels of inflammatory cytokines [59]. In contrast to TNF-α and IL-6, plasma levels of PGE_2 were only slightly elevated 2 h after hemorrhagic shock, while a significant rise was detected after 24 h. Since PGE_2 is known from several in vitro studies to block mRNA expression of TNF [33], this may explain the reduction in TNF synthesis and release 24 h after hemorrhage.

These results clearly demonstrate that hemorrhagic shock results in an activation of the cascade of inflammatory mediators even without a significant rise in serum endotoxin levels. The complex cascade of mediators released following hemorrhage appears to be activated in a very similar manner to sepsis and septic shock, although endotoxin does not appear to play a major role in activating the release of inflammatory mediators following hemorrhage. TNF-α is the first cytokine which is produced and released in significant amounts into the blood and is elevated very early after the onset of hemorrhage. Other inflammatory mediators, such as IL-6 or PGE_2, were found much later in the time course after the induction of hemorrhagic shock. This may indicate that TNF represents the pivotal cytokine in the cascade of inflammatory mediators which is responsible for inducing the synthesis and release of the other inflammatory mediators.

To further study the biological significance of increased TNF plasma levels on the synthesis and release of IL-6, circulating TNF was neutralized by preimmunization with a hamster antimurine TNF antibody in the same hemorrhagic shock model. Anti-TNF antibody-treated hemorrhaged mice demonstrated a significant reduction in TNF-α plasma levels at 2 and 24 h which were in the range of sham-operated animals [60]. Thus, the hemorrhagic shock-induced increase of circulating IL-6 could be attenuated by preimmunization with the anti-TNF antibody [60]. Similarly, in vitro Kupffer cell cultures from the anti-TNF antibody-treated group released less IL-6 following hemorrhagic shock than Kupffer cells from the vehicle-treated group [60]. These data indicate that TNF is able to up-regulate IL-6 production and release in vivo, confirming previous in vitro studies which demonstrated an enhancing effect of TNF on IL-6 mRNA expression and synthesis [30, 31]. Moreover, these data are in agreement with the results of Fong et al. [38], who reported the regulatory role of TNF in vivo on IL-6 release in an endotoxin model. The neutralization of circulating TNF via the anti-TNF antibody, however, further enhanced the release of IL-1 and TNF by macrophages [60], which suggests that circulating TNF, either directly or indirectly by some second mediator(s), controls the release of not only IL-1, but also its own release. This is supported by studies by Kindler et al. [47], who injected recombinant TNF into the peritoneal cavity of mice and measured TNF mRNA expression. The injection of TNF significantly enhanced peritoneal macrophages to express mRNA for TNF. Since in vitro studies clearly demonstrated that TNF is not an inhibitor but a potent stimulator of IL-1 release [61] and the blockade of TNF with monoclonal antibodies led to enhanced IL-1 and TNF release by macrophages [60], it appears unlikely that increased circulating TNF following hemorrhage directly regulates macrophage IL-1 release. It is more likely that secondary mediators, which are up-regulated by TNF, are involved in the regulation of macrophage cytokine release. In this regard, several studies have shown that TNF not only induces the synthesis of IL-1 [61, 62], but also up-regulates, as demonstrated above, the synthesis and release of IL-6 [30, 31] and PGE_2 [63–65]. This is of great biological significance for the regulation of the cytokine cascade, since IL-6, as shown by Schindler et al. [4], has an inhibitory effect on TNF and IL-1 release by peripheral blood monocytes. PGE_2 on the other hand, dramatically inhibits the synthesis of IL-1 on a posttranscriptional level [66] and of TNF on a transcriptional level through a negative feedback mechanism [67–70].

Based on previous studies concerning the close relationship between TNF and PGE_2, which may represent the pivotal regulatory mechanism for the cytokine cascade, in vitro and in vivo studies were carried out using a cyclooxygenase inhibitor to block PGE_2 synthesis. Kinetic studies of TNF release by peritoneal macrophages obtained from hemorrhaged mice showed a marked decrease in TNF levels in supernatants obtained from 48-h cultures in comparison to 24-h cultures [71]. These alterations in TNF release correlated with a significant elevation in PGE_2 release by these peritoneal macrophages [71]. However, the decrease in TNF release in 48-h cultures could be completely abolished by the addition of the cyclooxygenase inhibitor ibuprofen to these macrophage cultures [71]. These data further indicate that TNF release by macrophages is affected by arachidonic acid metabolites of the cyclooxygenase pathway. The major mechanism for the suppressive effect of eicosanoids, predominantly PGE_2, on TNF synthesis is probably caused by an elevation in intracellular cyclic adenosine monophosphate (cAMP) [70]. Although other prostaglandins were not tested in this study, it can be suggested that the observed effects are mainly caused by PGE_2, since Renz et al. [72] demonstrated that PGE_2, and, partially, PGE_1 at high concentrations, but not $PGE_{2\alpha}$, thromboxane B_2 (TXB_2), or arachidonic acid, suppress lipopolysaccharide (LPS)-induced TNF release by macrophages. Renz et al. [72] further described a dose-dependent effect of PGE_2 on TNF release by LPS-stimulated peritoneal macrophages with an 80% suppression of TNF release in the presence of 100 ng/ml PGE_3. The PGE_2 levels in peritoneal macrophage cultures from hemorrhaged animals following incubation with LPS were in a range of 80–100 ng/ml PGE_2, which is similar to the amounts of PGE_2 used by Renz et al. [72]. The measurements of PGE_2 plasma levels revealed a slight increase at 2 h and a significant rise at 24 h after induction of hemorrhagic shock. Animals were treated in vivo with ibuprofen immediately after resuscitation and the effect of cyclooxygenase blockade on cytokine release by peritoneal macrophages studied. The ibuprofen treatment significantly increased the release of IL-1 and TNF-α while the secretion of IL-6 by macrophages was reduced [73]. This further confirms the negative regulatory role of cyclooxygenase metabolites on the synthesis and release of TNF-α and IL-1 not only in vitro, but also in vivo. It should be mentioned that the suppression of essential macrophage (antigen presentation, Ia-expression) as well as splenocyte functions (proliferation, lymphokine synthesis), observed following hemorrhagic shock, were not seen in ibuprofen-treated animals despite elevated TNF production [73, 74]. These data may indicate that TNF activates the cytokine cascade with positive and negative regulatory mediators, but does not directly cause immunosuppression. Cytokines and arachidonic acid metabolites elicit the release of other mediators and/or each other and are likely to be important in propagating the host mediator cascade during shock, trauma, and sepsis. As demonstrated in Fig. 1, TNF-α seems to be the trigger cytokine in the cascade which is released early during the insult. This cytokine then activates various populations of macrophages to release IL-1, IL-6, and the arachidonic acid metabolite PGE_2. While TNF and IL-1 seem to be positive regulatory mediators in view of stimulating the host defense system, IL-6 and PGE_2 may be negative regulators. Both mediators suppress the synthesis and/or the release of TNF-α and IL-1. Although previous studies have described additional cytokines (up to IL-12), TNF, IL-1, IL-6, and PGE_2 represent the pivotal and central regulatory

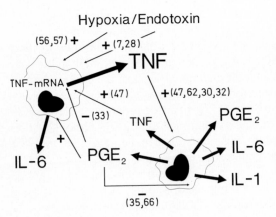

Fig. 1. The cascade of inflammatory mediators following hemorrhagic shock. The *bold arrows* illustrate the release of soluble mediators. The *thin arrows* indicate the effects of mediators on cytokine release by cells. The nature of impact is illustrated by (–) or (+). *TNF*, tumor necrosis factor-α; *IL-1*, interleukin-1; *IL-6*, interleukin-6; *PGE_2*, prostaglandin E_2; *numbers in parentheses*, references; *mRNA*, messenger ribonucleic acid

hormones of the cytokine cascade. However, it should be emphasized that the cytokine cascade may be triggered and amplified in a complex and inter-dependent manner. Hence, the entire milieu of hormonal and cytokine medi-ators must be considered in the assessment of biological response to injury.

References

1. Wilmore DW, Long JM, Mason AD et al. (1974) Catecholamines: mediators of the hyper-metabolic response to thermal injury. Ann Surg 180:653–668
2. Calvano SE, Chiao J, Reaves LE et al. (1984) Changes in free and total levels of plasma cortisol and thyroxine following thermal injury in man. J Burn Care Rehabil 5:143–151
3. Wilmore DW, Lindsey CA, Moylan JA et al. (1974) Hyperglucagonaemia after burns. Lancet 1:73–75
4. Schindler R, Mancilla J, Endres S, Ghorbani R, Clark SC, Dinarello CA (1990) Correlations and interactions in the production of interleukin-6 (IL-6), IL-1 and tumor necrosis factor (TNF) in human blood mononuclear cells: IL-6 suppresses IL-1 and TNF. Blood 75:40–47
5. Ayala A, Perrin MM, Kisala JM, Ertel W, Chaudry IH (1992) Polymicrobial sepsis selectively activates peritoneal but not alveolar macrophage to release inflammatory mediators (IL-1, IL-6 and TNF). Circ Shock (in press)
6. Hesse DG, Davatelis G, Felsen D et al. (1987) Cachectin/tumor necrosis factor gene expression in Kupffer cells. J Leukoc Biol 42:422
7. Beutler B, Krochin N, Milsark IH et al. (1986) Control of cachectin (tumor necrosis factor) synthesis: mechanism of endotoxin resistance. Science 232:977–980
8. Aggarwal BB, Kohr W, Hass PE et al. (1985) Human tumor necrosis factor, production, purification, and characterization. J Biol Chem 260:2345–2354
9. Tracey KJ, Lowry SF, Fahey TJ et al. (1987) Cachectin/tumor necrosis factor induces lethal septic shock and stress hormone responses in the dog. Surg Gynecol Obstet 164:415–422
10. Ferrari-Baliviera E, Mealy K, Smith RJ, Wilmore DW (1989) Tumor necrosis factor induces adult respiratory distress syndrome in rats. Arch Surg 124:1400–1405
11. Zechner R, Newman TC, Sherry B et al. (1988) Recombinant human cachectin/tumor necrosis factor but not alpha downregulates lipoprotein lipase gene transcription in mouse 3T3-L1 adipocytes. Mol Cell Biol 8:2394–2401
12. Feingold KR, Grunfeld C (1987) Tumor necrosis factor-alpha stimulates hepatic lipogenesis in the rat in vivo. J Clin Invest 80:184–190
13. Tracey KJ, Beutler B, Lowry SF et al. (1986) Shock and tissue injury induced by recombinant human cachectin. Science 234:470–474
14. Waage A, Halstensen A, Espevik T (1987) Association between tumor necrosis factor in serum and fatal outcome in patients with meningococcal disease. Lancet 1:355–357
15. Dinarello CA (1988) Biology of interleukin 1. FASEB J 2:108–115
16. Vyth Dreese FA, De Vries JE (1984) Induction of IL-2 production, IL-2 receptor expression and proliferation of T3-T-P11 cells by phobol ester. Int J Cancer 34:831–838
17. Ulich TR, Castillo JD, Keys M et al. (1987) Kinetics and mechanisms of recombinant human interleukin 1 alpha and tumor necrosis factor alpha induced changes in circulating numbers of neutrophils and lymphocytes. J Immunol 139:3406–3415
18. Chen L, Novick D, Rubinstein M, Revel M (1988) Recombinant interferon-beta 2 (interleukin-6) induces myeloid differentiation. FEBS Lett 239:299–304
19. Walter JS, Meyers P, Krüger JM (1989) Microinjection of interleukin-1 into brain: separation of sleep and fever responses. Physiol Behav 45:169–176
20. Watson ML, Lewis GP, Westwick J (1989) Increased vascular permeability and polymorpho-nuclear leucocyte accumulation in vivo in response to recombinant cytokines and supernatant from cultures of human synovial cells treated with interleukin-1. Br J Exp Pathol 70:93–101
21. Nawroth PP, Handley DA, Esmon CT, Stern DM (1986) Interleukin-1 induces endothelial cell procoagulant while suppressing cell surface anticoagulant activity. Proc Natl Acad Sci USA 83:3460–3464
22. Van Snick J (1990) Interleukin-6: an overview. Annu Rev Immunol 8:253–278

23. Hirano T, Toga T, Nakano N et al. (1985) Purification to homogeneity and characterization of human B-cell differentiation factor (BCDF or BSFp-2). Proc Natl Acad Sci USA 82:5490–5494

24. Ritchie DG, Fuller GM (1983) Hepatocyte-stimulating factor: a monocyte-derived acute phase regulatory protein. Ann NY Acad Sci 408:490–502

25. Castell JV, Gomez-Lechon MJ, David M et al. (1989) Interleukin-6 is the major regulator of acute phase protein synthesis in adult human hepatocytes. FEBS Lett 242:237–239

26. Helfgott DC, Fong Y, Moldawer LL et al. (1989). Human interleukin-6 is an endogenous pyrogen. Clin Res 37:564A

27. Nijsten MWN, DeGroot ER, Ten Duis HJ et al. (1987) Serum levels of interleukin-6 and acute phase responses. Lancet 2:921

28. Michie HR, Manogue KR, Spriggs DR et al. (1988) Detection of circulating tumor necrosis factor after endotoxin administration. N Engl J Med 318:1481–1486

29. Dinarello CA, Cannon JG, Wolff SM et al. (1986) Tumor necrosis factor (cachectin) is an endogenous pyrogen and induces production of interleukin-1. J Exp Med 163:1433–1450

30. Kasid A, Director EP, Rosenberg SA (1989) Regulation of interleukin-6 (IL-6) by IL-2 and TNF-alpha in human peripheral blood mononuclear cells. Ann NY Acad Sci 557:564–566

31. Zhang Y, Lin JX, Yip YK, Vilcek J (1989) Stimulation of interleukin-6 mRNA levels by tumor necrosis factor and interleukin-1. Ann NY Acad Sci 557:548–550

32. Bachwich PR, Chensue SW, Larrick JW et al. (1986) Tumor necrosis factor stimulates IL-1 and PGE_2 production in resting macrophages. Biochem Biophys Res Commun 136:94–101

33. Kunkel SL, Spengler M, May MA, Spengler R, Larrick J, Remick D (1986) Prostaglandin E_2 regulates macrophage-derived tumor necrosis factor gene expression. J Biochem 263:5380–5384

34. Mizel SB, Dayer JM, Krane SM, Mergenhagen SE (1981) Stimulation of rheumatoid synovial cell collagenase and prostaglandin production by partially purified lymphocyte-activating factor (interleukin-1). Proc Natl Acad Sci USA 78:2474–2477

35. Kunkel SL, Chensue SW, Phan SH (1986) Prostaglandins as endogenous mediators of interleukin-1 production. J Immunol 136:186–192

36. Tracey KJ, Lowry SF, Cerami A (1987) Physiological responses to cachectin. In: Tumour necrosis factor and related cytokines. Ciba Found Symp 131:88–108

37. Tracey KJ, Fong Y, Hesse DG et al. (1987) Anti-cachectin/TNF monoclonal antibodies prevent septic shock during lethal bacteremia. Nature 330:662–664

38. Fong Y, Tracey KJ, Moldawer LL et al. (1989) Antibodies to cachectin/TNF reduces interleukin-1 beta and interleukin-6 appearance during lethal bacteremia. J Exp Med 170:1627–1633

39. Uehara A, Gottschall PE, Dahl RR, Arimura A (1987) Interleukin-1 stimulates ACTH release by an indirect action which requires endogenous corticotropin releasing factor. Endocrinology 121:1580–1582

40. Beach JE, Smallridge RC, Kinzer CA et al. (1989) Rapid release of multiple hormones from rat pituitaries perfused with recombinant interleukin-1. Life Sci 44:1–7

41. Scarborough DE, Lee SL, Dinarello CA, Reichlin S (1989) Interleukin-1 stimulates somatostatin biosynthesis in primary cultures of fetal rat brain. Endocrinology 124:549–551

42. Sandler S, Bentzen K, Borg LAH et al. (1989) Studies on the mechanisms causing inhibition of insulin secretion in rat pancreatic islets exposed to human interleukin-1 beta indicate a perturbation in the mitochondrial function. Endocrinology 124:1492–1501

43. Roh MS, Drazenovich KA, Barbose JJ et al. (1987) Direct stimulation of the adrenal cortex by interleukin-1. Surgery 102:140–146

44. Garman RD, Jacobs KA, Clark SC, Raulet DH (1987) B-cell stimulatory factor 2 (beta$_2$ interferon) functions as a second signal for interleukin 2 production by mature murine T cells. Proc Natl Acad Sci USA 84:7629–7633

45. Strieter RM, Remick DG, Lynch JP et al. (1989) Interleukin-2 induced tumor necrosis factor-alpha (TNF-alpha) gene expression in human alveolar macrophages and blood monocytes. Am Rev Respir Dis 139:335–342

46. Nedwin GE, Svedersky LP, Bringman TS et al. (1985) Effect of interleukin-2, interferon-gamma, and mitogens on the production of tumor necrosis factor-alpha and beta. J Immunol 135:2492–2497

47. Kindler V, Sappino AP, Grau GE, Piguet PF, Vassalli P (1989) The inducing role of tumor necrosis factor in the development of bactericidal granulomas during BCG infection. Cell 56:731–740

48. Le J, Vilcek J (1987) Biology of disease: tumor necrosis factor and interleukin 1: cytokines with multiple overlapping biological activities. Lab Invest 56:234–248

49. Sugarman BJ, Aggarwal BB, Hass PE et al. (1985) Recombinant tumor necrosis factor alpha: effects on proliferation of normal and transformed cells in vitro. Science 230:943–945
50. Djeu JY, Blanchard DK, Halkias D et al. (1986) Growth inhibition of *Candida albicans* by human polymorphonuclear neutrophils: activation by interferon-gamma and tumor necrosis factor. J Immunol 137:2980–2984
51. Weinberg JR, Wright DJM, Guz A (1988) Interleukin-1 and tumour necrosis factor cause hypotension in the conscious rabbit. Clin Sci 75:251–255
52. Faist E, Mewes A, Strasser T et al. (1988) Alteration of monocyte function following major injury. Arch Surg 123:287–292
53. Fong Y, Moldawer LL, Shires GT, Lowry SF (1990) The biological characteristics of cytokines and their implicaiton in surgical injury. Surg Gynecol Obstet 170:363–378
54. Baker CC, Oppenheimer L, Lewis FR, Truncey DD (1980) The epidemiology of trauma death. Am J Surg 140:144–150
55. Stephan RN, Conrad PJ, Janeway CA, Geha AS, Baue A, Chaudry IH (1986) Decreased interleukin-2 production following simple hemorrhage. Surg Forum 37:73–75
56. Ayala A, Perrin MM, Meldrum DR, Ertel W, Chaudry IH (1990) Hemorrhage induces an increase in serum TNF which is not associated with elevated levels of endotoxin. Cytokine 2:170–174
57. Ertel W, Morrison MH, Ayala A, Chaudry IH (1991) Chloroquine attenuates hemorrhagic shock induced suppression of Kupffer cell antigen presentation and MHC class II antigen expression through blockade of tumor necrosis factor and prostaglandin release. Blood 78:1781–1788
58. Deitch EA, Ma L, Ma WJ et al. (1989) Inhibition of endotoxin-induced bacterial translocation in mice. J Clin Invest 84:34–42
59. Ayala A, Perrin MM, Ertel W, Chaudry IH (1992) Differential effects of hemorrhage on Kupffer cells: decreased antigen presentation despite increased inflammatory cytokine (IL-1, IL-6, and TNF) release. Cytokine (in press)
60. Ertel W, Morrison MH, Ayala A, Perrin MM, Chaudry IH (1991) Anti-TNF monoclonal antibodies prevent hemorrhage-induced suppression of Kupffer cell antigen presentation and MHC class II antigen expression. Immunology 74:290–297
61. Libby P, Ordovas JM, Auger KR, Robbins AH, Birinyi LK, Dinarello CA (1986) Endotoxin and tumor necrosis factor induce interleukin-1 gene expression in adult human vascular endothelial cells. Am J Pathol 124:179–185
62. Dayer JM, Beutler B, Cerami A (1985) Cachectin/tumor necrosis factor stimulates collagenase and prostaglandin E_2 production by human synovial cells and dermal fibroblasts. J Exp Med 162:2163–2168
63. Baud L, Perez J, Friedlander G, Ardaillou R (1988) Tumor necrosis factor stimulates prostaglandin production and cyclic AMP levels in rat cultured mesangial cells. FEBS Lett 239:50–54
64. Campbell IK, Piccoli DS, Hamilton JA (1990) Stimulation of human chondrocyte prostaglandin E_2 production by recombinant human interleukin-1 and tumour necrosis factor. Biochem Biophys Acta 1051:310–318
65. Atkinson YH, Murray AW, Krilis S, Vadas MA, Lopez AF (1990) Human tumour necrosis factor-alpha (TNF-alpha) directly stimulates arachidonic acid release in human neutrophils. Immunology 70:82–87
66. Dinarello CA, Marnoy SO, Rosenwasser LJ (1983) Role of arachidonate metabolism in the immunoregulatory function of human leukocyte pyrogen/lymphocyte activating factor/interleukin 1. J Immunol 130:891–895
67. Scales WE, Chensue SW, Otterness I, Kunkel SL (1989) Regulation of monokine gene expression: Prostaglandin E_2 suppresses tumor necrosis factor but not interleukin-1 alpha or beta-mRNA and cell-associated bioactivity. J Leukoc Biol 45:416–421
68. Kunkel SL, Wiggins RC, Chensue SW, Larrick J (1986) Regulation of macrophage tumor necrosis factor production by prostaglandin E_2. Biochem Biophys Res Commun 137:404–410
69. Karck U, Peters T, Decker K (1988) The release of tumor necrosis factor from endotoxin-stimulated rat Kupffer cells is regulated by prostaglandin E_2 and dexamethasone. J Hepatol 7:352–361
70. Lehmann V, Benninghoff B, Dröge W (1988) Tumor necrosis factor-induced activation of peritoneal macrophages is regulated by prostaglandin E_2 and cAMP. J Immunol 141:587–591
71. Ertel W, Morrison MH, Ayala A, Chaudry IH (1991) Eicosanoids regulate tumor necrosis factor synthesis after hemorrhage in vitro and in vivo. J Trauma 31:609–616

72. Renz H, Gong JH, Schmidt A et al. (1988) Release of tumor necrosis factor from macrophages: enhancement and suppression are dose-dependently regulated by prostaglandin E_2 and cyclic nucleotides. J Immunol 141:2388–2393
73. Ertel W, Morrison MH, Ayala A, Perrin MM, Chaudry IH (1991) Blockade of prostaglandin production increases cachectin synthesis and prevents depression of macrophage functions following hemorrhagic shock. Ann Surg 213:265–271
74. Ertel W, Morrison MH, Meldrum DR, Ayala A, Chaudry IH (1992) Ibuprofen restores cellular immunity and decreases susceptibility to sepsis following hemorrhage. J Surg Res (in press)

The Response of Interleukin-1 and Interleukin-6 in Patients Undergoing Major Surgery

R. J. Baigrie, P. M. Lamont, M. J. Dallman and P. J. Morris

Introduction

Tumour necrosis factor alpha (TNF), interleukin-1 beta (IL-1) and interleukin-6 (IL-6) are regarded as major mediators of the acute phase response (APR) in humans. While TNF and IL-1 are thought to be primarily responsible for the non-hepatic manifestations of the response e.g. fever, prostaglandinaemia, tachycardia, catabolism [1], IL-6 has been shown in vitro to be primarily responsible for the hepatic component of the APR, resulting in the synthesis of acute phase proteins (APP [2, 3]). Nonetheless IL-1 and TNF also induce synthesis of APPs, in particular C-reactive protein (CRP [4–6]). The transcription and production of IL-6 in fibroblasts, endothelial cells, keratinocytes and monocytes has been shown to be enhanced in vitro by IL-1 and TNF [7–10]. Therefore there is evidence that IL-1 and TNF may be partly responsible for the induction of IL-6, and all three of these cytokines then mediate the APR.

The measurement of cytokines in the peripheral blood has proved difficult and circulating cytokines in humans have largely been detected only in unusual clinical and experimental situations. Most reports have been of sporadic detections involving single or daily measurements of cytokines and there have been very few attempts to assay cytokines longitudinally over a predetermined series of time points during an acute illness or after a severe insult. TNF has seldom been consistently detected except after endotoxin administration, which however, does not induce a detectable IL-1 response in vivo [11]. Recently however, Shenkin detected a consistent rise in the serum IL-6 elective surgical patients but was unable to detect a consistent rise in IL-1 or TNF [12]. All these patients had uncomplicated clinical courses and the difference therefore between a pathological and a physiological IL-6 response remains far from clear.

The aim of this study was to sample patients intensively before, during and after major surgery, and to explore the association between cytokine levels in their plasma and their clinical course and CRP response. We have assessed the levels of IL-1, IL-6, TNF and interferon gamma (IFN-γ) in patients undergoing elective aortic aneurysm surgery. These patients are tumour free and have a

Nuffield Department of Surgery, University of Oxford, John Radcliffe Hospital, Oxford, OX3 9DU, UK

Host Defense Dysfunction
in Trauma, Shock and Sepsis
Eds. Faist/Meakins/Schildberg
© Springer-Verlag, Berlin Heidelberg 1993

relatively low risk of bacterial contamination and sepsis, thus allowing the impact of major surgical trauma on cytokine levels to be evaluated without the conflicting influence of bacterial contamination or malignancy.

Methods

Subjects. Twenty-one patients (18 men and three women) aged between 59 and 83 years were studied. All underwent elective aortic aneurysm repair. Operative and postoperative details were recorded, including the durations of operation, aortic clamping and ventilation, as well as blood transfusion volume, postoperative temperatures, white cell count (WCC), APACHE scores and duration of admission. APACHE scoring was performed on the basis of the initial and worst physiological parameters during the first 24 h postoperatively.

Samples. Cold spun plasma was prepared from venous blood collected in pyrogen-free tubes containing ethylenediaminetetraacetate (EDTA) and the proteinase inhibitor aprotinin. Aliquots of plasma were stored at $-70\,°C$. During the course of the study, a comparison was made of results obtained when blood was collected into tubes with and without aprotinin. This showed no variation in cytokine levels and thereafter aprotinin was not used.

Sample times. Samples were taken the day before surgery and a preoperative sample was taken after induction of anaesthesia. Thereafter patients were sampled after incision at 0.5, 1.0, 1.5, 2.0, 2.5, 3.0, 3.5, 4.0, 6, 8, 12, 24, 48 and 72 h and selected times thereafter.

Cytokine Assays. Commercially available 'sandwich' enzyme-linked immunosorbant assays (ELISA) were used throughout. (IL-6 and TNF assays from British Biotechnology Ltd, Oxford, UK; IL-1 and IFN-γ assays from Medgenix Diagnostics, High Wycombe, Bucks, UK). In each assay a standard curve using recombinant cytokine was constructed and each sample was assayed in duplicate. The minimum sensitivity of the assays was 4 pg/ml.

CRP assay. This was measured using flow nephelometry (Array Protein System, Beckman Instruments Ltd., High Wycombe, Bucks, UK) with a minimum detectable level of 6 mg/l.

Results

Clinical Results. Fourteen patients had an uncomplicated postoperative course. Three patients had minor postoperative problems including chest and urinary tract infections, however, none were serious enough to delay their discharge from hospital. Three patients suffered profound complications including irreversible renal failure requiring dialysis, adult respiratory distress syndrome, peripheral embolisation resulting in infarction and requiring distal amputations, infarction of the colon and gallbladder and bleeding gastric ulceration. One patient died at 17 days, the other two eventually left hospital after several months. None of these problems were anticipated during surgery or in the immediate postoperative period, one patient was thought not to warrant admission to the Intensive Therapy Unit (ITU) and was returned directly to the ward, another was discharged from the ITU at 22 h. The third was thought to be progressing well until about 40 h when he unexpectedly developed septic shock.

Interleukin-6. This cytokine was detectable in all patients before surgery (Fig. 1). This basal level did not change until a continuous increase began at 90–120 min after skin incision in all patients. IL-6 peaked at 4–48 h after the commencement of the operation and had fallen rapidly by 48–72 h in all patients who had an uncomplicated postoperative course. The three patients who suffered serious complications had a significantly greater IL-6 response (Fig. 2). In each case this response began during surgery or within 6 h of incision, which was well in advance of clinical signs of complications. The IL-6 response in the other three patients who had less serious complications did not differ significantly from the patients without complications.

Interleukin-1. IL-1 was not detected preoperatively in any patient (Fig. 3). However an early short-lived rise in IL-1 was detected in 17 patients. In each case it preceded the IL-6 response by several hours and disappeared rapidly. An example of this sequential pattern is given in Fig. 4. There was no significant difference in the peak IL-1 response of complicated and uncomplicated patients.

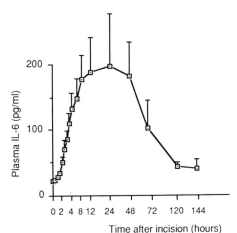

Fig. 1. The plasma IL-6 response in patients undergoing abdominal aortic aneurysm surgery. *Squares,* mean values (*n* = 20) and *standard error bars*

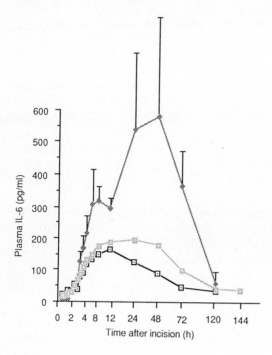

Fig. 2. The plasma IL-6 response in patients subgroups undergoing abdominal aortic aneurysm surgery. *Solid squares*, patients without complications (*n* = 17); *diamonds*, patients with complications (*n* = 3); *stippled squares*, all patients (*n* = 20)

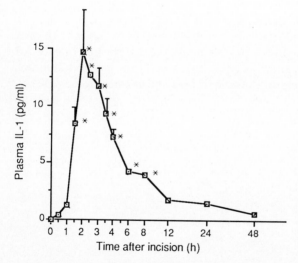

Fig. 3. The plasma IL-1 response in patients undergoing abdominal aortic aneurysm surgery. *Squares*, mean values (*n* = 20); *asterisks*, significantly different with respect to time 0.5 h (*p* ≤ 0.001 by Mann-Whitney U test)

Tumour Necrosis Factor and Interferon-γ. TNF and IFN-γ were not detected in any samples either before, during or after surgery.

C-reactive Protein. In all patients plasma CRP was noted to increase between 8 and 24 h and to peak around 48 h after the first incision, mean = 200 mg/l

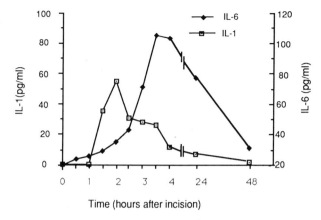

Fig. 4. An example in one patient of the plasma IL-1 response preceding IL-6 after major surgery

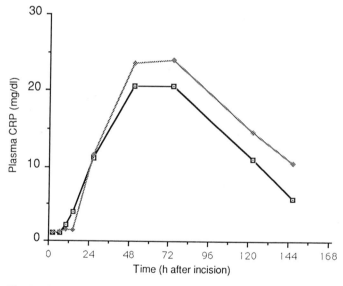

Fig. 5. The plasma CRP response in patients undergoing abdominal aortic aneurysm surgery. *Squares*, patients without complications; *diamonds*, patients with complications

(Fig. 5). Although the CRP values were slightly higher in the complicated patient group, the difference was not apparent until 48 h, by which time the complications were clinically evident.

Correlations. These were sought between various clinical data and the cytokine responses. The integrated IL-6 response as derived from the area under the IL-6 curve has previously been shown to correlate extremely accurately with the peak IL-6 value and we have therefore used peak values for correlation analysis [13].

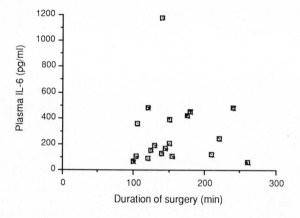

Fig. 6. Correlation between peak IL-6 response and duration of surgery in patients undergoing abdominal aortic aneurysm surgery. $r = 0.19$; $p = 0.49$

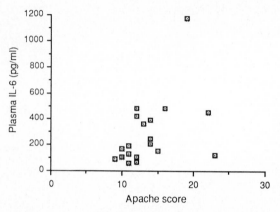

Fig. 7. Correlation between peak IL-6 response and APACHE scores in patients undergoing abdominal aortic aneurysm surgery. $r = 0.48$; $p < 0.05$

There was no correlation between the IL-1 and IL-6 response nor between either of these cytokines and the durations of operation (Fig. 6), aortic clamping and ventilation. Nor was any correlation observed between the cytokine responses and blood transfusion volume, postoperative temperatures and WCC. The most significant correlation was between the IL-6 response and the APACHE scores (Fig. 7).

Discussion

We have shown an early and brief IL-1 response to major surgical injury. This always preceded the IL-6 response in any individual patient. This data would seem to provide in vivo evidence consistent with the in vitro observation that IL-1 induces IL-6 synthesis and release [7–10]. While the absence of any correlation between the IL-1 and IL-6 response could be viewed as less consistent with this conclusion, it would be simplistic to imagine that cytokine induction might be reflected quantitatively in the peripheral circulation.

IL-1 has only occasionally been detected in the peripheral plasma, for example in four patients with meningococcal septicaemia [14], but these were only daily samples and the period when detectable IL-1 was present in these patients could easily have been missed. Furthermore, when human volunteers were administered TNF and endotoxin, IL-1 was not detected [11, 15], but no samples were taken between 1 and 3 h when our results suggest IL-1 might have been briefly present. It is clear from our results that an IL-1 response will be detected only by frequent sampling of the intra-operative or equivalent period after a major insult, as represented by major aortic surgery.

The IL-6 response seen in our uncomplicated patients is similar to those published in two recent reports [13, 16], but of interest are the patients who had a complicated postoperative course. Their IL-6 levels rose above the mean within a few hours of incision, preceding their subsequent complications. In each case there was no suspicion of poor progress until 24–48 h had passed. Their IL-6 response not only preceded their clinical signs by 12–36 h, but was also significantly greater and persisted longer than the response seen in the uncomplicated group.

The CRP response confirms that described in previous studies [17, 18]. Moreover the 20–30 h delay between the appearance of the cytokines and the CRP response, supports the hypothesis of IL-1 and IL-6 being mediators of APP synthesis.

There have been many attempts to correlate isolated cytokine levels with patient prognosis, the most notable of these being the detection of TNF. Although the increases have not been consistent, circulating levels of TNF have been associated with poor clinical outcome in septic or burn patients [14, 19, 20]. However serum levels of TNF have also been shown to have a negligible impact on the prediction of outcome when assessed in conjunction with simple clinical and laboratory variables [21]. Despite intensive sampling and the use of a sensitive immunoassay, TNF was not detected in our patients nor in a similar study of trauma patients [16]. Nonetheless TNF has been detected in plasma 90–120 min after insult [11], which corresponds to the period of IL-1 appearance in this study. It is possible therefore, that a very low concentration of TNF may be present, and along with IL-1, involved with IL-6 induction at this time.

This study has provided evidence concomitant with a primary role for IL-1 and IL-6 in the APR and synthesis of APPs, and has explored further the association between cytokine levels in blood and clinical outcome as previously reported [22]. Although our patient numbers are small, these results also suggest that the IL-6 response after major injury may predict the development of significant complications. IL-6 is released by most tissues in the body and its plasma level may therefore reflect the degree of tissue damage during injury. The surgeon is unable to assess tissue damage at the cellular level, due to harmful influences such as ischemia and pH change, which may induce the observed early rise of IL-6 either directly or via IL-1 mediation. Tissue damage obviously has a major influence on patient outcome and the use of IL-6 as a clinical marker, either alone or as part of a scoring system, deserves further evaluation.

References

1. Dinarello CA (1984) Interleukin-1. Rev Infect Dis 6:51–95
2. Castell JV, Andus T, Kunz D, Heinrich PC (1989) Interleukin-6. The major regulator of acute-phase protein synthesis in man and rat. Ann NY Acad Sci 557:87–99
3. Gauldie J, Richards C, Harnish D, Lansdorp P, Baumann H (1987). Interferon b2/B cell stimulatory factor 2 shares identity monocyte-derived hepatocyte-stimulating factor and regulates the major acute phase protein response in liver cells. Proc Nat Acad Sci USA 84:7251–7255
4. Hasselgren PO, Pederson P, Sax HC, Warner BW, Fischer JE (1988) Current concepts of protein turnover and amino acid transport in liver and skeletal muscle during sepsis. Arch Surg 123:992–999
5. Perlmutter DH, Dinarello CA, Punsal PI, Colten HR (1986) Cachectin/tumor necrosis factor regulates hepatic acute phase gene expression. J Clin Invest 78:1349–1353
6. Baumann H, Gauldie J (1990) Regulation of hepatic acute phase plasma protein genes by hepatocyte stimulating factors and other mediators of inflammation. Mol Biol Med 7:147–159
7. Bauer J, Ganter U, Geiger T, Jacobshagen U, Hirano T, Matsuda T, Kishimoto T, Andus T, Acs G, Gerok W, Ciliberto G (1988) Regulation of interleukin-6 expression in cultured human blood monocytes and monocyte-derived macrophages. Blood 72:1134–1140
8. Kohase M, Henriksen B, DeStefano D, May LT, Vilcek J, Sehgal P (1986) Induction of beta 2-interferon by tumour necrosis factor: a homeostatic mechanism in control of cell proliferation. Cell 45:659–666
9. Tosatu G, Jones KD (1990) Interleukin-1 induces interleukin-6 production in peripheral blood monocytes. Blood 75:1305–1310
10. Shalaby MR, Waage A, Aarden L, Espevik T (1989) Endotoxin, tumour necrosis factor-alpha and interleukin-1 induce interleukin-6 production in vivo. Clin Immunol Immunopathol 53:488–498
11. Michie HR, Manogue KR, Spriggs DR, Revhaug A, O'Dwyer ST, Dinarello CA et al. (1988) Detection of circulating tumour necrosis factor after endotoxin administration. N Engl J Med 318:1481–1486
12. Shenkin A, Fraser WD, Series J, Winstanley FP, McCartney AC, Burns HJG, van Damme J (1989) The serum interleukin-6 response to elective surgery. Lymphokine Res 8:123–127
13. Cruickshank AM, Fraser WD, Burns HJG, van Damme J, Shenkin A (1990) Response of serum interleukin-6 in patients undergoing elective surgery of varying severity. Clin Science 79:161–165
14. Girardin E, Grau GE, Dayer JM, Roux-Lombard P, Lambert P-H (1988) Tumour necrosis factor and interleukin-1 in the serum of children with severe infectious purpura. N Engl J Med 319:397–400
15. Michie HR, Spriggs DR, Manogue KR, Sherman ML, Revhaug A, O'Dwyer ST et al. (1988) Tumour necrosis factor and endotoxin induce similar metabolic responses in human beings. Surgery 104:280–286
16. Pullicino EA, Carli F, Poole S, Rafferty B, Malik STA, Elia M (1990) The relationship between the circulating concentrations of interleukin 6 (IL-6), tumour necrosis factor (TNF) and the acute phase response to elective surgery and accidental injury. Lymphokine Res 9:231–238
17. Colley CM, Fleck A, Goode AW, Muller BR, Myers MA (1983) Early time course of the acute phase protein response in man. J Clin Path 36:203–207
18. Stahl WM (1987) Acute phase protein response to tissue injury. Crit Care Med 15:545–550
19. Hack CE, De Groot ER, Felt-Bersma RJF, Nuijens JH, Strack Van Schijndel RJM, Eerenberg-Belmer AJM et al. (1989) Increased plasma levels of interleukin-6 in sepsis. Blood 74:1704–1710
20. Debets JMH, Kampmeijer R, van der Linden M, Buurman WA, van der Linden CJ (1989) Plasma tumour necrosis factor and mortality in critically ill septic patients. Crit Care Med 17:489–494
21. Calandra T, Baumgartner J-D, Grau GE, Wu M-M, Lambert P-H, Schellekens J, Verhoef J, Glauser MP (1990) Prognositc values of tumour necrosis factor/cachectin, interleukin-1, interferon alpha, and interferon gamma in the serum of patients with septic shock. J Infect Dis 161:982–987

Possible Role of Cytokines in the Stress Response of the Hypothalamo-Pituitary-Adrenal Axis During Upper Abdominal Surgery

Y. Naito[1], S. Tamai[1], K. Shingu[1], K. Shindo[2], T. Shichino[2], T. Matsui[1], O. Ebisui[3], J. Fukata[3], K. Yone[4], and K. Mori[2]

Introduction

It is well known that surgical invasion activates the hypothalamo-pituitary-adrenal (H-P-A) axis and induces marked elevation in plasma adrenocorticotropic hormone (ACTH) and cortisol levels during and after surgery. The stress response of plasma ACTH and cortisol levels cannot be totally suppressed by epidural [1] or subarachnoid anesthesia [2], especially in upper abdominal surgery [3], which suggests the involvement of some factor(s) other than afferent neural output arising from the injury site [4]. Some cytokines have recently been suspected to play important roles in the activation of the H-P-A axis at the times of infectious challenge and other stressful conditions [5–7]. To assess the possible involvement and role of cytokines in the stress response of the H-P-A axis during surgical procedures, we observed changes in the levels of plasma ACTH, cortisol, endotoxin, tumor necrosis factor-alpha (TNF-α), interleukin-1 (IL-1), and interleukin-6 (IL-6) in patients undergoing upper abdominal surgery. We then investigated the ACTH-releasing activities of these cytokines using an in vivo experimental system.

Materials and Methods

Clinical Experiments. We observed changes of plasma ACTH, cortisol, endotoxin, TNF-α, IL-1α, IL-1β, and IL-6 levels in eight patients undergoing pancreatoduodenectomy. Plasma samples were collected just before skin incision (0 h) and 2, 4, 6 and 8 h after skin incision. Plasma ACTH levels were determined using the ACTH IRMA kit Mitsubishiyuka (Mitsubishi Petrochemical, Tokyo). Plasma cortisol levels were determined as previously described [8]. Plasma endotoxin levels were assessed using a modified limulus test kit,

[1] Division of Emergency Medicine and Clinical Care Medicine, Kyoto University School of Medicine Sakyo-Ku Kyoto 606, Japan
[2] Department of Anesthesia, Kyoto University School of Medicine, Kyoto 606, Japan
[3] Second Division, Department of Internal Medicine, Kyoto University School of Medicine, Kyoto 606, Japan
[4] Biotechnology Research Laboratories, Teijin Tokyo Research Center, Teijin Limited, Hino, Tokyo 191, Japan

Host Defense Dysfunction
in Trauma, Shock and Sepsis
Eds. Faist/Meakins/Schildberg
© Springer-Verlag, Berlin Heidelberg 1993

Endotoxin-D (Seikagaku Kogyo, Tokyo). Plasma TNF-α levels were determined as previously described [9]. Plasma IL-1α and -β levels were determined
using the Human Interleukin-1α ELISA Kit and the Human Interleukin-1β
ELISA Kit (Otsuka Pharmaceutical, Tokushima). Plasma IL-6 levels were
determined using the Human Interleukin-6 ELISA Kit (Toray Fuji Bionix,
Tokyo).

Animal Experiment. Adult male rats of the Wistar strain, each weighing
300–350 g, were used in this experiment. A silastic cannula was inserted through
the jugular vein into the right atrium several days before blood sampling. At
least 12 h prior to blood sampling, cannulated animals were moved to a special
sampling cage in which blood could be drawn from the rats under conscious,
freely moving conditions without apparent stress throughout the experimental
period [5]. The recombinant human (rh) IL-1α, rhIL-1β, and rhIL-6 used in this
study are described elsewhere [5, 7]. rhTNF-α was a gift from Dainippon
Pharmaceutical (Osaka). Blood samples (0.5 ml) were immediately cooled on ice
and then centrifuged to obtain plasma samples. Red blood cells were resuspended in physiologic saline and returned to rats after each sampling.
Determination of plasma ACTH levels was described previously [6].

Statistical Analysis. Statistical analysis was performed by analysis of variance
and subsequent Bonferroni method; differences of $p < 0.05$ were considered
significant. Results were expressed as the mean ± SEM of each group.

Results

Changes in Plasma Hormone and Cytokine Levels. Figure 1 presents the changes
in plasma endotoxin, cytokine, and hormone levels during pancreatoduodenectomy. After skin incision, plasma ACTH and cortisol levels increased rapidly
and achieved their maximal levels within 6 h. While plasma endotoxin and
TNF-α levels increased significantly after skin incision, plasma IL-6 levels
remained unchanged for 2 h and then increased gradually. Plasma levels of these
two cytokines reached their maximal levels 4–6 h after skin incision. In all
patients, plasma IL-1α and IL-1β levels before skin incision were under the
minimal detectable limits of our assay systems. While plasma IL-1α levels
increased in some patients after skin incision (Table 1), no detectable changes
occurred in the remaining patients during the surgical procedure. In all patients,
plasma IL-1β levels remained almost undetectable throughout the surgical
procedure.

ACTH-Releasing Activities of Cytokines. Figure 2 presents the effects of rhTNF-
α, rhIL-1α, rhIL-1β, and rhIL-6 on the plasma ACTH levels of conscious, freely
moving rats. Plasma ACTH levels increased promptly after intravenous administration of these cytokines, and maximal values of plasma ACTH concentra-

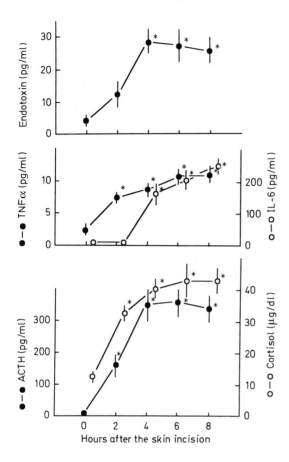

Fig. 1. Changes in plasma endotoxin, TNF-α, IL-6, ACTH, and cortisol levels during pancreatoduodenectomy. Each point represents the mean ± SEM of eight patients. *,$p < 0.05$ compared to the control value before skin incision (0 h).

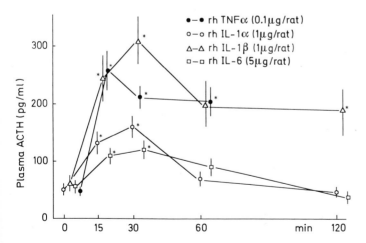

Fig. 2. Time-course changes of plasma ACTH levels in response to intravenous administration of rhTNF-α, rhIL-1α, rhIL-1β, or rhIL-6 in conscious, freely moving rats. Each point represents the mean ± SEM of ACTH determination from five rats. *,$p < 0.05$ compared to the control value

Table 1. Changes in plasma endotoxin and cytokine levels in patient 2

	0 h	2 h	4 h	6 h	8 h
Endotoxin (pg/ml)	4.0	15.0	37.4	39.8	49.2
TNF-α (pg/ml)	3.9	15.4	15.1	14.7	18.3
IL-1α (pg/ml)	< 7.8	8.6	15.8	20.8	23.4
IL-1β (pg/ml)	< 20	< 20	< 20	< 20	< 20
IL-6 (pg/ml)	90	80	140	300	340

tions were usually observed 15–30 min after the injection. Under the same experimental conditions, vehicle injection did not alter plasma ACTH levels.

Discussion

Injury and infection associated with surgical procedures stimulate the production of a variety of endogenous mediators, and these mediators in turn initiate immune, hematologic, and metabolic alterations that are integral to the response of the host to injury. Among these alterations, the stress response of the H-P-A axis seems to be most important in maintaining homeostasis and to be essential for survival [4]. The present study demonstrates that surgical invasion activates the H-P-A axis and induces a marked elevation in plasma ACTH and cortisol levels. Moreover, we observed an elevation in plasma endotoxin and cytokine levels, which suggests that the circulating endotoxin induces a generalized stimulation of cytokine production during surgical procedures. Recently, increasing evidence suggests the existence of bidirectional communication between the immune and neuroendocrine systems. Our recent studies have revealed that not only IL-1 but also TNF-α and IL-6 activate the H-P-A axis at the levels of the brain, pituitary, and adrenal glands and stimulate ACTH and glucocorticoid secretion [5–7, 10 11]. These findings strongly suggest that some classes of cytokine participate in the development of stress-induced activation of the H-P-A axis during surgery.

References

1. Schulze S et al. (1988) Surgery 103:321
2. Moller IW et al. (1984) Acta Anaesthesiol Scand 28:266
3. Naito Y et al. (1990) In Matsuki A et al. (eds) Endocrine response to anesthesia and intensive care Elsevier, Amsterdam, p 123
4. Weissman C (1990) Anesthesiology 73:308
5. Naito Y et al. (1990) Biochem Biophys Res Commun 167:103
6. Naito Y et al. (1989) Biochem Biophys Res Commun 164:1262
7. Naitoh Y et al. (1988) Biochem Biophys Res Commun 155:1459
8. Naito Y et al. (1989) Can J Anaesth 36:633
9. Yone K et al. (1990) Clin Chem Enzym Comms 3:1
10. Fukata J et al. (1989) J Endocrinol 122:33
11. Tominaga T et al. (1991) Endocrinology 128:526

The Synthesis of Stress Proteins in Cultured Cardiac Myocytes Is Induced by the Interleukins and Tumor Necrosis Factor

I. Löw-Friedrich[1], D. Weisensee[2], P. Mitrou[3], and W. Schoeppe[1]

Introduction

Mortality is very high in septic shock patients mainly due to cardiovascular failure. Clinical trials describe an acute septic cardiomyopathy with the typical features of severe cardiac insufficiency [1]. Several findings reported in the literature suggest a direct influence of immune mediators on the heart. The therapeutic use of interleukin (IL) 2 in oncology is frequently accompanied by severe cardiac complications resembling those observed in septic shock [2]. Patients on maintenance hemodialysis suffer from cardiac impairment; recently, increased IL-1 and tumor necrosis factor (TNF) serum levels have been documented in these patients [3]. In vitro studies indicate a direct effect of the cytokines on heart cell metabolism [4]. Our study was performed to investigate specific cardiotoxic effects of immune mediators on cultured cardiac myocytes. The detection of stress protein formation was employed as a test system to monitor cardiotoxicity [5].

Stress Proteins. The cellular stress response was first described in 1962 by Ritossa [6] in heat-shocked salivary glands of *Drosophila melanogaster*. Today it is generally agreed that cells of all species respond to toxic environmental conditions causing protein denaturation with the de novo synthesis of stress proteins. These are polypeptide families of constant molecular weight, especially 30 and 70 kDa. Scientific interest has focused on the function of stress proteins which regulate cellular protein turnover in detrimental situations. Stress proteins are involved in the degradation of denatured proteins, in the transmembrane transport of proteins, and in the stabilization of the cytoskeleton [7].

Methods and Materials

Fetal mouse cardiac myocytes were prepared by trypsin digestion [5]. The cell number was adjusted to 5×10^5 cells per dish. As fibroblasts and endothelial

[1] Abteilungen für Nephrologie, Klinikum der Johann Wolfgang Goethe-Universität, Theodor-Stern-Kai 7, 6000 Frankfurt, FRG
[2] Arbeitskreis für Kinematische Zellforschung, Fachbereich Biologie, Johann Wolfgang Goethe-Universität, Senckenberganlage 27, 6000 Frankfurt, FRG
[3] Abteilung für Hämatologie/Onkologie, Klinikum der Johann Wolfgang Goethe-Universität, Theodor-Stern-Kai 7, 6000 Frankfurt, FRG

cells adhere very early to the culture surface, whereas the myocytes remain in the supernatant, the different cell types could be separated by transferring the supernatant to new dishes after 1 h of incubation. The cardiac myocytes were kept for 2 days in alpha-medium supplemented with 20% fetal calf serum in a water-saturated atmosphere with 5% CO_2 which was afterwards replaced by Dulbecco's minimum Eagle's medium with 10% fetal calf serum. The experiments were performed after 7 days of cell culture. Incubation of the cultured heart cells with the test substances lasted 2 h; afterwards 0.05 mCi L-[^{35}S] methionine was added for a further 2 h. The myocytes were dissolved in O'Farrell's sample buffer, the protein was precipitated [8], and 150 000 cpm was applied per slot. Sodium dodecyl sulfate polyacrylamide gels (7.5% acrylamide) were run at 160 V for 4 h. The dried gels were fixed to a high-resolution film for autoradiography.

Cell culture compounds and media were obtained from Biochrom (FRG). The cytokines were provided by British Biotechnology (UK). All chemicals were of the highest purity available. L-[^{35}S] methionine was purchased from NEN (USA). The electrophoresis equipment was from Höfer Instruments (USA). The films for autoradiography (β-max) were supplied by Amersham (FRG), commercial sets with developer and fixer by Kodak (FRG). The pregnant mice were from the NMRI strain.

Results

A temperature shock (42 °C for 5 min) administered to investigate the effects of a fever condition induced two proteins of the 70 kDa family. Hydrogen peroxide (0.05%–0.001%) stimulated the de novo synthesis of a 30-kDa stress protein. The results obtained for the cytokines are displayed in Table 1.

Conclusions

Our investigation confirms a direct interference of the interleukins and TNF with myocardial stress protein formation. We conclude from the results of our

Table 1. Effects of cytokines on stress protein formation in cultured cardiac myocytes

Cytokine	Concentration (U/ml)	70 kDa	30 kDa
IL-1	5 000–500	2 Proteins	1 Protein
IL-2	50 000–6000	–	1 Protein
IL-3	10 000–300	–	1 Protein
IL-6	20 000–2500	–	1 Protein
TNF	2 000–250	–	1 Protein

study that the cytokines directly exert toxic effects on cultured heart cells. The induction of stress proteins makes cells more tolerant toward a second otherwise lethal stress [9]. Therefore, the stress protein formation might be involved in the protective mechanisms activated in trauma, shock, and sepsis. The expression of additional 70-kDa stress proteins by IL-1 might indicate that at least part of the stress protein response is specifically regulated.

References

1. Ognibene FP, Parker MM, Natanson C, Shelhamer JH, Parrillo JE (1988) Depressed left ventricular performance. Response to volume infusion in patients with sepsis and septic shock. Chest 93:903–910
2. Lee RE, Lotze MT, Skibber JM, Tucker E, Bonow RO, Ognibene FP, Carrasquillo JA, Shelhamer JH, Parrillo JE, Rosenberg SA (1989) Cardiorespiratory effects of immunotherapy with interleukin-2. J Clin Oncol 7:7–20
3. Herbelin A, Nguyen AT, Zingraff J, Urena P, Descamps-Latscha B (1990) Influence of uremia and hemodialysis on circulating interleukin-1 and tumor necrosis factor alpha. Kidney Int 37:116–125
4. Wagenknecht B, Hug M, Hübner G, Werdan K (1989) Myokardiale Wirkungen von Mediatoren. Intensivmed 26 [Suppl 1]:32–40
5. Löw I, Friedrich T, Schoeppe W (1989) Synthesis of shock proteins in cultured fetal mouse myocytes. Exp Cell Res 181:451–459
6. Ritossa F (1962) A new puffing pattern induced by temperature shock and DNP in *Drosophila*. Experientia 18:571–573
7. Schlesinger MJ (1990) Heat shock proteins. J Biol Chem 265:12111–12114
8. Wessel D, Flügge UI (1984) A method for the quantitative recovery of protein in dilute solution in the presence of detergents and lipids. Analyt Biochem 138:141–143
9. Spitz DR, Dewey WC, Li GC (1987) Hydrogen peroxide or heat shock induces resistance to hydrogen peroxide in Chinese hamster fibroblasts. J Cell Physiol 131:364–373

Effects of Tumor Necrosis Factor on the Hypothalamic–Pituitary–Adrenal Axis

K. Mealy, B. G. Robinson, J. A. Majzoub, and D. W. Wilmore

Introduction

Stimulation of the hypothalamic–pituitary–adrenal (HPA) axis is a central feature of the response to critical illness. The regulation of this response is unclear; afferent cortical and peripheral stimuli undoubtedly lead to HPA axis stimulation, but recently it has become apparent that cytokines are potent stimulators of this response. The purpose of this study was to examine the effects of tumor necrosis factor (TNF), a major cytokine mediator of endotoxic shock, on HPA axis gene expression and peptide release.

Methods

Thirty-six male Wistar rats (175–200 g) had central venous catheters inserted under phenobarbital anesthesia [1]. Following operation the animals received 0.9% saline (25 ml/24 hr) via the catheters and were allowed to recover for 72 hours. Prior to each study they were randomly allocated into two groups and received either 0.9% saline or TNF (rhTNF, 4 x 10^5 units/kg rat over 24 h, Asachi Chemical Industry, New York, NY) at a rate of 25 ml/24 h. The rats were allowed rat chow and water ad libitum throughout the study. Following 6, 12, and 24 h of infusion, animals were sacrificed by decapitation within 20 s of injection of sodium pentobarbital (40 mg/kg) down the central line. Trunk blood was collected into sodium heparin and ethylenediaminetetraacetic acid (EDTA) tubes for measurement of plasma corticotropin releasing hormone (CRH), arginine vasopressin (AVP), adrenocorticotropic hormone (ACTH), and corticosterone. Rat hypothalamus and anterior pituitaries were removed and stored at $-70\,°C$ for measurement of CRH, AVP, and proopiomelanocortin (POMC, the precursor of ACTH) mRNA levels. Adrenal glands were also removed and weighed.

RNA was prepared on frozen tissue according to the method of Chirgwin et al. [2]. Hybridizations were performed using $[\alpha\text{-}^{32}P]$ UTP-labeled antisense

Department of Surgery, Brigham and Women's Hospital and Endocrine Division, Children's Hospital, Harvard Medical School, Boston, MA 02115, USA

Host Defense Dysfunction
in Trauma, Shock and Sepsis
Eds. Faist/Meakins/Schildberg
© Springer-Verlag, Berlin Heidelberg 1993

complementary RNA probes. Riboprobe templates included the 700 base pair (bp) RsaI fragment of a rat CRH cDNA encoding bases 451–1838 of the rat CRH gene, the 350-bp fragment encoding bases 2158–2500 of the rat AVP gene, the actin cDNA, and a 900-bp fragment of the mouse POMC cDNA. Blots were washed as previously described [3] and RNA was quantified by densitometric scanning of autoradiograms and corrected for amounts of actin mRNA or 18S rRNA. ACTH and corticosterone levels were determined by radioimmunoassay (Nicols Institute Diagnostics, San Juan, Capistrano, CA, and Radioassay Systems, Carson, CA, respectively). Plasma CRH and AVP were measured as previously described [4].

Results are expressed as mean $\pm$ SEM. Two-way ANOVA was used for comparison of means; the Dunnett t test was used for post hoc comparisons. Differences were considered significant when $p < 0.05$.

Results

Thirty-six animals were entered into the study, evenly divided between the two groups. All animals survived to harvest with no apparent distress. One 12 h control animal, however, was excluded because of a catheter thrombus. Adrenal weight and plasma hormone levels in the TNF- and saline-infused animals are shown in Fig. 1. Adrenal weight was elevated in the TNF-infused group ($p < 0.05$). Plasma corticosterone was also significantly elevated in the TNF-infused group ($p < 0.0001$). The maximal increase occurred at 6 h (38.3 ± 10.7 vs 10.6 ± 5.4 µg/dl) and although the level diminished with time, it was still elevated above the controls at 12 and 24 h. Plasma ACTH also increased with TNF ($p < 0.0007$). There was no difference in plasma CRH between the TNF- and saline-infused animals. Plasma AVP was diminished in the TNF-infused group at 6 and 12 h; this difference was significant at 6 h (0.84 ± 0.14 vs 2.32 ± 0.62 pg/ml, $P < 0.05$).

Quantification of mRNA results is shown in Fig. 2. Pituitary POMC mRNA levels were significantly elevated in the TNF-infused animals at 6 h in comparison to controls (5.6 ± 1.2 vs 3.2 ± 1.0 arbitrary units, $p < 0.005$). POMC mRNA levels were lower in the TNF-infused group at both 12 and 24 h, the difference at 24 h being significant (3.2 ± 0.5 vs 3.8 ± 0.3 arbitrary units, $p < 0.02$). Whole hypothalamic CRH mRNA was significantly diminished in the TNF-infused animals at all time points ($p < 0.002$). There was no difference in hypothalamic AVP mRNA levels between the two groups.

As alterations in CRH mRNA levels could have occurred prior to 6 h, further studies were carried out in another 36 animals using an identical protocol with TNF infusion over 15 min and 1 and 3 h. Maximal increases in both plasma ACTH and corticosterone occurred within the first hour (Fig. 3). Plasma CRH and AVP did not increase with TNF infusion. Neither hypothalamic CRH nor pituitary POMC mRNA levels increased with TNF (Fig. 4);

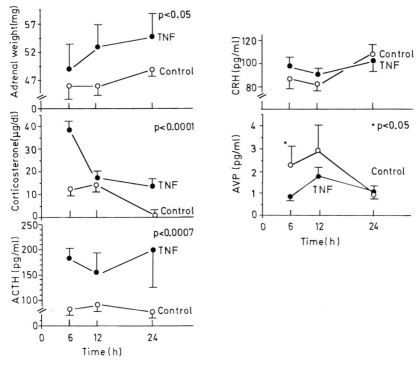

Fig. 1. Adrenal weight and plasma corticosterone, ACTH, CRH, and AVP in the TNF-infused and control groups at 6, 12 and 24 h

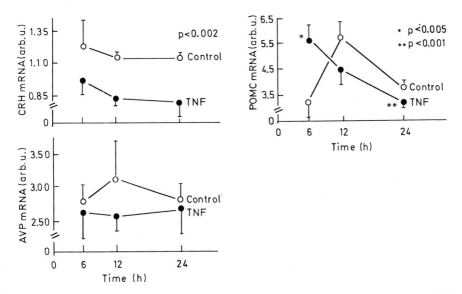

Fig. 2. CRH, AVP, and POMC mRNA in the TNF-infused and control groups at 6, 12 and 24 h

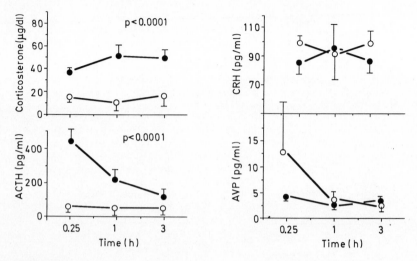

Fig. 3. Plasma corticosterone, ACTH, CRH, and AVP in the TNF-infused and control groups at 15 min and 1 and 3 h

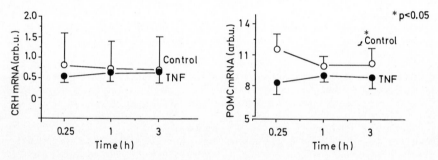

Fig. 4. CRH and POMC mRNA in the TNF-infused and control groups at 15 min and 1 and 3 h

in fact, at 15 min control POMC mRNA was greater than in the TNF-infused group, leading to a significant difference over this earlier period ($p < 0.05$).

Discussion

TNF gave rise to rapid activation of the HPA axis as reflected in increased POMC mRNA, plasma ACTH, and corticosterone levels and adrenal weight.

Both plasma ACTH and corticosterone was maximally increased within the first hour of TNF infusion and tended to diminish with time. Control ACTH and corticosterone levels remained within the basal range and demonstrated circadian changes throughout the study period. Plasma CRH levels were not significantly different between TNF and control groups, although at 6 h AVP levels were significantly diminished in the TNF group. Peripheral plasma peptide levels, however, may not correlate with peptide levels in the hypo-thalamic-portal circulation.

Despite rapid release of ACTH and corticosterone within 15 min, increased HPA axis gene expression only occurred at the level of the pituitary following 6 h of TNF infusion. POMC mRNA levels were increased at 6 h, whereas at 12 and 24 h POMC mRNA levels were diminished in comparison to controls. The initial increase in control POMC mRNA levels at 15 min is difficult to explain but is likely to be due to inherent differences in the two groups of animals prior to commencement of the study. It is unclear why saline-infused controls had POMC mRNA levels greater than TNF-infused animals following 12 h of infusion. This variation in control POMC mRNA may reflect the normal circadian changes observed in plasma ACTH and corticosterone. Also, this later decrease in POMC mRNA levels in response to TNF may represent negative feedback to elevated corticosterone levels. However, the exact relationship between POMC mRNA and plasma ACTH levels remains to be determined. It is possible that the magnitude of the POMC mRNA response to stress may be less important than temporal changes.

Hypothalamic CRH mRNA levels were diminished between 6 and 24 h following TNF infusion in comparison to controls. Diminished CRH mRNA levels also suggest that normal regulatory feedback mechanisms to increase ACTH and corticosterone exist following TNF infusion. The failure to demon-strate increased CRH mRNA in response to TNF infusion at any time, in addition to the earlier suppression of hypothalamic CRH mRNA in comparison to pituitary POMC mRNA, supports the contention that TNF has a direct effect on the pituitary. These results are in keeping with the in vitro data demonstrating direct effects of TNF on ACTH release from dispersed pituitary cells in culture [5]. Rothwell [6] found that the CRH antagonist α-helical CRH (9-41) did not modify the thermogenic effects of TNF, thus providing further evidence of a direct pituitary effect of TNF. In contrast in this study, the thermogenic effects of interleukin-1β (IL-1β) were found to be inhibited by α-helical CRH(9-41), indicating direct IL-1β effects on the hypothalamus. A direct IL-1β effect on the hypothalamus is supported by Suda et al. [7], who demonstrated that in the rat intraperitoneal IL-1β injection leads to increased hypothalamic CRH mRNA levels at 3 h. It is interesting to note that at this time period we found no TNF-induced increase in CRH mRNA levels. Evidence to date therefore suggests two different sites of action for TNF and IL-1 on the HPA axis; an explanation for this is not readily available.

This study demonstrates that TNF gives rise to a rapid and transient stimulation of the HPA axis. Our results suggest that TNF-induced increases in ACTH and corticosterone lead to feedback inhibition of hypothalamic CRH mRNA expression and furthermore TNF may directly stimulate pituitary POMC mRNA and ACTH release in vivo.

References

1. O'Dwyer ST, Smith RJ, Hwang TL, Wilmore DW (1986) Maintenance of small bowel mucosa with glutamine-enriched parenteral nutrition. J Parenter Enteral Nutr 13:579–585
2. Chirgwin JM, Przybyla AE, MacDonald RJ, Rutter WJ (1979) Isolation of biologically active ribonucleic acid from sources enriched in ribonuclease. Biochemistry 18:5294–5299
3. Adler GH, Smas CM, Majzoub JA (1988) Expression and dexamethasone regulation of the human corticotropin-releasing hormone gene in a mouse anterior pituitary cell line. J Biol Chem 263:5846–5852
4. Robinson BG, Emaneul RL, Frim DM, Majzoub JA (1988) Glucocorticoid stimulates expression of corticotropin-releasing hormone gene in human placenta. Proc Natl Acad Sci USA 85:5244–5248
5. Milenkovic L, Rettori V, Snyder GD, Beutler B, McCann SM (1989) Cachectin alters anterior pituitary hormone release by a direct action in vitro. Proc Natl Acad Sci USA 86:2418–2422
6. Rothwell NJ (1989) CRF is involved in the pyrogenic and thermongenic effects of interleukin 1β in the rat. Am J Physiol 256:E111–E115
7. Suda T, Tozawa F, Ushiyama T, Sumitomo T, Yamada M, Demura H (1990) Interleukin-1 stimulates corticotropin-releasing factor gene expression in rat hypothalamus. Endocrinology 126:1223–1228

Interleukin-2-Modulated Cytokine Secretion in Thermally Injured Patients

J. Teodorczyk-Injeyan[1], B. Sparkes[2], and Walter Peters[3]

Introduction

Interleukin-2 (IL-2), initially described as a T lymphocyte growth factor [1], also acts as a potent mediator of other immune cells' function, e.g., natural killer (NK) and B cells [2, 3] and as the regulator of heterogeneous secretory activity of normal human mononuclear phagocytes [4, 5]. IL-2-exposed monocytes augment the secretion of cyclooxygenase-derived metabolites including prostaglandin E_2 (PGE_2) [6] and increase the production and/or spontaneous secretion of interleukin-1 (IL-1) [7] and tumour necrosis factor α (TNF-α) [8].

In the burn patient both significant monocytosis and increased secretion of biologically active mediators of the immune and inflammatory responses have been reported [9]. We have recently described that sera from patients with major burns contain high levels of immunoreactive IL-2 [10]. This suggests that in the burn patient biological responses of the circulating monocytes will be affected by IL-2. The present study compares the effect of exogenous IL-2 on the spontaneous secretion of monocyte-derived IL-1, PGE_2, and TNF-α in thermally injured patients and normal donors.

Materials and Methods

Ten patients (nine males and one female) aged from 22 to 41 years, with full-thickness burns ranging from 25% to 40%, and partial injuries from 2% to over 30% total body surface area (TBSA), were studied. The blood samples used in this study were collected at 7- to 9-day intervals from 1 to 8 weeks postburn. Controls included seven healthy donors (all males) of comparable age. Peripheral blood monocytes were prepared from Ficoll-Hypaque-fractionated mononuclear cells by adherence to plastic (60–90 min, 37 °C). The adherent cell (AC) concentration per plate was determined for each experimental condition.

[1] Sunnybrook Research Centre and Department of Surgery, University of Toronto, Toronto, Ontario, Canada M4N 3M5
[2] Defence and Civil Institute of Environmental Medicine, North York, Ontario, Canada
[3] The Ross Tilley Burn Centre, Wellesley Hospital, Toronto, Ontario, Canada

Host Defense Dysfunction
in Trauma, Shock and Sepsis
Eds. Faist/Meakins/Schildberg
© Springer-Verlag, Berlin Heidelberg 1993

Patients' and control AC were then cultured for 24–30 h in the presence or absence of human purified IL-2 (Pharmacia) at concentrations ranging from 10 to 200 U/ml. Concentrations giving the highest responses were taken as optimal. At the conclusion of the culture period culture supernatants were collected and AC were removed from the plates for enumeration and dual immunofluorescence staining with a monoclonal anti-M3 (CD14) and anti-Tac (CD25) antibodies. The levels of IL-1 (α and β), TNF-α, and PGE$_2$ secreted in patients' and parallel control cultures were determined by a specific radioimmunoassay (RIA; Amersham). The content of the soluble form of IL-2 receptor α(IL-2Rα) was assessed by a commercial (T Cell Sciences) kit.

Results and Discussion

Two of the studied patients with injuries over 50% TBSA died at 14 and 89 days postburn. All patients had at least two (range two to six) studies completed over their hospitalization period. Spontaneous secretion of immunoregulatory mediators, i.e., IL-1, TNF-α, and PGE$_2$, was significantly ($P < 0.01$–0.05) elevated in burn patients compared with controls (Table 1). Particularly evident were increases in the level of TNF-α (up to 500% of control) and PGE$_2$ (up to tenfold). Optimal concentrations of IL-2, for altering the release of the factors both in patients and controls, were found to range from 100 to 200 U/ml. In normal AC cultures IL-2 demonstrated an overall stimulatory effect on the production of IL-1β and TNF-α, but somewhat reduced the secretion of PGE$_2$ (Table 1). This effect of IL-2 was reversed in AC preparations from burn patients (Table 1), for in the majority of IL-2-supplemented patients' AC cultures, the spontaneous secretion of IL-1β and TNF-α was markedly and significantly ($P < 0.05$) reduced compared with IL-2-free preparations (Table 1). As a result, optimal levels of IL-2 appeared to normalize the secretion of IL-1β in cultures from burn patients, but the levels of TNF-α, although diminished, still remained significantly elevated over controls (Table 1). Also in contrast to controls, the

Table 1. Effect of IL-2 on the secretion of IL-1, TNF-α, and PGE$_2$ by peripheral blood adherent monocytes from thermally injured patients and controls

Source	IL-2[a]	IL-1α (f mol/ml)	IL-1β (f mol/ml)	TNF-α (f mol/ml)	PGE$_2$[a]
Patients ($n = 10$)	–	41.4 ± 9	141 ± 32	382 ± 112	5268 ± 2241
	+	33.2 ± 11	88 ± 31	259 ± 88	8965 ± 2720
Controls ($n = 7$)	–	19.3 ± 3	64 ± 14	104 ± 15	745 ± 150
	+	18.1 ± 8	87 ± 12	130 ± 22	527 ± 199

Results represent means of levels in experiments carried out in individual patients over the postinjury period (up to 50 days post burn).
[a] Optimal IL-2 concentrations ranged from 100 to 200 U/ml.

Table 2. Surface expression and secretion of IL-2Rα by adherent monocytes (Leu M3$^+$) from thermally injured pateints and controls.

Source	IL-2Rα	
	Surface (%)	Secreted (U/ml)
Patients ($n = 10$)		
At 1 h	4.6 ± 3	ND
After 24 h	41 ± 15	142 ± 130
Controls ($n = 7$)		
At 1 h	< 1	ND
After 24 h	24 ± 7	< 50

The percentage of IL2Rα-expressing Leu M3$^+$ cells was determined immediately after isolation by plastic adherence (1 h) and after 24 h of culture.
ND, not determined.

already high synthesis (and secretion) of PGE$_2$ by patients' AC was significantly augmented by IL-2, frequently reaching levels up to 20-fold over normal (Table 1). To determine whether this disparate effect of IL-2 on the cytokine secretion by monocytes could result from these cells' altered capacity for interaction with the available lymphokine, the expression of IL-2 surface receptor (IL-2Rα or Tac) and its secretion were examined in thermally injured patients and controls. Following 24 h incubation 24% ± 7% (range 12%–32%) of LeuM3-positive normal AC were found to be also Tac-positive. The percentage of Tac-positive AC in cultures from burn patients was significantly higher (41% ± 15%, range 28%–63%; Table 2). Furthermore, in contrast to controls, the majority of patients' AC culture supernatants contained detectable concentrations of soluble IL-2Rα (range < 100–400 U/ml; Table 2).

Existing reports indicate that direct regulation of the secretory activity of normal human monocytes/phagocytes, by IL-2, requires high concentrations of this lymphokine (> 1000 U/ml) [6]. IL-2 may then augment the secretion of PGE$_2$ and IL-1β directly [4, 6] or through the induction of, and the subsequent action of, TNF-α [11]. However, concentrations of IL-2 utilized in the present study did not exceed 200 U/ml. Predictably we observed marginal to significant increases in the production of IL-1β and TNF-α and relatively unaltered PGE$_2$ secretion in IL-2-treated control AC cultures (Table 1). However, in AC cultures from burn patients the same concentrations of IL-2 significantly and inversely affected the secretion of the above mediators (Table 1), indicating that thermal injury specifically altered mediator sensitivity.

The precise mechanism of this IL-2 effect in the burn patient is not clear. However, the response of patients' AC to IL-2 could be determined by their state of activation. Resting normal monocytes/macrophages do not secrete significant amounts of immune and inflammatory mediators. Consequently, highly elevated spontaneous release of such molecules by patients' AC alone (Table 1) is an indication that activation of these cells had already occurred. Since high levels of lipopolysaccharide (LPS) [12] and other burn-induced factors [13] are present in the patient their interaction with circulating monocytes can be expected. The observed effect of IL-2 on patients' AC cultures (Table 1) might therefore reflect alteration in IL-1 or TNF-α secretion manifested by monocytes activated by such factors [7, 14, 15]. Furthermore, IL-2-triggered PGE$_2$ release, with associated increases in cAMP levels, could eventually contribute to reduction of IL-1, and indirectly, to TNF-α synthesis [14, 16]. The involvement of other macrophage-derived immune and inflammatory mediators (IL-6, TGF-β) on AC/IL-2 interaction cannot be excluded. Levels of such mediators are significantly elevated postburn [17], and their autocrine effect may enhance activity of IL-2 [18].

A second factor instrumental in an IL-2-effected secretory capacity of AC derives from an improved interaction between this lymphokine and the monocytes, since AC cultures from burn patients contain significantly greater numbers, compared to controls, of IL-2Rα-expressing cells (Table 2). The process of adherence alone induces surface IL-2Rα-expression only on a relatively low number of monocytes [19], and so elevated levels of membrane-associated and secreted Tac, with burn patients' AC, suggest its constitutive expression. IL-2Rα expression on normal human monocytes may be induced in vitro by activated T cell products such as IL-2 and interferon-γ [20], and IL-2Rα expression and secretion have both been described in patients with clinical conditions involving activation of the T cell compartment [21]. High levels of serum IL-2 and IL-2Rα indicate that T cell activation occurs also in the burn patient [10]. In conclusion the present study demonstrates that in the burn patients sequential action of the key immune lymphokine IL-2 may activate both positive and negative feedback circuits in monocyte/T cell interaction and directly or indirectly influence monokine-regulated inflammatory and metabolic responses.

Acknowledgements. The authors thank the nursing staff of the Ross Tilley Burn Centre for blood sample collection and for their unique commitment to burn care. Supported by contracts nos. DSS W7711-8-7053 and W7711-0-7098 from the Defence and Civil Institute of Environmental Medicine and by the International Association of Fire Fighters Burn Foundation.

References

1. Smith KA (1980) T-cell growth factor. Immunol Rev 51:337–357
2. Suzuki R, Handa K, Itoh K et al. (1983) Natural killer (NK) cells as a responder to interleukin 2 (IL 2). I. Proliferative response and establishment of cloned cells. J Immunol 130:981–987
3. Calvert JE, Johnstone R, Duggan-Keen MF et al. (1990) Immunoglobulin G subclasses secreted by human B cell in vitro in response to interleukin-2 and polyclonal activity. Immunol 70:162–167
4. Numerof RP, Aronson FR, Mier JW (1988) IL-2 stimulates the production of IL-1α and IL-1β by human peripheral blood mononuclear cells. J Immunol 141:4250–4257
5. Tilden AB, Dunlop NE (1989) Interleukin-2 augmentation of interleukin-1 and prostaglandin E$_2$ production. J Leukocyte Biol 45:474–477

6. Remick DG, Larrick JW, Nguyen DT et al. (1987) Stimulation of prostaglandin E_2 and thromboxane B_2 production by human monocytes in response to interleukin 2. Biochem Biophys Res Comm 147:86–93
7. Danis VA, Kulesz AJ, Nelson DS et al. (1990) Cytokine regulation of human monocyte interleukin-1 (IL-1) production in vitro. Enhancement of IL-1 production by interferon (IFN) gamma, tumour necrosis factor-alpha, IL-2 and IL-1, and inhibition by IFN-alpha. Clin Exp Immunol 80:435–443
8. Strieter RM, Remick DG, Lynch JP et al. (1989) Interleukin-2-induced tumor necrosis factor-alpha (TNF-alpha) gene expression in human alveolar macrophages and blood monocytes. Am Rev Respir Dis 139:335–342
9. Miller-Graziano CL, Fink M, Wu JY et al. (1988) Mechanism of altered monocyte PGE_2 production in severely injured patients. Arch Surg 123:293–299
10. Teodorczyk-Injeyan JA, Sparkes B, Mills G et al. (1991) Soluble interleukin 2-receptor α secretion is related to altered interleukin 2 production in thermally injured patients. Burns 17:290–295
11. Burchett SK, Weaver WM, Westfall JA et al. (1988) Regulation of tumor necrosis factor/cachectin and IL-1 secretion in human mononuclear phagocytes. J Immunol 140:3472–3481
12. Guo Y, Dickerson C, Chrest FJ et al. (1990) Increased levels of circulating interleukin 6 in burn patients. Clin Immunol Immunopathol 54:361–371
13. Sparkes BG, Monge G, Marshall SL et al. Plasma levels of cutaneous burn toxin and lipid peroxides in thermal injury. Burns 16:118–123
14. Hart PH, Whitty GA, Piccoli DS et al. (1989) Control by IFN-γ and PGE_2 of TNFα and IL-1 production by human monocytes. Immunology 66:376–383
15. Monge G, Sparkes BG, Allgöwer M et al. (1991) Influence of burn-induced lipid-protein complex on IL-1 secretion by PBMC in vitro. Burns 17:269–275
16. Hurme M (1990) Modulation of interleukin-1β production by cyclic AMP in human monocytes. FEBS Lett 263:35–37
17. Miller-Graziano CL, Szabo G, Kodys K et al. (1990) Aberrations in post-trauma monocyte subpopulation: role in septic shock syndrome. J Trauma 30:S86–87
18. Ruppert J, Peters JH (1991) IL-6 and IL-1 enhance the accessory activity of human blood monocytes during differentiation to macrophages. J Immunol 146:144–149
19. Herrmann F, Cannistra SA, Lindermann A et al. (1989) Functional consequences of monocyte IL-2 receptor expression. Induction of IL-1β secretion by IFNγ and IL-2. J Immunol 142:139–143
20. Hancock WW, Muller WA, Cotran RS (1987) Interleukin 2 receptors are expressed by alveolar macrophages during pulmonary sarcoidosis and are inducible by lymphokine treatment of normal lung macrophages, blood monocytes, and monocyte cell lines. J Immunol 138:185–191
21. Toossi L, Sedor JR, Lapurga JP et al. (1990) Expression of functional interleukin 2 receptor by peripheral blood monocytes from patients with active pulmonary tuberculosis. J Clin Invest 85:1777–1784

Cytokine Treatment of Radiation-Induced Hemopoietic Suppression: Results of Interleukin-6 and Granulocyte Colony-Stimulating Factor in a Murine Radiation Model

M. L. Patchen[1], T. J. MacVittie[1], B. D. Solberg[1], R. Fischer[1], and L. M. Souza[2]

Introduction

Following accidental radiation exposure or intensive radiotherapy severe hemopoietic depression often results from damage to hemopoietic stem and progenitor cell populations. The major risks of mortality following radiation exposure are sepsis (resulting from a lack of granulocytes) and hemorrhage (resulting from a lack of platelets). In recent years a variety of recombinant cytokines have been shown to possess hemopoietic activity [1, 2]. In particular, the ability of interleukin-6 (IL-6) to stimulate multilineage stem cell production [3–5] and the ability of granulocyte colony-stimulating factor (G-CSF) to enhance granulocyte production and function [6–8] have been demonstrated in vitro. Based on these effects, we hypothesized that in vivo IL-6 administration may amplify multilineage stem cell production, which if followed by G-CSF administration to induce multilineage cells towards granulocyte production, could provide an effective treatment for radiation- or drug-induced hemopoietic suppression. Before beginning such studies, however, it was necessary to evaluate the in vivo effects of each cytokine. The studies presented in this paper describe the ability of IL-6 and G-CSF to individually stimulate hemopoietic regeneration in vivo following radiation- induced hemopoietic injury in mice.

Methods and Materials

C3H/HeN female mice were purchased from Charles River Laboratories (Raleigh, NC). Mice were maintained in microisolator cages on hardwood-chip contact bedding and were provided commercial rodent chow and acidified (pH 2.5) water ad libitum. Upon arrival, all mice were tested for Pseudomonas and quarantined until test results were obtained. Only healthy mice were released for experimentation. Recombinant human IL-6 and G-CSF were provided by AMGen (Thousand Oaks, CA). Endotoxin contamination was less

---

[1] Department of Experimental Hematology, Armed Forces Radiobiology Research Institute, Bethesda, MD, USA
[2] AMGen, Thousand Oaks CA, USA

Host Defense Dysfunction
in Trauma, Shock and Sepsis
Eds. Faist/Meakins/Schildberg
© Springer-Verlag, Berlin Heidelberg 1993

than 0.5 ng/mg protein based on the Limulus amebocyte lysate assay. IL-6 was administered subcutaneously (s.c.) at a dose of 1000 µg/kg per day in a 0.1-ml volume from days 1–3 postirradiation. G-CSF was administered s.c. at a dose of 125 µg/kg per day in a 0.1-ml volume from days 3–12 postirradiation. IL-6 administration was initiated soon after irradiation and continued for only a short period in hopes of enhancing the production of multilineage progenitor cells without "burning out" the stem cell population from which these cells are derived. In contrast, G-CSF administration was delayed until 3 days postirradiation and continued through the majority of the expected period of myelosuppression in hopes of inducing regenerated multipotent progenitor cells to differentiate into granulocyte progenitors, and ultimately to enhance granulocyte production. IL-6 and G-CSF doses were chosen based on previous dose-response studies performed in our laboratory.

A theratron-80 source was used to administer unilateral total-body ^{60}Co radiation. Mice were placed in ventilated Plexiglas containers and irradiated at a dose rate of 0.4 Gy/min. Dosimetry was performed using ionization chambers [9]. Hemopoietic recovery studies were performed following sublethal 6.5-Gy irradiation and survival studies following an ∼ 75% lethal 8-Gy irradiation. Endogenous spleen colony-forming units (E-CFU) were used to evaluate multipotent hemopoietic progenitor cell recovery [10]. Mice were exposed to 6.5-Gy of total-body radiation in order to only partially ablate endogenous multipotent progenitor cells. Twelve days after irradiation, the spleens were removed, fixed in Bouin's solution, and the spleen colonies formed by the proliferation of surviving multipotent progenitor cells were counted. Five mice were evaluated in each treatment group in each experiment. Hemopoietic progenitor cells committed to granulocyte and/or macrophage development were assayed in vitro using a double-layer agar granulocyte-macrophage colony-forming cell (GM-CFC) assay [11]. Mouse endotoxin serum (5% v/v) was added to feeder layers as a source of colony-stimulating factor and colonies (> 50 cells) were counted after 10 days incubation in a 37 °C humidified environment containing 5% CO_2. Triplicate plates were cultured for each cell suspension in each experiment. The bone marrow and spleen cell suspensions used for each GM-CFC assay represented tissues from three normal, irradiated, or treated and irradiated mice and were prepared as previously described [11]. The number of nucleated cells in the suspensions was determined by Coulter counter. Blood to perform peripheral blood cell counts was obtained from halothane-anesthetized mice via cardiac puncture. White blood cell (WBC), red blood cell (RBC), and platelet (PLT) counts were determined by Coulter counter. Results of replicate experiments were pooled and are represented as the mean + / − standard error of pooled data. Student's t test was used to determine statistical differences. Significance level was set at $p < 0.05$.

Results

Compared to saline treatment, both IL-6 and G-CSF treatments accelerated hemopoietic recovery in irradiated mice. The E-CFU assay was used as a measure of the ability of IL-6 and G-CSF to stimulate postirradiation recovery of multipotent hemopoietic progenitor cells (Fig. 1). Compared to only 4.6 +/− 0.6 colonies observed in saline-treated mice, 9.3 +/− 1.3 and 12.5 +/− 1.4 colonies were observed in IL-6-treated and G-CSF-treated mice, respectively. To evaluate the ability of IL-6 and G-CSF to specifically induce recovery of granulocytes and macrophages, bone marrow and splenic GM-CFC recovery was also assayed in mice following a 6.5 Gy irradiation. Signs of GM-CFC regeneration in saline-treated mice were generally absent until 17 days postexposure, while GM-CFC recovery became evident as early as 14 days postirradiation in IL-6-treated and G-CSF-treated mice. Both bone marrow (Fig. 2) and splenic (Fig. 3) GM-CFC numbers in IL-6-treated and G-CSF-treated mice were significantly greater than in saline-treated mice on days 14, 17, and 20 postirradiation. IL-6-treated and G-CSF-treated mice also exhibited

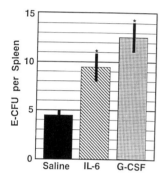

Fig. 1. Effect of saline interleukin 6 (IL-6), and granulocyte colony-stimulating factor (G-CSF) on endogenous spleen colony formation (E-CFU) in C3H/HeN mice irradiated with 6.5 Gy. Mice received IL-6 (1000 μg/kg. s.c.) on days 1–3 postirradiation and G-CSF (125 μg/kg, s.c.) on days 3–12 postirradiation. Data represent mean +/− standard error of values obtained from two to three experiments. *, $p < 0.05$ with respect to saline values

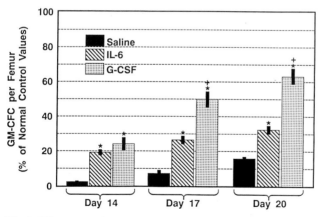

Fig. 2. Effect of saline, IL-6, and GCSF on femoral granulocyte-macrophage colony-forming cell (GM-CFC) recovery in C3H/HeN mice irradiated with 6.5 Gy on day 0. Data represented as a percentage of femoral GM-CFC content in nonirradiated control mice. Mice received IL-6 (1000 μg/kg, s.c.) on days 1–3 postirradiation and G-CSF (125 μg/kg s.c.) on days 3–12 postirradiation. Data represent the mean +/− standard error of values obtained from two to three experiments. *, $p < 0.05$ with respect to saline values; +, $p < 0.05$ with respect to IL-6 values.

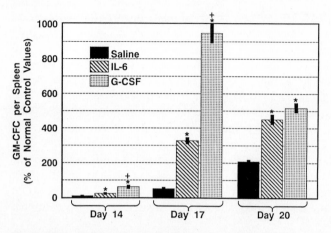

Fig. 3. Effect of saline, IL-6, and GCSF on splenic GM-CFC recovery in C3H/HeN mice irradiated with 6.5 Gy on day 0. Data represented as a percentage of splenic GM-CFC content in non-irradiated control mice. Mice received IL-6 (1000 µg/kg, s.c.) on days 1–3 postirradiation and G-CSF (125 µg/kg, s.c.) on days 3–12 postirradiation. Data represent the mean + / − standard error of values obtained from two to three experiments. *, $p < 0.05$ with respect to saline values; + , $p < 0.05$ with respect to IL-6 values

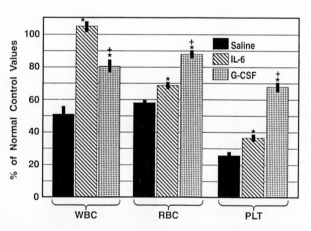

Fig. 4. Effect of saline, IL-6, GCSF on peripheral blood white cells (WBC), red cell (RBC) and platelet (PLT) recovery in C3H/HeN mice irradiated with 6.5 Gy on day 0 and assayed on day 20. Data represented as a percentage of WBC, RBC, and PLT counts in nonirradiated control mice. Mice received IL-6 (1000 µg/kg, s.c.) on days 1–3 postirradiation and G-CSF (125 µg/kg, s.c.) on days 3–12 postirradiation. Data represent the mean + / − standard error of values obtained from two to three experiments. *, $p < 0.05$ with respect to saline values; + , $p < 0.05$ with respect to IL-6 values

significantly accelerated peripheral WBC, RBC, and PLT recovery compared to saline-treated animals (Fig. 4). In general, the 10-day G-CSF treatment produced greater effects than the 3-day IL-6 treatment. Extending IL-6 treatment for 6 days increased GM-CFC, WBC, RBC, and PLT responses beyond those

Table 1. Comparison of hemopoietic responses induced by 3-day and 6-day IL-6 treatment in irradiated C3H/HeN Mice[a] as a percent of normal control values

	Saline	IL-6 × 3 days	IL-6 × 6 days	G-CSF
GM-CFC/femur	15.8 ± 0.9	32.6 ± 2.7^b	44.7 ± 3.7^b	$62.6 \pm 5.1^{b,c}$
GM-CFC/spleen	204.0 ± 8.3	455.6 ± 26.0^b	562.4 ± 33.0^b	508.6 ± 30.0^b
Peripheral blood WBC/ml	50.6 ± 5.1	113.5 ± 13.5^b	140.6 ± 8.6^b	$79.8 \pm 4.9^{b-d}$
RBC/ml	57.7 ± 2.4	69.1 ± 2.0^b	73.7 ± 1.2^b	$87.6 \pm 2.5^{b-d}$
PLT/ml	26.3 ± 1.3	36.3 ± 0.7^b	$42.6 \pm 0.8^{b,c}$	$67.5 \pm 3.2^{b-d}$

[a] Mice were irradiated with 6.5 Gy on day 0, administered IL-6 (1000 µg/kg, s.c.) on days 1–3 or on days 1–6 postexposure and assayed on day 20 postexposure.
[b] $p < 0.05$, with respect to saline values.
[c] $p < 0.05$, with respect to IL-6 × 3-day values.
[d] $p < 0.05$, with respect to IL-6 × 6-day values.
IL, interleukin; G-CSF, granulocyte colony-stimulating factor; GM-CFC, granulocyte-macrophage colony-forming cell; WBC, white blood cells; RBC, red blood cells; PLT, platelets

observed with 3-day IL-6 treatment (Table 1); however, most responses did not surpass those induced by the 10-day G-CSF treatment. In additional experiments, the ability of IL-6 and G-CSF to enhance survival in mice exposed to a more lethal dose of irradiation (8 Gy) was evaluated. At this radiation dose, only 24% of saline-treated mice survived 30 days postexposure. Interestingly, enhanced survival was not observed with IL-6 treatment, while G-CSF treatment increased survival to 57% ($p < 0.05$).

Discussion

These studies demonstrate the ability of both IL-6 and G-CSF to accelerate multilineage hemopoietic recovery in vivo following radiation-induced hemopoietic suppression. It is known that hemopoietic regeneration requires pluripotent stem cells capable of self-renewing, as well as differentiating into multipotent and committed progenitors capable of giving rise to mature cells with specialized functions (1). These processes are regulated by a variety of specific hemopoietic factors (1, 2). The E-CFU data presented here demonstrate that IL-6 is capable of regulating multilineage progenitor cell proliferation in vivo. However, our data also suggest that G-CSF is capable of amplifying this progenitor cell population in vivo. Likewise, both IL-6 and G-CSF enhanced GM-CFC recovery in irradiated mice. The accelerated recovery of peripheral WBCs, RBCs and PLTs observed in IL-6-treated and G-CSF-treated mice appeared to result from the ability of these cytokines to accelerate recovery of multipotent progenitor cells capable of "seeding" the various progenitor cell compartments necessary to reconstitute all hemopoietic lineages. Clearly, both the IL-6 treatment strategy and the G-CSF treatment strategy used in our studies resulted in accelerated hemopoietic regeneration in irradiated mice.

Although G-CSF therapy produced the greatest E-CFU and GM-CFC responses, both treatments resulted in multilineage hemopoietic repopulation. Currently studies in which IL-6 therapy on days 1–3 postirradiation is being followed by G-CSF therapy on days 3–12 postirradiation are underway in our laboratory. These studies should provide additional information concerning selective regulation of the hemopoietic hierarchy and assist in designing even better treatments for radiation- and drug-induced hemopoietic suppression.

Acknowledgments: We are grateful to Ms. B. Calabro and Ms. S. Reilly for excellent technical assistance. This work was supported by the Armed Forces Radiobiology Research Institute, Defense Nuclear Agency, under Research Work Unit 00132. Views presented in this paper are those of the authors; no endorsement by the Defense Nuclear Agency has been given or should be inferred. Research was conducted according to the principles enunciated in the Guide for the Care and Use of Laboratory Animals prepared by the Institute of Laboratory Animal Resources, National Research Council.

References

1. Robinson BE, Quesenberry PJ (1990) Review: hematopoietic growth factors: overview and clinical applications, part I. Am J Med Sci 300:163
2. Robinson BE, Quesenberry PJ (1990) Hematopoietic growth factors: overview and clinical applications, part II. Am J Med Sci 300:237
3. Ikebuchi K, Wong GG, Clark SC, Ihle JN, Hirai Y, Ogawa M (1987) Interleukin 6 enhancement of interleukin 3-dependent proliferation of multipotential hemopoietic progenitors. Proc Natl Acad Sci USA 84:9035
4. Okano A, Suzuki C, Takatsuki F, Akiyama Y, Koike K, Ozawa K, Hirano T, Kishimoto T, Nakahata T, Asano S (1989) In vitro expansion of the murine pluripotent hemopoietic stem cell population in response to interleukin 3 and interleukin 6. Application to bone marrow transplantation. Transplantation 48:495
5. Ishibashi T, Kimura H, Uchida T, Kariyone S, Friese P. Burstein SA (1989) Human interleukin 6 is a direct promoter of maturation of megakaryocytes in vitro. Proc Natl Acad Sci USA 86:5953
6. Metcalf D (1985) Colony stimulating factors. Science 229:16
7. Souza LM, Boone TC, Gabrilove J, Lai PH, Zsebo KM, Murdock DC, Chazin VR, Bruszewski J, Lu H, Chen KK, Barendt J, Platzer E, Moore MAS. Mertelsmann R, Welte K (1986) Recombinant human granulocyte colony-stimulating factor: effects on normal and leukemia myeloid cells. Science 232:61
8. Lopez AF, Nicola NA, Burgess AW, Metcalf D, Battye FL, Sewell WA, Vodas M (1983) Activation of granulocyte cytotoxic function by purified mouse colony-stimulating factors. J Immunol 131:2983
9. Schulz J, Almond PR, Cunningham JR, Holt JG, Loevinger R, Suntharalingam N, Wright KA, Nath R, Lempert D (1983) A protocol for the determination of absorbed dose from high energy proton and electron beams. Med Phys 10:741
10. Till J, McCulloch E (1963) Early repair processes in marrow cells irradiated and proliferating in vivo. Radiat Res 18:96
11. Patchen ML, MacVittie TJ (1985) Stimulated hemopoiesis and enhanced survival following glucan treatment in sublethally and lethally irradiated mice. Int J Immunopharmacol 7:923

Circulating Tumour Necrosis Factor in Active Inflammatory Bowel Disease

K. R. Gardiner[1], M. I. Halliday[1], F. Lloyd[2], S. Stephens[3], and B. J. Rowlands[1]

Introduction

Enteric bacteria and their products (endotoxins) have attracted attention as luminal antigens that may initiate or contribute to the enterocolitis and associated systemic illness of inflammatory bowel disease (IBD). It has been proposed that endotoxins originating from these intestinal flora cross the disrupted intestinal mucosal barrier of patients with IBD to enter the portal circulation [1]. If the hepatic capacity to eliminate endotoxins is exceeded, spillover into the systemic circulation occurs (Fig. 1). Systemic endotoxaemia has been demonstrated in ulcerative colitis and Crohn's disease and shown to correlate positively with disease activity [1, 2].

We put forward the hypothesis that these circulating endotoxins activate monocytes with the production of cytokines such as tumor necrosis factor (TNF) and interleukin-6 (IL-6). These would in turn activate more monocytes and neutrophils with the release of inflammatory mediators leading to the systemic clinical and biochemical features of IBD. We tested this hypothesis by: (a) measuring circulating levels of the cytokine TNF in patients with clinically active inflammatory bowel disease; (b) investigating for a correlation of the plasma TNF concentrations in these patients with biochemical indices of disease activity.

Materials and Methods

Patients. Included in the study were 33 patients with ulcerative colitis ($n = 20$) or Crohn's disease ($n = 13$), diagnosed on the basis of standard clinical, radiological and histological features, and hospitalised with a clinical relapse of their disease. Patients discharged or undergoing surgery within 5 days of admission

[1] Department of Surgery, The Queen's University of Belfast, Institute of Clinical Science, Grosvenor Road, Belfast BT12 6BJ, UK Belfast, UK
[2] Protein Laboratory, Clinical Chemistry, Belfast City Hospital, Lisburn Road, Belfast, BT9 7AB, UK
[3] Celltech Research, Celltech Ltd., 216 Bath Road, Slough, SL1 4EN UK

Host Defense Dysfunction
in Trauma, Shock and Sepsis
Eds. Faist/Meakins/Schildberg
© Springer-Verlag, Berlin Heidelberg 1993

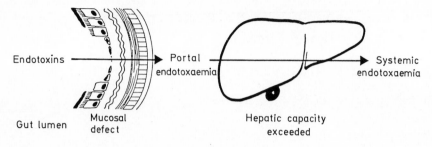

Fig. 1. Schematic representation of events leading to IBD

were excluded from this study. There were 18 men and 15 women; mean age was 38.9 years (range 19–72). Controls consisted of healthy volunteers.

Sample Collection and Analysis. Venous blood was collected aseptically into endotoxin-free glassware containing pyrogen-free heparin (20 U/ml), at the same time daily for 5 consecutive days after admission. Plasma from patients and healthy volunteers was separated by centrifugation (2000 rpm for 10 min), aliquoted into sterile cryotubes (Nunc 363401, Intermed, Denmark) and stored at − 80 °C until assayed for TNF using an enzyme-linked immunosorbent assay (ELISA) with neutralising monoclonal antibody CB0006 (Celltech, Slough, UK). Blood was simultaneously collected for measurement of the erythrocyte sedimentation rate (ESR), plasma viscosity (Coulter Viscometer II, Coulter Electronics, Luton, UK), C-reactive protein (CRP) by precipitin quantitation (Technicon 500, Technicon Instruments, New York, USA) and alpha-1 acid glycoprotein (aGP) using rate nephelometry (Beckman-Array analyser).

Statistics. The Mann-Whitney test for non-parametric data was used for analysis. The level of significance was $p < 0.05$.

Results

Blick et al. [3] have shown that the plasma half-life of TNF is short (15–17 min) in humans. In addition Michie et al. [4] have demonstrated that a bolus injection of endotoxin in healthy volunteers releases a brief pulse of TNF with a peak at 90 min and disappearance within 3–4 h. Therefore as the appearance of TNF is episodic and short-lived, we present our results as the peak plasma TNF level measured during the 5-day study periods in each patient.

Peak Plasma TNF Concentration. Nineteen patients (58%) with IBD were TNF positive (peak TNF > 10 pg/ml; range 12–140), of whom ten had Crohn's

Table 1. Disease activity in TNF-negative and TNF-positive patients (median ± SE)

	TNF negative (< 10 pg/ml)	TNF positive (10–150 pg/ml)
Alpha-1 glycoprotein (g/l)	1.06 ± 0.12	1.17 ± 0.01
C-reactive protein (mg/l)	22.2 ± 6.5	32.5 ± 9.9
ESR (mm/h)	47.0 ± 6.5	64.4 ± 6.1[a]
Plasma viscosity (mPas)	1.64 ± 0.03	1.74 ± 0.03[a]
Platelet concentration ($\times 10^3$/µl)	409.3 ± 50.6	479.6 ± 29.9
White cell count ($\times 10^3$/µl)	8.5 ± 0.7	9.0 ± 0.7
Albumin (g/l)	35.1 ± 6.4	5.4 ± 1.2

[a] $p < 0.05$.

Table 2. Alpha-1 glycoprotein concentration and TNF measurements

Group aGP concentration	TNF (pg/ml) (mean ± SE)	(peak TNF) (mean ± SE)	Positive TNF Patients	Days
1 ($n = 6$) 0.33–0.88 g/l	4.1 ± 2.2	14.2 ± 9.9	2 (33%)	4 (13%)
2 ($n = 19$) 0.89–1.76 g/l	9.0 ± 2.1[a]	26.1 ± 8.8	11 (52%)	27 (28%)
3 ($n = 8$) 1.77–2.64 g/l	14.2 ± 4.0[b]	41.2 ± 15.3	6 (75%)	15 (40%)

[a] Groups 1 versus 2, $p < 0.19$.
[b] Groups 1 versus 3, $p < 0.007$.

disease, and eight had ulcerative colitis. None of the healthy volunteers ($n = 100$) had a plasma TNF level greater than 10 pg/ml.

Plasma TNF Concentration and Disease Activity. The disease activity in the two groups of patients (TNF positive and negative) was compared using biochemical and haematological factors; the results are presented in Table 1. All the measures of disease activity were raised in the TNF-positive patients, but there were a significant differences only in ESR and plasma viscosity. Patients were also startified into three groups on the basis of their peak aGP concentration, which has been described as the best measure of disease activity in IBD [5]. Results are presented in Table 2 and Fig. 2. Plasma TNF was significantly higher in more active IBD (groups 2 and 3).

Discussion

There is increasing evidence that TNF, produced by the macrophages and monocytes of the host, acts as the primary afferent signal in the cascade of events leading to life-threatening sepsis [6]. These findings have stimulated interest in

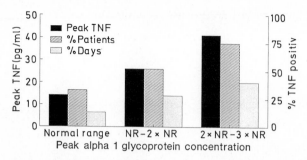

Fig. 2. Peak circulating TNF, percentage of patients, and percentage of days in three groups of patients defined by peak aGP concentration: 0.33–0.88 g/l (*normal range*), 0.89–7.76 g/l (*NR–2 × NR*), 1.77–2.64 g/l (*2 × NR–3 × NR*)

the role of TNF and other cytokines in the development of septic complications in other conditions such as major trauma, obstructive jaundice, and IBD.

We have demonstrated that circulating levels of TNF can be detected in 58% patients with a relapse of their IBD, and that higher levels are found in patients with more active disease. Sategna-Guidetta [7] reported increased serum TNF levels in 13 of 16 patients with ulcerative colitis using a technique of TNF-specific cytotoxicity but found no correlation with disease activity. MacDonald et al. [8] using ELISA detected plasma TNF levels of 10 pg/ml in two of five children with Crohn's disease and two of four with ulcerative colitis (range 18–150 pg/ml). They also demonstrated elevated frequencies of TNF-secreting cells in colonoscopic biopsies from children with Crohn's disease and ulcerative colitis when compared with normal intestine using spot ELISA. Mahida et al. [9] reported enhanced production of TNF by mononuclear cells, isolated from biopsies of inflamed colonic mucosa, on stimulation with lipopolysaccharide in comparison with normal mucosa in patients with colitis.

This study raises two important issues. The first concerns the contribution of TNF of the intestinal inflammation and/or the systemic illness in IBD. The gastrointestinal tract is known to be a prime target of TNF, accumulating 10% of a systemically administered dose [10]. At low doses, TNF causes diarrhoea, delayed gastric emptying and a mild enteritis [11]. Higher doses cause more extensive bowel necrosis and haemorrhage [12]. Michie et al. [13] have shown that administration of TNF to volunteers resulted in nausea, myalgia, fever, tachycardia and an acute phase protein response. In view of these known effects of TNF it is possible that TNF has a pathogenetic role in inflammatory bowel disease. However raised plasma TNF levels in these patients may just be a non-specific measure of immune activation in IBD. Brynskov and Tvede [14] have reported that plasma IL-2 and IL-2 receptors are also raised in patients with active Crohn's disease. In addition, Ligumsky et al. [15] have demonstrated that there is increased colonic mucosal IL-1 content and production in IBD.

The second issue raised is the origin of the TNF. It is probable that there is both an increased mucosal production of TNF [8, 9] with absorbtion into the portal circulation and also endotoxin-stimulated TNF secretion from circulating mononuclear cells.

References

1. Aoki K (1978) A study of endotoxaemia in ulcerative colitis and Crohn's disease. I. Clinical study. Acta Med Okayama 32:147–158
2. Colin R, Grancher T, Lemeland J-F et al (1979) Endotoxaemia in patients with inflammatory entercolitis. Gastroenterol Clin Biol 3:15–19
3. Blick M, Sherwin, Rosenblum M, Gutterman J (1987) Phase I study of recombinant TNF in cancer patients. Cancer Res 47:2986–2989
4. Michie HR, Manogue KR, Spriggs DR et al (1988) Detection of circulating TNF after endotoxin administration. N Engl J Med 318:1481–1486
5. Andre C, Descos L, Landais P, Fermanian J (1981) Assessment of appropriate laboratory measurements to supplement the Crohn's disease activity score. 22:571–574
6. Michie HR, Guillou PJ, Wilmore DW (1989) TNF and bacterial sepsis. Br J Surg 76:670–671
7. Sategna-Guidetta C (1989) Increased production of TNF in patients with ulcerative colitis. 2nd international frontiers in gastroenterology meeting on inflammatory bowel disease. March 1989, Dublin, Ireland
8. MacDonald TT, Hutchings P, Choy M-Y, Murch S, Cook A (1990) TNF and interferon gamma production measured at the single cell level in normal and inflamed human intestine. Clin Exp Immunol 81:301–305
9. Mahida YR, Wu K, Lamming CED et al. (1989) Human colonic TNF alpha production. Gastroenterology 96:A313
10. Beutler BA, Milsark IW, Cerami A (1985) Cachectin/TNF: production, distribution and metabolic fate in vivo. J Immunol 135:3972–3977
11. Patton JS, Peters PM, McCabe J et al. (1988) Development of partial tolerance to the gastrointestinal effects of high doses of recombinant TNF alpha in rodents. J Clin Invest 80:1587–1596
12. Sun X-M, Hsueh W (1988) Bowel necrosis induced by TNF in rats is mediated by platelet-activating factor. J Clin Invest 81:1328
13. Michie HR, Spriggs DR, Manogue KR et al. (1988) TNF and endotoxin induce similar metabolic responses in human beings. Surgery 104:280–286
14. Brynskov J, Tvede N (1990) Plasma IL-2 and soluble/shed IL-2 receptor in serum of patients with Crohn's disease, effect of cyclosporin. Gut 31:795–799
15. Ligumsky M, Simon PL, Karmeli F, Rachmilewitz D (1990) Role of IL-1 in inflammatory bowel disease enhanced production during active disease. Gut 31:686–689

Interleukin-1 and Tumor Necrosis Factor-α Suppress Hypoxia-Induced Production of Erythropoietin In Vitro

M. Wolff, W. Jelkmann, and J. Fandrey

Introduction

The glycoprotein growth factor erythropoietin (EPO) is primarily produced by the fetal liver and by the kidney in adults. EPO specifically stimulates the proliferation and maturation of erythroid precursor cells, especially colony and burst forming units-erythroid in the bone marrow [17]. Stimuli for EPO synthesis and secretion can be various kinds of lowered O_2 supply to a still poorly defined sensor mechanism [2]. Human EPO serum levels increase in response to hypobaric hypoxia [9] or hypoxic hypoxia [14]. Acute hemorrhage in humans results in a transient elevation of EPO production [5, 28, 32]. In chronic anemia there is an inverse relationship between hemoglobin concentration and the serum EPO level [10, 18]. Thus, EPO production would be expected to be greatly stimulated following surgical or accidental blood loss or in septicemia with respiratory failure. However, EPO is inappropriately low for the degree of anemia in patients with chronic renal failure [25], inflammatory [4, 19] and malignant disease [29], or in acute renal allograft rejection [3]. A common feature among these anemia-associated conditions, that is shared with severe trauma, burning, and sepsis [11], is the release of cytokines by activated monocytes [1, 8, 15, 16, 24, 34]. These monokines, namely, interleukin-1 (IL-1), interleukin-6 (IL-6), and tumor necrosis factor-α (TNF-α), have been shown to evoke systemic reactions in critically ill patients known as acute-phase response [11]. Therefore, a causal link between elevated cytokines and impaired erythropoiesis has been suggested [33]. TNF-α and IL-1 exert an antiproliferative effect on erythroid precursor cells [21, 35]. In contrast, IL-6 seems to stimulate erythropoiesis and leads to reticulocytosis [38]. These studies have mainly focused on erythropoiesis at the bone marrow level. Relatively little is known about the effects of monokines on the production of EPO, which can be regarded as the most potent stimulatory cytokine for red blood cell formation.

To address this question, we used a human hepatoma cell line as an in vitro model of EPO synthesis. We first established that EPO formation in these cells is stimulated by pericellular hypoxia. Second, we studied the effects of various monokines on hypoxia-induced EPO production.

Physiologisches Institut I, Rheinische Friedrich-Wilhelms-Universität Bonn, Bonn, FRG

Host Defense Dysfunction
in Trauma, Shock and Sepsis
Eds. Faist/Meakins/Schildberg
© Springer-Verlag, Berlin Heidelberg 1993

Material and Methods

The studies were carried out using the human hepatoma cell line HepG2 (American Type Culture Collection, HB 8065). The cells were routinely cultured in medium RPMI (Flow; Irvine, Scotland) supplemented with 10% fetal bovine serum (Gibco BRL; Eggenstein, FRG). The cultures were grown to confluent monolayers (approx. 0.5×10^6 cells/cm^2) either in 24-well polystyrol dishes with a 1.9 cm^2 bottom area (Falcon, Becton-Dickinson; Heidelberg, FRG) or in dishes with a gas-permeable 20.6 cm^2 FEP-Teflon bottom (Petriperm, Bachofer; Reutlingen, FRG). For cell propagation and all experiments described herein the cultures were incubated at 37 °C in humidified room air with 5% CO_2. Experiments were started by medium replacement (either 1 ml or 11 ml) resulting in a standard fluid layer of 0.53 cm.

Measurement of Pericellular Oxygen Tension. Pericellular PO_2 was continuously determined by polarographic, O_2-sensitive probes of a solid-state type (Neocath, Biomedical Sensors; Shiley, Irvine, USA). In polystyrol and in FEP-teflon dishes the probe tip was positioned at the monolayer level via boreholes through the lids. Prior to and after insertion the probes were calibrated at 37 °C in RPMI medium equilibrated by alternating bubbling with room air and nitrogen. The data were processed on a microcomputer (LICOX, GMS; Kiel-Mielkendorf, FRG). After 24 h the culture medium was harvested and frozen aliquots were analyzed for EPO, glucose, and lactate concentration. EPO was measured by a sensitive ELISA method (Medac; Hamburg, FRG). Glucose and lactate were determined by commercial UV kits (Boehringer Mannheim, FRG). Following rinsing with saline the cell layers were lysed with sodium dodecyl sulfate (5 g/l in 0.1 M NaOH). The amount of cellular protein was measured by the micro Lowry method (Sigma Diagnostics; Taufkirchen, FRG).

Cytokine Treatment. Human recombinant cytokines IL-1α, IL-β, IL-6, TNF-α, and interferon-γ (IFN-γ) were purchased from Boehringer Mannheim (FRG). The cytokines were diluted in culture medium and added to confluent monolayers of HepG2 cells, grown in polystyrol dishes under diffusion limited O_2 supply. Following 24 h of incubation the supernatants were collected for assay of EPO and the cell layers lysed for protein determination. EPO was measured by radioimmunoassay as described previously [19]. In addition, the production of α-fetoprotein (α-FP) was measured to rule out nonspecific effects on protein synthesis by the cytokines used. α-FP was determined by radioimmunoassay (Pharmacia; Uppsala, Sweden). Comparisons between groups treated with the respective cytokine and untreated controls were made with Dunnett's test assuming significance at $p < 0.05$.

Results

Figure 1 shows that confluent HepG2 cells cultured under conventional conditions, i.e., incubation in polystyrol dishes under room air with 5% CO_2, were

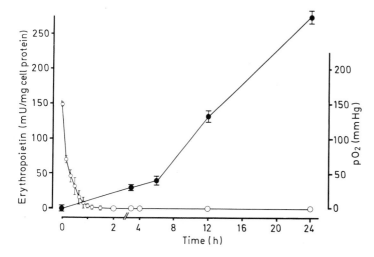

Fig. 1. Time course of erythropoietin production (●---●, $n = 4$) and pericellular PO_2 (○---○, $n = 8$) of HepG2 cells grown in polystyrol dishes under a medium layer of 0.53 cm and incubated in room air containing 5% CO_2. Values are means $\pm$ SD

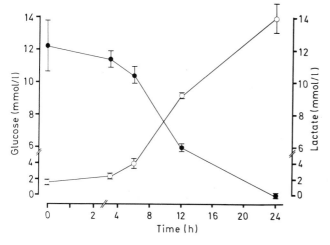

Fig. 2. Glucose consumption (●---●, $n = 4$) and lactate production (○---○, $n = 4$) of HepG2 cells under the conditions described in Fig. 1. Values are means $\pm$ SD

exposed to a remarkably low oxygen tension. Within 1 h after medium replacement the pericellular PO_2 dropped to < 1 mmHg. In this almost anoxic situation, EPO production was stimulated to 269 ± 9 mU/mg cell protein in 24 h. Moreover revealing the anaerobic conditions of those cultures, glucose is almost entirely utilized in 24 h and lactate is produced in an equimolar ratio (Fig. 2). In contrast, when the cells were cultivated in dishes with a gas-permeable bottom (Fig. 3), PO_2 was maintained at 127 mmHg on the cellular level. Here, EPO production was only 42 ± 5 mU/mg cell protein in 24 h

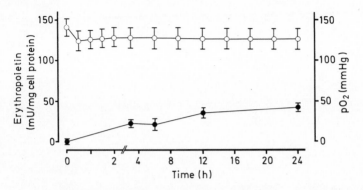

Fig. 3. Time course of erythropoietin production ($\bullet$---$\bullet$, $n = 4$) and pericellular PO$_2$ ($\circ$---$\circ$, $n = 8$) of HepG2 cells maintained in gas-permeable dishes with a FEP-teflon bottom. Otherwise same conditions as described in Fig 1. Values are means $\pm$ SD

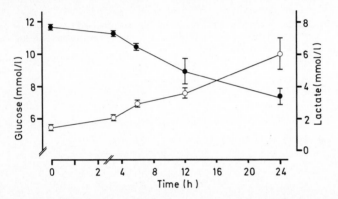

Fig. 4. Glucose consumption ($\bullet$---$\bullet$, $n = 4$) and lactate production ($\circ$---$\circ$, $n = 4$) of HepG2 cells cultured under the conditions corresponding to Fig 3. Values are means $\pm$ SD

(Fig. 3). Glucose consumption and lactate production under these conditions were rather low (Fig. 4).

With addition of IL-1, a dose-dependent, significant decrease of hypoxia-induced EPO production was observed (Fig. 5). IL-1β was slightly more effective than IL-1α. A similar effect could be demonstrated by addition of TNF-α (Fig. 6). In contrast, treatment with IL-6 and IFN-γ did not result in a significant decrease of EPO production (data not shown). α-FP synthesis was found to be unaffected by IL-1 and TNF-α.

Discussion

There is still lack of a reliable kidney cell culture model for controlled production of EPO. This is in part due to the fact that the precise cell type which

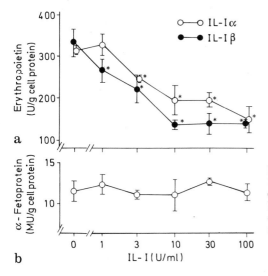

Fig. 5a,b. Effects of recombinant human IL-1α and IL-1β on the production of erythropoietin (**a**) and α-feto-protein (**b**) by HepG2 cells. Values are means ± SD of 24-h rates in 4 parallel cultures. *Asterisk*, significant difference from control

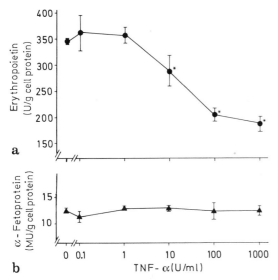

Fig. 6a,b. Effects of recombinant human TNF-α on the production of erythropoietin (**a** and α-fetoprotein (**b**) in HepG2 cultures. Values are means ± SD of 24-h rates in 4 parallel cultures. *Asterisk*, significant difference from control

produces EPO in the kidney is still a matter of controversy. Recently, two hepatoma cell lines have been identified which produce increased amounts of EPO when exposed to hypoxia [12]. This effect, however, could be demonstrated only by incubating low-density cultures in hypoxic-gas mixtures [12, 37]. In contrast, when confluent cultures were exposed to a oxygen-depleted atmosphere, EPO production was diminished [30]. This apparent discrepancy can be explained by our measurements of PO_2 on the cellular level. Even when incubated under room air with 5% CO_2, confluent HepG2 cells grown in gas-impermeable supports live under severe hypoxia with a $PO_2 < 1$ mmHg. This can be ascribed to a misproportion between the high O_2 consumption of the liver tumor cells and insufficient O_2 supply, which is limited by the culture dish and the depth of the medium layer. Our findings are consistent with the theoretical considerations made by McLimans et al. [26] regarding O_2 diffusion in cell culture systems, which indicate that a medium layer of more than 1.2 mm will rapidly lead to pericellular anoxia in primary hepatocyte cultures. In such cultures energy production is maintained by glycolysis which results in a high rate of lactate production. When confluent HepG2 cultures are incubated in a low oxygen gas phase, as Nielsen et al. did [30], the pericellular PO_2 will fall below the critical PO_2 for oxidative phosphorylation [39], thus leading to impaired protein and EPO synthesis. Adjustment of the pericellular PO_2 in a physiological range becomes possible, however, by reduction of the O_2 consumption of HepG2 cells, as achieved by using nonconfluent cultures [12, 37].

To cope with the problem of O_2 diffusion we used dishes with a gas-permeable bottom to control pericellular PO_2 [20]. A confluent monolayer of HepG2 cells grown in room air with 5% CO_2 ($PO_2 = 141$ mmHg) creates a relatively small PO_2 gradient of about 14 mmHg across the FEP-teflon bottom. The "constitutive" production of EPO in these dishes is only 25% compared to the production under diffusion-limited O_2 supply.

EPO formation thus stimulated by hypoxia could be suppressed by IL-1 and TNF-α, but not by IL-6 or IFN-γ. Despite marked differences in the primary structure of TNF-α and IL-1, which are also recognized by distinct cell surface receptors, both monokines are known to elicit similar effects on hepatic gene expression [7, 22]. In the human hepatoma cell lines HepG2 and Hep3B, TNF-α and IL-1 have been reported to stimulate the biosynthesis of several acute-phase proteins and to decrease the synthesis of albumin and transferrin. These effects of TNF-α and IL-1 on hepatic acute-phase gene expression were independent, dose related, and mainly regulated on a pretranslational level [6, 31]. Similarly, our results show that TNF-α and IL-1 decrease the synthesis of immunoreactive EPO, which is known to be regulated at the EPO mRNA level [12]. It could be presumed that the regulation of several discrete genes by TNF-α and IL-1 in a similar manner is accomplished by identical or different second messengers which trigger a common transcriptional or posttranscriptional mechanism, thus changing mRNA synthesis or mRNA turnover. However, further studies are necessary to prove which intracellular pathway can be implicated for the effects of IL-1 and TNF-α on EPO production.

There is strong evidence from recent in vivo and in vitro studies that IL-1 and TNF-α are involved in the pathogenesis of anemia in chronic disease [21, 33, 35, 36]. Nevertheless, it has to be determined whether these pleiotropic monokines act preferentially on the bone marrow level by inhibition of the EPO effects, or to what extent the suppression of EPO formation described herein contributes to the development of anemia or delays the recovery from anemia. The latter hypothesis is supported by increasing evidence for inappropriately low EPO serum levels in anemia of chronic infectious and noninfectious inflammatory disease, malignant disorders, and renal graft rejection [3, 4, 19, 25, 29]. Furthermore, there are indications that recombinant human EPO (rhuEPO) may overcome this relative EPO deficiency in inflammatory disease [27]. Little data, however, are available concerning erythropoiesis and EPO production after major injury or in septicemia [13]. As these patients in particular are depending on a sufficient oxygen transport capacity, relatively low EPO levels would provide a rational basis for the administration of rhuEPO. The beneficial effects of that replacement therapy may result from a reduced need for heterologous blood transfusions with its drawbacks of sensitization and immunosuppression [23].

Conclusions

First, the data presented here suggest that HepG2 cells are a useful model for oxygen-controlled EPO production. It should be emphasized, however, that metabolically active cells like the HepG2 cell line already live under severe hypoxia even when cultured conventionally in an atmosphere with 20% oxygen. Second, IL-1 and TNF-α suppress hypoxia-induced EPO formation in this in vitro model. Further studies are required to prove whether the increase in EPO production, which would be expected in response to anemia or hypoxia in critically ill patients, may be suppressed by these cytokines in vivo.

Acknowledgments. The authors wish to thank Dr. W. Fleckenstein for helpful advice concerning oxygen measurements and Mrs. Isenberg for secretarial assistance. This work was supported in part by DFG Grant Je 95/6-2.

References

1. Balkwill F, Osborne R, Burke F, Naylor S, Talbot D, Durbin H, Tavernier J, Fiers W (1987) Evidence for tumor necrosis factor/cachectin production in cancer. Lancet II:1229–1232
2. Bauer C, Kurtz A (1989) Oxygen sensing in the kidney and its relation to erythropoietin production. Annu Rev Physiol 51:845–856
3. Besarab A, Caro J, Jarrell BE, Francos G, Erslev AJ (1987) Dynamics of erythropoiesis following renal transplantation. Kidney Int 32:526–536
4. Birgegard G (1989) Erythropoiesis and inflammation. Contrib Nephrol 76:330–341
5. Cotes PM (1989) Physiological studies of erythropoietin in plasma. In: Jelkmann W, Gross AJ (eds) Erythropoietin. Springer, Berlin Heidelberg New York, pp 57–79
6. Darlington GJ, Wilson DR, Lachman LB (1986) Monocyte-conditioned medium, interleukin-1, and tumor necrosis factor stimulate the acute phase response in human hepatoma cells in vitro. J Cell Biol 103:787–793
7. Dinarello CA (1987) The biology of interleukin 1 in comparison to tumor necrosis factor. Immunol Lett 16:227–232
8. Eastgate JA, Symons JA, Wood NC, Grinlinton FM, Di Giovine FS, Duff GW (1988)

Correlation of plasma interleukin-1 levels with disease activity in rheumatoid arthritis. Lancet II:706–709

9. Eckhardt KU, Boutellier U, Kurtz A, Schopen M, Koller EA, Bauer C (1989) Rate of erythropoietin formation in humans in response to acute hypobaric hypoxia. J Appl Physiol 66:1785–1788

10. Erslev AJ, Wilson J, Caro J (1987) Erythropoietin titers in anemic, nonuremic patients. J Lab Clin Med 109:429–433

11. Faist E, Ninnemann J, Green D (eds) (1989) Immune consequences of trauma, shock, and sepsis. Mechanisms and therapeutical approaches. Springer, Berlin Heidelberg New York

12. Goldberg MA, Glass GA, Cunningham JM, Bunn HF (1987) The regulated expression of erythropoietin by two human hepatoma cell lines. Proc Natl Acad Sci USA 84:7972–7976

13. Gould SA, Rosen AI, Sehgal LR, Sehgal HL, Rice CL, Chamberlin WH, Moss GS (1985) Depressed red cell recovery following acute blood loss. Fed Proc 44:1265

14. Haga P, Cotes PM, Till JA, Minty BD, Shinebourne EA (1987) Serum immunoreactive erythropoietin in children with cyanotic and acyanotic congenital heart disease. Blood 70:822–826

15. Herbelin A, Nguyen AT, Zingraff J, Urena P, Decamps-Latscha B (1990) Influence of uremia and hemodialysis on circulating interleukin-1 and tumor necrosis factor α. Kidney Int 37:116–125

16. Imagawa DK, Millis JM, Olthoff KM, Derus LJ, Clna D, Sugich LR, Ozawa M, Dempsey RA, Iwaki Y, Levy PJ, Terasaki PI, Busuttil RW (1990) The role of tumor necrosis factor in allograft rejection. Transplantation 50:219–225

17. Jelkmann W (1986) Renal erythropoietin: properties and production. Rev Physiol Biochem Pharmacol 104:139–215

18. Jelkmann W, Wiedemann G (1990) Serum erythropoietin level: relationship to blood hemoglobin concentration and erythrocytic activity of the bone marrow. Klin Wochenschr 68:403–407

19. Jelkmann W, Wolff M, Fandrey J (1990) Modulation of the production of erythropoietin by cytokines: in vitro studies and their clinical implications. Contrib Nephrol 87:68–77

20. Jensen MD (1976) Diffusion in tissue cultures on gas-permeable and gas-impermeable supports. J Theor Biol 56:443–458

21. Johnson RA, Waddelow TA, Caro J, Oliff A, Roodman GD (1989) Chronic exposure to tumor necrosis factor in vivo preferentially inhibits erythropoiesis in nude mice. Blood 74:130–138

22. Le J, Vilcek J (1987) Tumor necrosis factor and interleukin 1: cytokines with multiple overlapping biological activities. Lab Invest 56:234–248

23. Levine EA, Gould SA, Rosen AL, Sehgal LR, Egrie JC, Sehgal HL, Revine HD, Moss GS (1989) Perioperative recombinant human erythropoietin. Surgery 106:432–438

24. Maury CPJ, Teppo AM (1988) Serum immunoreactive interleukin 1 in renal transplant recipients. Transplantation 45:143–147

25. McGonigle RJS, Wallin JD, Shadduck RK, Fisher JW (1984) Erythropoietin deficiency and inhibition of erythropoiesis in renal insufficiency. Kidney Int 25:437–444

26. McLimans WF, Blumenson LE, Tunnah KV (1968) Kinetics of gas diffusion in mammalian cell culture systems: II. Theory. Biotechnol Bioeng 10:741–763

27. Means RT, Olsen NJ, Krantz SB, Dessypris EN, Graber SE, Stone WJ, O'Neil VL, Pincus T (1989) Treatment of the anemia of rheumatoid arthritis with recombinant human erythropoietin: clinical and in vitro studies. Arthritis Rheum 32:638–642

28. Miller ME, Cronkite EP, Garcia JF (1982) Plasma levels of immunoreactive erythropoietin after acute blood loss in man. Br J Haematol 52:545–549

29. Miller CB, Jones RJ, Piantadosi S, Abeloff MD, Spivak JL (1990) Decreased erythropoietin response in patients with the anemia of cancer. N Engl J Med 322:1689–1692

30. Nielsen OJ, Schuster SJ, Kaufman H, Erslev AJ, Caro J (1987) Regulation of erythropoietin production in a human hepatoblastoma cell line. Blood 70:1904–1909

31. Perlmutter DH, Dinarello CA, Punsal PI, Colten HR (1986) Cachectin/tumor necrosis factor regulates hepatic acute-phase gene expression. J Clin Invest 78:1349–1354

32. Rhyner K, Egli F, Niemöller M, Wieczorek A, Greminger P, Vetter W (1989) Serumerythropoietinwerte bei verschiedenen Krankheitszuständen. Nephron 51 (Suppl 1):39–46

33. Roodman G (1987) Mechanisms of erythroid suppression in the anemia of chronic disease. Blood Cells 13:171–184

34. Saxne T, Palladino A, Heinegard D, Talal N, Wollheim A (1988) Detection of tumor necrosis

factor α but not tumor necrosis factor β in rheumatoid arthritis synovial fluid and serum. Arthritis Rheum 31:1041–1045

35. Schooley JC, Kullgren B, Allison AC (1987) Inhibition by interleukin-1 of the action of erythropoietin on erythroid precursors and its possible role in the pathogenesis of hypoplastic anemias. Br J Haematol 67:11–17

36. Tracey KJ, Wei H, Manogue KR, Fong Y, Hesse DG, Nguyen HT, Kuo GC, Beutler B, Cotran RS, Cerami A, Lowry SF (1988) Cachectin/tumor necrosis factor induces cachexia, anemia, and inflammation. J Exp Med 167:1211–1227

37. Ueno M, Seferynska I, Beckman B, Brookins J, Nakashima J, Fisher JW (1989) Enhanced erythropoietin secretion in hepatoblastoma cells in response to hypoxia. Am J Physiol, 257:C743–C749

38. Ulich TR, del Castillo J, Guo KZ (1989) In vivo hematologic effects of recombinant interleukin-6 on hematopoiesis and circulating numbers of RBCs and WBCs. Blood 73:108

39. Wilson DF, Rumsey WL, Green TJ, Vanderkooi JM (1988) The oxygen dependence of mitochondrial oxidative phosphorylation measured by a new optical method for measuring oxygen concentration. J Biol Chem 263:2712–2718

Neopterin, Interferon-γ, and Immunodeficiency States*

D. Fuchs, A. Hausen, G. Reibnegger, G. Weiss, E. R. Werner,
G. Werner-Felmayer, and H. Wachter

Neopterin as an Immunological Marker In Vitro and In Vivo

Concentrations of neopterin (D-erythro-6-trihydroxypropylpterin) in body fluids indicate the activation of cellular immunity in patients. In vitro, human macrophages release large amounts of neopterin on stimulation with interferon-γ (IFN-γ) [1, 8]. Other cytokines, e.g., tumour necrosis factor-α (TNF-α) are capable of further enhancing the IFN-γ-induced formation of neopterin. Neopterin concentrations correlate with the extent and the activity of disorders in which cell-mediated immune stimulation has a role (Table 1). In allograft recipients, neopterin concentrations rise early during the course of rejection episodes. Increasing neopterin is among the first signs of infections by viruses, occurring days or weeks before antibody seroconversion becomes measurable. In autoimmune disorders such as rheumatoid arthritis, neopterin levels correlate with the extent and activity of the disease. Neopterin levels are of predictive significance in patients with, for example, certain types of malignancy, multiple trauma, and human immunodeficiency virus (HIV) infection.

Correlation Between Endogenous Interferon-γ and Neopterin Formation In Vitro and In Vivo

Sensitive assays for neopterin (e.g., radioimmunoassay, high pressure liquid chromatography) easily allow neopterin concentrations in patients to be measured. In contrast, bioassays used for measurement of IFN-γ in T-cell cultures are usually not sensitive enough for measurements in serum from patients. Even radioimmunoassays allow a normal range of IFN-γ to be established only if optimized protocols are employed to increase the analytical sensitivity. Using sensitive techniques, significant positive correlations between serum levels of neopterin and IFN-γ were established (Table 2), e.g., in patients with haematological neoplasias and infections with viruses including HIV [2].

*This work was supported financially by the Fonds zur Förderung der Wissenschaftlichen Forschung, p 7910.
Institut für Medizinische Chemie und Biochemie, Universität Innsbruck, und Ludwig Boltzmann Institut für AIDS-Forschung, Innsbruck, Austria

Table 1. Neopterin as diagnostic tool in clinical immunology [1, 8]

	Value of neopterin monitoring
Transplantation	Indicates allograft rejection, predicts graft survival
Infectious diseases	Correlates with severity of infection; is of prognostic significance (e.g. HIV infection); rises before antibody seroconversion
Blood donor screening	Detects a variety of hazardous clinical conditions early (e.g. virus infections)
Autoimmune diseases	Correlates with extent and activity of disease; differentiates from noninflammatory disorders; valid for therapy monitoring
Malignant diseases	Correlates with extent and activity of disease; is of prognostic value at diagnosis and during follow-up
Immunomodulatory therapy	Rises during therapy with cytokines, e.g. IFN, interleukin-2, TNF; used for definition of bioactive dose

Table 2 Association between neopterin and interferon-γ in vitro and in vivo [2]

In vitro	
Monocytes/macrophages	IFN-γ induces neopterin formation and degradation of tryptophan
In vivo	
HIV infection	Increased neopterin correlates with increased serum IFN-γ; neopterin and IFN-γ correlate with increased kynurenine and decreased tryptophan in serum; increased neopterin in cerebrospinal fluid correlates with reduced tryptophan
Haematological neoplasias, sarcoidosis, virus infections	Increased neopterin correlates with increased serum IFN-γ
Therapy with immune response modifiers	Neopterin increase is paralleled by degradation of tryptophan

Association Between Chronic Immune Activation and Impaired T-Cell Response In Vitro

The list of disorders where immune stimulation can be detected by, for example, increased neopterin and IFN-γ (Tables 1, 2) in general covers those diseases where impaired T-cell response is common [2]. A diminished proliferative response of T-cells and reduced production of IFN-γ in vitro (on stimulation with antigens or mitogens) as well as skin test anergy correlate with enhanced circulating IFN-γ and neopterin levels in patients. Even in the early asymptomatic stage of HIV infection neopterin concentrations are higher in patients showing reduced T-cell proliferation in response to soluble antigens, compared with those showing a normal response. From these data it appears that chronic stimulation of T-lymphocytes and macrophages and release of cytokines, particularly release of IFN-γ, may have a role in inducing tolerance, resulting in skin test anergy and diminished T-cell responsiveness.

Endogenous Interferon-γ and Anaemia

Chronic inflammatory disorders are often associated with the development of anaemia, and neopterin concentrations correlate negatively with haemoglobin concentrations [4]. The finding of increased circulating neopterin and IFN-γ in patients with anaemia provides an in vivo correlate to in vitro data which show that cytokines such as IFN-γ and TNF-α are potent inhibitors of erythroid progenitor cells. Thus, endogenously released IFN-γ and TNF-α may be involved in haematopoietic suppression.

Endogenous Interferon-γ and Neurological/ Psychiatric Symptoms

In vitro, neopterin formation by stimulated human macrophages is paralleled by depletion of tryptophan from the culture medium and the formation of kynurenine [9]. Similarly, in patients with HIV infection strongly decreased serum tryptophan concentrations were found and correlated with neurological/psychiatric symptoms such as polyneuropathy and dementia [3]. In parallel, kynurenine levels were found to be increased. Several significant associations were shown to exist between neopterin, tryptophan metabolism, and IFN-γ in these patients [5]. Analogous metabolic changes were observed in cancer patients during treatment with immune response modifiers. It therefore appears that endogenous IFN-γ may contribute indirectly to precipitating neurological/psychiatric symptoms in patients with chronic inflammatory disorders, when the disorder is severe enough and the duration of the disease is long enough so that tryptophan degradation cannot be compensated by diet. Reduced availability of serotonin may result from low tryptophan levels. In addition, certain degradation products of tryptophan are potent neurotoxins.

Immune Stimulation in Patients with Multiple Trauma

Neopterin and IFN-γ data indicate a relationship between chronic immune stimulation and reduced T-cell responsiveness in patients. Depending on the degree and the duration, chronic immune stimulation may precipitate anaemia and neurological/psychiatric symptoms. Similar observations were made in patients with multiple trauma: Serum neopterin levels were significant predictors of sepsis [7]. In addition, neopterin concentrations correlated inversely with haemoglobin levels and the number of blood transfusions required [6].

In summary, the sequence of events which can be deduced from immunological profiles obtained in patients with multiple trauma [6, 7] appears to be as follows: Multiple trauma and blood loss initiate a peak production of cytokines within a few hours; this is followed by increased neopterin release. A higher degree of immunoactivation is associated with a higher risk of developing septic complications, and also risk of death. In agreement with other clinical conditions, immune stimulation causes reduced immunocompetence, which in turn allows invasion and spread of pathogens. In addition, haematopoiesis is inhibited by specific cytokines such as IFN-γ and TNF-α, causing anaemia and consequently the requirement for blood transfusion. Further studies will show whether tryptophan metabolism is also abnormal in such patients.

References

1. Fuchs D, Hausen A, Reibnegger G, Werner ER, Dierich MP, Wachter H (1988) Neopterin as a marker for activated cell-mediated immunity: application in HIV-1 infection. Immunol Today 9:150–155
2. Fuchs D, Malkowsky M, Reibnegger G, Werner ER, Forni G, Wachter H (1989) Endogenous release of interferon gamma and diminished response of peripheral blood mononuclear cells to antigenic stimulation. Immunol Lett 23:103–108
3. Fuchs D, Möller AA, Reibnegger G, Stöckle E, Werner ER, Wachter H (1990) Decreased serum tryptophan in patients with HIV-1 infection correlates with increased serum neopterin and with neurologic/psychiatric symptoms. J AIDS 3:873–876
4. Fuchs D, Hausen A, Reibnegger G, Werner ER, Werner-Felmayer G, Dierich MP, Wachter H (1991) Immune activation and the anaemia associated with chronic inflammatory disorders. Eur J Haematol 46:65–70
5. Fuchs D, Möller AA, Reibnegger G, Werner ER, Werner-Felmayer G, Dierich MP, Wachter H (1991) Increased endogenous interferon-gamma and neopterin correlate with increased degradation of tryptophan in human immunodeficiency virus type 1 infection. Immunol Lett (in press)
6. Robin B, Fuchs D, Koller W, Wachter H (1991) Course of immune activation markers in patients after severe multiple trauma. Pteridines (in press)
7. Strohmaier W, Redl H, Schlag G, Inthorn D (1987) D-erythroneopterin plasma levels in intensive care patients with and without septic complications. Crit Care Med 15:757–760
8. Wachter H, Fuchs D, Hausen A, Reibnegger G, Werner ER (1989) Neopterin as marker for activation of cellular immunity: immunologic basis and clinical application. Adv Clin Chem 27:81–141
9. Werner ER, Bitterlich G, Fuchs D, Hausen A, Reibnegger G, Szabo G, Dierich MP, Wachter H (1987) Human macrophages degrade tryptophan upon induction by interferon-gamma. Life Sci 41:273–280

Systemic Cytokine Response to Strenuous Exercise

H. Northoff[1], M. W. Baumstark[2], W. A. Flegel[1], and A. Berg[2]

The aim of this article is to summarize current knowledge on the modulation of systemic cytokine levels following exercise and to add some new information on interleukin 6 (IL-6) and IL-6-like activity in postexercise sera.

Cytokines

Cytokines are important immunomodulators, hormone-like mediator molecules, which transport signals for growth, function, or regulation among various cells of the immune system. They are generally small peptides or glycopeptides with molecular weights in the range of 13–30 kDa. Cytokines virtually govern the immune response, and there are few functions in which they are not involved. This holds true for the specific and the unspecific branches of the immune system and for interactions between the two. Cytokines includes lymphokines, monokines, interleukins, colony-stimulating factors, and other molecules.

Cytokines are produced by a host of different cells, including endothelial cells and fibroblasts. Lymphocytes and cells of the monocyte/macrophage lineage seem, however, to be the most important source of cytokines.

Apart from their eminent role in the immune response, cytokines also have pleiotropic effects. Thus, IL-1 has been shown to lead to the expression of adhesion molecules, bone resorption, destruction of cartilage, growth stimulation of fibroblasts, synovial cells, and epithelial cells, and induction of prostaglandins and to have many more functions [6, 13–16]. Hence, cytokines play key roles in many clinical settings such as acute phase reaction, wound healing, rheumatoid diseases, and septic shock syndrome.

Cytokines can be measured using bioassays, enzyme-linked immunosorbent assays (ELISA) or radioimmunoassays (RIA). Today, bioassays are still important. Many of these entail the disadvantage of interference by serum-borne inhibitors, but they can be very sensitive. Some bioassays, such as fever induction assays in rats or rabbits and the thymocyte costimulator assay, detect several lymphokines (IL-1 and IL-6). Others are more specific, such as the CTLL

[1] German Red Cross Blood Center and Department of Transfusion Medicine, University of Ulm, Obever Eselsberg 7900 Ulm, FRG
[2] Department of Physical Performance Medicine, University of Freiburg, 7800 Freiburg, FRG

Host Defense Dysfunction
in Trauma, Shock and Sepsis
Eds. Faist/Meakins/Schildberg
© Springer-Verlag, Berlin Heidelberg 1993

cell line growth assay (for IL-2), the combined assay with EL4 and CTLL cell lines (for IL-1), and the 7TD1 hybridoma growth assay (for IL-6). Immunochemical detection of cytokines using ELISA or RIA is quite specific, although these may produce false-positive results. Many ELISAs or RIAs are less sensitive than bioassays. ELISAs often function better with plasma than with serum.

Reports on Cytokines After Strenuous Exercise

There is an increasing number of reports showing elevated cytokine levels in serum or plasma after strenuous exercise. As early as 1969 an acute-phase reaction in athletes was described after strenuous, exhaustive exercise by Haralambie [10]. As we know today, this results from an increased production of cytokines since the production of acute-phase proteins by liver cells is induced by IL-6 and to a lesser extent by IL-1 and tumor necrosis factor (TNF) [2, 3].

In 1983 Cannon et al. found cytokine activity in postexercise serum using fever induction and costimulation of thymocyte growth as assays [4]. According to the state of knowledge at that time, the demonstrated cytokine activity was assumed to be IL-1 (endogenous pyrogen). As we now know, however, the assays used were not specific for IL-1 and included detection of IL-6. The latter was identified as an entity of its own, separate from IL-1, by Gauldie et al. in 1987 [2,1,9]. One year later our group found elevation of IL-6-like activity in the sera of marathon runners, using the 7TD1 hybridoma growth assay [11, 12]. Further results from this investigation are described below. In 1989 Dufaux et al. reported elevated TNF, soluble IL-2 receptor (IL-2R), and neopterin in plasma after strenuous exercise [7]. In the same year, TNF elevation was also shown by Espersen et al. [8]; this group also showed modulation of IL-2 levels in plasma.

The kinetics of the cytokine reaction after strenuous exercise are presented in Table 1. TNF and IL-6 are elevated shortly after the exercise and are usually back to about normal levels 24 h later. IL-2 shows an opposite behavior, with decreased values shortly after exercise and elevated values 2 days later. Soluble

Table 1. Systemic cytokine levels after strenuous exercise (From [7, 8, 11])

Time after exercise	Change in serum levels relative to baseline			
	TNF	IL-6	IL-2	IL-2R
0–3 h	Elevated	Elevated	Decreased	Normal
24 h	Normal	Some elevated	Some elevated	Normal
48 h	Normal	Normal	Elevated	Elevated

IL-2R was also elevated 1–2 days after exercise. TNF and IL-6 are most likely of monocyte/macrophage origin and therefore indicate an activation of the unspecific branch of the immune system. Local release of IL-1β in human muscle tissue has also been reported in association with exercise [5]. However, we were unable to detect systemic serum IL-1 by ELISA [12].

Modulation of IL-2 and IL-2R point to an activation of the specific branch of the immune system (lymphocytes). Increased consumption of IL-2 by activated natural killer cells or T cells must be considered as a cause of the observed early decrease in IL-2 levels.

New Findings on IL-6 and IL-6-like Activities After Strenuous Exercise

Previously we have shown elevated IL-6 in 16 marathon runners immediately after running [12]. In most cases IL-6 was normal again 24 h later. In addition, we compared these data with clinical chemistry data from the same set of runners and found that exercise-induced IL-6 after the run was positively correlated with total leukocytes ($p = 0.01$), monocytes ($p = 0.02$), NH_3 ($p = 0.01$), and iron ($p = 0.02$). Persistence of elevated IL-6, 24 h after the run was positively correlated with lactate at the aerobic threshold ($p = 0.05$) and negatively with VO_2:4 mmol lactate ($p = 0.01$). We were intrigued to find persistence of IL-6 correlating with performance markers. Unfortunately, we did not reproduce this finding when we tried to show the observed correlations with an independent set of tests from a different run under fairly comparable conditions. The data from the second run did, however, clearly confirm that IL-6 activity as measured by 7TD1 hybridoma growth is elevated in sera drawn immediately after running.

We feel that our first observation indicates an important feature of the cytokine reaction after strenuous exercise. The measurement of cytokine activity in serum as performed in our studies, however, may not be a reliable way to demonstrate the correlation with performance markers. Individual kinetics of release, clearance of cytokines, and inhibitors must be taken into account and may require more detailed investigations to be conclusive.

To corroborate that we were really dealing with IL-6 we conducted inhibition studies with a specific antibody in the 7TD1 assay. Polyclonal sheep antihuman IL-6 (kindly provided by Dr. L. Aarden, Amsterdam) inhibited the IL-6 activity partially while anti-IL-1 was inactive (Fig. 1). The anti-IL-6 inhibited up to 50% of the IL-6 activity in the serum. Controls showed that the antibody used was extremely potent and was able completely to inhibit large amounts of recombinant human IL-6 and natural IL-6 (supernatants from lipopolysaccharide-stimulated human monocytes). We conclude that, although there is clearly IL-6 in the sera, there is also some IL-6-like activity present which cannot be inhibited by anti-IL-6.

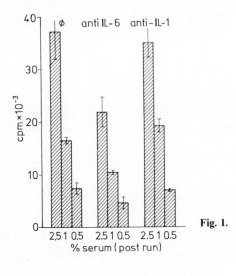

Fig. 1.

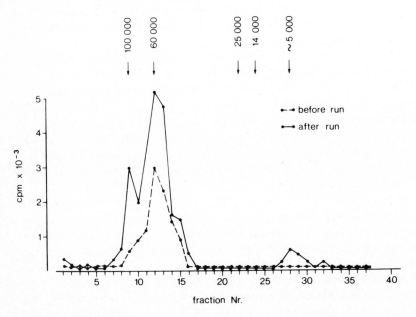

Fig. 2.

Elevation of IL-6 in sera following the run was also demonstrated by ELISA. Eight runners had low levels of IL-6 detectable before the run (10.2 ± 3.8 pg/ml) which were elevated (17.9 ± 8.4 pg/ml) immediately after the run. The other nine sera were negative before the run; six of these, however, were marginally positive after the run. Thus, while we confirmed the presence of IL-6 and the elevation of

IL-6 levels after the run, the ELISA results are compatible with the assumption that some IL-6-like activity is also present in the sera.

Finally, we performed an analysis of serum pooled from three runners by a Superose 12 column using a physiological salt concentration. The fractions were tested by the 7TD1 assay (Fig. 2). All bioactivity of IL-6 was recovered in the high molecular weight region (50–200 kDa) except a very minor portion at about 5 kDa. The latter, probably representing degradation products, was detectable only in serum from after the run. Sera following the run clearly contained more IL-6 bioactivity than that from before the run. There was, however, no IL-6 activity detectable in the range of 20–30 kDa, where free IL-6 would be expected. Therefore, we conclude that IL-6 or IL-6-like activity in postexercise sera occurs mainly bound to high molecular weight molecules in bioactive form.

In summary, there is accumulating evidence in the literature that systemic levels of cytokines such as IL-2, IL-6, TNF and IL-2R are modulated after strenuous exercise. The changes are, however, mild. Correlation with clinical or performance parameters may require more detailed investigations than are presently available. In postexercise sera, elevation of levels of IL-6 and of an IL-6-like activity can be shown. These activities are associated with high molecular weight molecules.

Acknowledgements. We thank, Mrs. Hilde Wintersinger and Mrs. Andrea Kuner for the excellent technical assistance.

References

1. Andus T, Geiger T, Hirano T, Northoff H, Ganter U, Bauer J, Kishimoto T, Heinrich PC (1987) Recombinant human B cell stimulatory factor 2 (BSF-2/IFN-beta2) regulates beta-fibrinogen and albumin mRNA levels in Fao-9 cells. FEBS Lett 221:18–22
2. Andus T, Heinrich PC, Bauer J, Tran-Thi TA, Decker K, Männel D, Northoff H (1987) Discrimination of hepatocyte-stimulating activity from human recombinant tumor necrosis factor alpha. Eur J Immunol 17:1193–1197
3. Andus T, Geiger T, Hirano T, Kishimoto T, Heinrich PC (1988) Action of recombinant interleukin 6, interleukin 1β and tumor necrosis factor α on the mRNA induction of acute phase proteins. Eur J Immunol 18:739–746
4. Cannon JG, Kluger MJ (1983) Endogenous pyrogen activity in human plasma after exercise. Science 220:617–619
5. Cannon JG, Fielding RA, Fiatarone MA, Orencole SF, Dinarello CA, Evans WJ (1989) Increased interleukin 1β in human skeletal muscle after exercise. Am J Physiol 257:R451–R455
6. Dinarello CA (1989) Interleukin-1 and its biologically related cytokines. Adv Immunol 44:153–205
7. Dufaux B, Order U (1989) Plasma elastase-α1-antitrypsin, neopterin, tumor necrosis factor, and soluble interleukin-2 receptor after prolonged exercise. Int J Sports Med 10:434–438
8. Espersen GT, Elbaek A, Ernst E, Toft E, Kaalund S, Jersild C, Grunnet N (1990) Effect of physical exercise on cytokines and lymphocyte subpopulations in human peripheral blood. APMIS 98:395–400
9. Gauldie J, Richards C, Harnish D, Lansdorp P, Baumann H (1987) Interferon β2/B-cell stimulatory factor type 2 shares identity with monocyte-derived hepatocyte-stimulating factor

and regulates the major acute phase protein response in liver cells. Proc Natl Acad Sci USA 84:7251–7255

10. Haralambie G (1969) Serum glycoproteins and physical exercise. Clin Chim Acta 26:287–291
11. Northoff H, Berg A (1991) Immunologic mediators as parameters of the reaction to strenuous exercise. Int J Sports Med 12:
12. Northoff H, Flegel WA, Männel DN, Baumstark M, Berg A (1990) Increased levels of interleukin-6 (IL-6) and/or IL-7 in sera of long-distance runners, In: Powanda MC, Oppenheim JJ, Kluger MJ, Dinarello CA (eds) The physiological and pathological effects of cytokines. Wiley, New York, pp 75–79
13. O'Garra A (1989) Interleukins and the immune system 2. Lancet I:1003–1005
14. O'Garra A (1989) Interleukins and the immune system 1. Lancet I:943–947
15. Oppenheim JJ, Gery I (1982) Interleukin 1 is more than an interleukin. Immunol Today 4:113–119
16. Oppenheim JJ, Kovacs EJ, Matsushima K, Durum SK (1986) There is more than one interleukin 1. Immunol Today 7:45–56

Section 9

The Mediator Role of TNF in Sepsis

Activation of Neutrophils by Tumor Necrosis Factor-α During Sepsis

G. Rothe[1], W. Kellermann[2], J. Briegel[2], B. Schaerer[2], and G. Valet[1]

Introduction

Endotoxin exposure of macrophages during the onset of bacterial infections leads to the sequential production of the cytokines tumor necrosis factor-α (TNF-α), interleukin-1β and interleukin-6 [1]. These cytokines are thought to enhance the local anti-bacterial immune response. TNF-α, the most potent modulator of neutrophil function, induces in vitro the inhibition of neutrophil chemotaxis [2], the expression of CD11/CD18 integrins resulting in the adherence of neutrophils to matrix proteins with the release of oxidants [3] and specific granule constituents [4], extravasation [5, 6], and increased phagocytosis [7].

Topical TNF-α administration in vivo induces localized vascular hyperpermeability and extravasation [8]. Systemic TNF-α exposure, in contrast, is experimentally associated with neutrophil-mediated oxidative and proteolytic tissue destruction [9]. This deleterious role of systemic neutrophil activation is confirmed by the correlation of the initial plasma levels of TNF-α during infection with the incidence of the adult respiratory distress syndrome and with the mortality rate [10].

The significance of TNF-α as a determinant for the prolonged neutrophil-mediated oxidative and proteolytic tissue destruction during the sepsis syndrome is, however, uncertain due to rapidly decreasing TNF-α plasma levels [10] and the experimental observation of cellular deactivation towards TNF-α following repeated in vitro exposure of neutrophils to TNF-α or cross-deactivation following cellular contact with bacterial agents [11]. This cross-deactivation has been shown to include shedding of the TNF-α receptors leading to an increase in the plasma TNF-α binding capacity and to an inhibition of TNF-α actions on other cells. [12]. The data showing deactivation of neutrophils towards TNF-α were generated with neutrophils from healthy normal individuals. Neutrophils from septic patients are, however, in a different functional state as visible from the flow cytometric measurement of cell biochemical

[1] Arbeitsgruppe Zellbiochemie, Max-Planck-Institut für Biochemie, Am Klopferspitz 18a, 8033 Martinsried, FRG
[2] Institut für Anästhesiologie, Klinikum Großhadern, Ludwig-Maximilians-Universität München, Marchioninistr. 15, 8000 Munich 70, FRG

Host Defense Dysfunction
in Trauma, Shock and Sepsis
Eds. Faist/Meakins/Schildberg
© Springer-Verlag, Berlin Heidelberg 1993

parameters of neutrophil function such as the activation of the oxidative burst cascade or the activation of the Na^+/H^+-antiport leading to alkalinization of the intracellular pH and an increase in cell volume [13, 14]. The goal of this study was, therefore, to characterize TNF-α effects on neutrophils from septic individuals in comparison with healthy normals. This was done by comparing in vitro effects of TNF-α on neutrophils from healthy normals with the functional state of in vivo activated neutrophils from septic patients, and their responses to addition of TNF-α or neutralizing anti-TNF-α antibodies.

Materials and Methods

Patients. Seventy-two venous blood samples were obtained from intensive care patients with or without bacterial infection or sepsis. Sepsis was assumed in the presence of a defined bacterial focus and secondary systemic effects of sepsis [15]. The 32 patients without infection had multiple organ failure scores, as defined by Goris et al. [16], of 1.87 ± 0.55 (mean $\pm$ standard error), in contrast to a score of 2.81 ± 0.31 for the 26 bacterially infected patients, and 6.71 ± 0.19 for the 14 patients with sepsis.

Cells. A suspension of leukocytes in autologous plasma was prepared by overlaying heparinized blood samples from intensive care patients and seven healthy normals on an erythrocyte-aggregating medium (Histopaque-1077, Sigma, Deisenhofen, FRG) for 30 min at 22 °C and 1 g [17]. The plasma supernatant is depleted of erythrocytes through accelerated sedimentation at the plasma-medium interface. This procedure induces no measurable prestimulation of the cells as contact of the neutrophils with the separation medium, centrifugation, or lysis of erythrocytes are avoided.

Staining. The cell suspension in autologous plasma (20 µl) was preincubated in 1 ml of Hank's balanced salt solution (HBSS, without phenol red or bicarbonate, Sigma; with 10 mM HEPES, pH 7.35) for 5 min at 37 °C either with 1 µl of the fluorogenic substrate dihydrorhodamine 123 (DHR, Molecular Probes, Eugene, OR, USA; 1 mM in N,N-dimethylformamide, DMF) for the quantitation of the hydrogen peroxide production by the intracellular oxidation of nonfluorescent DHR to green fluorescent rhodamine 123 [17, 18] or with 1 µl of the fluorogenic pH indicator 1,4-diacetoxy-2,3-dicyanobenzene (ADB, Calbiochem, Frankfurt, FRG; 50 mM in DMF) for the measurement of the intracellular alkalinization during cellular activation [13].

Stimulation. The cells loaded with the fluorogenic substrates were primed by a 5-min incubation with 10 ng/ml of human recombinant TNF-α (Sigma, produced in yeast, specific activity 2×10^7 U/mg protein) at 37 °C or incubated without TNF-α as a control. Direct effects of TNF-α were measured after 15 min of incubation without further stimulation, whereas effects of TNF-α on the response of neutrophils to stimulation were measured after additional 15 min of incubation with $10^{-7} M$ of the bacterial peptide N-formyl-Meth-Leu-Phe (FMLP, Sigma; stock 1 mM in DMF). Alternatively, samples were maximally stimulated with $10^{-7} M$ of the tumor promoter phorbol 12-myristate 13-acetate (PMA, Sigma; stock 1 mM in DMF) as a positive control.

Flow cytometry. 10 000 cells per sample were analyzed after counterstaining of dead cells with propidium iodide (PI, 30 μM, stock 3 mM in HEPES-buffered saline). The rhodamine 123 green fluorescence (515–545 nm), the PI red fluorescence (> 650 nm) and the cellular forward and right-angle light scatter of the DHR-stained cell samples were measured with 488-nm argon laser excitation on a FACScan flow cytometer (Becton Dickinson, San José, CA, USA). The cellular blue (420–440 nm) and green and red fluorescence (> 500 nm) of the ADB-stained cell samples was measured with 365-nm excitation by a high-pressure mercury arc lamp together with electrical determination of the cell volume on a FLUVO-II flow cytometer (Heka-Elektronik, Lambrecht/Pfalz, FRG). The list mode data were evaluated by DIAGNOS1 software using automated batch-processing with fixed gates and windows [19].

Results

Oxidative Burst Activity

A low oxidative burst activity with only 11.4% ± 2.6% of the neutrophils (mean ± SEM, $n = 7$) showing a high oxidative burst response was induced by incubation of the blood samples from healthy normals with $10^{-7} M$ FMLP (Fig. 1a). A similar low response was seen when the cells were incubated with 10 ng/ml TNF-α alone. A 5-min priming of neutrophils with TNF-α, in contrast, led to a high all-or-none-response to FMLP in a subpopulation of 32.0% ± 2.5% of the neutrophils with a mean fluorescence 23.6-fold (± 3.9) over the fluorescence of nonstimulated cells (Fig. 1b). The percentage of highly responsive neutrophils increased upon stimulation with increasing amounts of FMLP (up to $5 \times 10^{-6} M$) suggesting a wide heterogeneity of the thresholds controlling the FMLP-stimulated oxidative burst response. PMA stimulation by contrast induced a homogeneously high response in 96.8% ± 0.8% of the neutrophils showing that all neutrophils can react with oxidative burst activity.

   Neutrophils from septic patients following incubation under the same conditions showed a high oxidative burst response in a large subpopulation of neutrophils already in the presence of $10^{-7} M$ FMLP alone, indicating that these cells had been primed in vivo (Figs. 2a, 3). These cells also showed a higher response to exogenously added TNF-α suggesting that no deactivation towards TNF-α had occurred. Endogenous TNF-α was directly identified as a mediator

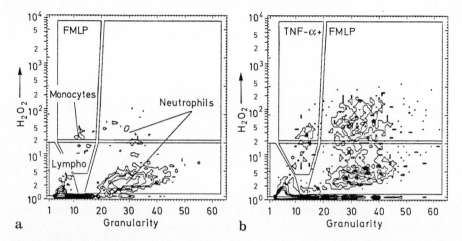

Fig. 1a, b. Effect of TNF-α on the oxidative burst response of neutrophils stimulated with the bacterial peptide FMLP. The intracellular production of hydrogen peroxide by peripheral blood leukocytes from a healthy individual was measured by flow cytometry by the intracellular oxidation of nonfluorescent DHR to the green fluorescent rhodamine 123 following stimulation with 10^{-7} M FMLP for 15 min **a** without or **b** with pretreatment of the cells with 10 ng/ml TNF-α for 5 min. Lymphocytes, monocytes and neutrophils are distinguished by the cellular side scatter

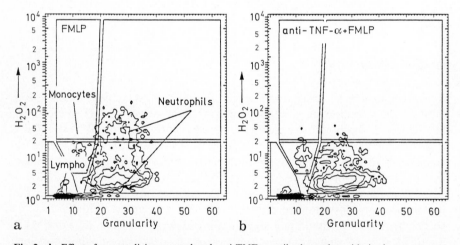

Fig. 2a, b. Effect of a neutralizing monoclonal anti-TNF-α antibody on the oxidative burst response of neutrophils to the bacterial peptide FMLP during sepsis. The intracellular production of hydrogen peroxide was measured as described in Fig. 1. Leukocytes from a patient with sepsis were stimulated with 10^{-7} M FMLP for 15 min **a** without or **b** with a 20-min preincubation in the presence of 200 ng/ml anti-TNF-α

of the in vivo priming of neutrophils in a subset of the blood samples obtained during sepsis by inhibition of the highly reactive subpopulation after a 20-min preincubation with a neutralizing anti-TNF-α antibody (clone 195, Boehringer Mannheim, Mannheim, FRG; Fig. 2b).

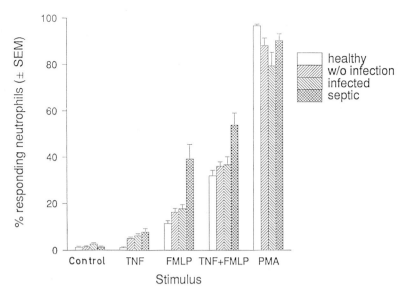

Fig. 3. Percentage of neutrophils responding with a high oxidative burst to stimulation with TNF-α or FMLP in blood samples from healthy normals ($n = 7$), and intensive care patients without ($n = 32$) or with bacterial infection ($n = 26$) or with sepsis ($n = 14$). The percentage of responsive neutrophils is calculated from the number of neutrophils in the upper right analysis window (Figs. 1 and 2), when related to the total number of neutrophils

Na$^+$/H$^+$-Antiport Activation

An increase of neutrophil cell volume, mediated by the activation of amiloride-sensitive Na$^+$/H$^+$ exchange, is already observed upon minor stimulation, in contrast to an oxidative burst response only upon stimulation above a certain threshold. Thus TNF-α alone induced a 11.2% ($\pm$ 3.3%) increase in neutrophil cell volume (Fig. 4) compared to a 27.8% ($\pm$ 2.9%) increase of cell volume

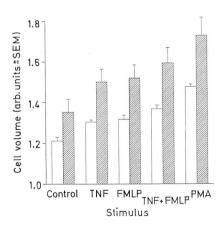

Fig. 4. Cell volume of neutrophils from healthy individuals ($n = 4$; *no hatching*) and patients with sepsis ($n = 4$; *hatched*). The leukocytes were stimulated for 15 min with 10^{-7} *M* FMLP or 10^{-7} *M* PMA with or without a 5-min pretreatment with 10 ng/ml TNF-α. The cell volume was measured by electrical sizing of cells hydrodynamically focused through the center of a cylindrical orifice (80 μm in diameter)

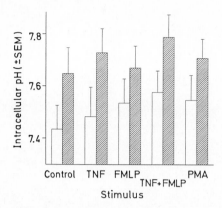

Fig. 5. Intracellular pH of neutrophils from healthy individuals ($n = 4$; *no hatching*) and patients with sepsis ($n = 4$; *hatched*). The leukocytes were stimulated for 15 min with $10^{-7} M$ FMLP or $10^{-7} M$ PMA with or without pretreatment with 10 ng/ml TNF-α for 5 min. The intracellular pH was measured by the ratio of the blue to green fluorescence of the pH indicator 2,3-dicyanohydroquinone loaded into the cells by the intracellular cleavage of ADB by cellular esterases

induced by maximal stimulation of the cells with PMA. Furthermore, the alkalinization of the intracellular pH was a sensitive indicator of TNF-α effects on neutrophils with a similarly high response to the combination of TNF-α and FMLP as to PMA alone (Fig. 5).

Neutrophils from patients during sepsis were in an activated state as shown by an increased cell volume (Fig. 4) and a more alkaline intracellular pH (Fig. 5). TNF-α alone and in combination with FMLP induced significant increases in neutrophil cell volume and pH confirming the high responsiveness of the neutrophils from septic patients to exogenous TNF-α observed in the oxidative burst measurements.

Discussion

This study shows that the in vitro priming of neutrophils by TNF-α leads to the graded recruitment of a previously unresponsive subpopulation of neutrophils to a high oxidative burst response towards FMLP. Neutrophils from patients with bacterial infections in combination with the systemic organ dysfunction of the sepsis syndrome were already highly stimulated in vivo as visible from a large FMLP-responsive subpopulation, in contrast to a low systemic neutrophil activation in patients with focal bacterial infection. This suggests that local neutrophil activation is sufficient to control a focal bacterial infection. When neutrophils are, however, systemically activated as shown by a primed oxidative burst response (Figs. 2, 3), this is tightly correlated to systemic and unspecific tissue destruction suggesting a deleterious role of the "activated" neutrophil in the peripheral circulation. The participation of endogenous TNF-α in neutrophil activation was demonstrable only in a subset of the septic samples by inhibition of the primed subpopulation of neutrophils with a neutralizing anti-TNF-α antibody. This is in agreement with the detection of increased plasma levels of TNF-α only in a subset of septic patients [10]. Neutrophil activation during sepsis is, therefore, either due to additional priming factors or to a relative lack of inhibitory macromolecules like the acute phase protein serum amyloid A [20].

The modulation of the size of the FMLP-responsive subpopulation of neutrophils by TNF-α suggests a modulation of the thresholds for the response to stimulation of the specific neutrophil receptor for bacterial proteins in form of an all-or-none event. Such a heterogeneous all-or-none response to FMLP stimulation has been previously suggested by flow cytometric assays of membrane depolarization [21]. The mechanism of the interaction of TNF-α with the FMLP response is not understood. The magnitude of the FMLP response is tightly regulated by the expression of the FMLP receptor, which is low in unstimulated cells, but rapidly upregulated upon stimulation [22]. TNF-α may potentially affect the termination of the cellular response to FMLP by the lateral redistribution of the FMLP receptor on the plasma membrane leading to a decreased signal transduction [23] and by receptor internalization [24], or may enhance responses at a postreceptor level [25, 26].

Neutrophil activation, independently of the oxidative burst cascade, leads to an increase in the pH and cell volume mediated by the amiloride-sensitive Na^+/H^+-antiport [27]. The extent of this alkalinization modulates the respiratory burst response to stimulation of the FMLP receptor of neutrophils [28]. The alkalinization of the intracellular pH and an increase of the neutrophil cell volume induced by TNF-α alone in this study was associated with an increased oxidative burst response upon further FMLP stimulation. Also samples from septic patients had a more alkaline pH and an increased cell volume when compared with samples from healthy controls confirming an earlier study in our laboratory, which included a total of 225 blood samples [13]. The increases in the intracellular pH and cell volume, therefore, seem to be indicators of an increased stimulation of the neutrophils which is associated with a decreased threshold for the induction of the all-or-none regulated oxidative burst response.

In conclusion, the correlation of the intravascular activation of neutrophils, visible from a highly FMLP-responsive subpopulation, with the systemic organ dysfunction of the sepsis syndrome, in contrast to no activation of circulating neutrophils in patients with focal bacterial infection, suggests a deleterious role of systemic neutrophil activation. A similar activation of neutrophils is inducible by a 5-min treatment of neutrophils from healthy normals with TNF-α. The activation of neutrophils from septic patients could be increased by in vitro exposure to TNF-α and partially reversed by anti-TNF-α antibodies in a subset of the samples. The pharmacological modulation of TNF-α effects on neutrophils by agents such as adenosine-analogs, which reverse the TNF-α-induced inhibition of neutrophil chemotaxis [29], should, therefore, be helpful in the inhibition of tissue destruction during sepsis. The flow cytometric parameters can be used for the detection of neutrophil activation predisposing to tissue destruction [13] as well as for the monitoring of the effects of therapeutic intervention.

References

1. Fong Y, Tracey KJ, Moldawer LL, Hesse DG, Manogue KB, Kenney JS, Lee AT, Kuo GC, Allison AC, Lowry SF, Cerami A (1989) Antibodies to cachectin/tumor necrosis factor reduce interleukin 1β and interleukin 6 appearance during lethal bacteremia. J Exp Med 170:1627–1633
2. Otsuka Y, Nagano K, Nagano K, Hori K, Oh-Ishi JI, Hayashi H, Watanabe N, Niitsu Y (1990) Inhibition of neutrophil migration by tumor necrosis factor. Ex vivo and in vivo studies in comparison with in vitro effect. J Immunol 145:2639–2643
3. Nathan C, Srimal S, Farber C, Sanchez E, Kabbash L, Asch A, Gailit J, Wright SD (1989) Cytokine-induced respiratory burst of human neutrophils: dependence on extracellular matrix proteins and CD11/CD18 integrins. J Cell Biol 109:1341–1349
4. Richter J, Olsson I, Andersson T (1990) Correlation between spontaneous oscillations of cytosolic free Ca^{2+} and tumor necrosis factor-induced degranulation in adherent human neutrophils. J Biol Chem 265:14358–14363
5. Moser R, Schleiffenbaum B, Groscurth P, Fehr J (1989) Interleukin 1 and tumor necrosis factor stimulate human vascular endothelial cells to promote transendothelial neutrophil passage. J Clin Invest 83:444–455
6. Furie MB, McHugh DD (1989) Migration of neutrophils across endothelial monolayers is stimulated by treatment of the monolayers with interleukin-1 or tumor necrosis factor-α. J Immunol 143:3309–3317
7. Klebanoff SJ, Vadas MA, Harlan JM, Sparks LH, Gamble JR, Agosti JM, Waltersdorph AM (1986) Stimulation of neutrophils by tumor necrosis factor. J Immunol 136:4220–4225
8. Abe Y, Sekiya S, Yamasita T, Sendo F (1990) Vascular hyperpermeability induced by tumor necrosis factor and its augmentation by IL-1 and IFN-γ is inhibited by selective depletion of neutrophils with a monoclonal antibody. J Immunol 145:2902–2907
9. Stephens KE, Ishizaka A, Wu Z, Larrick JW, Raffin TA (1988) Granulocyte depletion prevents tumor necrosis factor-mediated acute lung injury in guinea pigs. Am Rev Respir Dis 138:1300–1307
10. Marks JD, Marks CB, Luce JM, Montgomery AB, Turner J, Metz CA, Murray JF (1990) Plasma tumor necrosis factor in patients with septic shock. Mortality rate, incidence of adult respiratory distress syndrome, and effects of methylprednisolone administration. Am Rev Respir Dis 141:94–97
11. Schleiffenbaum B, Fehr J (1990) The tumor necrosis factor receptor and human neutrophil function. Deactivation and cross-deactivation of tumor necrosis factor-induced neutrophil responses by receptor down-regulation. J Clin Invest 86:184–195
12. Porteu F, Nathan C (1990) Shedding of tumor necrosis factor receptors by activated neutrophils. J Exp Med 172:599–607
13. Rothe G, Kellermann W, Valet G (1990) Flow cytometric parameters of neutrophil function as early indicators of sepsis- or trauma-related pulmonary or cardiovascular organ failure. J Lab Clin Med 115:52–61
14. Rothe G, Valet G (1990) Flow cytometric analysis of respiratory burst activity in phagocytes with hydroethidine and 2',7'-dichlorofluorescin. J Leukocyte Biol 47:440–448
15. Elebute EA, Stoner HB (1983) The grading of sepsis. Br J Surg 70:29–31
16. Goris RJA, te Boekhorst TPA, Nuytinck JKS, Gimbrère JSF (1985) Multiple-organ failure. Generalized autodestructive inflammation? Arch Surg 120:1109–1115
17. Rothe G, Oser A, Valet G (1988) Dihydrorhodamine 123: a new flow cytometric indicator for respiratory burst activity in neutrophil granulocytes. Naturwissen Schaften 75:354–355
18. Rothe G, Emmendörffer A, Oser A, Roesler J, Valet G (1991) Flow cytometric measurement of the respiratory burst activity of phagocytes using dihydrorhodamine 123. J Immunol Methods (in press)
19. Valet G, Warnecke HH, Kahle H (1987) Automated diagnosis of malignant and other abnormal cells by flow cytometry using the DIAGNOS1 program system. In: Burger G, Ploem JS, Goerttler K (eds) Clinical cytometry and histometry. Academic, London, pp 58–65
20. Linke RP, Bock V, Valet G, Rothe G (1991) Inhibition of the oxidative burst response of neutrophils by serum amyloid A. Biochem Biophys Res Comm (in press)
21. Fletcher MP, Gasson JC (1988) Enhancement of neutrophil function by granulocyte-macrophage colony-stimulating factor involves recruitment of a less responsive subpopulation. Blood 71:652–658

22. Norgauer J, Eberle M, Fay SP, Lemke HD, Sklar LA (1991) Kinetics of N-formyl peptide receptor up-regulation during stimulation in human neutrophils. J Immunol 146:975–980
23. Jesaitis AJ, Tolley JO, Bokoch GM, Allen RA (1989) Regulation of chemoattractant receptor interaction with transducing proteins by organizational control in the plasma membrane of human neutrophils. J Cell Biol 109:2783–2790
24. van Epps DE, Simpson S, Bender JG, Chenoweth DE (1990) Regulation of C5a and formyl peptide receptor expression on human polymorphonuclear leukocytes. J Immunol 144:1062–1068
25. McColl SR, Beauseigle D, Gilbert C, Naccache PH (1990) Priming of the human neutrophil respiratory burst by granulocyte-macrophage colony-stimulating factor and tumor necrosis factor-α involves regulation at a post-cell receptor level. Enhancement of the effect of agents which directly activate G proteins. J Immunol 145:3047–3053
26. Yuo A, Kitagawa S, Suzuki I, Urabe A, Okabe T, Saito M, Takaku F (1989) Tumor necrosis factor as an activator of human granulocytes. Potentiation of the metabolisms triggered by the Ca^{2+}-mobilizing agonists. J Immunol 142:1678–1684
27. Swallow CJ, Grinstein S, Rotstein OD (1990) Regulation and functional significance of cytoplasmic pH in phagocytic leukocytes. Curr Top Membr Transp 35:227–247
28. Simchowitz L (1985) Intracellular pH modulates the generation of superoxide radicals by human neutrophils. J Clin Invest 76:1079–1089
29. Sullivan GW, Linden J, Hewlett EL, Carper HT, Hylton JB, Mandell GL (1990) Adenosine and related compounds counteract tumor necrosis factor-α inhibition of neutrophil migration: implication of a novel cyclic AMP-independent action on the cell surface. J Immunol 145:1537–1544

Distinct Subpopulations of Human Peripheral Blood Monocytes Characterized by Absence of the CD14 Surface Marker, and Distinguished by High or Low Intracellular Glutathione

R. L. Rabin[1], F. J. Staal[2], M. Roederer[2], M. M. Beiber[1], L. A. Herzenberg[2], and N. H. Teng[2]

Introduction

The tripeptide glutathione (GSH) is the most prevalent intracellular thiol [1]. Among its many functions, GSH serves as a reducing agent and an antioxidant, absorbing intracellular reactive oxygen intermediates (ROI) which result from physical or chemical insults to cells [1]. ROI are also believed to be the toxic element of tumor cell cytotoxicity produced in response to tumor necrosis factor (TNF) [2–4]. Indeed, increased intracellular GSH protects otherwise sensitive murine fibroblasts from TNF cytotoxicity, in vitro [5], and N-acetytcysteine (NAC), a synthetic precursor of GSH, abrogates TNF cytotoxicity in rats [3].

In addition to modulating the cellular response to TNF, NAC has been demonstrated to modulate murine TNF secretion in vivo in response to endotoxemia [6]. Since NAC modulates HIV replication in human T cell [7, 8] by downregulating the activity of the transcriptional factor nuclear factor κB (NF-κB) [9], and since TNF synthesis is mediated by NF-κB [9], it is likely that NAC modulates TNF synthesis at the transcriptional level via NF-κB. Furthermore, GSH itself regulates HIV synthesis at the posttranscriptional level (independent of NF-κB), and thus may have additional mechanisms of regulation of TNF synthesis as well.

Although TNF was first recognized for its cachexia-inducing and antineoplastic activities [10], many studies now implicate this cytokine as central to the pathogenesis of a variety of disease states, including septic shock [11–14], cerebral malaria [15], and inflammatory arthritis [16]. The peripheral blood monocyte (PBM) is the major source of TNF [10]. However, TNF is almost undetectable in sera from healthy individuals, and monocytes do not secrete detectable levels of TNF, in vitro unless they are activated [17]. One very potent PBM activator is lipopolysaccharide (LPS) [18], the causative agent of gram-negative septic shock [19]. Other PBM activators that stimulate TNF-α secretion are PMA (phorbol 12-myristate 13-acetate diester), interleukin-1, and TNF itself [20]. Since TNF synthesis and secretion is linked to intracellular

---

[1] Departments of Gynecology and Obstetrics and [2] Genetics, Stanford University Medical School, Standford, CA, USA

Host Defense Dysfunction
in Trauma, Shock and Sepsis
Eds. Faist/Meakins/Schildberg
© Springer-Verlag, Berlin Heidelberg 1993

GSH, we first sought to define the distribution of GSH in purified human PBMs.

Materials and Methods

Purification of Human PBMs

Human mononuclear cells were isolated from buffy coat preparations which were obtained fresh from the Stanford University Medical Center Blood Bank. Mononuclear cells were isolated from the buffy coats over a Ficoll-Hypaque gradient. We then purified monocytes from mononuclear cells by counter-current centrifugal elutriation according to the method of Turpin et al. [21]. All media and solutions were negative for endotoxin by the limulus lysate amoebo-cyte assay (E-toxate, Sigma), sensitive to 10 pg/ml.

Analysis of Purified Human PBMs

In order to assess GSH concentration, we used the fluorochrome mono-chlorobimane (MCB, Molecular Probes, Eugene, OR, USA). MCB is conjugated to GSH via GSH S-transferase; only the stable GSH-MCB conjug-ate fluoresces upon exposure to UV light (ex/em 380/420 nm [22, 23]). PBMs were stained at room temperature for 15 min with MCB at a final concentration of 25 µM. After centrifuging through 0.5 ml of underlaid serum to remove unreacted MCB, monocytes were placed in ice.

In order to assess subpopulations of monocytes relative to CD14, the MCB-stained monocytes were stained with fluorescein isothiocyanate conjugated anti-CD14 (FITC-Leu M3, Becton-Dickinson, Mountain View, CA, USA) as well as phycoerythrin (PE) conjugated antibodies to the B, T, and natural killer (NK) markers, CD19, CD3, and either CD7 or CD56 (PE anti-Leu 12, PE anti-Leu 4, and PE anti-Leu 9 or 19, respectively ; Becton-Dickinson) for 15 min. After washing, the PBMs were also stained with propidium iodide (PI, Molecular Probes). The PBMs were then analyzed on a dual laser flow cytometer (Facstar Plus, Becton-Dickinson) after first gating out the PE$^+$ (B, T, and NK cells) and PI$^+$ (dead) cells.

To better define the subpopulation of monocytes, they were stained with FITC-Leu M3 in combination with PE conjugated monoclonal antibodies to other myeloid surface markers, CD33 (PE-Leu M9) and CD11c (PE-Leu M5).

Results

Purified monocytes (> 95% nonspecific esterase, NSE, positive) were stained with MCB and phenotypic markers conjugated with FITC or PE, and analyzed by multiparameter flow cytometry. As demonstrated in Fig. 1B, the CD14⁻ monocytes segregate into two subpopulations, distinguished by GSH levels. Subsequent cell sorting via fluorescence-activated cell sorter (FACS) and NSE staining demonstrates the CD14⁻, low GSH population to be 80% monocytes, and the CD14⁻, high GSH population to be 90% monocytes (results not shown). Furthermore, cell sorting on the basis of anti-Leu M5 (CD11c) demonstrates that CD11c⁺ cells are 100% monocytes, independent of CD14 expression. Figure 2 demonstrates that the CD14⁻, CD11c⁺ population contains both the high and low GSH subpopulation of monocytes.

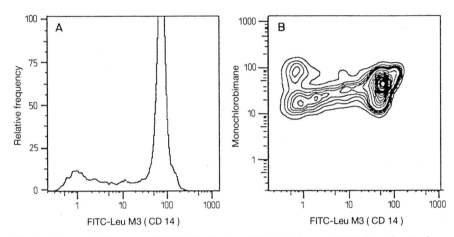

Fig. 1. A Log scale histogram of CD14 distribution of elutriated human PBMs. Lymphocytes have been excluded from this analysis with PE-Leu 4,16, and 19 (CD3, 20, and 56 respectively), and polymorphonuclear neutrophil (PMN) contamination was negligible (< 1%) **B** Log-log contour plot of the same population of monocytes demonstrating the two subpopulations of CD14⁻ monocytes distinguished by GSH concentration, as determined by the specific fluorochrome MCB. The difference in GSH concentration between the high and low subpopulations is fourfold.

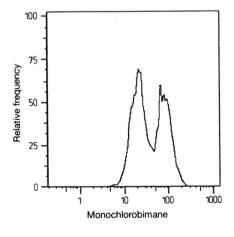

Fig. 2. Histogram of GSH distribution within the population of CD14⁻, CD11c⁺ monocytes. This population is demonstrated to be virtually 100% monocytes by nonspecific esterase staining of sorted cells.

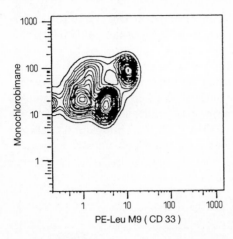

Fig. 3. A Histogram of CD33 distribution of elutriated PBMs. **B** Log-log contour plot of CD14⁻ monocyte subpopulation; CD33 vs MCB. Note that most, but not all of the low MCB cells are CD33 dim

Analysis of these CD14⁻ monocytes for the surface marker CD33 with PE-Leu M9 demonstrates the CD14⁻, low GSH population to be almost exclusively CD33dim, while the CD14⁻, high GSH population is exclusively CD33⁺.

Discussion

The surface marker CD14 is a 55-kDa glycoprotein (gp55) which is highly expressed on mature monocytes and macrophages, dimly expressed on PMNs and some monocytes, and, except for a small subpopulation of B cells, absent on lymphocytes. CD14 is phosphoinositol linked and upon activation with such substances as LPS or formyl peptides is cleaved from the surface membrane [24]. Recently, CD14 has been defined as a receptor for LPS when complexed with a specific binding protein of hepatocyte origin [25].

CD33 is a gp67 restricted to myeloid cells, expressed heavily on early granulocyte macrophage progenitors. It is expressed weakly on some granulocytes and increases with maturity. There is no reported effect on CD33 expression by activation [26]. All CD14⁺ monocytes are CD33⁺, but the converse is not true. Indeed, our results demonstrate that intracellular GSH concentration delineates the CD14⁻ population such that low CD33 are low GSH, and vice versa.

One interpretation of these results is that the CD14⁻, CD33dim, low GSH population is relatively immature, and would naturally progress to CD14⁺, CD33⁺, high GSH population. The CD14⁻, CD33⁺, high GSH population, then, may represent an intermediate stage of maturation, or activation, either in vivo, prior to blood donation, or in vitro, during purification. We have attempted to minimize monocyte activation during purification. Countercurrent centrifugal elutriation (CCE) purifies monocytes by negative selection; elutriated monocytes, by enzymatic criteria, are not activated [27]. Furthermore, all media are pyrogen free by the limulus lysate amoebocyte assay, and monocytes isolated by CCE do not produce TNF unless LPS (or other activators) are added (results not shown).

Alternatively, the CD14$^-$, CD33dim, low GSH subpopulation may represent activated monocytes. Recently published studies involving HIV-infected T cells [6], as well as murine endotoxemia in vivo, demonstrate that raising the GSH level protects against TNF secretion [7], thus supporting this second interpretation. Mature (CD14$^+$) monocytes are all CD33$^+$, however, and CD33 expression is reported not to change with activation. Furthermore, we would expect that monocytes would decrease their GSH level (a shift from the high to low GSH population) in response to activation with LPS, and that this decrease would correlate with TNF secretion.

In conclusion, we report subpopulations of human peripheral blood monocytes as determined by absence of CD14, and high or low GSH concentration, which correlates with the level of expression of CD33. As with previous reports of monocyte heterogeneity, we suggest that the differences in subpopulations are due to maturity, level of activation, or both, rather than a distinct phenotype. That the level of GSH is inherent in defining these subpopulations, and since GSH appears to regulate TNF secretion, these subpopulations of monocytes may be of particular importance in the pathophysiology of septic shock.

References

1. Deneke SM (1989)
2. Yaauchi NH (1989)
3. Zimmerman RJ (1989)
4. Larrick JW (1990)
5. Zimmerman RJ (1989)
6. Peristeris PA (1991)
7. Staal FJ (1991)
8. Roederer M (1990)
9. Baltimore D (1991)
10. Beutler B (1987)
11. Beutler B (1985)
12. Tracey KJ (1987)
13. Tracey KJ (1990)
14. Michie MB (1988)
15. Grau GE (1987)
16. Yocum DE (1989)
17. Kornbluth RS (1986)
18. Gifford GE (1986)
19. Braude AI (1986)
20. Philip R (1986)
21. Turpin J (1986)
22. Lee FYF (1989)
23. Rice GC (1986)
24. Goyert SML (1989)
25. Wright S (1990)
26. Koller U (1989)
27. Kelley JL (1987)

The Role of Endotoxins in Burns: Anomalies in Cytokine Regulation of Immunity*

R. A. Winchurch, D. Zhou, and A. M. Munster

Traumatic injury elicits a complex series of metabolic changes affecting almost all of the body's systems. Ultimately, survival depends upon marshaling a concerted response to injury such that homeostasis is restored, tissue injury is repaired, and the host's defense network responds to invasive pathogens. Often the immediate response to injury can set in motion a cascade of reactions that may eventually compromise later events such as responses to infection. The immunologic sequelae to acute traumatic injury have been studied extensively. These studies have shown that burn and trauma victims suffer from an impairment of almost all immunologic functions. Paramount among those functions compromised by injury is cell-mediated immunity. Thus, traumatic injury inhibits delayed-type hypersensitivity responses [1], and increases the rejection time of skin allografts [2]. Lymphoproliferative responses to mitogens [3] and recall antigens [4] are suppressed as are lymphocytotoxic responses [5]. A major defect following thermal injury is the decrease in T helper functions [6] and this decrease is reflected in a reduced representation of $CD4^+$ lymphocytes [7]. Regulatory cytokines and growth factors are also affected by trauma such that interleukin-2 (IL-2) production and the expression of IL-2 receptors (IL-2R) are impaired [8, 9]. In contrast, there are early increases in both interleukin-1 (IL-1) and tumor necrosis factor (TNF), and consequent to these increases interleukin-6 (IL-6) levels are elevated. B cell functions are affected less dramatically and consistently and both increases and decreases in B cell activities have been reported. The net effect of these changes on immunity is an increased susceptibility of infection such that even opportunistic pathogens pose a serious threat to the trauma patient.

The Role of Endotoxins

The mechanisms whereby trauma suppresses the immune system have not been clearly defined, although a number of hypotheses have been advanced. Recent

---

* This work was supported in part by funding from the Baltimore Firefighters Research Foundation.

Department of Surgery, Baltimore Regional Burn Center, Johns Hopkins University, School of Medicine, Baltimore, MD, USA

evidence indicates that a major cause of the immune aberrations consequent to trauma is an increase in circulating bacterial endotoxins (ET). These increases are evident even in the absence of gram-negative bacterial sepsis and in the burn victim these increases are related to the extent of the injury [10]. Endotoxins elicit a variety of physiologic effects including activation of the acute phase response [11]. A number of cytokines and growth factors are activated by endotoxin exposure including IL-1, TNF-α and IL-6 [12–14] and these factors play an important role in the acute phase response in addition to their immunoregulatory properties. Endotoxins activate B cells and induce both mitogenic activity and nonspecific production of immunoglobulins, notably IgM. Although it has been studied less extensively, endotoxins can also affect T cell activity and the net result is usually an inhibitory effect. In vivo exposure to endotoxin inhibits graft rejection, depresses in vitro reactivity to concanavalin A (Con A) [15] and inhibits cell-mediated anti-*Listeria* immunity [16]. Endotoxin can activate suppressor cells both in vivo and in vitro [17, 18].

Over the past several years we have studied the efficacy of endotoxin-neutralizing regimens of polymyxin B administration in the burn victim. Polymyxin B not only reduces the endotoxin burden but restores the proportion of CD4/CD8 T cells and improves T cell immune functions [19]. Moreover, the increased concentrations of IL-6 which are often evident in burn patient sera are also reduced by polymyxin B treatment [20].

IL-6 in Traumatic Injury

IL-6 is a regulatory cytokine which is often elevated in association with pathologic conditions characterized by abnormalities in immunity. Elevations in this factor are apparent in CSF of patients suffering from acute infection of the central nervous system [21], and are evident in patients with meningococcal septic shock [22] and gram-negative bacteremia [23]. IL-6 is also produced by monocytes exposed to either live or attenuated HIV [24]. Physical trauma also affects IL-6 levels and Ertel et al. have observed increases of over 2000 units/ml in T cell supernatants from patients suffering from major physical trauma [25].

While abnormal increases in IL-6 have been demonstrated in a variety of pathologic conditions the role, if any, of this cytokine in downregulating the immune defense network has not been studied. Previous studies of lymphocyte subsets of burn patients indicated a significant correlation between the levels of circulating IL-6 and a decrease in the representation of peripheral blood CD3[+] cells [20] (Fig. 1). The decrease in T cells was a reflection of decreases in both CD4[+] and CD8[+] cells. Concomitant with this decrease was an increase in the representation of CD19[+] B cells. This relationship suggested that IL-6 may similarly affect T cell functions. Using an in vitro murine model the effects of IL-6 on cell-mediated immunity were investigated. Con A activated lymphocytes were incubated in the presence of concentrations of IL-6 ranging from 50

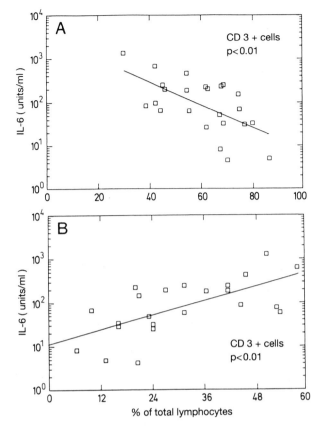

Fig. 1 A,B. Correlation analysis showing the relationships between serum IL-6 levels and the representation of **A** CD3+ cells, and **B** CD19+ cells in peripheral blood of burn patients

to 4000 units/ml. The upper limits of the concentration range were chosen to mimic the levels found in burn patient sera. Proliferative responses measured after 3 days revealed that IL-6 inhibited the Con A response in log dose-dependent fashion (Table 1). The maximum inhibition was on the order of 40% –60% but only rarely did it exceed 60%. Surprisingly, the same population of cells activated by the B cell mitogen lipopolysaccharide (LPS) responded to increases in IL-6 concentration with increased proliferation and this increase was also log dose-dependent. The effects of IL-6 on lymphocyte proliferation were similar to the relationships between IL-6 and the representation of T and B cell subsets in burn patient peripheral blood suggesting that these phenomena were somehow related.

The inhibitory effect of IL-6 on T cell-mediated responses was dependent upon the presence of macrophages and on the time of exposure. If IL-6 was added to the cultures later than 18 h or if it was removed prior to an exposure of 24 h proliferation proceeded normally. When macrophages were removed by

Table 1. Effects of IL-6 on proliferative responses to Con A and LPS

	IL-6 concentration (units/ml)					
	50	100	500	1000	2000	4000
Activator (Percent of control)						
Con A	97	91	76	62	45	37
LPS	117	133	176	202	213	255

Cells were incubated for 72 h in vitro with 2. µg/ml Con A or 20 µg/ml LPS 055:B5 in the presence or absence of graded concentrations of IL-6. Proliferation was determined by the incorporation of tritiated thymidine. In the absence of IL-6, Con A proliferation was 33 000 cpm and LPS proliferation was 25 000 cpm.

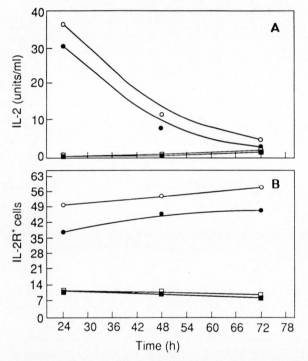

Fig. 2. A Comparison of IL-2 production in cultures exposed to Con A and Con A plus 2000 units IL-6. B Expression of cell-bound IL-2R in cultures exposed to Con A and Con A plus 2000 units IL-6. ●—●, Con A alone; ○—○, Con A plus IL-6, □—□, IL-6 alone; ■—■, medium control

depletion of adherent cells IL-6 no longer inhibited T cell proliferation and in fact there was an apparent enhancement of proliferation. These findings indicated that IL-6 or macrophage products induced by IL-6 affected the activation stage of T cell proliferation. However, further studies indicated that the activation steps affected by IL-6 were independent of IL-2. When the levels of IL-2 produced in the cultures containing Con A plus IL-6 were compared

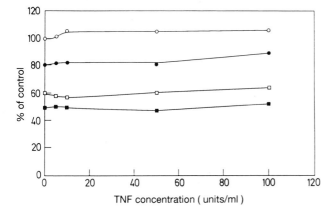

Fig. 3. Con A activated cells were incubated with varying concentrations of IL-6. Graded amounts of recombinant TNF-α was added at time 0 and the incubated continued for 72 h. Proliferative responses were determined by tritiated thymidine incorporation. ○ — ○, no IL-6; ● — ●, 100 units IL-6; □ — □, 500 units IL-6; and ■ — ■, 1000 units IL-6

with the IL-2 produced by Con A stimulated control cultures there was no diminution of IL-2 production. In fact, the IL-2 produced by the cultures containing IL-6 was slightly increased over that elicited by Con A alone. Similarly, the expression of the IL-2 receptor on T cells treated with Con A plus IL-6 was also increased (Fig. 2). In addition, IL-6 did not affect IL-2 signal transduction. Cells incubated for 48 h with Con A to induce the expression of IL-2R and treated with 50 units/ml IL-2 in the presence of increasing concentrations of IL-6 proliferated normally.

The involvement of macrophages suggested that TNF-α may play some role in the inhibition of the T cell responses. TNF has come under sharp scrutiny in recent years as a mediator of the body's response to infection [26]. It is produced by macrophages and is believed to play an increasingly important regulatory role in the response to trauma. Moreover, endotoxins are potent activators of TNF production [27]. The first question addressed in the study of TNF involvement concerned whether TNF, of itself, could inhibit Con A activated lymphoproliferative responses. The second question was whether TNF could synergize with IL-6 in suppressing responses. The data illustrated in Fig. 3 show that TNF over a broad concentration range had no effect on lymphocyte proliferative responses to Con A. Moreover, these data also show that concentrations of TNF from 0 to 100 units/ml did not enhance or abrogate the ability of IL-6 to suppress the response.

The Role of Transforming Growth Factor Beta

Macrophages also produce transforming growth factor beta (TGF-β), a cytokine known to be a potent regulator of a T cell-mediated proliferative responses.

Table 2. Effect of anti-TGF-β antisera on IL-6 suppression of Con A response (μl antisera/well)

	Medium	Control sera	Anti-TGF-β1			Anti-TGF-β2		
		10	1	5	10	1	5	10
Con A (cpm/culture)	32 870	38 708	–	–	52 011	–	–	55 090
Con A + IL-6 (cpm/culture)	12 109	22 677	14 103	49 464	50 820	14 687	23 346	59 393

Cells were cultured for 72 h with 2 μg/ml Con A in the presence or absence of 2000 units murine recombinant IL-6. Antisera in the amounts indicated were added at time 0.

TGF-β has been shown to impair both T cell and thymocyte proliferative responses [28]. When IL-6-suppressed cultures were incubated in the presence of antibodies specific for TGF-β there was a dramatic reversal of the suppression. The data in Table 2 show that 5 µl/well of anti-TGF-β1 and 10µl/well of anti-TGF-β2 completely reversed the inhibition induced by 2000 units/ml of IL-6. The neutralizing potency of the antisera indicated that the levels of TGF-β1 ranged from 4 to 20 ng/ml and that of TGF-β2 ranged from 2 to 4 ng/ml. TGF-β is known to be present in both active and latent forms and may also be complexed with α_2-macroglobulin [29]. The antibodies employed in these studies only recognized the active forms of TGF-β. The fact that both antisera abrogated IL-6-induced suppression indicated that IL-6 either induced production of active TGF or activated latent TGF already present in Con A activated cultures.

Conclusions

The present findings suggest that the increases in endotoxin evident in trauma victims may compromise the host's immune defenses by activating the synthesis of IL-6. Under ordinary circumstances IL-6 is usually associated with activation of T cells, thymocyte proliferation, and hematopoietic stem cell growth [9]. The extraordinary levels of IL-6 found in burn and trauma patients and in other pathologic conditions may in fact suppress immunity. This suppressive effect is specific in that it only affects certain T cell responses. The effect appears to be indirect in that it is dependent on macrophages and is mediated by the induction of TGF-β.

References

1. Munster AM, Winchurch RA, Keane RM et al. (1981) The 'in vitro skin test': a reliable and repeatable assay of immune competence in the surgical patient. Ann Surg 194:345–360
2. Ninnemann JL, Fisher JC, Frank HA (1978) Prolonged survival of human skin allografts following thermal injury. Transplantation 25:69–72
3. Miller CL, Baker CC (1979) Changes in lymphocyte activity after thermal injury. J Clin Invest 63:202–210
4. Munster AM, Winchurch RA, Birmingham WJ, Keeling P (1980) Longitudinal assay of lymphocyte responsiveness in patients with major burns. Ann Surg 192:772–778
5. Antonacci AC, Gupta S, Good RA, Shires GT, Fernandes G (1983) Natural killer and antibody-dependent cytotoxicity following thermal injury in humans. Curr. Surg 40:20–23
6. Antonacci AC, Good RA, Gupta S (1982) T-cell subpopulations following thermal injury. Surgery 155:1–8.
7. O'Mahony JB, Wood J, Rodrick ML et al. (1985) Changes in T lymphocyte subsets following injury. Ann. Surg. 202:580–586
8. Rodrick MK, Wood JJ, O'Mahony JB et al. (1986) Mechanisms of immunosuppression with severe thermal traumatic injuries in man: production of interleukin 1 and 2. J Clin Immunol 6:310–318

9. Theorczyk-Injeyan JA, Sparkes BG, Mills GB, Falk RE, Peters WJ (1987) Impaired expression of interleukin 2 receptor (Il-2R) in the immunosuppressed burned patient: reversal by exogenous Il-2. J Trauma 27:180–187

10. Winchurch RA, Thupari JN, Munster AM (1987) Endotoxemia in burn patients: levels of circulating endotoxins are related to burn size. Surgery 102:808–812

11. Wolpe SD, Cerami A (1989) Macrophage inflammatory proteins 1 and 2: members of a novel superfamily of cytokines. FASEB J 3:2565–2573

12. Ku G, Doherty NS, Schmidt LF, Jackson RL, Dinerstein RJ (1990) Ex vivo lipopolysaccharide-induced interleukin-1 secretion from murine peritoneal macrophages inhibited by probucol, a hypocholesterolemic agent with antioxidant properties. FASEB J 4:1645–1653

13. Kiener PA, Marek F, Rodgers G, Pin-Fang L, Warr G, Desiderio J (1988) Induction of tumor necrosis factor, IFN and acute lethality in mice by toxic and non-toxic forms of lipid A J Immunol 141:870–874

14. Fong Y, Moldawer LL, Marano M, Wei H, Tatter SB, Clarick RH, Santhanam U, Sherris D, May LT, Sehgal PB, Lowry SF (1989) Endotoxemia elicits increased circulating $b2$-IFN/IL-6 in man. J Immunol 142:2321–2324

15. Winchurch RA, Hilberg C, Birmingham W, Munster AM (1982) Inhibition of graft rejection by LPS: further evidence for effects on T lymphocytes. J Reticuloendothel Soc 31:31–42

16. Newborg MF, North RJ (1979) Suppressive effect of bacterial endotoxin on the expression of cell-mediated anti-Listeria immunity. Infect Immun 24:667–672

17. Winchurch RA, Hilberg C, Birmingham W, Munster AM (1982) Lipopolysaccharide-induced activation of suppressor cells: reversal by an agent which alters cyclic nucleotide metabolism. Immunology 45:147–153

18. Persson U (1977) Lipopolysaccharide-induced suppression of the primary immune response to a thymus-dependent antigen. J Immunol 118:789–793

19. Munster AM, Thupari JN, Winchurch RA, Ernst CB (1986) Reversal of post burn immunosupp-ression with low dose of polymyxin B J Trauma 26:995–998

20. Guo Y, Dickerson C, Chrest FJ, Adler WH, Munster AM, Winchurch R (1990) Increased levels of circulating interleukin 6 in burn patients. Clin Immunol Immunopathol 54:361–371

21. Houssiau FA, Bukasa K, Sindic CJM, Van Dammes J, Van Snick J (1988) Elevated levels of the 26K human hybridoma growth factor (interleukin 6) in cerebrospinal fluid of patients with acute infection of the central nervous system. Clin Exp Immunol 71:320–323

22. Waage A, Brandtzaeg P, Halstensen A, Kierulf P, Espevik T (1989) The complex pattern of cytokines in serum from patients with meningococcal septic shock. J Exp Med 169:333–338

23. Helfgott DC, Tatter SB, Santhanam U, Clarick RH, Bhardwaj N, May LT, Sehgal PB (1989) Multiple forms of IFN-beta2/IL-6 in serum and body fluids during acute bacterial infection. J Immunol 142:948–953

24. Nakajima K, Martinez-Maza O, Hirano T, Breen EC, Nishanian PG, Salazar-Gonzalez JF, Fahey JL, Kishimoto T (1989) Induction of IL-6 (B cell stimulatory factor-2/IFN-$b2$) production by HIV. J Immunol 142:531–536

25. Ertel W, Faist E, Hueltner L, Storck M, Schildberg FW (1990) Kinetics of interleukin-2 and interleukin-6 synthesis following major mechanical trauma. J Surg Res 48:622–628

26. Tracey KJ, Fong Y, Hesse DG et al. (1987) Anti-cachectin/TNF monoclonal antibodies prevent septic shock during lethal bacteraemia. Nature 330:662–664

27. Kornbluth RS, Edgington TS (1986) Tumor necrosis factor production by human monocytes is a regulated event: induction of TNF-mediated cellular cytotoxicity by endotoxin. J Immunol 137:2585–2590

28. Lotz M, Kekow J, Carson DA (1990) Transforming growth factor-B and cellular immune responses in synovial fluids. J Immunol 144:4189–4194.

29. O'Connor-McCourt MD, Wakefield LM (1987) Latent transforming growth factor beta in serum. J Biol Chem 262:14090–14099

Role of Tumor Necrosis Factor on *Pseudomonas aeruginosa* Infection and on Antitumor Activity in Relation to Arachidonic Cascade

N. Satomi, A. Sakurai, R. Haranaka, and K. Haranaka

Introduction

Pseudomonas aeruginosa infection is observed mostly under immunosuppressive conditions. We have clarified that the combined use of antibiotics and specific antibodies is effective against *P. aeruginosa* infection in vivo. Tumor necrosis factor (TNF) exerts strong antitumor activities against transplanted tumors. We must consider the strong toxicity associated with the combined effect of TNF and lipopolysaccharide (LPS). In the present experiments, the participation of TNF and LPS in *P. aeruginosa* infection was examined from the standpoint of preventing the lethality and elucidating the relationship with the arachidonic cascade.

Materials and Methods

P. aeruginosa NC5 strain was inoculated i.p. into each group of mice administered antibiotics, leukotriene (LT) inhibitor (ONO 1078), platelet-activating factor (PAF) antagonist (WEB 2086) or Japanese-modified traditional Chinese medicine (Sho-saiko-to). TNF and/or LPS were administered i.v. to Meth A sarcoma-bearing mice. Arachidonic cascade products were measured using a $[^3H]$ assay system.

Results

Antitumor effect and disadvantageous action in the combined use of TNF and LPS. With a combination of TNF and LPS the antitumor activity was synergistically enhanced. However, with this combination the lethality was also enhanced. Pretreatment with ONO 1078 and WEB 2086 revealed a preventive effect against the lethality of TNF and LPS ($p < 0.005$, $p < 0.0001$) as could pre-

Oohata General Hospital and Institute, 352 Kido, Sekijo, Ibaraki 308-01, Japan

Host Defense Dysfunction
in Trauma, Shock and Sepsis
Eds. Faist/Meakins/Schildberg
© Springer-Verlag, Berlin Heidelberg 1993

Table 1. Therapeutic effect of several treatments against *P. aeruginosa* infection

	LD_{50} of *P. aeruginosa* challenge
Experiment 1	
Control	7.5×10^3
ASTM	7.4×10^3
CBPZ	5.5×10^3
ASTM + CBPZ	5.0×10^4
Experiment 2	
Control	9.1×10^3
TNF	1.8×10^3
Anti-TNF antibody	2.1×10^5
Experiment 3	
Control	1.3×10^4
Polymyxin B	2.1×10^4
ONO 1078	4.7×10^4
WEB 2086	1.3×10^4
Sho-saiko-to	1.1×10^5

Astromicin (300 µg/mouse) and/or cefbuperazone (1.5 mg/mouse) were administered s.c. at the same time as and at 12 h after inoculation of *P. aeruginosa*. TNF (1000 U/mouse) or anti-TNF antibody (300 U/mouse) was administered s.c. at the same time as the bacterial challenge. Polymyxin B (0.5 mg/mouse), ONO 1078 (0.1 mg/mouse), or WEB 2086 (10 µg/mouse) was injected s.c. at 1 h prior to the bacterial challenge. Sho-saiko-to (50 mg/mouse) was administered p.o. for 2 weeks before the bacterial challenge. *P. aeruginosa* NC5 strain was suspended in 2.5% mucin and inoculated i.p.
LD_{50}, lethal dose for 50% of group; ASTM, astromicin; CBP2, cefbuperazone; TNF, tumor necrosis factor.

treatment with Sho-saiko-to ($p < 0.005$). Even such treatment did not inhibit the antitumor activity of TNF and LPS.

Protective effect of drugs against P. aeruginosa infection. Astromicin sulfate (ASTM) or Cefbuperazone sodium (CBPZ) revealed no therapeutic effect against *P. aeruginosa* infection at the present dosage. However, with a combination of these antibiotics synergistic effects were observed. Polymyxin B sulfate (PMB) exhibited a protective effect against experimental *P. aeruginosa* infection; even in in vitro experiments *P. aeruginosa* is resistant to PMB. Administration of TNF increased the lethality of the *P. aeruginosa* challenge. In contrast, administration of anti-mouse TNF antibody showed a strong protective activity against the lethal bacterial challenge. Pretreatment with ONO 1078 also exerted a protective effect. In contrast, WEB 2086 revealed no protective effect against *P. aeruginosa* infection, but pretreatment with Sho-saiko-to demonstrated a protective effect (Table 1).

Changes in serum levels of arachidonic cascade products following administration of TNF and/or LPS. With a combination of TNF and LPS, there was a synergistic increment in prostaglandins (PGs), thromboxane, and LTs. On pretreatment with Sho-saiko-to, suppression of the release of PGs and LTs was observed.

Conclusion

The lethal challenge of *P. aeruginosa* or TNF and LPS injection could be prevented by pretreatment with anti-TNF antibody, PMB, ONO 1078, or Sho-saiko-to. The combined effects of TNF and LPS may be deeply related to the lethality of *P. aeruginosa* infection. The activities of LT $C_4/D_4/E_4$ or PAF were also related to the lethality of *P. aeruginosa* infection, but this was probably due to the TNF which was subsequently produced and which acts in combination with LPS.

Survival from Cecal Ligation and Puncture and the Formation of Fibrous Adhesions in the Peritoneal Cavity Depend on Endogenous Tumor Necrosis Factor

B. Echtenacher[1, 2], W. Falk[1, 3], D. N. Männel[1, 2], and P. H. Krammer[1]

The purpose of this study was to clarify the role of tumor necrosis factor (TNF) in the recovery from peritonitis caused by sublethal cecal ligation and puncture (CLP). TNF is thought to play a beneficial role because pretreatment of mice with lipopolysaccharide (LPS) or TNF increased the survival rate of injected animals [1, 2]. To investigate the contribution of endogenous TNF to recovery from peritonitis we tested the effect of a neutralizing rat anti-mouse TNF monoclonal antibody (V1q) [3]. We showed that as little as 20 µg V1q/mouse effectively prevented lethal shock of the animals caused by subsequent injection of 400 µg LPS, demonstrating the in vivo efficacy of the antibody. Lethal bolus injections of LPS or bacteria are used as sepsis models by many investigators [4]. In these models the potentially lethal reactions (production of large amounts of interleukin-1 and TNF) of the organism may develop faster than the regulatory inflammatory reactions (e.g., acute-phase proteins, glucocorticoids). Therefore, these models may represent only part of the whole inflammatory repertoire [5]. We preferred CLP as a sepsis model because of its slower development and the presence of a septic focus [6, 7].

For sublethal CLP 10- to 14-week-old C3H/HeN mice were anesthetized, and the abdominal skin was shaved. A 0.7-cm midline incision was made. The cecum was exteriorized and filled with feces by milking stool back from the ascending colon. The cecum was ligated below the ileocecal valve and punctured once with a 0.9×40 mm needle. Gentle pressure was applied on the ligated cecum to exteriorize a small amount of feces. The cecum was then returned to the peritoneal cavity and the incision closed with clamps and Histoacryl blue (enbucrilate) tissue glue. Mice were observed for at least 2 weeks.

In sublethal CLP intraperitoneal injection of 0.1 mg V1q directly and up to 8 h after induction of experimental peritonitis lead to death of the animals within 1–3 days. Only if V1q was injected 16 h after CLP about half of the mice survived (Fig. 1). To correlate this result with production of endogenous TNF the serum of untreated CLP mice was tested for biologically active TNF. During the first 20 h no TNF was detectable. This may be explained by the assumption

---

[1] German Cancer Research Center, Im Neuenheimer Feld 280, 6900 Heidelberg, FRG
[2] New address: Klinik der Universität Regensburg, Pathologie/Tumorimmunologie, Franz-Josef-Strauß-Allee, 8400 Regensburg, FRG
[3] Medizinische Klinik I, Universität Regensburg, Franz-Josef-Strauß-Allee, 8400 Regensburg, FRG

Host Defense Dysfunction
in Trauma, Shock and Sepsis
Eds. Faist/Meakins/Schildberg
© Springer-Verlag, Berlin Heidelberg 1993

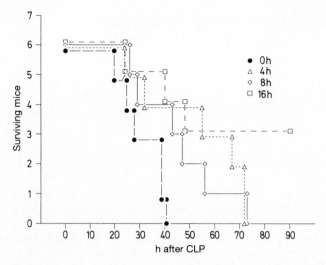

Fig.1. Requirement of TNF for survival from CLP during the first 8 h of peritonitis: 0 (●), 4 (△), 8 (◇), and 16 h (□) after CLP mice were injected with 100 µg monoclonal antibody V1q in 0.2 ml phosphate-buffered solution. These injections were repeated 24 h after CLP

that TNF is produced and consumed only locally at the punctured cecum. This was in line with findings by other investigators who also did not detect TNF after CLP even when they used lethal CLP or related models [8].

Surviving mice that were killed 2 weeks after CLP showed an encapsulated cecum and strong fibrous adhesions. Examination of mice that had died from CLP after V1q injection showed no fibrous adhesions to the cecum 1–3 days after CLP. To determine any correlation between the time of declining lethality after V1q injection and the occurrence of fibrous adhesions treated mice were killed at different times after CLP. There were no adhesions seen after 10 h. After 15 h fibrous adhesions became visible, and after 18 h such adhesions were pronounced (Fig. 2).

The lethal effect of monoclonal antibody V1q was prevented by injection of recombinant mouse TNF (rmTNF). V1q was injected immediately after CLP and rmTNF 1 h later. Remarkably, the same amount of rmTNF that saved CLP mice from lethal V1q injection killed CLP mice if rmTNF was injected without previous V1q administration. Therefore, a certain beneficial TNF concentration during CLP-induced peritonitis may have to be maintained because elimination of endogenous TNF or additional exogenous TNF would be lethal.

These observations may be explained by known properties of TNF. During the early phase of peritonitis endogenous TNF may stimulate nonlymphoid cells such as granulocytes and macrophages to ingest bacteria. TNF may enhance the procoagulant activity of the endothelium and mesothelium [9]. In addition, TNF may inhibit fibrinolysis [10]. Thus, adhesions of surrounding tissue (omentum, intestines) to the cecum are favoured by TNF. TNF production must

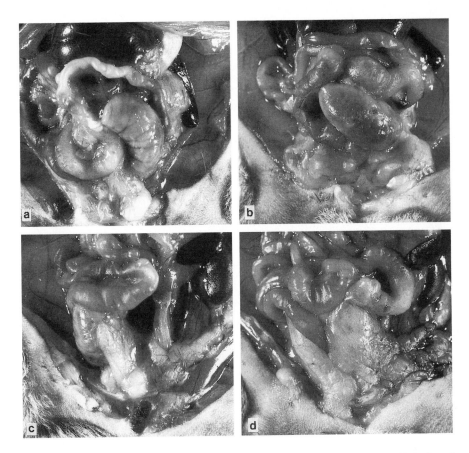

Fig.2a–d. The cecum of C3H/HeN mice at different times after CLP and intraperitoneal injection of anti-TNF monoclonal antibody V1q or Phosphate-buffered solution (PBS) only. **a** 18 h after CLP and injection of 100 µg V1q. No adhesions at the cecum. **b** 42 h after CLP and injection of 100 µg V1q. No adhesions at the cecum. **c** 18 h after CLP and injection of 100 µl PBS. Adhesions (intestine, omentum) at the cecum. **d** 42 h after CLP and injection of 100 µg V1q. The cecum is covered completely by adhesions of the intestine and omentum

be tightly controlled in order to avoid disseminated intravascular coagulation and vascular leakage. One possibility is the control of TNF secretion through protease inhibitors which may prevent the cleavage of membrane TNF from the cell surface [11]. TNF increases interleukin-6 concentration in the blood, and this cytokine enhances synthesis of acute-phase proteins, some of which are protease inhibitors [12]. This mechanism may also be effective in other cases in which serum TNF was not detectable but essential for survival because anti-TNF antibodies caused or accelerated the death of the infected animals (e.g. *Listeria, bacille Calmette-Guérin, Leishmania*) [13, 14, 15, 16]. In summary, these data indicate that the administration of anti-TNF antibodies in sepsis may be deleterious rather than beneficial.

References

1. Urbaschek B, Ditter B, Becker K-P, Urbaschek R (1984) Protective effects and role of endotoxin in experimental septicemia. Circ Shock 14:209
2. Sheppard BC, Fraker DL, Norton JA (1989) Prevention and treatment of endotoxin and sepsis lethality with recombinant human tumor necrosis factor. Surgery 106:156
3. Echtenacher B, Falk W, Männel DN, Krammer PH (1990) Requirement of endogenous tumor necrosis factor/cachectin for recovery from experimental peritonitis. J Immunol 145:3762
4. Beutler BA, Milsark IW, Cerami A (1985) Passive immunization against cachectin/tumor necrosis factor (TNF) protects mice from the lethal effects of endotoxin. Science 229:869
5. Luedke CE, Cerami A (1990) Interferon-γ overcomes glucocorticoid suppression of cachectin-/tumor necrosis factor biosynthesis by murine macrophages. J Clin Invest 86:1234
6. Wichterman KA, Baue AE, Chaudry IH (1980) Sepsis and septic shock—a review of laboratory models and a proposal. J Surg Res 29:189
7. Moss NM, Gough DB, Jordan AL, Grbic JT, Wood JJ, Rodrick ML, Mannick JA (1988) Temporal correlation of impaired immune response after thermal injury with susceptibility to infection in a murine model. Surgery 104:882
8. Evans GF, Snyder YM, Butler LD, Zuckerman SH (1989) Differential expression of interleukin-1 and tumor necrosis factor in murine septic shock models. Circ Shock 29:279
9. Van Hinsbergh VW, Kooistra T, Scheffler MA, Van Bockel JH, Van Muijen GN (1990) Characterization and fibrinolytic properties of human omental tissue mesothelial cells. Comparison with endothelial cells. Blood 75:1490
10. Medcalf BL, Kruithof EKO, Schleuning W (1988) Plasminogen activator inhibitor 1 and 2 are tumor necrosis factor/cachectin-responsive genes. J Exp Med 168:751
11. Niehoerster M, Tiegs G, Schade UF, Wendel A (1990) In vivo evidence for protease-catalysed mechanism providing bioactive tumor necrosis factor alpha. Biochem Pharmacol 40:1601
12. Heinrich PC, Castell JV, Andus T (1990) Interleukin-6 and the acute phase response. Biochem J 265:621
13. Nakane A, Minigawa T, Kato K (1988) Endogenous tumor necrosis factor (cachectin) is essential to host resistance against *Listeria monocytogenes* infection. Infect Immun 56:2563
14. Havell EA (1987) Production of tumor necrosis factor during murine listeriosis. J Immunol 139:4225
15. Kindler V, Sappino A-P, Grau GE, Piguet P-F, Vassalli P (1989) The inducing role of tumor necrosis factor in the development of bactericidal granulomas during BCG infection. Cell 56:731
16. Titus RG, Sherry B, Cerami A (1989) Tumor necrosis factor plays a protective role in experimental murine cutaneous leishmaniasis. J Exp Med 170:2097

The Cellular Mechanisms of Tumor Necrosis Factor-Induced Mortality: A Possible Role for Platelet Activating Factor and/or the Eicosanoids

J. M. Moore[1], M. Hubbard[1], M. Earnest[1], P. Williams[1], A. DiSimone[1], N. Abumrad[1], and J. R. Fletcher[2]

Introduction

Tumor necrosis factor (TNF) is hailed as the seminal mediator in endotoxemia and/or sepsis in animals and humans [1, 2]. Of particular interest recently has been the reported role of eicosanoids (PGS) and platelet activating factor (PAF) in mediating many of the events in the pathophysiology of endotoxemia/sepsis in animals [3, 4]. Interestingly, the putative effects of PAF and the eicosanoids alone or in endotoxemia/sepsis are very similar to those attributed to TNF. To make the situation even more complex, TNF stimulates endothelial cells or fibroblasts to synthesize PAF [5], prostacyclin [6], or PGE_2 [7] as well as many other potent cellular effectors.

The reported myriad effects of TNF stimulated a study to determine the interrelationships of PAF and the eicosanoids to the cellular events induced by TNF in vivo.

Methods and Materials

Male Sprague-Dawley rats (250–300 g; Charles River Laboratories) were stabilized from 2 to 4 days before experimentation. They were maintained in a 12-h light-dark sequence and allowed water and antibiotic-free chow ad libitum. On the day of the experiment, animals were placed in individual cages. Each animal was lightly anesthetized with halothane/oxygen mixture, had an anterior neck incision, followed by insertion of catheters (PE50) into the left carotid artery and left jugular vein. Catheters were flushed with heparinized saline, tunneled to the dorsal neck, and secured. The jugular vein catheter was used for injections. Rats were allowed to recover from the effects of the anesthesia for at least 1 h before baseline parameters were measured. At death or at the end of the survival period, animals were sacrificed and tissues removed for histological examination.

Hemodynamic measurements were obtained by connecting the carotid catheters to a Gould Brush physiograph (RS2300) via a PE23 transducer

---

[1] Vanderbilt University, Nashville, TN, USA
[2] Department of Surgery, University of South Alabama, Mobile, AL

Host Defense Dysfunction
in Trauma, Shock and Sepsis
Eds. Faist/Meakins/Schildberg
© Springer-Verlag, Berlin Heidelberg 1993

(Statham, Oxnard, CA, USA) and measured continuously for 4 h. Mean arterial pressure and heart rate were then compared between the groups.

Synthetic TNF (Peninsula Laboratories, CA, USA) was suspended in sterile nonpyrogenic saline and infused for 5 min. PAF (Bachem, Switzerland) was diluted in 0.25% bovine serum albumin/saline (sterile) and given as an infusion. Specific PAF receptor antagonists (BN52021 and SRI-63-675) were supplied by Dr. P. Braquet, IHB, France, and Sandoz Laboratories, USA, respectively. BN52021 was suspended in a phosphate solution (pH 7.3) and SRI-63-675 was suspended in sterile saline. Solutions were prepared on the day of the experiments.

All solutions utilized were examined for the presence of endotoxin utilizing the *Limulus* lysate method. Only the bovine serum albumin had any measurable amount of endotoxin (0.5 ng/ml).

Pilot studies had been conducted without randomization to determine the merits of the hypotheses. All other experiments conducted were designed by random number selection.

Histopathological evaluation was performed in a blind fashion utilizing hematoxylin and eosin stain. Standard criteria were utilized to determine ischemia, necrosis, edema, or other features of tissue specimens.

Data analysis was accomplished with paired t tests in the same group or ANOVA for repeated measures within groups or between groups. Differences in survival were determined by the χ^2 square method. A value of less than 0.05 was considered significant.

Results

Synthetic TNF doses that produced $\sim 90\%$ mortality had variable effects on hemodynamic parameters during the observation period. The most consistent finding was a gradual increase in the heart rate until there was a sudden change (slowing rhythm) then hypotension and death. In most animals there was a modest decrease in PaO_2 and in serum bicarbonate as well as a slight decrease in pH. Pretreatment with specific PAF receptor antagonists alone had minimal effects on the hemodynamic parameters, however, the animals died at ~ 2 h with similar events as those with TNF alone. Treatment with a cyclooxygenase inhibitor and with PAF infusion attenuated the dramatic hemodynamic events seen with TNF alone. In the PAF infusion/TNF animals, the MAP (mean arterial pressure) was generally lower than with TNF/saline, however, a greater percentage survived.

Histological abnormalities were seen only in the liver and the lung of animals receiving TNF. These findings consisted of microvascular edema and ischemia with cell death. Treatment with monoclonal antibody to TNF prevented these changes. Exogenous PAF and ibuprofen did not consistently reverse or prevent these histopathological findings.

Table 1. Mechanisms of TNF-induced mortality in rats (percentage survival)

		Time (h)			
		2	4	24	72
I	TNF Alone	30	13 (4/30)	–	–
II	PAF Receptor/TNF	17^+	17 (4/24)	–	–
III	IBU/TNF	89*	89* (25/28)	–	89*
IV	Vehicles/TNF	28	28 (5/18)	–	–
V	PAF/TNF	90*	90* (36/40)	–	90*

$^+ P < 0.01$ vs TNF alone
$* P < 0.001$ vs TNF alone at 2 h

Survival data are shown in Table 1. Preliminary studies demonstrated no deaths with TNF 60 ng/kg IV, 5 min, and produced no deaths in 24 h, whereas 600 ng/kg IV, 5 min, produced 100% mortality in 1–2 h; consequently, we elected to use 150 ng/kg IV, 5 min, which produced ~ 90% mortality in 4 h. The doses of the PAF receptor antagonist and cyclooxygenase inhibitor were based on pilot studies that demonstrated protection from exogenous PAF effects and effects on eicosanoid synthesis with exogenous TNF.

Discussion

The present study demonstrates: (1) that TNF produces metabolic acidosis, hemodynamic alterations, histological abnormalities in the liver and lungs, and predictable mortality within 4 h; (2) that two chemically different specific PAF receptor antagonists when administered before TNF enhanced TNF effects, producing death in half the time that was seen with TNF alone; (3) that infusion of exogenous PAF protected the animals from TNF-induced mortality; and (4) that a cyclooxygenase inhibitor, ibuprofen, protected animals from TNF-induced mortality.

Additional studies not reported in this report demonstrated that murine monoclonal antibody to whole TNF would provide 100% protection against all doses of TNF utilized (50–600 ng/kg) in this mortality study. These studies were done to ensure the conserved portion of TNF (115–130 amino acids) was recognized by the monoclonal antibody.

Our observation that TNF produces many of the pathophysiological events in endotoxemia/sepsis is similar to that reported by others [1, 2]. One unexplained observation is that our animals had minimal histological changes in the colon and kidneys when compared with other reports.

The effects of PAF receptor antagonists on TNF-induced mortality were just the opposite of what we expected. To ensure there was no endotoxin in the preparations of these agents, Limulus lysate studies were performed and no significant evidence of endotoxin was found. Several pilot studies were done before the present randomized study was performed. We are unable to explain these findings except to speculate that doses of PAF which have little observable effect on the intact animal may stimulate mediators or homeostatic mechanisms that alter TNF-induced effects. It is known that PAF, like endotoxin and TNF, induces eicosanoid synthesis [1]. It is possible that the agents which bind the PAF receptor may directly neutralize the TNF. That exogenous PAF infusions protected against TNF-induced mortality indicates that the enhanced effects of TNF in the presence of PAF receptor antagonists is a valid observation.

The improved survival with a cyclooxygenase inhibitor, ibuprofen, is consistent with the reports of Kettelhut et al. [8]. They demonstrated that two different cyclooxygenase inhibitors (indomethacin, 3 mg/kg; ibuprofen, 20 mg/kg) when administered 2 h before TNF substantively decreased mortality to 25% versus a 100% mortality in the TNF alone group. Further, they demonstrated that TNF produced a tenfold increase in PGE_2 (control, 0.40 ± 0.05 ng/ml; 3 h, 5.8 ± 0.51 ng/ml). Of particular interest in their study were the data that even when indomethacin was injected 1 h after TNF there was a decrease in mortality. Indomethacin also decreased the severity of the metabolic acidosis in their animals. The present study did not explore other potential benefits of cyclooxygenase inhibitors with TNF-induced effects, however if TNF is important in endotoxemia/sepsis, previous data from our laboratory has clearly demonstrated that indomethacin improves the survival in rats, dogs, and baboons subjected to severe endotoxemia [9]. Recently, others have reported that cyclooxygenase inhibitors decrease TNF-induced toxicity [10, 11]. The present findings and those of others suggest that the eicosanoids may have an important role in mediating the cellular TNF effects.

Mechanisms that are operative in endotoxemia/sepsis are complex. Similarly, TNF-induced cellular toxicity may be related to many divergent homeostatic or pathophysiologic mechanisms. Because of this complexity, it is imperative that interrelationships between known mediators that are recognized as important be explored carefully. Indeed, with the discovery of more specific inhibitors and monoclonal antibodies, these interrelationships can be better defined. Hopefully, better treatment options for patients with sepsis will emerge.

References

1. Beutler BA, Melsark IW, Cerami A (1985) Science 229:869–871
2. Waage A, Holstensen A, Espevik T (1987) Lancet 1:355–357
3. Fletcher JR, DiSimone AG, Earnest M (1990) Ann Surg 211:312–316
4. Moore JA, Earnest MA, DiSimone AG, Abumrad NN, Fletcher JR (1991) Circ Shock (in press)
5. Camussi G, Bussolino F, Salvidio G, Baglioni C (1987) J Exp Med 166:1390–1404
6. Kawakami M, Ishibashi S, Ogawa H, Murase T, Takaku F (1986) Biochem Biophys Res Commun 141:482–487
7. Oayer JM, Beutler B, Cerami A (1985) J Exp Med 162:2163–2168
8. Kettelhut IC, Fiers W, Goldberg AL (1987) Proc Natl Acad Sci USA 84:4273–4277

 9. Fletcher JR (1985) Biological protection with prostaglandins, vol 1. CRC, Boca Raton, pp 65–72
10. Talmadge JE, Bowersox O, Tribble H, Lee SH, Shepard HM, Ligitt D (1987) Am J Pathol 128:410–425
11. Evans DA, Jacobs DO, Revhaug A, Wilmore DW (1989) Ann Surg 204:312–321

Section 10

Endotoxin—Mechanisms of Action and Protection from Shock

Molecular Mechanisms of Lipopolysaccharide-Induced Cytokine Production by Monocytes

R. R. Schumann[1], J. C. Mathison[2], P. S. Tobias[2], and R. J. Ulevitch[2]

Introduction

Gram-negative sepsis is a greatly feared complication that occurs predominantly in patients that are traumatized, immune-suppressed, or under chemotherapy. Little effective therapy is available as now, and the overall mortality of septic shock is approximately 50%. The course of events starting with the undetectable entry of gram-negative bacteria into the organism and leading to the symptoms of full sepsis is so rapid that antibiotic treatment is usually of little use. Scientific interest thus has been focused lately on the host reaction that is triggered during the event of septic shock so that therapeutic intervention might become possible. It is known that endotoxin and its biologically active compound lipid A that enters the bloodstream in the event of sepsis is the cause of the complications of hypotension, disseminated intravascular coagulation (DIC), multiorgan failure, and eventually death [1, 2]. An important mediator in the cascade of events has recently been identified with tumor necrosis factor (cachectin/TNF), secreted by cells of monocytic origin (Mo) [3]. In vitro experiments confirm that lipopolysaccharide (LPS) can stimulate Mo to produce TNF and other monokines, so the Mo is considered to be a key cell in septic shock and related diseases.

Whenever a soluble substance has a specific effect on a certain cell the existence of a receptor on the cell membrane of that cell type or alternatively a soluble receptor or binding protein that is able to identify the activating substance is postulated. The search for LPS receptors on Mo and the investigation of proteins binding to LPS thus has been extensive, and there have been several candidates for the LPS receptor. However, no membrane molecule or protein could be identified to be the LPS receptor until recently, but interactions of plasma proteins with LPS have been found, involving high density lipoproteins (HDL) [4] and apolipoproteins [5].

[1] Innere Medizin I, Universitätsklinik, Institut für molekulare Biologie, c/o gödecke AG, Mooswaldallee 1-9, 7800 Freiburg i. Br., FRG
[2] Scripps Clinic and Research Foundation, Department of Immunology, La Jolla, CA, USA

Host Defense Dysfunction
in Trauma, Shock and Sepsis
Eds. Faist/Meakins/Schildberg
© Springer-Verlag, Berlin Heidelberg 1993

Identification and Biological Properties of Lipopolysaccharide-Binding Protein

Studies comparing acute phase serum with normal serum recently led to the discovery of a serum protein that is present at much greater quantities in acute phase serum than in normal serum [6]. This protein was found to bind to the lipid A moiety of LPS with high affinity [7] and consequently was named lipopolysaccharide-binding protein (LBP). It is produced in hepatocytes with a molecular mass of 50 kDa and is secreted into the bloodstream as a 60-kDa glycosylated protein. In many species LBP is present in normal serum at concentrations less than 0.5 μg/ml, rising to 50 μg/ml during the acute phase. After isolation and amino-terminal sequence analysis of LBP it was found that another protein that was discovered recently and that had LPS binding ability had a high degree of homology with LBP [8]. This protein, named bactericidal/permeability increasing protein (BPI), is found in the granules of neutrophil granulocytes, has a size of 50 kDa, and in contrast to LBP is toxic for gram-negative bacteria [9]. Cloning and sequence analysis of the cDNAs revealed a homology of 40% of LBP with BPI throughout the whole molecule [10]. Also, to a lesser degree, homology was found to cholesterol ester transport protein (CETP) and the existence of a protein family with the function of binding lipid structures and carrying them in an aqueous environment was postulated [11]. An overview of the three related proteins and a comparison of their function is shown in Table 1.

Functional studies about LBP revealed that it enhances the biological effects that LPS has on leukocytes. LBP/LPS complexes are far more active than LPS alone in stimulating Mo for TNF production [10] or in priming of granulocytes [12]. When working with subthreshold levels of LPS in vitro, which are much closer to levels found in vivo than the high LPS doses generally used in experiments, addition of LBP induces a cellular response (i.e., TNF production). LPS effects in whole blood where LBP is naturally present can be blocked with anti-LBP antibodies [10]. Furthermore, addition of LBP induces an LPS response in macrophages that were rendered unresponsive by an "LPS-adaptation" treatment [13]. LBP also acts as an opsonin for LPS-bearing particles

Table 1.

Protein	Amino acids			Localization	Binding function	
	Number	Homology			N-terminus	C-terminus
LBP	452			Serum	Lipid A	CD14
		44%				
BPI	456		23%	Granula of neutrophils	Lipid A	Membrane
		22%				
CETP	476			Serum	Phospholipid	Triglyceride

Table 2.

Target cell	LPS effect	LBP enhancement
Mo	TNF production	Yes
	LPS binding, phagocytosis	Yes (opsonin)
THP-1 (CD14 +)	IL-1 production	Yes
Neutrophils	"Priming"	Yes
Murine B-cells	Membrane IgG synthesis	No
(70 Z/3 cells)	Mitogenic	Not measured

such as LPS-coated erythrocytes and for gram-negative bacteria [14]. Addition of LBP also enhances the LPS-induced interleukin-1(IL-1) response of the myeloid cell line THP-1 when the cells have been pretreated with Vitamin D_3 and subsequently express CD14 on the surface (T.R. Martin and R.J. Ulevitch, manuscript in preparation).

To summarize, LBP does not act as a buffer or neutralizing protein against LPS but enhances the defense mechanisms of the host by forming complexes with LPS. These complexes are much more effective than LPS alone in triggering the immune response cascade, and LBP might function as a tool of the organism in helping to detect small amounts of LPS locally. The enhancement of LPS effects by LBP is shown in Table 2.

The Cellular Receptor for LPS/LBP Complexes CD14

Antibodies against the cell surface molecule CD14 are able to inhibit several of the specific effects LBP/LPS complexes have on cells. The strong TNF production that is observed when monocytes are stimulated with LBP/LPS can be suppressed when these cells are pretreated with monoclonal anti-CD14 antibodies, while treatment with other antibodies did not have this effect [15]. The same suppression was observed regarding the opsonic function of LBP. CD14 was known only as a "differentiation antigen" present in high quantities on monocytes/macrophages and in smaller numbers on neutrophils and B-cells. As these are the cells LPS has specific effects on, it appears that CD14 is the cellular receptor for LBP/LPS complexes.

CD14 is a 55-kDa glycoprotein that is detected by commercially available monoclonal antibodies named MO-2, My-4, Leu-M3, 3C10, and others. It is attached to the cellular membrane via a phospatidylinosityl-glycosyl (PIG or PI) anchor [16]. So far it is not known if signals can be transduced into the cell by a molecule that is PI anchored. Thus it appears likely that another membrane molecule is involved in the cellular LPS response or that CD14 presents LPS to another receptor on the cell surface. Our present model of LPS-mediated stimulation of cells for TNF production is shown in Fig. 1.

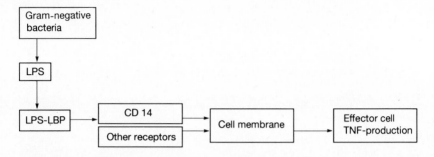

Fig. 1. Simplified model of LPS-mediated Mo stimulation. When LPS from gram-negative bacteria is released into the bloodstream it binds to the serum protein LBP and forms the LBP/LPS complex. This complex is recognized by the cell surface molecule CD14, which is a PI-linked membrane-bound protein. As signal transduction via the PI anchor is unlikely, another (unknown) membrane protein might be involved and finally lead to immune responses of the cell, i.e., TNF production.

Clinical Consequences

When in an experimental setup LPS is added to whole blood the monocytes are stimulated to produce large quantities of TNF. Pretreatment of the blood with antibodies against LBP reduced the LPS-induced TNF production dramatically [10]. The experiments that led to the discovery of the CD14 protein as receptor for LPS/LBP complexes, as mentioned earlier, also showed blocking of LPS-induced TNF production by using the anti-CD14 antibodies. Intervention at these two points of the LPS/LBP-CD14 pathway seems to suppress the host response, and antibodies might be candidates for animal experiments and clinical trials during septic shock. Measuring serum levels of LBP and soluble CD14 in patients during sepsis and also in other diseases could be very helpful too in understanding the pathomechanisms of phenomena that this ligand-receptor pathway is involved in.

CD14 is a membrane-bound protein that can be quantitatively measured on cells by fluorescence-activated cell sorter (FACS) analysis but also exists in relatively high quantities in soluble form in the serum. Measurements of soluble CD14 have shown that it is elevated in patients with different malignancies, in AIDS patients and in polytraumatized patients [17]. In the paroxysmal nocturnal hemoglobinemia (PNH) disease CD14, like all other PI-linked proteins, is missing entirely. The group of proteins that is connected to the cell membrane via a PI anchor includes the surface molecules Thy-1, CEA, and T-cell activating factor, adhesion molecules such as LFA-1 and N-CAM, and hydrolytic enzymes such as acetylcholinesterase and alkaline phosphatase.

Certain leukemias lack the q23-q31 region of chromosome 5 that includes the gene for CD14. Fifty percent of therapy-related acute non-lymphocytic leukemia (tANLL), 10% of ANLL, and 5%–10% of myelodysplastic syndrome (MDS) patients lack this genetic region that also encodes cytokine and cytokine receptor genes, i.e., IL-3, granulocyte-macrophage colony-stimulating factor

(GM-CSF), M-CSF, the human c-*fms* protooncogene FMS, endothelial cell growth factor (ECGF) and platelet-derived growth factor (PDGF) receptor. A possible role of the missing CD14 gene in the etiology of diseases has to be investigated and experiments involving measurement of serum levels of LBP and CD14 and the ability of cells to respond to LPS/LBP stimulation are underway.

Conclusions

In the attempt to understand the molecular mechanisms of gram-negative sepsis as ligand-receptor pair has been discovered with the LPS/LBP complex and the CD14 surface molecule that seems to be of high importance in LPS-mediated cell response. There is evidence that this discovery does not answer all the questions involved in septic shock but that there may be other elements involved in endotoxin-mediated cell activation as well. Both elements, the "adapter-protein" LBP and the cellular receptor CD14 (membrane bound and in soluble form), need further investigation and in vivo measurements of those proteins in different diseases will be of great interest.

Continuation of the basic molecular studies might also bring new insights into a newly discovered protein family, and expression of the recombinant proteins might aid in carrying out therapeutically aimed experiments. Monoclonal antibodies against LBP or CD14 are candidates for clinical trials as well as mutated forms of LBP. LBP mutants that are being constructed should maintain the binding function to LPS but lack the stimulatory binding capacity to CD14 or vice versa and so lose the adapter function and act as a blocking agent in the mechanisms that lead to septic shock.

Acknowledgments. Supported by USPHS grants AI-15136, GM-28585, and GM-37696.

References

1. Rietschel ET, Wollenweber H-W, Brade H et al. (1984) In: Rietschel ET (ed) Handbook of endotoxin: I. Chemistry of endotoxin. Elsevier, New York, pp 187–214
2. Mathison JC, Wolfson N, Ulevitch RJ (1988) Participation of tumor necrosis factor in the mediation of Gram-negative bacterial lipopolysaccharide induced injury in rabbits. J Clin Invest 81:1925–1937
3. Beutler B, Milsark IW, Cerami AC (1985) Passive immunization against cachectin/tumor necrosis factor protects mice from lethal effect of endotoxin. Science 29:869–871
4. Ulevitch RJ, Johnston AR (1978) The modification of biophysical and endotoxic properties of bacterial lipopolysaccharides by serum. J Clin Invest 62:1313–1324
5. Flegel WA, Wolpl A, Männel DN et al. (1989) Inhibition of endotoxin-induced activation of human monocytes by human lipopoteins. Infect Immun 57:2237–2245
6. Tobias PS, McAdam KPW, Soldau K, Ulevitch RJ (1985) Control of lipopolysaccharide-high density lipoprotein interactions by an acute phase reactant in human serum. Infect Immun 50:73–76

7. Tobias PS, Soldau K, Ulevitch RJ (1989) Identification of a lipid A binding site in the acute phase reactant lipopolysaccharide binding protein. J Biol Chem 64:10867–10871
8. Gray PW, Leong SR, Flaggs GW et al. (1989) Cloning of the cDNA of a human neutrophil bactericidal protein. Structural and functional correlations. J Biol Chem 264:9505–9509
9. Weiss, Elsbach P, Olsson I, Odeberg H (1978) Purification and characterization of a potent bactericidal and membrane active protein from the granules of human polymorphonuclear leukocytes. J Biol Chem 253:2664
10. Schumann RR, Leong SR, Flaggs GW et al. (1990) Structure and function of lipopolysaccharide binding protein. Science 249:1429– 1431
11. Tobias PS, Mathison JC, Ulevitch RJ (1988) A family of lipopolysaccharide binding proteins involved in responses to Gram-negative sepsis. J Biol Chem 263:13479–13481
12. Vosbeck K, Tobias PS, Mueller H et al. (1990) Priming of polymorphonuclear granulocytes by lipopolysaccharides and its complexes with lipopolysaccharide binding protein and high density lipoprotein. J Leukocyte Biol 47:97–104
13. Mathison JC, Virca GD, Wolfson N et al. (1990) Adaptation to bacterial lipopolysaccharide (LPS) controls LPS-induced tumor necrosis factor production in rabbit macrophages. J Clin Invest 85:1108–1118
14. Wright SD, Tobias PS, Ulevitch RJ et al. (1989) Lipopolysaccharide (LPS) binding protein opsonizes LPS-bearing particles for recognition by a novel receptor on macrophages. J Exp Med 170:1231
15. Wright SD, Ramos RA, Tobias PS et al. (1990) CD14, a receptor for complexes of lipopolysaccharide (LPS) and LPS binding protein. Science 249:1431–1433
16. Haziot C, Chen S, Ferrero E et al. (1988) The monocyte differentiation antigen, CD14, is anchored to the cellmembrane by a phosphatidylisonitol linkage. J Immunol 141:547–552
17. Krüger C, Schütt C, Obertacke U et al. (1991) Serum CD14 levels in polytraumatized and severely burned patients. Clin Exp Immunol 85:297–301

Natural Endotoxic Shock Protection by Soluble CD14

C. Schütt[1], C. Krüger[1], W. Schönfeld[2], U. Grunwald[1], and T. Schilling[1]

Introduction

Endotoxins and even anti-CD14 monoclonal antibodies (mAb) in an analogous reaction [1] induce monocyte activation, resulting in defense mechanisms mediated by oxygen radicals, tumor necrosis factor (TNF), interleukin-1 (IL-1), and interleukin-6 (IL-6). Recently, Wright et al. [2] described the function of the phosphoatidylinositol (PI)-anchored 53-kDa glycoprotein CD14 on monocyte membranes (mCD14) as a receptor for lipopolysaccharide (LPS). The binding of LPS is mediated by LPS-binding protein (LBP), a newly defined plasma protein present in high concentrations in human serum during acute phase responses. On the other hand, endotoxin-induced TNF, IL-6 and even reactive oxygen species are mediators of multiorgan failure and septic shock [3].

Therefore, it would be of great interest to look for soluble CD14 (sCD14) and its possible physiological function. sCD14 is a plasma protein of 48 kDA [4]. We detected the concentration of sCD14 in the human serum of healthy volunteers by means of a capture enzyme-linked immunosorbant assay (ELISA): 3.98–0.22 µg/ml ($n = 102$). We studied the role of affinity column-purified sCD14 during LPS-induced oxidative burst responses of human monocytes.

Luminol-Enhanced Chemoluminescence

Human mononuclear cells (MNC) were studied under serum-free conditions for response to different stimuli: anti-CD14 mAb RoMo-1 [1], LPS *Escherichia coli* 055:B5 (DIFCO), *E. coli* 0127:B8 (SIGMA), *E. coli* 04:K4 (SIFIN), and zymosan A (SIGMA), measured by luminol-enhanced chemoluminescence (LECL) using a Berthold luminometer (LB950).

Whereas LECL responses were measured after the addition of 10 µg/ml mAb RoMo-1 or opsonized zymosan, all LPS-tested charges were unable to induce LECL in MNC suspensions under serum-free conditions, but could do it

[1] Department of Medical Immunology, Ernst-Moritz-Arndt University, 2200 Greifswald, FRG
[2] Department of Microbiolgy and Immunology, Ruhr University, 4630 Bochum, FRG

Host Defense Dysfunction
in Trauma, Shock and Sepsis
Eds. Faist/Meakins/Schildberg
© Springer-Verlag, Berlin Heidelberg 1993

in whole-blood cultures. The preincubation of LPS stock solutions in human serum also results in LECL responses of MNC suspensions (Figs. 1, 2). If we use acute phase serum for "opsonization" we could observe a much more intensive free radical production (Fig. 3).

In earlier experiments we described a monocyte-activating ability of anti-CD14 mAb RoMo-1 [1] postulating a receptor nature of CD14. Therefore, it seems to be possible that LPS acts after opsonization by an LPS-binding protein of human serum via the mCD14 molecule according to Wright et al. [2].

Our experiments using CD14-negative monocytes of patients suffering from paroxysmal nocturnal hemiglobinuria (PNH) demonstrate that opsonized LPS can activate CD14-negative monocytes. Patients' cells respond to LPS to a

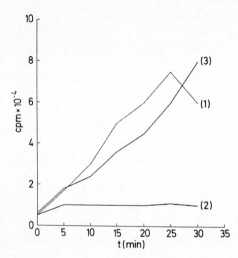

Fig. 1. LECL signals (cpm × 10⁻⁴) after activation of MNC under serum-free conditions by 5 µg/ml opsonized zymosan (*1*), 10 µg/ml LPS (*E. coli* 055:B5) (*2*), or activation of whole-blood suspensions by 10 µg/ml LPS (*E. coli* 055:B5; *3*)

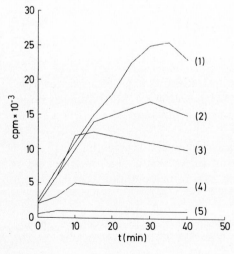

Fig. 2. LECL responses of MNC after activation by 1 µg/ml opsonized Zymosan (*1*), 10 µg/ml of different opsonized LPS charges (*E. coli* 055:B5; *2*), *E. coli* 0127:B8 (*3*), and *E. coli* 04:K4 (*4*) in comparison to NaCl control (*5*)

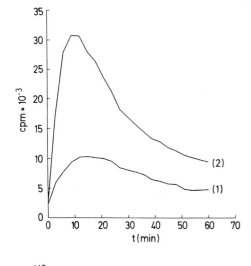

Fig. 3. LECL response of MNC after activation by 1 μg/ml LPS (*E. coli* 055:B5), opsonized by normal human serum (*1*) or acute phase serum (*2*)

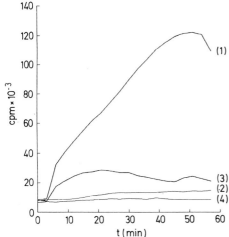

Fig. 4. LECL response of CD14-negative MNC from PNH patient after the addition of 10 μg/ml LPS (*E.coli* 055:B5), opsonized by normal human serum (*1*), or with addition of NaCl (*2*), in comparision to the response of CD14-positive MNC from a healthy donor (*3* and *4*, respectively)

greater extent than normal CD14-positive monocytes (Fig. 4). In control LECL experiments using anti-CD14 mAb, we could support the fluorescence-activated cell sorter (FACS) analysis (data not shown) of completely CD14-negative monocytes in PNH in two cases which were tested (Fig. 5).

Role of sCD14 in Endotoxin-Induced Free Oxygen Radical Production

Purified sCD14 prepared by ammonium sulfate precipitation and affinity chromatography using mAb RoMo-1 was used in the LECL model of monocyte

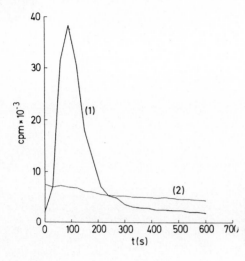

Fig. 5. Oxidative burst response after the addition of 10 µg/ml anti-CD14 mAb RoMo-1 to normal MNC (*1*) and PNH-MNC (*2*)

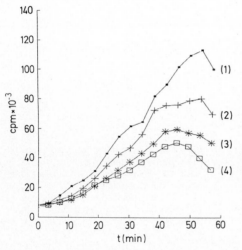

Fig. 6. Prevention of LPS (*E. coli* 055:B5)-induced free oxygen radical production by soluble CD14, (*1*), without the addition of purified sCD14 to the opsonizing serum; (*2*) + 3 µg/ml sCD14; (*3*) + 15 µg/ml sCD14; (*4*) + 30 µg/ml sCD14

activation by LPS as described above. Different sCD14 concentrations were added to the opsonizing serum before use. LPS stock solutions were incubated with this serum for 30 min at room temperature. In control experiments bovine serum albumin (BSA) was added to the serum used for opsonization. Figure 6 demonstrates that sCD14 is able to interfere in a dose-dependent manner with the LPS-induced monocyte activation mediated by serum proteins. The concentration of sCD14 in the opsonizing serum ranged from 4 µg/ml (without the addition of external sCD14) to 30 µg/ml. High dilution of LPS stock solutions excludes the quenching effects of serum proteins in the LECL system. The suppressive effect was mediated by sCD14 only, but not by other serum proteins, e.g., BSA (Fig. 7).

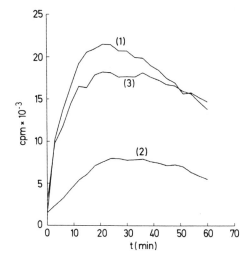

Fig. 7. LECL responses to opsonized LPS without (*1*) or with addition of 20 µg/ml sCD14 (*2*) in comparison to addition of 20 µg/ml BSA (*3*) to the opsonizing serum

Conclusions

Serum components are necessary for the LPS-activating capacity of free oxygen radical production by human monocytes in vitro. Our experiments demonstrate that acute-phase serum proteins express a stronger LPS-opsonizing capacity. Using CD14-negative monocytes, we could document that LPS-induced activation of monocytes was not necessarily mediated by LBP via membrane-bound CD14 molecules. From this point of view the dose-dependent sCD14-mediated suppression of reactive oxygen release induced by LPS — even at higher concentrations of LPS — suggests an overall interference of sCD14 in possibly different LPS-activating pathways.

Therefore the plasma protein sCD14 seems to be a natural protector against excessive mediator release from endotoxin-activated monocytes. This could be of relevance in preventing ongoing septic shock.

References

1. Schütt C, Ringel B, Nausch M, Bazil V, Horejsi V, Neels P, Walzel H, Jonas L, Siegl E, Friemel H, Plantikow A (1988) Human monocyte activation induced by an anit-CD14 monoclonal antibody. Immunol Lett 19:321
2. Wright DS, Ramos AR, Tobias SP, Ulevitch JR, Mathison CJ (1990) CD14, a receptor for complexes of lipopolysaccharide (LPS) and LPS-binding protein. Science 249:1431
3. Schlag G, Redl H (1989) Wandel im Sepsisverständnis der klinischen Medizin. Dtsch Med Wochenschr 114:475
4. Haziot A, Chen S, Ferrero E, Low GM, Silber R, Goyert MS (1988) The monocyte differentiation antigen, CD14, is anchored to the cell membrane by a phosphatidylinositol linkage. J Immunol 141:547

Use of Monophosphoryl Lipid A as a Prophylactic for Sepsis and Shock

J. A. Rudbach[1], J. T. Ulrich[1], K. B. Von Eschen[1], and J. D. Beatty[2]

Of patients who ultimately develop gram-negative sepsis and shock, many can be identified for inclusion into high-risk groups [1–3]. These groups include patients subjected to certain types of surgeries, some with traumatic injuries, and those with depressed immune systems. Appropriate immunomodulation of patients in these groups should be able to prevent or ameliorate septic shock.

A concerted effort has been underway for several years to develop a chemically modified and biologically attenuated form of lipopolysaccharide (LPS)/endotoxin as a prophylactic for septic shock [4]. This highly refined and defined material is monophosphoryl lipid A (MPL), and a 3-0-deacylated derivative of MPL (Fig. 1) is the form in current use.

In experimental animal models MPL can stimulate macrophages and trigger the production of lymphokines like interferon, interleukin-1, and interleukin-2 [5–8]. Animals pretreated with MPL are protected against challenge with a lethal dose of gram-negative bacteria (Table 1), as well as against gram-positive bacteria [9], viral [9, 10], protozoan [9], and fungal (J. A. Rudbach, et al., unpublished observations) agents.

The most serious clinical sequelae occur in cases of septic shock caused by gram-negative bacteria [2]; endotoxin is a major pathogenic factor in these cases of fatal "gram-negative shock." Data in Table 2 show that prophylactic use of MPL induces tolerance to a subsequent challenge with endotoxin. In addition to a reduction in lethality, this tolerance can be measured by refractivity of cells in vitro (G. L. Gustafson, unpublished observations), reduction in hemodynamic changes [11, 12], and amelioration of endotoxin-induced fevers (J. T. Ulrich, unpublished observations). Furthermore, MPL given prior to a lethal endotoxin challenge synergistically enhances the therapeutic value of monoclonal antibodies directed to endotoxin (J. T. Ulrich, unpublished observations).

In vitro MPL also stimulates human leukocytes and induces cytokine production [13]. In a clinical trial MPL was also shown to have bioactivity in vivo for human subjects. As shown in Fig. 2, increases in interleukin-6 were noted; also very small amounts of tumor necrosis factor alpha (TNF-α) were detected in sera of patients treated with MPL. The increases in serum neopterin

[1] Ribi ImmunoChem Research, Inc., Hamilton, MT 59840, USA
[2] Division of Surgery, City of Hope National Medical Center, 1500 East Duarte Road, Duarte, CA 91010, USA

Host Defense Dysfunction
in Trauma, Shock and Sepsis
Eds. Faist/Meakins/Schildberg
© Springer-Verlag, Berlin Heidelberg 1993

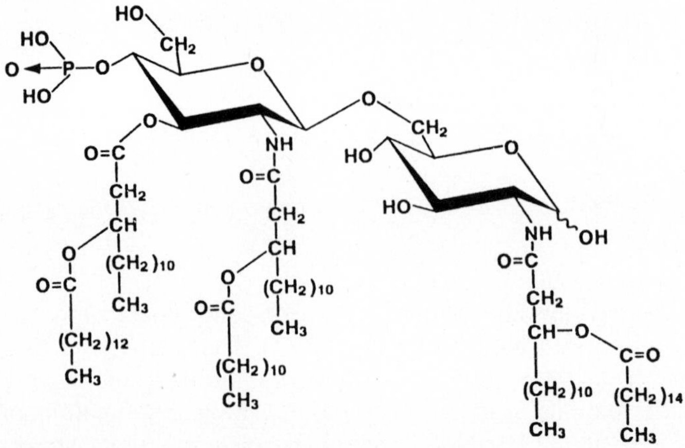

Fig. 1. Structure of hexacyl form of 3-0-deacylated MPL

Table 1. Prophylaxis with an appropriate dose of MPL protects mice from a lethal challenge with live *Escherichia coli*

Pretreatment			
Material	Dose (µg)	Day[a]	Survival %
Saline	–	– 2	11
MPL	10	– 2	44
MPL	50	– 2	100
MPL	100	– 2	100

[a] Treatment groups of 10–20 mice were challenged on day 0 with 5×10^8 viable *E. coli*.

Table 2. MPL induces early tolerance to lethal doses of endotoxin

	LD_{50}^a µg		
	Saline/LPS	MPL/LPS	LPS/LPS
Experiment 1[b]	258	1156	972
Experiment 2	588	843	–
Experiment 3	327	870	1054
Experiment 4	512	794	–
Experiment 5	250	755	–

Groups of mice were injected on day – 3 with saline, MPL (100 µg-/mouse), or *E. coli* LPS (25 µg/mouse). On day 0 the mice were challenged with various amounts of *E. coli* LPS. Survival was recorded and 50% lethal dose (LD_{50}) determinations calculated.
[a] LD_{50} calculated by method of Reed and Muench.
[b] Courtesy of Madonna et al. [6].

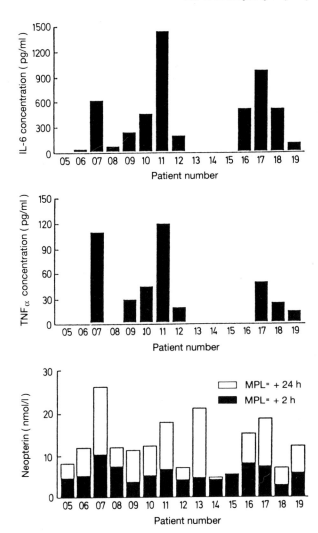

Fig. 2. Serum levels of IL-6 and TNF-α (both at 2 h) and neopterin at 2 and 24 h after patients received 100 μg/m² MPL i.v.. For Il-6 and TNF-α, "normal" values are below the baseline. The 2-h neopterin values are considered "normal" values. *Open bars*, MPL + 24 h; *Solid bars*, MPL + 2 h

showed that MPL stimulated macrophages in these trials (Fig. 2). Thus, MPL, which has been proved in animal models to have a prophylactic value for the prevention or reduction in severity of experimental sepsis and endotoxic shock, stimulates human cells in a similar manner. The clinical trials to date have shown that MPL can be used safely in humans, while exhibiting immunostimulatory activities. This unique approach constitutes one of the newer advances for intervention in septic shock.

References

1. Kreger BE, Craven DE, Carling PC, McCabe WR (1980) Gram-negative bacteremia. IV. Re-evaluation of clinical features and treatment in 612 patients. Am J Med 68:344–355
2. Luce JM (1987) Pathogenesis and management of septic shock. Chest 91:883–888
3. Bone RC, Fisher CJ Jr, Clemmer TP, Slotman GJ et al. (1989) Sepsis syndrome: a valid clinical entity. Crit Care Med 17:389–393
4. Rudbach JA, Cantrell JL, Ulrich JT, Mitchell MS (1990) Immunotherapy with bacterial endotoxins. In: Friedman H, Klein TW, Nakaro M, Nowatny A (eds) Endotoxin. Plenum, New York, pp 665–676
5. Henricson BE, Benjamin WR, Vogel SN (1990) Differential cytokine induction by doses of lipopolysaccharide and monophosphoryl lipid A that result in equivalent early endotoxin tolerance. Infect Immun 58:2429–2437
6. Madonna GS, Peterson JE, Ribi EE, Vogel SN (1986) Early-phase endotoxin tolerance: induction by a detoxified lipid A derivative, monophosphoryl lipid A. Infect Immun 52:6–11
7. Kiener PA, Mark F, Rodgers G et al. (1988) Induction of tumor necrosis factor, IFN-α, and acute lethality in mice by toxic and non-toxic forms of lipid A. J immunol 141:870–874
8. Bennett JA, Peter JH, Chudacoff R, McKneally MF (1988) Endogenous production of cytotoxic factors in serum of BCG-primed mice by monophosphoryl lipid A, a detoxified form of endotoxin. J Biol Response Mod 7:65–76
9. Ulrich JT, Mashihi KN, Lange W (1988) Mechanisms of nonspecific resistance to microbial infections induced by trehalose dimycolate (TDM) and monophosphoryl lipid A (MPL). Adv Biosci 68:167–178
10. Mashihi KN, Lange W, Brehmer W, Ribi E (1986) Immunobiological activities of nontoxic lipid A: enhancement of nonspecific resistance in combination with trehalose dimycolate against viral infection and adjuvant effects. Int J Immunopharmacol 8:339–345
11. Rackow EC, Astiz ME, Kim YB, Weil MH (1989) Monophosphoryl lipid A blocks the hemodynamic effects of lethal endotoxemia. J Lab Clin Med 113:112–117
12. Astiz ME, Rackow EC, Kim YB, Weil MA (1989) Hemodynamic effects of monophosphoryl lipid A compared to endotoxin. Circ Shock 27:193–198
13. Carozzi S, Salit M, Cantaluppi A et al. (1989) Effect of monophosphoryl lipid A on the in vitro function of peritoneal leukocytes from uremic patients on continuous ambulatory peritoneal dialysis. J Clin Microbiol 27:1748–1753

Hemodynamic and Pulmonary Response to Treatment with On-Line Adsorption on Polymyxin B During Endotoxemia in Pigs

B. Strittmatter, W. Schneider, K. Massarrat, A. Eckhardt, and B. U. von Specht

Introduction

Endotoxin can be neutralized by the antibiotic polymyxin B. However, the systemic use of this substance is limited due to its organ toxicity. Through extracorporal plasmapheresis and the binding of polymyxin B to a stationary phase it was possible to adsorb the endotoxin from the circulatory plasma. Cohen, using this method, markedly improved the mortality rate among rats due to endotoxemia. Using the pig as experimental animal, we examined the influence of the plasmapheresis with polymyxin B on the hemodynamics and pulmonary gas exchange.

Our experiments asked the following questions: (a) What changes do the circulation of the experimental animals show during the extracorporal circulation. (b) In what form are the signs of septic shock visible in our model? (c) What kind of influence does the therapeutic use of polymyxin B have on the course of septic shock?

Materials and Methods

Young hybrid pigs were treated with polymyxin B fixed with Sepharose through extracorporal circulation and plasmapheresis. Before this, endotoxin (*Salmonella abortus equi* S form) was given by perfusor in linearly increasing doses. The dose of endotoxin was increased until a plateau was achieved in the increase in pulmonary arterial pressure, the most sensitive parameter. After reaching this plateau, infusion of this dose was then continued for another hour. The following parameters were then measured: heart rate, arterial blood pressure, cardiac index, total peripheral resistance, pulmonary arterial pressure, pulmonary vascular resistance, pulmonary capillary wedge pressure, and pulmonary function.

There were five hybrid pigs in the experimental group (EP) and in the control group (EA).

Department of Surgery, University Hospital, Hugstetter Strasse 55, 7800 Freiburg, FRG

Host Defense Dysfunction
in Trauma, Shock and Sepsis
Eds. Faist/Meakins/Schildberg
© Springer-Verlag, Berlin Heidelberg 1993

Results

Heart Rate. The heart rate increased continuously in the experimental and control group until a maximum of 143 beats per minute was reached. Both groups reacted with a sharp increase in the heart rate after the administration of endotoxin. After a leveling off of the endotoxin was reached, however, there were no significant differences between the two groups (Fig. 1).

Arterial Blood Pressure. After administration of endotoxin, there was a weak initial increase in arterial blood pressure in both groups followed by a sharp drop to a level of 77 mmHg, substantially below the initial systolic pressure values (Fig. 2).

Cardiac Index. The baseline values of the cardiac index were $114 \, \text{ml min}^{-1} \text{kg}^{-1}$. The cardiac index of both experimental groups fell continuously to $77 \, \text{ml min}^{-1} \, \text{kg}^{-1}$ (Fig. 3).

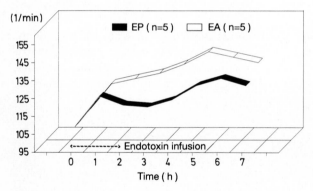

Fig. 1. Heart rate

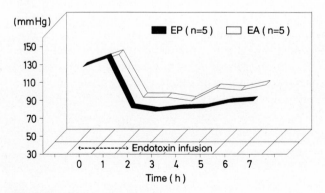

Fig. 2. Systolic arterial pressure

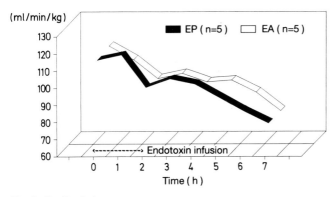

Fig. 3. Cardiac index

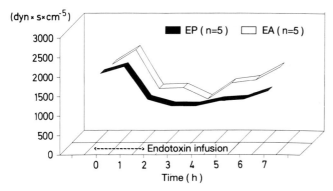

Fig. 4. Total peripheral resistance

Total Peripheral Resistance. The total peripheral resistance dropped markedly, especially after the first 1–2 h of the experiment and remained constant from the third to the fifth hour. Then a gradual increase was noted (Fig. 4).

Pulmonary Arterial Pressure. This, the most sensitive parameter for the effect of endotoxin, increased within the first hour of the experiment in both groups from 26 to 67 mmHg, dropped in the third hour to a value of 39 mmHg, and then followed a gradual increase to 50 mmHg. There was no significant difference between groups (Fig. 5).

Pulmonary Vascular Resistance. The pulmonary vascular resistance in both groups increased 4.5 times the baseline value within 8 h (Fig. 6).

Pulmonary Capillary Wedge Pressure. The pulmonary capillary wedge pressure remained at about 5 mmHg throughout the entire experiment in both groups (Fig. 7).

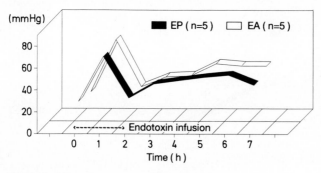

Fig. 5. Systolic pulmonary arterial pressure

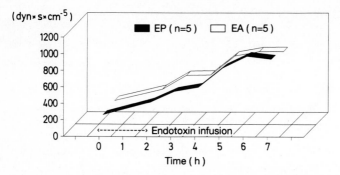

Fig. 6. Pulmonary vascular resistance

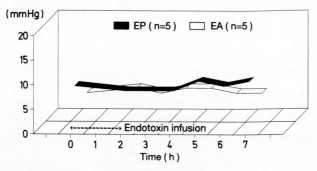

Fig. 7. Pulmonary capillary wedge pressure

Pulmonary Function. The arterial oxygen tension fell continuously in both experimental groups. At the same time there was a continuous rise in the CO_2 partial pressure. The oxygen carrier capacity dropped continuously in both groups due to the decreasing cardiac output and arterial oxygen content (Fig. 8). The mixed venous lactate rose in both groups from 1.8 mmol/l to 2.65 mmol/l.

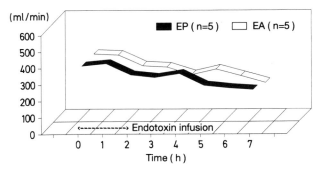

Fig. 8. Oxygen transport capacity

Mortality. Two of the animals in the group treated with polymyxin B (EP) survived the entire observational period of 7 h; the animals died after 3, 5, and 6 h, respectively. In the control group (EA) four animals survived; one animal died after 4 h.

Conclusion

The experimental animals (EP) displayed an intense, hypodynamic shock after the intravenous introduction of endotoxin. We observed a drop in the cardiac index, total peripheral resistance, and blood pressure in the general circulatory system. There was a two-peaked increase in pulmonary arterial pressure occurring in the pulmonary circulation. The occurrence of shock was also seen during the experiment by an increasing degeneration of the pulmonary gas exchange and decrease in the oxygen-carrying capacity. At no time was a difference between the experimental and control groups seen using the observed parameters. The extracorporal circulation without administration of endotoxin has no influence on the hemodynamics or gas exchange.

Contrary to the reports from Cohen and Issekutz we did not influence the endotoxemia with plasmapheresis and polymyxin B adsorption and did not prevent septic shock. This seems to indicate that endotoxin induces a multifactorial process with the activation of mediators which initiate septic shock and in which the endotoxin elimination alone has no further influence.

Further experiments should show how mediators (tumor necrosis factor, interleukin) behave, and what effect endotoxin elimination has on these mediators.

Apolipoprotein A-I-Enriched Lipoprotein Attenuates Tumor Necrosis Factor Production and Shock in an Anesthetized Rabbit Endotoxemia Model

A. P. Hubsch, J. E. Doran, P. G. Lerch, G. Hodler, J. J. Morgenthaler, and H. J. Heiniger

Introduction

When bacterial lipopolysaccharide (LPS) is exposed to plasma or serum it loses part of its activity through the formation of LPS-lipoprotein complexes (reviewed in [1]). In vitro studies have shown that lipoprotein-bound LPS is less potent than parent LPS in the induction of tumor necrosis factor (TNF) and other cytokines by macrophages. These complexes are also less potent in vivo: LPS-induced pathophysiologic changes are reduced.

In our laboratories an artificial lipoprotein, made of human apolipoprotein A-I and phosphatidylcholine, referred to as ApoLipo, has recently been produced. In in vitro studies ApoLipo depressed endotoxin-induced TNF production by macrophages. The purpose of the present study was to investigate whether prophylactic infusion of ApoLipo reduces TNF production and the pathophysiologic manifestations of shock in a rabbit endotoxemia model.

Materials and Methods

Rabbits were randomly assigned to one of four experimental groups. The test groups, designated 75-ApoLipo-LPS ($n = 6$) and 250-ApoLipo-LPS ($n = 3$) received a prophylactic infusion of ApoLipo (either 75 or 250 mg protein/kg of body weight dissolved in 50 ml saline, given over a 25-min period), followed after 15 min by a 6-h continuous LPS infusion (rate: 4.17 µg/kg h). LPS from *Escherichia coli O111-B5* was a generous gift from Professor B. Urbaschek, Mannheim, FRG. In the positive control group, designated Control-LPS ($n = 4$), the prophylactic infusion was replaced by a modified gelatin solution (Physiogel SRK, 250 mg protein/kg of body weight). The negative control group, referred to as 75-ApoLipo-Control ($n = 4$), received 75 mg/kg ApoLipo and pyrogen-free saline instead of endotoxin.

The animals were anesthetized throughout the procedure with a combination of pentobarbital sodium and fentanyl and were artifically ventilated with a constant respiratory volume. Pancuronium bromide was injected as needed.

Central Laboratory, Swiss Red Cross Blood Transfusion Service, CH-3000 Bern 22, Switzerland

Host Defense Dysfunction
in Trauma, Shock and Sepsis
Eds. Faist/Meakins/Schildberg
© Springer-Verlag, Berlin Heidelberg 1993

Catheters were inserted into the left carotid artery and right jugular vein for monitoring blood pressure and drawing arterial blood samples; and for drug infusion respectively. After surgery, the animals were heparinized (1500 U i.v.).

Arterial blood samples (3.5 ml) for blood gas analysis, hematocrit, leukocyte and thrombocyte count, determination of TNF activity (L929 cytotoxicity assay), human apolipoprotein A (nephelometry), antithrombin-III (Kabi), and total protein (Lowry) were drawn at specific times. Arterial blood pressure, heart rate, body temperature, and respiratory parameters were monitored continuously, in order to assess the effects of LPS infusion and also to adapt the infusion of anesthetics to the requirements of the individual animals. This animal study was approved by the Animal Protection Committee of the Canton of Bern, Bern, Switzerland.

Data are presented as mean $\pm$ standard error of the mean of replicate samples (the number is given in text). Statistical differences between groups were determined using Student's t test or Mann-Whitney U test for small samples as appropriate. Probabilities less than 0.05 were considered significant. Cell counts have been normalized with respect to their value at the beginning of LPS infusion (% baseline).

Results

The initial concentrations of human apolipoprotein A-I in the rabbits' plasma were 1.45 mg/ml and 5.16 mg/ml for doses of ApoLipo of 75 mg/kg and 250 mg/kg, respectively. The apparent distribution space of ApoLipo is 50 mg/kg which is consistent with the plasma space. The plasma half-life of human ApoA-I was 6 h (range 5.0–7.8 h, $n = 10$) in the animals treated with 75 mg/kg and 11 h (range 9.3–18.3 h, $n = 3$) in those receiving 250 mg/kg. LPS infusion had no significant influence on the circulatory half-life of ApoLipo.

Plasma TNF levels are shown in Fig. 1a. While no significant TNF production occurred in the non-LPS-treated animals, a TNF peak with a maximum of 29.4 $\pm$ 6.5 ng/ml 2 h after the beginning of LPS infusion was seen in the Control-LPS group. Only a slight, though still significant TNF production (peak value 1.2 $\pm$ 0.2 ng/ml at 1 h) was detected in the animals pretreated with 75 mg/kg of ApoLipo. No significant TNF production was observed in the animals treated with 250 mg/kg.

Figure 1b shows results of the arterial blood gas analyses. At baseline, there were no significant differences between groups, base excess was 0.5 $\pm$ 0.5. No significant changes in acid-base status were observed in the Apo-Control group during the experiment. In the Control-LPS group, base excess began to drop 30 min after the beginning of endotoxin infusion, reaching $- 8.8 \pm 2.0$ at the end of endotoxin infusion. The animals treated with ApoLipo had only a mild metabolic acidosis (final base excess $- 3.7 \pm 1.9$ and $- 2.8 \pm 1.2$ for 75 and 250 mg/kg, respectively).

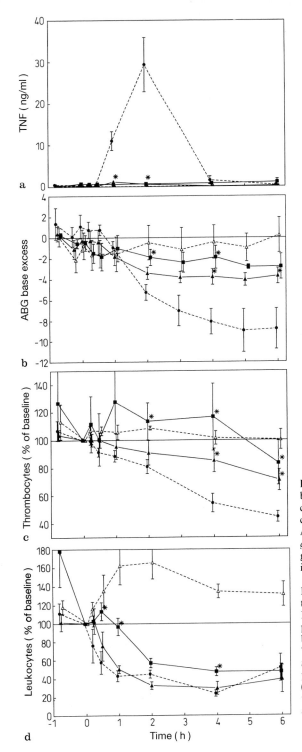

Fig.1.a. Serum TNF **b**, arterial blood gas (*ABG*) analyses base excess, **c** thrombocyte, and **d** leukocyte counts in rabbits. In the 75-ApoLipo-LPS group (*filled triangles*) and in the 250-ApoLipo-LPS group (*filled squares*), ApoLipo was infused prophylactically from time = − 0.75 h to time = − 0.25 h, LPS was infused continuously from t = 0 to t = 6 h. In the Control-LPS group (*filled circles*), the prophylactic infusion was replaced by modified gelatin solution. In the 75-ApoLipo-Control group (*open triangles*), the LPS infusion was replaced by saline. Significant (*p* < 0.05) differences (ApoLipo treated versus Control-LPS group) are indicated by *

The changes in leukocyte count are shown in Fig. 1d. Baseline leukocyte count was $6.3 \pm 0.4 \times 10^6$/ml. In the 75-ApoLipo-Control group, the leukocyte count did not stay at baseline level, but rose to $165 \pm 18\%$ of the baseline count after 2 h of saline infusion (2 h 15 min after the ApoLipo infusion), then slowly decreased towards baseline levels. In the Control-LPS group, the leukocyte count dropped immediately upon the start of endotoxin infusion, reaching a minimum of $24 \pm 3\%$ at 4 h. Significant differences from Control-LPS animals were only observed with 250 mg/kg of ApoLipo, where leukocyte counts at 30 min and 1 h of LPS infusion were significantly higher.

The patterns of thrombocyte count are shown in Fig. 1c. Baseline thrombocyte count was $524 \pm 31 \times 10^6$/ml. In contrast to the leukocyte count, the Apo-Control group showed no significant change from baseline count throughout the experiment. In the Control-LPS group, thrombocyte count decreased steadily with endotoxin infusion, reaching $44 \pm 4\%$ of the baseline count at 6 h. The thrombocyte count also dropped in the 75-ApoLipo group, but significantly less ($71 \pm 8\%$ of baseline at 6 h). The 250-ApoLipo-LPS showed no significant change in thrombocyte count as compared to baseline; at 2-, 4- and 6 h it was significantly higher than in the Control-LPS group.

Other measured parameters showed no significant differences between groups. Pyrogenicity and the classic hemodynamic changes mediated by LPS were not observed, since these parameters are markedly influenced by anesthesia.

Discussion

The TNF profiles observed in this study are consistent with values reported by Mathison [2] after bolus injections of parent- and plasma-altered LPS. The depression of TNF production by prophylactic infusion of ApoLipo was associated with an attenuation of the acidosis, confirming the role of TNF in the metabolic changes leading to acidosis in endotoxemia [3, 4]. Prophylactic infusion of ApoLipo also decreased the LPS-induced thrombocytopenia, either by a direct effect on the thrombocytes or by inhibiting the vascular changes leading to thrombocyte adherence. Though the endotoxin-induced leukopenia was not reduced, it was delayed by high doses of ApoLipo. Since LPS was infused continuously, this suggests that a higher amount of LPS was required. ApoLipo seems to be more efficacious in preventing the stimulation of macrophages and thrombocytes by LPS than that of polymorphonuclear neutrophils (PMNs) and other leukocytes. In contrast, the inactivation of LPS by high-density lipoprotein (HDL) is particularly efficacious for preventing neutropenia [1].

The inactivation of LPS by the formation of LPS-HDL complexes is a slow phenomenon generally requiring 3–6 h incubation [5], though Harris [6] observed a loss of LPS activity (statistically not significant) when an LPS lipoprotein mixture was injected into mice without any incubation. In the present study, the inactivation of LPS by ApoLipo did not require a prolonged incubation, which is consistent with all our in vitro data [7]. It remains to be investigated whether the mechanism of LPS inactivation by ApoLipo is the rapid formation of LPS-ApoLipo complexes (which are then slightly different from LPS-HDL complexes) or if an entirely different mechanism is operative. Studies investigating the interaction between ApoLipo, LPS, and various cell types are currently in progress.

In the present study, using a fully anesthetized model and a small number of animals, we were able to show a significant amelioration in some clinically important pathophysiologic changes associated with endotoxemic or septic shock by prophylactic infusion of ApoLipo. Further studies are needed to determine its effects on survival and to assess if it can also be used as a curative treatment, before it can be considered for clinical use.

References

1. Ulevitch RJ and Tobias PS (1988) Interactions of bacterial lipopolysaccharide with serum proteins. In: Levin J, ten Cate JW, Büller HR, vanDeventer SJ, Sturk A (eds) Bacterial endotoxins: pathophysiological effects, clinical significance, and pharmacological control. New York, Liss, pp 319–325
2. Mathison JC, Wolfson E, Ulevitch RJ (1988) Participation of tumor necrosis factor in the mediation of gram-negative bacterial lipopolysaccharide-induced injury in rabbit. J Clin Invest 81:1925–1937
3. Tracey KJ, Lowry SF, Fahey TJ, Albert JD, Fong Y, Hesse D, Beutler B, Manogue KR, Calvano S, Wei H, Ceramy A, Shires GT (1987) Cachectin/tumor necrosis factor induces lethal shock and stress hormone responses in the dog. Surg Gynecol obstet 164:415–422
4. Tredget EE, Yu YM, Zhong S, Burini R, Okusava S, Gelfand JA, Dinarello CA, Young VR, Burke JF (1988) Role of interleukin-I and tumor necrosis factor on energy metabolism in rabbit. Am J Physiol 255:E706–E768
5. Flegel WA, Wölpl A, Männel DN, Northoff H (1989) Inhibition of endotoxin-induced activation of human monocytes by human lipoproteins. Infect Immun 57:2237–2245
6. Harris HW, Grunfeld C, Feingold KR, Rapp JH (1990) Human very low density lipoproteins and chylomicrons can protect against endotoxin-induced death in mice. J Clin Invest 86:696–702
7. Doran JE, Lerch PG, Hubsch AP, Hodler, Morgenthaler JJ, Heiniger HJ (1991) In vitro modulation of tumor necrosis factor alpha production by an artificial lipoprotein enriched in apolipoprotein A-I but not by apolipoprotein A-I alone. 2nd international congress on the immune consequences of trauma, shock and sepsis, Munich

Escherichia coli-Induced Septic Shock in the Baboon: An Animal Model for the Evaluation of Neutralising Monoclonal Antibodies to Phospholipase A$_2$

R. Buchta[1], J. A. Green[1], G. M. Smith[1], C. Gabelish[1], D. Cairns[1], C. Salom[1], M. Conte[1], P. Mackie[1], R. Sublett[2], F. B. Taylor[3], I. A. Rajkovic[1], and K. F. Scott[1, 4]

Introduction

Phospholipase A$_2$ (PLA$_2$) is a soluble enzyme which is present in both intra- and extracellular compartments (Van den Bosch 1980; Vadas and Pruzanski 1986). A secretory phospholipase A$_2$ activity is clinically associated with onset and progression of sepsis and septic shock in humans (Vadas 1984; Vadas et al. 1988). We have identified this enzyme as a low molecular weight PLA$_2$, identical to that associated with rheumatoid arthritis (Green et al. 1991). The enzyme is proinflammatory and when infused into the circulation of animals induces the haemodynamic effects characteristic of severe bacterial infection and septic shock (Vadas and Hay 1983). It is therefore a potential target for monoclonal antibody therapy directed towards later stages of sepsis and shock.

We have expressed PLA$_2$ in mammalian cells and used this recombinant material to raise monoclonal antibodies for screening in inhibition assays. To establish the efficacy of these antibodies in vivo, prior to initiation of clinical trials, a suitable preclinical animal model would be of great value. The model of choice is limited by the species specificity of the monoclonal antibodies.

Materials and Methods

Blood samples were taken at regular intervals from anaesthetised baboons which have been infused with *Escherichia coli* organisms.

Murine monoclonal antibodies were raised against recombinant human inflammatory PLA$_2$ using standard immunisation and fusion protocols. Hybridomas were initially screened for production of specific monoclonal antibodies with a direct ELISA procedure.

[1] Pacific Biotechnology Ltd., 74 McLachlan Ave, Rushcutters Bay, NSW 2011, Australia.
[2] R. W. Johnson Pharmaceutical Research Institute, 4245 Sorrento Valley Boulevard, San Diego, CA 92121, USA
[3] Oklahoma Medical Research Foundation, 825 Northeast 13th St., Oklahoma City, OK 73104, USA
[4] New address: Garvon 'Institute of Medical Research, 384 Victoria Street, Darlinghurst, NSW 2010, Australia

Host Defense Dysfunction
in Trauma, Shock and Sepsis
Eds. Faist/Meakins/Schildberg
© Springer-Verlag, Berlin Heidelberg 1993

PLA$_2$ enzymatic activity in plasma samples was measured using either ^{14}C-labelled synthetic substrate or ^{14}C-labelled *E. coli* membrane preparations. The activity was expressed as a percentage of hydrolysis (Green et al., 1991).

Level of immunoreactive PLA$_2$ in plasma samples (1/10 dilution) was measured by a specific two-site ELISA using monoclonal antibodies which recognize distinct epitopes on the PLA$_2$ molecule (Smith et al., 1992).

The ability of monoclonal antibodies to inhibit PLA$_2$ activity in baboon serum was assessed by incubating serial dilutions of baboon plasma for 1 h with excess concentration of selected antibodies. The residual PLA$_2$ activity in these samples was then measured using the enzyme activity assay described above.

Results and Discussion

Candidate-neutralising antibodies have been identified based on their ability to inhibit recombinant PLA$_2$ in both the mixed-micelle activity assay, using a ^{14}C-labelled synthetic substrate (data not shown), and the *E. coli* membrane hydrolysis assay. Importantly, the selected antibodies were also able to neutralise the PLA$_2$ activity in human septic shock plasma (Green et al. 1991).

We have assessed the binding of our monoclonal antibodies to PLA$_2$s from human and porcine pancreas and snake venom (*Crotalus atrox* and *Crotalus durissus*) and found no cross-reactivity (Table 1). While the tertiary structure of PLA$_2$ is conserved across species, there is sufficient primary sequence variability between species to explain the unique specificity of antibodies described here for human inflammatory PLA$_2$.

Using a two-site ELISA system, developed for measuring PLA$_2$ levels in human plasma, we have assayed immunoreactive PLA$_2$ levels in an *E. coli*-induced septic shock model in baboons. In this model our antibodies were able

Table 1. Specificity of monoclonal antibodies to PLA$_2$

Different PLA$_2$s	Monoclonal antibodies					
	1	2	3	4	5	6
riPLA$_2$	+	+	+	+	+	+
Porcine pancreatic PLA$_2$	−	−	−	−	−	−
C. atrox PLA$_2$	−	−	−	−	−	−
C. durissus PLA$_2$	−	−	−	−	−	−
Human pancreatic PLA$_2$	−	−	−	−	−	−
Isotype	G$_1$	G$_1$	G$_1$	G$_1$	G$_1$	M

The ability of monoclonal antibodies (1–6) raised against recombinant human inflammatory PLA$_2$ (riPLA$_2$), to bind to different PLA$_2$ was assessed in a direct ELISA system using alkaline phosphatase-conjugated anti-murine second antibody.

to detect immunoreactive PLA$_2$ in the plasma. A time course analysis shows that both PLA$_2$ activity, as measured by the mixed-micelle assay (data not shown), and PLA$_2$ concentration, as measured by the ELISA (Fig. 1), became elevated from 3 to 10 h after *E. coli* infusion and remained elevated over the entire course of shock. Those monoclonal antibodies which neutralised human inflammatory PLA$_2$ also showed inhibition of baboon PLA$_2$ in both the mixed-micelle assay (data not shown) and the *E. coli* membrane assay (Fig. 2).

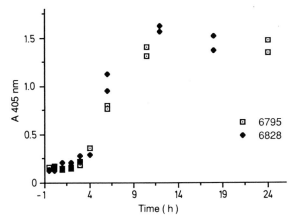

Fig. 1. Profile of plasma PLA$_2$ in the baboon model. Immunoreactive PLA$_2$ levels were measured in samples of baboon plasma over a period of 24 h. Monoclonal antibodies raised against recombinant human inflammatory PLA$_2$ were used in a specific two-site ELISA system. Relative levels of plasma PLA$_2$, shown here for two baboons (*6795* and *6828*), are expressed in ELISA absorbance units at 405 nm

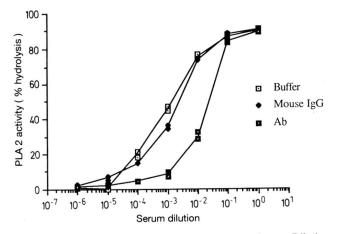

Fig. 2. Neutralisation of PLA$_2$ activity in baboon plasma. Dilutions of baboon plasma were incubated for 1 h with excess concentrations of antibodies (100 µg/ml). The residual PLA$_2$ activity in the samples was then measured in the ^{14}C-labelled synthetic substrate activity assay. Control mouse IgG was used at the same concentration as the test antibody

We conclude from these studies that neutralising antibodies raised to human inflammatory PLA_2 are capable of binding to and neutralising the PLA_2 activity generated in the plasma of baboons infused with *E. coli*. Measurement of PLA_2 activity and relative concentration in baboon plasma over the time course of septic shock establishes that PLA_2 activity is detectable after the onset of tumour necrosis factor elevation and prior to the tissue damage phase of shock in this model. The baboon will, therefore, provide a suitable preclinical model for the evaluation of monoclonal antibody therapy targeted towards neutralising the PLA_2 activity associated with septic shock.

References

Green JA, Smith GM, Buchta R, Lee R, Ho KY, Rajkovic IA, Scott KF (1991) The circulating phospholipase A_2 activity associated with sepsis is indistinguishable from that associated with rheumatoid arthritis. Inflammation 15:355–367

Smith GM, Ward RL, McGuigan L, Rajkovic IA, Scott KF (1992) Measurement of human phospholipase A_2 in arthritis plasma using a newly developed sandwich ELISA. Br J Rheumatol 31:175–178

Vadas P (1984) Plasma phospholipase A_2 levels correlate with the hemodynamic and pulmonary changes in Gram negative septic shock in man. J Lab Clin Med 104:873–881

Vadas P, Hay JB (1983) Involvement of circulating phospholipase A_2 in the pathogenesis of the hemodynamic changes in endotoxin shock. Can J Physiol Pharmacol 61:561–566

Vadas P, Pruzanski W (1986) Biology of disease. Role of secretory phospholipase A_2 in the pathobiology of disease. Lab Invest 55:391–404

Vadas P, Pruzanski W, Stefanski E (1988) Pathogenesis of hypotension in septic shock: correlation of circulatory phospholipase A_2 levels with circulatory collapse. Crit Care Med 16:1–7

Van den Bosch H (1980) Intracellular phospholipase A. Biochim Biophys Acta 606:191–246

Leukotriene Inhibitor and Antagonist Prevent Endotoxin Lethality in Carrageenan-Pretreated Mice

O. Masanori[1], K. Masayuki[1], Y. Shin-Ichi[2], M. Yasuo[2], and A. Shigematsu[1]

Introduction

Tumor necrosis factor (TNF) is a major cytokine which mediates endotoxin shock and causes multiple organ damage. Carrageenan (CAR), a sulfated polygalactose, is used as a macrophage blocker. We found that CAR pretreatment can enhance both lipopolysaccharide (LPS) induced TNF production and the rate of lethality in mice [1]. We postulated that inflammation plays a role in the mechanism of enhanced LPS-induced TNF production and lethality by CAR pretreatment because CAR is used not only as a macrophage blocker but also as an inflammatory agent. Recently it has been reported that leukotriene (LT) inhibitors suppress the LPS-induced TNF production and lethality in galactosamine-treated mice [2]. We therefore investigated the effect of 5-lipooxygenase inhibitor and LTC_4D_4 antagonist on LPS-induced TNF production and lethality in CAR-pretreated mice.

Materials and Methods

The ddY mice (6–7 weeks old) were injected intraperitoneally with CAR (5 mg/head). The various doses of 5-lipooxygenase inhibitor (AA-861, Takeda Pharmacoceutical), LTC_4D_4 antagonist (ONO 1078, Ono Pharmacoceutical), or saline (control) were administrated subcutaneously 23 h after CAR pretreatment. LPS was injected intravenously 24 h after CAR pretreatment. Two hours after LPS injection, sera were obtained from the mice for TNF assay in which L929 cytotoxicity was used. The lethality of mice was recorded up to 72 h.

Results

Either AA-861 (20 mmol/kg) or ONO-1078 (40 mmol/kg) significantly increased the survival rate after LPS (50 µg) administration in comparison with the control group. (Table 1); the Kaplan-Meier statistical method showed

[1] Department of Anesthesiology and [2] Department of Microbiology, School of Med., Univ. of Occup. and Envir. Health, 1-1 Jscigaoka Yahatanishiku, Kitakyushu 807, Japan

Host Defense Dysfunction
in Trauma, Shock and Sepsis
Eds. Faist/Meakins/Schildberg
© Springer-Verlag, Berlin Heidelberg 1993

$p < 0.001$ for AA-861 and $p < 0.01$ for ONO-1078 (Fig. 1). A 50% lethal dose (LD_{50}) of LPS in the control mice was 30 µg/head, and this increased to 83 µg/head with AA-861 (20 mmol/kg) and to 59 µg/head with ONO-1078 (40 mmol/kg) (Fig. 2). The lethality in mice was significantly improved by AA-861 (χ^2 test, $p < 0.01$) or ONO-1078 ($p < 0.05$) (Table 1). However, we did not find a significant difference in serum TNF activity between control mice and those treated with AA-861 or ONO-1078 (Fig. 3).

Table 1. Protective effect of LT inhibitor or antagonist against the lethality of 50 µg LPS

	Lethality (dead/total)		
	1	2	Total
AA-861			
20 mmol/kg	0/10	1/10	1/20
10 mmol/kg	3/10	3/10	6/20
5 mmol/kg	4/10	4/10	8/20
ONO-1078			
40 mmol/kg	3/10	1/10	4/20
20 mmol/kg	4/10	2/10	6/20
10 mmol/kg	4/10	4/10	8/20
Indomethacin			
40 mmol/kg	9/10		9/10
Saline	8/10	7/10	15/20

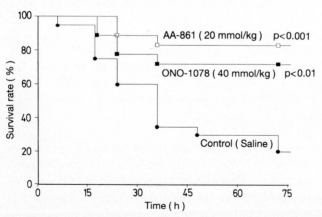

Fig. 1. Effect of LT inhibitor or antagonist on survival rate of CAR-pretreated mice after LPS (50 µg) injection. Either AA-861 (20 mmol/kg) or ONO-1078 (40 mmol/kg) increased significantly the survival rate in comparison with the control group (AA-861, $p < 0.01$; ONO-1078, $p < 0.05$; by the Kaplan Meier statistical method)

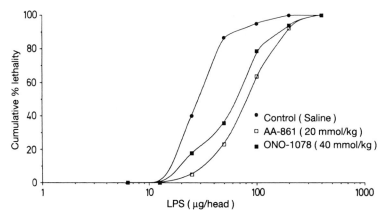

Fig. 2. Effect of LT inhibitor or antagonist on cumulative percentage lethality of CAR-pretreated mice by LPS injection. The lethality was determined 72 h after LPS administration. Each group consisted of ten ddY mice

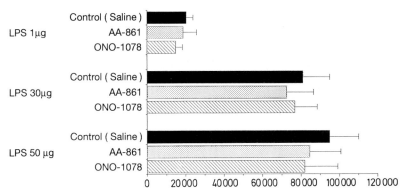

Fig. 3. Effect of LT inhibitor or antagonist on TNF activity stimulated by LPS in CAR-pretreated mice. The doses of AA-861 or ONO-1078 were 20 and 40 mmol/kg. The results are expressed as the mean $\pm$ SE for eight determinations

Discussion

We reported that CAR pretreatment can enhance both endotoxin-induced TNF production and the rate of lethality in mice. High TNF activity in sera is thought to be one of the causes that enhances the mortality rate in CAR-pretreated mice. Our results showed that AA-861 or ONO-1078 significantly suppresses the rate of LPS-induced mortality in CAR-pretreated mice. This finding is in accordance with that of Hagmann et al. who reported that LT antagonist prevents endotoxin lethality [3]. We therefore examined whether AA-861 or ONO-1078 reduces the LPS-induced TNF activity in sera of CAR-pretreated mice. Lipooxygenase products are involved in the synthesis of TNF because lipooxygenase inhibitors suppress the formation of TNF. However, our present data show that lipooxygenase inhibitor (AA-861) or LTC_4D_4 antagonist (ONO-1078) does not suppress TNF activity in serum 2 h after LPS injection. LTB_4 is one of the most potent chemoattractants of polymorphonuclear neutrophils. Granulocyte adhesion and emigration by endotoxin are considered to be due to LTB_4. On the other hand, LTC_4D_4 is well known as one of the mediators of bronchoconstriction, vascular leakage, cardiac depression. It has been shown that LPS induces production of LTs in vivo [4]. Recently it was shown that rhTNF-α directly stimulates arachidonic acid release in human neutrophil [5]. Thus LTB_4 and LTC_4D_4 are the most potent mediators of endotoxin shock. We believe that AA-861 or ONO-1078 prevents the LPS-induced lethality of CAR-pretreated mice by mainly attenuating the effect of LTB_4 and LTC_4D_4, the production of which are induced by LPS or TNF.

Conclusion

Both LT inhibitor and antagonist prevented endotoxin lethality in CAR-pretreated mice. However, we found no significant difference in serum TNF activities between control mice and those treated with AA-861 or ONO-1078. We suggest that LT is one of the important mediators in causing endotoxin shock.

References

1. Ogata M, Yoshida S, Kamochi M, Shigematsu A, Mizuguchi Y (1991) Enhancement of lipopolysaccharide-induced tumor necrosis factor production in mice by carrageenan pretreatment. Infect Immun 59:679–683
2. Schade UF, Ernst M, Reinke M, Wolter DT (1989) Lipooxygenase inhibitors suppress formation of tumor necrosis factor in vitro and in vivo. Biochem Biophys Res Commun 159:748–754
3. Hagmann W, Keppler D (1982) Leukotriene antagonists prevent endotoxin lethality. Naturwissenschaften 69:594–595
4. Hagmann W, Denzlinger C, Keppler D (1985) Production of peptide leukotrienes in endotoxin shock. FEBS Lett 180:309–313
5. Atkinson YH, Murray AW, Krilis S, Vadas MA, Lopez AF (1990) Human tumor necrosis factor-alpha (TNF-α) directly stimulates arachidonic acid release in human neutrophils. Immunology 70:82–87

Effect of Type-Specific Antiserum on the Pulmonary Hypertensive Response to Group B *Streptococcus* in Piglets

J. B. Philips, M. Chwe, J. X. Li, B. M. Gray, D. G. Pritchard, J. R. Oliver, K. Grantham, and W. Mena

Introduction

Group B streptococcal (GBS) organisms are a major cause of serious bacterial infections in newborns. Both clinical and laboratory studies have shown that GBS infection is associated with circulatory disturbances including pulmonary hypertension, which may lead to the persistent pulmonary hypertension of the newborn syndrome. Previous studies in our laboratories have shown that pretreatment of GBS organisms premixed with rabbit polyclonal type-specific antibody will augment the pulmonary hypertension seen with GBS organisms alone [1]. Since passive immunotherapy is being used clinically to treat infected infants, we thought it important to further evaluate the interaction of type-specific antigen and antibody in the cardiovascular disturbances induced by GBS sepsis. Availability of a mutant GBS organism which expresses no detectable type-specific antigen [2] allowed us to study the effect of antibody, with and without its antigen, on the cardiovascular hemodynamics of GBS infusion. We tested the hypotheses that (1) administration of encapsulated GBS organisms premixed with type-specific antibodies exacerbates the adverse effects caused by injection of GBS organisms alone, and (2) type-specific antibodies do not alter hemodynamic responses to the injection of a capsule-deficient mutant GBS organism

Materials and Methods

Six juvenile (2–4 week) piglets were acutely instrumented under halothane anesthesia for measurement of pulmonary, systemic, left atrial, and central venous pressures, along with pulmonary artery flow. Following surgery, halothane was discontinued and sedation was maintained with intermittent phenobarbital (10 mg/kg every hour).

The GBS type-Ib strain used was isolated from an infant with late onset sepsis and meningitis. This organism expresses a large amount of capsular type-

---

Departments of Pediatrics and Microbiology, University of Alabama at Birmingham, Birmingham, AL 35233-7335, USA

specific antigen, as determined by density gradient centrifiguration [3]. A capsule-deficient mutant was created from this strain by transposon insertion mutagenesis [4]. This mutant organism lacks detectable type-specific capsular polysaccharide as determined by immunodiffusion. Both organisms were grown to late-log phase in chemically defined media [5], were heat killed at 80 °C for 30 min, were washed twice, and resuspended in phosphate-buffered saline to a concentration of 1×10^9 colony forming units (cfu)/ml. Aliquots were frozen until the day of study when they were thawed and vortex mixed before use.

Antibody was made using classical methods in rabbits. This antiserum contains 2.0 mg/ml of type Ib-specific antibody as determined by enzyme-linked immunosorbant assay (ELISA) and has no hemodynamic effect when given alone (1).

For study, four different suspensions of GBS organisms were prepared. Two infusates consisted of the encapsulated and nonencapsulated GBS organisms alone; the other two were made by premixing the appropriate dose with 0.2 ml of the rabbit antiserum for 5 min with gentle shaking before injection. Each piglet was injected with 1×10^8 cfu/kg of each preparation in random order. Values were allowed to stabilize at least 5 min before the next injection.

For each variable, the preinjection value and the postinjection value at the peak of the pulmonary hypertensive response were recorded. The change (post minus pre) in each variable was calculated. The t-test was used to compared the effect of each antibody pretreated organism with its respective nontreated organism. Significance was accepted with $p \leqslant 0.05$.

Results

Addition of antibody to the encapsulated GBS organism significantly increased the intensity of the hemodynamic responses (Figs. 1 and 2). Pulmonary artery pressure was augmented by antibody, while pulmonary artery flow was reduced, and pulmonary vascular resistance increased markedly. No significant changes in systemic arterial, left atrial, or central venous pressures (not shown) were noted. Because of the large decrease in cardiac output, systemic vascular resistance increased significantly. Addition of antibody to the capsule-deficient mutant had no effect on the hemodynamic responses, when compared to the mutant alone.

Discussion

Preincubation of normally encapsulated GBS organisms with a polyclonal rabbit antiserum was found to significantly exacerbate the cardiovascular disturbances associated with bolus injection of the encapsulated GBS organisms

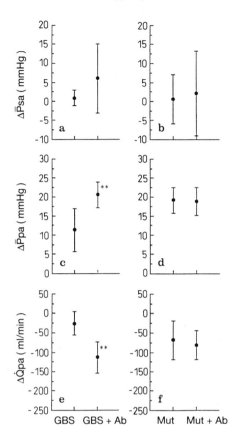

Fig. 1a–f. Effect of encapsulated infant's GBS and capsule deficient mutant GBS (*Mut*), with and without antibody (*Ab*), on the changes in mean systemic arterial pressure (*Psa*), pulmonary artery pressure (*Ppa*), and pulmonary artery flow (*Qpa*). **, $p \leqslant 0.01$ vs respective non-antibody pretreated organisms

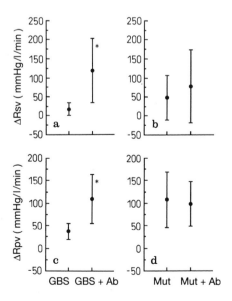

Fig. 2a–d. Effect of encapsulated infant's GBS and capsule deficient mutant GBS (*Mut*), with and without antibody (*Ab*) on the changes in mean systemic vascular resistance (*Rsv*) and pulmonary vascular resistance (*Rpv*). *, $p \leqslant 0.05$

into acutely instrumented piglets. Addition of the antiserum to a capsule-deficient mutant did not result in significant changes when compared to the effects of the mutant alone. Thus, antigen/antibody complexes appear to play a role in the intensity of the pulmonary hypertension seen with GBS sepsis, since antibody augmented the adverse effects of encapsulated GBS organisms, yet had no effect on the response to capsule-deficient organisms.

The mutant capsule-deficient organisms alone caused a pulmonary hypertensive response greater than that caused by encapsulated GBS organisms alone and similar to that caused by the encapsulated GBS organisms preincubated with antibody. This difference in responsiveness has been noted previously by us [2] and is consistent with our hypothesis that the capsular type-specific antigen partially obscures a hemodynamically active component(s) on the GBS surface.

The observation that type-specific antibody may augment the adverse effects noted with encapsulated organisms, raises the possibility that passive immunotherapy may have adverse side effects in infants with GBS sepsis. Antigen/antibody complex formation is a vital step in host defenses against bacterial invasion. Passive immunization may assist in this process, however, it remains possible that such therapy in septic infants could exacerbate ongoing circulatory derangements. Further studies will be required to determine the hemodynamic effects of administration of type-specific antibodies and other opsonins in animal models and, ultimately, in humans with established GBS sepsis.

References

1. Philips JB, Lyrene RK, Godoy G, Graybar G, Barefield E, Sams JEP, Gray BM (1988) Hemodynamic responses of chronically instrumented piglets to bolus injections of Group B Streptococci. Pediatr Res 23:81–85
2. Li J-X, Gray BM, Pritchard DG, Oliver JR, Reese JF, Philips JB (1990) Role of capsular polysaccharide in pulmonary hypertension induced by Group B Streptococcus. Pediatr Res 27:273A
3. Hakansson S, Holm S (1986) Influence of polysaccharide capsule and ionic strength on buoyant density of group B streptococci. Acta Pathol Microbiol Immunol Scand [B] 94:139–143
4. Rubens CE, Heggen LM (1988) Tn916 E: a Tn916 transposon derivative expressing erythromycin resistance. Plasmid 20:137–142
5. Van de Rijn I, Kessler RE (1980) Growth characteristics of Group A Streptococci in new chemically defined medium. Infect Immun 27:444–448

Detection of IgE Reactive With Lipopolysaccharide in Plasma of Traumatically Injured Patients

J. T. DiPiro[1], R. G. Hamilton[2], T. R. Howdieshell[1], D. Callaway[1], and N. F. Adkinson, Jr.[2]

Introduction

Gram-negative sepsis occurs commonly in patients who have sustained major traumatic injury. The study of the pathogenic mechanisms of gram-negative sepsis has focused on activation of macrophages by lipopolysaccharide and subsequent release of mediators such as interleukin-1 and tumor necrosis factor. These cytokines are believed to initiate processes which then lead to sepsis. The potential for allergic mechanisms participating in the sepsis syndrome has not been well studied. Anaphylaxis produces some manifestations that are similar to those with the sepsis syndrome. IgE-dependent activation of basophils and mast cells could potentially be involved in the sepsis syndrome. Recently, Jacobs and associates (1989) reported that blood histamine concentrations were not elevated in humans with septic shock. However, the presence of IgE reactive with bacterial products (such as lipopolysaccharide) may indicate the involvement of allergic mechanisms in this syndrome. This report presents data on anti-lipopolysaccharide IgE and total IgE in plasma of patients after major traumatic injury.

The objectives of this study were (a) to develop an enzyme immunoassay to detect IgE in plasma that is reactive with lipopolysaccharide, (b) to determine whether anti-lipopolysaccharide IgE can be detected in the plasma of patients who have sustained major traumatic injury, (c) if detected, to compare the frequency of detection of anti-lipopolysaccharide IgE in traumatically injured patients with that in healthy volunteers and patients with high total plasma IgE (> 200 ng/ml), and (d) to determine total IgE in plasma of selected patients who have sustained major traumatic injury.

Methods

Clinical Material. Plasma from three groups of subjects were selected from plasma banks of the investigators for study. The three groups included 35 healthy control subjects, 270 nontrauma patients known to have elevated total

---

[1] University of Georgia College of Pharmacy and the Medical College of Georgia, Room F1-1087 Department of Surgery, 1120 Fifteenth St., Augusta, GA 30912, USA
[2] Johns Hopkins University Asthma and Allergy Center, Baltimore, MD 21218, USA

Host Defense Dysfunction
in Trauma, Shock and Sepsis
Eds. Faist/Meakins/Schildberg
© Springer-Verlag, Berlin Heidelberg 1993

IgE (range 200–1700 ng/ml), and 32 patients who had sustained major traumatic injury (American College of Surgeons Trauma Score of greater than or equal to 10).

Assays of IgE. The enzyme immunoassay used to detect anti-lipopolysaccharide reactive IgE consisted of a murine monoclonal capture antibody (HP 6061) specific for human IgE (Fc) which was added at a dilution of 1:1000 to polystrene microtiter plates (Immulon 4, Dynatech) and incubated overnight. The antibody was nonreactive with human IgG and IgM. The plate was blocked with 0.5% bovine serum albumin; then subject plasma was added for 1 h. Biotinylated lipopolysaccharide (prepared by the investigators with lipopolysaccharide from the *Escherichia coli* J5 mutant) was then added and incubated at room temperature for 2 h. The system was developed with streptavidin-peroxidase conjugate and 2,2′-azinobis(3-ethylbenz) thiazoline sulfonic acid (ABTS) as substrate. The wells were read at 410 nm. Values were reported as absorbance and titers. A highly reactive anti-lipopolysaccharide IgE serum sample from a non-trauma patient (C-8097) was used as the positive control. The intraday coefficient of variation was less than 8%.

Inhibition of the anti-lipopolysaccharide IgE enzyme immunoassay with nonbiotinylated lipopolysaccharide was tested using sera from three patients (two traumatically injured patients and one nontrauma patient; Fig. 1). Immunoreactivity of biotinylated lipopolysaccharide was confirmed using two murine monoclonal anti-lipopolysaccharide antibodies (supplied courtesy of Dr. Martin Evans and Dr. Matthew Pollack, Uniformed Services University, Bethesda, MD). One antibody (J18-8D2) is known to be reactive with lipopolysaccharide core and lipid A regions while the other (042E1) is specific for the O chain of *E. coli*—0111 B4 (Fig. 2).

Total IgE in plasma was determined using an automated microparticle enzyme immunoassay (IMx, Abbott Diagnostics). Determinations were performed to ten trauma patients only.

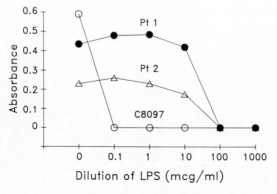

Fig. 1. Inhibition test of selected plasma determined to be positive for anti-lipopolysaccharide reactive IgE. Patients 1 and 2 were traumatically injured patients while C-8097 was a nontrauma patient with high total IgE

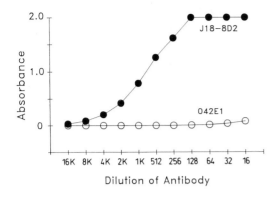

Fig. 2. Demonstration of the immunoreactivity of biotinylated lipopolysaccharide. Plates were coated with monoclonal antibody J18-8D2 which is known to be reactive with core and lipid A regions or with 042E1 which is known to be O chain specific

In the 32 traumatically injured patients who were studied, the mean age was 33 years ($\pm$ 8.2 years); there were 29 men and 3 women. Sepsis was observed in 17 patients.

Results

Anti-lipopolysaccharide reactive IgE was detected in serum from 17 of 32 trauma patients (53%), one of 35 healthy control subjects (3%), and three of 270 nontrauma patients with high total plasma IgE (1%). In subjects that had plasma positive for anti-lipopolysaccharide IgE the titers ranged from 1:2 to 1:32 in the trauma patients and healthy control patient, and from 1:2 to 1:28 in the nontrauma patients with high IgE.

The presence of anti-lipopolysaccharide IgE was not predictive of sepsis as it was detected in 47% of septic and 60% of nonseptic trauma patients. Also, it was not related to age or admission trauma score. In most patients, when anti-lipopolysaccharide IgE was detected it was positive within the first 48 h after admission.

Plasma from ten traumatically injured patients (4 samples each) was submitted for total plasma IgE determination. Of these samples, one patient had total IgE concentration less than 100 ng/ml (under the 75th percentile) while three patients had concentrations of 100–500 ng/ml (76th–98th percentiles), and six had concentrations greater than 500 ng/ml (over the 99th percentile).

Conclusions

IgE immunoreactive with lipopolysaccharide (*E. coli* J5 mutant) was detected in plasma from 53% of patients after major traumatic injury. Also, high total IgE concentrations (above the 99th percentile) were determined in six of ten trauma patients. The presence of lipopolysaccharide-specific IgE in some trauma patients and high total IgE in others presents the possibility that allergic/anaphylactic mechanisms may be activated following injury or sepsis and may participate in pathophysiologic syndromes experienced by trauma patients. Association of IgE activity with clinical events requires analysis of additional information including determinations of anti-lipopolysaccharide IgG and IgM and indicators of basophil and mast cell activation.

Reference

Jacobs R, Kaliner M, Shelhamer JH, Parrillo JE (1989) Blood histamine concentrations are not elevated in humans with septic shock. Crit Care Med 17:30–35

Altered Guanine Nucleotide Protein Function: Potential Role in Endotoxin Tolerance

K. Coffee[1], P. V. Halushka[2], W. C. Wise[1], and J. A. Cook[1]

Endotoxin stimulates macrophages to synthesize and release a number of monokines including tumor necrosis factor (TNF), colony stimulating factor, platelet-activating factor, interleukin-1 (IL-1) and arachidonic acid metabolites [1–8]. In recent years arachidonic acid metabolites or eicosanoids, a group of inflammatory mediators, have generated considerable interest [9–14]. Arachidonic acid is esterified in the 2-position of specific cellular phospholipids including phosphatidylcholine (PC), phosphatidyl-ethanolamine (PE), and phosphatidylinositol (PI) [15–19]. The generation of free arachidonic acid from phospholipids is thought to be a rate-limiting step in the formation of arachidonic acid metabolites [20]. Endotoxin-stimulated cells mobilize their phospholipids through at least two major pathways [21]. In the first pathway, phospholipase C cleaves phosphatidylinositol 4,5-biphosphate, yielding inositol-1,4,5-triphosphate (IP_3) and 1,2-diacylglycerol, both of which are second messengers [22–25]. IP_3 mobilizes cytoplasmic calcium while 1,2-diacylglycerol stimulates protein kinase C [26–28]. A separate diglyceride lipase cleaves arachidonic acid from the diacylglycerol molecule [29, 30]. In the second pathway, phospholipase A_2 (PLA_2) directly releases arachidonic acid and other unsaturated fatty acids from phospholipids including PC, PE, and PI. Rogers et al. [31, 32] observed significant depletion of [^{14}C] arachidonic acid from PC, PI, and PE phospholipid pools in endotoxin-stimulated macrophages, suggesting that endotoxin either directly or indirectly stimulates PLA_2. Free arachidonic acid is further metabolized by fatty acid cyclooxygenase, forming several metabolites including thromboxane A_2 (TXA_2), prostaglandins E and F (PGE_2, $PGF_{2\alpha}$), and prostacyclin (PGI_2). The other major pathway of arachidonic acid metabolism gives rise to the lipoxygenase products [33].

The mechanisms linking extracellular endotoxin to arachidonic acid metabolism remain unclear. A putative cell surface endotoxin receptor has been postulated [34–37]. Indications are, however, that the cell receptor is not directly linked to phospholipid turnover, but acts through an intermediate guanine nucleotide binding protein. These G regulatory proteins, cellular membrane proteins which hydrolyze guanosine triphosphate, serve as transducers of external signals [38]. The G regulatory proteins participate in a

Departments of Physiology[1], Pharmacology and Medicine[2], Medical University of South Carolina, 171 Ashley Avenue, Charleston, SC 29425, USA

Host Defense Dysfunction
in Trauma, Shock and Sepsis
Eds. Faist/Meakins/Schildberg
© Springer-Verlag, Berlin Heidelberg 1993

number of cellular activation states including hormonal stimulation or inhibition of adenylate cyclase, transducin coupled light activation of rhodopsin to stimulation of cGMP phosphodiesterase activity, and ligand-receptor interactions leading to increased arachidonic acid metabolism [39–41]. Certain GTP-binding proteins are targets of bacterial exotoxin-induced ADP ribosylation. Cholera toxin, using NAD as a substrate, ADP-ribosylates an arginine residue in the α subunit of G_S rendering it irreversibly active, whereas pertussis toxin ADP-ribosylates a cysteinyl residue close to the carboxy end of the α subunit of G_i resulting in loss of function [42]. In addition to G_S and G_i, G_T is ADP-ribosylated by cholera toxin [43], and G_o and G_T are the substrates of pertussis toxin [39, 44, 45].

Evidence of G protein involvement in phospholipase activation stems from studies reporting inhibition of arachidonic acid release from a variety of cells. Specifically, pretreatment with pertussis toxin reduces the release of arachidonic acid by compound 48/80 in mast cells [46], fMet-Leu-Phe in neutrophils [47, 48], thrombin in fibroblasts [49], and norepinephrine in FRTL5 thyroid cells [50]. In addition, evidence for G protein involvement in endotoxin activation is suggested from pertussis toxin inhibition of endotoxin-induced PGE_2 formation in mesangial cells [51] and IL-1 release in P388D1 cells [52] and U937 cells [53]. Many of these stimuli which activate PLA_2 induce the release of arachidonic acid from phospholipids, which results in the formation of metabolites derived from the cyclooxygenase and lipoxygenase pathways. These data are highly suggestive of G protein involvement in the transduction of signals that activate phospholipase C and/or PLA_2 [52, 54].

One experimental approach used to delineate important host defense mechanisms to endotoxin has been through the induction of endotoxin tolerance [55]. Endotoxin tolerance, induced by administering increasing sublethal injections of endotoxin, results in an acquired resistance to otherwise supralethal doses of endotoxin [56–60]. Within 24 h after a single dose of endotoxin, animals exhibit a marked cross-tolerance to a variety of other forms of shock including drum trauma, hemorrhagic shock, epinephrine shock, and oxygen toxicity [61–65]. This early tolerance does not seem to be associated with any humoral factor since it cannot be transferred passively [57, 59, 64, 65].

Previous studies have demonstrated increased plasma thromboxane B_2 (TXB_2) and 6-keto-$PGF_{1\alpha}$ in rats in response to endotoxin [66]. Tolerant rats, however, exhibit reduced plasma levels of these eicosanoids. Macrophage arachidonic acid metabolism is also altered during endotoxin tolerance. Endotoxin stimulation of TXB_2 and 6-keto-$PGF_{1\alpha}$ in vitro by peritoneal macrophages synthesis from tolerant rats is significantly suppressed (Fig. 1). The decreased endotoxin stimulation of arachidonic acid metabolism in peritoneal macrophages from tolerant rats cannot be attributed to decreased arachidonic acid substrate [67]. Macrophages from tolerant rats stimulated with calcium ionophore (A23187) produce increased amounts of TXB_2, PGE_2, and leukotrienes LTC_4/LTD_4 but decreased amounts of 6-keto-$PGF_{1\alpha}$ compared with cells from control rats (Figs. 2, 3). The desensitized response to endotoxin, thus,

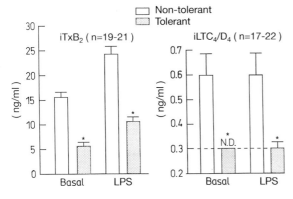

Fig. 1. Endotoxin (LPS, 50 µg/ml)-stimulated iTXB₂ and iLTC₄/D₄ production by endotoxin-tolerant and nontolerant rat peritoneal macrophages. *Bars* represent mean ± SEM. *Numbers in parentheses* represent number of plates per group. Cells were diluted to 1×10^6/ml and incubated for 3 h with endotoxin. *$P < 0.05$ compared with nontolerant macrophages. (From [32])

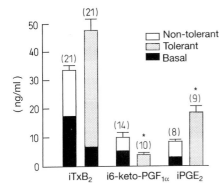

Fig. 2. A23187-stimulated iTXB₂·, i6-keto-PGF₁ₐ·, and iPGE₂ production by endotoxin-tolerant and nontolerant rat peritoneal macrophages. *Bars* represent mean ± SEM. *Numbers in parentheses* represent number of plates per group. Cells were diluted to 1×10^6/ml and incubated for 3 h in A23187 (1µM). *$P < 0.05$ compared with nontolerant macrophages. (From [32])

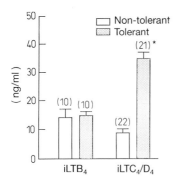

Fig. 3. A23187-stimulated immunoreactive (i)LTB₄ and iLTC₄/D₄ production by endotoxin-tolerant and nontolerant rat peritoneal macrophages. *Bars* represent mean ± SEM. *Numbers in parentheses* represent number of plates per group. Cells were diluted to 1×10^6/ml and incubated for 3 h in A23187 (1µM). *$P < 0.05$ compared with nontolerant macrophages. (From [32])

may be due to changes in endotoxin receptors or early postreceptor coupling events. These results bear similarities to reports of endotoxin desensitization leading to decreased TNF production. Zuckerman et al. [68] reported that murine macrophages exposed to endotoxin either in vivo or in vitro respond to an initial challenge with endotoxin by producing significant amounts of TNF; whereas macrophages exposed to a second endotoxin stimulus are refractory, exhibiting significantly reduced amounts of TNF release [68]. This refractory response was not evident when zymosan was used as a stimulus. Virca et al. [69] also demonstrated reduced endotoxin-stimulated TNF production from RAW 264.7 cells pretreated with a low concentration (10 ng/ml) of endotoxin.

We examined the potential role of G proteins in endotoxin-stimulated arachidonic acid release and metabolism in control macrophages and in macrophages from endotoxin-tolerant rats. Specifically, the effect of the modulators of G protein function, cholera and pertussis toxins, and the stable GTP analogue GTP-[γ-S], on endotoxin-stimulated macrophage arachidonic acid metabolism to intracellular TXB_2 ($iTXB_2$) was assessed.

Endotoxin stimulated a seven fold increase in $iTXB_2$ and a four fold increase in intracellular 6-keto-$PGF_{1\alpha}$ (i6-keto-$PGF_{1\alpha}$) concentrations compared with basal values ($P < 0.05$) in control macrophages (Fig. 4a,b).Pretreatment of control macrophages with pertussis toxin at concentrations of 0.1, 1.0, and 10 ng/ml resulted in a 55%, 44%, and 19% inhibition of endotoxin $iTXB_2$ synthesis, respectively ($P < 0.05$). Pertussis toxin produced a 64%, 77%, and 62% inhibition of endotoxin-stimulated i6-keto-$PGF_{1\alpha}$ synthesis at concentrations of 0.1, 1.0, and 10.0 ng/ml, respectively ($P < 0.05$). In tolerant macrophages, endotoxin stimulated only a 2.5-fold increase in $iTXB_2$ concentrations compared with basal values ($P < 0.05$;Fig. 4a), and stimulated significantly less $iTXB_2$ synthesis compared with control macrophages in response to endotoxin (15.6 ± 2.7 ng/ml vs 1.6 ± 0.09 ng/ml; $P < 0.05$). Pretreatment of tolerant macrophages with pertussis toxin at 0.1, 1.0, and 10 ng/ml resulted in minimal inhibition of $iTXB_2$ synthesis, respectively ($P < 0.05$). This inhibition observed

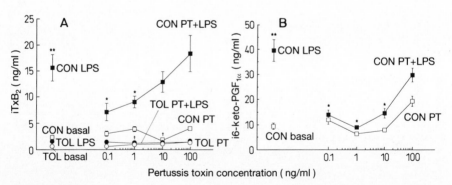

Pertussis toxin concentration (ng/ml)

Fig. 4.A. $iTXB_2$ concentrations from endotoxin-stimulated control (*CON*) and tolerant (*TOL*) macrophages pretreated with varying doses of pertussis toxin. Cells were stimulated with endotoxin following 4-h pretreatment with pertussis toxin. Macrophages were exposed to media (*BASAL*), endotoxin (*LPS*;50 µg/ml), pretreatment with pertussis toxin (*PT*;0.1–100 ng/ml), or pertussis toxin pretreatment plus endotoxin (*PT + LPS*). Data are expressed as Mean ± SEM, $n = 5$/group. *$P < 0.05$ compared with CON LPS as determined by Fisher's PLSD; **$P < 0.05$ compared with CON BASAL and TOL LPS as determined by Fisher's PLSD; †$P < 0.05$ compared with TOL LPS as determined by Fisher's PLSD. **B** i6-keto-$PGF_{1\alpha}$ concentrations from endotoxin-stimulated control (*CON*) and tolerant (*TOL*) macrophages pretreated with varying doses of pertussis toxin. See legend for Fig. 1A for details. (From [81])

in tolerant macrophages at pertussis toxin concentrations of 0.1, 1.0, and 10 ng/ml represents a decrease of only 0.2, 0.5, and 0.4 ng/ml versus 8.6, 6.7, and 2.9 ng/ml, respectively, in control macrophages.

Cholera toxin did not alter the basal concentrations of iTXB$_2$ or i6-keto-PGF$_{1\alpha}$ in control macrophages (Fig. 5a,b). Cholera toxin at 100 ng/ml and 1000 ng/ml enhanced endotoxin-stimulated iTXB$_2$ and i6-keto-PGF$_{1\alpha}$ concentrations in control macrophages ($P < 0.05$). Cholera toxin pretreatment did not alter the basal concentrations of iTXB$_2$ in tolerant macrophages at any of the concentrations employed. Cholera toxin at 100 ng/ml and 1000 ng/ml also enhanced endotoxin-stimulated iTXB$_2$ concentrations in tolerant macrophages ($P < 0.05$). However, the increase was significantly less ($P < 0.05$) in tolerant macrophages compared with control macrophages (15.4 ng/ml and 18.7 ng/ml increase in iTXB$_2$ in control cells at cholera toxin concentrations of 100 ng/ml and 1000 ng/ml respectively vs 3.19 ng/ml and 2.87 ng/ml increase in iTXB$_2$ in tolerant macrophages). Pretreatment with the B protomer of cholera toxin, which binds nonspecifically to the cell membrane, at the same concentration as the holotoxin had no effect to endotoxin-stimulated i6-keto-PGF$_{1\alpha}$ or iTXB$_2$ (data not shown). Since i6-keto-PGF$_{1\alpha}$ paralleled iTXB$_2$ production in control macrophages, only iTXB$_2$ was determined in subsequent studies involving control and tolerant macrophages treated with GTP-[γ-S].

In control macrophages, GTP-[γ-S] (100 μM) incorporation significantly ($P < 0.05$) stimulated iTXB$_2$ synthesis (Fig. 6). This concentration of GTP-[γ-S] used in the present study has been reported to have a stimulatory effect on G proteins and supports other data reporting GTP-[γ-S]-induced release of

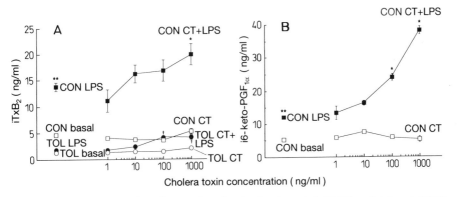

Cholera toxin concentration (ng/ml)

Fig. 5.A. iTXB$_2$ concentrations from endotoxin-stimulated control (*CON*) and tolerant (*TOL*) macrophages pretreated with varying doses of cholera toxin. Cells were stimulated with endotoxin following 4-h pretreatment with cholera toxin. Macrophages were exposed to media (*BASAL*), endotoxin (*LPS*;50 µg/ml), pretreatment with cholera toxin (*CT*;1.0–1000 ng/ml), or CT pretreatment plus endotoxin (*CT + LPS*). Data are expressed as Mean $\pm$ SEM, $n = 5$/group. *$P < 0.05$ compared to CON LPS as determined by Fisher's PLSD; **$P < 0.05$ compared to CON BASAL and TOL LPS as determined by Fisher's PLSD; †$P < 0.05$ compared to TOL LPS as determined by Fisher's PLSD. B i6-keto-PGF$_{1\alpha}$) concentrations from endotoxin-stimulated control (*CON*) and tolerant (*TOL*) macrophages pretreated with varying doses of cholera toxin. See legend for Fig. 2 for details. (From [81])

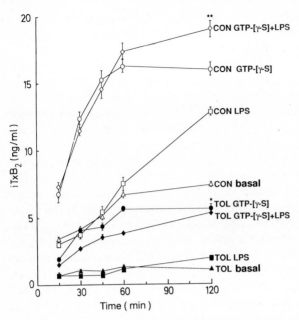

Fig. 6. GTP-[γ-S]-induced iTXB$_2$ synthesis in control (*CON*) and tolerant (*TOL*) macrophages following endotoxin stimulation. Macrophages underwent hypo-osmotic shock treatment (*BASAL*) containing GTP-[γ-S] (100 μM). Cells were stimulated with endotoxin (50 μg/ml) (*LPS*, GTP-[γ-S] + LPS) and aliquots taken at the designated time intervals for iTXB$_2$ quantitation by radioimmunoassay. Data are expressed as mean ± SEM, $n = 5$–8/group. *$P < 0.05$, control vs tolerant as determined by analysis of variance; **$P < 0.05$ GTP-[γ-S] + LPS vs GTP-[γ-S] as determined by Fisher's PLSD. (From [81])

arachidonic acid [70, 71]. The rate of GTP-[γ-S]-stimulated iTXB$_2$ synthesis was significantly greater in control compared with tolerant macrophages. The GTP-[γ-S]-stimulated amounts of iTXB$_2$ were also significantly higher in control macrophages compared with tolerant macrophages ($P < 0.05$). There was no significant difference in iTXB$_2$ concentrations from 15 to 60 min between macrophages treated with GTP-[γ-S] alone and macrophages treated with GTP-[γ-S] and stimulated with endotoxin (Fig. 6). However, endotoxin in combination with GTP-[γ-S] significantly ($P < 0.05$) increased iTXB$_2$ levels above cells treated with GTP-[γ-S] or endotoxin alone at 120 min in control macrophages but not in tolerant macrophages.

This study provides evidence that:(1) endotoxin-induced arachidonic acid metabolism in resident rat peritoneal macrophages may be mediated via G protein(s), and (2) endotoxin tolerance alters arachidonic acid metabolism in response to modulators of G protein activity. Pertussis toxin blocked endotoxin-stimulated production of iTXB$_2$ and i6-keto-PGF$_{1\alpha}$ whereas cholera toxin enhanced endotoxin-stimulated iTXB$_2$ and i6-keto-PGF$_{1\alpha}$ synthesis in control macrophages. The effects of pertussis and cholera toxin and GTP-[γ-S] on arachidonic acid metabolism were significantly decreased in tolerant macrophages compared with control macrophages.

The rate of iTXB$_2$ synthesis in response to GTP-[γ-S] suggests that the activation of the G protein regulating PLA$_2$ activity is rapid. In contrast, endotoxin-stimulated iTXB$_2$ synthesis demonstrates a lag phase and requires de novo protein synthesis [72]. Significantly decreased iTXB$_2$ release was observed in tolerant compared with control macrophages in response to GTP-[γ-S]. In addition, preliminary experiments indicate that GTPase activity, the hydrolysis of ^{32}P from GTP, is significantly reduced in tolerant macrophage membranes. In light of these results, the current data suggest that G protein activity may be altered in endotoxin tolerance.

The G proteins involved in endotoxin-induced arachidonic acid metabolism have not been identified. Endotoxin and the exotoxins may exert their effects through G proteins which are independent of one another, e.g., G$_i$ and G$_S$, or that they may produce effects through a single transducin-type G$_T$ protein. Recent data have shown that neutrophils, lymphocytes, and monocytes contain G$_{i2}$ and G$_{i3}$ [73, 74]. Daniel-Issakani et al. [53] have reported that endotoxin-induced IL-1 production in U937 cells is linked to a pertussis toxin-sensitive G protein which has been identified as G$_{i2}$ [75]. Whether this is the same G protein subtype involved in endotoxin-stimulated signal transduction events leading to PLA$_2$ activation is uncertain.

Aside from the biochemical and physiological importance of G proteins, there is growing evidence of possible altered G protein expression in several clinical disorders. These include hypo-or hyperthyroidism [76, 77], diabetes mellitus [78], and certain types of cardiovascular abnormalities [79]. Our results extend these observations by demonstrating that chronic endotoxemia leading to development of endotoxin tolerance is associated with decreased expression of G protein function. This depressed G protein function may play a role in the cross-tolerance to other noxious stimuli in this condition. The present data do not discern whether such decreased G protein function is specific for G protein subtypes or is indiscriminate. The determination of the cellular signal transduction events initiated by endotoxin and alterations induced by endotoxin tolerance merits further investigation.

Acknowledgements. This work was supported by NIH GM 27673. We appreciate the excellent typing and editorial assistance of Ms. Janie Nelson.

References

1. Adams DO, Hamilton TA (1984) The cell biology of macrophage activation. Annu Rev Immuno 2:283–318
2. Ruco LP, Meltzer MS, Rosenstreich DL (1978) Macrophage activation for tumor cytotoxicity: control of macrophage tumoricidal capacity by the LPS gene. J Immunol 121/2:543–548
3. Moore RN, Steeg PS, Mannel DN, Mergenhagen SE (1980) Role of lipopolysaccharide in regulating colony-stimulating factor-dependent macrophage proliferation in vitro. Infect Immun 30/3:797–804

4. Hamilton TA, Adams DO (1987) Molecular mechanisms of signal transduction in macrophages. Immunol Today 8/5:151–158
5. Bonney RJ, Humes JL (1984) Physiological and pharmacological regulation of prostaglandin and leukotriene production by macrophages. J Leukocyte Biol 35:1–10
6. Unanue ER (1976) Secretory function of mononuclear phagocytes. Am J Pathol 83/2:396–417
7. O'Flaherty Joseph T (1987) Phospholipid metabolism and stimulus-response coupling. Biochem Pharmacol 36/4:407–412
8. Morrison DC, Rudbach JA (1981) Endotoxin-cell-membrane interactions leading to trans-membrane signaling. Contemp Top Mol Immunol 81:187–218
9. Fink MP (1985) Role of prostaglandins and related compounds in the pathophysiology of endotoxic and septic shock. Semin Respir Med 7(1):17–23
10. Bull H, Herman AG (1982) Prostaglandins in circulatory shock. In: Herman AG et al. (eds) Cardiovascular pharmacology and the prostaglandins. Raven, New York, pp 327–345
11. Fletcher JR (1982) The role of prostaglandins in sepsis. Scand J Infect Dis [Suppl] 31:55–67
12. Needleman P, Turk J, Jakschik BA, Morrison AR, Lefkowith JB (1986) Arachidonic acid metabolism. Annu Rev Biochem 55:69–102
13. Wise WC, Cook JA (1980) Ibuprofen improves survival from endotoxic shock in the rat. J Pharmacol Exp Ther 215:160–168
14. Samuelsson B, Goldyne M, Granstrom E, Hamber M, Hammarstrom S, Malmsten C (1978) Prostaglandins and thromboxanes. Annu Rev Biochem 47:997–1029
15. Blackwell GJ, Duncombe WG, Flower RJ, Parsons MF, Vane JR (1977) The distribution and metabolism of arachidonic acid in rabbit platelets during aggregation and its modification by drugs. Br J Pharmacol 59:353–366
16. Mahadevappa VG, Holub BJ (1982) The molecular species composition of individual diacyl phospholipids in human platelets. Biochim Biophys Acta 713:73–79
17. Billah MM, Lapetina EG (1982) Evidence for multiple metabolic pools of phosphatidylinositol in stimulated platelets. J Biol Chem 257/20:11856–11859
18. Bills TK, Smith JB, Silver MJ (1977) Selective release of arachidonic acid from the phospholipids of human platelets in response of thrombin. J Clin Invest 60:1–6
19. Purdon AD, Smith JB (1985) Turnover of arachidonic acid in the major diacyl and ether phospholipids of human platelets. J Biol Chem 260/23:12700–12704
20. Irvine RF (1982) How is the level of free arachidonic acid controlled in mammalian cells? Biochem J 204:3–16
21. Lapetina EG (1982) Regulation of arachidonic acid production: role of phospholipases C and A2. Trends Pharmacol 3:115–118
22. Berridge MJ (1984) Inositol triphosphate and diacylglycerol as second messengers. Biochem J 230:345–360
23. Berridge MJ, Irvine RF (1984) Inositol triphosphate, a novel second messenger in cellular signal transduction. Nature 312:315–321
24. Majerus PW, Connolly TM, Deckmyn H, Ross TS, Bross TE, Ishii H, Bansal VS, Wilson DB (1986) The metabolism of phosphoinositide-derived messenger molecules. Science 234:1519–1526
25. Prpic V, Weiel JE, Somers SD, DiGuiseppi J, Gonias SL, Pizzo S, Hamilton TA, Herman B, Adams DO (1987) Effects of bacterial lipopolysaccharide on the hydrolysis of phospha-tidylinositol-4,5-bisphosphate in murine peritoneal macrophages. J Immunol 139:526–533
26. Cockcroft S (1984) Contrasting roles for receptor-stimulated inositol lipid metabolism in secretory cells. Biochem Soc Trans 17:966–968
27. Kukita M, Jirata M, Koga T (1986) Requirement of Ca^{2+} for the production of degradation of inositol 1,4,5-triphosphate in macrophages. Biochem Biophys Acta 885:121–128
28. Nomura H, Nakanishi H, Ase K, Kikkawa U, Nishizyka Y (1986) Inositol phospholipid turnover in stimulus-response coupling. Prog Hemost Thromb 143–158
29. Bell RL, Kennerly DA, Stanford N, Majerus PW (1979) Diglyceride lipase: a pathway for arachidonate release from human platelets. Proc Natl Acad Sci USA 76:3238–3241
30. Moscat J, Herrero C, Garcia-Barreno P, Municio AM (1986) Phospholipase C-diglyceride lipase is a major pathway for arachidonic acid release in macrophages. Biochem Biophys Res Comm 141/1:367–373
31. Rogers TS, Halushka PV, Wise WC, Cook JA (1986) Differential alteration of lipoxygenase and cyclo-oxygenase metabolism by rat peritoneal macrophages induced by endotoxin tolerance. Prostaglandins 31:639–650

32. Rogers TS, Halushka PV, Wise WC, Cook JA (1988) Arachidonic acid turnover in peritoneal macrophages is altered in endotoxin-tolerant rats. Biochim Biophys Acta 1001:169–175
33. Luderitz T, Schade U, Rietschel ET (1986) Formation and metabolism of leukotriene C_4 in macrophages exposed to bacterial lipopolysaccharide. Eur J Biochem 155:377–382
34. Haeffner-Cavaillon N, Chaby R, Cavaillon J, Szabo L (1982) Lipopolysaccharide receptor on rabbit peritoneal macrophages: I. Binding characteristics. J Immunol 128/5:1950–1954
35. Cavaillon J, Fitting C, Hauttencoeu B, Haeffner-Cavaillon N (1987) Inhibition by gangliosides of the specific binding of lipopolysaccharide (LPS) to human monocytes prevents LPS-induced interleukin-1 production. Cell Immunol 106:293–303
36. Jacobs DM (1984) Structural features of binding of lipopolysaccharides to murine lymphocytes. Rev Infect Dis 6/4:501–505
37. Larsen NE, Sullivan R (1984) Interaction of radiolabeled endotoxin molecules with human monocyte membranes. Biochim Biophys Acta 774:261–268
38. Spiegel AM, Gierschik P, Levine MA, Downs RW (1985) Clinical implications of guanine nucleotide-binding proteins as receptor-effector couplers. N Engl J Med 312/1:26–33
39. Ui M (1984) Islet-activating protein, pertussis toxin: a probe for functions of the inhibitory guanine nucleotide regulatory component of adenylate cyclase. Trends Pharmacol 5:277–279
40. Gilman AG (1984) G proteins and dual control of adenylate cyclase. Cell 36:577–579
41. Bourne H, Stryer L (1986) G proteins: a family of signal transducers. Annu Rev Cell Biol 2:391–429
42. Okajima F, Datada T, Ui M (1985) Coupling of the guanine nucleotide regulatory protein to chemotactic peptide receptors in neutrophil membranes and its uncoupling by islet-activating protein, pertussis toxin. J Biol Chem 260/10:6761–6768
43. Cassel D, Pfeuffer T (1978) Mechanism of cholera toxin action: covalent modification of the guanyl nucleotide-binding protein of the adenylate cyclase system. Proc Natl Acad Sci USA 75/6:2669–2673
44. Bokoch GM, Katada T, Northup JK, Hewlett EL, Gilman AG (1983) Identification of the predominant substrate for ADP-ribosylation by islet activating protein. J Biol Chem 258/4:2072–2075
45. Schleifer LS, Kahn RA, Hanski E, Northup JK, Sternweis PC, Gilman AG (1982) Requirements for cholera toxin-dependent ADP-ribosylation of the purified regulatory component of adenylate cyclase. J Biol Chem 257/1:20–23
46. Nakamura T, Ui M (1985) Simultaneous inhibitions of inositol phospholipid breakdown, arachidonic acid release, and histamine secretion in mast cells by islet-activating protein, pertussis toxin (a possible involvement of the toxin-specific substrate in the Ca mobilizing rece). J Biol Chem 260/6:3584–3593
47. Ohta H, Okajima F, Ui M (1985) Inhibition by islet-activating protein of a chemotactic peptide-induced early breakdown of inositol phospholipids and Ca^{2+} mobilization in guinea pig neutrophils. J Biol Chem 260/9:15771–15780
48. Bokoch GM, Gilman AG (1984) Inhibition of receptor-mediated release of arachidonic acid by pertussis toxin. Cell 39:301–308
49. Murayama T, Ui M (1985) Receptor-mediated inhibition of adenylate cyclase and stimulation of arachidonic acid release in 3T3 fibroblasts. J Biol Chem 260/12:7226–7233
50. Burch RM, Luini A, Axelrod J (1986) Phospholipase A_2 and phospholipase C are activated by distinct GTP-binding proteins in reponse to α_1-adrenergic stimulation in FRTL5 thyroid cells. Proc Natl Acad Sci USA 83:7201–7205
51. Wang J, Kester M, Dunn MJ (1988) Involvement of a pertussis toxin-sensitive G-protein-coupled phospholipase A_2 in lipopolysaccharide-stimulated prostaglandin E_2 synthesis in cultured rat mesangial cells. Biochem Biophys Acta 963:429–435
52. Jakway JP, DeFranco AL (1986) Pertussis toxin inhibition of B cell and macrophage responses to bacterial lipopolysaccharide. Science 234:743–746
53. Daniel-Issakani S, Spiegel AM, Strulovici B (1989) J Biol Chem
54. Chedid L, Parant M (1971) In: Kadis S, Weinbaum G, Ajl SJ (eds) Microbial Toxins Academic, New York, pp 415–456
55. Mulholland JH, Wolff SM, Jackson AL, Landy M (1965) Quantitative studies of febrile tolerance and levels of specific antibody by bacterial endotoxin. J Clin Invest 44/6:920–928
56. Greisman SE, Hornick RB, Carozza FA, Woodward TE (1964) The role of endotoxin during typhoid fever and tularemia in man: II. Altered cardiovascular responses to catecholamines. J Clin Invest 43/5:986–999

57. Greisman SE, Young EJ, DuBuy B (1973) Mechanisms of endotoxin tolerance: V. Specificity of the early and late phases of pyrogenic tolerance. J Immunol 103/6:1223–1236
58. Greisman SE, Young EJ, DuBuy B (1973) Mechanisms of endotoxin tolerance: VIII: specificity of serum transfer. J Immunol 111/5:1349–1360
59. Colditz IG, Movat HZ (1984) Desensitization of acute inflammatory lesions to chemotoxins and endotoxin. J Immunol 133/4:2163–2168
60. Chernow B, Roth BL (1986) Pharmacologic manipulation of the peripheral vasculature in shock: clinical and experimental approaches. Circ Shock 18:141–155
61. Howes EL, Rosenbaum JT (1985) Lipopolysaccharide tolerance inhibits eye inflammation: II. Preliminary studies on the mechanism. Arch Opthalmol 103:261–265
62. Bhattacherjee P, Parke A (1986) The reduction of inflammatory responses in lipopolysaccharide-tolerant eyes. Am J Pathol 122:268–276
63. Rosenbaum JT, Mandell RB (1983) The effect of endotoxin and endotoxin tolerance on inflammation induced by mycobacterial adjuvant. Yale J Biol Med 56:293–301
64. Beeson PB (1947) Tolerance to bacterial purogens: I. Factors influencing its development. J Exp Med 86:29–41
65. Freedman HH (1958) Passive transfer of tolerance to pyrogenicity of bacterial endotoxin. J Exp Med 92:453–463
66. Wise WC, Cook JA, Halushka PV (1983) Arachidonic acid metabolism in endotoxin tolerance. Adv Shock Res 10:131–142
67. Rogers TS, Halushka PV, Wise WC, Cook JA (1988) Differential alterations of lipoxygenase and cyclooxygenase metabolism by rat peritoneal macrophages induced by endotoxin tolerance. Prostaglandins 31/4:639–650
68. Zuckerman SH, Evans GF, Snyder YM, Roeder WD (1989) Endotoxin-macrophage interaction: post-translational regulation of tumor necrosis factor expression. J Immunol 143:1223–1227
69. Virca GD, Kim SV, Glaser KB, Ulevitch RJ (1989) Lipopolysaccharide induces hyporesponsiveness to its own action in RAW 264.7 cells. J Biol Chem 264:21951–21956
70. Virca GD, Kim SV, Glaser KB, Ulevitch RJ (1989) Role of guanine nucleotide binding protein in the activation of polyphospholinositide phosphodiesterase. Nature 314:534–536
71. Pfaffinger PJ, Martin JM, Hunter DD, Nathanson NM, Hille B (1985) GTP-binding proteins couple cardiac muscarinic receptors to a K channel. Nature 317:536–554
72. Geisel J, Cook JA, Ashton SH, Wise WC, Halushka PV (1990) De novo protein synthesis is required for endotoxin stimulation of arachidonic acid metabolism. Circ Shock (abstr) 31/1:57
73. Didsbury JR, Snyderman R (1987) Molecular cloning of a new human G protein: evidence for two $G_{i\alpha}$-like protein families. FEBS Lett 219:259–263
74. Beals CR, Wilson CB, Perimutter RM (1987) A small mutigene family encodes G_i signal-transduction proteins. Proc Natl Sci USA 84:7886–7890
75. Axelrod J, Burch RM, Jelsema CL (1988) Receptor-mediated activation of phospholipase A_2 via GTP-binding proteins: Arachidonic acid and its metabolites as second messengers. Trends Neurosci 11:117–123
76. Malbon CC, Rapiejko PJ, Watkins DC (1988) Permissive hormone regulation of hormone-sensitive effector systems. TIPS 9:33–36
77. Ransnäs L, Hammond HK, Insel PA (1988) Increased G_S in myocardial membranes from hyperthyroid pigs. Clin Res 36:552A
78. Gawler D, Milligan G, Spiegel AM, Unson CG, Houslay MD (1987) Abolition of the expression of inhibitory guanine nucleotide regulatory protein G_i activity in diabetes. Nature 327:229–231
79. Insel PA, Ransnäs LA (1988) G proteins and cardiovascular disease. Circulation 78:1511–1513
80. Coffee et al. (1990) Biochim Biophys Acta 1035:201–205

Section 11

**Clinical Aspects
of Multiple Organ Failure**

The Pattern of Organ Failure Following Severe Trauma-A Postmortem Study

H. C. Pape[1], G. Regel[1], W. Kleemann[2], J. A. Sturm[1], and H. Tscherne[1]

Introduction

In recent years, multiple organ failure (MOF) has gained increasing importance as a cause of death after severe trauma [1]. Subsequently, there have been more efforts to differentiate pathophysiological changes in the late phase after trauma.

From clinical observations it has become obvious that a close relationship exists between acute respiratory distress syndrome (ARDS) and MOF. Therefore it has been suggested that the mechanisms leading to posttraumatic pulmonary failure in the early phase might continue when the patient survives this complication [2]. If these mechanisms persist, this might be the cause of continuous damage to other organs and finally lead to MOF.

As of now, the research dealing with MOF has not succeeded in developing a clear-cut model for the pathogenesis of MOF. Several theories are currently under discussion, such as a prolonged activation of the complement system, the release of lysosomal enzymes, and toxic oxygen radicals [3]. Bacterial translocation from the gut and subsequent infection have also been made responsible. Another theory favors generalized inflammatory reactions as a response to the activation of several cascade systems.

We thus might be able to compare histological postmortem findings and changes in organ weight to clinical parameters of organ function.

Materials and Methods

Studies undertaken so far were done in heterogenous patient populations with limited numbers of patients. We therefore looked at histological specimens from all organs in patients dying from multiple trauma only. Parallel to histological data, clinical parameters indicative of organ function were documented on a retrospective basis. Clinical data of patients dying from severe trauma only were collected. In addition to general data, complications during the hospital stay were recorded, as well as parameters representative of clinical organ function of

Departments of [1]Trauma Surgery and [2]Forensic Medicine, Hanover Medical School, Konstanty Gutschowstrasse 8, 3000 Hannover 61, FRG

Host Defense Dysfunction
in Trauma, Shock and Sepsis
Eds. Faist/Meakins/Schildberg
© Springer-Verlag, Berlin Heidelberg 1993

organs known to be involved in MOF. Recording was done on a daily basis from the day of admission until death.

After death, all organs were weighed and sections were obtained in a standardized manner from the lung (bilaterally, upper middle and lower lobes), the liver (left and right lobes, middle portion), the heart (left ventricle and septum), and the kidney (cortex and medulla laterally from both sides).

The histological examination concerning cellular necrosis was evaluated in a semi-quantitative manner:
- Grade 0. No cell necrosis
- Grade I. Slight cell necrosis
- Grade II. Moderate cell necrosis
- Grade III. Severe cell necrosis

The patients were divided into three groups according to the time of death: group A, death within 48 h posttrauma; group B, death within 6 days posttrauma; and group C, death after 6 days posttrauma.

Results

Between 1983 and 1990 a total of 86 patients matched the criteria described above. Of these, in addition to the clinical data the organs of 59 patients were available for morphological evaluation. Of group A, 32.56 years in the patients 55 were male and 31 were female. The mean age was 32.93 years in group A, 32.56 years in group B, and 45.79 years in group C. The mean severity of injury as determined by the ISS (Baker) was 21.67 in group A, 25.25 in group B, and 27.55 in group C.

Lung. Clinical lung function was almost normal at day 1 in groups A and C. In group B, Horovitz ratio was lower initially and then deteriorated rapidly from

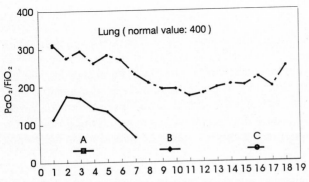

Fig. 1. Clinical lung (PaO_2/FiO_2) function as determined daily in groups A, B, and C

day 2. In group C lung function remained stable and deteriorated only in the very late phase (Fig. 1). Lung weight showed increasing values from group A to C. In all cases the organs weighed more than normal. The amount of cell necrosis was highest in groups A and C, showing damage up to grade III (Fig. 2).

Liver. The clinical function of the liver as measured by bilirubin values was within the normal limits in all groups. In group B bilirubin remained normal until death and in group C bilirubin remained normal until late and increased continuously until death (Fig. 3). Concerning organ weight, there was only a small difference between groups A and B, however, a greater difference between groups B, and C. In all groups the organ weight was significantly above normal levels. Between groups A, B and C we found increasing levels of cell necrosis (Fig. 4).

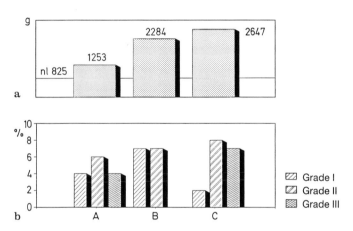

Fig. 2a, b. Lung morphology in groups A, B, and C. **a** Organ weight. **b** Cell necrosis *nl*, normal value

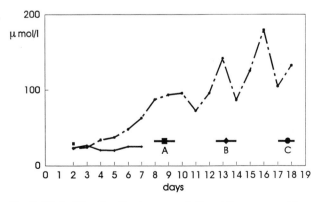

Fig. 3. Clinical liver function in groups A, B, and C as measured by serum bilirubin concentrations

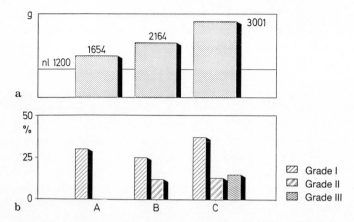

Fig. 4a, b. Liver morphology in groups A, B, and C. **a** Organ weight. **b** Cell necrosis. *nl*, normal value

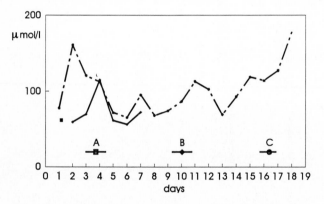

Fig. 5. Clinical kidney function in groups A, B, and C as measured by serum creatinine levels

Kidney. There was no significant difference in serum creatinine levels at day 1. Between days 2 and 4 a slight increase in creatinine levels was seen; this reduced to normal levels subsequently. In group C a late increase was seen as an indicator of organ failure (Fig. 5); however, the organ weight was highest in group B. Cell necrosis was less than in other organs but it increased in patients who survived longer (Fig. 6).

Heart. In the heart, as in other organs, the initial function was comparable in all groups. It then remained within normal limits until the late phase and then deteriorated until death in group C (Fig. 7). As in the kidney, organ weight was highest in group B and above normal limits in all organs. Grade 1 cell necrosis was highest in group B and the severest amount of necrosis was seen in group C (Fig. 8).

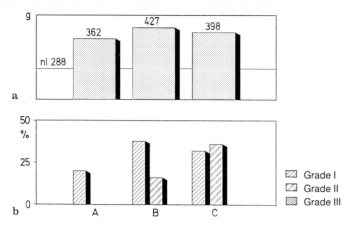

Fig. 6a, b. Kidney morphology in groups A, B, and C. **a** Organ weight. **b** Cell necrosis. *nl*, normal value

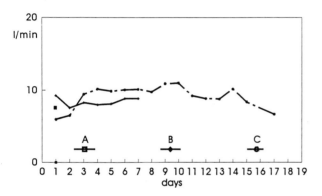

Fig. 7. Clinical heart function in groups A, B, and C as measured by cardiac output

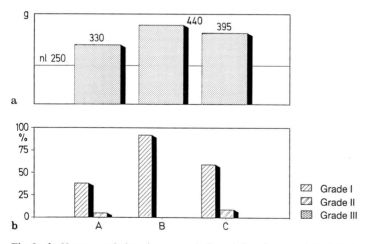

Fig. 8a, b. Heart morphology in groups A, B, and C. **a** Organ weight. **b** Cell necrosis. *nl*, normal value

Discussion

The aim of this study was to answer the following questions:

1. What is the sequence of organ failure in patients dying after multiple trauma?
2. What is the relationship between organ weight and cell necrosis?
3. Is there a correlation of clinical and histological findings in failing organs?

Since the development of definitions of MOF by Baue about 15 years ago, several authors have described patterns of organ failure. As one of the pertinent facts in most studies, the lung was the first organ to fail after severe trauma. Concerning the further sequence, variations have been found: While in the initial description Baue described the kidney as one of the organs involved early on, in studies done by Goris and Border the liver was involved next [1, 2, 6]. Fry saw sepsis as the major cause of the generalization of a problem that was initially limited to the lung. Border described disturbed generalized organ oxygenation due to cardiac impairment as the main problem [5]. Faist was the first to differentiate clearly between early and late functional impairment, i.e., the so-called "two-phase-MOF" [4]. According to this, early death results from fulminant organ failure due to hemorrhagic shock, whereas late organ failure is closely associated with infection, i.e., sepsis, a theory which has also been favored by Border [2]. In recent years, Goris has favored still another concept according to which infection is also present in MOF. However, sepsis is judged merely as an accompanying phenomenon and not as the definite cause of organ failure [6, 7]. Currently, there is active discussion about the representative sequence of organ failure following severe trauma. It is often related to different patho-physiological mechanisms, thus a clear-cut solution cannot be expected in the near future.

However, all authors agree that the lung represents an organ playing an outstanding role. This fact has been explained by the severity of permeability edema, which supposedly occurs in all organs, but causes most of the damage in the lung. In our study we also found that the lung fails early after trauma. Pulmonary function is the only parameter showing early sustained differences between the groups. This correlated with the amount of organ weight but not with cell necrosis. Thus, concerning cell death, a huge potential seems to be present in the lung.

In our study clinical liver function deteriorates late, but earlier than other organs. There was a clear-cut relationship: clinical organ function deteriorates late, as does organ weight and cell necrosis. In the kidney and heart, increasing cell necrosis does not correlate to organ weight. Both organs showed very late signs of clinical organ failure.

The reasons for this might be due to the different construction of organ tissues. In the lung, for example, there is a huge potential for the accumulation of the interstitial fluid, thus compensatory mechanisms of interstitial edema lead to only low-grade necrosis. In the liver, however, fluid cannot be stored and tissue necrosis is much more extensive and probably dependent upon organ weight.

The heart and kidney are both organs in which increasing necrosis in the late phase does not correlate to organ weight. If these findings are due to chronic hypoxia, inflammation of the whole body or other factors cannot be judged from our results.

We can currently draw the following conclusions concerning the pathomechanisms of MOF:

1. The sequence of organ failure seen clinically in our study was: early pulmonary failure and subsequent liver, kidney, and finally cardiac failure.
2. A relationship between organ weight and cell necrosis was mainly seen in the lung and liver. The kidney and heart appear to react with less edema despite a comparable fluid uptake.
3. A correlation between clinical and histological findings was seen in all organs except the lung. This organ shows differences from other internal organs regarding the function as well as the timing of failure—this might be due to its special morphological structure.

References

1. Baue AE (1975) Multiple progressive or sequential systems failure. Arch Surg 110:779
2. Border JR, Chenier R, Mc Menamy RH (1976) Multiple systems organ failure. Muscle fuel deficit with visceral protein malnutrition. Surg Clin North Am 56:1147
3. Dwenger A, Regel G, Neumann C, Schweitzer G (1986) Pathomechanisms of the adult respiratory distress syndrome (ARDS)—elastase contents of polymorphonuclear leucocytes and elastase release during passage across the blood-brain barrier Fresenius. Z Anal Chem 324:359
4. Faist E, Baue AE, Dittmer H, Heberer G (1983) Multiple organ failure in polytrauma patients. J Trauma 23:9
5. Fry DE, Pearlstein L, Fulton RL (1980) Multiple systems organ failure. Arch Surg 115:136
6. Goris JA, te Boekhorst TP, Nuytinck JKS (1985) Multiple organ failure—generalized autodestructive inflammation? Arch Surg 120:1109
7. Nuytinck JKS, Xavier JM, Ottermanns MW, Goris JA (1988) Whole body inflammation in trauma patients—an autopsy study. Arch Surg 123:1519

Hypertonic Volume Therapy: A Feasible Regimen to Contribute to the Prevention of Multiple Organ Failure?

U. Kreimeier[1], L. Frey[1], A. Pacheco[2], and K. Messmer[2]

Introduction

Trauma remains the leading cause of morbidity and mortality in patients under 45 years of age [2, 39]. Efforts to reduce trauma deaths focus on the improvement of prehospital care by rapid resuscitation from hypovolemia and systemic hypotension. Besides ventilatory assistance, primary resuscitation from severe trauma and shock aims at cardiocirculatory support by vigorous volume therapy and eventually vasoactive drugs to ensure peripheral oxygen delivery.

Systemic sepsis and multiple system organ failure are the most frequent and often fatal complications after trauma and major surgery [7, 12, 51]. The recognition that the failure of the gut and of distant organs may be causally related has led to heralding the gut as the "motor" of multiple system organ failure [8, 13]. Severe trauma and shock provoke a significant reduction in splanchnic blood flow and ischemic injury of the intestinal mucosa [16, 32]. Shock and hypoperfusion, by causing mucosal injury, result in the subsequent translocation of bacteria and endotoxins from the gut lumen into the systemic circulation [3]. The generation of oxygen free radicals via the enzyme xanthine oxidase, the concentration of which is highest in the villous tip of the intestinal mucosa, has been identified as the key determinant in the process of bacterial and endotoxin translocation [16, 19].

The primary factor rendering patients at risk of developing multiple system organ failure after shock and trauma is the persistence of impaired microcirculation with its sequelae for cellular and organ function [6, 40]. As a consequence of hypovolemia and low perfusion pressure, associated with severe blood loss and tissue trauma, nutritional blood flow is compromised and tissue hypoxia develops. The lumen of the capillaries becomes narrowed due to swelling of the endothelial cells and the adhesion of activated polymorphonuclear leukocytes (PMNL) to the vascular endothelium, phenomena which may completely abolish local flow. In addition, the interaction of PMNL with the venular endothelium is followed by the release of vasoactive mediators [26] and toxic oxygen species [20], promoting further redistribution of tissue perfusion and impediment of nutritional flow [6, 40].

---

[1] Institute of Anesthesiology and [2] Institute of Surgical Research, Ludwig-Maximilians University Munich, Klinikum Grosshadern, 8000 Munich 70, FRG

Host Defense Dysfunction
in Trauma, Shock and Sepsis
Eds. Faist/Meakins/Schildberg
© Springer-Verlag, Berlin Heidelberg 1993

On the other hand, microcirculatory failure present during established sepsis and endotoxemia is caused and sustained by the direct action of endotoxin and the release of vasoactive mediators [21]. Cytokines such as interleukin-1 and interleukin-6 and tumor necrosis factor are able to elicit many of the systemic effects characteristically seen during endotoxemia [17, 43]; these cytokines have also recently been shown to occur in the bloodstream in response to hemorrhage and tissue trauma [14]. The ensuing activation of cascade systems and PMNL-endothelial interaction favor a significant redistribution of capillary perfusion within the microvascular network with the end result of a critical overall reduction in nutritional blood flow [9, 41, 50]. Microcirculatory failure is thus regarded as a predominant mechanism for inadequate oxygen extraction from the tissues, which develops as early as the initial, hyperdynamic phase of septic shock [5, 41, 48].

Concept of "Small-Volume Resuscitation"

In 1980, Velasco and co-workers published their experimental data on the resuscitation of dogs subjected to severe hemorrhagic shock, which was lethal in animals treated with isotonic saline [52]. They demonstrated that 7.5% saline infused in a volume equivalent to only 10% of the shed blood volume rapidly increased systemic pressure and restored cardiac output, and allowed 100% long-term survival of dogs. In the same year, De Felippe et al. reported on 12 intensive care patients in hypovolemic shock refractory to conventional treatment [15]. These patients responded to intravenous injections of 100–400 ml of 7.5% sodium chloride—given as 50 ml portions—by a rise in arterial pressure, resumption of urine flow, recovery of consciousness, and thus reversal of the shock state.

In the past few years, the novel concept of primary resuscitation by means of hypertonic saline solution has been elaborated and various research groups have demonstrated that, even in the presence of a 50% blood loss, a volume as small as 4 ml/kg body weight of 7.2%–7.5% sodium chloride is sufficient to instantaneously restore cardiac output and to significantly increase systemic pressure [27, 30]. During "small-volume resuscitation" the hypertonic saline solution is given within 2–5 min through a peripheral vein; this mode of administration results in a rapid and pronounced increase in the plasma sodium concentration and thereby initiates a steep transmembraneous osmotic gradient. The most important mechanism of action of hypertonic solutions is the instantaneous mobilization of endogeneous fluid along the osmotic gradient with an increase in intravascular volume [27, 38]; in addition, direct myocardial stimulation, central nervous system (CNS) stimulation, neurogenic reflex mechanisms, enhanced sympathetic discharge, hormone release, improvement of blood fluidity, reestablishment of spontaneous arteriolar vasomotion, and peripheral arterial vasodilatation are involved ([27]; Fig. 1); most recent results

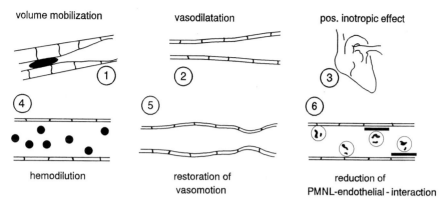

Fig. 1. Schematic view of the mode of action during small-volume resuscitation using hypertonic-hyperoncotic dextran solution (the numbers refer to Table 2)

suggest that the rapid cardiovascular response to hypertonic solutions might be partly mediated by the release of eicosanoids [36].

In severe hypovolemia, bolus infusion of 4 ml/kg body weight 7.2%–7.5% saline solution has been shown to lead to an increase in plasma volume by 8–12 ml/kg body weight [45, 49]. Mazzoni et al. have calculated that, after a 20% blood loss, 7.5% saline solution given over 10 sec in an amount equivalent to one seventh of the actual blood loss reestablishes normal blood volume within 1 min [38]. These authors ascribe the instantaneous volume effect to the rapid influx of fluid from the microvascular endothelium, red blood cells, and the interstitium.

Hypertonic Saline/Dextran Resuscitation

Several authors have reported on the transience of the cardiovascular response after small-volume resuscitation using exclusively hypertonic sodium chloride [27]. In order to preserve the intravascular volume gain, 7.2%–7.5% saline solution has been combined with colloids, i.e., dextran 60/70 or hydroxy-ethylstarch, to elicit a synergistic effect by increasing plasma osmolality and providing high plasma oncotic pressure [18, 24, 27]. Animal studies have revealed that, compared with hypertonic sodium chloride alone, hypertonic saline/6% dextran 70 causes a slightly better initial, but clearly more sustained circulatory response and increased survival [25, 34, 49, 53]. Based on the original work published by Smith et al. [49], Kramer and co-workers recently reported that hypertonic sodium chloride mixed with 6% dextran 70 given after severe hemorrhage over 2 h restored cardiac output for at least 180 min, which was significantly longer than hypertonic saline solution alone or 6% dextran 70 in isotonic saline [25].

The concept of applying small volumes of hypertonic saline/dextran solution for primary resuscitation from severe hypovolemia has proven effective in a prospective randomized study of trauma patients. As compared to Ringer's lactate, bolus infusion of 250 ml 7.5% NaCl/4.2% dextran 70 at the site of the accident resulted in a higher systemic pressure (49 mmHg vs 19 mmHg) and a higher survival rate (8/10 patients vs 3/10 patients) [22]. In an extension of their first study, in 1989 Holcroft et al. reported on 60 trauma patients entered into a randomized, prospective double-blind trial [23]. The administration of 7.5% saline/dextran resulted in higher blood pressure when the patients reached the emergency room as compared to Ringer's lactate given in the same amount (250 ml) and followed by conventional fluid therapy. The 30-day-survival rate was significantly higher after small-volume resuscitation using hypertonic saline/dextran. Most recently, the data from the multicenter trial in the United States on prehospital hypertonic saline/dextran infusion for posttraumatic hypotension have been published [37]. The 359 patients analyzed had a mean Injury Severity Score (ISS) of 19, and received either 250 ml 7.5% saline in 6% dextran 70 or Ringer's lactate, followed by conventional therapy. There was no difference in overall survival within the first 24 h; however, in the subgroup of patients requiring surgery and those with penetrating injury, hypertonic saline/-dextran infusion proved superior to Ringer's lactate ($p < 0.02$ and $p < 0.01$, respectively); in addition, there were fewer complications (acute respiratory distress syndrome renal failure, coagulopathy) than in the standard treatment group. The use of hypertonic saline/dextran solutions has proven safe in patients, as Holcroft et al. [23], Maningas et al. [35], and Mattox et al. in the USA multicenter trial [37] did not encounter any adverse effect, in particular no anaphylactoid reactions or dextran-related coagulopathies were observed.

Effect of Small-Volume Resuscitation on the Microcirculation in Trauma and Shock

The primary factor rendering patients at risk of developing multiple system organ failure after resuscitation from severe trauma is the persistence of microcirculatory failure with its sequelae for cellular and organ function. Kramer et al. demonstrated an increase in oxygen consumption in unanesthetized adult sheep resuscitated from severe hemorrhage by 7.5% saline/6% dextran 70 in a dose equivalent to 10% of blood loss [24]. In addition, Nakayama et al. reported on the reversal of cellular abnormalities after hemorrhagic shock in rats [46]. These laboratory findings corroborate the positive results from the above cited preclinical trials, and have received substantial support from recent experimental studies on the effect of small-volume resuscitation with hypertonic solutions on organ and nutritional blood flow [29, 30, 33, 47] (Table 1). The experimental data from our own group, based

Table 1. Established effects of small-volume resuscitation using 7.2%–7.5% saline/dextran solution

Systemic pressure	↑
Cardiac output	↑↑
Vascular resistance	↓
Nutritional blood flow	↑↑
Urinary output	↑
Survival rate	↑

Table 2. Comparative evaluation of the operational mechanisms of small-volume resuscitation using 7.2%–7.5% saline and 6%–12% dextran 60/70 solution

	7.2%–7.5% NaCl	6%–12% Dextran 60/70
1. Restoration of plasma volume	+ + +	+ +
2. Vasodilatation	+ +	+
3. Myocardial stimulation	+ +	+
4. Hemodilution with improvement in blood fluidity	+ +	+ + +
5. Restoration of spontaneous arteriolar vasomotion	+ +	+
6. Reduction of leukocyte/endothelial interaction	0	+ +

on studies employing radioactive microspheres in protracted traumatic-hemorrhagic shock with a 50% blood loss, have demonstrated that nutritional blood flow significantly increases within 5 min of i.v. bolus infusion of only 4 ml/kg body weight 7.2% saline, while the peripheral shunt flow remains far below prehemorrhage levels [29]. The addition of hyperoncotic (10%) dextran 60 not only prolongs but also significantly enhances the microcirculatory effect of 7.2% saline alone (Table 2): infusion of 4 ml/kg body weight of 10% dextran 60 in 7.2% saline solution in our experiments completely restored nutritional blood flow in kidney, gastric mucosa, small intestine, colon, and pancreas. Despite similar changes of the central hemodynamic parameters (systemic pressure, cardiac output), blood flow to these organs remained significantly lower after hypertonic saline resuscitation without dextran [29].

One reason for the superiority of the hypertonic-hyperoncotic saline/dextran solution appears to be the high oncotic power and water binding capacity of concentration dextran solution: the 25 g dextran infused with, e.g., 250 ml 10% dextran 60, will have the ability to keep 500–625 ml water in the intravascular space, which preserves the circulatory effect elicited by the hypertonic saline solution as compared to the addition of a less concentrated, i.e., 6% dextran 60, solution (water binding capacity 300–375 ml/250 ml 6% dextran solution). Furthermore, Bayer and co-workers have recently presented their data on the microcirculatory effects of hypertonic-hyperoncotic dextran solution after ischemia/reperfusion injury in the hamster dorsal skin fold model [4]. These authors demonstrated upon 4 h ischemia and reperfusion of striated muscle that the number of leukocytes adhering to the endothelium of postcapillary venules was significantly reduced over 24 h postreperfusion after bolus infusion of hypertonic saline/dextran solution, whereas the hypertonic saline alone did not exhibit a significant protective effect on postischemic leukocyte/endothelial interaction. Based on laboratory investigations on uncontrolled hemorrhage performed in anesthetized rabbits, hypertonic saline/dextran has been suggested to increase "intrinsic" microvascular reactivity, and thus lead to more efficient cardiodynamic improvement than conventional resuscitation with Ringer's lactate given even at 8.5 times the infusion volume of hypertonic saline/dextran [11].

Hypertonic Solutions in Sepsis and Endotoxin Shock

The concept of small-volume resuscitation by means of hypertonic solutions was originally designed for the primary treatment of severe hypovolemia occurring in hemorrhagic shock and trauma. After the initial experimental work by Velasco and co-workers [52] and the clinical observations of De Felippe et al. on intensive care patients [15], various research groups started to investigate the circulatory effect of hypertonic solutions in standardized animal models of hemorrhagic shock, whereas data on its effect on experimental models of sepsis and endotoxin shock have remained scarce.

The infusion of hypertonic solutions with an osmolality of 2400 mosmol/kg containing 50% glucose, insulin and potassium (GIK) is known to improve myocardial performance in septic shock in dogs [10]. Mullins and Hudgens reported that a small volume of hypertonic saline—1.2 ml/kg of 1080 mmol sodium/l (= 6.3% NaCl solution) given over 90 min—resuscitated dogs in endotoxin shock to the same extent as the identical amount of sodium given as isotonic Ringer's lactate [44]. Treatment with hypertonic saline was associated with a smaller increase in skin and subcutaneous tissue lymph flow, indicating less interstitial edema formation. Recently, Armistead et al. compared the effect of 10 ml/kg body weight hydroxyethylstarch (HES 450/0.7) in 0.9% NaCl with hydroxyethylstarch in 7.5% NaCl given over 30 min for initial fluid resuscitation in septic shock in dogs [1]. Arterial pressure, cardiac filling pressures, cardiac output, stroke volume, oxygen delivery, and oxygen consumption reached higher values after administration of the hypertonic saline/hydroxyethylstarch as compared to isotonic hydroxyethyl starch; however, the fluid requirements during the subsequent 3 h were not significantly different between the two groups.

Based on the favorable results obtained in our previous studies on small-volume resuscitation from hemorrhagic [30] as well as traumatic-hemorrhagic hypotension [29], we have analyzed the efficacy of hypertonic (7.2%) saline as well as of hyperoncotic (10%) dextran 60 solution in a standardized model of acute porcine endotoxemia. Our model is characterized by a high cardiac output/low peripheral resistance circulatory state during sustained i.v. infusion of endotoxin with vigorous volume support in order to preserve normal left ventricular filling pressure [28]. In these experiments 4 ml/kg body weight of hypertonic (7.2%) saline combined with hyperoncotic (10%) dextran 60 solution were given as bolus infusion over 2 min after 30 min of hyperdynamic endotoxemia [31]. Small-volume resuscitation with hypertonic saline/dextran solution led to a significant increase in cardiac index within less than 5 min, while systemic pressure remained unaffected. The hyperdynamic circulatory state was maintained throughout the ensuing 3-h observation period, during which only a fraction of the amount of conventional dextran 60 (6%) had to be substituted as compared to a control group without preinjection of hypertonic saline/dextran. Systemic oxygen delivery as well as blood flow to heart, kidneys, and splanchnic organs remained high [31].

Operational Mechanisms for Microcirculatory Resuscitation in Sepsis

When using small-volume resuscitation with hypertonic saline solution in hyperdynamic sepsis and endotoxin shock the following mechanisms are operational:
1. Maintenance of high cardiac output (direct myocardial stimulation; increase in preload)
2. Maintenance of peripheral vasodilatation (direct effect of hyperosmolarity; volume effect)
3. Reduction of tissue edema (shifting tissue water)

These three mechanisms promote the restoration of the severely impaired microcirculation. Furthermore, small-volume resuscitation reduces blood viscosity due to the concurrent hemodilution, thereby improving the fluidity of blood through the capillaries, an effect that is even more pronounced when hypertonic saline is combined with a colloid which itself exhibits positive rheologic properties, e.g., dextran 60. The specific action of hypertonic saline resuscitation at the microcirculatory level has been emphasized by Mazzoni and co-workers [38], who concluded from their model analysis on blood volume restoration after hemorrhage that mobilization of fluid out of the endothelium is most pronounced in those capillaries with swollen endothelium, a condition that is frequently observed after sustained periods of even focal ischemia. This shift of fluid from the endothelium increases the luminal diameter and thus reduces the hydraulic resistance of capillaries. The same authors demonstrated reopening of shock-narrowed capillaries upon infusion of 7.5% NaCl/6% dextran 70 in the tenuissimus muscle of rabbits in hemorrhagic shock [42].

Clinical Application of Small-Volume Resuscitation

The promising reports from preclinical studies about the efficacy of small-volume resuscitation using hypertonic saline/dextran solutions for primary treatment of severe trauma and hemorrhage [22, 23, 35] and the potentially favorable mechanisms operational, particularly at the level of the micro-circulation, have initiated clinical investigations in intensive care patients [27, 42]. Recently, Hannemann and co-workers reported on preliminary data obtained from critically ill patients with sepsis or acute respiratory distress syndrome. The authors demonstrated the efficacy of 2–4 ml/kg body weight of 7.5% hypertonic saline—combined with 6% hydroxyethylstarch—on central hemodynamics and oxygen metabolism [42]; at the end of the 15-min infusion period, the cardiac index had increased, as had pulmonary capillary wedge pressure, mean pulmonary artery pressure oxygen delivery, and oxygen consumption, while peripheral resistance was found to have decreased. At this moment, in Germany, a prospective, randomized multicenter trial is being performed in which the effect of small-volume resuscitation using 4 ml/kg body weight of 7.2% saline/10% dextran 60 solution is being compared to conventional fluid therapy for its efficacy in the hyperdynamic state of septic shock.

Conclusion

The novel concept of small-volume resuscitation using hypertonic solutions has been validated in various experimental models of severe hypovolemia and shock. Data from these experiments have demonstrated the efficacy of hypertonic saline/dextran solution with regard to the restoration of central hemodynamics and the normalization of compromised microcirculation. Besides the rapid restoration of macrohemodynamics and the prevention of early deaths, small-volume resuscitation particularly aims at the prevention of late complications, such as sepsis and multiple systems organ failure, on the basis of persisting microcirculatory disturbances.

The novelty of hypertonic saline/dextran resuscitation lies in its operational mechanisms at the microcirculatory level; these include the mobilization of fluid preferentially from swollen endothelium, the reduction of postischemic leukocyte adherence to the endothelium of postcapillary venules, and the restoration of spontaneous arteriolar vasomotion. Reopening of shock-narrowed capillaries and restoration of nutritional blood flow is thus promoted. Before this novel concept gains entrance into medical textbooks, however, more detailed information on the positive and perhaps hazardous effects of small-volume resuscitation in patients has to be accumulated.

References

1. Armistead CW, Vincent JL, Preiser JC, Debacker D, Minh TL (1989) Hypertonic saline solution-hetastarch for fluid resuscitation in experimental septic shock. Anesth Analg 69:714–720
2. Baker CC (1986) Epidemiology of trauma: the civilian perspective. Ann Emerg Med 15:1389–1390
3. Baker JW, Deitch EA, Li M, Berg RD, Specian RD (1988) Hemorrhagic shock induces bacterial translocation from the gut. J Trauma 28:896–906
4. Bayer M, Nolte D, Lehr HA, Kreimeier U, Messmer K (1991) Hypertonic-hyperoncotic dextran solution reduces postischemic leukocyte adherence in postcapillary venules. Langenbecks Arch Chir [Suppl]:375–378
5. Bihari DJ (1987) Mismatch of the oxygen supply and demand in septic shock. In: Vincent JL, Thijs LG (eds) Septic shock. Springer, Berlin Heidelberg New York, pp 148–160 (Update in intensive care and emergecy medicine vol 4)
6. Bihari DJ (1989) Multiple organ failure: role of tissue hypoxia. In: Bihari DJ, Cerra FB (eds) Multiple organ failure. Society of Critical Care Medicine, Fullerton, pp 25–36
7. Bone RC, Fisher CJ, Clemmer TP, Slotman GJ, Metz CA, Balk RA, The methylprednisolone severe sepsis study group (1989) Sepsis syndrome: a valid clinical entity. Crit Care Med 17:389–393
8. Border JR, Hassett J, LaDuca J, Seibel R, Steinberg S, Mills B, Losi P, Border D (1987) The gut origin septic states in blunt multiple trauma (ISS = 40) in the ICU. Ann Surg 206:427–448
9. Brigham KL, Meyrick B (1986) Endotoxin and lung injury. State of the art. Am Rev Respir Dis 133:913–927
10. Bronsveld W, van Lambalgen AA, van den Bos GC, Thijs LG, Koopman PA (1984) Effects of glucose-insulin-potassium (GIK) on myocardial blood flow and metabolism in canine endotoxin shock. Circ Shock 13:325–340
11. Bruttig SP, Discher D, Doherty TJ, Borgstroem P, Arfors KE (1991) Hypertonic saline dextran (HSD) improves peripheral microvascular performance following massive uncontrolled hemorrhage. Circ Shock 34:36
12. Carmona R, Catalano R, Trunkey DD (1984) Septic shock. In: Shires GT (ed) Shock and related problems. Churchill Livingstone, Edinburgh, pp 156–177
13. Carrico CJ, Meakins JL, Marshall JC, Fry D, Maier RV (1986) Multiple-organ-failure syndrome. Arch Surg 121:196–208
14. Chaudry IH, Ayala A, Ertel W, Stephan RN (1990) Hemorrhage and resuscitation: immunological aspects (editorial review). Am J Physiol 259:R663–R678
15. De Felippe J Jr, Timoner J, Velasco IT, Lopes OU (1980) Treatment of refractory hypovolaemic shock by 7.5% sodium chloride injections. Lancet ii:1002–1004
16. Deitch EA, Bridges W, Ma L, Berg R, Specian RD, Granger DN (1990) Hemorrhagic shock-induced bacterial translocation: the role of neutrophils and hydroxyl radicals. J Trauma 30:942–952
17. Fong Y, Moldawer LL, Shires GT, Lowry SF (1990) The biologic characteristics of cytokines and their implication in surgical injury. Surg Gynecol Obstet 170:363–378
18. Frey L, Kreimeier U, Pacheco A, Messmer K (1990) Effect of 7.2% saline/10% dextran-60 vs. 7.2% saline/10% hydroxyethylstarch on macro- and microhemodynamics in traumatic-hemorrhagic hypotension. Eur Surg Res 22:297 (Abstract)
19. Granger DN, Rutili G, McCord JM (1981) Superoxide radicals in feline intestinal ischemia. Gastroenterology 81:22–29
20. Granger DN, Benoit JN, Suzuki M, Grisham MB (1989) Leukocyte adherence to venular endothelium during ischemia-reperfusion. Am J Physiol 20:G683–G688
21. Hack CE, Thijs LG (1991) The orchestra of mediators in the pathogenesis of septic shock. In: Vincent JL (ed) Update in intensive care and emergency medicine. Update 1991. Springer, Berlin Heidelberg New York, pp 233–241
22. Holcroft JW, Vassar MJ, Turner JE, Derlet RW, Kramer GC (1987) 3% NaCl and 7.5% NaCl/Dextran 70 in the resuscitation of severely injured patients. Ann Surg 206:279–286
23. Holcroft JW, Vassar MJ, Perry CA, Gannaway WL, Kramer GC (1989) Perspective on clinical trials for hypertonic saline/dextran solutions for the treatment of traumatic shock. Braz J Med Biol Res 22:291–293

24. Kramer GC, Perron PR, Lindsey DC, Ho HS, Gunther RA, Boyle WA, Holcroft JW (1986) Small-volume resuscitation with hypertonic saline dextran solution. Surgery 100:239–247
25. Kramer GC, English TP, Gunther RA, Holcroft JW (1989) Physiological mechanisms of fluid resuscitation with hyperosmotic/hyperoncotic solutions. In: Passmore JC, Reichard SM, Reynold DG, Traber DL (eds) Perspectives in shock research, metabolism, immunonology, mediators and models. Alan R Liss, New York, pp 311–320
26. Kreimeier U, Frey L (1991) Schock. In: Hierholzer K, Schmidt RF (eds) Pathophysiologie des Menschen. VCH, Winheim, pp 1735–1745
27. Kreimeier U, Messmer K (1988) Small-volume resuscitation. In: Kox WJ, Gamble J (eds) Fluid resuscitation. Baillière's Clinical Anaesthesiology, vol 2. Baillière Tindall, London, pp 545–577
28. Kreimeier U, Yang Z, Messmer K (1988) The role of fluid replacement in acute endotoxin shock. In: Kox W, Bihari D (eds) Shock and the adult respiratory distress syndrome. Springer, Berlin Heidelberg New York, pp 179–190
29. Kreimeier U, Brückner UB, Niemczyk S, Messmer K (1990) Hyperosmotic saline dextran for resuscitation from traumatic-hemorrhagic hypotension: effect on regional blood flow. Circ Shock 32:83–99
30. Kreimeier U, Brückner UB, Schmidt J, Messmer K (1990) Instantaneous restoration of regional organ blood flow after severe hemorrhage: effect of small-volume resuscitation with hypertonic-hyperoncotic solutions. J Surg Res 49:493–503
31. Kreimeier U, Frey L, Dentz J, Herbel T, Messmer K (1991) Hypertonic saline dextran resuscitation during the initial phase of acute endotoxemia: effect on regional blood flow. Crit Care Med 19: (in press)
32. Kvietys PR, Granger DN (1989) Hypoxia: its role in ischemic injury to the intestinal mucosa. In: Marston A, Bulkley GB, Fiddian-Green RG, Haglund UH (eds) Splanchnic ischemia and multiple organ failure. Arnold, London, pp 127–134
33. Maningas PA (1987) Resuscitation with 7.5% NaCl in 6% dextran-70 during hemorrhagic shock in swine: effects on organ blood flow. Crit Care Med 15:1121–1126
34. Maningas PA, de Guzman LR, Tillman FJ, Hinson CS, Priegnitz KJ, Volk KA, Bellamy RF (1986) Small-volume infusion of 7.5% NaCl in 6% Dextran 70 for the treatment of severe hemorrhagic shock in swine. Ann Emerg Med 15:1131–1137
35. Maningas PA, Mattox KL, Pepe PE, Jones RL, Feliciano DV, Burch JM (1989) Hypertonic saline-dextran solutions for the prehospital management of traumatic hypotension. Am J Surg 157:528–534
36. Marti-Cabrera M, Ortiz JL, Durá JM, Cortijo J, Barrachina MD, Morcillo E (1991) Hemo-dynamic effects of hyperosmotic mannitol infusion in anesthetized open-chest dogs: modifica-tion by cyclooxygenase inhibition. Res Surg 3:29–33
37. Mattox KL, Maningas PA, Moore EE, Mateer JR, Marx JA, Aprahamian C, Burch JM, Pepe PE (1991) Prehospital hypertonic saline/dextran infusion for post-traumatic hypotension – the USA multicenter trial. Ann Surg 213:482–491
38. Mazzoni MC, Borgstroem P, Arfors KE, Intaglietta M (1988) Dynamic fluid redistribution in hyperosmotic resuscitation of hypovolemic hemorrhage. Am J Physiol 255:H629–H637
39. McCabe CJ (1990) Trauma: an annotated bibliography of the recent literature. Am J Emerg Med 8:446–463
40. Messmer KFW (1990) Mechanisms of traumatic shock and their consequences. In: Border JR, Allgöwer M, Hansen ST, Jr., Rüedi TP (eds) Blunt multiple trauma – comprehensive patho-physiology and care. Dekker, New York, pp 39–49
41. Messmer K, Kreimeier U, Hammersen F (1988) Multiple organ failure: clinical implications to macro- and microcirculation. In: Manabe H, Zeifach BW, Messmer K (eds) Microcirculation in circulatory disorders. Springer, Berlin Heidelberg New York, pp 147–157
42. Messmer K, Kreimeier U, Frey L, Pacheco A (1990) Abstracts of the 4th International Symposium on Hypertonic Resuscitation (Salt IV). Garmisch-Partenkirchen, FRG, June 17–19, 1990. Eur Surg Res 22:291–316
43. Michie HR, Manogue KR, Spriggs DR, Revhaug A, O'Dwyer S, Dinarello CA, Gerami A, Wolff SM, Wilmore DW (1988) Detection of circulating tumor necrosis factor after endotoxin administration. N Engl J Med 318:1481–1486
44. Mullins RJ, Hudgens RW (1987) Hypertonic saline resuscitates dogs in endotoxin shock. J Surg Res 43:37–44
45. Nakayama S, Sibley L, Gunther RA, Holcroft JW, Kramer GC (1984) Small-volume resuscit-ation with hypertonic saline (2,400 mosm/liter) during hemorrhagic shock. Circ Shock 13:149–159

46. Nakayama S, Kramer GC, Carlsen RC, Holcroft JW (1985) Infusion of very hypertonic saline to bled rats. Membrane potentials and fluid shifts. J Surg Res 38:180–186
47. Prough DS, Whitley JM, Taylor CL, Deal DD, DeWitt DS (1991) Small-volume rescuscitation from hemorrhagic shock in dogs: effects on systemic hemodynamics and systemic blood flow. Crit Care Med 19:364–372
48. Shoemaker WC (1986) Hemodynamic and oxygen transport patterns in septic shock: physiologic mechanisms and therapeutic implications. In: Sibbald WJ, Sprung CL (eds) Perspectives on sepsis and septic shock. Society of Critical Care Medicine, Fullerton, pp 203–234
49. Smith GJ, Kramer GC, Perron P, Nakayama S, Gunther RA, Holcroft JW (1985) A comparison of several hypertonic solutions for resuscitation of bled sheep. J Surg Res 39:517–528
50. Thijs LG, Groeneveld ABJ (1987) The circulatory defect of septic shock. In: Vincent JL, Thijs LG (eds) Septic shock. Springer, Berlin Heidelberg New York, pp 161–178 (Update in intensive care and emergency medicine, vol 4)
51. Trunkey DD (1983) Trauma. Sci Am 249:20–27
52. Velasco IT, Pontieri V, Rocha e Silva RM Jr, Lopes OU (1980) Hyperosmotic NaCl and severe hemorrhagic shock. Am J Physiol 239:664–673
53. Velasco IT, Oliveira MA, Rocha e Silva M (1987) A comparison of hyperosmotic and hyperoncotic resuscitation from severe hemorrhagic shock in dogs. Circ Shock 21:338–338

A New Sepsis Scale for Burns: Correlation with Endotoxin and Host Response

A. M. Munster, M. Meek, R. A. Winchurch, and C. Dickerson

The measurement of surgical sepsis remains an unsolved problem. The use of positive blood cultures or would cultures has never been particularly satisfactory, except perhaps as an end point for the treatment of septicemia of surgical origin. With the realization that the host response, rather than the mere presence of bacteria, contribute to what is clinically seen as "the septic picture", attempts have been made to develop sepsis scores which are based on measures of the host response as well as bacteriologic information. The additional measurement, using the new chromogenic Limulus lysate assay, of plasma endotoxin concentration adds another dimension to the evaluation of sepsis. The correlation between the induction of tumor necrosis factor and endotoxemia is well documented [1, 2, 3]. We have shown that burn size is well correlated with plasma endotoxin concentration [4], but the correlation of endotoxin concentration to the occurrence of sepsis in these patients has never been clearly shown. Border [5] used a sepsis scale to document the effect of enteral nutrition in intensive care patients. The popular APACHE II system [6] has been used by some authors for correlation with sepsis [7] but the APACHE II system was not designed for continuous measurement of sepsis, and although an excellent prognostic tool, it does not allow for some of the finer differential aspects seen in clinically septic patients.

The scale about to be described was drawn largely around Border's original measurements, but with some modifications. We added to our study measurements of plasma endotoxin concentration, interleukin-6 (IL-6) as an expression of the host response, and microbiologic data from patients. In addition, patients were administered polymyxin B in a prospective randomized fashion, as polymyxin B reduces the serum endotoxin concentration [8] and we sought, by reducing endotoxin concentration, to further illuminate the effect of this intervention on the sepsis score.

The details of the microbiologic data and the effect of polymyxin therapy will be detailed in another report. This report concerns the relationship between the sepsis score, the induction of IL-6 and the plasma endotoxin concentration.

Baltimore Regional Burn Center, Francis Scott Key Medical Center and the Department of Surgery, Johns Hopkins University, Baltimore, Maryland, USA

Host Defense Dysfunction
in Trauma, Shock and Sepsis
Eds. Faist/Meakins/Schildberg
© Springer-Verlag, Berlin Heidelberg 1993

Table 1. Baltimore sepsis score: Daily × 14 days; use most deviant score of day

PATIENT DATA

Name ———————————————— Hospital # ———————— Adm. ————

% Burn ————— % 3rd ————— Age ————— DOB ————— PB ————

S ————— Outcome ————— CON ————— D

Dates of Surgery ————————————————— # Days on Respir-

ator

Dates of +VE B.C. (Gur + or −, indicate) ——————————————

Inhalation injury   Y   N   MSO₄ ———— Day 3 ———— Day 10 ————

DATA——

PBD	TACHY	SBP	T MAX T MIN	BDEF	PLATS	WCC	CREAT	SVR	U/O	PEEP	O₂	COMA	A/B	TOT
0														
1														
2														
3														

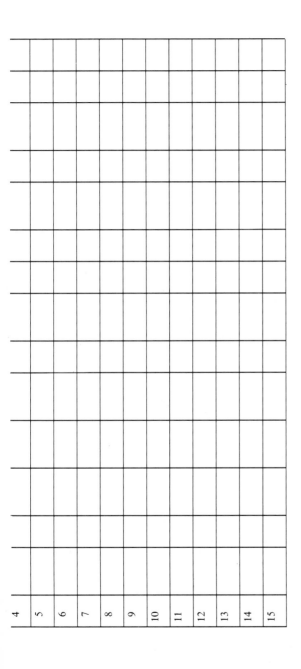

Materials and Methods

Forty-one adult patients with burns over 20% total body surface were enrolled in the study. After obtaining informed consent, patients were randomized to receive or not to receive polymyxin B. Following enrollment, daily for 14 days postburn, blood was obtained for endotoxin and IL-6 measurement, and the sepsis scale administered.

The Sepsis Scale

The scale is shown in Table 1 and the interpretation and scoring in Table 2. This system makes allowances, in a quantitative fashion, for patients on various pressor agents for the maintenance of blood pressure, and the dose required to do so; it also makes allowances for the fine changes in mentation and sensorium that septic burn patients undergo, as observed by the nursing staff. Briefly, the scale indicates: 0–10 points, an injured patient doing very well; 11–20 points, the

Table 2. Baltimore sepsis scale: scoring system

	Points	Maximum
Tachycardia	1 each 10 > 120	None
Systolic BP	1 each 10 < 90	None
	or 1 each cummulative 10 mg pressors	
Temperature = (Tmax/min)	1 each °C > 38.5	None
	or < 36.0	
Base deficit	1 each 3 mM > 5	None
Platelets	1 each 5K < 35K	None
White cell count	1 each 5K > 15K	None
Creatinine	1 each 2 mg > 2 mg	5 points/day
	or patient on dialysis	
SVR	1 each 100 < 800	None
Urine output	1 each 50 ml < 500/day	None
PEEP	1 each 3 mm > 5	None
O$_2$ (PaO$_2$/FIO$_2$ ratio)	1 each .30 < 2.0	None
Coma: Modified Glasgow Scale		6 points/day
Oriented × 3 and cooperative	1	
Occasional confusion, but mostly oriented	2	
Frequent confusion but cooperative tries to help with dressings,recognizes family and staff	3	
Semiconscious or delirious most of the time, cannot help with dressings, does not recognize family or friends	4	
Expresses pain response to stimulation, no other response	5	
Coma, no pain response	6	
Antibiotics	1 for each in use	3

PEEP, positive end respiratory pressure

patient is having problems; 21–30 points, the patient is gravely ill; and, over 30 points, usually in multiple organ failure and critical.

Chromogenic *Limulus* Lysate Assay

In principle, the assay depends on activation of a proenzyme in the *limulus* lysate of endotoxins. The activated enzyme catalyzes the hydrolysis of p-nitroanaline (pNA) from the colorless substrate Ac-Ile-Glu-Arg-pNA, is directly proportional to the concentration of endotoxin, and is quantitated by absorbance at 405 nm. With the use of well-defined endotoxin standards, a curve is generated from which the concentration of endotoxin in unknown samples can be determined. For the assay, 100-μl samples are dispensed into pyrogen-free borosilicate tubes and brought to 37 °C. One hundred microliters of freshly reconstituted *limulus* lysate is added, and the incubation is then continued for 10 min. Substrate (200 μl) is added, and the incubation is continued for an additional 3 min. The reaction is stopped by adding 200 μl of 50% acetic acid. The absorbance of standards and samples is measured at 405 nm. Background absorbance of reagent blanks and diluted plasma are subtracted and the endotoxin concentration is computed from a linear equation derived from measuring absorbencies of standards ranging from 0.1 to 1.0 endotoxin IU/ml. The levels of endotoxin in the samples are corrected for dilution, and the endotoxic concentration is expressed as units per milliliter.

IL-6 Measurements Determination

The levels of IL-6 were determined using the B9 assay as described by Aarden [9]. The IL-6-dependent B9 cells were obtained from Dr. Rick Nordan, NCI, National Institutes of Health, and were maintained by serial passage in culture.

For the assay, 10 IU of standard IL-6 (Endogen Laboratories, Boston, MA, USA) or serum samples were serially diluted in $\log_2$ increments in microtiter plates in duplicate. Log-phase B9 cells were added at a final concentration of 1×10^4 in 50-μl volumes and the plates were incubated for 3 days at 37 °C. Tritiated thymidine was added for the final 4 h of incubation and proliferation was determined by scintillation counts. The data were analyzed by weighted probit analysis using the computer program described by Sette et al. [10].

Statistical Analysis

Age, burn size, and sepsis score (mean daily score for 14 days of study) were compared between deaths and survivors by use of the t test. Correlation analysis between the scores, IL-6, and endotoxin concentrations was performed by Pearson's r coefficient, and checked by the Mann-Whitney test.

Table 3. Baltimore sepsis scale: clinical data ($n = 41$)

	Deaths ($n = 7$)	Survivors ($n = 34$)	p
Age	40.42 ± 6.0	32.82 ± 1.4	NS
Burn size	41.07 ± 6.3	40.06 ± 3.1	NS
Score[a]	23.77 ± 3.2	7.30 ± 1.1	< 0.001

[a] Mean daily score first 14 days postburn.
t test.

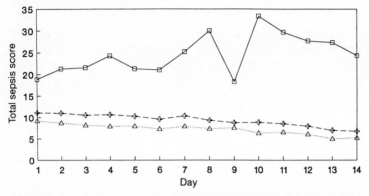

Fig. 1. Average total sepsis score for all patients (–♦–), survivors (⋯△⋯), and deaths (–▫–)

Results

Basic clinical data are shown in Table 3. Age and burn size were well matched in the two groups. The main daily score between deaths and survivals was statistically highly significantly different.

Polymyxin therapy reduced the serum endotoxin concentration from a mean of 0.38 IU to a mean of 0.33 IU. This difference is not statistically different because of variation in the range of endotoxin concentration. There was no significant correlation between the sepsis score (mean 10.35) and the endotoxin concentration (mean for all patients 0.35 IU). There was, however, a highly significant correlation between the IL-6 level, 211.288 IU, and the sepsis score. Although this relationship was significant, the relationship was not linear. A striking difference, illustrated in Fig. 1, is noted between the sepsis scores of deaths and survivors.

Discussion

The reduction of endotoxin concentration from treatment with polymyxin B is smaller than we had previously reported [8], but in this series of patients the incidence of gram-negative sepsis (15 out of a total of 68 positive cultures) was much smaller than usual. The vast majority of patients with positive blood cultures in this study grew out gram-positive organisms, and we attribute to this the lack of statistically significant reduction in endotoxin concentration by the polymyxin therapy. Similarly, because of this relatively small number of gram-negative isolates from blood, the correlation between endotoxemia and either IL-6 concentration or the sepsis score does not reach levels of statistical significance. Of far greater interest is the close correlation between the level of IL-6 and the sepsis score. The prognostic significance of other cytokines induced during the septic response, in particular IL-6 and tumor necrosis factor has been well documented [11]. IL-6 is a consistent marker of the host response in burns [12] and this relationship is confirmed in the current study. It would thus appear that the current sepsis scale meets the requirements of measuring the host side of the equation. The most valuable use of such a scale is obviously to measure intervention, whether this be surgical, antibacterial, or biological, to modify the host response. The next logical step will be the employment of this scale to measure the result of interventions.

References

1. Michie HR, Manogue KR, Spriggs DR, Revhaug A, O'Dwyer S, Dinarello CA, Cerami A, Wolff SM, Wilmore DW (1988) Detection of circulating tumor necrosis factor after endotoxin administration. New Eng J Med 318:1481
2. Schirmer WJ, Schirmer JM, Fry DE (1989) Recombinant human tumor necrosis factor produces hemodynamic changes characteristic of sepsis and endotoxemia. Arch Surg 124:445
3. Sanchez-Cantu L, Rode HN, Christou NV (1989) Endotoxin tolerance is associated with reduced secretion of tumor necrosis factor. Arch Surg 124:1432
4. Winchurch RA, Thupan JN, Munster AM (1987) Endotoxemia in burn patients: levels of circulating endotoxins are related to burn size. Surgery 102:808
5. Border JR, Hassett J, LaDuca J, Seibel R, Steinberg S, Mills B, Losi P, Border D (1987) The gut origin septic states in blunt multiple trauma (ISS = 40) in the ICU. Ann Surg 206:427
6. Knaus WA, Draper EA, Wagner DP, Zimmerman JE (1985) APACHE II: a severity of disease classification system. Critical Care Med. 13:818
7. Bohnen JMA, Mustard RA, Oxholm SE, Schouten BD (1988) APACHE II score and abdominal sepsis. Arch Surg 123:225 (1988)
8. Munster AM, Xiao GX, Guo T, Wong LA, Winchurch RA (1989) Control of endotoxemia in burn patients by use of Polymyxin B. JBCR 10:327
9. Aarden LA, DeGrot ER, Schaap OL, Lansdrop PM (1987) Production of hybridoma growth factor by human monocyter. Eur J Immunol 17:1411
10. Sette A, Drorini L, Marubini E, Doria G (1988) A microcomputer program for probic analysis of Interleukin-2 (IL-2) titration data. J Immunol Methods 86:265
11. Waage A (1989) Brandtzaeg P, Halstensen A, Kierulf P, Espevik T (1989) The complex pattern of cytokines in serum from patients with meningococcal septic shock. J Exp Med 169:333
12. Guo Y, Dickerson C, Chrest FJ et al. (1990) Increased levels of circulating interleukin-6 (IL-6) in burn patients. Clin Immunol Immunopath. 54:361

Multiple Organ Failure: Clinical Characteristics of Gut-Origin Septic States

J. R. Border

Multiple organ failure is a stereotyped cumulative sequence of organ failures. These septic organ failures may be grouped. The first group is a failure of pulmonary oxygen transport in association with a failure of peripheral oxygen extraction, high cardiac output, and low total peripheral resistance. The second group is muscle atrophy in association with gut hepatic failure. This is commonly associated with high-output renal failure. Finally, we have disorders of blood coagulation followed by terminal biventricular myocardial failure, pulmonary edema, and death.

The major variation in the septic organ failures is in the time from insult to death. That time varies widely depending upon pre-existing disease, the magnitude and reversibility of the insult, and the care given in the intensive care unit (ICU). In the ICU support of oxygen transport at a high level is required for the rest of the organ failures to be observed. If this cannot be achieved death occurs early from progressive cardiopulmonary failure. Our patients have generally received fluid volume support to maintain a urine output of about 100–150 ml/h in the operating room and ICU in order to maintain maximum cardiac output. We also try to maintain an arterial oxygen tension of 100–150 mmHg in the first 3 days to maximize oxygen transport. Oliguric renal failure is not a normal component of multiple organ failure and reflects inadequate circulatory support. The gut hepatic failure that occurs is significantly alleviated if a protein nutritional support is maintained between 2 and 4 g/kg per day. On average we have used 2.38 g/kg but that includes very septic patients receiving 4 g/kg and not very septic ones receiving 1.5 g/kg. This is given both enterally and parenterally with mixed calories only slightly in excess of expenditure.

It has now become apparent in blunt multiple trauma that surgical management on the night of injury that allows an upright chest position and the rapid attainment of a mobile patient is very important in preventing or reducing the duration of the septic organ failures. These statements are clearly true for femur fractures, spine fractures, and weight-bearing pelvis fractures. These studies of blunt multiple trauma, plus studies of burn and penetrating trauma and a wide variety of experimental trauma, are all consistent with enteral protein being a key ingredient in reducing the bacteriologic and septic organ failure manifestations of multiple organ failure.

University of Buffalo, 462 Gaider Street, Buffalo, NY 14215, USA

Host Defense Dysfunction
in Trauma, Shock and Sepsis
Eds. Faist/Meakins/Schildberg
© Springer-Verlag, Berlin Heidelberg 1993

The essential point is that for a long period of time we viewed multiple organ failure as being due to bacterial complications in wounds, blood, urine, and lung and therefore searched for stronger and better antibiotics. It appears very probable that antibiotics are not very helpful. To the extent that the systemic antibiotics utilized kill the gut commensal bacteria they support the growth of pathogenic, antibiotic-resistant bacteria and are thus harmful. Selective gut decontamination clearly reduces the bacteriologic manifestations of multiple organ failure without reducing the septic organ failures and mortality rate.

A New View of the Physiology Involved

The septic response is clearly due to normal systemic release by the activated leukocyte systems of cytokines and their effect on the hypothalamus. The septic organ failures are due to abnormal systemic release of destructive products by the activated leukocyte systems. The primary activators of the leukocyte systems are damaged devitalized tissue, bacteria, and bacterial toxins alone or in some combination.

Wounds

The normal business of the leukocyte system (polymorphonuclear leukocytes, monocytes-macrophages, lymphocytes, endothelium, mast cells, etc.) is to clear damaged devitalized tissue, bacteria, and bacterial toxins from a wound. A wound may be defined as a volume of devitalized tissue set in a larger volume of marginally viable tissue surrounded by normal tissue. The septic response is the body's way of mobilizing oxygen transport and energetic and synthetic substrates to support both the wound activities and the body's systemic response to the wound. The systemic response is based upon supporting protein synthesis for cellular replication or maintenance in the bone marrow, lymph nodes, gut mucosa, liver, and the working muscles. Resting muscle is the source of the amino acids required. This source is limited and easily exhausted. The systemic septic response and the protein synthesis and cellular replication that occur are regulated by the cytokines in very complex ways. The septic response also shuts off ketogenesis, leaving glutamine as the only gut mucosa energetic fuel to support enterocyte replication. The glutamine utilized comes largely from muscle and the lung. Since the devitalized tissue involved is self, a high degree of local wound immune suppression is always present.

The leukocyte system active in tissue may be divided into largely immobile and mobile elements. The mobile elements are primed in the plasma, adhere to the endothelium, and migrate to the area of damaged devitalized tissue. In the wound a second solid-phase activation produces a high rate of release of destructive products. These are oxidants, lysosomal enzymes, split complement products, coagulation factors, prostaglandins, leukotrienes, thromboxanes, kinins, histamine, and a large number of other products. These destructive agents are active extracellularly to prepare damaged and devitalized material for phagocytosis and intracellularly in the phagolysosome to kill bacteria and digest phagocytized material. These destructive products can clearly convert marginally viable tissue to devitalized tissue and damage fully viable tissue. In addition to the destructive products released by the activated leukocyte systems, both skin wounds (burns) and ischemic reperfused gut mucosa have tissue systems (xanthine oxidase and histamine) that can release oxidants to further devitalize tissue in the local wound and damage distant organ function. This tissue system normally works in conjunction with the leukocyte systems. This is the ischemia reperfusion injury that occurs in association with a wound or independent of a wound.

The essential point is that the wound produced by the initial agent has a given volume of devitalized tissue and marginally viable tissue. The leukocyte and tissue systems then release destructive products that expand the volume of devitalized tissue. The volume of devitalized tissue is yet further expanded if oxygen transport is limited to the marginally viable tissue of the wound. The volume of devitalized tissue is also dependent upon the techniques and timing of local wound management. It is this final volume of devitalized tissue that provides a diffusion barrier that limits destructive product access to circulating blood and antibiotic access to any bacteria in the wound, and provides nutrient to support bacterial growth.

The Gut Wound

If oxygen transport is limited enough there will be acute ischemia reperfusion injuries in organs not affected by direct trauma such as the gut mucosa. In addition, if protein nutritional support is inadequate or given only intravenously, this will also impair enterocyte replication and hepatic protein synthesis. Finally, acute respiratory distress syndrome (ARDS) limits pulmonary output of glutamine and thus also limits enterocyte replication, in this way further contributing to the gut-origin septic states. It has now become apparent that there is, in addition, a gut wound due not only to original failures of oxygen transport but also to subsequent failures of management in the intensive care unit. Traumatic wounds have diffusion barriers that limit access of leukocyte destructive products to the circulation. This is not at all true for the destructive products released by the gut hepatic leukocyte system when it is activated by translocated bacteria and bacterial toxins. Activation of this system is followed by direct release of destructive products into the circulating blood. The hepatic leukocyte system may limit systemic access for a while but is soon overcome. It appears true that release of these destructive products is the major cause of the pulmonary failure observed. Peritonitis would also activate this system. These destructive products then produce sufficient pulmonary damage (pulmonary wound) that the pulmonary leukocyte system is activated. This causes release of destructive products directly into arterial blood that damage the function of the systemic organs. Concurrently, this type of pulmonary damage plus any damage from the primary injury provides nutrient to support bacterial growth, while the changes in the gut bacterial flora plus orotracheal intubation provide pathogenic bacterial access so that nosocomial pneumonia adds yet another pulmonary leukocyte system activation.

One essential point here is that all such patients have their known wounds plus a gut wound. The second essential point is that, though the ischemic tissue, bacteria, and bacterial toxins are not per se very important, the leukocyte systems' activation with output of destructive products that they produce is. The third essential point is that the septic organ failures are much more likely to be produced by gut hepatic leukocyte systems' activation than by the wound leukocyte system, given our present day methods of systemic support and of wound and antibiotic management.

Conclusion

Multiple organ failure is synonymous with the gut origin septic states. The primary problem is systemic release of leukocyte destructive products. A second problem is release of oxidants from damaged tissue. This also contributes to the organ failure. Our primary therapies in the past have been aimed at removing the leukocyte activation produced by damaged devitalized tissue and bacteria in various combinations. We must now add two therapeutic aims to this basic approach. The first has as its primary aim removal of gut hepatic leukocyte system destructive products by supporting the normal antibacterial and antibacterial toxin mechanisms of the gut. The second has as its basic aim control of the destructive products released by the leukocyte system.

To support the gut mucosa as a barrier we must deliver adequate nutritional protein both enterally and parenterally in association with proper gut mucosa energetic fuels and the hormones and vitamins that modulate enterocyte replication. The nutritional protein required is some where between 2 and 4 g/kg per day. At least a quarter of this should be delivered enterally. At the very least, ketone bodies and glutamine are required as gut mucosa energetic fuels while at the very least, epidermal growth factor is required as a hormone, and vitamins A and C as the required vitamins. One of the primary antipathogenic bacterial properties of the gut is provided by the commensal bacteria. Our past therapies by use of stomach alkalinization and indiscriminate use of the broad spectrum antibiotics have grossly interfered with the function of the commensal bacteria. The primary antibacterial toxin mechanism of the gut has been binding the endotoxin to bile salts. We should probably be giving bile salts and investigating other neutralizing agents.

To the preceding changes in therapy we may now add antidestructive product therapy such as antioxidants, anti-eicosanoic acid products, antiproteinases, anti-histamine release agents and a variety of other such materials.

Intraperitoneal Infections and Multiple Organ Failure

T. Hau

Secondary bacterial peritonitis is always a polymicrobial infection. The bacteria originate from the intestinal tract whose wall is disrupted either by traumatic perforation or by a disease process. The bacteria causing peritonitis are, therefore, members of the normal gastrointestinal flora. Even though several hundred bacterial species colonize the gut, the number of bacteria cultured from patients with intraperitoneal infections is much smaller. This may in part be due to technical reasons, but Onderdonk et al. [1] has shown that only a few bacteria of a fecal inoculum persist after escape from the gut into the peritoneal cavity. Thus, the bacteriology of intraperitoneal infections is relatively uniform: the commonly found organisms are listed in Table 1 [2]. The data contained in this table apply primarily to patients with disease processes of the colon and distal ileum. Even though the bacteriologic findings in perforations of the upper gastrointestinal tract are initially different, they will be identical to those of lower intestinal perforations if the peritonitis is allowed to go on untreated. The reason for this is that the paralytic ileus developing during peritonitis will eventually lead to colonization of the upper gastrointestinal tract with colonic bacteria, and translocation of bacteria from the gut through the intact bowel wall into the peritoneal cavity, abdominal lymph nodes, parenchymatous organs, and peritoneal abscesses has been described [3, 4].

Bacteria elicit a response in the peritoneal cavity either by direct action on the mammalian cells or by means of endotoxin, exoenzymes, or as yet unknown mediators. Of the anaerobic gram-negative organisms, only fuso-bacteria possess a biologically active endotoxin. Most other anaerobic bacteria exert their pathogenic potential through other mechanisms. The production of super-oxide dismutase seems to be essential. Other factors of pathogenicity are exoenzymes and capsular polysaccharides. Even though it is generally felt that those factors produce local tissue damage essential for the formation of abscesses, it has also been shown that anaerobic bacteria can induce the same pathophysiologic changes as do endotoxin-containing bacteria [6]. However, endotoxin remains the best-studied toxin elaborated by bacteria in peritonitis. Endotoxins or lipopolysaccharides are high molecular weight compounds and part of the outer layer of the cell wall of many bacteria. The molecule consists of a lipid moiety, an R-core, and an O-polysaccharide and is released when the cell

Department of Surgery, Nordwest-Krankenhaus Sanderbusch, Sande, FRG

Host Defense Dysfunction
in Trauma, Shock and Sepsis
Eds. Faist/Meakins/Schildberg
© Springer-Verlag, Berlin Heidelberg 1993

Table 1. Bacteriology of intraperitoneal infections ($n = 383$)

Bacteria	No. of infections	Percentage
Aerobic		
Staphylococci	29	8
Streptococci	108	28
Escherichia coli	235	61
Klebsiella/Enterobacter	101	26
Proteus	87	23
Pseudomonad	30	8
Serratia marcescas	–	
Anaerobic		
Bacteroides	288	75
Anaerobic cocci	97	25
Clostridia	67	18
Fusobacteria	34	9
Eubacteria	94	25
Yeasts/fungi		
Candida	6	2
Others	–	

dies. The classical effects of endotoxin have been fever, either by action on the central nervous system or caused by the release of endogenous pyrogen from phagocytotic cells, neutropenia caused by a rapid margination of granulocytes, followed by granulocytosis, platelet aggregation and shock due to the release of vasoactive substances.

The local host defense in the peritoneal cavity consists of the direct absorption of bacteria into the lymphatics through stomata in the diaphragmatic peritoneum, the phagocytosis of bacteria either by resident macrophages or by granulocytes attracted through the peritoneal cavity, the killing of bacteria by complement, and, finally, the localization of the infection in form of abscesses. Many of the events necessary for host defense can be initiated by endotoxin, as we will see below, especially the activation of macrophages, the migration of bacteria into the peritoneal cavity, and the killing of bacteria by the phagocytes or complement [2]. However, simultaneously, a systemic septic state is induced.

The effects of endotoxin important in patients with peritonitis will be summarized briefly, based on a review by Morrison and Ryan [7]. These effects are not only due to the lipid moiety, as quantified by the *Limulus* amebocyte lysate assay, but also to other parts of the molecule. Most of the actions of endotoxin are conveyed by mediators. The lipid region of endotoxin activates the classical pathway of complement, whereas the alternative pathway is activated via the polysaccharide region. The activation of the complement system generates anaphylatoxins which are essential for the chemotaxis of mononuclear and polymorphonuclear cells but also induce vasodilatation and smooth muscle contraction. Endotoxin also activates arachidonic acid metabolism via the cyclooxygenic pathway, with subsequent release of prostaglandins, and the lipooxygenic pathway, with the release of leukotrienes. The most important substances, prostaglandins E_2 and $F_{2\alpha}$ (PGE_2; $PGF_{2\alpha}$), leukotriene C_4 (LTC_4), are necessary for the production of interleukins and other mediators produced by macrophages and the modulation of macrophage effector function. They cause vasodilatation, vasoconstriction, and chemotaxis. That this mechanism is operational in sepsis is shown by the fact that the hemodynamic changes induced by endotoxemia can be reduced by arachidonic acid metabolite antagonists, i.e., indomethacin or ibuprofen [8]. Endotoxin also causes the release of platelet-activating factor by neutrophils, macrophages, platelets, and endothelial cells, causing platelet aggregation, degranulation of neutrophils, increased vascular permeability, hypotension, and death. Intervascular thrombosis observed during endotoxemia is mediated by factor XII and tissue factor of the coagulation cascade. Endotoxin also leads to the secretion of interleukin-1 and tumor necrosis factor by macrophages, with their known secondary effects, but it is not the only substance to do so. It also leads to secretion of colony-stimulating factor by macrophages and B-lymphocytes, interferon, and endorphins.

The signs of systemic sepsis during peritonitis can become important for the diagnosis of the disease. While under ordinary circumstances the diagnosis of an intraperitoneal infection is obvious due to the typical abdominal findings, it might be difficult to make in patients who develop peritonitis postoperatively. Intraperitoneal infections develop after 0.7% of elective abdominal operations and carry a mortality of over 40%. This dreaded complication occurs most frequently after total gastrectomy and colonic resection. On the other hand, approximately half of all intraabdominal abscesses are sequelae of intraabdominal surgery [10]. As already mentioned, local signs are lacking in many of these patients or are difficult to distinguish from the normal postoperative condition. Fry et al. [11] reported that relaparotomy was indicated in 29% of patients on the basis of X-ray findings, in 23% on the basis of signs of systemic sepsis, in 15% because of wound problems, in 11% because of multiple organ failure, in 8% because of purulent secretion from drains, and in only 7% because of typical local findings. The most common clinical signs of postoperative peritonitis are fever, absent bowel sounds, wound infections, and a palpable mass. Even if there are no local signs, a postoperative intraperitoneal infection should be suspected if signs of systemic sepsis are present. The physiologic basis for the clinical picture of the early stages of generalized sepsis is increased cardiac index, decreased peripheral resistance, and decreased arteriovenous oxygen difference. The pulmonary wedge pressure is normal. The diagnosis of this pathophysiological state can be made most accurately by invasive monitoring. However, this is only feasable in high-risk patients. Therefore, a clinical diagnosis should be made before organ dysfunction develops.

Carrico et al. [12] have divided the septic state and multiple organ failure into four stages: (1) Increased fluid requirements and respiratory alkalosis with normal kidney and liver function. (2) The typical hemodynamic changes of sepsis, slight hypoxia, and occasionally a marginal elevation of bilirubin. (3) Signs of shock with low blood pressure, increased heart rate, severe hypoxia, and increase of creatinine as well as clinical jaundice. (4) Need for ionotropic drugs, CO_2 retention, oliguria, and hepatic encephalopathy. From this it is clear that one can diagnose the septic state in the early stages by close clinical observation. Whether laboratory tests, i.e., determination of endotoxin and acute phase protein levels, allow an earlier diagnosis remains controversial.

While typical local signs lead to early reexploration, the suspicion of a postoperative intraperitoneal infection on the basis of signs of systemic sepsis requires further investigations. The nature and location of the infection should be ascertained by ultrasound or computed tomography. However, one should keep in mind that the sensitivity and specificity of both methods is decreased in the postoperative phase [13]. A fluid collection diagnosed either by computed tomography or ultrasonography, the nature of which is undetermined, should be aspirated and examined for the presence of bacteria by gram staining [14].

If modern imaging methods give no hint of intraperitoneal infections, one should not proceed to relaparotomy but rather look for another septic focus. If, however, an intraabdominal abscess or a localized peritonitis is found, leakage of the anastomosis should be documented or ruled out by contrast studies. If the anastomosis is intact, the infection may be drained percutaneously [14]. Local drainage is also indicated if an anastomotic leak has been documented by contrast study and the anastomosis can be defunctionalized, for example by a completely diverting colostomy. However, if there is a massive anastomotic leak, reexploration is mandatory. The diagnostic and therapeutic systems are summarized in Fig. 1.

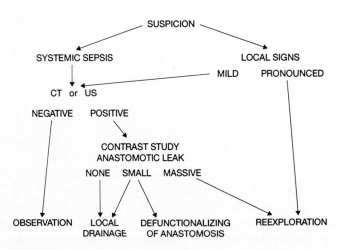

Fig. 1. Decision making in diagnosis and treatment of postoperative intraperitoneal infections

References

1. Onderdonk A, Weinstein W, Sullivan N (1974) Experimental intraabdominal abscess in rats: quantitative bacteriology of infected animals. Infect Immunol 10:1256
2. Hau T, Ahrenholz DH, Simmons RL (1979) Secondary bacterial peritonitis: the biological basis of treatment. Curr Probl Surg 16:1
3. Wells CL, Rotstein OD, Pruett TL, Simmons RL (1986) Intestinal bacteria translocate into experimental intraabdominal abscesses. Arch Surg. 121:102
4. Deitch EA, Berg R, Specian R (1987) Endotoxin promotes the translocation of bacteria from the gut. Arch Surg 122:185
5. Hofstad T (1984) Pathogenicity of anaerobic gram-negative rods: possible mechanisms. Rev Infect Dis 6:189
6. Wiles JB, Cerra FB, Siegel JH, Border JR (1980) The systemic response: Does the organism matter? Crit Care Med 2:55
7. Morrison DC, Ryan JL (1987) Endotoxins and diseases mechanisms. Annu Rev Med 38:417
8. Fink PM, MacVittie TJ, Casey LC (1984) Inhibition of prostaglandin synthesis restores normal hemodynamics in canine hyperdynamic sepsis. Ann Surg 200:619
9. Förster E, Hau T (1989) Die postoperative Peritonitis. 11th Chirurgisches Charité-Symposium, Berlin, pp 53–58
10. Aeder MI, Wellmann JL, Haaga JR, Hau T (1983) Role of surgical and percutaneous drainage in the treatment of abdominal abscesses. Arch Surg 118:273
11. Fry DE, Pearlstein L, Fulton RL, Polk HC (1980) Multiple system organ failure. Arch Surg 115:136
12. Carrico JC, Meakins JL, Marshall JC, Fry D, Maier RV (1986) Multiple organ failure syndrome. Arch Surg 121:196
13. Norwood SH, Civetta JM (1985) Abdominal CT scanning in critically ill surgical patients. Ann Surg 202:166
14. Hau T, Haaga JR, Aeder MI (1984) Pathophysiology, diagnosis, and treatment of abdominal abscesses. Curr Probl Surg 21:1

The Role of Empirical Laparotomy in the Management of Sepsis and Multisystem Organ Failure

H. C. Polk[1], P. Burgess[2], and W. G. Cheadle[1]

A major diagnostic dilemma in the management of the critically ill surgical patient is the confirmation and identification of sources of occult infection as a cause of multisystem organ failure (MSOF). This condition currently accounts for 73% of all deaths after major operative procedures and trauma [1] and is the main cause of death and morbidity for all surgical intensive care unit patients [2, 3].

To date, the pathophysiologic causes of MSOF are still not fully understood. The syndrome is manifested in patients who have sustained major injury, shock, or hypoxia. It has, however, required the experience of two decades and several wars for the various presentations of the syndrome to be recognized as a single disease complex [4].

The role of infection in the initiation of MSOF in a surgical patient is widely but not exclusively accepted. Some regard the presence of MSOF in a postoperative surgical patient to be an absolute indication for empirical laparotomy [5], while others argue that even in the presence of drainable pus, the high mortality of MSOF makes surgical intervention futile [6].

MSOF syndrome is characterized by the progressive deterioration of respiratory, renal, and hepatic function, in addition to gastrointestinal mucosal failure. Mortality is directly related to the number of organ systems involved and the age of the patient.

In the lung, there is a characteristic basement membrane injury, with endothelial cell damage, destruction of type 1 alveolar pneumocytes, and deposition of platelets and fibrin aggregates [7, 8].

Renal function deteriorates with the progressive decrease in glomerular filtration, presumably secondary to renal cortical ischemia. Changes in renal perfusion are probably due to the action of circulating vasoactive agents including catecholamines, angiotensin II, and prostaglandins.

Hepatic failure is reflected in the progressive deterioration of liver function tests. Hypoalbuminemia indicates the nutritional effects of the hypermetabolism state associated with MSOF [2]. The basal metabolic rate may be raised twofold, with increased proteolysis and decreased protein synthesis [9].

In the gut, enforced enteral starvation and splanchnic vasoconstriction contribute to bacterial colonization of the upper gastrointestinal tract. Colonic

[1] Department of Surgery, University of Louisville School of Medicine, Louisville, KY 40292, USA
[2] Department of Surgery, University of Newcastle-Upon-Tyne, UK

Host Defense Dysfunction
in Trauma, Shock and Sepsis
Eds. Faist/Meakins/Schildberg
© Springer-Verlag, Berlin Heidelberg 1993

flora migrate proximally and may be aspirated into the respiratory tract to initiate gram-negative commensal pneumonia. The loss of normal gut function probably allows the translocation of bacteria and endotoxins into lymphatics and portal blood due to the failure of gastrointestinal barrier function, and, hence, loss of containment of intestinal flora. As a result, the reticuloendothelial systems of the gut and liver are gradually overwhelmed, permitting distant foci of gut-derived organisms at the sites of tissue hypoxia, necrosis, or foreign body/prosthetic implants.

Gastrointestinal hemorrhage is the most overt indicator of gut involvement in MSOF. It is often a terminal event for the patient, due to loss of intestinal mucosal integrity related to ischemia, coupled with hepatic failure and coagulopathy.

The specific mechanism of these physiological changes appears to be due to a primary cellular injury. The formation of serum-immune complexes has been proposed to account for the systemic, multiorgan spectrum of the syndrome [10]. A fibronectin deficiency has been alleged to allow microcirculatory injury by endotoxins and immune complexes [11]. Basement membrane injury may also occur due to changes in cellular redox potential [12]. Recent studies suggest that MSOF may be a further manifestation of a general stress response to tissue injury or sepsis, the basis of which is dependent upon macrophage-derived cytokines such as tumor necrosis factor acting on cells mediated by local prostaglandins [13].

The dilemma for the surgeon who is caring for the patient who has undergone major surgery is whether clinical deterioration due to the onset of MSOF can be accounted for by the presence of occult infection or by abscess within the abdominal cavity, which can be drained effectively.

The diagnosis of intraabdominal collections requiring drainage is still dependent on clinical suspicion, supported by localization techniques such as ultrasound, computerized tomography, or radionuclide imaging. Radiological confirmation of the presence of intraabdominal collections is associated with high specificity and sensitivity. Ultrasound examination alone has reportedly detected 57%–90% of intraabdominal abscesses [14–16]. Computerized tomography has detected 90% [17] and similar accuracy has been reported for gallium-67 [18, 19]. Some studies have shown equal effectiveness independent of the method of imaging used [20]. However, the incidence of false negative investigations may be high [5].

When identified, collections may be percutaneously drained to allow microbiological cultures to be performed, antibiotic lavage instituted, and subsequent contrast studies via the drain performed to document the resolution of the abscess. This can be achieved successfully in 80% of definable collections, with the subsequent resolution of the abscess in 85% of cases. Morbidity and mortality related to the procedure is low in experienced centers [21]. Reexploration of the abdominal cavity for suspected sepsis, however, is associated with mortality rates of 33%–71% [5]. If performed on the basis of MSOF alone, these patients have a mortality rate of 81%. If a drainable focus of sepsis is identified, the mortality rate is still high at 67% [5].

Death as a result of MSOF is related to the number of systems involved, but a consistent theme is that better mechanical control of infection has the greatest probability for the resolution of the organ failure cascade [1]. Varying reports of reversible MSOF after drainage of an intraabdominal abscess [22] conflict with accounts of poor salvage rates in trauma patients subjected to empirical laparotomy for sepsis [6].

A negative laparotomy in patients with MSOF is associated with a high mortality, but in patients explored on the basis of MSOF alone, more than half will often have a drainable pus collection not detected by radiological investigation [5]. It is clear that clinical suspicion alone is often as accurate and reliable as sophisticated imaging techniques when assessing a patient with MSOF. Special studies should be used selectively to help indicate the site of incision and route of drainage. However, these studies never exclude the presence of intraabdominal pus.

The very high mortality associated with MSOF dictates that until absolute methods of excluding intraabdominal sepsis are established, patients who develop MSOF after previous abdominal surgery or injury should be considered for empirical laparotomy. This is mandatory for patients with demonstrable signs of peritoneal tenderness, regardless of the results of imaging studies [5]. A negative laparotomy rate of up to 50% can be expected [22], but an equal number of patients will have a drainable collection of pus. There is, as yet, no clear evidence of the percentage of patients who may be saved by this approach.

Increased survival in surgical patients acquiring MSOF necessitates improvements in the management of the syndrome and the development of other biological markers of sepsis. The fact that MSOF is initiated at a cellular level with changes in host metabolism that induce autocannibalism has led to the search for specific mediators of MSOF. In the case of markers of sepsis and outcome, monocyte antigen-presenting capacity appears to reflect an innate immune ability to withstand major sepsis and appears to predict which patients exhibit a poor outcome from sepsis [23].

Intraabdominal sepsis is still associated with a high morbidity and mortality after major operative procedures or trauma. In patients sustaining penetrating abdominal injuries, intraabdominal abscess formation is the most common complication encountered. This alone has a mortality rate of 25%, but when coupled with MSOF, mortality is over 90%. Research is required to guide logical management of MSOF and to reduce this unacceptable mortality.

References

1. Fry DE, Pearlstein L, Fulton RL, Polk HC Jr (1980) Multiple system organ failure: the role of uncontrolled infection. Arch Surg 115:136–140
2. Barton R, Cerra FB, (1989) The hypermetabolism multi-system organ failure syndrome. Chest 96:1153–1160
3. Baue AE, Chaudry IH (1980) Prevention of multiple system organ failure. Surg Clin North Am 60 (5):1167–1178

4. Trunkey DD (1988) Inflammation and trauma. Arch Surg 123:1517 (editorial)
5. Hinsdale JG, Jaffe BM (1984) Re-operation for intra-abdominal sepsis: indications and results in modern critical care setting. Ann Surg 199:31–36
6. Norton LW (1985) Does drainage of intraabdominal pus reverse multiple organ failure? Am J Surg 149:347–350
7. Hohn DC, Myers AJ, Gherini ST, Beckman A, Markison RE, Churg AM (1980) Production of acute pulmonary injury by leukocytes and activated complement. Surgery 88:48–58
8. Thorne LJ, Kuenzig M, McDonald HM, Schwartz SI (1980) Effect of denervation of a lung on pulmonary platelet trapping associated with traumatic shock. Surgery 88:208–214
9. Clowes GH Jr, George BC, Villee CA Jr, Saravis CA (1983) Muscle proteolysis induced by a circulating peptide in patients with sepsis or trauma. N Engl J Med 308:545–552
10. Eiseman B, Sloan R, Hansbrough J, Mcintosh R (1980) Multiple system organ failure: clinical and experimental. Am Surg 46:14–19
11. Saba TM, McCafferty MH, Lansey ME (1983) Depressed reticuloendothelial function in the surgical patient. Infect Surg 2:124–133
12. Ozawa K, Aoyama H, Yasuda K, Shimahara Y, Nakatani T, Tanaka J, Yamamoto M, Kamiyama Y, Tobe T (1983) Metabolic abnormalities associated with postoperative organ failure: a redox theory. Arch Surg 118:1245–1251
13. Michie HR, Eberlein TJ, Spriggs DR, Manogue KR, Cerami A, Wilmore DW (1988) Interleukin-2 initiates metabolic responses associated with critical illness in humans. Ann Surg 208:493–503
14. Doust BD, Doust VL (1976) Ultrasonic diagnosis of abdominal abscess. Am J Dig Dis 21:569–576
15. Richardson R, Norton LW, Eule J, Eiseman B (1975) Accuracy of ultrasound in diagnosing abdominal masses. Arch Surg 110:933–939
16. Hill BA, Yamaguchi K, Flynn JJ, Miller DR (1975) Diagnostic sonography in general surgery. Arch Surg 110:1089–1094
17. Robison JG, Pollock TW (1980) Computed tomography in the diagnosis and localization of intraabdominal abscesses. Am J Surg 140:783–786
18. Caffee HH, Watts G, Mena I (1977) Gallium 67 citrate scanning in the diagnosis of intraabdominal abscess. Am J Surg 133:665–669
19. Damron JR, Beihn RM, Deland FH (1976) Detection of upper abdominal abscesses by radionuclide imaging. Radiology 120:131–134
20. Korobkin M, Callen PW, Filly RA, Hoffer PB, Shimshak RR, Kressel HY (1978) Comparison of computed tomography, ultrasonography, and gallium-67 scanning in the evaluation of suspected abdominal abscess. Radiology 129:89–93
21. Mandel SR, Boyd D, Jaques PF, Mandell V, Staab EV (1983) Drainage of hepatic, intraabdominal and mediastinal abscesses guided by computerized axial tomography: successful alternative to open drainage. Am J Surg 145:120–125
22. Polk HC Jr, Shields CL (1977) Remote organ failure: a valid sign of occult intraabdominal infection. Surgery 81:310–313
23. Polk HC, Wellhausen SR, Regan MP, George CD, Cost K, Borzotta AP, Davidson PR (1986) A systematic study of host defense processes in badly injured patients. Ann Surg 204:282–299

Management of the Wound as Therapy for Multiple Organ Failure

L. Flint

The wound, defined in its broadest sense, is the common beginning feature of all injured patients. Trauma surgeons have, for the past two decades, sought to influence the subsequent course of injured patients by shortening the interval between the creation of the injury (wound) and definitive therapy: by achieving early wound closure to minimize the metabolic effects of the wound and lessen the chance for bacterial infection; and by aggressive management of the complex or infected wound to minimize the opportunity for wound-related complications. In this report, I will review the available evidence that wound management can prevent, alter, or ameliorate the multiple organ failure syndrome (MSOF).

In order to evaluate the available reports of experience with patients at risk for or overtly manifesting the MSOF, it is necessary to review the various methods of establishing the clinical diagnosis. Diagnosis of MSOF may be made by several methods including evaluation of the clinical status of the patient, measuring various laboratory manifestations of this condition, and measuring mediators which may indicate the presence of MSOF as well as produce its effects.

In our surgical intensive care unit we distinguish between three forms of organ failure. Type I, "typical" multiple organ failure is found in patients with hyperdynamic cardiovascular systems as well as hepatic, respiratory, or renal failure. These patients usually pass through the various stages of organ failure as defined by Carrico et al. [1]. A second group of patients will have single organ failure (type II), usually without hepatic insufficiency. A third group of patients will have early, reversible organ failure (type III) accompanied by hyperdynamic cardiovascular changes but this "septoid" state does not progress. The laboratory diagnosis of MSOF is typically documented by measuring the functional status of various organs which are failing. Hemodynamic and oxygen transport measurements, and pulmonary, hepatic, and renal function measurements are typically made. Also in this category are various assessments of the immune system which may have diagnostic and prognostic value.

Cytokines, such as tumor necrosis factor (TNF) and the interleukins, have recently caught the interest of clinicians because of the potential diagnostic value as well as because of their roles in mediating MSOF. TNF has been

Tulane University School of Medicine, 1430 Tulane Avenue, New Orleans, LA 70112, USA

Host Defense Dysfunction
in Trauma, Shock and Sepsis
Eds. Faist/Meakins/Schildberg
© Springer-Verlag, Berlin Heidelberg 1993

recovered from experimental animals in shock, and when injected into animals produces a septic shock syndrome [2]. In addition, TNF has been recovered from the sera of volunteers injected with endotoxin [3]. Patients with burns, infectious purpura, parasitic infestation, and meningococcemia have had positive assays for TNF and the level recovered has correlated with mortality [4–7]. Interleukins have not been regularly recovered and cannot be depended upon as a diagnostic marker.

Where the clinical diagnosis of MSOF has been established or is known to be a significant risk, prevention and treatment with various wound management techniques have been studied. Bone, in a prospective study, and Seibel, in a retrospective review, have documented that MSOF can be prevented by aggressive fixation of long bone fractures within the first 12–24 h after injury [8, 9]. Other fractures, such as pelvic fracture, which are important precursors of MSOF have not been as carefully studied, although we showed that the vast majority of patients with pelvic fracture could be resuscitated, have definitive hemostasis, and be made ready for open reduction within 24 h of injury [10].

Early excision and grafting of burns has been an area of interest and several investigators have suggested that MSOF can be prevented with this approach [11, 12]. Randomized, prospective approaches, focusing on large burns (20%–40% of body surface area BSA) have not confirmed this belief [13]. Once MSOF due to burn wound sepsis is established, débridement and coverage has salvaged some patients.

Drainage of intra-abdominal abscess has been a major method of controlling and reversing MSOF. This approach has been controversial, however [14, 15]. We believe that localized abdominal infection, if adequately treated, is beneficial to patients with early, compensated MSOF. Once the syndrome is established and decompensation occurs, laparotomy is seldom helpful.

References

1. Carrico J, Meakins J, Marshall J, Fry D, Maier R (1986) Multiple organ failure syndrome. Arch Surg 121:196–197
2. Sherry B, Cerami A (1988) Cachectin/tumor necrosis factor exerts endocrine, paracrine, and autocrine control of inflammatory responses. J cell Biol 107:1269–1277
3. Fong Y, Marano M, Moldawer L, Calvano S et al. (1990) The acute splanchnic and peripheral tissue metabolic response to endotoxin in humans. J Clin Invest 85:1896–1904
4. Marano M, Fong Y, Moldawer L, Wei H et al. (1990) Serum cachectin/tumor necrosis factor in critically ill patients with burns correlates with infection and mortality. Surg Gynecol Obstet 170:32–38
5. Girardin E, Grau G, Dayer J, Roux-Lombard P et al. (1988) Tumor necrosis factor and interleukin 1 in the serum of children with severe infectious purpura. New Engl J Med 319:397–400
6. Scuderi P, Sterling K, Lam K, Finley P et al. (1986) Raised serum tumour necrosis factor in parasitic infections. Lancet 12/13:1364–1365
7. Waage A, Halstensen A, Espevik T (1987) Association between tumor necrosis factor in serum and fatal outcome in patients with meningococcal disease. Lancet 2/14:355–357

8. Bone L, Bucholz R (1986) The management of fractures in the patient with multiple trauma. J Bone Joint Surg [Am] 68:945–949
9. Seibel R, LaDuca J, Hassett J et al. (1985) Blunt multiple trauma (ISS 36), femur traction and the pulmonary failure-septic state. Ann Surg 202:283–289
10. Flint L, Brown A, Richardson JD et al. Definitive control of mortality in pelvic fracture. Ann Surg (in press)
11. Tompkins R, Schoenfeld D, Behringer G et al. (1986) Prompt eschar excision: a treatment system contributing to reduced burn mortality. Ann Surg 204:272–280
12. Gray D, Pine R, Harnar T et al. (1982) Early surgical excision versus conventional therapy in patients with 20 to 40 percent burns. Am J Surg 144:76–79
13. Sorensen B, Fisker N, Steensen J, Kalaja E (1984) Acute excision or exposure treatment. Scand J Plast Reconstr Surg 18:87–93
14. Hinsdale J, Jaffe B (1984) Re-operation for intra-abdominal sepsis. Ann Surg 199:31–36
15. Norton L (1985) Does drainage of intra-abdominal pus reverse multiple organ failure? Am J Surg 149:347–350

Aggressive Enteral Nutrition Reduces Sepsis in the Hypercatabolic Injured Patient

E. E. Moore and F. A. Moore

Metabolic support is an integral component of surgical critical care. While prompt restoration of oxygen availability is clearly essential, timing, composition, and route of nutritional support may be important factors in patients at risk for multiple organ failure (MOF). The ensuing discussion will focus on: (a) timing of substrate delivery and (b) route of administration based on our clinical investigation over the past decade. The acutely injured patient was selected as a model of hypermetabolism because of relative homogeneity with respect to age, comorbid factors, and stress level.

Early Nutritional Support

The postinjury stress response peaks at 3–4 days and, if not driven by another insult, subsides in 7–10 days [1]. The immutable associated hypercatabolism, however, can produce significant protein malnutrition in this relatively short period. In 1976, Border et al. [2] suggested that acute protein malnutrition is an insidious risk factor for MOF, i.e., when oxidative amino acid demands cannot be met by skeletal muscle proteolysis, the "autocannibalism" progresses to erode crucial visceral protein. Recently, Souba et al. [3] documented enhanced glutamine release from the lung as well as skeletal muscle in stressed animals, suggesting an early sacrifice of functional protein to support metabolic demands. Thus, it is conceivable that failure to provide adequate nutritional support in the first 3–5 days after major trauma predisposes the patient to MOF. This concept has been supported by experimental work [4, 5], and clinical evidence is beginning to emerge [6].

Our first clinical investigation, therefore, was designed to ascertain whether early nutritional support would influence patient outcome after severe trauma. In 1979, stimulated by the success of needle catheter jejunostomy (NCJ) after elective gastrointestinal (GI) surgery reported by Page et al. [7], we completed a prospective trial to confirm the feasibility of NCJ in patients who had sustained major abdominal trauma. Immediate enteral feeding was categorically successful despite extensive injuries in the small bowel and colon [8]. Convinced of the

Department of Surgery, Denver General Hospital and the University of Colorado Health Sciences Center, Denver, Colorado, USA

Host Defense Dysfunction
in Trauma, Shock and Sepsis
Eds. Faist/Meakins/Schildberg
© Springer-Verlag, Berlin Heidelberg 1993

efficacy and safety of the NCJ, and prepared with the abdominal trauma index (ATI) [9] to identify the high-risk patients, we then initiated a study to ascertain the impact of immediate postinjury nutritional support [10]. During a 2.5-year period, all patients undergoing celiotomy at the Denver General Hospital (DGH) with an ATI score of more than 15 were enrolled in this prospective study; 75 (20%) of the 371 injured patients requiring abdominal exploration met this criterion. Such patients were randomized to either a control or enteral-fed group. Control patients received conventional dextrose (5%) in water (D5W; approximately 100 g/day IV) during the first 5 postoperative days, and then high-nitrogen total parenteral nutrition (TPN; nonprotein, NP, nonprotein; calories:N_2 = 133:1) by central vein if they were not tolerating a regular diet at that time. The enterally fed group had an NCJ placed at initial laparotomy. Infusion of an elemental diet (Vivonex HN, Norwich Eaton Pharmaceuticals, Norwich, NY, USA; NP calorie:N_2 = 150:1) was begun via the NCJ within 12 h postoperatively, and advanced to meet metabolic demands within 72 h.

Results of this study are summarized in Table 1. The control (n = 31) and enteral-fed (n = 32) groups were comparable with respect to age, injury mechanism, shock at admission, colonic disruption, splenectomy, and ATI score. Twenty of the enteral-fed patients were maintained on the elemental diet for more than 5 days (range 5–20, mean 9 days), while four (12%) received TPN. Nine (29%) of the 31 controls developed septic abdominal abscess. Moreover, the mean ATI score of patients developing septic complications in the control group was 31, while in the enteral group it was 48. Finally, the cost savings based on a review of actual hospital bills exceeded U.S. $3000/patient in the enteral-fed group. Thus, this prospective randomized study demonstrated a statistically significant reduction in septic morbidity after major abdominal trauma as a result of immediate postinjury nutritional support in previously well-nourished individuals.

Table 1. Clinical benefits of early postinjury nutritional support

Study group	Total lymphocyte count (cell/mm^3)	N_2 balance (g/day)	Major sepsis	Hospital cost/patient (U.S.$)
Control (n = 31)			9 (29%)	
Day 1	1408 ± 158	− 13.2 ± 0.5		19 636
Day 4	1175 ± 176	− 11.4 ± 0.7		
Day 7	1482 ± 138	− 11.1 ± 0.7		
Enteral (n = 32)			3 (9%)	
Day 1	1831 ± 206	− 13.7 ± 0.7		
Day 4	1344 ± 166	− 3.9 ± 1.6*		16 280
Day 7	2054 ± 164*	− 5.2 ± 1.3*		

* $p ± < 0.05$

Total Enteral Nutrition Versus Total Parenteral Nutrition

Acknowledging the benefit of early nutrition in the high-risk patient, the next question we addressed was the optimal route of substrate delivery, i.e., enteral nutrition (TEN) or parenteral nutrition (TPN). Safety, convenience, and cost have been commonly stated advantages of enteral nutrition, but theoretical physiologic benefits are far more compelling. Recent work has established that the gut is metabolically active [11, 12], immunologically important [3, 13], and bacteriologically decisive in the stressed patient. Central to this concept is an emerging consensus that gut-derived bacteria or endotoxin are primary factors in the genesis of postinjury MOF [14, 17]. Endotoxin is known to recruit, prime, and activate neutrophils; damage endothelium and alter receptors; induce cytokine release; and trigger the complement and clotting cascades. The vast hepatic sinusoidal network, lined with Kupffer cells, is strategically located to interact with gut-derived endotoxin. In addition to clearing endotoxin, Kupffer cells are a rich source of inflammatory mediators, e.g., tumor necrosis factor, interleukins, platelet-activating factor, and arachidonic acid metabolites, which are strongly implicated in the systematic response to critical illness [18, 19]. Viewed collectively, the malnourished, dysfunctional gut has been invoked as the "motor of MOF."

Our second series of investigations, therefore, were designed to question whether gut preservation via TEN would confer an advantage compared to early TPN [20]. Fifty patients with an ATI score of more than 15 and less than 40 were randomized at laparotomy to receive either TEN (Vivonex TEN) or TPN (Freamine HBC 6.9% and Trophamine 6%; Kendall-McGaw Laboratories, Irvine, CA, USA); both regimens contained 2.5% fat and 33% branched-chain amino acid (BCAA) and had a NP calorie:N_2 ratio of 150:1. Nutritional support was initiated within 12 h postinjury and advanced to achieve positive N_2 balance within 48 h. The study groups (TEN, 23; TPN, 27) were comparable in age (28.3 ± 1.9 vs 31.4 ± 2.4 years), ATI (24.5 ± 1.3 vs 24.2 ± 1.2), injury severity score (ISS; 28.8 ± 2.8 vs 25.8 ± 2.0), and initial metabolic stress (day 1 urine urea N_2 UUN_2 13.0 ± 1.5 vs 12.4 ± 0.7 g). The TPN group received a slight advantage in overall protein-calorie intake, but N_2 balance remained equivalent throughout the study period (day 5—TEN 0.4 ± 1.6 g//day vs TPN 0.8 ± 1.0 g/day). Of note, standard visceral protein markers (total protein, albumin, transferrin, and retinol-binding protein) all increased over the study period in the TEN group, while decreasing in TPN patients (Fig. 1).

To test the hypothesis that enteral nutrition reduces bacterial translocation, we examined prioritization of hepatic protein synthesis, defined as the relative balance of acute-phase proteins compared with constitutive proteins (nonacute phase). Specific serum protein levels were profiled by crossed immunoelectrophoresis. When segregated by treatment groups, divergent patterns emerged. A representative constitutive protein, α_2-macroglobulin (α_2-M), and a representative acute-phase protein, α_1-antitrypsin (α_1-AT), are shown. There was equivalent

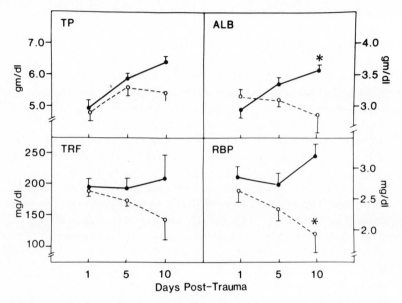

Fig. 1. The TEN (*solid line*) vs TPN (*dashed line*) clinical study demonstrated consistent improvement in standard visceral protein markers (*TP*, total protein; *ALB*, albumin; *TRF*, transferrin; *RBP*, retinol-binding protein) in enterally fed patients; *$p < .05$

depression of α_2-M levels in the TPN and TEN groups on day 1, but on day 10 the α_2-M level in the TEN group returned to normal while remaining depressed in the TPN group (Fig. 2). In contrast, serum levels of the α_1-AT increased to a greater degree in the TPN group. Baseline levels were similar for both groups but, on day 5, α_1-AT levels in the TPN group increased more than in the TEN group (Fig. 3). These data suggest that TEN ameliorates reprioritization of hepatic protein synthesis after major torso trauma. Although speculative, we believe this reflects a reduction in bacterial translocation via preservation of gut mucosal integrity.

In view of these findings, we continued this study to ascertain the clinical impact [21]. Ultimately, 75 (39 TEN, 36 TPN) of 407 patients undergoing emergent laparotomy were prospectively randomized; 16 patients were subsequently excluded from the study, leaving 59 evaluable subjects (29 TEN 30 TPN). The study groups were comparable at presentation with respect to age (TEN 28 ± 2 vs TPN 32 ± 2 years), injury mechanism (28% vs 36% blunt), ISS (28.7 ± 2.3 vs 25.1 ± 1.0), ATI (24.7 ± 1.1 vs 24.0 ± 1.0), and physiologic status (revised trauma score, RTS, 6.9 ± 0.2 vs 6.9 ± 0.3). On day 5, caloric and N_2 intake were higher in TPN patients than in the patients receiving TEN. But again, no significant differences for N_2 balance were noted at day 5 ($- 0.3 \pm 1.0$ vs 0.1 ± 0.8 g/day). As shown previously, albumin, transferrin, and retinol-binding protein levels remained more depressed throughout the study in patients receiving TPN. Additionally, bilirubin, alkaline phosphatase, and

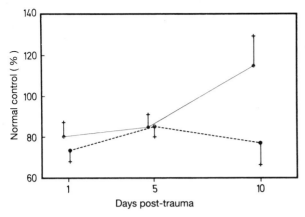

Fig. 2. Constitutive proteins, represented by α_2-macroglobulin, normalized in the TEN group (*solid line*) but remained depressed in the TPN patients (*dashed line*)

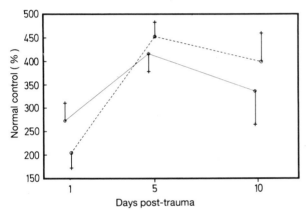

Fig. 3. Acute-phase proteins, represented by α_1-antitrypsin, remained elevated to a greater extent in the TPN group (*dashed line*) compared with the TEN patients (*solid line*)

glucose levels were higher in patients receiving TPN, and exogenous insulin was required in five (17%) of the TPN group compared with one (3%) of the TEN group.

Complications occurred in ten enteral patients (34%) compared to 17 TPN patients (57%). Seven patients in the TPN groups and six patients in the TEN group experienced nonseptic complications including pancreatitis (five patients), atelectasis (three patients), recurrent pneumothorax (one patient), biliary fistula (one patient), breakdown of exteriorized colon repair (one patient), and cerebrospinal fluid leak (one patient). Septic complications are summarized in Table 2. The overall incidence of septic morbidity was five (17%) patients in the TEN group and 11 (37%) patients in the TPN group. There was a significant

Table 2. Septic complications of TEN versus TPN study groups after major abdominal trauma

Complications	Group TEN (n = 29)	TPN (n = 30)	p value
Major infections			
Abdominal abscess	1	2	0.03
Pneumonia	0	6	
Total	1 (3%)	6 (20%)	
Minor infections			
Wound	3	1	
Catheter	0 4 (14%)	2	NS
Urinary	0	1	
Miscellaneous	1	2	
Total	4 (14%)	5 (17%)	
Total patients	5 (17%)	11 (37%)	

difference with respect to major infections (pneumonia and intra-abdominal abscess), i.e., one (3%) patient in the TEN group compared with six (20%) in the TPN group. All six pneumonias were in the TPN group. The mechanism of injury for these patients was blunt in three and gunshot wound in three; the mean ATI score was 27.8 ± 2.2, and the mean ISS was 25.0 ± 3.7. Pathogens identified by sputum culture included two *Staphylococcus aureus*, and one each *E scherichia coli*, *Streptococcus pneumoniae*, *Pseudomonas aeruginosa*, *Proteus mirabilis*, *Serratia marcescens*, and *Citrobacter* sp. In summary, this prospective, randomized study demonstrated a statistically significant reduction in septic morbidity in high-risk patients receiving early TEN compared with early TPN.

Finally, we have performed a meta-analysis to examine the question of TEN versus TPN in a large, contemporary surgical experience [22]. During a 4-year period ending June 1988, a series of nine prospective trials were conducted to compare the utility of Vivonex TEN (Norwich Eaton Pharmaceuticals, Inc., Norwich, NY, USA) with nutritionally similar TPN solutions in moderately to severely stressed postoperative patients. One study was excluded from analysis because patients had either extensive preoperative nutritional support or were septic at study entry. The remaining eight sites enrolled 230 patients (19–59 patients each) who received early postoperative nutritional support: 118 were randomized to receive TEN and 112 were randomized to receive TPN. The various trials were not identical because they were not based upon a standardized multinuclear study protocol; however, study designs were remarkably similar. Four sites enrolled trauma patients only: entry criteria included an ATI of 16–40 or an ISS of 9–40. The remaining four sites enrolled trauma or other surgical patients who would normally require postoperative nutritional support. Eligible patients received TEN by NCJ (n = 81), or nasoenteric tube (n = 37). All enterally fed patients received Vivonex TEN. The TPN solutions used in seven studies were prepared by the hospital pharmacies to be nutritionally

Table 3. Meta-analysis of eight prospective studies comparing TEN versus TPN in hypercatabolic surgical patients

Complications	Blunt trauma		Penetrating trauma		Nontrauma surgery		Total patients	
	TEN (n = 48)	TPN (n = 44)	TEN (n = 38)	TPN (n = 40)	TEN (n = 32)	TPN (n = 28)	TEN (n = 118)	TPN (n = 112)
Abdominal abscess	2	1	2	6	1	0	5	7
Pneumonia	4	10	1	2	1	3	6	15
Wound infection	0	2	3	1	1	0	4	3
Bacteremia	1	4	0	1	0	0	2	5
Urinary infection	1	1	0	1	0	1	1	3
Line sepsis	0	4	0	1	0	2	0	7
Other	5	4	1	1	0	1	6	6
Total events	13	26	7	13	4	7	24	46
Number of patients	10	22*	6	11	3	6	19	39*

* $p < .05$

comparable to Vivonex TEN. Four sites used a combination of Trophamine 6.0% and Freamine 6.9% (Kendall-McGaw Laboratories, Inc., Irvine, CA, USA), while three mixed Travasol 10% and Branchamine 4% (Travenol Laboratories, Deerfield, IL, USA). The salient features of this meta-analysis are summarized in Table 3. Nearly twice as many TPN as TEN patients developed infections (TEN, 16%; TPN, 35%; $p = 0.01$). On average, each of these TPN patients developed 1.1 septic complications compared to 1.0 for each of these TEN patients. Breakdown of septic complications by patients subgrouping indicated the most significant differences were among trauma patients (TEN, 19%; TPN, 39%; $p = 0.02$). Moreover, the rate of septic complications remained significantly different when patients with line sepsis were excluded: 33% of TEN patients compared with 19% of TEN trauma patients ($p = 0.04$) and 41% of blunt trauma TPN patients compared with 21% of TEN patients ($p = 0.05$). In conclusion, this meta-analysis corroborated a significant reduction in septic morbidity attributable to early TEN in the stressed surgical patient.

References

1. Cerra FB (1987) Hypermetabolism, organ failure, and metabolic support. Surgery 101:1–14
2. Border JR, Chenier R, McMenamy RH, La Duca J, Seibel R, Birkholm R, Yn L (1976) Multiple systems organ failure: muscle fuel deficit with visceral protein malnutrition. Surg Clin North Am 56:1147–1167
3. Souba WW, Klinberg US, Plumley DA, Salloum RM, Flynn TC, Bland TT, Copeland EM (1990) The role of glutamine in maintaining a healthy gut and supporting the metabolic response to injury and infection. J Surg Res 48:383–391
4. Kudsk KA, Stone JM, Carpenter G, Sheldon GF (1983) Enteral and parenteral feeding influences mortality after hemoglobin-*E. coli* peritonitis in normal rats. J Trauma 23:605–609
5. Saito H, Trocki O, Alexander JW, Kopcha R, Heya T, Jasse SN (1987) The effect of route of nutrient administration on the nutritional state, catabolic hormone secretion, and gut mucosal integrity after burn injury. JPEN 11:1–7
6. Alexander W, MacMillian BG, Stinnett JG, Ogle CK, Bozian RC, Fisher DE, Krummell R (1980) Beneficial effects of aggressive protein feeding in severely burned children. Ann Surg 192:505–517
7. Page CP, Carlton PK, Andrassy RJ, Feldtman RW, Shield CF: (1979) Safe cost-effective postoperative nutrition—defined formula diet via needle catheter jejunostomy. Am J Surg 138:939–945
8. Moore EE, Dunn EL, Jones TN (1981) Immediate jejunostomy feeding: its use after major abdominal trauma. Arch Surg 116:681–684
9. Moore EE, Dunn EL, Moore JB, Thompson JS (1981) Penetrating abdominal trauma index. J Trauma 21:439–445
10. Moore EE, Jones TN (1986) Benefits of immediate jejunostomy feeding after major abdominal trauma—a prospective randomized study. J Trauma 26:874–881
11. Souba WW, Roughneen PT, Goldwater DL, Williams JC, Rowland BJ (1987) Post-operative alterations interorgan glutamine exchange in exterectomized dogs. J Surg Res 42:117–125
12. Wilmore DW, Smith RJ, O'Dwyer ST, Jacobs DO, Ziegler TR, Wong XD (1988) A central organ following surgical stress. Surgery 104:917–923
13. Maddaus MA, Wells CL, Platt JL, Condie RM, Simmons RC (1988) Effect on T cell modulation on the translocation of bacteria from the gut and mesenteric lymph node. Ann Surg 207:387–398
14. Border JR, Hassett J, La Duca J, Seibel R, Steinberg S, Mills B, Losi P, Border D (1987) The gut origin septic states in blunt multiple trauma (ISS = 40) in the ICU. Ann Surg 206:427–448

15. Deitch EA, Winterton J, Berg R (1987) The gut as a portal of entry bacteremia. Ann Surg 205:681–692
16. Marshall JC, Christow NV, Horn R, Meakins JL (1988) The microbiology of multiple organ failure. Arch Surg 123:309–315
17. Rush BF, Sori AJ, Murphy TF, Smith S, Flanagan JJ, Machiedo GW (1988) Endotoxemia and bacteremia during hemorrhagic shock. Ann Surg 207:549–554
18. Faist E, Mewes A, Baker CC, Strasser T, Alkan SS, Rieber P, Heberer G (1987) Prostaglandin E (PGE)-dependent suppression of interleukin 2 (IL-2) production in patients with major trauma. J Trauma 27:837–848
19. Goris JA, Roekhorst TP, Nuytinch JK, Gimbrere JSF (1985) Multiple-organ failure, generalized autodestructive inflammation. Arch Surg 120:1109–1115
20. Moore FA, Moore EE, Jones TN, Peterson VM (1989) TEN versus TPN following major torso trauma—reduced septic morbidity. J Trauma 29:916–923
21. Peterson VM, Rundus C, Moore EE, Jones TN, Emmett M, Moore FA, Parsons P (1988) TEN versus TPN following major torso injury: attenuation of hepatic protein reprioritization. Surgery 104:199–207
22. Moore FA, Feliciano DV, Andrassy RJ, McArdle AH, Morgenstein TB, Kellum JM, Moore EE. Enteral feeding reduces postoperative septic complications — results of a meta-analysis. Ann Surg (manuscript submitted)

Clinical-Mediator Correlations of Multiple Organ Failure and Preventive/Therapeutic Strategies: To Block, Stimulate, or Replace? That is the Question

A. E. Baue

Introduction

Much has been learned about the factors, relationships, and mediators involved in multiple organ failure (MOF). In spite of this knowledge and better support of organ function, MOF remains a problem with high morbidity and mortality. We know that the mechanisms and mediators of an inflammatory response so necessary for survival after injury may initiate MOF. The questions now are: (a) Can we safely block parts of an inflammatory response?, (b) Is there failure of host defense or an excessive or uncontrolled host defense response, or both?, (c) Of what importance are the normal mechanisms of control of inflammation? (d) Is there benefit from stimulation of host defense and the use of growth factors? Much needs to be learned to answeer these questions. In the meanwhile, prevention of MOF is the key to better results.

The biologic conundrum I will review is whether an extensive inflammatory response, which should protect the individual, contributes to MOF and self-destruction. The answer seems to be yes, although the circumstances in which this occurs are still being elaborated. If it is true, can we block all or part of the response without doing harm?

Common Threads in MOF

The common threads in the development of MOF include the following:
1. Initially there is shock with circulatory instability after injury, which produces ischemia and the possibility of an ischemia-reperfusion injury in the early injury phase.
2. There are mechanical factors that contribute, including immobility in a forced supine position, pain, shallow breathing, and dependency.This is particularly accentuated if the patient has fractures and cannot be mobilized.
3. There are the humoral factors, the cellular mediators of tissue injury and inflammation so necessary for survival which, with overwhelming activation or systemic activation, may contribute to remote organ damage.

Department of Surgery, Saint Louis University Medical Center, 3635 Vista Avenue at Grand Boulevard, St. Louis, MO 63110-0250, USA

Host Defense Dysfunction
in Trauma, Shock and Sepsis
Eds. Faist/Meakins/Schildberg
© Springer-Verlag, Berlin Heidelberg 1993

4. Infection with further activation of mediators, interleukins, cachectin, and systemic activation of what should be a local response can be an over-whelming insult.
5. Gut failure and the gut-septic syndrome with bacterial translocation of organisms is very likely a problem. It remains to be determined in what clinical settings this reaches clinical significance.
6. Metabolic difficulties with muscle failure, liver failure, protein failure, septic auto-cannibalism, and sepsis overwhelm the individual as MOF begins to develop [1].

Injury and Inflammation: the Mediators

There is no doubt that the mediators of inflammation and the various enzyme cascades can be activated so extensively that they become toxins and produce tissue and organ damage. These include the interleukins IL-1, IL-2, IL-3, and IL-6, which have profound effects on the individual. Tumor necrosis factor (TNF) has been studied extensively and has been infused in normal human volunteers producing the symptoms of inflammation. Complement activation and the anaphylatoxins, particularly C3a and C5a, are necessary for inflammation but can also be damaging. While cells have a number of toxic materials which play a role in bacterial killing and also in breaking down necrotic tissue. Oxygen free radicals form one group and the proteases the other. It is proposed that production and release of these can damage surrounding tissue, particularly the endothelium of organs such as the lungs. The autocoids all participate in the inflammatory response contributing to the increased capillary permeability and other alterations. They include the eicosanoids (prostaglandins and leukotriene), kallikreins, histamine, serotonin, and somatomedin. The reticulo endothelial system with fibronectin and tuftsin is involved. Immune complexes can produce damage in a number of ways, including capillary obstruction. Endothelial factors can increase adherence, aggregation, and other problems. Other products of injury are involved. Thus the inflammatory response, if overly active, can produce the dolor, rubor, tumor, and calor that characterize the increased blood flow, increased capillary permeability, cell infiltration, phagocytosis, bacterial killing, and tissue breakdown so necessary to control bacterial or foreign antigen invasion and to heal the wound [2].

The five groups of cell adhesion molecules or receptors [3] are the integrins, the adherence molecules of immunoglobulins, the cadherins, the endothelial leukocyte adhesion molecules (ELAM), and lymphocyte homing receptors. They play a major role in cell-to-cell and cell-to-matrix communication. Many activities of these molecules may be a problem for the injured individual. They may be responsible for white cells aggregating in pulmonary capillaries and elsewhere to produce adult respiratory distress syndrome (ARDS) and other problems. However, there are diseases of adhesion, congenital abnormalities, which include ELAM and lactic acid dehydrogenase (LAD) deficiencies, both of which result in abnormal leukocyte function, severe infections, and death at an early age [3]. In addition, a disease of platelet adhesion produces a bleeding disorder called Glanzmann's thrombasthenia. Thus, interfering with these adherence molecules may produce serious problems. It has been documented, for example, that an anti-CD 18 (CD 18 human neutrophil adherence glycoprotein) antibody will protect an animal from hemorrhagic shock [4]. However, using this antibody to the adherence molecule CD 18 also increases the incidence and severity of subcutaneous abscess formation by *Staphylococcus aureus* in animals [5]. Thus we may not be able to have it both ways.

Inhibitors

A number of inhibitors or blocking agents of inflammatory mediators have been evaluated in experimental situations (Table 1). Antioxidants such as superoxide dismutase have been used to prevent accumulation or damaging effects of superoxide anions [6]. Allopurinol inhibits xanthine oxidase, which is a producer of superoxide anions. Monoclonal antibodies to TNF and IL-6 have been evaluated and are effective in animals if given before an insult produced either by TNF or by endotoxin [7–9]. Antibodies to the adherence molecules have been evaluated, as have myeloperoxidase inhibitors, cyclooxygenase inhibitors, platelet-activating factor antagonists, ACE inhibitors, leukotriene antagonists or inhibitors, and recombinant anti-proteases [10–12]. Platelet-activating factor receptor antagonists have also been developed. All of these inhibitors may be helpful in certain isolated circumstances: however, their use in the multiply injured patient could produce additional problems.

Biologic Regulation of Inflammation

For all biologic processes there are feedback loops or control mechanisms. Because the cytokines and their effects have been defined so recently their control mechanisms are only now being studied. There seem to be many such regulators (Table 2). Regulation of autoimmunity is one such control mechanism [13], as is the development of heat-shock proteins, which are protective for cells [14–16]. α_2-Macroglobulin is thought to bind cytokines [17]. Autoantibodies to cytokines, which may be common, could be carriers or inhibitors and thus could either facilitate or neutralize the effects of the cytokines [18]. The central nervous system, the endocrine system, and the immune system have very close interrelationships which form regulatory mechanisms [19]. Some cytokine inhibitors bind to cytokines and compete for binding sites [20]. IL-4, IL-8, and IL-10 are known to be inhibitors of other cytokines such as IL-1, IL-2, and IL-6.

Table 1 Inhibitors or blocking agents for inflammatory mediators

Antioxidants
Xanthine oxidase inhibitor, allopurinol
Monoclonal antibodies to:
   TNF
   IL-6
   Adherence molecules
Myeloperoxidase inhibitors
Cyclooxygenase inhibitors
Platelet-activating factor antagonist
ACE inhibition
Leukotriene antagonists-inhibitors
Recombinant-anti-proteinases
Platelet-activating factor receptor antagonist

Table 2 Biologic regulation of inflammation: the feedback loops and control mechanisms

Regulation ofautoimmunity
Heat-shock proteins
α_2-Macroglobulin
Autoantibodies to cytokines
   may be common in healthy individuals
   carriers or inhibitors? could facilitate or neutralize
Central nervous system–Endocrine immune system reationships
Cytokine inhibitors
   Binding to cytokines
   Competitors for binding sites
   IL-4, IL-8
   IL-10
Leukoprotease inhibitor
Human complement receptor type 1
Protective effects of cytokines (IL-1, TNF, TGF-β)
Other biologic control mechanisms
   Tachyphylaxis with endotoxin injection
   Continuous infusion of TNF: level peaks and
   disappears symptoms appear and disappear
   Bolus infusion: instant assault, no time for
   feedback loops or protective mechanisms

These seem to be feedback loops or control mechanisms. There is also a leukoprotease inhibitor and human complement receptor type 1, which seem to be regulatory mechanisms. It has also been demonstrated that IL-1, TNF, and transforming growth factor β will protect an animal if given in small quantities [20–22].

Other biologic control mechanisms also seem to be present. There is tachyphylaxis with repeated endotoxin injections. During continuous infusion of TNF, the circulating level of TNF peaks and disappears and symptoms appear and disappear [23]. Finally, a bolus infusion or a continuous or rapid

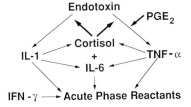

Fig. 1. Stimulation of production or release of cytokines by endotoxin is inhibited by cortisol and PGE$_2$

───▶ increases production or release
━━━▶ inhibits production

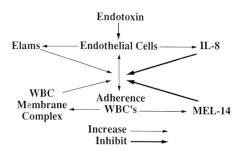

Increase ───▶
Inhibit ━━━▶

Fig. 2. Adherence of white cells to endothelial cells is increased by various receptor molecules and inhibited by others

intravenous infusion of these substances may overwhelm the individual and not allow the feedback loops or protective mechanisms to develop. Examples of these are shown in the feedback mechanisms for the production of TNF and IL-1 by endotoxin. There is the negative feedback loop of cortisol and prostaglandin E$_2$ with injury (Fig. 1). The effect of endotoxin on endothelial cells increases adherence of white blood cells (WBC) (Fig. 2), but there are both promoters and inhibitors of the adherence of white cells to endothelium. Although there may be self-destructive inflammatory responses developing, it may be difficult to block one of them. It may also be difficult to block the excesses without interfering with the basic process. Probably all cannot be blocked, and deleterious effects may be produced by blocking efforts.

Stimulation or Replacement

It would seem much more worthwhile to stimulate or replace. A number of growth factors have been evaluated, some clinically and others in experimental animals, which show positive effects with platelet-derived growth factor, epidermal growth factor, transforming growth factors, fibroblast growth factor, and insulin-like growth factor or somatomedin (Table 3). IL-2 may be helpful as a lymphocyte growth factor [24] along with colony-stimulating factors, granulocyte-macrophage colony-stimulating factor, growth hormone [25–27], and

Table 3. Growth factors

Platelet-derived growth factor (PDGF)
Epidermal growth factor (EGF)
Transforming growth factors (TGF$_\alpha$, TGF$_\beta$)
Fibroblast growth factor (FGR)
Insulin-like growth factor I (IGF-1 or
somatomedin C) and IGF-II
Interleukin-2
Colony stimulating factors (CSF-1, CSF-2,
multi-CSF, granulocyte-macrophage CSF)
Growth hormone
Erythropoietin

Table 4. Protective factors

Surface replacement
Prostaglandin E$_1$
Glutamine
Arginine
Sublethal dose of endotoxin
IL-1
IL-2

---

erythropoietin. Other protective factors are being evaluated and show some initial promise (Table 4). Surfactant replacement in newborns with respiratory difficulties seems to be helpful [28] and is now being evaluated in an adult population with ARDS. Prostaglandin E$_1$ was initially thought to be helpful in patients with ARDS [29] but is now being questioned [30] and requires further evaluation. Substrates such as glutamine [31, 32] and arginine may be helpful, as would sublethal doses of endotoxin, IL-1, and IL-2 [33]. Some of these have been described in my keynote address earlier in this book.

Prevention of MOF

Thus there is great excitement in this wonderful world of cytokines, monoclonal antibodies, and inhibiting agents. Much will be learned, and much will be accomplished. In the meanwhile, we must try to prevent MOF. The following strategies will help:

1. We must return to the basics with rapid transport, early definitive therapy, and an organized system to care for the injured. There must be careful assessment and fine-tuning for elective operations and a definitive, zero-defect operation or repair of injuries (no leaking anastomoses, collections, wound separations, etc.).

2. Early rapid resuscitation must be carried out to decrease the depth and duration of shock and improve microcirculatory blood flow to decrease

ischemia and reperfusion injury. This requires volume—warm and fast. Hypertonic solutions and other agents to improve the microcirculation, such as ATP-MgCl$_2$ and pentoxiphylline, a vasodilating agent, should be considered.

3. It is necessary to stop or control the injury by early definitive operation. This includes immobilization of long-bone and pelvic fractures, and repair of the liver, kidneys, spleen, and bowel. The body cavities must be clean and functional. The necrotic (injured) tissue burden must be decreased to lower the inflammatory quotient.

4. We must remove as much necrotic tissue as possible as soon as possible to decrease the inflammatory response (the weight of infected, injured, or ischemic tissue determines the extent of inflammatory activation).

5. We must recognize that support of the circulation and the kidneys may jeopardize the lungs.

6. Early organ support before failure occurs is necessary. The lungs may require intubation—intermittent mandatory ventilation with continuous positive airway pressure (CPAP) or positive end-expiratory pressure (PEEP). The circulation requires optimal cardiac output without acidosis, produced by increasing preload, inotropic agents, and/or afterload reduction. Circulatory and ventilatory support must be balanced by using ventricular function curves for optimal volumes and PEEP. Support of the kidneys requires an awareness of the relationship of sepsis, tissue necrosis, and inflammation to renal function and the need for polyuria, which indicates that sodium, but not water, is retained with sepsis. Oxygen consumption must be considered. It is recommended presently that oxygen consumption be driven to a higher than normal level by the use of both fluids (colloid) and inotropic agents. The work of Shoemaker suggests that oxygen transport greater than 600 ml/min.m^2 and oxygen consumption greater than 170 ml/min.m^2 will best contribute to the survival of the sick patient [34].

   For the gastrointestinal tract and metabolism, it is necessary to prevent ulceration and bleeding. This may best be done by early enteral feeding. Enteral nutrition with full nutrients is best for preserving the integrity of the gastrointestinal tract. Adjuvants which can be considered to maintain gut structure and function include glutamine or α-ketoglutarate, neurotension, and lipids. Growth hormone may be helpful to stimulate metabolism along with medium chain triglycerides, fish lipids (omega 3 fatty acids), and arginine. Selective gut decontamination for the possibility of colonization and pneumonia requires more evaluation.

7. We must recognize the presence or possibility of sepsis, such as peritonitis or acalculous cholecystitis, when MOF begins.

8. Steroids should be avoided and buffers used only when necessary.

9. Antibiotics should be used early and briefly for contamination.

10. For the contaminated peritoneal cavity, all modalities of therapy should be considered and the appropriate one selected for the individual patient. This

may include frequent reexploration, an open incision, continuous irrigation, or the use of mesh with a zipper for intermittent irrigation and exploration of the peritoneal cavity.

11. Along with this, we must continue to evaluate and study other approaches. Most important in this regard is the possibility of supporting host defense by the use of human monoclonal antibodies to endotoxin, recombinant IL-2, thymopentin, or interferon-γ. Growth factors should also be considered, particularly the platelet-derived factors for wounds, human growth hormone and insulin-like growth factor 1 and epidermal growth factors for wound healing, and granulocyte colony-stimulating factor for neutropenia or better white cell function. As we do this, certainly the care of the injured patient will improve and the incidence of MOF should decrease.

My answer to the question of whether to block, stimulate, or replace is this: blocking all the effects of the mediators of inflammation is not possible and may be harmful. One cannot fool Mother Nature. Stimulation or replacement of host defense activities seems sound, and such studies are under way. Support of the patient and prevention of infection, decrease in inflammation, and support of normal organ function should best prevent MOF. Although the philosopher-movie star Mae West said that too much of a good thing is wonderful, for the injured patient, too much of a good thing (host defense) may be deadly.

References

1. Baue AE (1990) Multiple organ failure: patient care and prevention. Mosby, St Louis
2. Baue AE (1991) The horror autotoxicus and multiple organ failure. Arch Surg (in press)
3. Albelda SM, Buck CA (1990) Integrins and other cell adhesion molecules. FASEB J 4:2868–2880
4. Vedder NB, Fouty BW, Winn RK, Harlan JM, Rice CL (1989) Role of neutrophils in generalized reperfusion injury associated with resuscitation from shock. Surgery 106:509–516
5. Sharar SR, Winn RK, Harlan JM, Rice CL (1991) Anti-CD18 antibody increases the incidence and severity of subcutaneous abscess formation after high dose *S. aureus* injection in rabbits. Surgery (in press)
6. Saez JC, Ward PH, Gunther B et al. (1984) Superoxide radical involvement in the pathogenesis of burn shock. Circ Shock 12:229–239
7. Tracey KJ, Fung Y, Hesse KR et al. (1987) Anti-cachetin/TNF monoclonal antibodies prevent septic shock during lethal bacteremia. Nature 330:6662–6624
8. Hinshaw LB, Tekamp-Olson P, Chang ACK et al. (1990) Survival of primates in LD_{100} septic shock following therapy with antibody to tumor necrosis factor (TNFz). Circ Shock 30:279–292
9. Yim JH, Tewari A, Pearce MK, Zou JC, Abrams JS, Starnes HF Jr (1990) Monoclonal antibody against murine interleukin-6 prevents lethal effects of Escherichia coli sepsis and tumor necrosis factor challenge in mice. Surg Forum 41:114–117
10. Weiss SJ (1989) Tissue destruction by neutrophils. N Engl J Med 300:365–376
11. Figdor CG, van Kooyk Y, Keizer GD (1990) On the mode of action of LFA-1. Immunol Today 11:227–280
12. Faist E, Ertel W, Cohnert T, Huber P, Inthorn D, Heberer G (1990) Immunoprotective effects of cyclooxygenase inhibition in patients with major surgical trauma. J Trauma 30:8–18
13. Schwartz R (1989) In Cohen IR: An electric summary of symposium on autoimmunity. Immunol Today 10:394–396
14. Ellis J (1987) Proteins as molecular chaperons. Nature 328:378–379
15. Polla BS, Young D (1989) Heat shock proteins and immunity. Immunol Today 10:393–394

16. Kaufman SH (1990) Heat shock proteins and the immune response. Immunol Today 11:129–136
17. James K (1990) Interactions between cytokines and A_2-macroglobulin. Immunol Today 11:163–166
18. Berdtzen K, Svenson M, Jonsson V, Hippe E (1990) Autoantibodies to cytokines: friends or foes? Immunol Today 11:167–169
19. Khansari DN, Margo AJ, Faith RE (1990) Effects of stress on the immune system. Immunol Today 11:170–175
20. Durum SK, Mealy K (1990) Hilton Head revisited: cytokine explosion of the 80's takes shape of the 90's. Immunol Today 11:103–107
21. Alexander HR, Fraker DL, Swendenborg JA, Norton JA (1991) Human recombinant inter-leukin-1 (IL-1) protection against lethality of endotoxin and experimental sepsis in mice. J Surg (in press)
22. Silver GM, Gamelli RL, O'Reilly M, Hebert JC (1990) The effect of interleukin-la on survival in murine model of burn wound sepsis. Arch Surg 125:922–925
23. Michie HR, Spriggs DR, Manogue RR et al. (1988) Tumor necrosis factor and endotoxin induce similar metabolic responses in human beings. Surgery 104:280–286
24. Gough DB, Moss NM, Jordan A, Gribic JT, Roderick ML, Mannick JA (1988) Recombinant interleukin-2 (rIL-2) improves immune response and host resistance to septic challenge in thermally injured mice. Surgery 104(2):292–300
25. Herndon DN, Barrow RE, Junkel KR, Broemeling L, Rutan RL (1990) Effects of recombinant human growth hormone on donor-site healing in severely burned children. Ann Surg 212:424–430
26. Zeigler TR, Young LS, Manson JM, Wilmore DW (1988) Metabolic effects of recombinant human growth hormone in patients receiving parenteral nutrition. Ann Surg 208:6–16
27. Manson JM, Smith RJ, Wilmore DW (1988) Growth hormone stimulates protein synthesis during hypocaloric parenteral nutrition. Ann Surg 208:136–149
28. Horbar JD, Soll RF, Sutherland JM et al. (1989) A multicenter randomized, placebo-controlled trial of surfactant therapy for respirator distress syndrome. N Engl J Med 320:959–966
29. Holcroft JW, Vasary MJ, Weber CJ (1986) Prostaglandin E_1 and survival in patients with the adult respiratory distress syndrome: a prospective trial. Ann Surg 203:371–380
30. Silverman HJ, Slotman G, Bone RC et al., the Prostaglandin E_1 Study Group (1990) Effects of prostaglandin E_1 on oxygen delivery and consumption in patients with the adult respiratory distress syndrome. Chest 98:405–410
31. Klimberg VS, Salloum RM, Kasper M et al. (1990) Oral glutamine accelerates healing of the small intestine and improves outcome after whole abdominal radiation. Arch Surg 125:1040–1045
32. Hinshaw DB, Ruger JM, Delius RE, Hysolp PA (1990) Mechanism of protection of oxidant-injured endothelial cells by glutamine. Surgery 108:298–305
33. Bensard DD, Brown JM, Anderson BO et al. (1990) Induction of endogenous tissue antioxidant enzyme activity attenuates myocardial reperfusion injury. J Surg Res 49:126–131
34. Shoemaker WC, Appel PL, Kram HB, Waxman K, Lee T-S (1988) Prospective trial of supranormal values of survivors as therapeutic goals in high risk surgical patients. Chest 94:1176–1186

Section 12

**The Pathophysiologic Impact of
Bacterial Translocation and
Strategies for its Prevention**

Bacterial Translocation Following Major Thermal Injury in Rats, Sheep, and Mini-Pigs

D. N. Herndon[1, 2], S. T. Zeigler[1, 2], T. C. Rutan[1], R. Saydjari[2], S. E. Morris[3], G. I. Beerthuizen[4], R. Tokyay[1], and C. M. Townsend[2]

While great strides have been made in the care of burn patients, there are still over 4000 deaths caused by burns annually in the United States. Sepsis remains a major cause of mortality and morbidity. Bacterial translocation has recently been suggested as a possible mechanism for allowing gut flora to escape into the systemic circulation and seed previously sterile organs [1]. The mucosa of the gastrointestinal tract serves as protection from caustic damage and prevents the egress of potentially harmful substances which could then penetrate across to other organ systems. Much evidence has shown that after a major thermal cutaneous injury the integrity of this mucosal barrier is compromised [2]. The mechanisms responsible for this mucosal damage have been investigated using three different models.

Methods

Sprague-Dawley rats ($n = 146$) were divided into three groups. Group I sham burn plus saline, Group II 50% total body surface area (TBSA) burn plus saline, Group III 50% TBSA burn plus 10μg/kg per day of bombesin [3]. Animals were pair fed chow and killed at four days. Mesenteric lymph nodes and blood were obtained aseptically at autopsy. Mucosal weights of the distal 20 cm of small bowel was taken to assess any trophic effects.

Twenty-three chronically instrumented ewes were divided into four groups [4]. All animals were prepared with arterial, venous, and pulmonary artery catheters along with ultrasonic flow probes placed around the cephalic mesenteric artery (CMA). Group I received sham ($n = 6$) burn, group II ($n = 5$) received 40% TBSA burn, group III ($n = 5$) had a mechanical occluder placed around the CMA with reduction in flow by 50% for the initial 8 h by an inflatable cuff, and group IV ($n = 7$) received 40% TBSA burn with selective infusion of nitroprusside into the CMA to maintain blood flow at preburn levels. Burn resuscitation consisted of lactated Ringer's and ovine plasma to maintain

[1] Shriners Burns Institute
[2] University of Texas Medical Branch, Galveston, TX, USA
[3] Department of Surgery, University of Utah, School of Medicine, Salt Lake City, Utah, USA
[4] University of Nijmegen, Nijmegen, The Netherlands

Host Defense Dysfunction
in Trauma, Shock and Sepsis
Eds. Faist/Meakins/Schildberg
© Springer-Verlag, Berlin Heidelberg 1993

cardiac output (CO) and urine output (UO) at preinjury levels. All groups were observed for 48 h then underwent aseptic harvesting of internal organs after sacrifice.

Twelve chronically instrumented miniature pigs were divided into two groups [5]. All animals had ultrasonic flow probes placed around the superior mesenteric artery (SMA) and portal venous catheters inserted. Each group received 40% TBSA burn and resuscitation via the Parkland formula. Group I received OKY046, a specific thromboxane synthetase inhibitor, 10 mg/kg bolus prior to burn and 100 µg/kg per minute following burn for 16 h. Group II received saline only. Animals were observed for 48 h then sacrificed.

An additional 12 chronically instrumented miniature pigs were divided into two groups [6]. Group I received sham burn and group II received 40% TBSA burn. After 48 h, animals were sacrificed and organs harvested aseptically for culture and intestinal segments taken for DNA, RNA, and ornithine decarboxylase (ODC) analysis.

Results

In the rat experiment, burn injury resulted in a decrease ($p < 0.05$) in mucosal weight compared with sham (Fig. 1). The burn group had 86% translocation ($p < 0.05$) of bacteria to mesenteric lymph nodes compared to 0% for sham. The bombesin group showed a normalization of mucosal weight and a decrease in translocation to 28% of mesenteric lymph nodes ($p < 0.05$) compared with burn alone.

In the chronically instrumented sheep experiments, the CMA blood flow decreased to 40% of baseline ($p < 0.05$) after thermal injury and returned to preinjury levels by 16 h. With the occluder inflated the CMA blood flow was

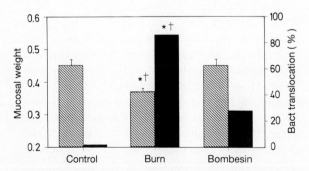

Fig. 1. The effects of a 50% TBSA burn and burn + bombesin on mucosal weight (g/100 g body weight) and bacterial translocation to mesenteric lymph nodes in the rat model. With administration of 10 µg/kg per day of bombesin, the loss of mucosal weight (*light hatching*) after burn is prevented ($p < 0.05$) and bacterial translocation (*dark hatching*) is decreased by 66% ($p < 0.05$). * + $p < 0.05$ versus control and bombesin

held at 50% of baseline for 4 h. With selective infusion of nitroprusside into the CMA following burn, there was no decrease seen in intestinal blood flow. The cultures of mesenteric lymph nodes showed that the burn and the occluder groups had significant quantitative increases in bacteria compared to sham and selective nitroprusside infusion as seen in Fig. 2.

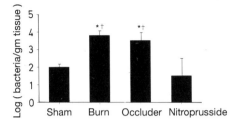

Fig. 2. Quantitative cultures of mesenteric lymph nodes following 40% TBSA burn in sheep are significantly increased when compared with sham burn ($*p < 0.05$). With selective infusion of nitroprusside into the CMA following burn, the quantitative cultures are no different than the sham ($+ p < 0.05$). Mechanically occluding the CMA to similar decreases in blood flow that occur following 40% TBSA burn in sheep results in increase in bacterial translocation. ($p < 0.05$)

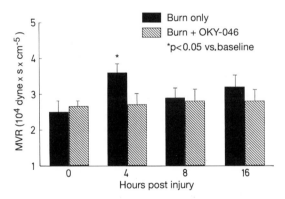

Fig. 3. In the mini-pig model a 40% TBSA burn results in increases in the mesenteric vascular resistance (MVR) seen at four h postinjury ($p < 0.05$). Blocking thromboxane synthesis with OKY-046, this increase in MVR is prevented

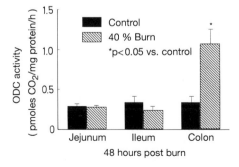

Fig. 4. Ornithine decarboxylase (ODC) is the rate-limiting step in polyamine synthesis in gut mucosa. Increased activity of ODC is used as a marker for gut mucosal regeneration. Following 40% TBSA burn in the mini-pig ODC activity is seen to be elevated within the colon ($p < 0.05$) 48 h after burn suggesting an earlier injury and ongoing repair

In the chronically instrumented pig experiments, SMA blood flow was significantly decreased within the first hours following burn by 33% ($p < 0.05$) of baseline with concomitant 100% incidence of translocation of bacteria to mesenteric lymph nodes despite maintenance of CO, UO, and mean arterial pressure with Parkland resuscitation. Following 40% burn there was an increase in ODC activity in the colon along with increases in DNA and RNA content in the small bowel and the colon (Fig. 3). With pretreatment with OKY046 the postburn increase in mesenteric vascular resistance was prevented ($p < 0.05$) as seen in Fig. 4.

Conclusions

The care of burn victims has improved tremendously over the last three decades with improvements in topical antimicrobial, early excision and grafting, improvement in intensive care, and proper resuscitation. Despite these impressive advances, sepsis associated with burns is still a leading cause of mortality and morbidity. Typically, the offending bacteria are of a type that generally resides in the gastrointestinal tract. The phenomenon of bacterial translocation is believed to be the nidus of subsequent seeding of sterile organs in this population.

We have clearly shown that with a major thermal injury there is a significant decrease in gastrointestinal blood flow. In both the pig and the sheep, this has been demonstrated. Also, by mechanically reducing the mesenteric blood flow to mimic the reduction seen after burn, we are able to reproduce similar rates of bacterial translocation. The rate of bacterial translocation can be lessened by selectively infusing nitroprusside into the mesenteric artery following thermal injury, thereby preventing vasoconstriction. In a similar fashion, we have blocked the increase in MVR after thermal injury by selectively blocking thromboxane synthesis. This suggests that the decrease in mesenteric blood flow is mediated primarily by thromboxane, a known potent vasoconstrictor.

We were also able to ameliorate the decrease in mucosal weight and thus decrease the rate of bacterial translocation following burns with the administration of an intestinal growth factor, bombesin. There also appears to be significant mucosal damage following thermal injury as shown by large increases in reparative markers seen in the colonic mucosa and small bowel. Therefore, there is a significant decrease in mesenteric blood flow after major thermal injury. This is associated with an increased incidence of bacterial translocation which can be perturbed by prevention of mesenteric vasoconstriction. With improvement in mucosal function, bacterial translocation is lessened.

References

1. Maejima K, Deitch EA, Berg RA (1984) Promotion by burn stress of the translocation of bacteria from the gastrointestinal tract of mice. Arch Surg 119:166–171
2. Carter EA, Tompkins RG, Schiffrin ES, Burke JF (1990) Cutaneous thermal injury alters macromolecular permeability of rat small intestine. Surgery 107:335–341
3. Coffey GA, Milhoan RA, Abdullah A et al. (1988) Bombesin inhibits bacterial translocation from the gut in burned rats. Surg Forum 39:109–110
4. Morris SE, Navaratnam N, Herndon DN (1989) Decreased mesenteric blood flow independently promotes bacterial translocation in the chronically instrumented sheep. Surg Forum 40:88–89
5. Tokyay R, Traber DL, Herndon DN (1990) Thromboxane synthetase inhibition prevents the increased mesenteric vascular resistance seen after major thermal burn in a chronic porcine model. Surg Forum 41:56–59
6. Saydjari R, Herndon DN, Beerthuizen GIJM et al. Bacterial translocation and its relationship to visceral blood flow, gut mucosal ornithine decarboxylase activity and DNA in pigs. J Trauma (in press)

Does Early Portal Bacteremia/Endotoxemia Prime for Postinjury Multiple Organ Failure?

F. A. Moore, E. E. Moore, R. S. Poggetti, and O. J. McAnena

There is an emerging consensus that gut-derived bacteria and endotoxin are prime etiologic factors in the genesis of postinjury multiple organ failure (MOF) [1–3]. Central to this evolving concept has been the documentation of bacterial translocation in animals subjected to a variety of noxious insults [2]. Although bacterial translocation has been consistently demonstrated in these experimental models, its occurrence in man is uncertain and its precise role and specific mechanisms of initiating distant organ dysfunction remain to be established [3]. Portal bacteremic or endotoxemic activation or priming of Kupffer cells is one plausible link [4–7]. In this study, we examined the gut–portal vein–liver axis during the early postinjury period to determine if gut-derived bacteria, endotoxin, or cytokines appear in the portal vein and if their presence correlates with the development of MOF.

Materials and Methods

During a 9- month period ending December 1989, 20 patients with known risk factors for MOF required emergency laparotomy following trauma and had placement of a portal vein catheter. Management of abdominal trauma was uniform throughout the study period. Patients were characterized by the Revised Trauma Score (RTS), Injury Severity Score (ISS), and Abdominal Trauma Index (ATI). In addition to tracking standard clinical outcome variables, MOF was quantitated by a scoring system that grades the dysfunction of eight individual organ systems: 1 for minimal derangement, 2 for moderate, and 3 for severe. The worst individual scores after 48 h were summed and a score greater than 8 was defined as MOF. Portal and systemic blood samples were obtained after placement of the portal vein catheter and then again at 6, 12, 24, 48 h and 5 days postoperatively. These samples were cultured for aerobic and anaerobic bacterial growth (Bactec NR-660). Endotoxin (LPS) was assayed using the chromogenic *Limulus* amoebocyte lysate test (QCL-1000, Whittaker Bioproducts, Walkersville, MD, USA). There was no detectable LPS in any of the normal controls ($n = 15$). Tumor necrosis factor (TNF) was assayed using a

Department of Surgery, Denver General Hospital, and the University of Colorado Health Sciences Center, Denver, CO 80204, USA

Host Defense Dysfunction
in Trauma, Shock and Sepsis
Eds. Faist/Meakins/Schildberg
© Springer-Verlag, Berlin Heidelberg 1993

radioimmunoassay specific for human TNF-α (Genzyme Corp, Boston, MA, USA). Normal control TNF levels ranged from 60 to 320 pg/ml (mean $\pm$ SEM 169 $\pm$ 16 pg/ml). Complement fragment C3a levels were measured by radioimmunoassay (Amersham International, Amersham, UK). Normal control C3a ranged from 184 to 376 ng/ml (mean $\pm$ SEM 318 $\pm$ 34 ng/ml). Interleukin-6 (IL-6) was assayed by a double "sandwich" enzyme-linked immunoabsorbant assay (Amgen Inc., Boulder, CO, USA). IL-6 was not detected in normal controls. For statistical analysis, analysis of variance was used to discern significant differences over time for the various assays and between portal and systemic samples at the same point.

Results

The ages of the 20 study patients ranged from 18 to 86 years (mean 34 $\pm$ 4) and 80% were men. Injury mechanism was blunt in 14 (70%) and penetrating in six. Twelve patients (60%) arrived in shock (systolic blood pressure $<$ 90 Torr); the mean RTS was 6.4 $\pm$ 0.4. Inclusion criteria included massive transfusion in 11 (23.8 $\pm$ 4.8 units blood in the first 24 h) and major abdominal trauma in six (ATI 31 $\pm$ 2), while three patients sustained multiple fractures (ISS 34 $\pm$ 4). Six patients (30%) developed MOF; in five this occurred later than postinjury day 5. Two of these MOF patients and single early positive portal cultures; one grew a coagulase-negative staphyloccocal species, the other was positive for *Propionibacterium acnes*. All patients with MOF were eventually treated for major pulmonary infections, but only one cases of pneumonia (*Staphyloccocus aureus*) occurred during the first 5 days. The remaining were late cases (after postinjury day 5); offending organisms included three *Enterobacter* species, two *Acinobacter* species, and one *Echerichia coli*. One of these patients was subsequently treated for systemic fungemia. There was one early death due to head injury and shock, while two of the six MOF patients succumbed at 16 and 34 days respectively.

Nine (2%) of 424 blood cultures obtained by protocol were positive. Breakdown by time, site, and organism is shown in Table 1. *P. acnes* is generally dismissed as a blood culture contaminant, while coagulase-negative staphylococci are generally ascribed to an intravenous catheter. Additionally, simultaneous portal and systemic blood samples obtained in the first 48 h were negative for endotoxin. These samples were run in triplicate and, to be certain that undetectable endotoxin was not simply due to increased levels of inhibitors, 100 randomly selected patient plasma samples were spiked with known amounts of LPS (0111:B4) prior to heat inactivation and 1:40 dilution. Percent recovery was 94.3 $\pm$ 2.5, and in 77 of these samples recovery exceeded 90%. Due to these negative portal studies, we began to sample ileocolic mesenteric lymph nodes (MLN) intraoperatively. Of the 12 samples obtained in this study, four (25%) were culture positive. *Enterobacter cloacae*, enterococcus,

Table 1. Blood culture surveillance in patients at risk for MOF

Blood sample	Time					
	0 h	6 h	12 h	24 h	48 h	5 days
Portal						
Positive cultures	1	1	1	0	3	2
	(P)	(S)	(P)		(S, S, A)	(S, S)
Total cultures	40	40	36	34	32	30
Systemic						
Positive cultures	0	0	0	0	0	1
						(SA)
Total cultures	40	40	36	34	32	30

Portal and systemic cultures were obtained in the operating room (0 h) and at 6, 12, 24, 48 h and 5 days postoperatively. P, *Propionibacterium acnes*; S, Coagulase-negative staphylococci, A, *Acinobacter* species; SA, *Staphyloloccus aureus*.

Table 2. Portal and systemic inflammatory marker's in patients at risk for MOF

Time	C3a (ng/ml) ($n = 18$)		TNF (pg/ml) ($n = 18$)		IL-6 (pg/ml) ($n = 14$)	
	Portal	Systemic	Portal	Systemic	Portal	Systemic
0 h	781 ± 107	802 ± 122	116 ± 17	118 ± 16	390 ± 85	414 ± 91
6 h	493 ± 76	434 ± 76	148 ± 17	141 ± 20	337 ± 49	373 ± 54
12 h	337 ± 47	370 ± 62	155 ± 23	149 ± 20	237 ± 46	269 ± 59
24 h	491 ± 67	412 ± 55	155 ± 20	166 ± 26	173 ± 40	180 ± 45
48 h	533 ± 64	503 ± 55	146 ± 24	139 ± 21	98 ± 38	94 ± 37

Portal and systemic levels (Mean ± SEM) of complement fragment (C3a), tumor necrosis factor (TNF), and interleukin-6 (IL-6) obtained in the operating room (0 h), and 6, 12, 24, and 48 h postoperatively.

α-hemolytic streptococci, and coagulase-negative *Staphylococcus* species were the individual organisms identified. Three of the four patients with positive MLN cultures arrived in shock, but there was no correlation with these positive MLNs and subsequent MOF. And finally, simultaneous portal and systemic blood levels of C3a, TNF, and interleukin-6 (IL-6) were nearly identical (Table 2) and, specifically, were not different in the MOF patients. Additionally, individual levels of C3a, TNF and IL-6 did not correlate with the development of MOF.

In a subsequent group of 61 patients requiring urgent trauma laparotomy, we obtained blood cultures in the emergency department. Three (7%) of the 43 patients whose systolic blood pressure (SBP) exceeded 90 Torr had positive culture results (*P. acnes* in 2, coagulose-negative staphylococci in 1), whereas six (33%) of 18 patients with a SBP less than 90 Torr had blood cultures positive for coagulase-negative staphylococci, α-hemolytic streptococci, *Enterococcus*, *E. coli*, and *Bacteroides fragilis*. Four of these patients with positive cultures exsanguinated shortly after hospitalization.

Discussion

Gut-derived bacteria and endotoxin have recently been involved as prime etiologic factors in postinjury MOF, and it has been postulated that the liver plays a pivatol role in regulating the systemic manifestations of this morbid syndrome [1–7]. Although the supporting basic research is logical and compelling, the clinical evidence that early bacteremia or endotoxemia play a significant role in the genesis of MOF is at best circumstantial. As a correlate to their animal shock model, Rush et al. sampled blood within 3 h of admission in 50 acutely injured patients: cultures were positive in 10 (56%) of the 18 patients with an initial SBP < 80 Torr [3]. Unfortunately, this gravely injured group of patients had little chance of developing MOF (13 of 18 died within 24 h). Indeed, our recent emergency department data confirm that 33% of patients arriving moribund had positive cultures, but again two-thirds exsanguinated early. On the other hand, the 20 study patients who survived laparotomy and who were at known risk for MOF had no evidence of early systemic bacterial translocation nor did we document any gut–portal vein–liver signalling. With the exception of contaminants, portal blood had only one pathogen emerge from 224 samples, and to our surprise, we could find no endotoxin. Cytokine levels, albeit elevated, were nearly identical to systemic levels and individual levels did not correlate with the development of distant organ dysfunction. Clearly our data do not exclude the lymphatics as a significant route of early bacterial translocation. The rare occurrence of systemic bacteremia as well as the nonspiking nature of the TNF levels, however, suggest that if early translocation is occurring to the MLN, it is a well contained process.

References

1. Wilmore DW, Smith RJ, O'Dwyer ST et al. (1988) The gut: a central organ after surgical stress. Surgery 104:917–923
2. Deitch FA, Winterton J, Berg R (1987) The gut as a portal entry bacteremia. Ann Surg 205:681–692
3. Rush BF, Sori AJ, Murphy TF et al. (1988) Endotoxemia and bacteremia during hemorrhagic shock. Ann Surg 207:549–554
4. Keller GA, West MA, Cerra FB et al. (1985) Modulation of hepatocyte protein synthesis by endotoxin activated Kupffer cells. Ann Surg 201:87–95
5. Peterson VM, Moore EE, Jones TN et al. (1988) TEN versus TPN following major torso trauma: attenuation of hepatic protein repriorization. Surgery 104:199–205
6. Marshall JC, Lee C, Meakins JL et al. (1987) Kupffer cell modulation of the systemic immune response. Arch Surg 122:191–196
7. Ogle CK, Arita H, Nagy H et al. (1989) The immunosuppressive effects of the invivo administration of endotoxin as influenced by macrophages. J Trauma 29:1015–1020

Prevention of Bacterial Translocation with Early Enteral Feeding—A Feasible Approach?*

J.W. Alexander

Infection is the leading cause of death in severely traumatized patients who spend more than 5 days in the intensive care unit, being responsible for approximately 75% of deaths. The reasons for this are multifactorial, but a major factor appears to be a failure of gut barrier function against translocation of endotoxin and microorganisms from the intestine which follows inadequate enteral nutrition. Thermal injury in experimental animals has been used as a model for studying this important problem.

Dominioni et al. [1] developed a model to study enteral feeding in guinea pigs with a 30% total body surface full-thickness burn. Gastrostomy tubes were placed for enteral feeding approximately 1 week before burn injury which allowed the delivery of pump-controlled continuous gastrostomy feedings that could be stringently regulated with regard to composition and amount. The model allowed the performance of complex metabolic studies with control of both nutritional and non-nutritional variables. These investigators initially used a feeding regimen to mimic what was being used clinically and this was associated with a 50%–70% increase in the resting energy expenditure 2–3 weeks following thermal burn. During the first 24 h animals received only lactated Ringer's solutions by gastrostomy. During the second 24 h they received one-third strength of a burn formula, during the third 24 h they received two-thirds strength formula, and after 72 h they received full-strength formula. This resulted in an approximate 15% loss of body weight initially and the weight could be stabilized by administering 175 kcal/kg per day. Weight gain was associated with an intake of 200 kcal/kg per day. When full-strength formula was given immediately after burn injury at 175 kcal/kg per day, the weight loss was only approximately 5% of the initial body weight. More surprisingly, the animals did not become as hypermetabolic with the increase in resting energy expenditure being approximately 80% less than animals fed with the delayed feeding regimen described above.

Mochizuki et al. [2] found that there was a dramatic (approximately 50%) reduction in the jejunal mucosal mass of burned guinea pigs receiving only lactated Ringer's in the first 24 h. In contrast, animals fed full-strength formula during the first 24 h had an insignificant loss of mucosal weight. Jejunal mucosal

* Supported in part by USPHS grant AI 12936.
Transplantation Division, University of Cincinnati College of Medicine, 231 Bethesda Avenue, Cincinnati, OH 45267-0558, USA

thickness was reduced approximately 30% in the first 24 h in animals given only lactated Ringer's, but there was no loss in thickness in animals fed full-strength formula. Atrophic changes in animals given only lactated Ringer's was confirmed by scanning electron microscopy. Plasma cortisol and glucagon rose significantly and dramatically in animals given only lactated Ringer's but did not rise significantly in animals fed immediately after burn injury. Perhaps of greatest interest was a highly significant inverse correlation between the jejunal mucosal weight and both plasma cortisol and plasma glucagon at 24 h.

The working hypothesis to explain these observations was that a lack of enteral nutrition following burn injury was associated with rapid atrophy of the gastrointestinal mucosal mas with loss of the barrier to translocation of endotoxin and intestinal microbes. When translocation of these substances occurred, it was associated with activation of macrophages both in the mesenteric lymph nodes and liver, with the release of cytokines including interleukin-1 (IL-1), IL-6, and tumor necrosis factor (TNF). Additionally, the arachidonic acid pathway was activated with the release of prostaglandin E_2 (PGE_2) and the complement pathway was activated with the release of a number of important activation products which were immunosuppressive including fluid phase C3b, C3a, C5a, C3c, C3d, and C3e. The cytokines, particularly IL-1 and IL-6, act centrally on the nervous system to stimulate the release of adrenocorticotropic hormone (ACTH), which stimulates the adrenal glands to produce cortisol, and other mediators which result in the release of norepinephrine and glucagon, which together are important mediators for the hypermetabolic response. It was further reasoned that biological effects of the prostaglandin, cytokine, and complement degradation products released were deleterious to the microcirculation and increased the likelihood of the development of multiple system organ failure.

Additional investigations by Inoue et al. [3] showed that translocation of *Candida albicans* occurred regularly following burn injury and the degree of translocation was related to the size of the burn. When translocation was measured as the recovery of viable organisms in the mesenteric lymph nodes, in animals given a gavage of *Candida albicans* just before burn injury, recovery of viable organisms was first seen 6 h following burn injury and reached a maximal degree 24 h after burn injury.

These studies lead to an investigation of the process by which *C. albicans* and *Escherichia coli* and endotoxin translocate across the intestinal barrier following thermal injury [4]. Both guinea pigs and rats were used for these studies in which the translocation probe was placed into a Thiry Vella loop of animals at the time of 50% total body surface area burn. The loop was excised at various intervals during the first 24 h and examined for translocation. *C. albicans* was seen to attach to the mucosal surface within 1 h and to become embedded in the microvillus layer. There was rapid transport of the organisms across the plasma membrane without evidence of classical phagocytosis. In particular, the internalized organisms were not surrounded by a plasma membrane. The candidal bodies moved progressively from the apical to the basal portions of the enterocytes, always passing through enterocytes and never between them. When they reached the basal layer, they were extruded into the lamina propria with bits of surrounding cytoplasm, a process also quite unlike classical exocytosis. Upon reaching the lamina propria, some of the *Candida* remained free, others were phagocytized by macrophages, some passed into the central lacteals and lymphatics, and others into venules. Plugs with *Candida* and associated phagocytic cells, cellular debris, and platelets were sometimes found in small venules and lymphatics. Organisms were carried to the lymphoid tissue in both Peyer's patches and regional lymph nodes, where they could be found in both medullary areas of the nodes and in germinal centers. In animals that were sacrificed at 24 h, small microabscesses could occasionally be seen in vessels with invasion of the vessel wall. Additionally, an endotoxin-specific monoclonal antibody was used to label translocated *E. coli* in tissue by fluorescent microscopy. *E. coli* were found to pass directly across the cytoplasm of the enterocyte in a manner similar to *C. albicans* and to enter the lamina propria, and endotoxin acted in a similar way. However, unlike *C. albicans*, the organisms and endotoxin were found to pass directly into and through the muscular layer, passing between rather than through the myocytes.

Subsequent studies in burned mice showed passage of both ^{14}C labeled endotoxin and intact ^{14}C-labeled *E. coli* directly through the intact bowel wall to enter the peritoneal cavity [5]. This transport occurred as early as 2 h following burn injury in mice gavaged with bacteria immediately before injury. When assessed by radioactive counts per gram of tissue, the translocation was greatest to the mesenteric lymph nodes, with significant amounts translocating to the spleen and lungs. The greatest amount of killing of translocated organisms occurred in the mesenteric lymph nodes and spleen with less efficient killing in the liver and lungs.

Rush et al. [6] showed that there was a significant correlation of positive blood cultures with the degree of hemorrhagic shock in patients. Patients with admission blood pressures less than 80 mmHg had a greater than 50% incidence of positive cultures compared to less than 10% of patients with an admission blood pressure greater than 110 mmHg. Other studies from that laboratory [7] showed that translocation associated with hemorrhagic shock was also associated with mortality. None of the animals demonstrating translocation with hemorrhagic shock survived, compared to 80% of animals not demonstrating translocation, although the severity of the shock was the same.

These studies and those of Beerthuizen et al. [8] strongly suggest that the intestinal blood flow is an important factor in the predisposition to translocation. Since it was well-known that enteral food can increase blood flow to the intestine, Inoue et al. [9] studied blood flow to the intestine in fed and starved animals subjected to a thermal injury. They were able to show that burn injury was associated with a decrease in intestinal blood flow, particularly to the jejunum and cecum 24 h following burn injury, even though cardiac output was normal or increased, and that administration of a diet significantly increased blood flow in both of these intestinal segments. This was an important observation since other experiments showed that administration of a single bolus of diet could significantly decrease the incidence of translocation of *C. albicans* from the intestinal tract of a burned guinea pig [10]. Those studies also demonstrated that ideal colonization was significantly associated with the degree of translocation, but only in starved and not in fed animals. Likewise, serum cortisol levels were associated significantly with the incidence of *Candida* translocation to the mesenteric lymph nodes.

Another interesting experiments by Inoue et al. [11] studies burned animals given either *C. albicans* or saline by gavage before burn injury and then either immediately fed or starved for 72 h. The mortality rate was significantly higher at 72 h in starved than fed animals that had been gavaged with *Candida*. The fed animals without *Candida* had a mortality of only 1 in 25 animals, and in fed animals with *Candida* there was a mortality of only 2 in 25 animals. Thus, starvation itself did not increase mortality but the presence of *Candida* in the intestinal tract associated with translocation resulted in a higher mortality in starved but not fed animals.

To further investigate the effect of early feeding in burn injury, 14 patients were prospectively randomized to receive enteral feeding within 12 h of burn injury or to receive intravenous fluids with a delay in enteral feeding for 72 h [12]. Patients with early feeding had a total of 6 infectious episodes compared to 12 in the controls, and there were 4 instances of diarrhea in the group fed early compared to 8 in the controls. Nitrogen balance, total serum protein, albumin, serum ceruloplasm, and serum immunoglobulin were all significantly higher during the first week in patients that were fed early compared to the controls. None of the patients had complications from early feeding. The safety of early, aggressive enteral feeding has been further supported by the studies of McDonald and Deitch [13] who gave immediate gastric feedings to 107 seriously burned patients with an average burn size of 40% with no instances of aspiration of pneumonia.

Perioperative enteral feedings can also be safely accomplished in burned patients, as reported by Buescher et al. [14] who fed 47 patients through operations with no complications. Jenkins et al. [15] had a similar experience, feeding 60 patients through 132 operative procedures with no incidence of aspiration. These studies all support the concept that nutritional therapy can be given to seriously injured patients with gastric atony by placing nasoduodenal tubes and feeding directly into the small intestine.

Intravenous feedings are associated with a much higher incidence of complications than enteral feedings. Saito et al. [16] placed both central venous catheters and gastrostomy tubes in animals 7 days before burn injury. They were then randomly allocated to receive either gastric feedings or intravenous feedings. Animals fed gastrically had significantly less weight loss than those fed intravenously. Furthermore, there was significant atrophy of the mucosa of the jejunum and ileum at both 1 and 14 days following burn injury in intravenously fed animals but not enterally fed animals. Similar to in animals not receiving any nutritional support, plasma cortisol and glucagon were elevated for the first 24 h in animals fed intravenously but not in those fed a nutritionally similar formulation by the intestinal tract. Similar to the previous studies of Mochizuki et al. [2], there was a significant correlation between plasma cortisol and plasma glucagon with jejunal mucosal weight. It is not surprising from these studies then that Alverdy et al. [17] found that total parenteral nutrition (TPN) promoted bacterial translocation from the intestine. Approximately 70% of animals fed intravenously developed translocation to the mesenteric lymph nodes compared to none of the animals fed regular chow. However, when the parenteral formulation was fed enterally, the incidence of translocation was decreased but was still significantly greater than control animals fed chow. Mochizuki et al. [18] demonstrated that animals fed with TPN following gastrectomy had an increase in the plasma endotoxin levels whereas animals fed enterally did not. Furthermore patients coming to the operating room fed with TPN had significantly higher portal vein endotoxin levels than did not patients with enteral feedings. Finally, Moore et al. [19] randomly divided patients with serious trauma into two groups, both fed within the 12 h following injury. One group was given TPN intravenously while the other was given the TPN formulation enterally. Those fed total enteral nutrition had significantly higher levels of transferrin on day 5 and a significant reduction in infections (9% compared to 37%).

Composition of the diet also influences outcome. Two groups of animals were given enteral diets of exactly the same composition with the exception that the source of nitrogen in one diet was an intact whey protein and the other diet had crystalline amino acids in the same concentrations that are found in whey protein [20]. Animals receiving the amino acid diet lost significantly more weight than the animals receiving whole protein. In addition, their gut mucosal mass was heavier, they had higher levels of serum albumin, C3, and transeferrin, and their nitrogen balance was improved. It was not surprising that Shou et al. [21] were able to show that a polypeptide diet prevented translocation in metho-trexate-induced colitis, whereas elemental diets with or without supplemental glutamine did not. On the other hand, Fox et al. [22] demonstrated that glutamine supplementation reduced blood endotoxin levels in a similar model of methotrexate induced enterocolitis and somewhat prolonged survival. Glutamine was also found to prevent translocation following abdominal radiation [23]. Indeed, there are several nutrients that might affect translocation besides glutamine. These include arginine, lipids (especially omega 6 fatty acids), and fibers which degrade to generate short-chain fatty acids. However, probably the most important factor in translocation of the gut in patients is luminal feeding.

In summary, intestinal atrophy occurs rapidly in the absence of enteral nutrition, and this process is greatly accelerated with increasing severity of traumatic injury. However, early enteral nutrition following trauma can prevent atrophy of the intestinal mucosa and decrease the incidence of septic complications and diarrhea. This effect may, in part, be because enteral nutrition increases blood flow to the intestine and decreases the translocation of microorganisms and endotoxins from the intestinal tract. In contrast, parenteral nutrition is associated with atrophy of the intestinal mucosa and increased microbial translocation. Translocation of microbes can occur without breaks in the mucosa or direct intestinal injury. Microbes pass directly through the enterocytes rather than between them. Translocation of bacteria and endotoxins can trigger the hypermetabolic response and induce a septic state, and failure of the gut barrier function leading to translocation may be an important contributing factor to the development of multiple system organ failure. Fortunatley, continuous enteral nutrition can be administered safely and effectively immediately after injury or operative procedure and in the presence of gastric atony and throughout anesthesia.

References

1. Dominioni L, Trocki O, Mochizuki H, Fang CH, Alexander JW (1984) Prevention of severe postburn hypermetabolism and catabolsim by immediate intragastric feeding. J Burn Care Rehabil 5:106–112
2. Mochizuki H, Trocki O, Dominioni L, Brackett KA, Joffe SN, Alexander JW (1984) Mechanism of prevention of postburn hypermetabolism and catabolism by early enteral feeding. Ann Surg 200:297–310
3. Inoue S, Wirman JA, Alexander JW, Trocki O, Cardell RR (1988) *Candida albicans* translocation across the gut mucosa following burn injury. J Surg Res 44:479–492
4. Alexander JW, Boyce ST, Babcock GF, Gianotti L, Peck MD, Dunn DL, Pyles T, Childress CP, Ash SK (1990) The process of microbial translocation. Ann Surg 212(4):496–512
5. Alexander JW, Gianotti L, Pyles T, Carey MA, Babcock GF (1991) Distribution and survival of *Escherechia coli* translocation from the intestine following therapy injury. Ann Surg (in press)
6. Rush BF Fr, Redan JA, Flanagan JJ Jr et al. (1989) Does the bacteremia observed in hemorrhagic shock have clinical significance? Ann Surg 210:342–347
7. Sori A, Rush BF, Lysz TW, Smith S, Machiedo G (1988) The gut as a source of sepsis after hemorrhagic shock. Am J Surg 155:187–192
8. Beerthuizen GIJM, Barrow RD, Curry B, Herndon DN (1990) Blood flow to the abdominal organs in a porcine model with a 40% third-degree burn. Proceedings of the American Burn Association, Abstr 159
9. Inoue S, Luke S, Alexander JW, Trocki O, Silberstein EB (1989) Increased gut blood flow with early enteral feeding in burned guinea pigs. J Burn Care Rehabil 10:300–308
10. Inoue S, Epstein MD, Alexander JW, Trocki O, Jacobs P, Gura P (1989) Prevention of yeast translocation across the gut by a single enteral feeding after burn injury. JPEN J Parenter Enteral Nutr 13(6):565–571
11. Inoue S, Peck M, Alexander JW (1991) Fungal translocation is associated with increased mortality after thermal injury in guinea pigs. J Burn Care Rehabil (in press)
12. Jenkins M, Gottschlich M, Alexander JW, Warden GD (1988) A preliminary evaluation of the effect of immediate enteral feeding on the hypermetabolic response following severe burn injury (Abstr). Proceedings of the American Burn Association
13. McDonald WS, Deitch EA (1991) Immediate enteral feeding in burn patients is safe and effective. Ann Surg 213(2):177–183
14. Buescher TM, Cioffie WG, Becker WK, McManus WF, Pruitt BA Jr (1990) Perioperative enteral feedings. Program Booklet of the American Burn Association, Abstr 162
15. Jenkins M, Gottschlich M, Baumer T, Khoury J, Warden GD (1991) Enteral feeding during operative procedures. Program Booklet of the American Society for Parenteral Nutrition, Abstr 31, p 406
16. Saito H, Trocki O, Alexander JW, Kopcha R, Heyd T, Joffe SN (1987) The effect of route of nutrient administration on the nutritional state, catabolic hormone secretion and gut mucosal integrity after burn injury. JPEN J Parenter Enteral Nutr. 11:1–7

17. Alverdy JC, Aoys E, Moss GS (1988) Total parenteral nutrition promotes bacterial translocation from the gut. Surgery 104:185–190
18. Mochizuki H, Yoshimura K, Ohsaki Y, Tamakuma S (1987) Endotoxemia in surgical patients. Prog Med 7:1105–1110
19. Moore FA, Moore EE, Jones TN et al. (1989) TEN versus TPN following major abdominal trauma: reduced septic morbidity. J Trauma 29:916–923
20. Trocki O, Mochizuki H, Dominioni L, Alexander JW (1986) Intact protein versus free amino acids in the nutritional support of thermally injured animals. JPEN J Parenter Enteral Nutr 10:139–145
21. Shou J et al. (1990) Polypeptide based diet prevents translocation in methatrexate induced enterocolitis. Meeting of the American Society of Parenteral and Enteral Nutrition, January 1990
22. Fox AD, Kripke SA, de Paula J et al. (1988) Effect of a glutamine-supplemented enteral diet on methotrexate-induced enterocolitis. JPEN J Parenter Enteral Nutr 12:325–331
23. Souba WW, Hautamaki D, Mendenhall W et al. (1990) Oral glutamine reduces bacterial translocation following abdominal radiation. J Surg Res 48:1–5

Gut-Derived Infectious-Toxic Shock Syndrome: Therapeutic Chances with Polyspecific Immunoglobulins

*H. Cottier, A. Hässig, and R. Kraft

Septic shock is probably the most feared complication of major surgery, especially of interventions in the abdominal cavity [1]. Frequently, but by no means always, bacteremia accompanies this condition, and gram-negative microbes predominate as causative agents. This points to the intestine as the main source of infection, i.e. it involves—at least in many cases—a gut-derived infectious-toxic shock (GITS). Despite considerable progress in antibiotic therapy and supportive care, the fatality rate has remained high [2]. There is thus a need for novel strategies.

At present, substantial effort is being centered on the use of immunological methods to improve results of prophylaxis and/or therapy in GITS. Septic shock leading to multiple organ failure has aptly been termed host defense failure disease. In fact, elderly patients with a reduced nutritional status and markedly diminished cell-mediated immune reactivity, tested on the skin, are particularly at risk of developing an infectious-toxic postoperative complication [4]. One would therefore wish to introduce prophylactic and/or possibly, therapeutic immunostimulation to the approaches aimed at preventing or combating GITS (for review [6]). Although animal experiments have shown that various possibilities exist for improving the capacity of the immune apparatus, there is an astounding scarcity of clinical reports dealing with this strategy.

Most efforts at present focus on *passive humoral immunization*, which can be subdivided into prophylactic and/or therapeutic *anti-infectious* versus *antitoxic* administration of antibodies. The latter comprises the use of poly- (review [6]) or monoclonal (see [7]) anti-core lipopolysaccharide (LPS) antibodies on the one hand, and monoclonal antibodies directed against proinflammatory mediators, for example, tumor necrosis factor-alpha (TNF-α) [8] and interferon-gamma [9], on the other. Anti-infectious passive immunization includes the administration of monoclonal antibodies [10] or polyclonal hyperimmune immunoglobulins [11] specific for certain epitopes—or groups thereof—on O-, K-, H-, and/or other surface antigens of gram-negative bacteria. Such preparations have been given with considerable success to patients infected by one or a few strain(s) of gram-negative bacteria, such as *Pseudomonas aeruginosa*.

* Zeutrallaboratorium Blutspendedienst SRK Wankdorfstr. 10, CH-3000 Bern 2, Central Laboratory Swiss Red Cross Blood Transfusion Service, and Institute of Pathology, University of Bern, Bern, Switzerland

Host Defense Dysfunction
in Trauma, Shock and Sepsis
Eds. Faist/Meakins/Schildberg
© Springer-Verlag, Berlin Heidelberg 1993

Another, probably complementary, strategy of passive anti-infectious immunization, which we discuss in some detail, is the use of *pooled, polyspecific human immunoglobulins, especially IgG, for intravenous use* (IVIG; review [12]).

In both small rodents [13] and humans [14], the lymph nodes draining the gut undergo an antigen-driven expansion in the first phase of postnatal life which by far exceeds that seen in lymph nodes of other locations, and which is not observed in "germ-free" (axenic) animals. This indicates that a large portion—if not the bulk—of antibodies constituting pooled IgG are directed against antigens of intestinal bacteria. It was, in fact, shown that IVIG contains antibodies against most enteric microorganisms tested [15], and that normal human serum often protects mice against otherwise lethal doses of gram-negative bacteria [16]. Therefore, IVIG can be regarded as a poly-specific antibody pool that is in a large part directed against enteric microbes.

It is now generally accepted that GITS often commences with an acute intestinal barrier failure (see [17]) caused by ischemia-reperfusion damage [18]. Depending on the severity of injury, this may result in a partial denudation of the gut mucosa and to a sudden exposure of subepithelial tissues to a massive multispecies bacterial attack. Success or failure of antimicrobial defense is often decided in the early phase of infection [19]. Neutrophils are specially suited for rapidly combating the invaders, and C3b-IgG heterodimers have been shown to be particularly effective opsonizers for microorganisms to be taken up by granulocytes [20]. This observation and the fact that this is a multispecies microbial challenge suggest that antibodies, also those of the IgG class, are rapidly consumed in such a situation. It has in fact been reported that levels of circulating IgG may fall, in the course of a septic shock, to about 50% of normal [21]. If this notion is correct, pooled, polyspecific immunoglobulins should be particularly beneficial if given to surgical at- risk patients preoperatively, i.e., shortly before intestinal barrier failure may occur or as early after such an event as possible.

Unfortunately, reports on animal studies in this field are scarce. By analogy, one may cite the finding that the prophylactic administration of 0.5 g/kg body weight of pooled human immunoglobulins to small rodents reduced the lethality after intraperitoneal inoculation of 2×10^{10} colony-forming units of *Salmonella typhimurium* from 80% to 0% [22].

Results of pilot studies and preliminary findings in extended, controlled clinical trials on *prophylactic/preoperative administration* of low or moderate doses of polyspecific IgG to patients at risk of developing septic shock are encouraging. In 1980, Duswald and colleagues [23] gave 20 g IVIG to each of the study patients shortly before surgical intervention. Compared to controls, this group experienced significantly fewer postoperative infectious complications. IVIG was also employed with considerable success to prevent the development of adult respiratory distress syndrome (ARDS) [24], one of the most reliable signs of an infectious-toxic process that threatens to become dangerous. By analogy to surgery, Bacigalupo and coworkers [25] administered IVIG to individuals undergoing allogeneic bone marrow transplantation. Both chemotherapy and whole-body irradiation used in this procedure are known to cause some degree of intestinal barrier failure. Such patients, each given a prophylactic dose of 0.5 g/kg IVIG experienced significantly fewer cases of ARDS than the controls. The authors feel that they benefit so much from this treatment that it has been maintained since 1983 (Bacigalupo, personal communication). Cafiero and his group [21] administered less than 0.2 g/kg body weight of IVIG prior to major intestinal surgery. They noticed a reduction in the frequency of postoperative infections from 78% in the controls to 41% in patients given preoperative IVIG. In the latest, and largest, controlled multicenter study, 0.4 g/kg IVIG prior to surgery, and postoperatively once a week as risk persisted, significantly reduced, compared to controls with placebo, the incidence of postsurgery local infections and pulmonary complications [26]. Thus, in all reports dealing with prophylactic, in particular preoperative, administration of IVIG, beneficial effects have been observed, although the doses given were moderate or even low.

A protective action of IVIG, depending on the dose, was also noticed when given from *early after major injury* on. Glinz et al. [27] treated polytraumatized patients with 12 g IVIG per person on admission to the hospital as well as 5 and 12 days later. Despite the rather low doses, these individuals suffered less frequently from pulmonary complications than controls. The incidence of late sepsis, however, was not significantly different between the two groups. A clearly measurable improvement in the condition was noticed in intensive care unit patients given moderate doses of IVIG (enriched with some IgM and IgA) on admission and 12, 24, and 36 h later [28]. Somewhat similar doses of IVIG, i.e., 0.4 g/kg given 1 day after admission to the intensive care unit, plus 0.2 g/kg 2 days thereafter, and "when needed" another 0.4 g/kg after 5 days, led to shortening of the fever period, a drop in the number of positive blood cultures from 40% to 8%, and a reduction in the need for antibiotics from 95% to 38%. The lethality of IVIG-treated patients was 58%, compared to 75% in the control group [29].

This—incomplete—account of clinical observations seems to indicate that to be optimally effective in prevention and/or therapy of GITS IVIG should already be given preoperatively in surgery patients at risk and at least as early as possible in polytraumatized individuals. The latter also pertains to patients with severe burns, which belongs to the almost established indications of IVIG [30]. In all these conditions, repetitive administration should be considered.

It also seems that the dose of IVIG, not only the time schedule of this type of passive immunization, may be of paramount importance. This view is based in part on the results of clinical pilot studies [31–33] that suggest a marked improvement following administration of large amounts of polyspecific, pooled immunoglobulins. In accordance with this concept, it was reported that patients in whom the concentration of igG in the blood plasma was kept above 10 g/l rarely developed postoperative infectious complications [21].

There is no solid evidence that pooled human IgG contains protective anti-core LPS antibodies [34]. It seems reasonable therefore to assume that the

beneficial effects mentioned above of prophylactic and early therapeutic administration of IVIG in surgical patients at risk of developing GITS rely on the
presence in these preparations of antibodies directed against serotype-specific
antigens on gram-negative and other bacteria. These, in sufficient amounts, are
known to be highly protective against the respective species and strains of
microorganisms.

If this assumption is valid, administration of IVIG would correspond to an
essentially anti-infectious prophylaxis and/or therapy. The polyspecificity of the
pooled antibodies contained in these preparations may well be most helpful at
the time of acute intestinal barrier failure, i.e. when the initial multispecies
bacterial attach takes place. We see no substitute for pooled human IgG to exert
a protective anti-infectious effect in this first phase of a process that may
ultimately lead to GITS. Possibly, IVIG may be supplemented with pooled
immunoglobulins given perorally or intraintestinally [35].

Since the use of IVIG in patients at risk of developing GITS represents an
approach that differs from the other above-mentioned strategies of passive
immunization, it may be viewed as complementing rather than replacing
alternative immunological means to prevent or at least counteract this group of
life-threatening disorders.

One is thus tempted to foresee a *combination of various immunological
treatments* to be adopted in the future, for example, immunostimulation some
time before surgery in elderly patients with reduced cell-mediated immune
reactivity in skin tests; polyspecific IVIG at the time of acute intestinal barrier
failure and for a limited period of time thereafter; monoclonal antibodies against
core LPS and/or, TNF before the onset of and during the infectious-toxic
process that may lead to GITS; and appropriate, serotype-specific hyperimmune
immunoglobulins (if available) as soon as one or a few bacterial species are
recognized as predominant in the infectious process, for example, in bacteremia
or septicemia.

Thus, in this tentative scheme, anti-infectious and antitoxic strategies are
complementary rather than mutually exclusive. It will be important, however, to
ask the question in any clinical situation of whether the infectious or the toxic
component of the process predominates. Accordingly, one should caution
against using the term "septic" in conditions that are primarily characterized by
an excessive cascade of proinflammatory mediators; here an antiphlogistic and
antiendotoxin treatment seems to be most important. Conversely, situations
with a predominance of gram-negative bacterial overgrowth in the tissues
confront us with a largely different problem. In such cases, for instance, the use
of certain antibiotics may be dangerous because of endotoxin release, and anti-
core LPS antibodies given prior to their administration may be indicated. In
bacteriemia/septicemia caused by one or a few microorganisms, corresponding
hyperimmune immunoglobulins are apt to offer the best chance of a beneficial
effect.

In conclusion, pooled human IVIG preparations have the unique property
of containing antibodies with innumerable specificities, many of them directed

against microbial antigens of the gut contents. IVIG therefore, appears, particularly well suited for supporting specific opsono-phagocytosis in the defense against the multispecies bacterial attach following intestinal barrier failure. Preliminary reports on beneficial effects of prophylactic/therapeutic application of IVIG in patients at risk of developing GITS tend to support this notion. The use of IVIG can be complementary to other immunological strategies to counteract GITS, i.e., preoperative immunostimulation in surgical patients at risk; anti-core LPS antibodies to neutralize endotoxin; monoclonal anti-TNF antibodies to dampen the excessive inflammatory cascade; and hyperimmune imunoglobulin, possibly also monoclonal antibodies, directed against particular microbial serotypes to combat severe infections/septicemia caused by the respective species/strains.

References

1. Shires GT (1986) Historical perspective. In: Gallin JL, Fauci AS (eds) Advances in host defense mechanisms. Raven, New York, pp 1–3
2. The Veterans Administration Systemic Sepsis Cooperative Study Group (1987) Effect of high-dose glucocorticoid therapy on mortality in patients with clinical signs of systemic sepsis. N Engl J Med 317:659–665
3. Siegel JH (1990) Multiple organ failure as a systemic disease of host-defense failure. In: Schlag G, Redl H, Siegel JH (eds) Shock, sepsis, and organ failure. Springer, Berlin Heidelberg New York, pp 627–638
4. Christou NV (1989) Relationship between immune function and post-trauma morbidity and mortality. In: Faist E, Ninnemann J, Green D (eds) Immune consequences of trauma, shock and sepsis. Mechanisms and therapeutic approaches. Springer, Berlin Heidelberg New York, pp 357–362
5. Faist E, Ertel W, Mewes A (1988) Möglichkeiten der Immunmodulation bei chirurgischen Patienten. In: Schmutzler W, Darlath W, Knopp J (eds) Immunstimulation, Dustri, Munich, pp 103–116
6. Baumgartner JD, Calandra T, Glauser MP (1988) Intervention on gram-negative bacterial disease by immunoglobulin therapy: reality or myth? In: Krijnen HW, Strengers PFW, van Aken WG (eds) Immunoglobulins. Central Laboratory of the Netherlands Red Cross Blood Transfusion Service, Amsterdam, pp 191–205
7. Baumgartner JD (1990) Monoclonal anti-endotoxin antibodies for the treatment of gram-negative bacteremia and septic shock. Eur J Clin Microbiol Infect Dis 9:711–716
8. Tracey KJ, Fong Y, Hesse DG, Manogue KR, Lee AT, Kuo GC, Lowry SF, Cerami A (1987) Anti-cachectin/TNF monoclonal antibodies prevent septic shock during lethal bacteraemia. Nature 330:662–664
9. Billiau A (1988) Not just cachectin involved in toxic shock. Nature 331:665
10. Kirkland TN, Ziegler EJ (1984) An immunoprotective monoclonal antibody to lipopolysaccharide. J Immunol 132:2590–2592
11. Kistler D, Kauhl W, Piert M, Hettich R (1989) Unterstützende Therapie mit einem Pseudomonas-Immunglobulin beim septischen Schock von Brandverletzten. Intensivmedizin 26 [Suppl 1]: 138–143
12. Hässig A, Cottier H (1988) The role of immunoglobulins in the control of inflammatory reactions. In: Krijnen HW, Strengers PFW, van Aken WG (eds) Immunoglobulins. Central Laboratory of the Netherlands Red Cross Blood Transfusion Service, Amsterdam, pp 77–86
13. Schwander R, Hess MW, Keller HU, Cottier H (1980) The postnatal development of lymph nodes in mice. Immunobiology 157:425–436
14. Luscieti P, Hubschmid T, Cottier H, Hess MW, Sobin LH (1986) Human lmyph node morphology a function of age and site. J Clin Pathol 33:454–461

15. Barandun S, Imbach P, Kindt H, Morell A, Nydegger UE, Römer J, Schneider T, Sidiropoulos D, Skvaril F (1981) Der Klinische Einsatz von Immunglobulin (Gammaglobulin). Sandoz, Basel
16. DeMaria A jr, Johns MA, Berberich H, McCabe WR (1988) Immunization with rough mutants of *salmonella minnesota*; initial studies in human subjects. J Infect Dis 158:301–311
17. Fiddian-Green RG (1988) Splanchnic ischaemia and multiple organ failure in the cirtically ill. Ann R Coll Surg 70:128–134
18. Deitch EA, Bridges W, Ma L, Berg R, Specian RD, Granger DN (1990) Hemorrhagic shock-induced bacterial translocation: the role of neutrophils and hydroxyl radicals. J Trauma 30:942–951
19. Meakins JL (1981) clinical importance of host resistance to infection in surgical patients. Adv Surg 15:225–255
20. Malbran A, Frank MM, Fries LF (1987) Interactions of monomeric IgG bearing covalently bound C3b with polymorphonuclear leukocytes. Immunology 61:15–20
21. Cafiero F, Gipponi M (1989) Profilassi delle infezioni in chirurgia per neoplasia dell'apparato digerente. IN: Rossi Ferrini P (ed) Impiego clinico delle immunoglobuline endo-vena: presente e futuro. Grafiche Mazzuchelli, Milano, pp 63–68
22. Emerson TE jr, Lurton JM, Collins MS (1985) Efficaciousness of immunoglobulin G prophylaxis on mortality and physiological variables in gram-negative peritonitis in rodents. Circ Shock 17:213–222
23. Duswald KH, Müller K, Seifert J. Ring J (1980) Wirksamkeit von i.v. Gammaglobulin gegen bakterielle Infektionen chirurgischer Patienten. Münch Med Wochenschr 122:832–836
24. Burkhardt A, Cottier H (1989) cellular events in alveolitis and the evolution of pulmonary fibrosis. Virchows Arch [B] 58:1–13
25. Bacigalupo A, Frassoni F, van Lint MT, Chierichetti S, Corbetta PD, Studer C, Marmont AM (1983) Prevention of ARDS, occurring after allogeneic marrow transplantation, with high-dose intravenous immunoglobulins. Exp Hematol 11 [Suppl 14]:135 (abstract)
26. Cometta A, Baumgartner JD, Lee M, Glauser MP, the Anti-Core LPS IVIG Collaborative Study Group (1990) Prophylaxis of infection in high risk surgical patients (pat) with standard intravenous immunoglobulin G (St-IVIG) or with antibody to core glycolipid (Co-IVIG). ICAAC abstr nr 476
27. Glinz W, Grob PJ, Nydegger UE, Ricklin T, Stamm F, Stoffel D, Lasance A (1985) Polyvalent immunoglobulins for prophylaxis of bacterial infections in patients following multiple trauma. Intensive Care Med 11:288–294
28. Just HM, Metzger M, Vogel W, Pelka RB (1986) Einfluss einer adjuvanten Immun-globulintherapie auf Infektionen bei Patienten einer operativen Intensiv-Therapie-Station. Klin Wochenschr 64:245–256
29. DeSimone C, Delogu G, Corbetta G (1988) Intravenous immunoglobulins in association with antibiotics: a therapeutic trial in septic intensive care unit patients. Crit Care Med 16:23–26
30. Garner RJ, Sacher RA (1988) Intravenous gammaglobulin therapy. Am Assoc Blood Banks, Arlington
31. Schedel I (1988) New aspects in the treatment of gram-negative bacteraemia and septic shock. Infection 16:8–11
32. Schedel I (1990) Invited comment. Vox Sang 58:319–321
33. Dominioni L, Benevento A, Zanello M. Gennari R, Besozzi MC, Hourcade M, Dionigi R (1991) Non specific immunotherapy and intravenous gammaglobulin administration in surgical sepsis. In: Imbach P, de Haes P, Morell A, Nydegger UE, Perret BA (eds) Immunotherapy with intravenous immunoglobulin. Academic, London (in press)
34. McCabe WR, DeMaria A jr, Berberich H, Johns MA (1988) Immunization with rough mutants of *Salmonella minnesota*: protective activity of IgM and IgG antibody to the R595 (Re chemotype) mutant. J Infect Dis 158:291–300
35. Tutschka PJ (1988) Gammaglobulin therapy in bone marrow transplantation. In: Garner RJ, Sacher RA (eds) Intravenous gammaglobulin therapy. Am Assoc Blood Banks. Arlington, pp 79–97

Maintenance of Gastrointestinal Integrity After Burn Injury with Specific Dietary Supplementation and Epidermal Growth Factor

R. L. Zapata-Sirvent, J. F. Hansbrough, M. C. Cox, and P. Wolf

Introduction

One of the primary functions of the gastrointestinal (GI) tract mucosa after digestion and absorption of nutrients is to exclude endotoxin and bacteria from reaching the systemic circulation and distal organs, thus creating the possibility of sepsis. However, this property may be altered by certain conditions such as the presence or absence of intraluminal nutrients [1], hormones, and various types of injury [2–5]. Alterations in GI mucosal structure and function may lead to bacterial translocation (BT), which may increase infectious morbidity and mortality in this group of patients [6].

The inflammatory response induced by translocating microorganisms in the systemic organs may be implicated in the pathogenesis of multiple organ failure [7]. Although clinically the BT phenomenon remains controversial, much direct evidence for BT has been accumulated from animal models of injuries. In critically injured patients, bacteremia may develop without a specific focus which can be identified clinically or at the autopsy table [8]. The majority of bacteria isolated in such cases are enteric gram-negative organisms, suggesting that the GI tract may be the possible source [4].

Alterations in structure and function of the GI tract after injury have been well described, and may relate to BT [2]. Alexander [7] has shown that early enteral feeding may preserve the gut barrier function against BT and also decrease the catabolic response seen after injury. Certain hormones, especially urogastrone–epidermal growth factor (EGF), stimulates maturation and proliferation of the enterocyte [9, 10]. EGF alone and in conjunction with glutamine has been shown to reduce gut atrophy in parenterally fed rats [11, 12].

The study presented here was designed to investigate the effects of enteral feeding, using three different types of diets, and the GI tract hormone EGF on burn-induced alterations of GI tract mucosa observed 24 h after injury.

Departments of Surgery and Pathology, University of California, San Diego Medical Center, San Diego, CA, 92103, USA

Host Defense Dysfunction
in Trauma, Shock and Sepsis
Eds. Faist/Meakins/Schildberg
© Springer-Verlag, Berlin Heidelberg 1993

Materials and Methods

Animals. Female outbred CF-1 mice, 8–12 weeks of age, from Charles River Laboratory, (Wilmingon, MA USA) were maintained in accordance with guidelines of the University of California, San Diego (UCSD) Animal Research Committee.

Thermal Injury. Animals were anesthetized with methoxyflurane vapor (Penthrane, Abbott Laboratories, North Chicago, IL, USA). A demarcated area on the shaved and depilated dorsum was burned by a 6-s exposure to steam, similar to described methods [13]. This produced a full-thickness burn of 25% total body surface area (TBSA). Animals were resuscitated with 2 cm^3 intraperitoneal (i.p.) normal saline, and one i.p. injection of morphine (15 mg/kg) for analgesia. Control animals received similar anesthesia, morphine, and i.p. saline (Fig. 1).

Enteral Diets. Three different diets were allowed immediately after injury. Normal chow (Harlan Sprague Dawley, WI, USA) contains crude protein, fat, and fiber. Traumacal, a commercial synthetic enteral feeding formulation (Mead Johnson, Evansville, IN, USA), contains a high protein and high lipid content. Impact is a defined diet containing arginine, nucleic acids, high protein, and mixed fats including fish oil (Sandoz Nutrition, Minneapolis, MN, USA). A burn control group was fasted for 24 h and allowed only water.

Epidermal Growth Factor. Human recombinant EGF (r-HuEGF, Amgen, Thousand Oaks, CA, USA) was administered by i.p. injection in a dose of 4 µg/0.5 ml at 1 and 12 h after injury. In this group of experiments the control and treated animals were fasted.

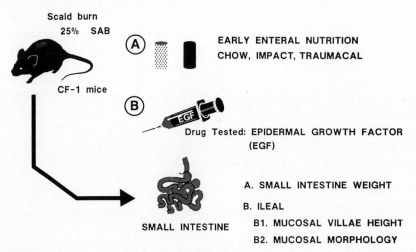

Fig. 1. Sequence of experimental steps in the animal model

Tissue Histology. At 24 h after injury, animals were sacrificed by cervical dislocation. The small bowel was removed and the lumen was washed with normal saline, removing all the intestinal contents; the bowel was then weighed. A segment from the distal ileum was placed in formalin. Tissue was embedded in paraffin, and 5-µm sections were stained with hematoxylin and eosin (H&E). Mucosal villae height and morphology were assessed by light microscopy.

Statistical Analysis. The data is reported as the mean $\pm$ SEM, and comparisons were made of the normal mucosal villae height for each group using Student's *t* test. Statistical significance was assumed at the 95% confidence level, or $p < 0.05$.

Results

The group of animals fasted after burn injury had to be separated to individual cages to inhibit cannibalism. Mortality after burn injury in fasted animals was not observed during the 24-h period of this study.

Significant alterations can be found after burn injury. A marked decrease in the small intestine weight was observed for 10 days after burn (Fig. 2). As early as 24 h postburn, distal mucosal morphology is altered, showing signs of degeneration, fragmentation, atrophy, widening between the villae, and shortening (Fig. 3). These changes were more prominent in the burned and fasted animals.

Animals allowed early enteral feeding with normal chow and Impact showed significantly improved mucosal villous height (Fig. 4) and mucosal morphology, but significant improvement in small intestine weight compared with fasted burned animals was not seen. Less degeneration, less villous fragmentation, and a more uniform mucosal pattern were seen in the chow and Impact groups. Traumacal-fed animals did not show signs of improvement.

The i.p. administration of EGF partially prevented the morphologic alterations in the GI tract mucosa following burn injury, and improved mucosal villous height (Fig. 5). The villae were thinner and longer, and although some

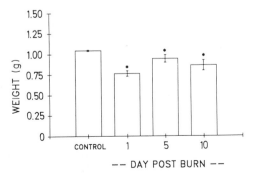

Fig. 2. Decrease in small intestine weight after burn injury in fed animals * $P < 0.05$ compared with control

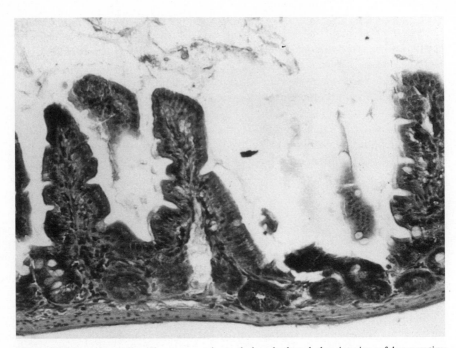

Fig. 3. At 24 h postburn, distal ileum mucosal morphology is altered, showing signs of degeneration, fragmentation, and atrophy

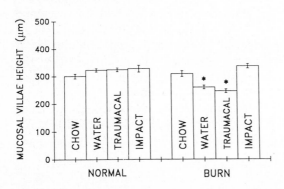

Fig. 4. Early enteral feeding with normal rodent diet chow and Impact showed improvement in mucosal villae height. *$P < 0.05$ compared with own control

fragmentation and degeneration were observed, the intestinal areas showed more intact and uniform villous morphology (Fig. 6).

Discussion

These experiments clearly identified the protective effect that early enteral feeding, specially defined diets, and certain GI tract hormones may have on burn-induced alterations of the GI tract mucosa.

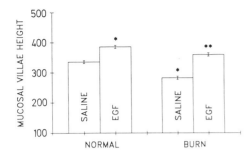

Fig. 5. The i.p. administration of EGF increased mucosal villae height in normal and burned animals. *$P < 0.05$ compared with normal + saline; **$P < 0.05$ compared with burn + saline

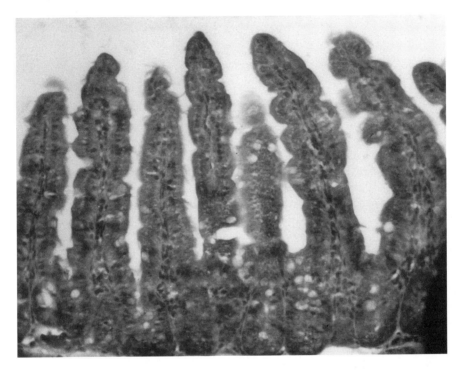

Fig. 6. The morphology of the GI tract improved after EGF administration. The villae were thinner and longer, although some degeneration was observed

It is well known that following burn injury the GI tract loses its barrier integrity, allowing endotoxin and bacteria to reach systemic organs through the lymphatic or the portal blood, creating the possibility of infection. BT may be one cause of the high incidence of morbidity and mortality in this special group of patients prone to develop infections, due to the alterations in their immune response [13].

As shown in Fig. 7, three factors play a role in the pathogenesis of the BT phenomenon: the gut mucosal barrier, the immune response, and the ecologic balance of the intestinal flora [14]. After burn injury, increases in small intestine

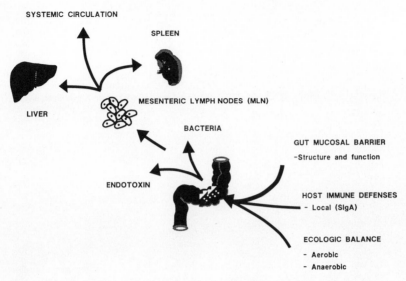

SYSTEMIC CIRCULATION

SPLEEN

LIVER

MESENTERIC LYMPH NODES (MLN)

BACTERIA

GUT MUCOSAL BARRIER

-Structure and function

ENDOTOXIN

HOST IMMUNE DEFENSES

- Local (SIgA)

ECOLOGIC BALANCE

- Aerobic
- Anaerobic

Fig. 7. Factors implicated in the etiopathogenesis of bacterial translocation (*SIgA*, Secretory immunoglobulin A)

permeability have been described [15, 16], and atrophy of the small bowel appears to correlate with BT [2]. In this study a clear alteration in the gut barrier property was observed, and as early as 24 h after injury, fragmentation, degeneration, and atrophy are apparent.

The role of early enteral feeding after burn injury has been emphasized by Alexander [7]; early feeding preserves the gut barrier and decreases the catabolic response in burned rats. Neglecting the GI tract after injury by waiting until the patient is "stable" before parenteral nutrition is initiated may aggravate GI tract alterations. Decreases in nutrient blood flow to the gut have been described after burn injury; it is possible that nutrients in the gut may increase blood flow and also provide necessary energy and stimuli to induce secretion of enterohormones which may stimulate cell division and repair processes. It is already known that parenteral nutrition induces gut atrophy and facilitates BT [17], and recent reports are beginning to show a difference in morbidity and mortality in critically injured patients when total parenteral nutrition (TPN) and enteral nutrition are compared [18]. Enteral nutrition is physiologic and induces preservation of the intestinal structure, boosts immune and endocrine functions, and also decreases the catabolic response after injury [7].

Certain key nutritional elements may need to be included in the formulation to obtain the desired level of protection of the GI tract. The intestinal mucosa has remarkably high cell turnover, and maintenance of intestinal cell growth and function requires a constant supply of energy. Some nonessential amino acids, such as arginine, may be indispensable in times of critical injury. Arginine, in a similar way to glutamine, may be used by the enterocyte [19]. Arginine may also stimulate the immune response, regulating a second important factor in the pathogenesis of BT. In addition, bulk-forming agents may modify the luminal content in the GI tract, may increase blood flow, and may stimulate production of GI secretions and hormones and prevent alterations in the ecologic flora [20, 21]. Fiber administered with oral TPN decreases BT and improves the gut barrier [22]. Impact contains arginine and mixed fats, including fish oil which blocks the generation of prostaglandin E_2 (PGE$_2$), a known immunosuppressant that is elevated after burn injury; PGE$_2$ may also induce muscle and body wasting after injury [23].

EGF is a 53-amino-acid polypeptide first isolated from mouse submandibular gland, and is one of the most biologically potent and best characterized growth factors in terms of its physical, chemical, and biologic properties [24]. EGF reduces the GI tract atrophy during TPN administration [11], and clearly increases enterocyte maturation and proliferation [9, 10, 11]. In our study EGF partially prevented alterations in morphology of the distal ileum, and although some derangements were observed a more homogeneous mucosal pattern was evident. In addition, EGF increased significantly the small intestine weight and the mucosal villae height.

In this study the protective effect of early enteral nutrition with specific diets, and the use of EGF in fasted burned animals, prevented the loss of mucosal integrity in the postburn period. Maintenance of structure and function of the GI tract mucosa after injury may help prevent BT, and the cascade of events observed in this phenomenon. The translocation of endotoxin and bacteria may induce severe inflammatory reaction, the liberation of important cytokines including TNF, interleukin-1 (IL-1), and interleukin-6 (IL-6), and may increase arachidonic acid metabolites such as PGE$_2$. Complement may be activated leading to a consumption state, which may aggravate immunosuppression. These multiple effects may lead to development of sepsis and multiple organ

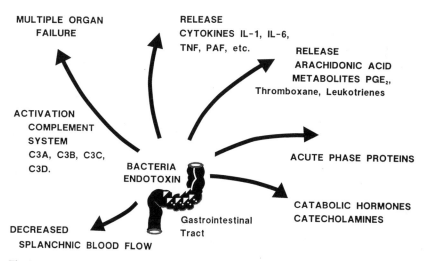

Fig. 8. Possible alterations induced by the translocation of bacteria and endotoxin from the GI tract

failure [7] (Fig. 8). Blocking BT may prevent this cascade of effects and may decrease infectious morbidity and mortality in this group of patients.

References

1. McManus JPA, Isselbacher KJ (1970) Effect of fasting versus feeding the rat small intestine. Gastroenterology 59:214–221
2. Jones WG, Minei JP, Barber AE, Rayburn JL, Fahey TJ, Shires T III, Shires T (1990) Bacterial translocation and intestinal atrophy after thermal injury and burn sepsis. Ann Surg 211:399–405
3. Maninous MR, Tso P, Berg R, Deitch E (1991) Studies of the route, magnitude and time course of bacterial translocation in a model of systemic inflammation. Arch Surg 126:33–37
4. Sori AJ, Rush BF, Lysz TW, Smith S, Machiedo GW (1988) The gut as source of sepsis after hemorrhagic shock Am J Surg 155:187–192
5. Guzman-Stein G, Bonsack M, Liberty J, Delaney JP (1989) Abdominal radiation causes bacterial translocation. J Surg Res 46:104–107
6. Deitch EA (1990) The role of intestinal barrier failure and bacterial translocation in the development of systemic infection and multiple organ failure. Arch Surg 125:403–404
7. Alexander JW (1990) Nutrition and translocation. JPEN 14:170S–174S
8. Kreger BE, Craven DE, Carling PC, McCabe WR (1990) Gram-negative bactermia: III. Reassessment of etiology, epidemiology and ecology in 612 patients. Am J Med 68:332–343
9. Thompson JS, Sharp JG, Saxena SK, McCullagh KG (1987) Stimulation of neomucosal growth by systemic urogastrona. J Surg Res 42:402–410
10. Ulsen MH, Lyn-Cook LE, Raasch RH (1986) Effect of intraluminal EGF on mucosal proliferation in the small intestine of adult rats. Gastroenterology 91:1134–1140
11. Bragg LE, Hollingsed TC, Thompson JS (1990) Urogastrone reduces gut atrophy during parenteral alimentation. JPEN 14:183–286
12. Jacobs DO, Evans DA, O'Dwyer ST, Smith RJ, Cullmore DW (1988) Combined effects of glutamine and epidermal growth factor on the rat intestine. Surgery 104:358–364
13. Hansbrough JF, Zapata-Sirvent RL, Hoyt D (1990) Postburn immune suppression: an inflammatory response to the burn wound. J Trauma 30:671–675
14. Maejima K, Deitch E, Berg R (1984) Promotion by burn stress of the translocation of bacteria from the GI tract of mice. Arch Surg 119:166–172
15. Carter EA, Tompkins RG, Schiffrin E, Burke JF (1990) Cutaneous thermal injury alters macromolecular permeability of the rat small intestine. Surgery 107:335–341
16. Epstein MD, Tchervenkov JI, Alexander JW, Johnson R, Vester JW (1991) Increased gut permeability following burn trauma. Arch Surg 126:198–200
17. Alverdy JC, Aoys E, Moss GS (1988) TPN promotes bacterial translocation from the gut. Surgery 104:185–190
18. Moore FA, Moore EE, Jones TN, McCroskey BL, Peterson V (1989) TEN vs TPN following abdominal trauma reduces septic morbidity. J Trauma 29:916–923
19. Kirk SJ, Barbul A (1990) Role of arginine in trauma, sepsis and immunity. JPEN 14:226S–229S
20. Topping DL, Illman RJ (1986) Bacterial fermentation in the human large bowel. Time to change from the roughage model of dietary fibre? Med J Aust 144:307–309
21. Savage DC (1978) Factors involved in colonization of the gut epithelial surface. Am J Clin Nutr 31:S131–S135
22. Spaeth G, Specian RD, Berg R, Deitch EA (1990) Bulk prevents bacterial translocation induced by the oral administration of TPN solution. JPEN 14:442–447
23. Alexander JW (1990) Gastrointestinal integrity in translocation and sepsis. Inf Surg [Suppl 1990]:31–36
24. Gregory H (1975) Isolation and structure of urogastrone and its relationship of epidermal growth factor. Nature 257:325–327

Selective Decontamination of the Digestive Tract: Open Questions and Controversies

L. L. Dever[1] and W. G. Johanson Jr.[2]

Hospital-acquired bacterial infections are common complications of severe illness and appear to cause adverse patient outcomes. Most of these "secondary" infections are preceded by colonization of one or more mucosal surfaces by newly acquired or translocated bacterial species. Selective decontamination of the digestive tract (SDD) is based on the rationale that prevention of such colonization will prevent subsequent infections. An additional rationale added in recent years is that reducing the bacterial population in the gut might reduce exposure of the host to circulating bacteria and/or bacterial products in circumstances in which gut permeability is abnormally high.

SDD has had a developmental history that is similar to other advances in medical technology. It was founded out of perceived medical necessity, for example, the high rate of infection in critically ill patients. Its major features, such as the concept of preserving the anaerobic flora, were based on basic science observations or animal studies. It has dramatic and easily observed effects on the bacterial flora of the host, inducing changes that appear to have intrinsic value (face validity). Its use has been championed by an ardent group of investigators, including its originators (an encouraging sign). Justification for the use of SDD has been largely based on its obvious effect on microbial flora and the apparent beneficial effects demonstrated in observational studies.

Inevitably, detractors have been present from the outset, suggesting that a number of flaws are present in the existing trials, for instance: (a) they are unblinded, with the investigator often being the treating physician himself; (b) no placebo treatment group is included; (c) controls, if used at all, are not concurrent; (d) the treatment confounds diagnostic criteria; and (e) patient groups are heterogeneous. In part, objections to SDD grew out of the experience with prophylactic administration of topical polymyxin B for pneumonia prevention reported from the Respiratory Intensive Care Unit (ICU) of Beth Israel Hospital in Boston in the early 1970s [1–3]. The conclusion of those investigators was that continuous administration of polymyxin B topically was inappropriate and dangerous because it led to the emergence of resistant organisms which caused lethal infections [3]. However, resistance was produced

[1] Infectious Diseases Division, Department of Medicine, University of Texas Health Science Center at San Antonio
[2] Pulmonary Diseases Division, Department of Medicine, University of Texas Medical Branch, 7135 Shearn Moody Plaza, Galveston TX 77550, USA

Host Defense Dysfunction
in Trauma, Shock and Sepsis
Eds. Faist/Meakins/Schildberg
© Springer-Verlag, Berlin Heidelberg 1993

only by selection of intrinsically resistant strains, i.e., there was no evidence that previously sensitive organisms had become resistant to polymyxin B during its use in the unit. Further, the investigators' initial goal of reducing pneumonias caused by *Pseudomonas aeruginosa* was achieved.

Another facet of this earlier work provides an important background for the more recent SDD studies. The Beth Israel polymyxin B trials were initiated because of a continuing respiratory ICU problem with pneumonia, especially that due to *P. aeruginosa*. A prevalence study performed just before the use of polymyxin B began found that 21% of patients developed pneumonia, 50% of which were caused by *P. aeruginosa* [4]. The incidence of pneumonia during the placebo cycles of the polymyxin B trial 3–5 years later had decreased to 8.1% in the same unit [2]. This observation illustrates the hazard in relying on historic controls, especially when many aspects of patient management and environmental measures are changed in addition to the administration of prophylactic drugs.

The early polymyxin B trials did not use concurrent controls. It was reasoned that the use of the drug in some, but not all, patients would increase the chances for drug resistance. An absence of concurrent controls has been virtually a constant feature of SDD research. The Munster investigators used this basic approach in each of two ICUs simultaneously so that treated and untreated subjects were studied concurrently but in different units [5]. However, the patient populations of the two units were very different, and this approach does not really alter the objection to the lack of concurrent controls. This objection is based on concerns that, over long study periods, patient populations change (seasonal or other effects), patient management schemes change (different physicians, new drugs), and so forth. Concurrent SDD and control, but not placebo, groups have been studied in some centers without obvious adverse effects [6, 7], and this approach should be encouraged.

It has been argued that the simultaneous presence of SDD and untreated patient groups in a single ICU might lead to a beneficial effect among untreated patients through an effect of SDD on the bacterial flora of the unit, not just that of individual patients [8]. This type of effect, where an intervention affects both treated and untreated groups, is often referred to as "contamination bias." It may be very difficult to separate from the effects of other modifications which are made consciously or unconsciously. For example, staff awareness of a study being performed on infections in a unit is likely to have an effect on a variety of behaviors, whether intended or not. Continuing reminders about hand-washing and other aspects of nosocomial infection prevention have been shown to reduce the incidence of infections. It might be expected, therefore, that the incidence of infections would diminish during periods of study, independently of any drug effect. This concern is the strongest argument for blinded, concurrent controlled studies.

None of the existing SDD trials have been performed in a blinded fashion. It is argued that such would be impossible since the buccal paste cannot be hidden. However, it would not be impossible to use placebo paste, gastric instillations, and intravenous infusions, although such would certainly add to the expense of the trial. Until placebo-controlled studies are performed, the results of SDD trials will be viewed with suspicion.

The dramatic effects of the SDD program on the bacterial flora of the host are readily apparent within a few days. Even if blinded as to drug versus placebo, clinicians caring for the patients would certainly know group designation if they were appraised of culture results. It seems essential that endpoints be defined that are independent of culture results so that individuals who are not involved in the care of the patients can make these determinations. Kerver et al. [6] used two types of outcomes—clinically defined infections and bacteriologically proven infections—and reported their results for both outcomes. However, when the clinicians involved in the care of the patient know the patient's treatment group and culture results, it is impossible to avoid bias in the interpretation of clinical findings.

All of the SDD studies have used formalized, prospectively defined criteria to diagnose infections, although there has been little uniformity among studies (Table 1). All studies required a new or advancing pulmonary infiltrate radiographically. Some investigators have required the presence of bacteria in cultures of tracheal aspirates as one of several criteria for respiratory infection. Others have used only the presence of purulent secretions, along with other evidence of lung infection. The reliability and validity of these approaches in detecting respiratory infection have been poor when studied rigorously [12, 13]. Among postoperative patients, fewer than 50% of those with clinical signs customarily associated with pneumonia have significant bacterial contamination of the distal lung that requires antimicrobial therapy [13]. It is reasonable to expect that these results would be applicable to many of the patients included in the published SDD trials as well. If so, it is possible that SDD prevents only unimportant febrile syndromes associated with proximal airway colonization but does not prevent actual pneumonia.

Perhaps the greatest concern about SDD, now that a reasonable amount of experience has been accumulated, is the lack of beneficial effect on mortality observed in most studies (Table 2). The obvious interpretations of this finding

Table 1. Diagnostic criteria for nosocomial pneumonia

Reference	Temperature	WBC	PaO$_2$	X-ray	Secretions	
					WBC	Bacteria
Ulrich et al. [9]	Yes	Yes	No	Yes	No	Yes
Ledingham et al. [10]	Yes	Yes	Yes	Yes	Yes	No
Kerver et al. [6]	Yes	Yes	No	Yes	No	Yes
Hartenauer et al. [5]	$+/-$	$+/-$	$+/-$	Yes	Yes	No
	(At least 1 of $+/-$)					
Unertl et al. [11]	$+/-$	$+/-$	$+/-$	Yes	Yes	No
	(At least 2 of $+/-$)					

Table 2. Patient characteristics and outcomes

	Controls				SDD			
Reference	n	Trauma (%)	NP (%)	Died (%)	n	Trauma (%)	NP (%)	Died (%)
Kerver et al. [6]	47	32	85	32	49	24	12[a]	28
Ledingham et al. [10]	161	14	11	24	163	11	1.2[a]	24
Ulrich et al. [9]	52	17	56	54	48	10	14[a]	31[a]
Hartenauer et al. [5]	101	10	45	45	99	10	10[a]	34
Unertl et al. [11]	20	35	45	30	19	32	5[a]	26
Stoutenbeek et al. [14]	59	100	59	–	63	100	8[a]	–

NP, Nosocomial pneumonia

are either that SDD does not prevent infections as the cultural data would suggest that it does, or that infections are not as important in determining outcomes for seriously ill patients as clinicians have thought. Several confounding factors render interpretation of the available data difficult at best. Infections occur most often among the most ill patients; these same patients are most likely to experience complications, prolonged hospitalizations, and even death [15]. Thus, there is an unavoidable association between nosocomial infections and various complications.

Physiologic indices have been used in SDD studies to group together patients with quantitatively similar abnormalities in bodily function. However, the predictive accuracy of these indices is highly disease specific so that an APACHE II score of 25 results in very different mortality estimates for a septic patient and a trauma victim. It is likely that the reason that trauma patients have been shown to benefit from SDD is the relative homogeneity of this patient group. Conversely, the lack of an effect on mortality in most studies may be the result of inapparent differences in patient groups, differences that are masked by similarities in acute physiology scores. As with all applications of this type, the predictive power for individual patients is poor, and the technique is most applicable to large patient groups. This limitation suggests that single-unit studies of SDD will never have sufficient power to answer questions about its efficacy with clarity. However, successful implementation of multi-unit trials of SDD will place an enormous burden on investigators to standardize clinical management, as well as to precisely define patient groups and diagnostic criteria.

SDD is a powerful tool with which important aspects of critical illness can be investigated. These questions include the Following: (a) Are bacterial infections major determinants of outcome for seriously ill patients? (b) Does SDD only obscure clinical findings of infection while not altering tissue effects? (c) Do only certain patient groups benefit from SDD? If so, what are their characteristics? (d) What components of the SDD regimen are important? Experience to date suggests that it is a reasonably safe procedure, at least when conducted in a controlled fashion. Proof of its efficacy, and further elucidation of the role of bacterial infection in determining outcomes from serious illness, will await larger clinical trials that incorporate appropriate controls.

References

1. Greenfield S, Teres D, Bushnell LS, Hedley-Whyte J, Feingold DS (1973) Prevention of gram-negative bacillary pneumonia using aerosol polymyxin as prophylaxis. I. Effect on the colonization pattern of the upper respiratory tract of seriously ill patients. J Clin Invest 52:2935–2940
2. Klick JM, DuMoulin GC, Hedley-Whyte J, Teres D, Bushnell LS, Feingold DS (1975) Prevention of gram-negative bacillary pneumonia using polymyxin aerosol as prophylaxis. J Clin Invest 55:514–519
3. Feeley TW, Du Moulin GC, Hedley-Whyte J, Bushnell LS, Gilbert JP, Feingold DS (1975) Aerosol polymyxin and pneumonia in seriously ill patients. N Engl J Med 293:471–475
4. Stevens RM, Teres D, Skillman JJ, Finegold DS (1974) Pneumonia in an intensive care unit. Arch Intern Med 134:106–111
5. Hartenauer U, Thulig B, Lawin P, Fegeler W (1990) Infection surveillance and selective decontamination of the digestive tract (SDD) in critically ill patients–results of a controlled study. Infection 18 [Suppl 1]:s22–s30
6. Kerver AJH, Rommes JH, Mevissen-Verhage EAE, Hulstaert PF, Vos A, Verhoef J, Wittebol P (1988) Prevention of colonization and infection in critically ill patients: a prospective randomized study. Crit Care Med 16:1087–1093
7. Flaherty J, Kabins SA, Weinstein RA (1989) New approaches to the prevention of infection in intensive care unit patients. In: Van Saene HKF, Stoutenbeek CP, Lawin P, Ledingham IM (eds) Infection control in intensive care units by selective decontamination. Springer, Berlin Heidelberg, New York, pp 184–188 (Update in intensive care and emergency medicine, vol 7)
8. Van Saene HKF, Stoutenbeek CP, Gilbertson AA (1990) Review of available trials of selective decontamination of the digestive tract (SDD). Infection 18 [Suppl 1]:s5–s9
9. Ulrich C, Harinck-de Weerd JE, Bakker NC, Doornbos L, de Ridder VA (1989) Selective decontamination of the digestive tract with norfloxacin in the prevention of ICU-acquired infections: a prospective randomized study. Intensive Care Med 15:424–431
10. Ledingham IM, Eastaway AT, McKay IC, Alcock SR, McDonald JC, Ramsay G (1988) Triple regimen of selective decontamination of the digestive tract, systemic cefotaxime, and microbiological surveillance for prevention of acquired infection in intensive care. Lancet I:785–790
11. Unertl K, Ruckdeschel G, Selbmann HK, Jensen U, Forst H, Lenhart FP, Peter K (1987) Prevention of colonization and respiratory infections in long-term ventilated patients by local antimicrobial prophylaxis. Intensive Care Med 13:106–113
12. Andrews CP, Coalson JJ, Smith JD, Johanson WG (1981) Diagnosis of nosocomial bacterial pneumonia in acute, diffuse lung injury. Chest 80:254–258
13. Fagon JY, Chastre J, Hance AJ, Guiguet M, Trouillet JL, Domart Y, Pierre J, Gibert C (1988) Detection of nosocomial lung infection in ventilated patients. Am Rev Respir Dis 138:110–116
14. Stoutenbeek CP, van Saene HKF, Miranda DR, Zandstra DF (1984) The effect of selective decontamination of the digestive tract on colonization and infection rate in multiple trauma patients. Intensive Care Med 10:185–192
15. Haley R, Hooton T, Culver D et al. (1981) Nosocomial infections in U.S. Hospitals, 1975–1976. Estimated frequency by selected characteristics of patients. Am J Med 70:947–959

Selective Decontamination of the Digestive Tract (SDD): Review of Available Clinical Studies

C. P. Stoutenbeek[1] and H. K. Van Saene[2]

Introduction

Selective decontamination of the digestive tract (SDD) is based on two observations: first, most infections in intensive care are endogenous, i.e. caused by potential pathogens carried in the throat and gastrointestinal tract; secondly, the indigenous, mostly anaerobic flora has a very low intrinsic pathogenicity and helps to prevent colonization by more pathogenic exogenous microorganisms. SDD aims to selectively eliminate pathogens from the oropharynx and gastrointestinal tract by high doses of topical nonabsorbable antibiotics, which affect the indigenous flora as little as possible.

The original SDD regimen [1] consists of a combination of polymyxin E, Tobramycin and Amphotericin (PTA regimen). This is applied topically to both the oropharynx (in a sticky paste) and to the gastrointestinal tract, throughout intensive care unit (ICU) stay. A parenteral agent (cefotaxime) is administered during the first 4 days, for two reasons: first, to eliminate potential pathogens such as pneumococci commonly present in the oropharyngeal flora of normal people and not covered by the nonabsorbable agents; and, secondly, to treat colonization/infection of the lower airways by potential pathogens acquired by many patients prior to admission to the ICU.

SDD has been described in many different ways, e.g. selective gut decontamination (SGD), selective bowel decontamination (SBD), selective parenteral and enteral antisepsis regimen (SPEAR). However, the essential elements of this infection prevention technique are:
1. Decontamination of the oropharynx
2. Decontamination of the gastrointestinal tract
3. A short-term systemic antibiotic prophylaxis
4. An intensive bacteriological monitoring

---

[1] Department of Intensive Care, Onze Lieve Vrouwe Gasthuis, 1e Oosterparkstraat 179, 1091 HA Amsterdam, The Netherlands
[2] Department of Medical Microbiology, University of Liverpool, P.O. Box 147, Liverpool L69 3BX, UK

Host Defense Dysfunction
in Trauma, Shock and Sepsis
Eds. Faist/Meakins/Schildberg
© Springer-Verlag, Berlin Heidelberg 1993

Analysis of Available Trials

Study Design. Sixteen SDD trials have been reported so far, two of them in preliminary form only [15, 16]. These studies vary greatly in study design, patient selection, the SDD regimen and the use of systemic cefotaxime (Table 1). Eight studies were designed as randomized controlled trials, two studies used concurrent controls in two seperate ICUs with cross-over of the treatment after a period of time [9, 11], one is an observational cohort study in liver transplantation [5] and five used consecutive groups.

SDD Regimen. Nine studies used the PTA regimen. Since tobramycin and amphotericin B are not available for oral use in the USA, gentamicin and nystatin have been used instead [5, 15, 16]. Two studies replaced tobramycin by norfloxacin (absorbable) for economical reasons [8, 10]. Brun Buisson et al. [7] used a totally different combination of low dose polymyxin E with neomycin and nalidixic acid. In two studies no oropharyngeal decontamination has been used [7, 11]. In five studies SDD has been used without cefotaxime prophylaxis. However, many patients did receive systemic antibiotics for perioperative prophylaxis or other reasons.

Patient Selection. Patient selection criteria vary greatly among these studies: in two studies all patients admitted to the ICU were included [3, 11], while in other studies only patients requiring mechanical ventilation for at least 3-4 days or prolonged ICU stay (> 4 days) were included. Only few trials studied a homogeneous, primarily noninfected patient population such as trauma patients or patients undergoing liver transplantation or oesophageal resection [1, 5, 12]. Most studies included a mixed medical/surgical population of both infected and noninfected patients. In some studies as many as 50%–75% of all patients were already infected on admission [3, 4, 8, 10].

Results

Colonization Rate

In most studies microbiological surveillance cultures of both throat and rectum were taken. However, in some studies only throat [2], or only rectum [7, 11], or neither throat nor rectum cultures were taken [13].

All trials using the PTA combination showed the efficacy of this decontamination regimen. Within 2–3 days after starting SDD the oropharynx was free of pathogens. Intestinal decontamination generally took more time (6–10 days) due to absence of peristalsis. However, secondary colonization of the gastrointestinal tract with new pathogens was almost completely prevented in these

Table 1. Published SDD trials in intensive care

Trials/authors	Design			Numbers		Inclusion criteria			Patients
	RCT	PTA	Ctx	C	SDD	ICU	MV	Inf	
Stoutenbeek et al. [1]	+	+	+	59	63	≥5	≥3	−	Trauma
Unertl et al. [2]		−	−	20	19		≥4	−	Trauma, neurological
Ledingham et al. [3]		+	+	161	163	−	−	+	
Kerver et al. [4]	+	+	+	47	48	≥5	+	+	Liver transplantation
Wiesner et al [5]		−	+		30	−	−	+	
Konrad et al. [6]		+	−	83	82		≥4	+	
Brun Buisson et al. [7]	+	−	−	50	36	>2	−	+	
Ulrich et al. [8]	X^a	−	+	52	48	>5	−	+	
Thülig et al. [9]	+	+	+	101	99	≥5	≥3	+	
Aerdts et al. [10]		−	−	39	17		≥5	+	
Godard et al. [11]	X^a	+	+	84	97	−	−	−	Oesophageal resection
Tetteroo et al. [12]	+	+	+	58	56	−	−	−	
McClelland et al. [13]		+	+	12	15	≥7	≥5	+	Renal failure
Sydow et al. [14]		+	+	48	45		≥4	−	
Flaherty et al. [15]	+	−	−	56	51	?	?	?	Cardiac surgery
Cockerill et al. [16]	+	−	+	50	45	>4	?	?	

RCT, randomized controlled trial; PTA, polymyxine E, tobramycin, amphotericin B; CTX, cefotaxime; C, control group; SDD, SDD-treated group; ICU, ICU stay in days; MV, duration of mechanical ventilation in days; Inf, infection present on admission; Patients, patient selection; X^a, Consecutive trial in two ICUs with cross-over of the treatment

studies. So far no studies are available evaluating gastrointestinal decontamination by regimens using gentamicin instead of tobramycin.

The decontamination regimen used by Brun Buisson et al. [7] was not effective in preventing secondary intestinal colonization by *Pseudomonas*.

Colonization of the respiratory tract has been evaluated in all except two studies [7, 11] and all found a significant decrease of colonization by gram-negative bacilli in the SDD-treated groups. All five studies that evaluated colonization of the urinary tract found a significant reduction by SDD [1, 8, 9, 12, 13].

Infection Rate

The infection rate was the end-point of all SDD trials. The results of the fully published controlled trials are summarized in Table 2. In all studies except one ([7]) a highly significant reduction of the bronchopulmonary infection rate was found in the SDD-treated group, in particular of gram-negative pulmonary infections. In 7 out of the 11 studies that evaluated the urinary tract infections, SDD significantly reduced the infection rate. In many studies SDD also reduced the wound infection rate and the septicaemia rate (Table 2). In six out of eight studies in which the total infection rate has been evaluated, SDD reduced the infection rate with more than 50%. The two studies that failed to show an effect of SDD, did not use oropharyngeal decontamination, did not use parenteral cefotaxime prophylaxis and used a different SDD regimen [7, 11].

Table 2. Acquired infection rates in SDD trials

Author	RTI (%)	UTI (%)	Wounds (%)	Bloods (%)	Total
Stoutenbeek et al. [1]	59–8	32–2	25–5	42–3	81–16
Unertl et al. [2]	70–21				
Ledingham et al. [3]	18–3	3–1	2–1	11–8	24–10
Kerver et al. [4]	40–6[a]	6–3[a]	17–2[a]	57–30	81–39
Konrad et al. [6]	42–6				
Brun Buisson et al. [7]	22–20	20–5	6–0	4–6	34–33
Ulrich et al. [8]	50–15	50–23	27–8	23–21	77–52
Thülig et al. [9]	46–10	24–9		7–8	
Aerdts et al. [10]	69–6	36–35	18–0	33–6	
Godard et al. [11]	15–2	25–19	5–1	12–11	35–26
Tetteroo et al. [12]	14–2	22–9	35–11	2–2	57–21
McClelland et al. [13]	50–7	50–13	17–7	25–20	83–33
Sydow et al. [14]	75–7	31–11	19–16	8–7	

Total, percentage of infected patients; RTI, respiratory tract infection rate; UTI, urinary tract infection rate.
[a] number of infections (infection rate not reported); since one patient can have more than one infection, the infection rate may be lower.

Mortality

The mortality data are summarized in Table 3. In four of the 13 studies a lower mortality was found in the SDD-treated group [1, 8, 9, 14]. In two other studies [4, 13] the infection-related mortality decreased, but not overall mortality. In some studies a difference in mortality has been found for subgroups of patients, e.g. trauma patients or patients requiring more than 7 days' intensive care [3] or with an ICU stay > 48 h [11]. However, in many studies the number of patients enrolled was too small for differences to reach significance.

The fact that the dramatic reduction in acquired infection rate is not accompanied by a significant reduction in mortality seems to challenge the widely accepted view that infection is one of the major causes of death in patients requiring prolonged intensive care. However, most of these studies included patients with severe infections present on admission: e.g. in the study of Kerver et al. [4], 23% of the control group and 39% of the SDD-treated patients were admitted to the ICU because of intra-abdominal sepsis. In these patients the prognosis is determined by the primary infection rather than by the ICU-acquired infections. In another study cerebral injury was the most common cause of death [2]. The effect of SDD on mortality can only be investigated in a controlled multicentre trial, in a homogeneous population of primarily non-infected patients in whom ICU-acquired infections are a major cause of death.

Table 3. Mortality rates in SDD trials (%)

Author	Center	Control		SDD	
		No.	%	No.	%
Stoutenbeek et al. [1]	Groningen	5/59	8	2/63	3
Unertl et al. [2]	Munich	6/20	30	5/19	26
Ledingham et al[3]	Glasgow	39/161	24	39/163	24
trauma			26		0
ICU stay ≥ 7 d			34		13
Kerver et al. [4]	Utrecht	15/47	32	14/48	29
infection-related			17		4
Konrad et al. [6]	Ulm	18/83	22	25/82	30
Brun Buisson et al. [7]	Paris	12/50	24	8/36	22
infection-related			10		9
Ulrich et al. [8]	The Hague	28/52	54	15/48	31
infection-related			15		0
Thülig et al. [9]	Münster	46/101	46	34/99	34
infection-related			23		7
Aerdts et al. [10]	Nijmegen	6/39	15	2/17	12
Godard et al. [11]	Lyon	15/84	18	12/97	12
ICU stay > 48 h			18		6
Tetteroo et al [12]	Rotterdam	2/58	3	3/56	5
McClelland et al. [13]	Liverpool	7/12	58	9/15	60
infection-related			50		27
Sydow et al. [14]	Göttingen	7/48	14	0/45	0
infection-related			6		0

Emergence of Resistance

The major problem in the ICU under conventional antibiotic treatment is colonization and superinfection with resistant gram-negative pathogens and yeasts. The SDD studies show without exception a remarkable absence of these superinfections, notwithstanding the systemic prophylaxis with cefotaxime.

A patient treated with SDD is successfully decontaminated when only anaerobes, streptococci and coagulase-negative staphylococci (i.e. indigenous flora) are isolated from cultures of throat, rectum or skin. Many of these coagulase-negative staphylococci are methicillin-resistant, and most of the streptococci are aminoglycosid and cephalosporin resistant. However, this should not be considered as selection of resistant strains, because these microorganisms are commensals with a very low intrinsic pathogenicity and do not generally necessitate antibiotic treatment. In case antibiotic therapy should be necessary, they can be treated with vancomycin or ampicillin.

So far there is no indication that SDD increases the risk of selection of resistant *pathogens* during many years of uninterrupted use of the same regimen. On the contrary, it has been shown that SDD is highly effective in controlling outbreaks with multiply resistant microorganisms in the ICU [7]. The gastrointestinal tract is the major reservoir of multiply resistant pathogens in intensive care patients. Elimination of these reservoirs by treating colonized patients with SDD decreases the risk of transmission of these pathogens to other patients. There is increasing evidence that SDD has a major impact on the ecology of the unit.

Indications for SDD

Based on the results of the available studies a tentative list of indications for SDD includes:
1. Prolonged mechanical ventilation (> 48 h)
2. Organ transplantation (liver, heart, lung and pancreas)
3. Preoperatively, in high risk operations (oesophageal resection, gastric resection etc)
4. Burns
5. Treatment of severe infections
6. Outbreaks of multiply resistant microorganisms

References

1. Stoutenbeek CP, van Saene HKF, Miranda DR, Zandstra DF (1984) The effect of selective decontamination of the digestive tract on colonisation and infection in multiple trauma patients. Intensive Care Med 10:185–192

2. Unertl K, Ruckdeschel G, Selbmann HK, Jensen U, Forst H, Lenhardt FP, Peter K ((1987) Prevention of colonization and respiratory infections in longterm ventilated patients by local antimicrobial prophylaxis. Intensive Care Med 13:106–113
3. Ledingham McAI, Alcock SR, Eastaway AT, McDonald JC, McKay IC, Ramsay G (1988) Triple regimen of selective decontamination of the digestive tract, systemic cefotaxime, and microbiological surveillance for prevention of acquired infection in intensive care. Lancet 1:785–790
4. Kerver AJH, Rommes JH, Verhage EAE (1988) Prevention of colonization and subsequent infection in surgical intensive care patients. A prospective randomized study. Crit Care Med 16:1087–1093
5. Wiesner RH, Krom RAF, Hermans P (1988) Selective bowel decontamination to decrease gram-negative aerobic bacterial and candida colonization and prevent infection after orthotopic liver transplantation. Transplantation 45:570–574
6. Konrad F, Schwalbe B, Heeg K, Wagner H, Wiedeck H, Kilian J, Ahnefeld FW (1989) Kolonisations-, Pneumoniefrequenz und Resistenzentwicklung bei langzeitbeatmeten Intensivpatienten unter selektiver Dekontamination des Verdauungstraktes. Anaesthesist 38:99–109
7. Brun Buisson C, Legrand P, Rauss A et al. (1989) Intestinal decontamination for control of nosocomial multiresistant gram-negative bacilli. Study of an outbreak in an intensive care unit. Ann Intern Med 10:873–881
8. Ulrich C, Harinck-de Weerd JE, Bakker NC, Jacz K, Doornbos L, de Ridder VA (1990) Selective decontamination of the digestive tract with norfloxacin in the prevention of ICU-acquired infections: a prospective randomized study. Intensive Care Med 15:424–431
9. Thülig B, Hartenauer U, Diemer, Lawin P, Fegeler W, Kehrel R, Ritzerfeld W (1989) Selektive Florasuppression Zur Infektionskontrolle in der operativen Intensivmedizin. Anaesth Intensivther Notfallmed 24:345–354
10. Aerdts SJA, Clasener HAL, van Dalen R, van Lier HJJ, Vollaard EJ, Festen J (1991) Prevention of bacterial colonization of the respiratory tract and stomach of mechanically ventilated patients by a novel regimen of selective decontamination in combination with initial systemic cefotaxime. J Antimicrob Chemother [Suppl] (in press)
11. Godard J, Guillaume C, Reverdy ME, Bachmann P, Bui-Xuan B, Nageotte A, Motin J (1990) Intestinal decontamination in a polyvalent ICU: a double-blind study. Intensive Care Med 16:307–311
12. Tetteroo GWM, Wagenvoort JHT, Castelein AL, Tilanus HW, Ince C, Bruining HA (1990) Selective decontamination to reduce gram-negative colonization and infection after oesophageal resection. Lancet 335:704–707
13. McClelland P, Murray AE, Williams PS, van Saene HKF, Gilbertson AA, Mostafa M, Bone JM (1990) Reducing sepsis in severe combined acute renal and respiratory failure by selective decontamination of the digestive tract. Crit Care Med 18:935–939
14. Sydow M, Buchardi H, Crozier TA, Rüchel R, Busse C, Seyde W (1990) Einfluβ der selektiven Dekontamination auf nosokomiale Infektionen, Erregerspektrum und Antibiotikaresistenz bei langzeitbeatmeten Intensivpatienten. Anaesth Intensivther Notfallmed 25:416–423
15. Flaherty J, Kabins SA, Weinstein RA (1989) New approaches to the prevention of infection in intensive care unit patients. In: van Saene HKF, Stoutenbeek CP, Lawin P, McALedingham I (eds) Update in intensive care and emergency medicine (Infection control by selective decontamination, vol 7) Springer, Berlin Heidelberg New York, pp 184–188
16. Cockerill FR, Muller SM, Anhalt JP, Thompson RL (1989) Reduction of nosocomial infections by selective digestive tract decontamination (SDD) in the ICU (Abstr). 29th ICAAC, Houston, American Society of Microbiology

Nonselective Gut Decontamination for Avoidance of Bacterial Translocation in Shock

J. Brand, A. Ekkernkamp, A. Helbig, and G. Muhr

Introduction

With a total mortality of about 20%, septic multiple organ failure (MOF) is the main cause of death in polytraumatized patients. Secondary organ failure usually begins 4–8 days after primary successful treatment. A septic focus can hardly ever be identified [5–7, 20]. The gut as a shock organ and a trigger of septic macrophage reaction has become the center of research interest. In traumatic shock the alpha-adrenergic potency in the gastointestinal tract leads to a reduction in the mesenterial blood flow to 15%–20% of normal [15]. Dysfunction of the intestinal mucosal barrier with a translocation of gram-negative bacteria can be shown in analogous shock situations in animal experiments [2, 3, 8, 10, 13, 19–21].

Until now few therapeutic or prophylactic steps have been taken in hospitals. Selective gut decontamination (SGD) led only to a decrease in infection and colonization, not in lethality [22–24]. As we know from elective surgery of the colon, orthograde gut lavage can reduce the number of germs by 95% [4, 18]. We attempted to eliminate this mechanism at the earliest possible time by non-selective gut decontamination (NSGD) with an effective orthograde lavage.

Patients and Methods

In a prospective study we examined 58 polytraumatized patients (ages 15–65 years) whose injury had occurred less than 6 h prior to admission and whose injury severity score (ISS) was over 24. Of the 58, 30 were randomized to standard intensive care plus orthograde gut lavage (mean age 32.4 years; mean ISS 30.9), and 28 received standard intensive care alone (mean age 29.9 years; mean ISS 29.3). The orthograde gut lavage was carried out at the earliest possible time, i.e., after vital stabilization and before any non-vital operation. We used Golitely's solution until a clear rinse was achieved. After 48 h all patients in the study group who did not show signs of definitive stabilization were subjected to another rinsing. Besides the routine clinical examinations we

Chirurgische Universitätsklinik Bergmannsheil, Gilsingstr. 14, 4630 Bochum, FRG

Host Defense Dysfunction
in Trauma, Shock and Sepsis
Eds. Faist/Meakins/Schildberg
© Springer-Verlag, Berlin Heidelberg 1993

analyzed serum elastase, c-reactive protein (CRP), and MOF-score, according to Marshall. None of the patients had suffered head injury, and there was no septic focus.

Results

The analysis of elastase (Fig. 1a) and CRP (Fig. 1b) revealed a peak directly after trauma and another between the fourth and tenth days after the injury occurred. The graphs of the NSGD group show a distinctly lower level especially at the

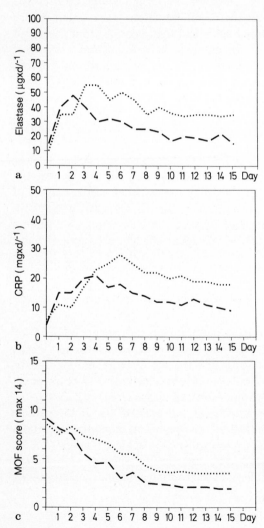

Fig. 1a-c. Results of laboratory measurements over a 15-day period in patients receiving NSGD (––– ; $n = 30$) and controls (····· ; $n = 28$). **a** Elastase. **b** c-reactive protein. **c** MOF score

time of the second peak and thereafter. The decrease in MOF scores was significantly faster in the study group (Fig. 1c). Mortality was 21% (6/28) in the control group and 16.6% (5/30) in the study group. Fatal septic MOF occurred in 5/28 patients (17.8%) in the control group; compared with this we achieved a significant improvement in the study group, in which 3/30 (10%) patients died of septic MOF. There were no complications as a result of lavage, no measurable increase in blood volume, and no electrolyte shift. Occasional regurgitation of the rinsing solution was not harmful as our patients were intubated and under mechanical ventilation. After severe trauma to the spine or pelvis lavage was less effective than otherwise, due to extensive retroperitoneal hematomae with secondary gut paralysis. After abdominal trauma we regularly carried out catheter jejunostomy; this served initially for the lavage and later for providing enteral nutrition. Rinsing was seen to be particularly effective in these patients.

Discussion

Septic MOF as a cause of bacterial and endotoxin translocation depends clearly on the quantity of the translocated matter [1, 2, 16, 17]. A first peak in translocation is reached after 2 h. In our test a plateau over 8 h was observed [10–13]. In the following 24 h the number of germs and the content of endotoxin doubled [25]. A reduction in translocated matter should theoretically be achieved by a drastic reduction in the number of germs in the gut at an early phase. In large clinical studies the number of germs, for example, in the respiratory tract, was reduced by SGD, as were the number of infections in intensive care units, especially in the case of pneumonia. A decrease in septic MOF, particulary of mortality, was not reported [3, 14, 22, 23]. Some have expressed critical opinions concerning the possible development of resistance by continuing SGD [6, 8, 14].

In both laboratory and clinical terms we observed significant differences in comparison of very early gut lavage for decontamination with our standard regimen. Our clinical observations show that all patients who received a particularly effective lavage (e.g., by catheter jejunostomy) had exceptionally good results. There were no complications from rinsing. On the basis of our experience we regard NSGD in the posttraumatic phase as suitable for the prevention of septic complication. Side effects are not likely, a development of resistance is not to be feared, and costs are low. NSGD leads to a reduction in the enteral bacteria reservoir. The clinical effectiveness of this method, based on good theoretical grounds, has also been established in animal experiments.

References

1. Alverdy J, Hoon Sang C, Sheldon GF (1985) The effect of parenteral nutrition on gastointestinal immunity. Ann Surg 85:681
2. Baker JW, Deitch EA, Berg R (1987) Hemorrhagic shock impairs the mucosal barrier, resulting in bacterial translocation from the gut and sepsis. Surg Forum 38:73
3. Baker JW, Deitch EA, Li M, Berg RD, Specian RD (1988) Hemorrhagic shock induces bacterial translocation from the gut. J Trauma 28:896
4. Beck DE, Mayo U, Harford FJ, Palma De J (1984) Comparison of cleansing methods in preparation for colon surgery. Dis Colon Rectum 7(28):491
5. Border JR (1982) Trauma and Sepsis. In: Worth MH (ed) Principles and practice of trauma care. Williams and Wilkins, Baltimore
6. Border JR, Hassett J, La Duca J, Seibel R, Steinberg S, Mills B, Losi P, Border D (1987) The gut origin septic states in blunt multiple trauma (ISS = 40) in the ICU. Ann Surg:427
7. Carrico CJ, Meakins JL, Marshall JC (1986) Multiple organ failure syndrome. Arch Surg 121:196
8. Deitch EA, Maejima K, Berg R (1985) Effect of oral antibiotics and bacterial overgrowth on the translocation of the GI-tract microflora in burned rats. J Trauma 25:385
9. Deitch EA, Winterton J, Berg R (1987) Effect of starvation, malnutrition and trauma on the GI-tract flora and bacterial translocation. Arch Surg 122:1019
10. Deitch EA, Winterton J, Li M et al. (1987) The gut as a portal of entry for bacteremia: role of malnutrition. Ann Surg 205:681
11. Deitch EA, Bridges RM (1987) Effect of stress and trauma on bacterial translocation from the gut. J Surg Res 42:536
12. Deitch EA, Berg R, Specian R (1987) Endotoxin promotes the translocation of bacterial from the gut. Arch Surg 122:185
13. Falk A, Redfors S, Myrvold H, Haglund U (1985) Small intestinal mucosa lesions in feline septic shock: a study of pathogenesis. Circ Shock 17 (4):327
14. Haralambie E, Mahmond HK, Linzemeier G, Wendt F (1983) The "clostridial effect" of selective decontamination of human gut with trimethoprim/sulfamethoxazolin in neutropenic patients. Infection 11 (4):201
15. Herfarth C (1988) Das Problem der Ischämie von Leber und Darm. Hefte Unfallheilkd 200:345
16. Maejima K, Deitch EA, Berg RD (1984) Bacterial translocation from the gastrointestinal tracts of rats receiving thermal injury. Infect Immun 43:6
17. Maejima K, Deitch EA, Berg R (1984) Promotion by burn stress of the translocation of bacteria from the gastrointestinal tracts of mice. Arch Surg 119:166
18. Pockros PJ, Foroozan P (1985) Golitely Lavage versus a standard colonoscopie preparation. Gastroenterology 88:545
19. Rush BF, Sori AJ, Murphy TF, Smith SL, Flanagan J, Machiedo GW (1988) Endotoxemia and bacteremia during hemorrhagic shock. The link between trauma and sepsis. Ann Surg 207:549
20. Saadia R, Schein M, MacFarlane C, Boffard KD (1990) Gut barrier function and the surgeon. Br J Surg 77:487
21. Schlag G, Redl H (1988) Neue Erkenntnisse des Schockgeschehens in der Traumatologie. Unfallchirurgie 14:3
22. Stoutenbeek CP, van Saene HK, Miranda DR, Zandstra DF (1984) The effect of selective decontamination of the digestive tract on colonisation and infection rate in multiple trauma patients. Intensive Care Med 10:185
23. Stoutenbeck CP, van Saene HK, Miranda DR et al. (1987) The effect of oropharyngeal decontamination using topical nonabsorbable antibiotics on the incidence of nosocomial respiratory tract infection in multiple trauma patients. J Trauma 27:3
24. Van Uffelen R, Rommes JH, Saene HK (1987) Preventing lower airway colonisation and infection in mechanically ventilated patients. Crit Care Med 15:99

Section 13

**Antibiotic Interactions
with Host Defenses**

Antibiotics and Phagocytic Cell Function: A Critical Review

P. Van der Auwera[1], M. Bonnet[1], M. Husson[1], and F. Jacobs[2]

Introduction

Interest in the interaction between antibiotics and professional phagocytes has focused on several aspects [1, 2]: intracellular penetration and bioactivity, direct enhancing or depressing effects (toxicological approach), or indirect functional effects through specific action of the antimicrobial on the pathogen (enhancement below the minimum inhibitory concentration, MIC, or post antibiotic leukocyte enhancement).

Intracellular Penetration and Bioactivity

This approach is useful since intracellular pathogens (either exclusive, as *Chlamydia* and mycobacteria; facultative-preferential as *Legionella*; or only occasional, as *staphylococcus aureus* and *Haemophilus influenzae*) can escape antibiotics which do not penetrate well into the cells (β-lactams and aminoglycosides). Furthermore, the intracellular site of sequestration may be specific for each pathogen and depends on the presence of appropriate virulence factors [3]. The most popular method is to incubate phagocytic cells (macrophages or neutrophils—PMNs) with the antimicrobial, wash it away rapidly, and measure the amount associated with the cell pellet (cell-associated drug) by HPLC, radioactive labeling, fluorimetry, or microbiologically [4]. For the new fluoroquinolones, all methods have provided very similar results with cell-associated/extracellular concentration of 3–15 depending on the cell type and the drug tested.

    Limitations and drawbacks are numerous. The antimicrobial may be bound to the surface of the cell (cholesterol and phospholipid binding is suspected for amphotericin B [5], phospholipid binding occurs with several antimalarial drugs [6], and protein binding is suspected for both vancomycin and teicoplanin

[1] Laboratoire de Microbiologie et Clinique des Maladies Infectieuses, Laboratoires d'Investigation Clinique H. J. Tagnon, Service de Médecine, Institut Jules Bordet, rue Héger-Bordet, 1 1000 Brussels, Belgium
[2] Cliniques des Maladies Infectieuses et Tropicales, Service de Médecine, Cliniques Universitaires de Bruxelles, Hôpital Erasme, route de Lennick 808, 1070 Brussels, Belgium

Host Defense Dysfunction
in Trauma, Shock and Sepsis
Eds. Faist/Meakins/Schildberg
© Springer-Verlag, Berlin Heidelberg 1993

[7]). The antimicrobial may leak rapidly out of the cell during washing and centrifugation (a few minutes for the new fluoroquinolones and most macrolides except azithromycin); the antimicrobial can be inactivated through binding to inner cell membranes (suspected for amphotericin B). The cell type is important as the duration of incubation with the antimicrobial. Macrophages use pinocytosis hence aminoglycosides and penicillins can be found intracellularly; PMNs do not use pinocytosis hence intracellular penetration of these antimicrobials is very low. Prolonged incubation (hours) allows aminoglycosides to be concentrated into lysosomes. Prestimulation of the test cells may increase the capture of several antimicrobials, probably by ingestion of the antimicrobial present in the extracellular fluid. Another possible effect of cell activation (in vivo) is exemplified by the very high concentrations of clindamycin and roxythromycin found in the alveolar macrophages of smokers by comparison with cells obtained from nonsmokers [8]. The group of Tulkens [8–10] has studied the subcellular distribution, including lysosomal association of several antimicrobials using resting macrophages and PMNs. Using this method, it was shown that almost one-third of the intracellular concentration of fluoroquinolones and macrolides and about 5% of intracellular concentration of clindamycin were found to be associated with the lysosomes.

The indirect method is to use phagocytic cells preloaded with test microorganisms. Intracellular bioactivity is measured either by colony counting after lysis of the phagocytic cells or alteration in intracellular growth measured by the accumulation of a radioisotopic substrate. Established lines of macrophages are convenient because their oxidative killing mechanism is poor, allowing intracellular survival or even growth. PMNs are less convenient due to their high killing efficacy (especially for the oxidative killing mechanisms) and their small survival time in vitro (24 h at the most) [11]. Conclusions from these studies are valid only in terms of intracellular bioactivity in the subcellular compartment in which the test bacteria is located. A major technical drawback of the indirect method is the adherence of the test organism to the surface of the phagocytic cells. Elimination of the adherent bacteria by lysis should be carried out, or controls at 4 °C (no ingestion allowed) should be included.

Toxicological Approach

The toxicological aspect represents a highly controversial area in the study of antibiotic-phagocyte interaction. Most studies have been limited to a single function such as chemiluminescence (see discussion of many artifacts in [12]), chemotaxis, superoxide generation, or ingestion and to the description of an "event" (significant difference by comparison to a control) without assessing the mechanism of interaction. The high variability linked to the origin of the cells (between-volunteer variability for neutrophils and possibly macrophages) has not been the subject of extensive work.

Figures 1 and 2 show the type of donor-dependent variability found with several PMNs functions and their responsiveness to antimicrobial agents. Discrepancies between investigators may be due to differences in cell preparation (all blood versus purified neutrophils, different methods of purification) and methods. Activation of neutrophils may occur during cell preparation and result in conflicting results [13]. The enhancement of neutrophil activity by several semisynthetic cephalosporins is probably due to indirect binding to monocytes or macrophages and release of activators [14]. It may be also the case for roxythromycin, as suggested by the priming of formyl-methionyl-leucyl-phenylalanine (fMLP)-induced chemiluminescence (Fig. 3) [15]. The key role of the plasma membrane as the target for polyfunctional depression (or activation) has been shown or suggested for several antimicrobials which are highly concentrated in phagocytic cells such as amphotericin B (associated with a decreased membrane fluidity) [16], coumermycin (associated with impairment of signal transduction; Fig. 2) [17], chloroquine, and analogs [18]. The "immunostimulating" effect of amphotericin B on macrophages has been associated with the capacity of binding to the cell membrane. Interaction with the cell membrane may result in different consequences on specific receptors. Amphotericin B (indirectly) decreases the affinity of fMLP receptor but can increase the

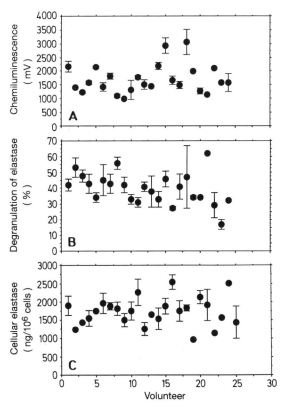

Fig. 1A–C. Variability of neutrophil functions among healthy human volunteers. Neutrophils were obtained from peripheral veinous blood by dextran sedimentation and Ficol-Hypaque centrifugation. **A** Chemiluminescence response (peak value) induced by PMA (3×10^{-6} M). Result for each volunteer (mean $\pm$ SEM) corresponding to 10^6 neutrophils. Each volunteer tested two to ten times. **B** Exocytic degranulation of elastase by neutrophils induced by fMLP (10^{-5} M). Degranulation response (mean $\pm$ SEM) as a function of the volunteer source of the cells. Each volunteer tested two to seven times. **C** Total cellular-associated elastase (immunoassay). Mean $\pm$ SEM for each of the 25 volunteers tested (one to seven assays for each volunteer) in ng/10^6 neutrophils

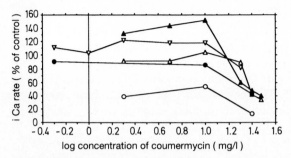

Fig. 2. Variability of toxicological response of neutrophil functions among healthy human volunteers: impairment of fMLP signal transduction by coumermycin (30-min preincubation) as measured by the rate of increase in cytoplasmic ionized calcium (Quin-2, fluorimetry). Each symbol corresponds to the PMNs obtained from a different volunteer

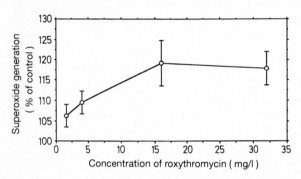

Fig. 3. Priming of fMLP-induced superoxide generation by preincubation (30-min) of human neutrophils with roxythromycin Mean ± SEM of duplicate experiments using the PMNs from three different volunteers

expression of Fc receptor (see discussion in [19]). Rifampicin, which specifically competes for the fMLP receptor without affecting C5a receptor dependent chemotaxis [20] increases adherence to polystyrene and decreases random migration by a nonspecific mechanism [21]. These remarks suggest that a multifunctional approach should be undertaken whenever possible, and that the mechanism responsible for any interaction be explored.

Indirect Effects: Preincubation of the Pathogen

Test bacteria should be described carefully to appreciate the presence of a capsule or several virulence determinants associated with resistance to serum killing, phagocytosis, or escape mechanisms from intracellular killing. Several experimental designs have been used, each with specific limitations and drawbacks. Preincubation of the test bacteria at sub-MIC levels can result in many different modifications: serum susceptibility, opsonic requirements either immune or non immune resulting in better ingestion, nonspecific adherence to

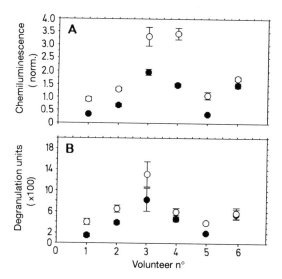

Fig. 4A, B. Preincubation of a b-capsulated strain of *Haemophilus influenzae* with MIC/2 concentration of antibiotics (60-min preincubation) increases the response of human PMNs in vitro. PMNs were obtained from six different volunteers. **A** Luminol-enhanced chemiluminescence (normalized units: rate of chemiluminescence in 10 µV/min normalized for a opsonized bacteria: PMN ratio of 1:1; range studied: 20–200, in triplicate). **B** degranulation of elastase (immunoassay) in percentage (normalized for a bacteria/PMN ratio of 1:1; range studied: 200–2000, in triplicate)

phagocytic cells, increased susceptibility to oxygen-dependent or -independent mechanisms either intra- or extracellularly. The preincubated bacteria may release substances which are able to directly stimulate or prime the phagocytic cells. Figure 4 shows that a b-capsulated strain of *H. influenzae* incubated for a short period of time (60 min) with MIC/2 of cefuroxime induces a stronger chemiluminescence and degranulation response by PMNs than untreated bacteria, even if the enhancement was quantitatively variable with the volunteer source of the cells. Selection of sub population during pretreatment is a potential risk in experiments using overnight preincubation. Preincubation of the test bacteria at levels above the MIC (or minimal bactericidal concentration) is even more difficult to standardize. Removal of the antimicrobial can be achieved by filtration, dilution, or inactivation of the antimicrobial (i.e., β-lactamase). When the bacterial inoculum is partially killed during the preincubation period, the presence of dead bacterial cells (not measured by viable counting!) contributes to phagocytosis and possibly to the activation of the neutrophils.

Clinical Relevance

Besides the issue of intracellular penetration, in many instances of toxicological and indirect effects studies in discriminant animal models are needed. As far as human studies are concerned, the impact of a phagocytic-enhancing (or depressing) antibiotic on a good baseline response rate (> 90%) obtained with a phagocytic-neutral control antimicrobiotic (with identical spectrum of activity and pharmacokinetic properties, e.g., cefodizime versus cefuroxime) would be almost impossible to measure in a double-blind prospective study because of the very high number of patients (thousands!) required to restrict to an acceptable β error. In selected subpopulations of patients with acquired deficit of phagocytic functions, smaller clinical studies might be able to show a difference in outcome related to phagocytic-modulation properties. Ex vivo studies have occasionally shown potentially clinically relevant effects.

We have recently studied the peripheral PMNs of patients receiving amphotericin β (Fungizone) to correlate with the very strong multifunctional inhibition found in vitro [19]. Five patients receiving amphotericin β (50 mg) have been studied so far. Blood samples were collected before and 1 h after the start of infusion. The following functions were found unchanged by amphotericin β administration: superoxide generation induced by fMLP, phorbol myristate acetate, and opsonized zymosan, ingestion of *Candida albicans* by adherent

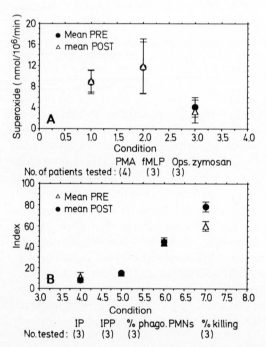

Fig. 5A, B. Ex vivo investigation of PMNs functions in patients receiving amphotericin β (50 mg) for deep fungal infection **A** Generation of superoxide induced by three different stimuli (phorb myristate acetate, fMLP, and opsonized zymosan). **B** Ingestion and intracellular killing of *C. albicans* by glass-adherent PMNs (300 PMNs counted). *Closed circles* before administration; *open triangles*, 1 h after the begining of amphotericin β, infusion; n, number of patients investigated, *IP*, mean number of ingested yeasts/adherent PMN; *IPP*, mean number of ingested yeast/adherent phagocytizing PMN; % *phago. PMNs* percentage of adherent PMNs, with intracellular yeast; % *Killing*, percentage of death yeast from intracellular yeasts. Mean $\pm$ SEM

neutrophils (Fig. 5), adherence to polystyrene, 3-(4,5-dimethylthiazol-2-yl)-2,5-diphenyl-tetrazinium-bromide reduction, degranulation of β-glucuronidase, vitamin B_{12} binding-protein, elastase, cellular content in β-glucuronidase, myeloperoxidase, and elastase. This in marked contrast to in vitro findings documenting a multifunctional inhibition at similar concentrations [19]. Intracellular killing of *C. albicans* by adherent PMNs was slightly enhanced (Fig. 5), suggesting that some of the cell-associated drug remains bioactive, as also shown in vitro [19]. Serum concentration (HPLC) was 0.8–1.5 mg/l and PMN-associated concentration was 10 mg/l or greater.

Conclusion

At present, among the numerous aspects of antibiotic-phagocytic cell interaction, only intracellular penetration and bioactivity are considered clinically relevant and beneficial for the treatment of infections due to intracellular pathogens such as *Legionella*, *Chlamydia*, and *Toxoplasma*. In addition, this may be also of clinical relevance in selected types of infections due to *S. aureus*, *H. influenzae*, *Brucella*, and *Salmonella*.

Acknowledgements. The authors acknowledge the help of the following collaborators from the Neutrophil Laboratory of Institut Jules Bordet: A. Vandermies, V. Duchâteau, W. Boumedian (technicians), T. Matsumoto, and N. Ogata, (postgraduate MDs from Kyushu University, Japan), G. Petrikkos, (Postgraduate MD from the University of Athens, Greece), G. Prinz (postgraduate MD from Lazlo Hospital, Budapest, Hungary) and A. M. Bourguignon (nurse).

References

1. Van der Auwera P (1989) The immunomodulation effects of antibiotics. Curr Opin Infect Dis 1:363–374
2. Van den Broek PJ (1989) Antimicrobial drugs, microorganisms and phagocytes. Rev Infect Dis 11:213–245
3. Moulder JW (1985) Comparative biology of intracellular parasitism. Microbiol Rev 49:298–337
4. Van der Auwera P, Matsumoto T, Husson M (1988) Intraphagocytic penetration of antibiotics. J Antimicrob Chemother 22:185–190
5. Collette N, Pascual-Lopez A, Heymans C, van der Auwera P, Meunier F (1989) Tissular concentration and bioactivity of amphotericin B in cancer patients treated with Fungizone. Antimicrob Agents Chemother 33:362–340
6. Chevli R, Fitch CD (1982) The antimalarial drug mefloquine binds too membrane phospholipids. Antimicrob Agents Chemother 21:581–586
7. Van der Auwera P, Bonnet M, Husson M (1990) Influence of teicoplanin and vancomycin on degranulation by PMNs stimulated by various agonists: an in vitro study. J Antimicrob Chemother 26:683–688
8. Carlier MB, Zenebergh A, Tulkens PM (1987) Cellular uptake and subcellular distribution of roxythromycin and erythromycin in phagocytic cells. J Antimicrob Chemother [Suppl B]: 47–56
9. Carlier MB, Scorneaux B, Zenebergh A, Tulkens PM (1987) Uptake and subcellular distribution of 4 quinolones (Pefloxacin; Ciprofloxacin; Ofloxacin; RO-236240) in phagocytes. Program and

abstracts of the 27th interscientific conference on antimicrobial agents and chemotherapy. American Society for Microbiology, New York, no 622, p 205

10. Zenebergh A, Bottcher P, Brison J, Tulkens PM (1987) Comparative uptake and subcellular distribution of 4 closely related lincosaminides, clindamycin, lincomycin, pirlimycin, and glycyl-pirlimycin in phagocytes. Program and abstracts of the 27th interscientific conference on antimicrobial agents and chemotherapy. American Society for Microbiology, New York no 1080, p 285

11. Van der Auwera P, Prinz G, Petrikkos G (1991) Activity of intracellular antibiotics. Infection (in press)

12. Briheim G, Dahlgren C (1987) Influence of antibiotics on formyl-methionyl-leucyl-phenyl-alanine-induced leukocyte chemiluminescence. Antimicrob Agents Chemother 31:763–767

13. Boogaerts MA, Vercelotti G, Roelant C, Eyssen M, Verwilghen RL, Jacobs HS (1986) Importance of platelet-free granulocyte preparations, as shown by improved cell separation techniques. Scand J Haematol 37:229–236

14. Onishi H, Kosuzume H, Inaba H, Okura M, Mochizuki H, Suzuki Y, Fuji R (1983) Effect of AC-1370, a new semisynthetic cephalosporin, on phagocyte functions. Antimicrob Agents Chemother 23:874–880

15. Bonnet M, Husson M, van der Auwera P (1989) Neutrophil priming by *Haemophilus influenzae*: influence of sub-MIC concentrations of antibiotics. 16th international congress on chemotherapy. Jerusalem, p 77

16. Yasui K, Masuda M, Masuoka T, Yamazaki M, Koniyama A, Akabane T, Murata K (1988) Miconazole and amphotericin B alter polymorphonuclear leukocyte functions and membrane fluidity in similar fashions. Antimicrob Agents Chemother 32:1864–1868

17. Van der Auwera P, Husson M, Brasseur R, Ruysschaert JM (1989) Interaction between the DNA-gyrase inhibitor coumermycin and the membrane of human neutrophils. In: Gilissen G, Opferkuch W, Peters G, Pulverer G (eds). The influence of antibiotics on the host-parasite relationship III. Springer, Berlin Heidelberg New York, pp 281–285

18. Labro MT, Babin-Chevaye C (1988) Effects of amodiaquine, chloroquine, and mefloquine on human polymorphonuclear neutrophil function in vitro. Antimicrob Agents Chemother 32:1124–1130

19. Van der Auwera P, Meunier F (1989) In vitro effects of cilofungin (LY 121019), amphotericin B and amphotericin B-deoxycholate on human polymorphonuclear leucocytes. J Antimicrob Chemother 24:747–763

20. Gray GD, Smith CW, Hollers JC, Chenoweth DE, Fiegel VD, Nelson RD (1983) Rifampin affects polymorphonuclear leukocyte interactions with bacterial and synthetic chemotaxins but not interactions with serum derived-chemotaxins. Antimicrob Agents Chemother 24:777–783

21. Van der Auwera P, Husson M (1989) Influence of rifampicin and ansamycin on motility and adherence of human neutrophils studied in vitro. J Antimicrob Chemother 24:347–353

Interaction of Antibiotics with the Phagocyte Oxidative Burst

M. T. Labro and J. El Benna

Introduction

The study of interactions between antibiotics and the host defense system dates virtually from the discovery of these therapeutic agents. However, it is only in recent years that the emerging concept of immunomodulation by antibacterial drugs has received worldwide interest with a view to the development of new strategies for the treatment of infectious diseases. Since phagocytes play a pivotal role in the immediate defenses against invading pathogens, it is thus of major importance to analyze the effects of antimicrobial agents on the functions of these cells [1]. A key step in phagocyte-mediated destruction of pathogens, referred to as the oxidative burst [2], lies in the ability of phagocytes to generate reactive oxygen species.

We present a brief overview of the published data concerning the interactions between antimicrobial agents—true antibiotics, synthetic antibacterial agents, antifungal and antiparasitic drugs—and the phagocyte oxidative burst. These interactions may be conveniently classified into five groups: (a) direct effects of antimicrobial drugs on the oxidative burst; (b) artifactual effects by interference of drugs with detection systems (although this scavenging or quenching action may or may not exist in vivo); (c) indirect effects via alterations of bacteria, leading to modifications of susceptibility to (and/or stimulation of) oxidant-generating systems; (d) synergy (or antagonism?) occurring between reactive oxygen species and antimicrobial drugs; and (e) modification of drugs by oxidants produced by phagocytes, leading to toxicity for the host. Before presenting the relevant data, it is necessary to describe briefly the mechanisms involved in oxidant generation by phagocytes and the technical approaches used to measure the effects of drugs on this function.

The Oxidative Burst

Among the phagocytes, polymorphonuclear neutrophils (PMN) display the most outstanding ability to mount an oxidative burst. The enzyme responsible for this exists as a membrane-associated NADPH oxidase which converts

INSERM U294, CHU Xavier Bichat, 46 rue Henri Huchard, 75018 Paris, France oxygen in the extracellular medium (or in the phagocytic vacuole) into super-oxide anion (O_2^-). The enzyme is dormant in resting neutrophils but becomes activated when PMN are stimulated by soluble factors (bacteria-derived products, phorbol myristate acetate, or PMA, leukotrienes, calcium, ionophores, etc.) or opsonized and unopsonized particles (zymosan, bacteria). The molecular mechanisms of activation remain unknown, but it is clear that different pathways can be operative depending on the stimulus. They involve various second messengers among which protein kinase C (PKC), membrane phospholipases, inositol phosphates, diacyl glycerol, and intracellular calcium play a prominent role. Once O_2^- has been formed, 80% of it is dismutated to hydrogen peroxide (H_2O_2); subsequent reactions involving the azurophilic granule enzyme myeloperoxidase (MPO) lead to the formation of other toxic agents including hydrochlorous acid (HOCl) and chloramines. Other possible reactive species generated by PMN are the hydroxyl radical (OH°) and singlet oxygen ($^1O_2$). Phagocytes of the monocyte-macrophage series and polymorphonuclear eosinophils are also able to produce oxidants during phagocytosis or after exposure to certain inflammatory mediators, but this oxidative burst is far less potent than that of PMN. In particular, monocyte-derived macrophages lack MPO, and do not thus produce the ultimate oxidant species. Other factors which affect the respiratory burst in phagocytes are the following: animal species, body site of harvest, state of the cell (normal, elicited—i.e., inflammatory—or activated), nature and concentration of the stimulus.

That oxidant production is crucial for bacterial killing is supported by the clinical evidence of dramatic propensity to infections in patients with a defective phagocyte oxidative burst, particularly chronic granulomatous disease. The mechanisms underlying bacterial killing via oxidative stress are unclear. Different roles have been attributed to the various species (O_2^-, H_2O_2, HOCl and OH°), and bacterial cell targets susceptible to them may include unsaturated lipids of the membrane and outer envelope, pyridine nucleotides, sulfhydril groups, heme enzymes, and nucleic acids. It should be pointed out that reactive oxygen radicals are not only involved in killing bacteria (as well as virus-infected and tumor cells) but can also be toxic to normal cells and tissues and cause various pathological changes, sometimes resulting in refractory inflammation, autoimmunity, and malignancies. Deeper insight into the mechanisms intervening in the activation and functioning of this oxidant production by phagocytes may be obtained from a number of excellent reviews [3–5].

Methods for studying the phagocyte oxidative burst are numerous, but none fully reflects in vivo conditions. Some analyze overall oxidant production (cyanide-insensitive O_2 consumption test, luminol-amplified chemiluminescence, or CL), whereas others specifically measure one or other reactive species. The most commonly used assays for O_2^- are the nitroblue tetrazolium reduction test (although the specificity of this technique has been questioned), the superoxide dismutase inhibitable reduction of cytochrome C, and lucigenine-amplified CL; for H_2O_2, the most common methods are the oxidation scopoletin in the presence of peroxidase and the generation of oxygen by catalase; the iodination assay is used for the MPO-H$_2$O$_2$-halide system. More sophisticated techniques involve the use of fluorescence-activated cell sorters, electron spin resonance, and gas chromatography.

Direct Effects of Antimicrobial Drugs on the Phagocyte Oxidative Burst

A critical review of the relevant data reveals a large degree of controversy, something common to the analysis of all drug–phagocyte interactions. Many of these conflicting results stem from the use of various techniques, incubation times and stimuli, the nature of the phagocyte, the drug concentrations, and sometimes the lack of appropriate controls. When attention is focused on these different points, a clearer picture emerges; a simplified, although nonexhaustive presentation of the recognized effects of some antimicrobial agents at therapeutic concentrations on the phagocyte oxidative burst is given in Table 1. Whereas most β-lactams do not seem to alter this phagocyte function directly, two cephalosporins (cefotaxime and cefpimizole) enhance the PMN oxidative burst [6–9].Cefotaxime primes the PMN response to a second stimulation by opsonized particles only, and the presence of an acetoxy at position 3 of the cephem ring is important for this effect [10]. Cefpimizole does not stimulate

Table 1. Direct effect of antimicrobial agents on the phagocyte oxidative burst in vitro

No effect	Increase	Decrease
Most β-lactams	Cefotaxime [6, 7]	Cefotaxime [11]^a
	Cefpimizole [8, 9]	
	Clofazimine [12–15]	
Spiramycin [16]	Josamycin [16, 20, 21]	Roxithromycin [16–18]
Oleandomycin [16]		Erythromycin [19]
Clindamycin [18]		Trimethoprim [18, 22, 23]
Chloramphenicol [18, 23, 26]		Sulfamethoxazole [22, 23]
Aminoglycosides [18, 22, 23]		Dapsone [12, 24, 25]
Vancomycin [33]		Cyclines [19, 23, 26]
Teicoplanin [33]		Rifampin [11a, 27]
Metronidazole [17]		Isoniazid [30]
Quinolones [11, 26]		Fusidic acid [28]^b
Fusidic acid [28]		
Miconazole [34]		Amphotericin B [26, 34, 35]
Fluconazole [34]		Ketoconazole [35]
Chloroquine [36]		Quinine [37]
Cinchonine [37]		Mefloquine [36, 38]
Amodiaquine [36]		M-desethyl amodiaquine [39]

The reported effects include those observed at therapeutic concentrations.
^{a} This effect was observed for monocytes only.
^{b} This effect was observed for PMN only

PMN directly but induces macrophages to release a factor which, in turn, activates various PMN functions [9]. Nielsen [11] has observed a decrease in O_2^- production by monocytes stimulated by PMA after incubation with cefotaxime (> 20 mg/l), contrary to our results obtained using human PMN [6, 7].

Other antimicrobial drugs which enhance the phagocyte oxidative burst are the dihydrophenazines, particularly clofazimine [12, 13]. This antileprosy drug displays an immunosuppressive activity which has been ascribed to its pro-oxidative effect on phagocytes. The mechanism of this enhancing effect could be mediated by an activation of phospholipase A_2 [14]. Interestingly, this drug also reversed the inhibitory effect of the 25 kDa *Mycobacterium tuberculosis* glyco-protein [15]. Adverse effects of antibacterial agents on the phagocyte oxidative burst concern those observed with some macrolides, in particular roxithromycin [16–18] and erythromycin [17–19]. Although the concentrations required to induce a depressive effect appear higher than those therapeutically achievable in the serum (> 10 mg/l), they may be clinically relevant when tissue concentrations are considered. Contrary to these 14-membered ring macrolides, josamycin (a 16-membered ring macrolide) has been reported to enhance the phagocyte oxidative burst [16], which could explain the immune suppressive activity of this drug [20, 21]. The precise mechanism supporting the effects of macrolides on the oxidative response of phagocytes is unclear but likely depends upon the intracellular concentration of these drugs. Furthermore, an inter-individual sensitivity to the depressive effect of roxithromycin has been reported [16]. Similarly, clindamycin, a cell-penetrating antibiotic decreases the phago-cyte oxidative burst, but the inhibitory concentrations are higher than those therapeutically achievable [18].

Other antibacterial drugs which are reported to depress the phagocyte oxidative burst are the following: trimethoprim and sulfamethoxazole [22, 23], dapsone [12, 24, 25], cyclines [19, 23, 26] and rifampin [11, 27]. Fusidic acid has been shown to depress PMN but not monocyte superoxide response [28] whereas it does not alter PMN-CL [28, 29]. Other examples of discrepancies between the results obtained with different techniques are found with erythro-mycin and isoniazid. Erythromycin does not modify the PMN-CL response or O_2^- production at concentrations below 100 mg/l [16, 19], whereas it does induce a dose-dependent inhibition of $OH°$ and H_2O_2 generation [19]. Similarly, isoniazid does not modify PMN-CL but significantly decreases the MPO-mediated iodination reaction [27]; this may be related to the irreversible inhibition of MPO by this drug resulting from heme loss and the formation of compound III [30]. This is likely related to its antimycobacterial activity, which relies mainly on its oxidative metabolism by mycobacterial peroxidases.

For all the agents mentioned above, the mechanisms of inhibition are largely unknown, with the exception of the cyclines whose depressive effects have been related to chelation of Ca^{2+} and Mg^{2+}, both cations involved in many cellular functions. Another mechanism suggested for cycline-induced inhibition is the likely production of $^1O_2$ by these drugs under light excitation which secondarily induces phagocyte self-damage [31, 32]. Aminoglycosides, polymyxin, chloramphenicol, metronidazole, teicoplanin, vancomycin and quinolones do not induce modifications of the phagocyte oxidative burst at therapeutic concentrations [17, 18, 22, 23, 26, 33]. Among the antifungal agents, there is agreement on a depressive but reversible effect of therapeutic concentrations of amphotericin B [26, 34, 35] and ketoconazole [35]. Lastly, antimalarial drugs generally impair human phagocyte responses although these effects appear at high (clinically irrelevant) concentrations except for mefloquine, quinine, and the amodiaquine metabolite monodesethyl amodiaquine [36–39]. Various mechanisms are involved, including cellular uptake with subsequent phagolysosomal alkalinization, as well as inhibition of PKC (El Benna and Labro, submitted for publication) and irreversible alteration of proteins by reactive quinone-imine species.

The clinical relevance of the drug-induced effects reported above is difficult to ascertain. Interindividual variability in sensitivity to drugs, sometimes reported in vitro, may be further amplified in vivo, particularly with regard to the functional status of phagocytes which largely depends on pathological conditions. For instance, some cephalosporins which do not modify the oxidative burst in vitro may restore this function when it is depressed. This has been observed for cefaclor in infected patients with an underlying MPO deficiency [40] and for cefodizime in chronic hemodialysis patients with impaired whole-blood chemiluminescence [41]. In accordance with the invitro data, cefpimizole increased PMN-CL ex vivo as well as superoxide anion production in healthy elderly volunteers and cancer patients [42]. Tetracyclines and erythromycin, which are reported to depress the phagocyte oxidative burst in vitro, also display anti-inflammatory properties in vivo [43, 44]. It is more difficult to explain the ex vivo effects of roxithromycin, which depresses oxidant production by PMN in vitro; 90 min after the ingestion of a single 300-mg dose the oxidative burst of PMN from six healthy volunteers was increased [45]. The overall invivo effect of any drug on phagocytes must take into account the possibility that other immune mediators may be responsible for the modifications observed ex vivo. Other possibilities explaining controversies between in vitro and ex vivo data may involve the removal of drugs during cell separation when the inhibition is reversible. This might explain the failure of Anderson et al. [46] to demonstrate an abnormal respiratory burst in PMN isolated from patients having ingested cotrimoxazole.

Artifactual Interference of Antimicrobial Drugs with Tests Used To Measure Phagocyte Oxidative Burst

The modification of oxidant production by phagocytes in the presence of antimicrobial agents in vitro may not always be ascribed to a direct effect of the drug on cell metabolism. Appropriate controls using cell-free oxidant-generating systems are required to exclude interference with the drug in the detection method. Various authors have found that due to its light-absorbing property, rifampin alters CL measurements [23, 27], and that O_2^{-} quenching by this drug could also result in an apparent decrease in O_2^{-} production by phagocytes [47]. Similarly, Briheim and Dählgren [48] reported that both penicillin G and ampicillin inhibited PMN-CL, whereas chloramphenicol increased it; however, these effects were also observed in cell-free systems. Recently, ampicillin has been shown to serve as an electron donor and/or superoxide generator, resulting in increased reduction of cytochrome C [49]. We have observed a similar effect on direct cytochrome C reduction by amodiaquine and its metabolite monodesethyl amodiaquine (manuscript in preparation), in agreement with the reported effects of quinones. These "artifactual" effects may have biological significance since reactive oxygen species participate in bacterial killing and tissue destruction. Quenching by a drug would thus result in decreased bactericidal function, whereas generation of oxidants could amplify tissue damage. Interestingly, Halliwell and Wasil [50] recently proposed that decreased collagenase activity, a beneficial effect of tetracyclines in patients with rheumatoid diseases, could be related to their powerful scavenging of HOCl, an activator of latent collagenase activity.

Consequences of Bacterial Alterations by Antimicrobial Agents on the Phagocyte Oxidative Burst

Numerous data refer to increased bacterial susceptibility to phagocyte killing after their exposure to subinhibitory concentrations of antibiotics. However, the underlying mechanisms are less clear. Most studies concerning the effect of β-lactams on sensitive bacterial strains show an increased susceptibility to nonoxidative killing [51, 52]. In contrast, Ono et al. [53] observed that pretreatment of *Klebsiella pneumoniae* by cefodizime or cefpimizole increased their susceptibility to hydrogen peroxide. Furthermore, these drug-altered pathogens had stronger stimulatory effect on the CL of PMN from healthy volunteers and patients with bacterial infections or lung cancer [54]. We observed similar modifications of sensitivity to O_2^{-}-dependent killing when *Pseudomonas aeruginosa* was exposed for 18 h to ceftriaxone (an antibiotic not active on this species) [55]; furthermore, the altered bacteria stimulated PMN-CL better than controls. This increased stimulating activity of antibiotic-treated *P. aeruginosa* was also obtained when this bacterium was exposed for 18 h to other cephalosporins (whether or not active on this species) and appeared to be mediated by alterations of the cell wall, particularly bacterial lectins, neo-antigens, and increased number of complement-binding sites [56]. In contrast, Ginsburg et al. [57] reported that *Staphylococcus aureus* and group A streptococci cultivated in the presence of penicillin below minimal inhibitory concentration (MIC) G and opsonized by various cationic and anionic agents, induced much lower PMN-Cl and O_2^{-} production than controls. The stimulating effect of antibiotic-treated bacteria on the phagocyte oxidative burst has also been observed with macrolide-altered *Haemophilus influenzae* [58] and quinolone-altered *S. aureus* [59]. We have analyzed the susceptibility of quinolone-treated *P. aeruginosa*; unexpectedly, bacteria surviving an overnight's exposure to sub-MIC ciprofloxacin, ofloxacin, and pefloxacin displayed an increased resistance to acellular oxidant-generating systems; this suggests that one of the bactericidal mechanisms of these molecules is related to oxidant-stress production [60].

Synergistic Interactions Between Antimicrobial Agents and the Phagocyte Oxidative Burst

With regard to the intracellular bioactivity of phagocyte-penetrating antibiotics, particularly quinolones, macrolides, or rifampin, some studies suggest that the intracellular/extracellular ratio may not alone be sufficient to explain the activity of such drugs on intracellular pathogens. Among possible mechanisms, and apart from the direct drug-mediated stimulatory activity on phagocyte functions (see "Direct Effects of Antimicrobial Drugs on the Phagocyte Oxidative Burst"), it is possible that cooperation occurs between reactive oxygen species and antibacterial agents, although few data are available. Van Rensburg et al. [61] have shown that various fluoroquinolones (difloxacin, ciprofloxacin, pefloxacin, and fleroxacin) exhibit good intraphagocytic activity in normal PMN. However, their intracellular bioactivity was substantially less marked in tests with PMN from patients with chronic granulomatous disease. Similarly, intracellular antibacterial effect obtained with amoxycillin, clindamycin, erythromycin and roxithromycin [62, 63] was significantly decreased when PMN with defective O_2^{-}-dependent killing mechanisms were used. Recently we have found a synergistic bactericidal cooperation between, on the one hand, josamycin and, to a lesser extent, erythromycin and, on the other, an oxidant stress obtained in vitro with acellular systems (xanthine plus xanthine oxidase or H_2O_2) [64]. This synergy was observed when *S. aureus* (a strain sensitive to macrolides) was the bacterial target but not with *P. aeruginosa* (a resistant strain). The phenomenon is poorly understood but could be due to chemical modifications of the unsaturated lactone rings. No such bactericidal synergy has been reported for rifampin, a drug effective against intracellular *S. aureus* phagocytosed by PMN from patients with chronic granulomatous disease [47].

Other data concerning possible cooperation between oxidant species and antimicrobial agents were recently presented by Malhotra et al. [65] who examined the potential interactions between antimalarial drugs (chloroquine, quinine and mefloquine) and oxygen-reactive species. Chloroquine and quinine (but not mefloquine) activity against *Plasmodium falciparum* was potentiated by the peroxidase–hydrogen peroxide system. The mechanism of this synergy was not explained.

Oxidant-Mediated Transformation of Antimicrobial Agents into Host-Toxic Species

While modifications of antimicrobial drugs by oxidant-producing phagocytes may result in increased antimicrobial activity (see "Consequences of Bacterial Alterations by Antimicrobial Agents on the Phagocyte Oxidative Burst"), the other side of the coin is the possible generation of molecules with increased toxicity for host tissues. Such effects are not generally mentioned in reviews of phagocyte–drug interactions, although they are of major therapeutic interest. Among these "negative" interactions, is the recently reported peroxidase-dependent oxidation of sulfonamides by monocytes and PMN from humans and dogs [66]. Adverse reactions to sulfonamides, with serious idiosyncratic reactions, are a major therapeutic problem; this toxicity appears to be mediated by N_4-oxidation of sulfonamides into the hydroxylamine and nitroso-metabolites. The liver is traditionally considered to be major source of reactive intermediates, but the study by Cribb et al. [66] suggests that phagocytes could be direct effectors of the formation of these toxic derivatives. This would explain, in particular, drug-induced agranulocytosis and generalized hypersensitivity syndromes. Similar mechanisms have been suggested for the toxicity of the arylamine dapsone [67] and are probably involved in that of amodiaquine [68, 69] and chloramphenicol [70].

Conclusion

In this short review, it emerges clearly that interactions between antimicrobial drugs and the phagocyte oxidative burst are multifaceted. Indeed, the optimal conditions for improving antibacterial therapy are far from evident. Direct or indirect stimulation of oxidant production by phagocytes, while increasing bacterial eradication, may also lead to undesirable side effects. Invitro artifacts complicate the analysis of drug-induced alterations of oxidant production, raising questions as to their role as scavengers or amplifiers of such reactions in vivo. Modifications of drugs under the influence of oxidants may result in bactericidal synergy or, alternatively, toxicity for the host. We have restricted this review to one of the multiple activities of phagocytes. The effects of drugs on oxidative metabolism in these cells should, however, be considered in the light of overall functions (i.e., chemotaxis, phagocytosis, O_2^--independent killing mechanisms, perhaps nitric oxide production, and numerous regulatory activities).

From an even wider approach, phagocyte activities must also be seen within the complex panorama of immune phenomena, including neuro-endocrine and chronobiologic regulation. When all these points are taken into account, it is clear that models suitable for studying phagocyte-drug interactions are lacking. Cooperation between scientists from all fields (chemistry, biochemistry, immunology, bacteriology, and medicine) is essential for piecing together the jig-saw puzzle of reactions occurring during infectious diseases and evolving new strategies in antimicrobial therapy for the future.

Acknowledgement We thank Miss F. Breton for her expert secretarial assistance. The authors regret not being able to cite all the excellent relevant work published to date.

References

1. Van den Broek PJ (1989) Antimicrobial drugs, microorganisms and phagocytes. Rev Infect Dis 11:213–245
2. Baldridge CW, Gerard RW (1933) The extra respiration of phagocytosis. Am J Physiol 193:235–236
3. Beaman L, Beaman BL (1984) The role of oxygen and its derivatives in microbial pathogenesis and host defense. Annu Rev Microbiol 38:27–48
4. Clark RA (1990) The human neutrophil respiratory burst oxidase. J Infect Dis 161:1140–1147
5. Babior BM (1978) Oxygen-dependent microbial killing by phagocytes. N Engl J Med 298:659–668; 721–725
6. Labro MT, Babin-Chevaye C, Hakim J (1986) Effects of cefotaxime and cefodizime on human granulocyte functions in vitro. J Antimicrob Chemother 18:233–237
7. Labro MT, Amit N, Babin-Chevaye C, Hakim J (1987) Cefodizime (HR221) potentiation of human neutrophil oxygen-independent bactericidal activity. J Antimicrob Chemother 19:331–341
8. Ohnishi H, Kosuzume H, Inaba H et al. (1983) Effects of AC-1370, a new semi-synthetic cephalosporin, on phagocyte functions. Antimicrob Agents Chemother 23:874–880
9. Ohnishi H, Inaba H, Mochizuki H, Kosuzume H (1984) Mechanism of action of AC-1370 on phagocyte functions. Antimicrob Agents Chemother 25:88–92
10. Labro MT, Bryskier A (1987) Interaction of cefotaxime versus desacetyl cefotaxime on human neutrophil functions. Chemioterapia 2 [Suppl]:234–236
11. Nielsen H (1989) Antibiotics and human monocyte function. II. Phagocytosis and oxidative metabolism. APMIS 97:447–451
12. Van Rensburg CEJ, Gatner EMS, Imkamp FMJH, Anderson R (1982) Enhancement by clofazimine and inhibition by dapsone of production of prostaglandin E2 by human polymorphonuclear leukocytes in vitro. Antimicrob Agents Chemother 21:693–697
13. Savage JE, O'Sullivan JF, Zuis BM, Anderson R (1989) Investigation of the structural properties of dihydrophenazines which contribute to their pro-oxidative interactions with human phagocytes. J Antimicrob Chemother 23:691–700
14. Anderson R, Beyers AD, Savage JE, Nel AE (1988) Apparent involvement of phospholipase A2 but not protein kinase C in the pro-oxidative interactions with human phagocytes. Biochem Pharmacol 37:3635–3641
15. Wadee AA, Anderson R, Rabson AR (1988) Clofazimine reverses the inhibitory effect of *Mycobacterium tuberculosis*-derived factors on phagocyte intracellular killing mechanisms. J Antimicrob Chemother 21:65–74
16. Labro MT, El Benna J, Babin-Chevaye C (1989) Comparison of the in-vitro effects of several macrolides on the oxidative burst of human neutrophils. J Antimicro Chemother 24:561–572
17. Anderson R (1989) Erythromycin and roxithromycin potentiate human neutrophil locomotion in vitro by inhibition of leukoattractant-derived superoxide generation and autooxidation. J Infect Dis 159:966–973

18. Hand WL, Hand DL, King-Thompson NL (1990) Antibiotic inhibition of the respiratory burst response in human polymorphonuclear leukocytes. Antimicrob Agents Chemother 34:863–870
19. Miyachi Y, Yoshioka A, Imamura S, Niwa Y (1986) Effects of antibiotics on the generation of reactive oxygen species. J Invest Dermatol 4:449–453
20. Villa ML, Valenti F, Mantovani M, Scaglione F, Clerici E (1988) Macrolidic antibiotics: effects on primary in vitro antibody responses. Int J Immunopharmacol 10:919–924
21. Villa ML, Valenti G, Scaglione F, Falchi M, Fraschini F (1989) In-vivo and in-vitro interference of antibiotics with antigen-specific antibody responses: effect of josamycin. J Antimicrob Chemother 24:765–774
22. Ono Y, Kunii O (1989) Influence of forty-two antimicrobial agents on the chemiluminescence response of human phagocytic cells. Chemotherapy (Tokyo) 37:583–589
23. Siegel JP, Remington JS (1982) Effect of antimicrobial agents on chemiluminescence of human polymorphonuclear leukocytes in response to phagocytosis J Antimicrob Chemother 10:505–515
24. Webster GF, Alexander JC, Mc Carthur WP, Leyden JJ (1984) Inhibition of chemiluminescence in human neutrophils by dapsone. Br J Dermatol 110:657–663
25. Stendahl O, Molin L, Dahlgren C (1978) The inhibition of polymorphonuclear leukocyte toxicity by dapsone. J Clin Invest 62:214–220
26. Duncker D, Ullmann V (1986) Influence of various antimicrobial agents on the chemilumescence of phagocytosing human granulocytes. Chemotherapy 32:18–24
27. Zeis BM (1988) Antimycobacterial drugs and the production of reactive oxidants by polymorphonuclear leukocytes in vitro. Chemotherapy 34:56–60
28. Kharazmi A, Nielsen H (1988) Fusidic acid and human phagocyte function. J Antimicrob Chemother 22:262–263
29. Naess A, Flo RW, Solberg CO (1990) Effect of fusidic acid on migration and chemiluminescence of polymorphonuclear leukocytes. Eur J Clin Microbiol Infect Dis 1:42–44
30. Van Zyl JM, Basson K, Uebel RA, van der Walt BJ (1989) Isoniazid-mediated irreversible inhibition of the myeloperoxidase antimicrobial system of the human neutrophil and the effect of thyronines. Biochem Pharmacol 38:2363–2373
31. Glette J,Sandberg S, Haneberg B, Solberg MO (1984) Effect of tetracyclines and UV light on oxygen consumption by human leukocytes. Antimicrob Agents Chemother 26:489–492
32. Glette J, Sandberg S, Hopen G, Solberg CO (1984) Influence of tetracyclines on human polymorphonuclear leukocyte function. Antimicrob Agents Chemother 25:354–357
33. Van der Auwera P, Petrikkos G, Husson M, Klastersky J (1986) Influence of various antibiotics on superoxide generation by normal human neutrophils. Arch Int Physical Biochim 94:S23–S28
34. Roilides E, Walsh TJ, Rubin M, Venzon D, Pizzo PA (1990) Effects of antifungal agents on the function of human neutrophils in vitro. Antimicrob Agents Chemother 34:196–201
35. Abruzzo GK, Gillinan DM, Capizzi TP, Fromtling RA (1986) Influence of six antifungal agents on the chemiluminescence response of mouse spleen cells. Antimicrob Agents Chemother 29:602–607
36. Labro MT, Babin-Chevaye C (1988) Effects of amodiaquine, chloroquine and mefloquine on human polymorphonuclear neutrophil functions in vitro. Antimicrob Agents Chemother 32:1124–1130
37. El Benna J, Labro MT (1990) Effect of quinine and cinchonine on human neutrophil functions in vitro. J Antimicrob Chemother 25:949–957
38. Ferrante A, Rowan-Kelly B, Seow WK, Thong YH (1986) Depression of human polymorphonuclear leucocyte function by antimalarial drugs. Immunology 58:125–130
39. Labro MT, El Benna J (1991) Effect of monodesethyl amodiaquine on human polymorphonuclear neutrophil functions in vitro. Antimicrob Agents Chemother 35:824–830
40. Grant M, Raeburn JA, Sutherland R, Harkness RA, Gormley IP, Kowolik MJ (1983) Effect of two antibiotics on human granulocyte activities. J Antimicrob Chemother 11:543–554
41. Vanholder R, van Landschoot N, Dagrosa E, Ringoir S (1988) Cefodizime: a new cephalosporin with apparent immune-stimulating properties in chronic renal failure. Nephrol Dial Transplant 2:221–224
42. Yagita A, Oda T, Tatekawa I et al. (1989) The influence of cefpimizole or latamoxef treatment on human neutrophil functions in cancer patients. Chemotherapy (Tokyo):1282–1289
43. Dalziel K, Dykes PJ, Marks R (1987) The effect of tetracycline and erythromycin in a model of acne-type inflammation. Br J Exp Pathol 68:67–70
44. Plewig G, Schöpf E (1976) Anti-inflammatory effects of antimicrobial agents. Drugs 11:472–473

45. Labro MT, Bryskier A, Babin-Chevaye C, Hakim J (1988) Interaction de la roxithromycine avec le polynucléaire neutrophile humain in vitro et ex vivo. Pathol Biol 36:711–714
46. Anderson R, Grabow G, Oosthuysen R, Theron A, van Rensburg AJ (1980) Effects of sulfamethoxazole and trimethoprim on human neutrophil and lymphocyte functions: in vivo effects of cotrimoxazole. Antimicrob Agents Chemother 17:322–326
47. Höger PH, Vosbeck K, Seger R, Hitzig WH (1985) Uptake, intracellular activity and influence of rifampin on normal function of polymorphonuclear leukocytes. Antimicrob Agents Chemother 28:667–674
48. Briheim G, Dahlgren C (1987) Influence of antibiotics on formylmethionyl-leucyl-phenyl-alanine-induced leukocyte chemiluminescence. Antimicrob Agents Chemother 31:763–767
49. Umeki S (1990) Ampicillin serves as an electron donor. Int J Biochem 22:1291–1293
50. Halliwel B, Wasil M (1988) Tetracyclines as antioxidants in rheumatoid arthritis: scavenging of hypochlorous acid. J Rheumatol 15:530
51. Labro MT, Pochet I, Babin-Chevaye C, Hakim J (1987) Effect of ceftriaxone-induced alterations of bacteria on neutrophil bactericidal function. J Antimicrob Chemother 20:857–869
52. Root RK (1981) Antibacterial properties of polymorphonuclear leukocytes and their inter-actions with antibiotics. In: Schlesinger D (ed) Microbiology ASM, Washington DC pp176–180
53. Ono Y, Ueda Y, Baba M, Nishiya H, Kunii O (1989) Influence of a subinhibitory concentration of antibiotics on opsono-phagocytic functions of Klebsiella pneumoniae by human phagocytes. Chemotherapy (Tokyo) 37:1487–1490
54. Ono Y, Ueda Y, Baba M, Nozue N et al. (1988) Effect of cefodizime (THR-221) on the function of human phagocytic cells. Chemotherapy (Tokyo) 36:140–148
55. Labro MT, Babin-Chevaye C, Hakim J (1988) Influence of subinhibitory concentrations of ceftriaxone on opsonization and killing of Pseudomonas aeruginosa by human neutrophils. J Antimicrob Chemother 22:341–352
56. Labro MT, El Benna J (1990) Comparison of cefodizime with various cephalosporins for their indirect effect on human neutrophil oxidative burst in vitro. J Antimicrob Chemother 26 [Suppl C]: 49–57
57. Ginsburg I, Borinski R, Sadovnik M, Shauli S, Wecke J, Giesbrecht P, Lahav M (1985) Antibiotics and polyelectrolytes modulate bacteriolysis and the capacity of bacteria to trigger an oxygen burst in neutrophils. In: Adam D, Hahn H, Opfenkuch W (eds) The influence of antibiotics on the host-parasite relationship II. Springer, Berlin Heidelberg New York, pp 141–151
58. Bonnet M, Duchateau V, Vandermies A, Husson W, van der Auwera P (1990) Chemilumines-cence and degranulation of human neutrophils by H. influenzae preincubated with sub-MIC erythromycin (E), roxithromycin (R), clarithromycin (C) and azithromycin (A). Proceedings of the ICAAC. Atlanta abstract 166
59. Roszkowski R, Ciborowski W, Ko HL, Schumacher-Perdreau F et al. (1985) The effect of subinhibitory concentrations of selected antibiotics on bacteria-phagocyte interaction. In: Adam D, Hahn H, Opferkuch W (eds) The influence of antibiotics on the host-parasite relationship II. Springer, Berlin Heidelberg New York, pp 179–187
60. Labro MT, Bryskier A, Babin-Chevaye C, Hakim J (1989) Pseudomonas aeruginosa: alterations induced by low concentrations of 4-quinolones. In: Gillissen G, Opferkuch W, Peters G, Pulverer G (eds) The influence of antibiotics on the host-parasite relationship III. Springer, Berlin Heidelberg New York, pp 26–37
61. Van Rensburg CEJ, Joone G, Anderson R (1990) Interactions of the oxygen-dependent antimicrobial system of the human neutrophil with difloxacin, ciprofloxacin, pefloxacin and fleroxacin in the intraphagocytic eradication of Staphylococcus aureus. J Med Microbiol 32:15–17
62. Anderson T, Joone G, van Rensburg CEJ (1986) An in-vitro investigation of the intracellular bioactivity of amoxycillin, clindamycin and erythromycin for Staphylococcus aureus. J Infect Dis 153:593–600
63. Anderson T, van Rensburg CEJ, Joone G, Lukey PT (1987) An in-vitro comparison of the intraphagocytic bioactivity of erythromycin and roxithromycin. J Antimicrob Chemother 20 [Suppl B]: 57–68
64. Labro MT, El Benna J (1990) Synergistic bactericidal interaction of josamycin with human neutrophils in vitro. J Antimicrob Chemother 26:515–524
65. Malhotra K, Salmon D, Le Bras J, Vilde JL (1990) Potentiation of chloroquine activity against Plasmodium falciparum by the peroxidase-hydrogen peroxide system. Antimicrob Agents Chemother 34:1981–1985

66. Cribb A, Miller M, Tesori A, Spielberg SP (1990) Peroxidase-dependent oxidation of sulfonamides by monocytes and neutrophils from human and dogs. Mol Pharmacol 38:744–751
67. Weetman RM, Boxer LA, Brown MP, Mantich NM, Baehner RL (1980) In vitro inhibition of granulopoiesis by 4-amino-4'-hydroxylamino-diphenyl sulfone. Br J Haematol 45:361–370
68. Christie G, Breckenridge AM, Park BK (1989) Drug-protein conjugates. XVIII. Detection of antibodies towards the antimalarial amodiaquine and its quinone imine metabolite in man and the rat. Biochem Pharmacol 38:1451–1458
69. Maggs JL, Tingle MD, Kitteringham NR, Park BK (1988) Drug-protein conjugates. XIV. Mechanisms of formation of protein-arylating intermediates from amodiaquine, a myelotoxin and hepatotoxin in man. Biochem Pharmacol 37:303–311
70. Teo S, Pohl L, Halpert J (1986) Production of superoxide anion radicals during the oxidative metabolism of amino-chloramphenicol. Biochem Pharmacol 35:4584–4586

Intraphagocytic Cell Penetration and Intracellular Bioactivity of Antibiotics

A. Pascual

The possibility that some antimicrobials may penetrate into phagocytic cells is of potential interest in determining the fate of organisms known to survive intracellularly. Among them we can include: *Salmonella spp*, *Brucella spp*, *Mycobacterium tuberculosis*, *Listeria monocytogenes*, *Legionella pneumophila*, and *Staphylococcus aureus*. This group of facultative intracellular organisms characteristically causes chronic debilitating infections, for which prolonged antimicrobial therapy is required to achieve adequate clinical control. Although it has not been clearly established whether it is the ability of these organisms to persist intracellularly that results in their chronicity, the study of antimicrobial penetration into phagocytic cells has been stimulated largely by the desire to improve therapy against these bacteria.

Basically, four different methods have been applied for measuring antimicrobial uptake by phagocytes. The radiometric assay described by Klempner and coworkers [1] is a sensitive and accurate method but requires radiolabeled antimicrobials which are expensive and sometimes difficult to obtain. Moreover, pitfalls have been described in testing drug uptake by leukocytes using radiolabeled drugs owing to radiolytic decomposition and loss of microbiologic activity [2]. Bioassay techniques are relatively insensitive, laborious, and generally inappropriate for kinetic studies [3]. High-performance liquid chromatography has also been applied to measure intracellular concentrations of antimicrobials but this method requires high extracellular concentrations, higher than the therapeutic ones, and large volumes of cells [4]. Finally, we have developed a fluorometric assay for measuring fluoroquinolone uptake by phagocytic cells. This method, based on the natural fluorescence of the quinolone nucleus is a sensitive and reproducible method [5, 6].

Regardless of the methodology and experimental conditions beta-lactams do not penetrate into phagocytes rendering cellular to extracellular concentration (C/E) ratio lower than 0.1–0.2 in different studies (Table 1). Aminoglycosides show a slightly higher penetration with C/E ratio values ranging from 0.3 to 0.7. Lincosamides and macrolide uptake by phagocytes is very high [7]. The C/E ratio goes from three for lincomycin to over 20 for clindamycin. The new macrolides, such as roxithromycin and azithromycin, show an extremely high penetration into different phagocytes offering C/E ratios greater than 30

Department of Microbiology, School of Medicine, Apdo 914, 41080 Sevilla, Spain

Host Defense Dysfunction
in Trauma, Shock and Sepsis
Eds. Faist/Meakins/Schildberg
© Springer-Verlag, Berlin Heidelberg 1993

Table 1. Beta-lactam and aminoglycoside uptake by human polymorphonuclear leukocytes

Antimicrobial	C/E[a]
Penicillin	0.01
Ampicillin	0.2
Cefazolin	0.1
Cefamandole	0.01
Ceftazidime	0.01
Imipenem	0.1–1.0
Gentamycin	0.7
Netilmicin	0.3

[a] Cellular to extracellular concentration. From different authors.

Table 2. Lincosamide and macrolide uptake by human PMN

Antimicrobials	C/E[a]
Lincomycin	3
Clindamycin	20
Erythromycin	10
Roxithromycin	30
Azithromycin	20–50

[a] Cellular to extracellular concentration. From different authors.

Table 3. Antimicrobial uptake by human phagocytes

Antimicrobial	C/E[a]
Rifampin	4–8
Chloramphenicol	4–10
Trimethroprim	6
Vancomycin	4
Teicoplanin	13–50
Pipemidic acid	5
Isoniazid	1.5
Ethambutol	2–4
Metronidazole	1

[a] Cellular to extracellular concentration. From different authors.

(Table 2) [8, 9]. Other antimicrobials that show good intraphagocytic penetration are shown in Table 3.

The new fluoroquinolones have also shown high intracellular penetration into phagocytes. As measured by fluorometry the C/E ratio values for norfloxacin ciprofloxacin, ofloxacin, and lomefloxacin were higher than four at extracellular concentrations of 2 mg/l (Fig. 1). Similar results have been observed using different methodology [4, 10]. Quinolones, as has been observed with other antimicrobials, reach high intracellular concentrations in other types of cells such as epithelial cells and fibroblasts (Table 4). This phenomenon may have some relevance to human infections produced by microorganisms that are able to survive and even multiply within epithelial cells.

It should be emphasized that the radiometric high-pressure liquid chromatography fluorometric methods measure the presence of the antimicrobial as a chemical, whereas microbiological methods measure its activity [3]. This fact may explain the discrepancy observed sometimes with the different methods. As an example, clindamycin and erythromycin showed a high penetration using a radiometric assay (C/E: 10.0 and 6.0 respectively) [1, 7] but a low one (C/E:1.0) when it was measured by microbiological assay [3].

At least four probable mechanisms for antimicrobial entry into phagocytic cells have been described. The entry of penicillin, which is limited to approximately 20% of the extracellular concentration, appears to occur during phagocytosis. When phagocytes ingest bacteria they also engulf some of the extracellular media that contain the antibiotic [11].

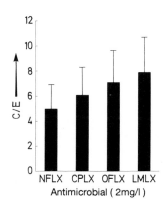

Fig. 1. Intracellular penetration of norfloxacin (*NFLX*), ciprofloxacin (*CPLX*), ofloxacin (*OFLX*), and lomefloxacin (*LMLX*) into human (*n* = 4). Extracellular concentrations: 2 mg/l. Experiments were carried out for 20 min at 37 °C.

Table 4. Penetration of different quinolones into epithelial and fibroblast culture cells

	Hep–2	McCoy	Vero
Ofloxacin	2.1 ± 0.2	3.9 ± 1.1	3.4 ± 1.2
(−) Ofloxacin	2.8 ± 0.6	4.7 ± 1.3	2.4 ± 0.6
Lomefloxacin	ND	2.0 ± 0.5	2.1 ± 0.6
Temafloxacin	ND	1.2 ± 0.3	2.7 ± 0.9

Experiments were carried out for 20 min (37 °C) at extracellular concentrations of 5 mg/l [6].
ND, not determined

Intracellular accumulation of the highly lipid-soluble antimicrobials, such as rifampin, appears to result from solubility partitioning. In fact, formalin-killed phagocytes concentrate rifampin to a similar degree as viable cells do [12].

In general, weak bases, such as macrolides, accumulate in highly acidic intracellular compartments (such as the lysosomes of phagocytic cells) and reach an equilibrium dependent upon the pH gradient between the lysosomes and the extracellular fluid. Other mechanisms, however, could also mediate the intracellular penetration of macrolides [9].

Finally, an active membrane transport system that requires cellular viability, physiological environmental temperature, metabolic energy, and the establishment of a large cellular–extracellular gradient has been described for some antimicrobials such as clindamycin and ofloxacin [1, 6, 13]. Ofloxacin uptake by human polymorphonuclear leukocytes (PMN) was significantly impaired at 4°C or when formalin-killed cells were used. In the same way, the presence of different metabolic inhibitors also impaired the penetration of this antimicrobial [6].

The aforementioned methods to evaluate the intracellular concentration of antimicrobials have an important limitation. What we are really measuring is the antimicrobial association to the phagocytes, but that does not really mean that the antimicrobial is intracellular. It could, for example, be bound to the membrane. Moreover, these studies cannot exclude the possibility that the drug may have been inactivated within the leukocyte or may have been accumulated in locations other than the lysosomes.

It is important then to complete the studies on antimicrobial penetration with studies on the intracellular activity of these antimicrobials. To evaluate it, PMNs or macrophages that contain intracellular bacteria are incubated in an antimicrobial—containing medium and the survival of intracellular bacteria is quantified.

Hand and coworkers [14] observed that a high intracellular concentration does not always mean good intracellular activity. Clindamycin and erythromycin, which achieved high cellular levels in PMN, failed to produce a significant reduction in viable intraphagocytic *S. aureus* during 3 h of antimicrobial exposure. In contrast, rifampin, which was concentrated severalfold by phagocytes, was able to kill intracellular staphylococci. Gentamicin and penicillin G penetrated rather poorly. However, while gentamicin demonstrated efficient intraphagocytic killing of bacteria penicillin had no intracellular effect against *S. aureus*.

Another example is teicoplanin. We observed a high intracellular penetration of teicoplanin (C/E > 40), reaching C/E ratios greater than 50 in both PMNs and peritoneal macrophages. Teicoplanin, however, failed to reduce the intracellular survival of *staphylococcus epidermidis* in a 3-h assay at a concentration of 1 × minimal inhibitory concentration (MIC). These observations show that the ability to enter phagocytes is only one of the factors which determines the intracellular antibacterial activity of an anitmicrobial [15].

In general, it can be said that beta-lactams have no intracellular activity (Table 5). Aminoglycosides that penetrate poorly have sometimes shown some

Table 5. Correlation between intraphagocytic penetration and activity of antimicrobials: general guidelines

Antimicrobial	Penetration	Activity
Beta-lactam	None	0
Aminoglycosides	Low	0/ +
Lincosamides	High	0/ + / + +
Macrolides	High	0/ + / + +
Rifampin	High	+ + +
Quinolones	High	+ +

intracellular activity. Lincosamides and macrolides are a bit controversial in the sense that in following extensive studies against different bacteria they have shown good activity on occasions, although this is not always the case.

Rifampin always offers a good intracellular activity and something similar occurs with the fluoroquinolones. In different studies, ciprofloxacin, enoxacin, norfloxacin, and ofloxacin have shown a good intracellular activity against different bacteria. In our experience, ofloxacin and ciprofloxacin, even at concentrations as low as $1 \times \text{MIC}$, significantly reduced the intracellular survival of *S. aureus* in a 3-h assay [16].

The clinical implications of antimicrobial entry into phagocytic cells must be viewed with great caution. Although in vitro studies have demonstrated that antimicrobials which enter phagocytes are better able to kill intracellular bacteria, substantial clinical experience has demonstrated the efficacy of antimicrobials that are excluded from these cells. For example, penicillinase-resistant penicillins are excluded from phagocytes and yet they are highly effective antimicrobials for the treatment of most *S. aureus* infections. Similarly, although ampicillin and gentamicin do not erradicate *E. coli* contained within macrophages in vitro, they are clearly effective antimicrobials for the treatment of infections due to *E. coli*. There is similar disparity between the failure of antimicrobials to penetrate phagocytes in vitro and their clinical usefulness against infections with such facultative intracellular bacteria as *Listeria* and *Legionella* species and mycobacteria.

Nevertheless, there may be specific circumstances in which antimicrobials that gain access to and kill intracellularly persisting bacteria play a role in determining the outcome of infections. The addition of rifampin to oxacillin or vancomycin may improve the clinical outcome in patients with severe staphylococcal infections. However, there is a need for controlled, double-blind studies to investigate this important question.

References

1. Klempner MS, Stirt B (1981) Clindamycin uptake by human neutrophils. J Infect Dis 144:472–475
2. Maderazo EG, Kripas CJ, Breaux SP, Woronick CL, Moore R (1989) Pitfalls in testing drug

uptake by leukocytes using radiolabeled drugs and an explanation of conflicting results with clindamycin. Chemotherapy 35:123–129

3. Van der Auwera T, Matsumoto T, Husson M (1988) Intraphagocytic penetration of antibiotics. J Antimicrob Chemother 22:185–192

4. Koga H (1987) High performance liquid chromatography measurement of antimicrobial concentrations in polymorphonuclear leukocytes. Antimicrob Agents Chemother 31:1904–1908

5. Pascual A, Garcia I, Perea EJ (1989) Fluorometric measurement of ofloxacin uptake by human polymorphonuclear leukocytes. Antimicrob Agents Chemother 33:653–656

6. Pascual A, Garcia I, Perea EJ (1990) Uptake and intracellular activity of an optically active ofloxacin isomer in human neutrophils and tissue culture cells. Antimicrob Agents Chemother 34:277–280

7. Hand WL (1988) Antibiotics and phagocytic cells. Antimicrob News lett 5:53–58

8. Hand WL, King-Thompson N, Holman JW (1987) Entry of roxithromycin (RU 965), imipenem, cefotaxime, trimethoprim and metronidazole into human polymorphonuclear leukocytes. Antimicrob Agents Chemother 31:1553–1557

9. Hand WL (1990) Uptake of antibiotics by human polymorphonuclear leukocyte cytoplasts. Antimicrob Agents Chemother 34:1189–1193

10. Zweerink MM, Edison AM (1988) The uptake of ^{3}H-norfloxacin by human polymorphonuclear leukocytes. J Antimicrob Chemother 21:266–267

11. Veale DR, Finch H, Smith H (1976) Penetration of penicillin into human phagocytes containing Neisseria gonorrhoeae. J Gen Microbiol 95:353–363

12. Höger PH, Vosbeck K, Seger R, Hitzig WH (1985) Uptake, intracellular activity and influence of rifampin on normal function of polymorphonuclear leukocytes. Antimicrob Agents Chemother 28:667–674

13. Hand WL, King-Thompson NL (1982) Membrane transport of clindamycin in alveolar macrophages. Antimicrob Agents Chemother 21:241–247

14. Hand WL, King-Thompson NL (1986) Contrast between phagocyte antibiotic uptake and subsequent intracellular bacterticidal activity. Antimicrob Agents Chemother 29:135–140

15. Pascual A, Tsukayama D, Kovarik J, Gekker G, Peterson PK (1987) Uptake and activity of rifapentine in human peritoneal macrophages and polymorphonuclear leukocytes. Eur J Clin Microbiol 6:152–157

16. Pascual A, Martinez Martinez L, Perea EJ (1989) Effect of ciprofloxacin and olfoxacin on human polymorphonuclear leukocyte activity against staphylococci. Chemotherapy 35:17–22

Extraphagocytic Killing
of Bacteria in the Presence of Antibiotics

P. J. van den Broek

Introduction

The antibacterial activity of antimicrobial drugs can be modulated by phagocytes in many ways [1]. This review focuses on how phagocytes influence the effect of antimicrobial drugs on nonphagocytized bacteria. Several mechanisms could be responsible for the influence of granulocytes or mononuclear phagocytes on the antibacterial effect of antibiotics on extracellular bacteria.

Phagocytes have two means of killing bacteria, the oxidative and the nonoxidative killing mechanisms. During phagocytosis of bacteria, the oxygen-dependent microbicidal system generates superoxide anions and hydrogen peroxide. More powerful microbicidal substances are formed from hydrogen peroxide and halide ions by the action of myeloperoxidase released from the lysosomes into the phagosomes. Stimulation of the cells is necessary for the production of oxidative microbicidal substances. Therefore, the effect of antibiotics on nonphagocytized bacteria is influenced only by the oxidative killing mechanism if the phagocytes are stimulated in some way. The non oxidative killing mechanism might modify antibiotic activity by the secretion of bactericidal substances by the cells. Phagocytes are known to release bactericidal substances from their lysosomes during phagocytosis. The synthesis and secretion of some of the lysosomal enzymes, for example, lysozyme, by mononuclear phagocytes is not dependent on external stimulation of the cells [2]. The microbicidal contents of the cells also reach the environment when the cells die and undergo lysis. Another way in which phagocytes might influence the activity of antibiotics is by lowering the pH of the environment. The pH has a profound influence on the activity of several antibiotics. β-Lactam antibiotics inhibit the growth of many bacteria at a pH below 6.5, but lysis does not occur at higher pH values. This phenomenon is called pH-dependent tolerance and can be abolished by cellular enzymes such as lysozyme [3]. The antibacterial activity of aminoglycosides is also pH dependent: the lower the pH, the less active the antibiotic.

University Hospital Leiden, Department of Infectious Diseases, P. O. Box 9600, 2300 RC Leiden, The Netherlands

Host Defense Dysfunction
in Trauma, Shock and Sepsis
Eds. Faist/Meakins/Schildberg
© Springer-Verlag, Berlin Heidelberg 1993

Extraphagocytic Killing of Bacteria by Antibiotics

For experimental data relevant to the influence of phagocytes on the antibacterial activity of antimicrobial drugs against extracellular bacteria, four types of experiments can be considered (Fig. 1A). Incubation of bacteria pretreated with antibiotics in the presence of phagocytes and serum results in phagocytosis and killing of the bacteria (Fig. 1A). The decrease in the number of viable bacteria is a measure of the combined activity of cells and antibiotic. Many species of bacteria pretreated with often subinhibitory concentrations of penicillins, cephalosporins, aminoglycosides, erythromycin, vancomycin, clindamycin, or lincomycin are killed more effectively by granulocytes, and the same has been shown for killing by mononuclear phagocytes after pretreatment with chloramphenicol erythromycin, rifampicin, or clindamycin (for review of literature see [1].

Another type of experiment in which the combined activity of phagocytes and antibiotic is determined is the simultaneous incubation of cells, bacteria, antibiotic, and serum (Fig. 1B). Impaired antibacterial activity of benzylpenicillin and vancomycin and unaltered activity of teicoplanin against *Staphylococcus aureus* was shown in the presence of serum and human monocytes [4]. A possible explanation for the negative effect on the antibacterial activity of antibiotics is the fact that serum induces phagocytosis and immediate killing of a large number of staphylococci by phagocytosis, whereas it takes some time before any effect of the antibiotics is seen. This means that fewer bacteria are left over for the antibiotic, which therefore contributes less to the total antibacterial effect. Increased phagocytosis and killing of *Escherichia coli* by peritoneal macrophages has been described in the presence of concentrations of streptomycin or polymyxin B below the minimal inhibitory concentration [5]. It is possible that in the experiments discussed above, the cells exert an extracellular effect on the killing of bacteria, but it is impossible to separate the extracellular and intracellular effects on bacteria.

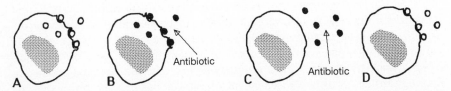

Fig. 1A-D. Four experimental conditions under which phagocytes might influence the extracellular killing of bacteria by antimicrobial drugs. **A** Antibiotic pretreated bacteria (○) are incubated in the presence of phagocytes and serum; the bacteria are phagocytized and killed by the cells. **B** Phagocytes, bacteria (●) and antibiotic are incubated together in the presence of serum, which induces phagocytosis and killing of bacteria by the phagocytes. **C** Phagocytes, bacteria, and antibiotic are incubated in the absence of serum; the cells do not phagocytose and kill the bacteria. **D** Antibiotic-pretreated bacteria are incubated in the presence of cytochalasin B-treated cells and serum; the bacteria attach to the plasma membrane of the cells but are not ingested.

Table 1. Antibacterial effect of antibiotics against extracellular *S. aureus* in the presence of granulocytes or monocytes

	Antibacterial effect after 3h of incubation		
	No cells	Granulocytes	Monocytes
Benzylpenicillin (0.1 mg/1)	0.59 ± 0.07	1.50 ± 0.22	1.72 ± 0.26
Vancomycin (0.5 mg/1)	0.41 ± 0.06	0.74 ± 0.10	0.95 ± 0.11
Teicoplanin (0.1 mg/1)	0.31 ± 0.10	ND	1.08 ± 0.15
Phosphonomycin (1 mg/1)	0.83 ± 0..23	1.39 ± 0.15	1.09 ± 0.30

The antibacterial effect is expressed as the logarithim of the ratio of the number of bacteria in the absence of antibiotic to that in the presence of antibiotic. The means and standard deviations of at least three experiments each are given.

To obtain information about extracellular killing, the results of experiments designed according to model C or D can be used (Fig. 1). Unlike the experiments of type A and B, these experiments do not reflect what happens at the site of an infection, however, they can teach us more about the mechanisms involved in the extracellular interaction between phagocytes, bacteria and antimicrobial drugs. The influence of human granulocytes or monocytes on the antibacterial activity of benzylpenicillin, vancomycin, teicoplanin, and phosphonomycin against extracellular *S. aureus* has been investigated by incubating cells, bacteria, and antibiotics without serum (Fig. 1C). In the absence of serum the bacteria do not adhere to the cells and are not phagocytized by the cells [6]. The effect of the antibiotics on *S. aureus* was enhanced by both granulocytes and monocytes. The increase in the effect of phosphonomycin by monocytes was the only one that was not statistically significant (Table 1) [4].

Root et al. [7] studied the effect of attachment of antibiotic-pretreated bacteria to the plasma membrane of granulocytes on the killing of these bacteria (Fig. 1D). Phagocytosis involves two steps, attachment of the bacteria to the surface of the phagocyte and ingestion. Opsonization of the bacteria by immunoglobulins and/or complement is mandatory for optimal phagocytosis. To ingest a bacterium the phagocyte extends pseudopods around it until the plasma membranes meet and fuse, thus forming a phagocytic vacuole. Ingestion can be blocked by treatment of the phagocytes with cytochalasin B. Pretreatment of *S. aureus* with subinhibitory concentrations of benzylpenicillin or vancomycin led to increased killing of bacteria attached to the cytochalasin B-treated granulocytes. Pretreatment of *S. aureus* with gentamicin did not augment killing [7].

The Role of the Oxygen-Dependent Microbicidal System

As stated above, stimulation of granulocytes or mononuclear phagocytes is necessary for the production of microbicidal substances by the oxygen-dependent killing system. In the experiments in which there is no attachment and ingestion of bacteria (Fig. 1C), stimulation of the cells is not likely to occur unless binding of the antibiotics to the cell membrane serves as a stimulus. To determine whether the oxidative killing mechanism is activated under these experimental conditions, the production of hydrogen peroxide was measured during incubation. No hydrogen peroxide production was found when granulocytes or monocytes were incubated alone, in the presence of *S. aureus* or benzylpenicillin (Table 2; data for monocytes are shown). Stimulation of the oxidative killing mechanism by preincubation of the cells with phorbol myristate acetate (PMA) resulted in hydrogen peroxide production but not in further enhancement of the antibacterial activity of benzylpencicillin or vancomycin

Table 2. H_2O_2 production by monocytes[a]

	H_2O_2 (nM/10^6 monocytes)			
	0 h	1 h	2 h	3 h
Monocytes	0	0	0	0
PMA-pretreated monocytes[b]	0	2.99	2.60	2.48
Monocytes in the presence of *S. aureus*	0	0	0	0
Monocytes in the presence of 0.1 mg/l benzylpenicillin	0	0	0.17	0.19
PMA-pretreated monocytes[b] in the presence of catalase	0	0	0	0

[a] The cells were incubated in Hank's balanced salt solution at 37 °C, and H_2O_2 production was measured.
[b] Monocytes were incubated in the presence of 100 ng/ml PMA for 5 min at 37 °C: the cells were then washed twice before re-incubation for measurement of H_2O_2 production.

Table 3. The influence of PMA pretreatment of monocytes on the enhancement of the antibacterial effect of benzylpenicillin and vancomycin on *S aureus*

	Antibacterial effect after 3h of incubation[a]	
	Benzylpenicillin (0.1 mg/l)	Vancomycin (0.5 mg/l)
S aureus	0.88 ± 0.21 (9)[b]	0.46 ± 0.13 (11)
S aureus in the presence of monocytes	1.72 ± 0.26 (3)	0.95 ± 0.11 (8)
S aureus in the presence of PMA-pretreated monocytes	1.80 ± 0.04 (3)	1.14 ± 0.08 (3)

[a] The antibacterial effect is expressed as the logarithm of the ratio of the number of bacteria in the absence of antibiotic to that in the presence of antibiotic.
[b] Figures in parantheses, number of experiments
[c] Monocytes were incubated in the presence of 100 ng/ml PMA for 5 min at 37 °C. The cells were then washed twice before reincubation with *S aureus* and antibiotic.

(Table 3). Therefore, it seems unlikely that the oxidative killing mechanism is involved in the extracellular enhancement of the antibacterial activity of antibiotics.

In the experiments with cytochalasin B-treated granulocytes in which antibiotic-treated bacteria attach to the granulocytes but are not ingested, stimulation of the oxidative killing mechanism can be expected. Indirect evidence for the role of this microbicidal system in the enhanced killing of penicillin-treated pneumococci and *S. sanguis* is the fact that inhibition of myeloperoxidase by azide abolishes the effect, moreover myeloperoxidase-deficient granulocytes and granulocytes from patients with chronic granulomatous disease (CGD) do not augment killing of pretreated streptococci. The oxygen-dependent killing mechanism did not appear to play a role in the augmented killing of penicillin or vancomycin-treated *S. aureus* attached to granulocytes [8].

The Role of the Oxygen-Independent Microbicidal System

The effect of the microbicidal products of the oxygen-independent killing mechanism on the antibacterial activity of antibiotics has been studied using cell lysates, granule extracts, and purified enzymes *S. aureus* bacteria treated with nafcillin are lysed by lysozyme more readily than the untreated staphylococci [9–11]; the same applies for penicillin-treated *S. sanguis* [3]. *S. aureus* treated with benzylpenicillin, cloxacillin, or nafcillin and benzylpenicillin-treated group A streptococci are more susceptible than untreated bacteria to lysis by leukocyte extracts and lysozyme [12, 13]. Cationic proteins from the phagocytes can influence the effect of hydrophobic antibiotics by enhancing the penetration of these antibiotics through the outer membrane of gram-negative bacteria. For example, polymyxin B nonapeptide, which exerts no antibacterial activity but is a polycationic protein, increases the activity of novobiocin, fusidic acid, erythromycin, clindamycin, nafcillin, and cloxacillin against *E. coli* and *Salmonella typhimurium* [14, 15]. Treatment of *E. coli*, *Klebsiella pneumoniae*, *Salmonella minnesota*, and *shigella sonnei* with chloramphenicol, tetracycline, gentamicin, or streptomycin makes the bacteria more sensitive to the microbicidal effect of a granule extract of granulocytes [16].

The role of the nonoxidative killing mechanism in the enhancement of the effect of benzylpenicillin on extracellular *S. aureus* by monocytes has been studied by using monocyte supernatant obtained by incubating monocytes in Hanks' balanced salt solution (HBSS) for 3 h at 37° C; the cells are then extracted from the medium by centrifugation and filtration. The effect of benzylpenicillin on *S. aureus* in this monocyte supernatant was greater than that in HBSS, indicating that the monocytes secrete a factor that enhances the effect of benzylpenicillin [6]. This monocyte factor has not been fully characterized as yet. Investigations with purified radiolabeled peptidoglycan extracted from *S. aureus* have shown that the monocyte supernatant contains a factor that degrades peptidoglycan. Peptidoglycan prepared from *S. aureus* cultured in the presence of a low concentration of benzylpencillin is degraded to a greater extent than peptidoglycan from untreated *S. aureus* [17]. This observation might offer an explanation for the enhancement of the activity of benzylpenicillin against extracellular *S. aureus*; benzylpenicillin causes changes in the structure of peptidoglycan, making the peptidoglycan more susceptible to degradation by the monocyte factor.

The nonoxidative killing mechanism was shown to play a role in the enhanced killing of benzylpenicillin or vancomycin-pretreated *S. aureus* attached to granulocytes while ingestion was blocked by treatment of the granulocytes with cytochalasin B [7]. Granulocytes from patients with CGD, which have an defective oxygen-dependent killing mechanism, caused enhanced killing of attached staphylococci. Heparin and alpha-1-trypsin, both of which interfere with microbicidal products of the nonoxidative killing system, reduced the killing of attached staphylococci pretreated with antibiotic.

Conclusions

The available data indicate that granulocytes and monocytes enhance the effect of antibiotics, which inhibit cell wall synthesis, on extracellular staphylococci and streptcocci. Microbicidal substances produced by the nonoxidative killing mechanism of phagocytes lead to augmentation of antibiotic activity. A possible explanation for the extraphagocytic synergism between antibiotics and cell-derived microbicidal substances is antibiotic-induced changes in the structure of the bacterial cell wall which then becomes more sensitive to degradation by the cellular enzymes. Microbicidal products of the oxidative killing mechanism can enhance the effect of antibiotics if the bacteria are attached to the plasma membrane of the phagocytes. This seems too be true for streptococci but not staphylococci.

References

1. Van den Broek PJ (1989) Antimicrobial drugs, microorganisms, and phagocytes. Rev Infect Dis 11:213–245
2. Henson PM (1980) Mechanisms of exocytosis in phagocytic inflammatory cells. Am J Pathol 101:494–511
3. Horne D, Tomasz A (1980) Lethal effect of a heterologous murein hydrolase on penicillin-treated *Streptococcus sanguis*. Antimicrob Agents Chemother 17:235–246
4. Van den Broek PJ, Boys LFM (1980) The influence of human monocytes on the antibacterial activity of vancomycin and teicoplanin against *Staphylococcus aureus*. J Antimicrob Chemother 25:787–795
5. Adam D, Philipp P, Belohradsky BH (1971) Studies on the influence of host defence mechanisms on the antimicrobial effect of chemotherapeutic agents. Effect of antibiotics on phagocytosis of mouse-peritoneal macrophages in vitro. Artzl Forsch 25:181–184

6. Van den Broek PJ, Buys LFM, Van den Barselaar MT, Leijh PCJ, van Furth R (1985) Interaction between human monocytes and penicillin G in relation to the anti-bacterial effect on *Staphylococcus aureus*. J Infect Dis 152:521–529

7. Root RK, Isturiz R, Molavi A, Metcalf JA (1981) Interactions between antibiotics and human neutrophils in the killing of staphylococci. Studies with normal and cytochalasin B-treated cells. J Clin Invest 67:247–258

8. Isturiz R, Metcalf JA, Root RK (1985) Enhanced killing of penicillin-treated gram-positive cocci by human granulocytes: role of bacterial autolysins, catalase, and granulocyte oxidative pathways. Yale J Biol Med 58:133–143

9. Warren GH, Gray J (1964) Production of a polysaccharide by *Staphylococcus aureus*. III. Action of penicillins and polysaccharides on enzymic lysis. Proc Soc Exp Biol Med 116:317–323

10. Warren GH, Gray J (1965) Effect of sublethal concentrations of penicillins on the lysis of bacteria by lysozyme and trypsin. Proc Soc Exp Biol Med 120:504–511

11. Warren GH, Gray J (1967) Influence of nafcillin on the enzymic lysis of *Staphylococcus aureus*. Can J Microbiol 13:321–328

12. Efrati C, Sacks T, Ne'eman N, Lahav M, Ginsberg I (1976) The effect of leukocyte hydrolases on bacteria. VIII. The combined effect of leukocyte extracts, lysozyme, enzyme "cocktails," and penicillin on the lysis of *Staphylococcus aureus* and group A streptococci in vitro. Inflammation 1:371–407

13. Ginsburg I, Lahav M, Bergner-Rabinowitz S, Ferne M (1982) Effect of antibiotics on the lysis of staphylococci and streptococci by leukocyte factors, on the production of cellular and extra-cellular factors by streptococci, and on the solubilization of cell-sensitizing agents from gram-negative rods. In: Eickenberg HU, Hahn H, Opferkuch W (eds). The influence of antibiotics on the host-parasite relationship. Springer, Berlin Heidelberg New York pp 219–227

14. Vaara M, Vaara T (1983) Polycations sensitize enteric bacteria to antibiotics. Antimicrob Agents Chemother 24:107–113

15. Vaara M, Vaara T (1983) Polycations as outer membrane-disorganizing agents. Antimicrob Agents chemother 24:114–122

16. Pruul H, Wetherall BL, McDonald PJ (1982) The susceptibility of antibiotic-pretreated gram-negative bacteria to the bactericidal activity of human neutrophil granule extract. In: Eickenberg HU, Hahn H, Opferkuch W (eds). The influence of antibiotics on the host-parasite relationship. (Springer) Berlin Heidelberg New York pp 208–217

17. Van den Broek PJ, van Furth R (1985) Influence of monocytes on the antibacterial activity of penicillin G on *Staphylococcus aureus*. In: van Furth R. (ed) Mononuclear phagocytes. Characteristics, physiology, and function. Nijhoff, Boston, pp 473–476

Cell Wall Inhibitors and Bacterial Susceptibility to Phagocytosis

A. M. Cuffini, N. A. Carlone, V. Tullio, and G. Cavallo

Clinical experience has shown that the efficacy of antibiotic therapy depends not only on the direct effect exerted by the antibiotic on a given microorganism (expressed in terms of the minimum inhibitory or minimum bactericidal concentration) but also on the functional activity of the immune system of the host. The literature reports evidence suggesting that many antimicrobial drugs can modulate host defenses in various ways. It thus follows that a possible influence (both negative and positive) of antibiotics on phagocyte functions should always be tested, especially when antibiotics are given for the treatment or prophylaxis of infections in immunocompromised patients. In these cases it would be logical to employ drugs enhancing rather than depressing host defenses.

β-Lactam antibiotics are widely used, both singly and in combination with other antibiotics, in the treatment and prevention of infections in immunocompromised patients [13]. This review summarizes the available information on the interaction of various cell wall inhibitors with phagocytosis by professional phagocytic cells, namely polymorphonuclear and mononuclear leukocytes and macrophages.

Data on the influence of these antibiotics on phagocytosis are abundant, contradictory and hard to compare because of the variations in methods used for assessing phagocytosis and the differences in experimental design. Several methods for quantitation of bacterial phagocytosis by phagocytic cells have been described.

Although visual evaluation of phagocytosis has frequently been used, this method is imprecise and limited by the inability either to differentiate between nonspecific attachment of bacteria to the cell membrane and ingested bacteria or to quantitate intracellular microbes [32]. Phagocytosis has also been assayed indirectly by measuring the microbicidal activity of the phagocytes. The disadvantage of this method is that it does not differentiate killing and ingestion and does not distinguish between bacteria killed outside and those killed inside the cell. The use of radiolabeled bacteria to measure cellular uptake has overcome some of these difficulties. The advantage of this assay is that is accurate and easy to perform [32].

These methodologic problems in estimation of phagocytosis are paralleled by problems in design variations, depending on different cell systems, the strain

Institute of Microbiology, University of Turin, Via Santena 9, 10126 Torino, Italy

Host Defense Dysfunction
in Trauma, Shock and Sepsis
Eds. Faist/Meakins/Schildberg
© Springer-Verlag, Berlin Heidelberg 1993

of organism, the antibiotic, its concentrations (therapeutic, subinhibitory, high doses, including those well outside the therapeutically attainable range), the duration and timing of antibiotic exposure of both phagocyte and micro-organism, the serum-opsonized bacteria, the in vitro and in vivo environment, etc. Comparisons of results obtained by different methods are therefore risky due to the lack of an appropriate, standardized experimental methodology. Nevertheless, despite all the difficulties and contradictions, there is a con-siderable measure of agreement about certain findings.

It is well known that antibiotics may act directly on the cells of the phagocytic system, or they may affect phagocytosis indirectly inducing changes in bacteria which render them more sensitive to subsequent phagocytosis. Table 1 shows most of the cell wall inhibitors investigated with respect to their interaction with phagocytosis.

There is fairly consistent evidence that antibiotics acting on the cell wall (penicillins, cephalosporins, monobactams, carbapenems, glycopeptides) do not seem to exert any relevant effect on the phagocytosis of various microorganisms, when phagocytes, bacteria and antimicrobial drugs are all present together in the experiment [24, 25, 30, 31], with the exception of ampicillin [10, 12, 25] and cefoperazone [31].

While most of these antibiotics do not directly affect phagocyte function, such drugs may indirectly alter bacterial susceptibilities to both phagocytosis and killing, interfering with some cellular mechanisms necessary for mainten-ance of the surface integrity of the microorganism without affecting viability. Sub-MIC levels of cell wall inhibitors can exert a profound effect on bacterial morphology and consequently on the bacterial surface [3, 4, 21], similar to the morphology of bacteria isolated from individuals under β-lactam therapy [22]. Such morphologic alteration could influence the interaction of bacteria with the cell of the host defense mechanism. Most studies on the effect of β-lactams and glycopeptides on phagocytosis have dealt with the results of pretreatment of bacteria with the drugs and thereafter exposing the bacteria to the phagocytes. It seems likely that if a bacterium is first altered by a cell wall inhibitor, resulting in a subtle but significant change in cell wall integrity, the phagocyte may react to the microorganism in a more positive manner.

Generally the β-lactam induced structural damage has been reported to increase susceptibility of bacteria to phagocytosis.

Griffin [14] suggested that changes on bacterial surface structures resulted in the rupture of a nonimmunological linkage between bacteria and phagocytes, depending on the interaction of specific molecules on the bacterial surface with receptors for these molecules on the phagocytic plasma membrane, rendering the bacteria more accessible to phagocytosis. Horne et al. [16] demonstrated that pretreatment of group B streptococci with penicillins, cephalosporins, and vancomycin increases the susceptibility of these bacteria to phagocytic functions. This sensitization is related to antibiotic-stimulated loss of capsular material or to some other alteration in the cell surface caused by the loss of membrane components, lipoteichoic acids, and lipids [16]. Exposure of gram-

Table 1. Cell wall inhibtors investigated with respect to their interaction with phagocytosis

Antibiotic	References
Penicillin	[23, 24, 25, 31, 35]
Methicillin	[23, 24, 35]
Benzylpenicillin	[23, 24, 31, 35]
Nafcillin	[23, 25, 31, 35]
Oxacillin	[21, 30, 31]
Amoxycillin	[11, 24, 35]
Ampicillin	[10, 12, 31, 33, 35]
Bacampicillin	[10]
Carbenicillin	[2, 23]
Ticarcillin	[2, 11, 23]
Piperacillin	[24, 25, 33]
Mezlocillin	[2, 23]
Azlocillin	[2, 23]
Aztreonam	[11, 20, 26]
Clavulanic acid	[11]
Imipenem	[1, 23]
Vancomycin	[30, 31]
Teicoplanin	[5, 30, 31]
Cefazolin	[7, 31]
Cephalexin	[17, 31, 33]
Cephradine	[11]
Cephalotin	[24, 31, 33]
Cefadroxil	[24, 31]
Cephaloridine	[16, 31]
Cefuroxime	[17, 34]
Cefoxitin	[16, 24]
Cefamandol	[11, 24]
Cefonicid	[29]
Cefotiam	[31]
Cefepime	[27]
Ceftriaxone	[13, 18, 19, 27, 28]
Ceftazidime	[8, 20, 24]
Cefotaxime	[9, 17, 20, 31]
Ceftizoxime	[18]
Cefoperazone	[20, 31]
Moxalactam	[15, 31]

negative bacteria to aztreonam enhances phagocytosis through modification of cell surface structures, mediated through an increase in surface hydrophobicity which enhances bacterial association with phagocyte membranes with subsequent phagocytosis [26]. Exposure of gram-negative bacilli to β-lactam antibiotics causes the bacilli to elongate into filamentous forms which are more susceptible to both phagocytosis and killing than bacillary forms [15, 18].

Altered cell surface characteristics of the cell wall inhibitor treated bacteria may increase the bacterial sensitivity to serum bactericidal mechanisms, the efficiency of opsonization, the bactericidal action of complement and antibody, with subsequent enhancement of the rate of phagocytosis. Adinolfi et al. [1] showed that prior treatment with sub-MIC imipenem results in an increased susceptibility of bacteria to the bactericidal activity of immune serum. Other investigators [17] evidentiated that the growth of encapsulated strains of *Klebsiella pneumoniae* in the presence of several cephalosporins results in reduced expression of the polysaccharide capsule together with increased exposure of various outer membrane protein antigens, so that a more efficient opsonization and enhanced phagocytosis occur. Williams [34] showed that sub-MIC β-lactam antibiotics modify K capsular antigens of *K. pneumoniae* so that complement factor C3b binds to their surface. Raponi et al. [27] showed that cell wall inhibitors interfere with the assembly of Ki capsular polysaccharide of encapsulated *Escherichia coli*, leading to a better access of complement components to receptors on the cell wall of antibiotic-treated bacteria, resulting in an enhanced complement consumption as well as phagocytosis. Cephalosporins and aztreonam preexposure of *E. coli* before IgG-opsonization give a much higher uptake than exposure after IgG opsonization, as shown by Lingass et al.[20]. These β-lactam antibiotics seem to modify the surface of bacteria in such a way that they enhance opsonization with IgG.

In the past 10 years the antibiotic modulation of the phagocytic cell functions has become the major subject of our investigations [6]. Our studies have dealt with the influence of several antimicrobial agents on macrophage functions. The macrophages play an important role in the host defense, since they either take part in the earliest and latest phases of the infection (by preparing and presenting the antigen for T cell recognition, by directly fighting the invader by phagocytosis, by cleaning up the debris, and by eliminating the cellular and metabolic breakdown products) or influence other phagocytic cells involved with release of specific factors.

The current state of our research on the interaction of various cell wall inhibitors with both mouse and human macrophage phagocytosis is reported in Tables 2–4. Phagocytosis was carried out by taking into account three distinct experimental conditions that more mimic in vivo conditions: phagocytosis with contemporary presence of macrophages, bacteria and antibiotic; phagocytosis of antibiotic-pretreated bacteria; and phagocytosis carried out by antibiotic pretreated macrophages. All the experiments were conducted in the presence of subinhibitory antibiotic concentration (half the MIC) and without bacterial opsonization.

If phagocytes, bacteria and antibiotic are all present together in the experiment (Table 2), both penicillins in subinhibitory doses impair the human macrophage phagocytosis, reducing the percentage of staphylococci ingested [6, 10]. These data confirm the results of other researchers who found that ampicillin depresses phagocytic activities at therapeutic concentrations [12, 25]. Our experiments carried out with sub-MIC cefazolin [7], cefonicid [29], cefotaxime [9], and ceftazidime [8] indicate that all four cephalosporins increase phagocytosis of both gram-positive and gram-negative bacteria by mouse and human macrophages, in comparison with the control systems

Table 2. Antibiotic effects on macrophage phagocytosis: bacteria exposed to antibiotics during macrophage attack

Antibiotic (1/2 MIC μg/ml)	Microorganism (10^7 cells)	Macrophages (10^6 cells)	Phagocytosis
Ampicillin			
0.25 μg/ml	*Staphylococcus aureus*	Human	Adverse
Bacampicillin			
0.12 μg/ml	*Staphylococcus aureus*	Human	Adverse
Cefazolin			
15 μg/ml	*Escherichia coli*	Mouse	Good
7.5 μg/ml	*Staphylococcus aureus*	Mouse	Good
0.5 μg/ml	*Bacillus subtilis*	Mouse	Good
Cefonicid			
1.5 μg/ml	*Klebsiella pneumoniae*	Human	Excellent
Cefotaxime			
4 μg/ml	*Staphylococcus aureus*	Mouse	Poor
Ceftazidime			
15 μg/ml	*Staphylococcus aureus*	Human	Excellent
2.5 μg/ml	*Pseudomonas aeruginosa*	Human	Excellent
Teicoplanin			
0.4 μg/ml	*Staphylococcus aureus*	Human	Good

(Table 2). At concentrations of half its MIC for bacteria, teicoplanin [5, 6] causes human macrophages to ingest staphylococci at a greater rate than do macrophages without drug (Table 2). Moreover, phagocytes harvested from mice receiving intravenous cefotaxime, ceftazidime, or teicoplanin show greater phagocytic activity than those from control mice, suggesting that potentiation of host defenses can occur in vivo [5, 8, 9].

Penicillin-pretreated bacteria show different patterns toward phagocytosis (Table 3): ampicillin-exposed organisms are more resistant, while bacampicillin-exposed organisms are highly susceptible. This different pattern has yet to be elucidated. Therefore, electron microscopy investigation seems to rule out the possibility that the enhanced sensitization of bacampicillin-treated bacteria is related to the direct damage induced by the drug on the microbe, since similar changes in cell surface and irregular, abnormal cross walls are detectable with both penicillins [10].

Cephalosprin and teicoplanin-pretreated gram-positive and gram-negative bacteria, undergoing morphologic and biochemical changes, become more sensitive to both mouse and human macrophage phagocytosis (Table 3), with increased susceptibility to the bactericidal activity of lysozime [5–28]. β-Lactam pretreatment of macrophages usually affects neither morphology nor efficiency of macrophages [7, 9, 28] since normal phagocytosis occurs, similar to that in controls (Table 4).

In conclusion, the failure of antibiotic therapy is often due to the inability of the patient's immune system to provide the support that antibiotics need for eradication of the infection. In the circumstances, a further depression by treatment with antibiotics with "anti-host" characteristics should be obviously

Table 3. Antibiotic effects on macrophage phagocytosis: bacteria exposed to antibiotics before macrophage attack

Antibiotic (1/2 MIC µg/ml)	Microorganism (10^7 cells)	Macrophages (10^6 cells)	Phagocytosis
Ampicillin			
0.25 µg/ml	*Staphylococcus aureus*	Human	Adverse
Bacampicillin			
0.12 µg/ml	*Staphylococcus aureus*	Human	Good
Cefonicid			
1.5 µg/ml	*Klebsiella pneumoniae*	Human	Good
Cefotaxime			
4 µg/ml	*Staphylococcus aureus*	Mouse	Good
Ceftazidime			
15 µg/ml	*Staphylococcus aureus*	Human	Good
2.5 µg/ml	*Pseudomonas aeruginosa*	Human	Good
Teicoplanin			
0.4 µg/ml	*Staphylococcus aureus*	Human	Good

Table 4. Antibiotic effects on macrophage phagocytosis: macrophages exposed to antibiotics before the assay

Antibiotic (1/2 MIC µg/ml)	Microorganism (10^7 cells)	Macrophages (10^6 cells)	Phagocytosis
Ampicillin			
0.25 µg/ml	*Staphylococcus aureus*	Human	No effect
Bacampicillin			
0.12 µg/ml	*Staphylococcus aureus*	Human	No effect
Cefazolin			
15 µg/ml	*Esherichia coil*	Mouse	No effect
7.5 µg/ml	*Staphylococcus aureus*	Mouse	No effect
0.5 µg/ml	*Bacillus Pneumoniae*	Human	No effect
Cefonicid			
1.5 µg/ml	*Klebsiella pneumoniae*	Human	No effect
Cefotaxime			
4 µg/ml	*Staphylococcus aureus*	Mouse	Good

avoided. As this review summarizes, general absence of phagocytic function impairment and synergism with phagocytes has been shown for cell wall acting antibiotics. Moreover, their great efficacy exhibited in the treatment of clinical infections, which substantially exceeds any expectations based on their activity and pharmacokinetic behavior in vitro [25], seems to confirm the ability of these antibiotics to "manipulate" the body immune defenses, improving the final outcome of infection.

The conclusion to be drawn is that the immunological side effects of antibiotics should be always taken into account in addition to the various potential side effects of antibiotics. These considerations underscore the necessity to design a standardized laboratory procedure to test the antibiotic immunomodulation, allowing either a better comparison of the results or the intelligent choice in prescribing antibiotics, particularly in special situations, such as the immunocompromised patient.

References

1. Adinolfi LE (1988) Antimicrob Agents Chemother 32:1012–1082
2. Burgaleta C (1985) Drug Res 35:603
3. Carlone NA (1984) Drugs Exp Clin Res 1:47–54
4. Carlone NA (1987) Drugs Exp Clin Res 10:623–629
5. Carlone NA (1989) J Antimicrob Chemother 23:849–859
6. Carlone NA (1991) J Chemother 3 [Suppl 1]:98–104
7. Cuffini AM (1982) Int J Tissue React 4:31–40
8. Cuffini AM (1987) J Antimicrob Chemother 20:261–271
9. Cuffini AM (1989) Microbios 58:147–154
10. Cuffini AM (1991) J Chemother 3 [Suppl 1]:122–127
11. Elhawary A (1984) Chemioterapia 3:354–357
12. Grant M (1983) J Antimicrob Chemother 11:543–554
13. Grassi G (1984) Am J Med 77 [Suppl 46]:37–41
14. Griffin FM (1982) In: Gallin JI, Fauci AS (eds) Phagocytic cells. Raven New York, pp 31–57 (Advances in hoist defense mechanisms, vol 1)
15. Hammer MC (1988) Antimicrob Agents Chemother 32:1565–1570
16. Horne D (1981) Antimicrob Agents Chemother 19:745–753
17. Kadurugamuwa JL (1985) Antimicrob Agents Chemother 28:195–199
18. Labro MT (1987) J Antimicrob Chemother 20:849–855
19. Labro MT (1988) J Antimicrob Chemother 22:341–352
20. Lingaas E (1989) J Antimicrob Chemother 23:701–710
21. Lorian V (1975) Antimicrob Agents Chemother 7:864–870
22. Lorian V (1982) J Clin Pathol 31:351–354
23. Milatovic D (1986) In:Peterson PK, Verhoef J (eds) The antimicrobial agents annual, no 1. Elsevier, New York, pp 446–457
24. Miler I (1990) Padiatr Grenzgeb 29:377–385
25. O'Grady F (1985) In: Greenwood D, O'Grady F (eds) The Scientific basis of antimicrobial chemotherapy Cambridge University Press, Cambridge, pp 341–365 (Society for general microbiology symposium, no 38)
26. Pruul H (1988) J Antimicrob Chemother 22:675–686
27. Raponi G (1990) Antimicrob Agents Chemother 34:332–336
28. Traub WH (1986) Zentralbl Bakteriol Mikrobiol Hyg [4] 85–94
29. Tullio V (1991) J Chemother [Suppl 4]:534–553
30. Van der Auwera P (1987) J Antimicrob Chemother 20:399–404
31. Van den Broek PJ (1989) Rev Infect Dis 12:213–245
32. Verhoef J (1985) Eur J Clin Microbiol 4:758–762
33. Welch WD (1981) Antimicrob Agents Chemother 20:15–20
34. Williams P (1987) Antimicrob Agents Chemother 31:758–762
35. Yourtee EL (1982) Gallin JI, Fauci AS (eds) Phagocytic cells. Raven, New York, pp 187–209 (Advances in host defense mechanisms, vol 1)

Protein Synthesis Inhibitors and Bacterial Susceptibility to Phagocytosis

C. G. Gemmell

It is well recognised that antibiotics can be either bactericidal or bacteriostatic and on this basis their therapeutic efficacy can be measured. In particular those drugs in the latter category may depend upon the underlying activity of the host's reticulo-endothelial system (RES) in order to demonstrate their full efficacy. Antibiotics whose mode of action is based upon bacterial ribosomal protein biosynthesis are usually bacteriostatic, and this article will concentrate on their bioactivity in concert with phagocytic cells.

Growth of various bacterial species in the presence of sub-growth-inhibitory concentration (sub-MIC) of various antibiotics has been shown to result in significant structural and topographic changes in the bacterial cell, including filamentation, increased numbers of thickened cross-walls and loss of surface appendages such as fimbriae or surface antigens. Such changes are likely to influence the outcome of the host–parasite relationship [3]. The possible consequences include an increase or decrease in chemotaxin expression and an increase or decrease in surface components which might alter the cell's requirement for serum opsonins and consequent changes in susceptibility to phagocytosis [2].

Several antibiotics which interfere with protein biosynthesis have been described with unique biological activity in this respect, including the lincosamines, fusidic acid and some of the macrolides. Why such drugs should express such activity whereas other drugs with a somewhat similar biochemical mode of action remain inactive may be related to differences in the specific stage of protein biosynthesis inhibited (Fig. 1). Consequently the expression of microbial virulence factors may or may not be impaired in the presence of each of these drugs.

The most obvious examples which have been examined in some detail by several groups of investigators include protein A expression by *Staphylococcus aureus*, M protein expression by *Streptococcus pyogenes*, K antigen expression by *Escherichia coli* and capsule antigen expression by *Bacteroides fragilis*.

Levels of protein A detectable on different strains of *S. aureus* are variable, but its presence is recognized to impair serum opsonisation through its ability to bind to the Fc fragment of immunoglobulin. Growth of protein A-rich strains in the presence of sub-MIC levels of clindamycin, fusidic acid and pseudomonic

Department of Bacteriology, Royal Infirmary, 86 Castle Street, Glasgow, UK

Host Defense Dysfunction
in Trauma, Shock and Sepsis
Eds. Faist/Meakins/Schildberg
© Springer-Verlag, Berlin Heidelberg 1993

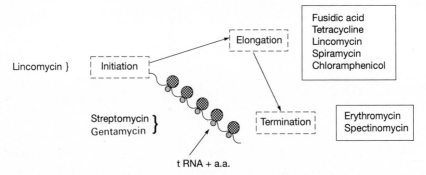

Fig. 1. Antibiotics and ribosomal protein biosynthesis. a.a., amino acids

acid modified the expression of protein A and by so doing increased complement activation via the alternative pathway and subsequent ingestion/killing by phagocytic cells in vitro (Table 1). The effect of one of these drugs, namely clindamycin, is more pronounced upon protein A-rich strains rather than upon protein A-poor strains [4, 10, 15]. In addition, *Staphyloccus epidermidis*, which lacks protein A is unaffected by exposure to the antibiotic.

Likewise, M protein expression by *Streptococcus pyogenes* grown in the presence of sub-MIC clindamycin was markedly reduced; loss of M protein could be measured serologically and recognised ultrastructurally. Changes in the expression of T antigen could also be demonstrated. These antigenic changes resulted in increased rates of chemotaxis by polymorphonuclear leucocytes (PMNL) towards the antibiotic-exposed bacteria, their isolated cell walls or cell wall antigens. The reduced amounts of M protein potentiated phagocytic ingestion (Table 2) and killing as a result of increased deposition of C3b on the streptococcal cells [5]. Nevertheless, other antibiotics which inhibit protein biosynthesis, namely chloramphenicol and erythromycin, did not display similar biological activity towards M antigen expression of *Streptococcus pyogenes* [6].

Table 1. Effect of different opsonic sources on susceptibility of *Staphylococcus aureus* grown in the presence and absence of clindamycin to phagocytosis. (Results adapted from [15])

Drug treatment	1% normal human serum	1% heated serum	10% serum from agammaglobulin- aemic patient
None	25	30	50
1/2 MIC clindamycin	90	55	95
1/4 MIC clindamycin	60	60	85

Numbers are perentages of bacteria ingested by human PMN after opsonsiz- ation with serum.
MIC, minimal inhibitory concentration

Table 2. Phagocytosis by polymorphonuclear leucocytes (PMNL) and monocytes (MN) of *Streptococcus pyogenes* exposed to sub-MIC clindamycin

Drug treatment	Ingestion by PMNL (%)	Ingestion by MN (%)
None	8 + 1.5	6 + 0.6
1/2 MIC	42 + 4.2	39 + 3.6
1/4 MIC	34 + 2.4	28 + 2.2
1/10 MIC	30 + 2.1	17 + 1.1

Values are MIC, minimal inhibitory concentration. mean + SD of at least three experiments

However, the foregoing examples are based upon gram-positive cocci and drugs which would normally be used in therapy of infections caused by these organisms. It is clear that certain protein synthesis inhibitors are capable of interfering with expression of proteinaceous virulence factors by pathogenic bacteria.

These studies have now been extended to gram-negative pathogens. In particular, two intestinal tract pathogens, *E. coli* and *B. fragilis*, have been examined with respect to their ability to express microcapsular antigen or full capsule in the presence of sub-MIC concentrations of certain antibiotics.

As far as *B. fragilis* is concerned, its pathogenicity is based upon its ability to elaborate a polysaccharide capsule. Animal-passaged strains are much more heavily encapsulated than those grown in vitro. Growth of *B. fragilis* in the presence of sub-MIC clindamycin resulted in cells deficient in capsule. Such cells were more easily phagocytosed by PMNL, elicited a greater chemiluminescent response and were more easily killed than their encapulated control [7, 8]. Addition of partially purified capsular polysaccharide (glycocalyx) to clindamycin-exposed *Bacteriodes* cells [13, 14] restored their resistance to opsonophagocytosis (Table 3). It is not yet clear why an antibiotic which owes its biological activity to inhibition of protein biosynthesis should be able to inhibit the biosynthesis of a polysaccharide which is polymerised on the surface of the

Table 3. Influence of exogenous glycocalyx on susceptibility of clindamycin-grown *Bacteroides fragilis* to phagocytosis by human PMNL (Adapted from [13])

Drug treatment	Bacteria ingested by PMNL (%)
None	15 ± 2
1/2 MIC clindamycin	68 ± 5
1/2 MIC clindamycin + 1 mg/l isolated glycocalyx	20 ± 1
1/2 MIC clindamycin + 0.1 mg/l isolated glycocalyx	69 ± 10

PMNL, polymorphonuclear leucocytes; MIC, minimal inhibitory concentration

Table 4. Phagocytosis of *Escherichia coli* strains exposed to 1/2 MIC netilmicin (From [12])

Drug treatment	Ingestion by PMNL of strains belonging to serotype (%)			
	01:K −	01:K1	07:K −	07:K1
None	52	8	75	4
1/2 MIC netilmicin	58	38	82	32

MIC, minimal inhibitory concentration; PMNL, polymorphonuclear leucocytes

bacterium. It is possible that the drug acts on a vital enzyme involved in biosynthesis of the macromolecule. Similar studies with the fluoroquinolones have revealed that these drugs can also potentiate opsonophagocytosis of *B. fragilis* [11], again suggesting that some fundamental enzyme involved in polysaccharide biosynthesis is impaired by drug action.

E. coli strains may or may not express K antigens on their surface. These antigens confer resistance to serum killing, resistance to phagocytosis and pathogenicity for man and experimental animals. Several drugs have been used to examine the biosynthesis of this antigen. Netilmicin at a sub-MIC is able to make K-positive strains of *E. coli* susceptible to opsonophagocytosis [12]. In contrast, K strains are not affected by exposure to the antibiotic (Table 4). Clindamycin is also able to potentiate phagocytic ingestion of *E. coli* [1, 9].

This presentation has sought to summarize the effect of antibiotics which interfere at different stages of protein biosynthesis on the expression of various bacterial virulence factors. It is clear that differences between each of these drugs may be related to their molecular mode of action. We are only beginning to understand these differences in terms of bacterial pathogenicity. Of relevance to this argument is the recognition that the lincosamines, chloramphenicol, the macrolides and the tetracyclines each act at different stages of protein biosynthesis including initiation, peptide bond formation and chain elongation and termination. A fuller understanding of the drug–bacterium interaction will require detailed investigation at the subcellular level.

References

1. Bassaris HP, Lianou PE, Papavassiliou JT (1988) Interaction of subminimal inhibitory concentrations of clindamycin and *Escherichia coli*: effects on adhesion and polymorphonuclear leukocyte function. J Antimicrob Chemother, Suppl B:25–32
2. Cialdella JI, Vavra JJ, Marshall VP (1986) Susceptibility of bacteria to serum lysis or phagocytosis following growth in subinhibitory levels of lincosaminide or spectinomycin related antibiotics. J Antibiot (Tokyo) 39:978–984

3. Gemmell CG (1985) Elaboration of structural and soluble virulence factors by antibiotic-damaged bacteria: consequences for host defences. Zentralbl Bakteriol Mikrobiol Hyg [A] 3, Suppl I 179–189

4. Gemmell CG, O'Dowd A (1983) Regulation of protein A biosynthesis in *Staphylococcus aureus* by certain antibiotics: its effect on phagocytosis by leukocytes. J Antimicrob Chemother 12:587–597

5. Gemmell CG, Peterson PK, Schmeling D, Kim Y, Mathews J, Wannamaker L, Quie PG (1981) Potentiation of opsonization and phagocytosis of *Streptococcus pyogenes* following growth in the presence of clindamycin. J Clin Invest 67:1249–1259

6. Gemmell CG, Peterson PK, Schemling D, Quie PG (1982) Studies on the potentiation of phagocytosis of *Streptococcus pyogenes* by treatment with various antibiotics. Drugs Exp Clin Res. 8:235–240

7. Gemmell CG, Peterson PK, Schmeling D, Mathews J, Quie PG (1983) Drug-induced modification of *Bacteroides fragilis* and its susceptibility to phagocytosis by human PMN. Eur J Clin Microbiol 2:327–334

8. Howard RJ, Soucy DM (1983) Potentiation of phagocytosis of *Bacteroides fragilis* following incubation with clindamycin. J Antimicrob Chemother 12, Suppl C:63–68

9. Lianou PE, Bassaris HP, Votta EG, Papavassiliou JT (1985) Interaction of subminimal inhibitory concentrations of clindamycin and Gram-negative aerobic organisms: effects on adhesion and polymorphonuclear leukocyte function. J Antimicrob. Chemother 15:481–487

10. Milatovic D, Braveny I, Verhoef J (1983) Clindamycin enhances opsonization of *Staphylococcus aureus*. Antimicrob Agents Chemother 24:413–417

11. Pulverer G, Peters G (1986) Investigations on ofloxacin: antibacterial activity and influence on the immune system. Infection 14:S245–247

12. Raponi G, Vreede RW, Rozenberg-Arska M, Hoepelman IM, Keller N, Verhoef J (1989) The influence of subminimal inhibitory concentrations on the interaction of *Escherichia coli* with host defences. J Antimicrob Chemother 23:565–576

13. Veringa EM, Ferguson DA, Lambe DW, Verhoef J (1989) The role of glycocalyx in surface phagocytosis of *Bacteroides* spp. in the presence and absence of clindamycin. J Antimicrob Chemother 23:711–720

14. Veringa EM, Lambe DW, Ferguson DA, Verhoef J (1989) Enhancement of opsonophagocytosis of *Bacteroides* spp. by clindamycin in subinhibitory concentrations. J Antimicrob Chemother 23:577–587

15. Veringa E, Verhoef J (1985) Influence of subinhibitory concentrations of clindamycin on the phagocytosis of *Staphylococcus aureus*. In: Adam D, Hahn H, Opferkuch W (eds) Influence of antibiotics on the host-parasite relationship. Springer, Berlin Heidelberg New York, pp 259–266

Section 14

The Role of Nutrition in Host Defense

Augmentation of Host Defense Reactivity with Special Nutrients*

J. W. Alexander

Introduction

Nutritional therapy has become an increasingly important component of therapeutic intervention for human disease, especially during critical illness. Recent studies have shown that the effects of nutritional therapy can extend well beyond the treatment and prevention of deficiencies of dietary components, partly because some nutrients have pharmacologic effects, i.e., when given in quantities different from that normally in the diet or in excess of that which will prevent deficiency, they may elicit biological responses in a manner similar to pharmacologic agents. Among these nutrients are the long-chain polyunsaturated fatty acids (PUFA), arginine, and, to a lesser extent, vitamins E, C, and A. The nucleotides, zinc, and selenium may have pharmacologic effects under certain conditions, but carbohydrates and proteins themselves probably do not. Among the above, the PUFA and arginine are the most important.

Arginine

In 1980, Barbul and his colleagues [1] reported that a 1% oral dietary supplement of arginine prevented thymolysis and T-cell dysfunction in injured rats. They also showed an increased thymic weight and T-cell mitogenic responses in rats without injury. A subsequent study [2] by the same group showed that supplementary dietary arginine would increase wound-healing strength and reparative collagen accumulation in implanted sponges. Further studies by Barbul et al. [3] used arginine in intravenous hyperalimentation for rats with fractured femurs. There was an improvement in nitrogen balance with a reduction in weight loss and an improvement in the immune responsiveness of lymphocytes.

A recent controlled, randomized study by Daly et al. [4] showed that dietary arginine (5% of energy) given to patients with major operative procedures was

---

* Supported in part by USPHS grant AI12936 and the Shriners of North America.
Transplantation Division, University of Cincinnati College of Medicine, Cincinnati, OH 45267-0558, USA

Host Defense Dysfunction
in Trauma, Shock and Sepsis
Eds. Faist/Meakins/Schildberg
© Springer-Verlag, Berlin Heidelberg 1993

able to improve the responsiveness of peripheral lymphocytes to phytomitogens. The mechanisms of action of arginine have been studied extensively but are still incompletely understood [5]. Arginine increases the synthesis and release of growth hormone and prolactin from the pituitary, both of which have positive influences on the immune response. Insulin release is also stimulated, along with glucagon and pancreatic polypeptides and adrenal catecholamines. At the biochemical level, arginine may be converted to citrulline or ornithine and may be the precursor for the putrescines which are important low-molecular-weight compounds that support cellular growth. Although cellular growth is stimulated by arginine, animal experiments have generally shown that arginine during wound repair is suppressive for growth of tumors.

Studies by Saito et al. [6] used a burned guinea pig to investigate the effect of arginine on outcome following thermal injury. Responsiveness in sensitized animals to dinitrofluorobenzene showed that arginine (1% and 2% of dietary energy) increased the delayed hypersensitivity responses in a dose-dependent manner, but 4% arginine was no better than control animals without supplemental arginine. In these studies, the delayed hypersensitivity response was inversely related to the ability of the animal to clear *Staphylococcus aureus* injected subdermally. Mortality was improved with supplemental arginine, being 28% in animals receiving 1% arginine, 22% in animals receiving 2% arginine, and 56% in animals receiving no supplemental arginine. The effect of arginine in improving resistance to infection was further demonstrated by Madden et al. [7], who showed that arginine could significantly reduce mortality in a cecal ligation and puncture model.

Lipids

Partly because of the relationship of the dietary fats to the development of cardiovascular disease, research on lipid metabolism has occurred at an increasing pace during the last two to three decades. It is generally accepted that the American diet contains too much lipid, averaging 48% of the nonprotein calories in 1980 [8]. Lipids are particularly important because they are rapidly absorbed by the intestinal tract and transported to the liver where they are processed and attached to carriers. Short- and medium-chain fatty acids are used primarily as energy sources. Long-chain fatty acids, particularly PUFA of the omega 3 and omega 6 families are incorporated into the lipid membranes of different cells at different rates and markedly influence their function including transport, receptor formation and function, fluidity, signaling, and enzyme activity. Kinsella [9] has provided a recent excellent review of the subject. The formation of membranes itself reflects the physical properties of the phospholipids (PL) which spontaneously associate to form bilayer structures. The plasma membranes of eukaryote cells contain up to 10^3 PL species as well as numerous protein species. Both the proteins and lipids are capable of rapid lateral mobility and there is constant remodeling. The uneven distribution of lipid types in inner and outer membranes support functional consequences. The PUFA may both stimulate membrane signaling and be released by membrane activation. Also, the amount and type of PUFA in membranes markedly affects secondary eicosanoid responses. Thus, lipids may play an extremely important role in cell physiology and cell-to-cell interactions. Further recent reviews of the role of lipids in immune responses can be found in articles by Hwang [10] and Kinsella et al. [11].

The role of lipids in nutritional support of thermal injury was investigated by Mochizuki et al. [12] in 1984. Animals were provided with a gastrostomy tube 1 week before a 30% thermal burn was inflicted. After the burn injury, animals received only lactated Ringer's for the first 24 h, increasing the caloric intake to 175 kCal/kg by 72 h and keeping the daily intake at this level for 14 days. The liquid diets provided were identical with the exception that lipid calories, provided by safflower oil (approximately 74% linoleic acid, omega 6), was varied at 0%, 5%, 15%, 30%, and 50% of nonprotein calories, reducing the carbohydrate component appropriately. Animals receiving 0%, 5%, and 15% of the calories maintained their body weight whereas animals receiving 30% and 50% of their nonprotein calories as lipids lost body weight even though their caloric intake was the same. The resting energy expenditure was not affected by the amount of fat in the diet. Liver weight was best maintained on diets with 0%–15% lipid calories and was significantly reduced by 30% lipid diets. Fatty infiltrates of the liver occurred with 50% iipid calories. Nitrogen content of the liver generally decreased with increasing amounts of lipids. Serum transferrin levels were highest in animals receiving 5% and 15% of lipids, as was C3. The carcass weight, representing the major skeletal muscle mass, was best maintained with no lipids and progressively decreased as the amount of lipid in the diet was increased. It was felt that the adverse effects of the safflower oil was a result of the generation of prostaglandins and leukotrienes through the arachidonic acid pathway. In particular, it was felt that prostaglandin E_2 (PGE_2) was an important mediator since it is profoundly immunosuppressive and can cause loss of muscle mass [10]. It was reasoned that substitution of omega 3 fatty acids for omega 6 fatty acids in the diet might result in a beneficial effect because the omega 3 fatty acids are converted to the less biologically potent trianoic prostaglandins compared to the dienoic prostaglandins. Therefore, a similar experiment was done using fish oil (rich in omega 3 fatty acid) as the sole source of lipids [13], varying the amount of lipid in the diet at 5%, 15%, 30%, and 50%. Animals receiving 15% of nonprotein calories as fish oil maintained body weight best and the most marked weight loss was found in animals receiving 50% fish oil. Resting energy expenditure was slightly but insignificantly better with animals receiving 15% of energy as fish oil. However, cell-mediated immunity was not significantly influenced by the amount of fish oil, nor was macrophage bactericidal index, although it was best in animals with 15% of fish oil. It was concluded that animals receiving lower levels of fish oil had better body weights, better carcass weights, higher liver weights, and higher liver nitrogen than did animals receiving 30% or 50% fish oil.

A further experiment [14] compared diets which were identical except for the composition of the lipids, which was held constant at 12% of energy. One group of animals received linoleic acid, a second group received safflower oil (74% linoleic acid), and a third group received fish oil (traces of linoleic acid but rich in omega 3 fatty acids, approximately 35% eicosopentanoic acid, EPA, and docosahexanoic acid, DHA). Two weeks following thermal injury, the animals were sacrificed. Body weight was significantly better in the animals receiving fish oil compared to linoleic acid, with safflower oil animals intermediate. The same was true for carcass weight and spleen weight, reflecting lymphoid mass. Adrenal weight was significantly greatest in the animals receiving the linoleic acid, reflecting stress. The amount of lipid had no effect on serum albumin, but serum transferrin levels were significantly higher in animals fed fish oil than linoleic acid or safflower oil. The opsonic index, a complex immune function, was significantly depressed in animals receiving linoleic acid; this was partially reversed by the administration of indomethacin, indicating that at least some of the effect was caused by arachidonic acid pathway products. Opsonic indexes were actually better than normal in animals receiving fish oil. In animals receiving safflower oil the opsonic index was slightly depressed, and in animals receiving linoleic acid it was markedly depressed. Somewhat surprisingly, the metabolic rate was reduced in animals receiving fish oil compared to those receiving safflower oil.

Studies in Humans

Using the immunopharmacologic principles related to dietary PUFA and arginine as noted above, a new burn diet was formulated which derived 20% of energy from whey protein, 2% of energy from arginine, and 12% of energy from lipids, with half of the lipid energy coming from safflower oil and half from fish oil. Using a prospective randomized trial in seriously burned patients, this diet was compared to two other dietary supplements which contained approximately the same amount of protein but higher amounts of lipids and no supplemental arginine [15]. The three groups, which had 21, 20, and 19 patients, were evenly distributed with regard to risk factors including age, the presence or absence of smoke inhalation, and the size of the burn injury. Patients receiving the new diet had a reduced length of stay when expressed as days of hospitalization per percentage of burn, and they had a significantly reduced incidence of wound infection. Daly et al. [16] recently compared a similar diet (Impact) with Osmolite HN in a preparation randomized trial of postoperative feeding in patients with upper gastrointestinal and pancreatic cancers. The use of Impact reduced infections and wound complications from 37% to 11% and shortened hospital stay from 20.2 days to 15.8 days ($p = 0.01$).

Lipids in Sepsis

The role of nutritional support in sepsis was also studied in an animal model of prolonged peritonitis. Previous models of experimental peritonitis, including injection of bacteria singly or in mixtures, alone or with adjuvants, in fecal pellets, capsules, or in fibrin clots, or models that used cecal ligation and puncture, all resulted in death of the experimental animals before nutritional intervention could be expected to have an effect. Because of this, a new model was developed which involved the implantation of a bacteria-filled osmotic pump into the peritoneal cavity of guinea pigs which had been previously provided with gastrostomy for controlled enteral feedings [17]. Subsequent studies using this model have shown that a caloric intake sufficient to prevent weight loss was associated with much higher mortality than a caloric intake associated with significant weight loss (100 kcal/kg per day). Caloric intake of 175 kcal/kg per day or even 150 kcal/kg per day, an amount barely sufficient to prevent weight loss in guinea pigs with a 30% burn, was associated with uniform death [17]. Even more surprising was the observation that protein deficient diets were protective in animals given 125 kcal/kg per day [18]. Specifically, animals receiving a 5% protein diet for the 2 weeks of the infection had a 45% survival compared to only 12% survival in animals given 15% protein in their diet. Also, in contrast to the findings in burn animals, arginine supplementation was found to be detrimental in a dose-related manner up to 6% [19]. On the other hand, increasing the total lipids in the diet to 56% of energy did not have an adverse effect. Indeed, there was no difference in overall survivals of animals receiving 3.5%, 14%, and 56% of their calories as lipids. The type of lipid did make a difference, however, with survival of more than 80% in animals receiving a 50:50 mixture of safflower oil and fish oil [20]. Survival in animals receiving only safflower oil was 18% and survival of animals receiving only fish oil was 36%.

In other experiments mice were fed ad libitum for 2 weeks with normal chow or diets which were high in lipid content (20% of total energy) or low in lipid content (5% of total energy), using either safflower oil or fish oil as sources of lipids. There was definite protection from infection with high levels of safflower oil but not low levels [21]. Fish oil was not protective at either level. A further experiment [22] comparing safflower oil with oleic acid, coconut oil, and fish oil, showed significantly better protection against acute bacterial infection in animals receiving safflower oil than fish oil, with oleic acid and coconut oil giving intermediate results. Also, in contrast to the experiments in septic guinea pigs, burned mice given *Pseudomonas* in the burn wound eschar had better survival when prefed diets high in protein levels but with restricted calories [23]. The reasons for these discrepant results in animals with acute infection compared to those with existing infection are still not entirely clear. However, additional in vitro experiments have shown that PGE_2 has counter-regulator effects on tumor necrosis factor (TNF) induction and release [10]. It is quite possible that TNF is the agent primarily responsible for mortality in acute infection experiments and that the acute elevation of PGE_2 (which rapidly down-regulates TNF) may be responsible for the protection in animals prefed with high levels of omega 6 fatty acids. In contrast, chronic immunosuppression may result from continued elevation of PGE_2 levels in individuals fed with high levels of omega 6 fatty acids following injury, thus making them more susceptible to the development of newly established spontaneous infections.

Conclusion

These observations suggest that nutritional support with special nutrients is highly effective needs to be disease specific using the emerging principals of nutritional pharmacology. Septic animals with prolonged peritonitis do poorly with high energy intakes and high-protein diets. In such animals, supplemental arginine may decrease mortality when given before a septic challenge, but it may increase mortality in the already septic animal. Relatively high caloric densities of lipids rich in both omega 3 and omega 6 fatty acids are beneficial in septic animals. However, diets rich in omega 6 fatty acids appear to be protective in animals with an acute bacterial challenge. The optimal nutritional formulation for treatment of sepsis in man has not yet been determined, but it will most certainly be different from the formulation currently in use and may be different for different types of infections.

References

1. Barbul A, Wasserkrug HL, Seifter E, Rettura G, Levenson SM, Efron G (1980) Immunostimulatory effects of arginine in normal and injured rats. J Surg Res 29:288–235
2. Barbul A, Rettura G, Levenson SM, Seifter E (1983) Wound healing and thymotropic effects of arginine: a pituitary mechanism of action. Am J Nutr 37:336
3. Barbul A, Wasserkrug HL, Yoshimura N, Tao R, Efron G (1984) High arginine levels in intravenous hyperalimentation abrogate post-traumatic immune suppression. J Surg Res 36:620–624
4. Daly JM, Reynolds J, Thom A, Kinsley L, Dietrick-Gallagher M, Shou J, Ruggieri B (1988) Immune and metabolic effects of arginine in the surgical patient. Ann Surg 208(4):512–523
5. Reynolds JV, Daly JM, Zhang S, Evantash E, Shou J, Sigal R, Ziegler MM (1988) Immunomodulatory mechanisms of arginine. Surgery 104:142–151
6. Saito H, Trocki O, Wang SL, Gonce SJ, Joffe SN, Alexander JW (1987) Metabolic and immune effects of dietary arginine supplementation after burn. Arch Surg 122:784–789
7. Madden HP, Breslin RJ, Wasserkrug HL, Efron G, Barbul A (1988) Stimulation T-cell immunity by arginine enhances survival in peritonitis. J Surg Res 44:658–663
8. Welsh SO, Marston RM (1982) Review of trends in food use in the United States, 1909 to 1980. J Am Diet Assoc 81:120–128
9. Kinsella JE (1990) Lipids, membrane receptors, and enzymes: effects of dietary fatty acids. JPEN J Parenter Enkral Nutr [Suppl]:200–217
10. Hwang D (1989) Essential fatty acids and immune response. FASEB J 3(9):2052–2061

11. Kinsella JE, Lokesh B, Broughton S, Whelan J (1990) Dietary polyunsaturated fatty acids and eicosanoids: potential effects on the modulation of inflammatory and immune cells: an overview. Nutrition 6(1):24–44
12. Mochizuki H, Trocki O, Dominioni L, Ray MB, Alexander JW (1984) Optimal lipid content for enteral diets following thermal injury. JPEN J Parenter Enteral Nutr 8:638–646
13. Trocki O, Heyd TJ, Waymack JP, Alexander JW (1987) Effects of fish oil on postburn metabolism and immunity. JPEN J Parenter Enteral Nutr 11:521–528
14. Alexander JW, Saito H, Trocki O, Ogle CK (1986) The importance of lipid type in the diet after injury. Ann Surg 204:1–8
15. Gottshlich MM, Jenkins M, Warden GD, Baumer T, Havens P, Snook JT, Alexander JW (1990) Differential effects of three enteral dietary regimens on selected outcome variables in burn patients. JPEN J Parenter Enteral Nutr 14(3):225–236
16. Daly JM, Lieberman M, Goldfine J, Shou J, Weintraub FN, Rosato EF, Lavin P (1991) Enteral nutrition with supplemental arginine, RNA, OMEGA-3 fatty acids: a prospective clinical trial. 15th Clinical Congress of the American Society for Parenteral and Enteral Nutrition, Abstr 17, p 308
17. Alexander JW, Gonce SJ, Miskell PW, Peck MD (1989) A new model for studying nutrition in peritonitis. The adverse effect of over-feeding. Ann Surg 209:332–340
18. Peck MD, Alexander JW, Gonce SJ, Miskell PW (1989) Low-protein diets improve survival from peritonitis in guinea pigs. Ann Surgery 209(4):448–454
19. Gonce SJ, Peck MD, Alexander JW, Miskell PW (1990) Arginine supplementation and its effect on established peritonitis in guinea pigs. JPEN J Parenter Enteral Nutr 14:237–240
20. Peck MD, Ogle CK, Alexander JW (1991) Composition of fat in enteral diets can influence outcome in experimental peritonitis. Ann Surg (in press)
21. Peck MD, Ogle CK, Alexander JW, Babcock GF (1990) The effect of dietary fatty acids in response to pseudomonas infection in burned mice. J Trauma 30:445–452
22. Peck MD, Ogle CK, Alexander JW, Babcock GF (1991) Dietary fat and infection in burned animals. J Burn Care Rehabil 12(1):43–45
23. Peck MD, Babcock GF, Alexander JW (1991) The role of protein and calorie restriction on outcome from *Salmonella* infection in mice. Nutrition (submitted)

The Role of Structured Lipids in Host Defense Interactions

R. A. Forse, G. L. Blackburn, and B. R. Bistrian

Lipids are important components in the host defense to injury and sepsis. They not only provide a necessary and preferred substrate but are important modulators of cellular response and function. Over the past several years the role of lipids in these two areas has been better clarified in the stressed state. It is the attempt to optimize lipid composition for use both as a fuel and a modulator of the cellular response that has led the development of the structured lipid.

In the nutritional support of host defense in injury and sepsis, exogenous lipids can be provided by either the enteral or parenteral route. Septic patients preferentially oxidize a mixed fuel and the optimal exogenous fuel should provide both lipid and carbohydrate substrate in a relatively narrow range [1, 2]. By the use of such mixtures, acclerated hepatic lipogenesis and resultant immunosuppression can be limited. In the septic patient provided with mixed fuel the lipid not only serves as a fuel but retards hepatic lipogenesis [3]. Typically lipids that have been used in the nutritional support have been long chain triglycerides (LCT) which were 14 carbons and longer. They were supplied as a soybean or safflower oil with a high percentage of the essential free fatty acid linoleic acid. Not only did the LCT decrease fatty infiltration of the liver but the fat improving nitrogen balance was equivalent to the carbohydrate [1, 2, 4]. The lipid source when provided in excess could have side effects (Table 1) including inhibition of neutrophil function, impaired macrophage phagocytosis, and depression or blockage of reticuloendothelial system (RES), all of which decrease the host defence [5–9] (Table 1). The latter dysfunction in animal experiments resulted in impaired bacterial clearance with increased bacterial sequestration in the lung [10]. Furthermore, there was evidence of decreased clearance and ultilization of these lipids during severe sepsis when lipoprotein

Table 1. Long chain triglycerides

1. Inhibition of neutrophil function
2. Inhibition of macrophage phagocytosis
3. Blocking the hepatic RES and thus impairing bacterial clearance
4. Decreasing clearance by lipoprotein lipase in sepsis
5. Dependent on carnitine oxidation which is decreased in sepsis

Department of Surgery and Medicine, Harvard Medical School, New England Deaconess Hospital, 194 Pilgrim Road, Boston, MA 02215, USA

Host Defense Dysfunction
in Trauma, Shock and Sepsis
Eds. Faist/Meakins/Schildberg
© Springer-Verlag, Berlin Heidelberg 1993

lipase activity was suppressed [11,12]. This resulted in decreased LCT oxidation with increased storage as fat. Finally there was evidence that a relative deficiency in carnitine often developed with sepsis, which would result in decreased oxidation of the LCT that was delivered to the cell as LCT oxidation is carnitine dependent [13].

Medium chain triglycerides (MCT) are currently thought to be an ideal substrate for the stressed and septic state. These lipids have chain lengths of 6–12 carbons, but commerical MCT are principally 8–10 carbons. The current sources for the MCT, palm kernel and coconut oils, have chain lengths of 8–10 carbons. There are several properties of the MCT that make them more efficient in injury and sepsis (Table 2). The MCT are hydrolysed in the brush border of the intestine or adsorbed intact and then predominantly transported to the liver by the portal circulation as medium chain fatty acids after intracellular hydrolysis [14]. More recent studies indicate that up to 15% of the MCT will be made into chylomicrons when the diet is predominantly MCT [15]. MCT adsorption does not require pancreatic lipase and the re-formation of the triglyceride into chylomicrons, which are transported by the thoracic duct. At the liver the medium chain fatty acids are efficiently used as a fuel, with the production of carbon dioxide, acetate, and ketone bodies [14]. MCT oxidization in the mitochondria uses a non-carnitine-dependent pathway which improves their oxidation in sepsis [16] and results in decreased adipose tissue storage. The ketone bodies formed from this efficient oxidation can be used as fuel by tissues such as the muscle, thereby reducing proteolysis, although ketogenesis is limited if carbohydrate is also provided. If used as the sole fuel source MCT can produce toxic effects in animals; however, these effects are limited by the use of mixtures of MCT and LCT as well as the provision of carbohydrate [17–19]. Studies employing protein kinetics and nitrogen balance have indicated that MCT/LCT solutions are associated with improved protein sparing in both animal and human studies. When administrated as a 75% MCT/25% LCT mixture the improved protein sparing is associated with an increased lipid oxidation and an increase in thermogenesis [20]. Improved protein sparing results in improved host defense with recent evidence of improved cellular immune function [21]. One of the alterations in host defense related to excessive infusions of LCT has been decreased phagocytosis by the RES system. This decrease in Kupffer cell function has been associated with increased mortality in septic animals [10]. Often animal studies have demonstrated increased bacteremia when large

Table 2. Medium chain triglycerides advantages

1. Hydrolyzed at the intestinal brush border and transported to liver by portal circulation
2. Efficiently oxidized to acetate, ketones and CO_2
3. Decreased adipose tissue storage
4. Oxidized by a carnitine-independent pathway
5. Decreased blockage of the RES and improved bacterial clearance

amounts (75% of nonprotein calories) of LCT are infused and have also demonstrated that when lipid was greater than 50% of the nonprotein calories the bacterial sequestration was increased in the lung and uptake in both the spleen and the liver decreased. The use of solutions containing MCT improved the host defense, particularly in terms of the RES function. In animals the hepatic clearance of radiolabeled pseudomonas was improved with the MCT solutions, with decreased bacteria being cleared by the lung [10]. In human studies the hepatic clearance of ^{99}Tc-sulfur was also improved with an MCT/LCT lipid infusion as compared to an LCT infusion (E. A. Mascioli, personal communication). In these patient trials the MCT/LCT mixture did not result in any significant ketotic or lactic acidosis [19].

These animal and human studies have clearly demonstrated improved substrate utilization and immune function with an MCT/LCT lipid mixture. Subsequently, a number of different mixtures of the lipids were investigated. The mixtures were either a physical mix of the MCT and LCT oils in various proportions, or a mixture of the lipids that was hydrolyzed and then allowed to reesterify. The result of the reesterification was randomly formed combinations of the MCT/LCT mixture on the glycerol backbone. These arranged triglycerides have been named structured lipids (SL). It was Jandacek et al. who demonstrated that MCT and LCT were efficiently absorbed from intestine when they were in the form of a SL [22]. In particular, it was the SL with the MCT on the 1 and 3 position and the LCT on the 2 position that the absorption of both lipids was most effective. These findings were confirmed by Hubbard and McKenna, and the SL concept was advanced [23]. The mechanism for blood clearance of a lipid emulsion is not completely understood. The lipid emulsions are supplied as triglycerides with a phospholipid to provide the emulsion. Once in the blood stream the emulsion particles adsorb apoproteins from the circulating lipoproteins and, the principle apoproteins adsorbed are A and C, which adhere to the outer surface of the particle. These apoproteins then provide the activation of the lipoprotein lipase needed for hydrolysis of the triglyceride. It has been noted that although MCT is rapidly cleared from the blood stream its clearance was delayed when the MCT was infused with LCT [24]. Other investigators have found that the co-infusion of MCT and LCT results in a faster clearance of the LCT [25, 26]. In vitro studies of LPL action on MCT, LCT, a SL, and a physical mix of the lipids found that the MCT was hydrolyzed more rapidly. In addition the study found that the hydrolysis of the SL was slower then the physical mix [27]. These in vitro assays did not correlate with the in vivo blood lipid profiles. However, the action of LPL on the lipids, particularly the SL in sepsis, maybe an important issue.

The use of MCT/LCT SL in stressed animal models showed improved nitrogen balance, higher serum albumins, and increased protein synthesis in liver and muscle [28–30] (Table 3). The sparing of body protein with both enteral and parenteral routes of administration of the SL was most evident with a mixture of 60%–75% MCT and 40%–25% LCT. When the mixture of MCT/LCT was on a 50:50 molar basis there was no improvement in the protein

Table 3. MCT/LCT SL effect in animals with thermal injury

Parameter	LCT	MCT	Physical mix	SL
Oxygen consumption (μmol/100g per hour)	4973 ± 312	4856 ± 287	5416 ± 394	5475 ± 562
Energy expenditure (kcal/kg per day)	134 ± 8	130 ± 8	147 ± 4	149 ± 15
Cumulative nitrogen balance (mg)	-12 ± 9	-29 ± 20	$37 \pm 11*$	$56 \pm 21*$
Rectus muscle fractional synthetic rate (%/day)	2.4 ± 0.8	2.60 ± 0.1	$3.3 \pm 0.1**$	$3.1 \pm 0.2**$
Liver fractional synthetic rate (%/day)	32 ± 4	28 ± 3	$46 \pm 3**$	$52 \pm 5*$

$*p < .05$ different from LCT and MCT; $** < .05$ different from LCT. Adapted from [30]

sparing effect. In addition, animal studies using an intravenous injection of radiolabeled pseudomonas indicated that the SL resulted in improved RES function as compared to the LCT and was similar to the MCT emulsion. In addition, the SL resulted in significantly less bacteria being sequestered in the lung [10] (Table 4). Thus the SL containing the MCT/LCT mix has proven to have several advantages in the injured state (Table 5).

There is increasing evidence that the type of LCT that is used in stressed states is important, particularly with host defence. The recent evidence is that omega-3, omega-9, and omega-6 must all be considered in the lipid support of the patient. Investigations using omega-3 polyunsaturated fatty acids (PUFA) have shown that there are alterations in the prostaglandin metabolites, and

Table 4. Organ sequestration in thermally injured animals intravenous administered isotope labeled pseudomonas

Lipid source	Liver	Spleen	Lung
LCT	31.4 ± 7.1	10.0 ± 2.7	4.5 ± 1.7
MCT	$43.5 \pm 3.1*$	7.0 ± 0.1	$2.4 \pm 0.3*$
SL	$41.5 \pm 1.5*$	7.0 ± 0.1	$2.9 \pm 0.5*$

$*p < .05$ versus the LCT.
The data are the percentage of infused counts per minute of the pseudomonas that were counted in the organ Adapted from [10].

Table 5. MCT/LCT SL: advantages

1. Have the advantages of the MCT
2. Reduce toxicity of the MCT
3. Improve LCT adsorption form the intestine
4. Improve LCT clearance form the blood
5. Improve protein sparing in injured animals
6. Decrease protein oxidation by leucine kinetics
7. Increase protein synthesis in the liver and muscle
8. Improve hepatic RES bacteria clearance
9. Decreased bacterial sequestration in the lung

changes in the physical characteristics of the cell membrane and in the function of membrane-based receptors [31–33]. These biological effects have been noted in both animal and human studies. The physical changes of the cell membrane resulting from omega-3 PUFA results in a cell membrane with more fluidity, resulting in alterations in cellular adherence. The result of the fluidity change is thought to change receptor function, but more investigation is needed in both of these areas. There is experimental evidence that the omega-3 is a competitive substrate for arachidonic acid cyclooxygenase and lipoxygenase pathways. Both the eicosapentaenoic and docosahexaenoic acid in omega-3 oils result is the now well described alterations in both leukotrienes and thromboxanes. With cell stimulation there is release of arachidonic acid by phospholipases. Arachidonic acid is then converted into the 2 series of prostaglandins including PGI_2, PGE_2, and PGF_2, as well as the 4 series of leukotrienes, including LTB_4 and LTC_4. These are all very biologically active in terms of immunosuppression, activation of the inflammatory response, increased vasopermeability, and increased neutrophil migration and activation. The omega-3 components, including both eicosapentaenoic and docosahexaenoic acid, result in production of the prostaglandin 3 series and the leukotriene 5 series, both of which are less biologically active. Consequently, there is less vasoconstriction and inflammatory stimulation. It appears that the regulation of the vasoactive tone and the state of regulation of the immune response is a balance between the biologically active components of the 2 series and the 4 series and the metabolites from the 3 series and the 5 series. By adjusting the amount of LCT in the diet, this balance can be regulated. Investigations in which the level of the prostaglandins in the 2 series and the 4 series were decreased using cyclooxygenase inhibitors resulted in improved immune function in thermally injured animals [34]. There is now good evidence that the key cells to the injury response, both neutrophils and macrophages, are altered by the use of the omega-3 PUFA. The omega-3 PUFA result in significantly less stimulation and cytokine production [31, 35]. The neutrophil oxidative burst and chemotaxis are reduced with increased omega-3 PUFA in the diet [36]. In addition, there is evidence that omega-3 PUFA can decrease the transmembrane signal and the prostaglandin response in isolated Kupffer cells [37]. These changes in cell function were associated with changes in the cell free fatty acid composition, reflecting the dietary intake. In animal studies in which the diet was 36% lipid calories a diet of omega-3 PUFA resulted in improved survival to endotoxemia [38]. This was associated with a significant decrease in membrane arachidonic acid. Studies using a similar diet of omega-3 PUFA demonstrated a decreased febrile response to interleukin-1 [39]. This is supported by the decreased cytokine response of isolated macrophages from animals and humans fed on diets high in omega-3 PUFA [31]. Emulsions of omega-3 have been infused into animals for short periods of time, resulting in improved survival with endotoxemia. This was associated with improved mixed venous oxidation and decreased lactic acidosis [40]. These results were possibly due to the alterations in prostaglandin metabolites but also due to the decreased cytokine production.

The subsequent generation of SL has attempted to take advantage of the omega-3 PUFA effects and the need for MCT to be infused with LCT. In animals fed with a SL of 60% MCT and 40% omega-3, and who received a thermal injury, the SL animals had improved nitrogen balance, increased protein synthesis, decreased protein oxidation, and a reduced energy expenditure as compared to LCT-fed animals [41] (Table 6). The results were explained as the improved protein sparing of the MCT-based SL with the decreased energy expenditure resulting from the omega-3. In animals infused with a SL of MCT/omega-3 PUFA there was an improved cardiovascular response to an endotoxemia with no significant acidemia and stable bicarbonate levels throughout the endotoxin exposure as compared to a LCT group [40, 42]. In animals fed on a SL of MCT and omega-3 PUFA and then starved for 48 h there was still evidence of a metabolic improvement to a thermal injury [43]. These data show that the dietary effect of the SL was maintained, indicating that the lipids had a lasting effect on the cell membrane composition. RES or other immune studies have not been conducted in these animal experiments.

There is some evidence that the use of SL will improve host defence with tumors [44, 45]. The SL used was based on MCT with omega-3 and its was compared intravenously with both a physical mix of the lipids and a LCT emulsion. Using isotope protein kinetics, the SL resulted in improved protein sparing as compared to the other infusions. The tumor protein turnover in the tumor was increased with the SL as compared to the other lipids; however, the tumor growth was reduced with the animals receiving the SL [44]. In a separate experiment rats with sarcoma was infused with a SL of MCT/omega-3. The animals were then treated with or without a tumor necrosis factor (TNF) infusion to determine both the tumor and host response. In animals who received both the TNF and the SL, the tumor volume was reduced the most, while the animal carcass weight and nitrogen balance were better maintained. Protein kinetic studies indicated that the host protein metabolism was best achieved with the combination of the TNF and the SL. These data suggest that a

Table 6. MCT/omega-3 SL effect in thermal injured animals

Parameter	LCT	SL
Oxygen consumption (μmol/100 per hour)	7691 ± 175	7168 ± 242*
Energy expenditure (kcal/kg per day)	208 ± 4	194 ± 7*
Total liver weight (g/100 g body weight)	4.14 ± 0.09	4.58 ± 0.21*
Total liver protein (mg/100g body weight)	833 ± 17	910 ± 30**
Cumulative nitrogen balance (mg)	28 ± 22	82 ± 18**
Whole body kinetics		
% Leucine flux oxidized	36.5 ± 1.5	28.5 ± 1.4***
S/Q	63.5 ± 1.5	71.5 ± 1.4***

*$p < .05$; **$p < .025$; ***$p < .0005$.
S/Q is the ratio of protein synthesis to leucine appearance.
Adapted from [41].

SL with omega-3 will promote cytokine tumor inhibition while reducing the associated host protein catabolism [45].

Other investigations looking at specific immune effects of SL have some conflicting data. Mice were raised on different diets of lipids including the physical mixes and SL. Although both the MCT and the omega-3 decreased prostaglandin production by stimulated isolated peritoneal macrophages, the SL was not as effective [31]. This has raised a question about the effectiveness of the free fatty acids from the SL and the possibility of different pools of substrate being available to the cyclooxygenase and the lipoxygenase enzymes. More recently a SL that was enzymatically prepared with MCT and omega-3 was used in animals studies of endotoxemia. The lipid emulsion was compared to a LCT emulsion. In vitro lymphocyte proliferation studies were done with concanavalin A stimulation (Tables 7, 8). The animals infused with the SL had a significant decrease in the lymphocyte proliferation as compared to the saline or LCT groups. Despite this there was evidence that the other biological effects of the SL with the omega-3 did not occur. Indeed the SL animals had increased levels of PGE_2, a lactic acidosis, and decreased survival. It is possible that the latter fact was related to the significantly decreased lymphocyte response.

The present evidence is that SL may play a role in the nutritional support of the critically ill patient and improve the host defence. Using SL decreases the

Table 7. Enzymatically prepared MCT/omega-3 SL infusion in endotoxemic rats: lymphocyte proliferation to concanavalin A stimulation

	Concanavalin A (µg/ml)	
	0	3.125
LCT	0.5 ± 0.1	43.6 ± 19.2
SL	0.4 ± 0.1	7.7 ± 2.1*

*Data are counts (× 1000) per minute.
Animals were infused with endotoxin 1 mg/kg per day.
*$p < .05$ versus LCT.

Table 8. Enzymatically prepared MCT/omega-3 SL infusion in endotoxemic rats: metabolic parameters

Parameter	LCT	SL
Mean arterial pressure (mmHg)	82.5 ± 8.40	66.2 ± 12.3*
Blood pH	7.51 ± 0.04	7.38 ± 0.06*
Blood lactate (mmol/l)	4.40 ± 0.90	8.00 ± 0.50*
Neutrophil count (× 1000/mm³)	4.70 ± 0.90	2.70 ± 1.00*
Thromboxane B2 (pg/ml)	185 ± 28	290 ± 38*

Data are based on final value after 12 h of endotoxin infusion (1 mg/kg per day).
*$p < .05$ versus LCT.

depression of host defences associated with LCT. The SL provide the opportunity to take advantage of the efficient MCT substrate utilization and the biological activity of specific LCT such as omega-3. Enterally, the SL results in a more efficient absorption of the LCT, while parenterally there is evidence of improved LCT clearance. The SL reduces the stress-induced protein catabolism, and improves net protein synthesis in the liver. Specifically the use of SL results in improved RES function and decreased bacterial sequestration in the lungs, which is an important host defence to endotoxin and in particular the loss of the gastrointestinal barrier function. The current state of research in structured lipids will need to determine the effect of these designer molecules in sepsis and injury, particularly with regard to specific host defence.

References

1. Mochizuki H, Trocki O, Dominioni L et al. (1984) Optimal lipid content for enteral diets following thermal injury. JPEN 8:638–646
2. Macfie J, Smith RC, Hill GL (1981) Glucose or fat as a nonprotein energy source. Gastroenterology 80:103–107
3. Stoner HB, Little RA, Frayn KN (1983) The effect of sepsis on the oxidation of carbohydrate and fat. Br J Surg 70:32–35
4. Yamazaki K, Maiz A, Sobrado J et al. (1984) Hypocaloric lipid emulsions and amino acid metabolism in injured rats. JPEN 8:361–366
5. Du Toit DF, Villet WT, Heydenrych J (1978) Fat-emulsion deposition in mononuclear phagocytic system. Lancet II:898
6. Forbes GB (1978) Splenic lipidosis after administration of intravenous fat emulsions. J Clin Path 31:765–771
7. Fischer GW, Wilson SR, Hunter KW et al. (1980) Diminished bacterial defences with Intralipid. Lancet II:819–820
8. van Haelst UJ, Sengers RC (1979) Effect of parenteral nutrition with lipids on the human liver. Arch Cell Pathol B 22:323–332
9. Alexander JW, Saito H, Trocki O et al. (1986) The importance of lipid type in the diet after burn injury. Ann Surg 204:1–8
10. Sobrado J, Moldawer LL, Pomposelli JJ et al. (1985) Lipid emulsions and reticuloendothelial system function in healthy and burned guinea pigs. Am J Clin Nutr 42:855–863
11. Robin AP, Greenwood MR, Askanazi J (1981) Influence of total parenteral nutrition on tissue lipoprotein lipase activity during chronic and acute illness. Ann Surg 194:681–686
12. Robin AP, Askanazi J, Greenwood MR (1981) Lipoprotein lipase activity in surgical patients: influence of trauma and infection. Surgery 90:401–408
13. Harris RL, Frenkel RA, Cotter R et al. (1982) Lipid mobilization and metabolism after thermal trauma. J Trauma 22:194–198
14. Babayan VK (1987) Medium chain triglycerides and structured lipids. Lipids 22:417–420
15. Swift LL, Hill JO, Peters JC et al. (1990) Medium-chain fatty acids: evidence for incorporation into chylomicron triglycerides in humans. Am J Clin Nutr 52:834–836
16. Sailer D, Muller M (1981) Medium chain triglycerides in parenteral nutrition. JPEN 5:115–119
17. Bach A, Guisard D, Debry G et al. (1974) Metabolic effects following a medium chain triglycerides load in dogs: V. Influence of the perfusion rate. Arch. Int Physiol Biochim 82:705–719
18. Cotter R, D'Alleinne C (1989) Medium-chain triglycerides. A Preclinical Perspective. In: Kinney JM, Borum PR (eds) Perspectives in clinical nutrition. Urban and Schwarzenberg, Baltimore
19. Mascioli EA, Porter KA, Randall S, Kater G, Ghosn SJ, Babayan VK, Bistrian BR, Blackburn GL (1989) Metabolic response to intravenous medium-chain triglycerides. In: Kinney JM, Borun PR (eds) Perspectives in clinical nutrition. Urban and Schwarzenberg, Baltimore

20. Mascioli EA, Randall S, Porter KA et al. (1991) Thermogenesis from intravenous medium-chain triglycerides. JPEN 15:27–31
21. Redmond HP, Shou J, Kelly CJ, Leon P, Cheng BA, Rush J, Daly JM (1991) Immune responses in mild and severe protein-calorie malnutrition. JPEN 15 [Suppl]:21S
22. Jandacek RJ, Whiteside JA, Holcombe BN et al. (1987) The rapid hydrolysis and efficient absorption of triglycerides with octanoic acid in the 1 and 3 positions and long-chain fatty acid in the 2 position. Am J Clin Nutr 45:940–945
23. Hubbard VS, McKenna MC (1987) Absorption of safflower oil and structured lipid preparations in patients with cystic fibrosis. Lipids 22:424–428
24. Heird WC, Grundy SM, Hubbard VS (1986) Structured lipids and their use in clinical nutrition. Am J Clin Nutr 43:320–324
25. Young SK, Johnson RC, Cotter R et al. (1984) Competitive interaction between medium- and long-chain lipid emulsions. Fed Proc 43:865
26. Cotter R, Taylor CA, Johnson R et al. (1987) A metabolic comparison of a pure long-chain triglyceride lipid emulsion (LCT) and various medium-chain triglyceride (MCT)-LCT combination emulsions in dogs. Am J Clin Nutr 45:927–939
27. Lutz O, Lave T, Meraihi Z et al. (1989) Activities of lipoprotein lipase on long- and medium-chain triglyceride emulsions used in parenteral nutrition. Metabolism 38:507–513
28. Mok KT, Maiz A, Yamazaki K et al. (1984) Structured medium-chain and long-chain triglyceride emulsions are superior to physical mixtures in sparing body protein in the burned rat. Metabolism 33:910–915
29. DeMichele SJ, Karlstad MD, Babayan VK et al. (1988) Enhanced skeletal muscle and liver protein synthesis with structured lipid in enterally-fed burned rats. Metabolism 37:787–795
30. DeMichele SJ, Karlstad MD, Bistrian BR et al. (1989) Enteral nutrition with structured lipid: effect on protein metabolism in thermal injury. Am J Clin Nutr 50:1295–1302
31. Kinsella JE, Lokesh B, Broughton S et al. (1990) Dietary polyunsatured fatty acids and eicosanoids: potential effects on the modulation of inflammatory and immune cells: an overview. Nutrition (London) 6(S):24–44
32. Kinsella JE (1990) Lipids, membrane receptors, and enzymes: effects of dietary fatty acids. JPEN 14:200S–217S
33. Kinsella JE, Lokesh B (1990) Dietary lipids, eicosanoids, and the immune system. Crit Care Med 18:S94–S113
34. Freeman TR, Shelby J (1988) Effects of anti-PGE antibody on cell mediated immune response in thermally injured mice. J Trauma 28:190–194
35. Lokesh BR, Black JM, Kinsella JE (1989) The suppression of eicosanoid synthesis by peritoneal macrophages is influenced by the ratio of dietary docosahexaenoic acid to linoleic acid. Lipids 24:589–593
36. Lee TH, Hoover RL, Williams JD et al. (1985) Effect of dietary enrichment with eicosapentaenoic and docosahexaenoic acids on in vitro neutrophil and monocyte leukotriene generation and neutrophil function. New Engl J Med 312:1217–1224
37. Bankey PE, Billiar TR, Wang WY et al. (1989) Modulation of Kupffer cell membrane phospholipid function by n-3 polyunsaturated fatty acids. J Surg Res 46:439–444
38. Mascioli E, Leader L, Flores E et al. (1988) Enhanced survival to endotoxin in guinea pigs fed IV fish oil emulsion. Lipids 23:623–625
39. Pomposelli JJ, Mascioli EA, Bistrian BR et al. (1989) Attenuation of the febrile response in guinea pigs by fish oil enriched diets. JPEN 13:136–140
40. Pomposelli JJ, Flores E, Hirschberg Y et al. (1990) Short-term TPN containing n-3 fatty acids ameliorate lactic acidosis induced by endotoxin in guinea pigs. Am J Clin Nutr 52:548–552
41. Teo TC, DeMichele SJ, Selleck KM et al. (1989) Administration of structured lipid composed of MCT and fish oil reduces net protein catabolism in enterally fed burned rats. Ann Surg 210:100–107
42. Teo TC, Selleck KM, Wan JMF et al. Long-term feeding with structured lipid composed of medium chain and n-3 fatty acids ameliorates endotoxic shock in guinea pigs (in press)
43. Swenson ES, Selleck KM, Babayan VK et al. Persistence of metabolic effects after long term oral feeding of a structured triglyceride derived from medium chain triglyceride and fish oil in burned and normal rats (in press)
44. Ling P, Istfan N, Babayan V et al. (1989) Effect of fish oil medium chain triglyceride structured lipid (FMS) on tumor growth and protein metabolism in Yoshida sarcoma-bearing rats. JPEN 13:5S
45. Mendez B, Crosby L, Babayan V et al. (1989) Metabolic effects of structured lipid (SL) composed of MCT and fish oil (MCT/FO) in sarcoma-bearing rats. JPEN 13:21S

Manipulation of Cytokine Synthesis Through Dietary Lipids*

S. Endres[1], S. N. Meydani[2], and C. A. Dinarello[3]

Aside from its pyrogenic effects, interleukin-1 (IL-1) influences a wide array of biological functions (reviewed in [1]). Originally described in purified material from monocyte supernatants, most effects have been confirmed using recombinant IL-1 [2]. To date the only known pharmacologic agents to reduce IL-1 synthesis are corticosteroids and cyclosporin A. We have completed a study to investigate whether dietary supplementation with n-3 fatty acids contained in fish oils affects the synthesis of IL-1 and tumor necrosis factor (TNF) [3]. The main forms of n-3 fatty acids are eicosapentaenoic acid and docosahexaenoic acid. They are scarce in a normal Western diet but occur in significant amounts in marine oils.

Since IL-1 and TNF are principal mediators of inflammation, reduced production of these cytokines may contribute to the amelioration of inflammatory symptoms in patients taking n-3 supplementation. Therefore, we decided to investigate the effects of n-3 fatty acids on the synthesis of the cytokines IL-1 and TNF.

Nine healthy volunteers added 16 g of fish-oil concentrate (MaxEPA) per day to their normal diet. In vitro production of IL-1 and TNF was determined by incubating peripheral blood mononuclear cells for 24 h with different stimuli. At the end of the incubation, the cells were lysed by freeze-thawing to obtain total cytokine, i.e., cell-associated plus secreted cytokine. IL-1β [4], IL-1α [5], and TNF [6] were measured by specific radioimmunoassays (RIA).

Figure 1 illustrates the production of IL-1β during the course of the study. Our findings demonstrate that n-3 fatty acid supplementation reduced the IL-1β production induced by endotoxin. The effect was most pronounced 10 weeks after stopping the supplementation and suggests prolonged incorporation of n-3 fatty acids into a pool of circulating mononuclear cells (MNC). The capacity of the MNC from these donors to synthesize IL-1β returned to the presupplement

* Supported by grants from the Deutsche Forschungsgemeinschaft (En 169/2-2) and the National Institutes of Health (al-15614)
[1] Medizinische Klinik, Klinikum Innenstadt der Universität München, Ziemssenstr. 1, 8000 Munich 2, FRG
[2] USDA Human Nutrition Research Center on Aging, Tufts University, New England Medical Center, Boston, MA 02111, USA
[3] Department of Medicine, Tufts University, New England Medical Center, Boston, MA 02111, USA

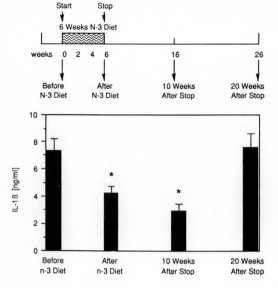

Fig. 1. Influence of *n*-3 fatty acids on production of IL-1β stimulated with endotoxin. Mononuclear cells were incubated for 24 h with 1 ng endotoxin/ml. IL-1β was determined by RIA. The *bars* represent the mean values for nine volunteers with *error bars* as the standard error of the mean. An *asterisk* indicates significant difference from the baseline (before *n*-3 diet) at $p < 0.05$

level 20 weeks after ending the supplementation. Similar results were observed when we measured IL-1α and TNF.

There are several clinical implications of these findings. They form a pathophysiologic rationale for therapeutic trials with *n*-3 fatty acids in certain diseases like rheumatoid arthritis [7] with documented involvement of inflammatory cytokines such as IL-1 and TNF.

Suppression of IL-1 and TNF-synthesis by *n*-3 fatty acids has been found in further studies in humans and in animal models. The study designs and results are compared in Table 1. While suppressive effects of *n*-3 fatty acids on neutrophil [13] and monocyte function have been demonstrated, little is known about the effect of *n*-3 fatty acids on the function of lymphocytes [14]. Recently, we determined formation of interleukin-2 (IL-2) in the samples of MNC stimulated with phytohemagglutinin (PHA) from the above-described study. In addition we studied the effect of oral *n*-3 fatty acids on PHA-induced proliferation of MNC, a functional parameter closely linked to IL-2 production and effect [15]. IL-2 synthesis from stimulated peripheral blood MNC was suppressed from 6.2 ng/ml at baseline to 2.2 ng/ml 10 weeks after the end of *n*-3 fatty acid supplementation (65% decrease; $p = 0.04$). At the same time, PHA-induced proliferation of MNC was suppressed by 70% from the presupplement level. IL-2 production returned to the premedication level at the end of the studies. These findings are in accordance with decreased IL-2 production after *n*-3 fatty acid supplementation in female volunteers found by Meydani et al. [12]. Both reduced IL-2 production and decreased MNC proliferation may be linked to the decreased production of IL-1 in the same cell population which we had previously found [4].

Table 1. In vivo studies examining the effect of *n*-3 fatty acids on cytokine production MNC, mononuclear cells.

Source	Model	Cells	Intervention (period in weeks)	Suppression (%)	
[3, 8]	Healthy volunteers	MNC	*n*-3 as triglyceride (6)	IL-1β	61
				TNF	40
[9]	Rats	Kupffer cells	*n*-3 as triglyceride (6)	IL-1	45
				TNF	81
[10]	Mouse, diabetic	Peritoneal macrophages	*n*-3 as ethylester (6)	IL-1	27
[11]	Patients with rheumatoid arthritis	MNC	*n*-3 as ethylester (24)	IL-1	41
[12]	Healthy volunteers	MNC	*n*-3 as triglyceride (12)	IL-1β	50
				TNF	52

Suppression of cytokine production by dietary *n*-3 fatty acid supplementation may have clinical implications. To date, a suppression of the magnitude we observed can only be achieved by administration of glucocorticoids or cyclosporin A, with their known side effects, particularly during long-term administration. In a recent study, *n*-3 fatty acids even enhanced cyclosporin A-induced immunosuppression in an animal transplant model [16].

Acknowledgements. The authors wish to acknowledge the help of Reza Ghorbani, Bhanu Sinha, and Doris Stoll in these studies.

References

1. Dinarello CA (1989) Interleukin-1 and its biologically related cytokines. Adv Immunol 44:153–205
2. Dinarello CA, Cannon JG, Mier JW, Bernheim HA, LoPreste G, Lynn DL, Love RN, Webb AC, Auron PE, Reuben RC, Rich A, Wolff SM, Putney SD (1986) Multiple biological activities of human recombinant interleukin-1. J Clin Invest 77:1734–1739
3. Endres S, Ghorbani R, Kelley VE, Georgilis K, Lonnemann G, van der Meer JW, Cannon JG, Rogers TS, Klempner MS, Weber PC, Schaefer EJ, Wolff SM, Dinarello CA (1989) The effect of dietary supplementation with *n*-3 fatty acids on the synthesis of interleukin-1 and tumor necrosis factor by mononuclear cells. N Engl J Med 320:265–271
4. Endres S, Ghorbani R, Lonnemann G, van der Meer JWM, Dinarello CA (1988) Measurement of immunoreactive interleukin-1β from human mononuclear cells: optimization of recovery, intrasubject consistency and comparison with interleukin-1α and tumor necrosis factor. Clin Immunol Immunopathol 49:424–438
5. Lonnemann G, Endres S, van der Meer JWM, Cannon JG, Dinarello CA (1988) A radioimmunoassay for human interleukin-1 alpha: measurement of IL-1 alpha produced in vitro by human blood mononuclear cells stimulated with endotoxin. Lymphokine Res 7:75–85
6. van der Meer JWM, Endres S, Lonnemann G, Cannon JG, Ikejima T, Okusawa S, Gelfand JA, Dinarello CA (1988) Concentrations of immunoreactive human tumor necrosis factor alpha produced by human mononuclear cells in vitro. J Leukocyte Biol 43:216–223

7. Krane SM, Dayer JM, Simon LS, Byrne S (1985) Mononuclear cell conditioned medium containing mononuclear cell factor (MCF), homologous with interleukin-1, stimulates collagen and fibronectin synthesis by adherent rheumatoid synovial cells: effects of prostagladin E_2 and indomethacin. Coll Relat Res 5:99–117

8. Endres S, Kelly VE, Dinarello CA (1987) Effects of dietary omega-3 fatty acids on the in vitro production of human interleukin-1. J Leukocyte Biol 42:617 (abstract)

9. Billiar T, Bankey P, Svingen B et al. (1988) Fatty acid intake and Kupffer cell function: fish oil alters eicosanoid and monokine production to endotoxin stimulation. Surgery 104:343–349

10. Linn T, Noke M, Woehrle M et al. (1989) Fish oil-enriched diet and reduction of low-dose streptozocin-induced hyperglycemia. Diabetes38:1402–1411

11. Kremer J, Lawrence D, Jubiz W et al. (1990) Dietary fish oil and olive oil supplementation in patients with rheumatoid arthritis. Clinical and immunological effects. Arthritis Rheum 33:810–820

12. Meydani SN, Endres S, Woods MM, Goldin BR, Soo C, Morrill-Labrode A, Dinarello CA, Gorbach SL (1991) Oral n-3 fatty acid supplementation suppresses cytokine production and lymphocyte proliferation: comparison in young and older women. J Nutr (in press)

13. Lee TH, Hoover RL, Williams JD, Sperling RI, Ravalese III J, Spur BW, Robinson DR, Corey EJ, Lewis RA, Austen KF (1985) Effect of dietary enrichment with eicosapentaenoic and docosahexaenoic acids on in vitro neutrophil and monocyte leukotriene generation and neutrophil function. N Engl J Med 312:1217–1224

14. Payan DG, Wong MYS, Chernov-Rogan T et al. (1986) Alterations in human leukocyte function induced by ingestion of eicosapentaenoic acid. J Clin Immunol 6:402–410

15. Endres S, Meydani SN, Ghorbani R, Schindler R, Dempsey RA, Dinarello CA (1991) Mononuclear cell proliferation and interleukin-2 production are suppressed by dietary n-3 fatty acids but enhanced by oral aspirin (manuscript submitted)

16. Kelly VE, Kirkman RL, Bastos M, Barrett LV, Strom TB (1989) Enhancement of immunosuppression by substitution of fish oil for olive oil as a vehicle for cyclosporine. Transplantation 48:98–102

Dietary Fish Oil Prevents Postischemic Leukocyte/Endothelium Interaction Through Inhibition of Leukotriene Biosynthesis

H. A. Lehr[1], D. Nolte[1], C. Hübner[2], and K. Messmer[1]

Introduction

The manifestations of reperfusion injury are characterized by the chemotactic accumulation, aggregation, and adhesion of circulating leukocytes to the microvascular endothelium [1]. Through the release of toxic degranulation products and oxygen metabolites, adherent leukocytes contribute to the final extent of reperfusion injury, characterized by the breakdown of capillary perfusion [2] and the loss of endothelial integrity [3]. The central role of leukocyte adhesion in the pathophysiologic sequelae of reperfusion injury has been inferred from experiments where ischemia/reperfusion injury was significantly reduced by neutrophil depletion with antineutrophil serum or by monoclonal antibodies directed towards leukocyte adhesion receptors [1].

Leukotrienes, metabolites of arachidonate (AA) produced in the 5-lipoxygenase pathway, initiate many of the microcirculatory manifestations of ischemia/reperfusion injury. While the cysteinyl leukotrienes affect microvessel permeability [4], leukotriene (LT) B_4 has been implicated in the process of leukocyte accumulation and adhesion to the microvascular endothelium [5].

This manuscript summarizes the results of two studies in which we demonstrate that the manifestations of ischemia/reperfusion injury can be effectively prevented by pharmacologic and dietary inhibition of leukotriene biosynthesis.

Methods

For intravital fluorescence microscopy, we used the dorsal skinfold chamber model in awake Syrian golden hamsters [6]. This model permits the microscopic quantification of leukocyte/endothelium interaction, functional capillary density, macromolecular leakage, and the microhemodynamic parameters, vessel diameter and red cell velocity, in postcapillary venules of a thin striated muscle contained within the observation window. Chamber implantation and intravital microscopy were performed as previously described in detail [7, 8, 9].

[1] Institute of Surgical Research, University of Munich, FRG
[2] Department of Pediatrics, University of Hamburg, FRG

Host Defense Dysfunction
in Trauma, Shock and Sepsis
Eds. Faist/Meakins/Schildberg
© Springer-Verlag, Berlin Heidelberg 1993

A 4-h ischemia was induced to the chamber tissue by gently pressing the skin muscle against the cover slip with a silicone pad and an adjustable screw, just sufficient to empty the blood vessels. Leukocyte/endothelium interaction, functional capillary density, and plasma extravasation (parameters described in the legends to the Figs. 1–3) were assessed in 4–6 postcapillary venules per chamber prior to ischemia and 0.5 h, 2 h, and 24 h after reperfusion. Four weeks prior to the experiments the animals were fed with either standard laboratory chow or a diet supplemented with 5% by weight of a fish oil concentrate (EICOSAPEN, Hormon Chemie Pharma, Munich, Germany). In a third group of animals, leukotriene biosynthesis was inhibited pharmacologically by MK-886 (10 mg/kg, i.v., starting 10 min prior to ischemia and until 2 h after reperfusion; MK-886 was kindly provided by Dr. A. W. Ford-Hutchinson, Merck Frosst, Canada).

Results

In control animals, ischemia/reperfusion elicited leukocyte adhesion to the microvascular endothelium with a maximum 0.5 h after reperfusion (Fig. 1). As a consequence, functional capillary density decreased to about 60% of the preischemic baseline situation (Fig. 2). Although a partial recovery of capillary perfusion was observed, about 30% of all capillaries were irreversibly excluded

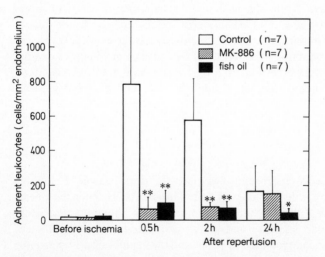

Fig. 1. Leukocyte/endothelium interaction in postcapillary venules before ischemia and 0.5 h, 2 h, and 24 h after reperfusion. For contrast enhancement leukocytes were stained in vivo with acridine orange (0.5 mg/kg per minute i.v.). Adherent leukocytes were defined as cells that did not move or detach from the endothelium within 1 min and expressed as number of cells per millimeter squared of endothelial surface. Measurements were performed on control hamsters ($n = 7$, *empty bars*), MK-886-treated hamsters ($n = 7$, *hatched bars*), and fish oil-fed hamsters ($n = 7$, *black bars*). Data given in the figure are means ± SD. *$p < 0.05$, **$p < 0.01$ vs control hamsters (Wilcoxon test)

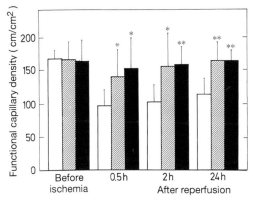

Fig. 2. Functional capillary density before ischemia and 0.5 h, 2 h, and 24 h after reperfusion. For contrast enhancement, plasma was stained in vivo with fluorescein-isothiocyanate-labeled dextran (FITC-dextran, M_r 150000; 5 µg in 100 µl saline, i.v.). Functional capillary density was assessed planimetrically as the total length of red cell-perfused capillaries per observation area. Measurements were performed in nine different sites per observation chamber in control hamsters ($n = 7$, *empty bars*) MK-886-treated hamsters ($n = 7$, *hatched bars*), and fish oil-fed hamsters ($n = 7$, *black bars*). Data given in the figure are means $\pm$ SD. *$p < 0.05$, **$p < 0.01$ vs control hamsters (Wilcoxon test)

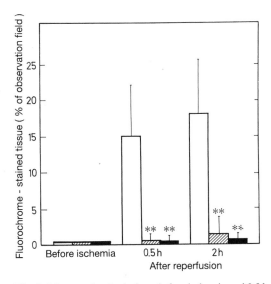

Fig. 3. Macromolecular leakage before ischemia and 0.5 h, 2 h, and 24 h after reperfusion. Macromolecular leakage was assessed by planimetric quantification of the area where fluorescein-labeled plasma (FITC-dex-tran, M_r 150000; 5 µg in 100 µl saline, i.v.), had extravasated across the functionally impaired endothelium of postcapillary venules into the interstitial space, given as percentage of the observation field. Measurements were performed in control hamsters ($n = 7$, *empty bars*), MK-886-treated hamsters ($n = 7$, *hatched bars*), and fish oil-fed hamsters ($n = 7$, *black bars*). Data given in the figure are means $\pm$ SD. *$p < 0.05$, **$p < 0.01$ vs control hamsters (Wilcoxon test)

from the circulation (Fig. 2). Endothelial integrity, assessed by the extravasation of fluorescein-labeled macromolecules, was impaired in the early reperfusion period (Fig. 3). In contrast to these results, the microvascular manifestations of ischemia/reperfusion injury were effectively reduced in animals treated with either MK-886 or dietary fish oil (Figs.1–3).

Discussion

These experiments demonstrate that pharmacologic leukotriene biosynthesis inhibition and dietary fish oil attenuate postischemic leukocyte adhesion to the endothelium of postcapillary venules (Fig. 1) and preserve postischemic capillary perfusion and endothelial integrity (Figs. 2, 3).

The concept that leukotrienes are involved in ischemia/reperfusion injury has been supported in the same animal model by the demonstration that (1) leukotrienes accumulate in the postischemic muscle tissue, and (2) the adhesion of circulating leukocytes to the endothelium and the extravasation of plasma into the interstitial space can be stimulated by topical superfusion onto the chamber tissue of LTB_4 and LTD_4, respectively [7].

The generation of biologically active leukotrienes from AA can not only be suppressed pharmacologically, but also by the incorporation into leukocyte membrane phospholipids of eicosapentaenoate (EPA), the major n-3 fatty acid contained in fish oil [10]. In fact, fish oil feeding to the hamsters in our study resulted in a drop in the AA/EPA weight percentage ratio in leukocyte lipids from 39.0 ± 9.9 to 1.8 ± 0.3 [8], which corresponds well with values reported in human subjects before and after 4–6 weeks on fish oil-supplemented diets and which resulted in a marked inhibition of leukotriene biosynthesis and leukocyte function [11]. Although dietary fish oil exerts a variety of further metabolic changes including inhibited generation of oxygen free radicals, platelet activating factor, interleukin-1, tumor necrosis factor, and endothelium-derived relaxing factor [12], which have all been implicated as mediators in postischemic leukocyte/endothelium interaction, the similarities between the results obtained for dietary fish oil and MK-886 suggest that under the conditions of our experiment, the efficacy of dietary fish oil can be attributed to the inhibition of leukotriene formation.

The demonstration that the microvascular manifestations of reperfusion injury can be effectively attenuated by pharmacologic leukotriene biosynthesis inhibition and dietary fish oil may open the way to novel prophylactic and therapeutic strategies in the clinical setting of localized or systemic ischemia.

References

1. Hernandez LA, Grisham MB, Twohig B et al. (1987) Role of neutrophils in ischemia-reperfusion-induced microvascular injury. Am J Physiol 253:H699

2. Schmid-Schönbein GW (1987) Capillary plugging by granulocytes and the no-reflow phenomenon in the microcirculation. Fed Proc 46:2397
3. Björk J, Hedqvist P, Arfors KE (1983) Increase in vascular permeability induced by leukotriene B_4 and the role of polymorphonuclear leukocytes. Inflammation 6:189
4. Hua XY, Dahlén SE, Lundberg JM, Hammarström S, Hedqvist P (1985) Leukotrienes C_4, D_4 and E_4 cause widespread and extensive plasma extravasation in the guinea pig. Naunyn-Schmiedebergs Arch Pharmacol 330:136
5. Dahlén SE, Björk J, Hedqvist P et al. (1981) Leukotrienes promote plasma leakage and leukocyte adhesion in post capillary venules: in vivo effects with relevance to the acute inflammatory response. Proc Natl Acad Sci USA 78:3887
6. Endrich B, Asaishi K, Götz A, Messmer K (1980) Technical report—a new chamber technique for microvascular studies in unanesthetized hamsters. Res Exp Med 177:125
7. Lehr HA, Guhlmann A, Nolte D, Keppler D, (Berl), Messmer K (1991) Leukotrienes as mediators in ischemia-reperfusion in a microcirculation model in the hamster. J Clin Invest 87:2036
8. Lehr HA, Hübner C, Nolte D, Kohlschütter A, Messmer K (1991) Dietary fish oil blocks the microcirculatory manifestations of ischemia/reperfusion injury in striated muscle in hamsters. Proc Natl Acad Sci USA 88:6726
9. Lehr HA, Guhlmann A, Nolte D, Keppler D, Messmer K (1991) Preservation of postischemic capillary perfusion by selective inhibition of leukotriene biosynthesis. Trans Proc 23:833
10. Lee TH, Mencia-Huerta JM, Shih C, Corey EJ, Lewis MA, Austen KF (1984) Effects of exogenous arachidonic, eicosapentaenoic, and docosahexaenoic acids on the generation of 5-lipoxygenase pathway products by ionophore-activated human neutrophils. J Clin Invest 74:1922
11. Endres S, Ghorbani R, Kelley VE, et al. (1989) The effect of dietary supplementation with n-3 polyunsaturated fatty acids on the synthesis of interleukin-1 and tumor necrosis factor by mononuclear cells. N Engl J Med 320:265
12. Leaf A (1990) Cardiovascular effects of fish oils. Beyond the platelet (editorial). Circulation 82:624

Dietary Requirement for Preformed Purine and Pyrimidine Bases for Intact Function of Cellular Immune Response: A Review

L. G. Kabbash and R. A. Forse

The nucleotides are involved with many biological pathways. They are precursors to both ribonucleic acid (RNA) and deoxyribonucleic acid (DNA) synthesis and are essential components for cellular energetics and metabolism.

A nucleotide is composed of a nitrogen base, a sugar molecule, and one or several phosphate groups. The major pyrimidine bases are uracil, cytosine, and thymidine while the major purines are adenine and guanine. With the sugar attached the base becomes a nucleoside, and the sugar involved is a pentose. Phosphate esters of the nucleoside make up the nucleotide. This paper will make reference to all of the above as a general source of purines and pyrimidines. The process for nucleotide biosynthesis is a complex interaction, and there is a dependency on amino acid metabolism for it to be effective. In addition, there is a salvage pathway for the reutilization of the nucleotides. The details for these systems can be reviewed elsewhere [1].

RNA and DNA synthesis is a fundamental component for cell proliferation. The transcription and translation associated with RNA is essential for protein synthesis and regulation of the cell metabolism. The energy needs of the cell are regulated by adenosine triphosphate which is a key component of energy transfer. Cyclic adenosine monophosphate (AMP) and guanosine monophosphate are very important mediators of hormone receptor transmembrane signals. The various forms of adenine nucleotides are components of coenzymes such as nicotinamide adenine dinucleotide (NAD), nicotinamide adenine dinucleotide phosphate (NADP), and coenzyme A. It is thus not unexpected that nucleotides should be very important in the immune system where there are several types of metabolically active cells.

The optimal growth and function of metabolically active cells requires nucleotides. It had previously been thought that dietary nucleotides were not the source of the needed nucleotides, rather that they came from de novo synthesis in the liver. Subsequently, dietary purines were shown to influence the purine pool and protein synthesis. An interesting observation is that intestinal epithelial cells lack the ability for de novo nucleotide synthesis and are dependent on the dietary source. Extensions of this observation have now established that a nucleotide-free diet will result in a significant decrease in intestinal and colonic messenger (m)RNA [2]. These nucleotide deprived mucosal cells may be

Department of Surgery, Harvard Medical School, New England Deaconess Hospital, 194 Pilgrim Road, Boston, MA 02215, USA

Host Defense Dysfunction
in Trauma, Shock and Sepsis
Eds. Faist/Meakins/Schildberg
© Springer-Verlag, Berlin Heidelberg 1993

susceptible to a maturation arrest. As a result of this dietary influence it has been well established that the breakdown product of purines, uric acid, can be altered by the dietary intake of purines. This issue with pyrimidines is much less as the breakdown products beta-alanine and beta-aminoisobutyric acid are not toxic. However, there is evidence that the dietary intake of the pyrimidines will decrease the de novo pyrimidine synthesis [3].

The first clue to the importance of nucleotides in the immune response was in the discovery of adenosine deaminase (ADA) deficiency. The loss of this enzyme results in increased adenosine and deoxyadenosine, however, there is a deficiency in deoxyguanosine triphosphate (dGTP), deoxycytidine triphosphate (dCTP), and deoxythymidine triphosphate (dTTP). This inborn error of metabolism results in severe combined immunodeficiency in which both cellular and humoral immunity are impaired [4]. The lymphoid tissues and cells from these patients are sensitive to changes in purine catabolism, whereas the other tissues and cells function normally. Another example of the importance of nucleotides is found in patients with purine nucleoside phosphorylase (PNP) deficiency. This enzyme cleaves inosine and deoxyinosine as part of the purine salvage pathway. A deficiency of this enzyme results in increased levels of inosine and deoxyinosine. In these patients this inborn error is associated with defective T cell function [5]. Finally, orotic aciduria is a hereditary disorder of pyrimidine metabolism due to the lack of orotidylate pyrophosphorylase and orotidylate decarboxylase. This defect can be overcome with dietary supplementation with uridine [1]. This illustrates the fact that dietary manipulation of the nucleotides can have an influence on nucleotide metabolism despite the long-held belief that dietary nucleotides are poorly utilized.

It is important to note that glutamine has an important role in nucleotide metabolism. Glutamine is involved with the rate-limiting step of de novo synthesis of purine and pyrimidine nucleotides. There is an increased need for glutamine in immune cells undergoing stimulation and proliferation. Inadequate levels of glutamine will result in decreased rates of lymphocyte proliferation with mitogen stimulation [6]. This may be related to the associated decreased availability of nucleotides. Thus protein malnutrition and dietary glutamine supplementation will have an influence on biosynthesis.

The effect of nucleotides on immune function was initially described in transplantation. Patients with renal allografts and who were provided with total parenteral nutrition (TPN) which was nucleotide free had a suppressed immune response to the allograft despite decreased levels of immunosuppressive drugs [7]. A number of animal models have been used to further describe the nucleotide effect on transplant survival. A model of cardiac allograft in BALB/c mice with a well-defined rejection curve was provided with different diets. Using this model, a diet which is nucleotide free produces a significant prolongation of the cardiac transplant. When the animals were provided with RNA, adenine, or uracil the cardiac allograft survival decreased, returning to the control values [8]. Additional studies looking for a synergistic effect found that a nucleotide-free diet and cyclosporine were synergistic. The combination provided the longest cardiac allograft transplant survival in the mice [7]. Of interest is that in vascularized cardiac allografts the effect of the nucleotide-free diet was only evident when combined with cylosporine. Again, the effect was synergistic, and this will be important for future transplant immunosuppression [9].

Another set of experiments has been carried out using the popliteal lymph node assay (PLNA) to measure the in vivo alloantigen lymphoproliferative response [10]. In animals the PLNA was decreased when the diet was nucleotide free. To further demonstrate this effect the animals were initially provided with a protein-free diet. This caused a decrease in the cell-mediated immune response. A number of diets were then provided to determine the ability of the diets to reverse the decreased cell-mediated immunity induced by the protein depletion. Diets with RNA or uracil produced an immune response similar to that in the animals which had not been protein depleted. Animals which had the nucleotide-free diet gained carcass weight on their diet but their cell-mediated response was still decreased. The important observation in this experiment is that although the animals were able to restore their body cell mass with the protein repletion, the absence of dietary pyrimidines resulted in a deficient immune response. More defined studies of the immune cells revealed that the lymphocytes from the animals restored on the diets with RNA and uracil had increased interleukin-2 (IL-2) receptors, as well as Mac-1 and Lyt-1 receptors. The results of these receptor analyses would indicate that the dietary nucleotides are involved with the macrophage activation of the T helper/inducer cell population [11].

The need for nucleotides is more evident in the cells which are rapidly proliferating. Experiments with lymphocytes reveal that mitogen stimulation increases both pyrimidine and purine biosynthesis. Stimulated lymphocytes will also increase the salvage of exogenous nucleotides [12]. Studies of both peripheral lymphocytes and thymocytes in the G_1 phase of the cell cycle indicate that there is no purine biosynthetic function; however, when the cells are in the S phase, de novo synthesis is present. This would suggest that cells in the G phase are dependent on the availability of exogenous nucleotides [13]. In addition, these studies suggest that the peripheral lymphocyte has decreased salvage of the pyrimidines in the G_1 phase [14]. It is the G_1 phase lymphocytes that are capable of producing the cellular mediators of the immune response [15]. In experiments with a nucleotide-free diet, there is an increase in the number of undifferentiated bone marrow cells and thymocytes [16]. These data indicate that there is a need for exogenous nucleotides for lymphocyte proliferation and differentiation. The data support the results from the cardiac allograft studies. Investigations on cyclosporine have found that the effect of the drug is to cause a T-lymphocyte G_1 phase arrest [17]. Thus it is possible to understand the synergistic effect of the nucleotide-free diet and the cyclosporine. The production of cytokines is altered by a deficiency of nucleotides. A nucleotide-free diet will result in a decrease in IL-1, IL-2, and IL-3 production. Addition of RNA or uracil restores the production of these cytokines, while adenine supplementation does not [18].

The enzymes involved with nucleotide metabolism are increased within lymphocyte subpopulations and have been used as cell markers of differentiation. Terminal deoxynucleotidyl transferase (TdT) is an example of such an enzyme for undifferentiated T cells. Investigators have identified that phytohemagglutinin (PHA) stimulation causes an increase in purine nucleotide biosynthesis and one-carbon metabolism [19]. There is substantial evidence that the enzymes related to nucleotide metabolism are regulated by cellular differentiation. ADA specific activity is increased in the cortical thymocytes as compared to the level in the lymph nodes, spleen, or the circulation [20, 21]. T helper/inducer cells express greater PNP and ADA activity as compared to the T-suppressor/cytotoxic lymphocytes [22, 23]. The activity of the enzyme ecto-5' nucleotidase (5'NT) is similar to the activity of PNP with increasing activity in mature lymphocytes. These enzyme data support the importance of nucleotide metabolism in the immune response.

Another area of investigation has been infection and systemic septicemia. This research has looked at the response to bacterial challenge as well as macrophage phagocytosis. When the mice were fed diets with RNA or uracil they had a significantly greater resistance to an intravenous challenge of *Staphylococcus aureus* and *Candida albicans* as compared to the animals fed on diets that were either nucleotide free or supplemented with adenosine [24, 25]. Of interest is the fact that the macrophages from the mice on the nucleotide-free diet had decreased phagocytosis as compared to those on the diets of RNA, uracil, or adenosine. This would suggest that, in contrast to lymphocytes, macrophage phagocytic activity can be restored with either purines or pyrimidines. In studies in which BALB/c and DBA/2 mice were fed nucleotide-free diets there was a significant decrease in their survival to a challenge of *Candida* [26]. There was also a greater survival of the *Candida* organism when isolated from the spleen of the mice. As with the previous studies, if the mice were fed with RNA or uracil but not adenine there was increased survival to the *Candida* challenge.

There has been some work in the area of tumor immunology. This work has specifically looked at the growth of tumors with a lack of nucleotides. In these experiments a deficiency of nucleotides resulted in decreased growth, and the authors concluded that nucleotides were necessary for optimal tumor growth. These tumors are derived from T lymphocytes, and this dependency on nucleotides was not demonstrated by other cell lines. Based on the previous work, it is not unexpected that this specific tumor line would be dependent on nucleotides. The work does suggest that certain tumors which are more nucleotide dependent could be treated with nucleotide metabolism manipulation.

This review indicates that the nucleotides are important in the immune response. They appear to play a key role in both lymphocyte and macrophage proliferation and function. This will result in a decrease in cell-mediated immunity with dietary depletion of nucleotides. Increased susceptibility to infections is one of the consequences. In terms of transplantation, a nucleotide-free diet decreases the allograft rejection and has a synergistic effect with cyclosporine. These effects are due to lymphocyte maturation arrest in the G_1 phase of the cell cycle. Of importance is the fact that much of this work has been done in animals, leaving future work in humans to determine the clinical relevance.

References

1. Montgomery R, Dryer RL, Conway TW et al. (1983) In: Montgomery R, Dryer RL, Convay TW, Spector AA, (eds) Biochemistry: a case-oriented approach. Mosby, St Louis, p 562
2. Leleiko NS, Martin BA, Walsh M et al. (1987) Tissue-specific gene expression results from a purine and pyrimidine free diet and 6 mercaptopurine in the rat small intestine and colon. Gastroenterology 93:1014
3. Zollner N, Grobner W (1977) Purine and pyrimidine metabolism. Elsevier, Amsterdam, p 165
4. Giblett ER, Anderson JE, Cohen F et al. (1972) Adenosine-deaminase deficiency in two patients with severely impaired collular immunity. Lancet 2:1067
5. Giblett ER, Ammann AJ, Sanderman R et al. (1985) Nucleoside-phosphorylase deficiency in a child with severely defective T-cell immunity and normal B-cell immunity. Lancet 1:1010
6. Parry-Billings M, Evans J, Calder PC et al. (1990) Does glutamine contribute to immunosuppression after major burns? Lancet 1:523
7. Van Buren CT, Kulkarni AD, Rudolph F (1983) Synergistic effect of a nucleotide-free diet and cyclosporine on allograft survival. Transplant Proc [Suppl] 1/2:2967
8. Van Buren CT, Kulkarni AD, Schandle VP et al. (1983) The influence of dietary nucleotides on cell-mediated immunity. Transplantation 36:350
9. Van Buren CT, Kim E, Kulkarni AD et al. (1987) Nucleotide-free diet and suppression of immune response. Transplant Proc [Suppl] 5:57
10. Twist VW, Barnes RD (1973) Popliteal lymph node weight gain assay for graft-versus-host reactivity in mice. Transplantation 15:182
11. Kulkarni A, Fanslow A, Higley H et al. (1989) Expression of immune cell surface markers in vivo and immune competence in mice by dietary nucleotides. Transplant Proc 21:121
12. Peters GJ, Veerkamp JH (1983) Purine and pyrimidine metabolism in peripheral blood lymphocytes. Int J Biochem 15:115
13. Cohen A, Barankiewicz J, Lederman HM et al. (1984) Purine metabolism in human T lymphocytes: role of the purine nucleoside cycle. Can J Biochem 62:577
14. Cohen A, Barankiewicz J, Gelfand EW (1985) Roles of alternative synthetic and catabolic purine pathways in T lymphocyte differentiation. Ann NY Acad Sci 451:26
15. Waldmann TA (1986) The structure, function, and expression of interleukin-2 receptors on normal and malignant lymphocytes. Science 232:727
16. Rudolph FB, Fanslow WC, Kulkarni AD, et al. (1985) Effect of dietary nucleotides on lymphocyte maturation. Adv Exp Med Biol 195A:497
17. Koponen M, Grieder A, Hauser R et al. (1985) Interference of cyclosporin with lymphocyte proliferation: effects on mitochondria and lysosomes of cyclosporin-sensitive or resistant cell clones. Cell Immunol 93:486
18. Van Buren CT, Kulkarni AD, Fanslow WC et al. (1985) Dietary nucleotides, a requirement for helper/inducer T lymphocytes. Transplantation 40:694
19. Rowe PB, Tripp E, Craig GC (1979) In: Kisluik RL, Brown GM (eds) Chemistry and biology of pteridines. Elsevier, Amsterdam, p 1001
20. Chechick BE, Schrader WP, Minowada J (1981) An immunomorphologic study of adenosine deaminase distribution in human thymus tissue, normal lymphocytes, and hematopoietic cell lines. J Immunol 126:1003
21. Freire-Moar JM, Rodriguez D, Rodriguez-Segadi S et al. (1984) The distribution of adenosine deaminase, purine nucleotide phosphorylase and 5'nucleotidase in subpopulations of thymocytes, bone marrow cells and other lymphoid organs in mice. Int J Biochem 16:225
22. Massaia M, Ma DDF, Sylwestrowicz TA et al. (1982) Enzymes of purine metabolism in human peripheral lymphocyte subpopulations. Clin Exp Immunol 50:148

23. Minkowski MD, Burdeira A (1985) Differential functional subsets of cultured murine T cells express characteristic levels of adenosine deaminase activity. Cell Immunol 95:380
24. Kulkarni AD, Fanslow WC, Rudolph FB et al. (1988) Modulation of delayed hypersensitivity in mice by dietary nucleotide restriction. Transplantation 44:847
25. Fanslow WC, Kulkarni AD, Van Buren CT et al. (1988) Effect of nucleotide restriction and supplementation on resistance to experimental murine candidiasis. JPEN 12:49
26. Rudolph FB, Kulkarni AD, Fanslow WC et al. (1990) Role of RNA as a dietary source of pyrimidines and purines in immune function. Nutrition [Suppl] 1:45

Relationship of Plasma Acute-Phase Protein to Amino Acid Levels During High-Dose Branched Chain Amino Acid Support in Sepsis

C. Chiarla[1], I. Giovannini[1], J. H. Siegel[2], and M. Castagneto[1]

Introduction

Acute-phase proteins (APP) play an important role in sepsis in the regulation of the inflammatory reaction, in the host defense against bacterial invasion, and in the related host protection from autoinjury. The whole spectrum of APP action is not fully understood; however, it is well established that changes in APP levels in sepsis mostly reflect increased protein synthetic activity. Therefore, it would be helpful to have more information about the relationship of APP to amino acid (AA) dose and plasma levels. This study was performed to assess the impact of high-dose branched chain amino acid (BCAA) support on several plasma APP and on AA patterns, with their reciprocal interactions.

Materials and Methods

Sixteen severely injured patients who developed sepsis were studied. Sepsis was diagnosed on the basis of the following: temperature over 38.3 °C, white blood cell count over 12 000 or under 3000 cells/mm^3, demonstration of a source of infection by a positive wound, abscess, blood culture, or by a positive sputum culture in the case of respiratory infections. Patients were prospectively, randomly assigned to receive a 49% BCAA parenteral solution ($n = 8$, BCAA enriched Mixture, Clintec Nutrition, Deerfield, USA) or a 16% BCAA solution ($n = 8$, Travasol, Clintec Nutrition) [1, 2]. There was no other difference between the 49% BCAA and 16% BCAA groups in nutritional regimens, with the same glucose (5.47 $\pm$ 1.01 versus 5.76 $\pm$ 1.58 g/kg per 24 h), fat (0.96 $\pm$ 0.47 versus 0.96 $\pm$ 0.68 g/kg per 24 h), total AA load (1.48 $\pm$ 0.26 versus 1.62 $\pm$ 0.60 g/kg per 24 h) and total AA gluconeogenic potential [3]. Injury and sepsis severity scores did not differ (Mann-Whitney test) in the two groups [4–6].

On an 8-h basis, 364 studies were performed for a maximum of 10 days after randomization or until death or recovery from sepsis. Blood samples were

---

[2] MIEMSS, University of Maryland, Baltimore (USA) [1] Centre of Study for Shock Physiopathology CNR, Department of Surgery, Catholic University School of Medicine, Via Val Pavara 119 00168 Rome

Host Defense Dysfunction
in Trauma, Shock and Sepsis
Eds. Faist/Meakins/Schildberg
© Springer-Verlag, Berlin Heidelberg 1993

drawn for measurements of plasma AA and APP: fibrinogen, c-reactive protein (CRP), transferrin, ceruloplasmin, α_1-antitrypsin, α_2-macroglobulin. Plasma cholesterol and lactate, and urinary 3-methylhistidine excretion were also sampled. Plasma AA and urinary 3-methylhistidine were determined using a Beckman AA analyzer, the plasma APP using radial immunodiffusion assay methodology. The total plasma input of each AA was calculated as the sum of the muscle-liberated AA (as estimated by 3-methylhistidine excretion, using the quantities of each AA shown to be released from septic muscle by Pearl et al. [7]) plus the quantity infused. The quantity obtained, divided by the AA plasma level and normalized by the extracellular fluid volume, represented the mean clearance of that AA, as previously described [1].

Statistical analysis and validation of the results were performed by Student's *t*-test and least-squares regression analysis using standard methods.

Results

In spite of the large APP variability caused by the multiple factors affecting their concentrations, including the timing of measurements, several definite correlations with AA doses and levels were found. Fibrinogen was directly related to BCAA dose ($R^2 = 0.14$, $p < 0.0001$; Fig. 1) and unrelated to total AA and non-BCAA doses. It was higher in the 49% BCAA group compared to the 16% BCAA group (11.98 ± 3.25 versus 9.31 ± 2.77 mg/ml; $p < 0.001$). It was inversely related to most AA levels, especially to the levels of all AA known to be transported intracellularly by the transport system A (TSA-AA). Among these, glycine level explained by itself 31% of the fibrinogen variability ($R^2 = 0.31$, $p < 0.0001$), while slightly weaker correlations were found between fibrinogen and serine, methionine, proline, and α-aminoisobutyric acid. Levels of these AA were directly and strongly interrelated; the level of α-aminoisobutyric acid could be predicted with an 87% control of its variance from the levels of glycine, serine and proline ($R^2 = 0.87$, $p < 0.0001$). Fibrinogen was directly correlated to most AA clearances and particularly to BCAA and TSA-AA clearances. Leucine clearance accounted for 18% of the fibrinogen variability ($R^2 = 0.18$, $p < 0.0001$).

It was noted that the infusion of 49% BCAA, compared to 16% BCAA, resulted in remarkably lower levels of proline (156 ± 53 versus 372 ± 323 µM/l; $p < 0.001$) and in a much flatter direct relationship of proline to leucine levels ($p < 0.0001$). The observation that the proline load was roughly equivalent in the 49% BCAA group, compared to the 16% BCAA group, while the leucine load was threefold, suggested an increased clearance of proline related to an increased clearance of leucine in the 49% BCAA group versus the 16% BCAA group; regression analysis with calculated clearances reconfirmed this finding. Similar paradoxical findings (changes in plasma AA levels dissociated from differences in AA load) were also found for serine (another TSA-AA) with a

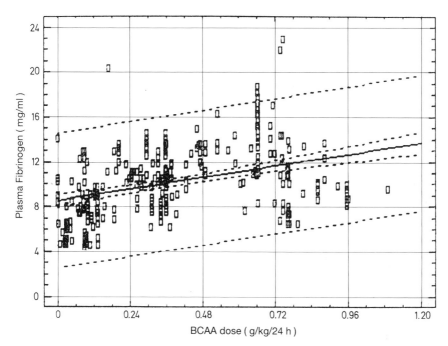

Fig. 1. Relationship between plasma fibrinogen levels and BCAA in all measurements, with 95% confidence limits. Plasma fibrinogen was unrelated to total amino acid and non-BCAA doses (see text)

significantly decreased plasma level in the 49% BCAA group versus the 16% BCAA group (101 ± 85 versus 122 ± 62 μM/l; $p < 0.001$), in spite of a significantly higher load (0.045 ± 0.01 versus 0 g/kg per 24 h; $p < 0.001$), and also for taurine, which had a significantly increased level in the 49% BCAA group compared to the 16% BCAA group (117 ± 98 versus 81 ± 53 μM/l; $p < 0.001$) in the absence of taurine infusion.

CRP, overall, was not significantly correlated with the total AA dose, the BCAA dose, or the non-BCAA dose. However, the 49% BCAA group had higher mean values compared to the 16% BCAA group (199 ± 115 versus 169 ± 124; $p < 0.001$) and showed higher initial increases in CRP and a more return toward normal. The pattern of correlation with plasma AA levels was similar to that found for fibrinogen. There were negative correlations with TSA-AA, lysine, arginine, threonine, hydroxyproline, and other AA ($p < 0.0001$); however, for any given plasma AA level, the 49% BCAA group tended to have lower CRP than the 16% BCAA group. This finding was statistically significant in several instances and was related to the more rapid decrease in CRP in measurements taken after the initial increase in the 49% BCAA group. Relationships of CRP to AA clearances were positive, as in the case of fibrinogen; they were stronger for lysine, arginine, threonine, asparagine plus aspartate, and hydroxyproline clearances and were weaker or not statistically significant for other AA.

Transferrin was directly related to the total AA dose, which explained 17% of its variance ($R^2 = 0.17$, $p < 0.0001$). The correlation was higher in the 16% BCAA group ($R^2 = 0.34$, $p < 0.0001$, Fig. 2); in both groups combined it became less strong because there were several high transferrin levels in the 49% BCAA group, also at low AA loads. Transferrin was directly related to plasma levels of serine, isoleucine, leucine, valine, alanine, lysine, arginine, threonine, and histidine. Less important relationships were found for other AA. Serine alone explained 31% ($R^2 = 0.31$, $p < 0.0001$) and leucine 16% ($R^2 = 0.16$, $p < 0.0001$) of the variance in transferrin. The relationships with calculated clearances were not particularly relevant. Mean values in the 49% BCAA group compared to the 16% BCAA group were not significantly different (1.53 ± 0.42 versus 1.58 ± 0.52.

Ceruloplasmin was not significantly related to total AA, BCAA, or non-BCAA doses; however, it was higher in the 49% BCAA group than in the 16% BCAA group (511 ± 79 versus 478 ± 119; $p < 0.01$). Poor correlations were found between ceruloplasmin and both AA levels and clearances. Similar results were obtained for $\alpha_1$antitrypsin and α_2-macroglobulin, which in the 49% BCAA group compared to the 16% BCAA group were higher (7.30 ± 1.19 versus 6.69 ± 2.90; $p < 0.05$) and lower (1.96 ± 0.44 versus 2.15 ± 0.63; $p < 0.01$),

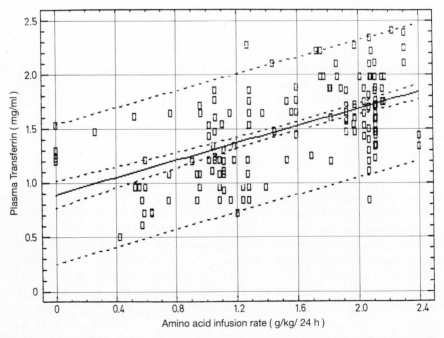

Fig. 2. Relationship between plasma transferrin levels and total amino acid doses in the 16% BCAA group, with 95% confidence limits (see text)

respectively. Changes in APP levels were correlated with BCAA-mediated changes in plasma cholesterol. Particularly remarkable was the direct correlation between transferrin and plasma cholesterol ($R^2 = 0.38$, $p < 0.0001$). There were lower lactate levels (1.22 ± 0.37 versus 1.93 ± 1.10 mmol/l; $p < 0.001$) for equivalent glucose and gluconeogenic loads, and lower α-aminoisobutyric acid (9.02 ± 5.16 versus 23.69 ± 23.00 μM/l; $p < 0.001$) and 3-methylhistidine (529 ± 205 versus 581 ± 253 μM/per 24 h; $p < 0.05$) in the 49% BCAA compared to the 16% BCAA group.

Discussion

The results in this study show that the characteristics of the APP response in posttraumatic sepsis are at least in part related to doses, plasma levels and clearances of AA and BCAA.

The fibrinogen level, in spite of multiple causes of variability, was found to be clearly related to BCAA dose (Fig. 1) and to levels and clearances of many AA. Roughly similar patterns were obtained for CRP, whose interactions with doses, levels, and clearances of AA and BCAA were also mediated by the timing of measurements along the biphasic temporal pattern of CRP evolution. Transferrin acted differently; it was less clearly related to BCAA doses than to total AA doses, and the relationships with plasma AA tended to be opposite to those found for fibrinogen and CRP. These results are consistent with previously published results [8] which indicated, in general, a good relationship between fibrinogen and CRP patterns, and a different action for transferrin. In this study there were less remarkable correlations with ceruloplasmin, α_1-antitrypsin, and α_2-macroglobulin.

Particularly relevant was the finding that most of the observed interrelationships between APP and AA involved changes in levels and clearances of AA known to be transported intracellularly by TSA. In sepsis intracellular AA transport is impaired in muscle as an effect of cytokines and circulating hormones, and in spite of a greater hepatic uptake some AA levels increase in plasma; this has also been observed for TSA-AA [9–11]. Increases in proline levels have also been related to the deterioration of central and peripheral septic metabolic abnormalities [12]. The BCAA-mediated decreases in TSA-AA and increases in clearance which were observed in this study were associated with decreases in lactate for equivalent exogenous gluconeogenic loads and with decreases in 3-methylhistidine excretion. These data imply an increased intracellular flux of AA and possibly a reversal of impaired TSA-AA transport in muscle, with reduced gluconeogenic use of AA and/or an improved metabolic utilization of gluconeogenesis products.

The results thus imply that changes in APP are associated with signs of increased intracellular flux of AA and of partial reversal of septic metabolic abnormalities. The BCAA-mediated increase in taurine level in the absence of taurine infusion (which is consistent with an improvement in hepatic trans-sulfuration) and the strong positive relationship between transferrin and cholesterol (which increased with BCAA dose) in the presence of decreasing lactate level for equivalent gluconeogenic loads also imply an increased hepatic synthesis activity with a reversal of impaired energy metabolism in the 49% BCAA group compared to the 16% BCAA group.

The clinical implications of these findings relate to the evidence that the pattern of APP response in sepsis may be influenced by the infused amino acid formula, and more specifically by the BCAA load. Such an effect takes place together with the signs of BCAA-mediated reduction in endogenous proteolysis, reversal of the pattern related to TSA impairment, improvement in protein synthesis activity, and restoration of energy metabolism, as evidenced in this study and in previous related studies [1, 2].

References

1. Chiarla C, Siegel JH, Kidd S et al. (1988) Inhibition of post-traumatic septic proteolysis and ureagenesis and stimulation of hepatic acute-phase protein production by branched-chain amino acid TPN. J Trauma 28:1145
2. Chiarla C, Giovannini I, Siegel JH et al. (1990) Relationship of plasma cholesterol level to doses of branch-chain amino acid in sepsis. Crit Care Med 18:32
3. Wolman SL, Fields LA, Cheema-Dhadli S et al. (1980) Protein conversion to glucose; an evaluation of the quantitative aspects. JPEN 4:487
4. Greenspan L, Mc Lellan B, Greig H et al. (1985) AIS and ISS: a scoring chart. J Trauma 25:61
5. Stevens LE (1983) Gauging the severity of surgical sepsis. Arch Surg 118:1190
6. Skau T, Nyström PO, Carlsson C (1985) Severity of illness in intra-abdominal infection. A comparison of two indexes. Arch Surg 120:152
7. Pearl R, Clowes GHA, Hirsch EF (1985) Prognosis and survival as determined by visceral amino acid clearance in severe trauma. J Trauma 25:777
8. Sganga G, Siegel JH, Brown G et al. (1985) Reprioritization of hepatic plasma protein release in trauma and sepsis. Arch Surg 120:187
9. Guidotti GG, Borghetti AF, Gazzola GC (1978) The regulation of amino acid transport in animal cells. Biochim Biophys Acta 515:329
10. Hasselgren PO, James JH, Fischer JE (1986) Inhibited muscle amino acid uptake in sepsis. Ann Surg 203:360
11. Bereta J, Kurdowska A, Koj A et al. (1989) Different preparations of natural and recombinant human interleukin-6 (IFN-β_2, BSF-2) similarly stimulate acute phase protein synthesis and uptake of α-aminoisobutyric acid by cultured rat hepatocytes. Int J Biochem 21:361
12. Cerra FB, Caprioli J, Siegel JH et al. (1979) Proline metabolism in sepsis, cirrhosis and general surgery. Ann Surg 190:577

Section 15

New Insights into the Mechanisms of Wound Healing

Wound Management and the Stress Response

D. N. Herndon[1,2], R. L. Rutan[1,2], T. C. Rutan[1,2], and J. M. Mlakar[2]

Thermal injury induces a more pronounced hypermetabolic stress response than seen following other trauma or infections, characterized by increased glucose catabolism, severe protein and fat wasting, negative nitrogen balance, and increased oxygen consumption [6, 25, 31]. As this catabolic state continues, weight loss, lean muscle mass loss, immunologic compromise, poor or delayed wound healing, and prolonged recovery time may result [1, 7, 13, 28, 32].

In our pediatric burn patients with greater than 60% total body surface area full-thickness burns, excisional therapy of burned tissues, excluding the face, within 48 h, resulted in improved survival [26]. Early excision and grafting of burns did not, however, change the metabolic rate, which remained elevated for over 60 days for patients treated with excisional or conservative therapy [23]. During the hypermetabolic phase, we have been able to maintain body weight to $\pm$ 3% of preadmission values using continuous feeding to meet 1600 kcal/m^2 body surface area per day plus 1500 kcal/m^2 body surface area burn per day [10]. However, this aggressive nutritional support does not reduce the exaggerated hypermetabolic response to major burn injury, and our patients continued to display evidence of peripheral wasting with central fat redistribution to the liver, ventricular hypertrophy with occasional cardiomyopathy, stunted growth, and delayed wound healing. We feel that a major aim of effective wound management in the acute postburn period is earlier reduction of the hypermetabolic response.

Following thermal injury, serum levels of catecholamines, corticosteroids, and glucagon are markedly increased [31], while levels of growth hormone and insulin-like growth factor 1 (IGF-1) are decreased [3]. Catecholamine-mediated hypermetabolism results in increased peripheral lipolysis and muscle catabolism with central fat redistribution, leading to fatty infiltration of the liver and increased morbidity [32]. Measured serum catecholamine levels are eight to ten times higher postburn [31], greatly in excess of the amount needed to effectively increase heart rate [2] and possible contractility. Although optimal cardiac output postburn has not yet been determined, it is probably greater than normal. Circulating catecholamines stimulate tachycardia and increase myocardial contractility as part of a compensatory mechanism to optimize oxygen

[1] University of Texas Medical Branch, Galveston, Texas, USA
[2] Shriners Burn Institute, Galveston, Texas, USA

Host Defense Dysfunction
in Trauma, Shock and Sepsis
Eds. Faist/Meakins/Schildberg
© Springer-Verlag, Berlin Heidelberg 1993

delivery [17]. Sustained levels of catecholamines have been shown, both clinic-ally and experimentally, to be harmful to the heart, and may induce ventricular hypertrophy, myocarditis, focal myocardial necrosis or cardiomyopathy, and may account for the postburn cardiomyopathy recognized in children [17, 19, 20, 27].

Wilmore et al. [31] demonstrated a reduction in metabolic rate with combined alpha- and beta- adrenergic blockade following large burn injuries. Adrenalectomy or catecholamine depletion by chronic reserpine administration lowered metabolic rates and increased mortality in rats with 60% total body surface area burns [5]. Use of beta-adrenergic blockers alone, however, remains attractive to reduce catecholamine-mediated hyperdynamic responses if overall cardiac function and metabolic rate are not adversely affected. Experimentally, propranolol has been shown to prevent the development of catecholamine-induced histologic changes in the myocardium of rats [16]. The effects of propranolol to reduce both heart rate and contractility are highly desirable since two of the primary determinants of myocardial oxygen consumption are simultaneously affected or decreased.

To test if chronic administration of propranolol in patients with massive thermal burns could be beneficial to decrease lipolysis and myocardial work without adversely affecting cardiac function or whole-body metabolism, a series of human trials was performed. First, twelve patients of similar age and burn size were given a 5-day propranolol infusion (0.7 mg/kg every 8 h) and divided into fed ($n = 6$) and fasted ($n = 6$) groups. The rate of urea production was $54\% \pm 12\%$ higher in fasted patients on the fifth day of propranolol infusion (experimental) than 24 h after cessation of propranolol (basal). This significant difference indicates an accelerated rate of net protein breakdown from pro-pranolol treatment [8]. This was attenuated, but not abolished, with feeding. Plasma glucose, total free fatty acid, insulin levels, metabolic rate and trigly-cerides showed no significant differences between basal and experimental levels for either group.

To test the effect of propranolol on postburn myocardial function, intra-venous propranolol (0.5 mg/kg per day or 1 mg/kg per day) was given at the height of the hypermetabolic response to six nonseptic adolescent patients with $82\% \pm 11\%$ total body surface area burn [15]. Two clinically derived indices of myocardial oxygen consumption were used to estimate the energy expenditure of the working heart. Both pressure-work index (PWI) and rate-pressure product (RPP) were decreased from baseline 30%–35% after 0.5 mg/kg or 1 mg/kg dosages ($p < 0.01$). Propranolol caused significant decreases in heart rate (157 ± 16–121 ± 18 beats/min) and left ventricular work index (7.6 ± 1.0–5.9 ± 1.4 kgm/min per square meter). Propranolol had no effect on cardiac output, pulmonary artery wedge pressure, and central venous pressure. Interestingly, cardiac output after propranolol treatment demonstrated a sub-maximal or hypoeffective response to endogenous circulating catecholamines and adequate myocardial oxygen delivery was maintained. A separate trial demonstrated that nonseptic, beta-blocked burn patients could appropriately respond to cold stress by increasing their resting energy potentials by as much as 41% ($p < 0.05$), suggesting that propranolol could be used safely in the management of hypermetabolic states without adversely affecting response to stress [11]. Finally, burn patients demonstrated a small but significant paradoxical increase in vascular resistance with propranolol infusion seems to help the postburn hyperdynamic heart without compromising ability to respond to stress.

Although the administration of propranolol has been shown to decrease the cardiac response to thermal trauma, the pediatric burn patient continues to demonstrate aberrant substrate metabolism and wound healing. Marked growth delays of both height and weight have been demonstrated in a group of postburn pediatric patients who had sustained greater than a 40% total body surface area burn. This growth delay persisted for as long as 3 years postinjury without any "catch-up" growth experienced [22]. Growth hormone (hGH) is a potent anabolic agent which stimulates amino acid entry into the cells for protein synthesis or gluconeogenesis, increases cell proliferation, mobilizes fats for lipolysis, promotes skeletal growth, regulates serum glucose levels and promotes positive nitrogen and calcium balances.

Thirty years ago, studies demonstrated that pituitary-derived hGH exerted a positive effect on protein metabolism and nitrogen balance in trauma and surgical patients [12, 20, 25]. The salutory effects noted included increased appetite, decreased nitrogen losses, increased retention of nitrogen and potassium, weight gain, more rapid wound healing, increased oxygen utilization and decreased respiratory quotient. Additionally, serum levels of IGF-1 were increased [12, 25]. At that time, studies were limited by the availability of natural hGH.

Biosynthetic hGH (rhGH) became commercially available about 5 years ago and is produced by recombinant DNA technology from an *E. Coli* host. Most of these early studies indicated that the salutory effects of hGH would occur only in the face of adequate nutrition, but McManson and Wilmore determined that the positive nitrogen balance could be achieved with as little as 140 gm/m^2 body surface area per day of carbohydrate and 1 g/kg per day protein in conjunction with 10 mg/day rhGH [15]. Despite hypocaloric nutrition, it appears that rhGH can induce a positive nitrogen balance, reduced protein oxidation, increase lipolysis, weight gain or maintenance, and positive mineral and trace element balance [14, 29, 30, 33]. In the surgical patient, unable to tolerate enteral nutrition, the administration of rhGH in conjunction with peripheral parenteral nutrition may supply sufficient exogenous calories and raw materials for anabolic activity, obviating the need, expense, and risk of total parenteral nutrition.

More recently, studies have attempted to quantitate the changes in wound healing by rhGH administration. In a double-blind, randomized study of 17 adult burn patients, a 2-day decrease in the length of time for split-thickness donor sites to heal was noted in the rhGH treated group [24]. Additionally, there was almost a four fold increase of circulating IGF-1 levels in the rhGH treated group. A similar study of 40 postburn pediatric patients showed a 2- to 4-day increase in the rate of donor site healing in rhGH treated patients, which ultimately resulted in a shorter hospital stay [9]. Pharmacokinetics of rhGH were also remarkable different in the hypermetabolic, hyperdynamic burn patient than in their hGH-deficient counterparts. Peak levels of rhGH appeared and disappeared more rapidly in the burned children. Again, increases in wound healing were associated with elevated levels of IGF-1.

The reduction of the hypermetabolic, hyperdynamic response to burn injury demonstrated with beta-adrenergic blockade, coupled with the increased anabolic activity of hGH may provide the ability to pharmacologically manipulate the stress response and funnel those energies into more salutory effects. Investigations into the clinical applications of both agents continues, including a more definitive measure of the synergistic effects produced when both are utilized.

References

1. Alexander JW (1986) Nutrition and infection-a new perspective on an old problem. Arch Surg 121:966–972
2. Clutter WE, Bier DM, Suresh SD et al. (1980) Epinephrine plasma metabolic clearance rates and physiologic thresholds for metabolic and hemodynamic actions in man. J Clin Invest 66:94–101
3. Doleck R (1990) The endocrine response to thermal injury. In: Dolecek R, Brizio-Molteni L, Molteni A, Traber DL (eds) Endocrinology of thermal injury. Lea and Febriger, Philadelphia
4. Gore DC, Honeycutt D, Jahoor F et al. Propranolol diminishes extremity blood flow in burned patients. Arch Surg (in press)
5. Herndon DN, Wilmore DW, Mason AD Jr et al. (1977) Humoral mediators of non-temperature dependent hypermetabolism in 50% burned adult rats. Surg Forum 28:37–39
6. Herndon DN, Wilmore DW, Mason AD (1978) Development and analysis of a small animal model stimulating the human postburn hypermetabolic response. J Surg Res 25:394–403
7. Herndon DN, Curreri PW, Abston S et al. (1987) Treatment of burns. Curr Prob Surg 2:347–397
8. Herndon DN, Barrow RE, Rutan TC et al. (1988) Effect of propranolol on hemodynamic and metabolic responses of burned pediatric patients. Ann Surg 208:94–100
9. Herndon DN, Barrow RE, Kunkle KR et al. (1990) Effects of recombinant human growth hormone on donor site healing in severaly burned children. Ann Surg 212/4:424–431
10. Hildreth MA, Herndon DN, Desai MH, Broemeling LD (1990) Current treatment reduces calories required to maintain weight in pediatric patients with burns. J Burn Care Rehabil 11/5:405–409
11. Honeycutt D, Barrow RE, Herndon DN Cold stress in severely burned patients after beta-blockade. Ann Surg (in press)
12. Liljadahl SO, Gemzell CA, Plantin LO, Birke G (1961) Effect of human growth hormone in patients with severe burns. Acta Chir Scand 122:1–4
13. Long CL, Spencer JL, Kinney JM et al. (1968) Carbohydrate metabolism in man: effect of elective operations and major injury. J Appl Physiol 31:110–119
14. McManson JM, Wilmore DW (1986) Positive nitrogen balance with human growth hormone and hypocaloric intravenous feeding. Surg 100/2:188–197
15. Minifee PK, Barrow RE, Abston S et al. (1989) Improved myocardial oxygen utilization following propranolol infusion in adolescents with postburn hypermetabolism. J Pediatr Surg 24/8:806–811.
16. Moncrief JA (1966) Effect of various fluid regimens and pharmacologic agents on the circulatory hemodynamics of the immediate postburn period. Ann Surg 164:94–100
17. Raab W (1960) Key position of catecholamines in functional and degenerative cardiovascular pathology. Am J Cardio 5/5:571–578

18. Raab W (1961) Sympathogenic origin and antiadrenergic prevention of stress-induced myocardial lesions. Am J Cardiol 8:203–211
19. Reichenbach DD, Benditt EP (1970) Catecholamines and cardiomyopathy: the pathogenesis and importance of myofibrillar degeneration. Hum Pathol 1/1:12–50
20. Roe CF, Kinney J (1962) The influence of human growth hormone on energy sources in convalescence. Surg Forum 13:369–371
21. Rona G (1985) Catecholamine cardiotoxicity. J Mol Cell Cardio 17:291–306
22. Rutan RL, Herndon DN (1990) Growth delay in postburn pediatric patients. Arch Surg 125 13:392–395
23. Rutan TC, Herndon ND, Abston S et al. (1986) Metabollic rate alterations to early excision and grafting versus conservative treatment. J Trauma 26/2:240–248
24. Sherman SK, Demling RH, Lalonde C et al. (1989) Growth hormone enhances re-epithelialization of human split thickness skin graft donor sites. Surg Forum 40:37–39
25. Soroff HS, Rozin RR, Mooty J et al. (1967) Role of human growth hormone in the response to trauma: 1. Metabolic effects following burns. Ann Surg 166/5:739–752
26. Thompson P, Herndon DN, Abston S et al. (1987) Effect of early excision on patients with major thermal injury. J Trauma 27:205–207
27. Todd GL, Baroldi G, Pieper GM et al. (1985) Experimental catecholamine-induced myocardial necrosis; I. Morphology, quantification and regional distribution of acute contraction band lesioins. J Mol Call Cardiol 17:317–338
28. Volenec FJ (1979) Metabolic profiles of thermal trauma. Ann Surg 190:694–698
29. Ward HC, Halliday D, Sim AJW (1987) Protein and energy metabolism with biosynthetic human growth hormone after gastrointestinal surgery. Ann Surg 206/1:56–61
30. Wilmore DW, Moylan JA Jr, Bristow BF et al. (1974) Anabolic effects of growth hormone and high caloric feedings following thermal injury. Surg Gynecol Obstet 138:875–884
31. Wilmore DW, Long JM, Mason AD Jr et al. (1974) Catecholamines: mediator of the hypermetabolic response to thermal injury. Ann Surg 180:653–666
32. Wolfe RR (1986) Nutrition and metabolism in burns. Crit Care (SOCOM) 7:19–63
33. Zeigler TR, Young LS, McManson JK, Wilmore DW (1988) Metabolic effects of recombinant human growth hormone in patients receiving parenteral nutrition. Ann Surg 208/1:6–16

The Role of the Wound in Posttraumatic Immune Dysfunction

M. C. Regan[1] and A. Barbul[2]

Despite the success of modern surgical treatment in decreasing the early death rates following traumatic injury, late morbidity and mortality, the majority of which are septic in origin, still represent a major problem [1–3]. The presence of alterations in host immune reactivity is associated with the persistence of septic complications following operative and accidental trauma [4]. Clinically and experimentally, trauma is associated with impaired response to delayed-type hypersensitivity skin tests [5, 6], decreased allograft rejection [7, 8], and enhanced tumor growth [9, 10], all of which depend, at least in part, on intact T-cell function. The exact nature of cellular immune defects remains undetermined. Various investigators have described the appearance of serum suppressive factors [11–15], circulating suppressor T cells [16, 17], or suppressor macrophages [18, 19] after accidental trauma, burns, or major surgical procedures. The incidence of posttraumatic immune suppression is related to the magnitude of the injury [10, 20–22], but even relatively minor degrees of trauma, including many routine operative procedures, result in a decreased immunocompetence [23, 24].

There is little agreement about the source of the serum immunosuppressive factors or the mechanism of their induction. It has been suggested that burn injury may cause immune alterations via the absorption of large amounts of damaged tissue components into the general circulation [14, 25]. Similarly, the release of large quantities of tissue constituents following traumatic tissue disruption may play a role in the immune alterations seen following nonburn trauma. There is normally a lag period between the time of injury and the appearance of immunological alterations, suggesting that other mechanisms may be proportionally more important.

A feature common to all these injured states is the presence of wounded tissue. Not only is there evidence to suggest that the incidence of posttraumatic immune suppression is related to the magnitude of the injury, but in addition there is a direct linear relationship between the extent of injury and the incidence of posttraumatic septic complications and mortality [1, 3]. Tissue disruption sets into motion a sequence of inflammation and repair aimed at restoration of tissue integrity and function. Achieving this goal necessitates the removal of dead and damaged tissue and the synthesis of new tissue to repair the damage.

---

[1] Department of Surgery, Sinai Hospital of Baltimore, MD 21215, USA
[2] Department of Surgery, John Hopkins Medical Institutions, Baltimore, MD 21205, USA

Host Defense Dysfunction
in Trauma, Shock and Sepsis
Eds. Faist/Meakins/Schildberg
© Springer-Verlag, Berlin Heidelberg 1993

The wound is becoming recognized as a site of intense immunological activity with both macrophages and lymphocytes playing an active role in the regulation of healing [26]. In vivo wounds display alterations in immune activity compared to other sites in the body. In guinea pigs, inoculation of small quantities of methylcholanthrene-induced liposarcoma cells, which do not normally give rise to tumors when inoculated into normal skin, lead to tumor formation and death when inoculated into 3-, 9-, and 11-week-old wounds [27]. Similar effects were observed with the KHT mouse tumor in C3H/He mice, B16 melanoma in C57BL mice, and the MethA sarcoma in BALB/c mice, where the number of cells necessary to induce a tumor was significantly reduced when the cells were injected into a surgical wound rather than into nonwounded tissue [28]. In a model of avian Rous sarcoma virus tumorigenesis it has been shown that, despite evidence of diffuse virus infiltration in normal tissues, tumors only develop at the site of initial inoculation and at wound sites remote from the inoculation site [29]. In addition, the secondary tumors arise de novo and not simply as a result of metastatic spread [30].

There is also evidence to suggest that the immune alterations observed in the wound environment are not necessarily confined to the healing site. Fisher and Fisher [31] showed that while injection of 50 Walker 256 carcinosarcoma intraportally via a celiotomy resulted in no detectable tumor formation, all animals developed tumors in the liver if subjected to laparotomy, as late as 3 months after the injection. Similar evidence of distant effects from operative wounds was observed by Gunduz et al. [32]. Surgical excision of one tumor resulted in an increase in the growth rate of the remaining tumor. Thus alterations in immune activity occur not only at the wound site, but also at sites remote from the wound. This suggests that in certain circumstances immune alterations found in the wound environment may not be confined to the wound alone. Many locally beneficial cellular interactions, including normal immune activities, may have a quite different and potentially detrimental effect outside the confines of their normal domain. Therefore it is possible that in the presence of major tissue damage and the need for extensive wound repair, alterations in immune activity, which are normally limited to the site of healing, could potentially overspill into the general circulation, resulting in multiple, possibly undesirable alterations in normal host immune function (Fig. 1). If indeed the wound is a potential source of factors which contribute to alterations in immune function, it might be expected that the extracellular wound fluid (WF) which collects at the site of repair, would be rich in such factors. Thus systemic administration of WF to normal subjects might be expected to parallel the effects of a natural overspill of such wound factors into the systemic circulation. Support for this hypothesis is provided by a number of in vivo studies examining the effect of parenterally administered extracellular WF in normal animals. Intraperitoneal administration of WF collected from 10-day-old wounds inhibited in vivo allogeneic responses as assessed by skin graft rejection. Daily injection of 0.5 ml (20 mg/ml protein) WF significantly enhanced graft survival to 27.3 ± 2.6 days when compared with autologous serum injection (16.7 ± 0.9

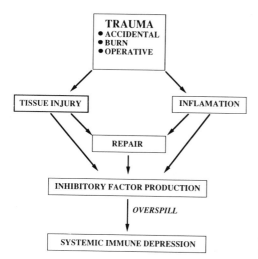

Fig. 1. A working hypothesis for the role of the wound in post-traumatic immune dysfunction

days; $p < 0.01$) and saline solution (14.7 ± 1.6 days; $p < 0.01$) [33]. Shimazu [34], using a comparable model, reports similar findings for allograft survival but was unable to show any survival advantage for xenografts.

In vivo administration of WF also impairs host immune responses to sepsis. In a model of sepsis, induced by cecal ligation and puncture, intravenous administration of 10-day-old WF (10 mg ml/protein) every 12 h resulted in a significantly higher mortality compared to control animals receiving serum prepared from nontraumatized rats (Fig. 2) [35]. These findings are similar to those obtained by parenteral administration of a suppressive factor obtained from the serum of either severely burned patients or patients undergoing aortic aneurysm repair. Injection of this low-molecular-weight fraction intraperitoneally in A/J mice infected with *Listeria monocytogenes* caused a significant increase in mortality compared to controls. The low-molecular-weight fraction was not intrinsically toxic, causing no mortality when administered to

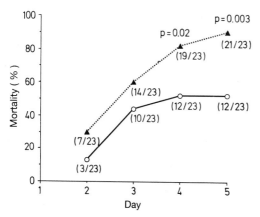

Fig. 2. Mortality curves after cecal ligation and puncture of wound fluid-treated (*broken line*) and control (*solid line*) serum-treated rats. *Numbers in parentheses* refer to the number of dead animals/total starting number

noninfected controls [36]. The WF and the low-molecular-weight fractions used in these in vivo studies had both been shown to inhibit the lymphocyte blastogenic response to mitogens in vitro.

The factors(s) in WF responsible for these effects are still not known. Many of the cytokines produced by cells for intercellular communication have immunosuppressive qualities. Transforming growth factor beta (TGF-β) [37] and (tumor necrosis factor-α) (TNF-α) [38], both known to be present in significant quantities at the site of healing, can suppress many macrophage and lymphocyte activities. It is conceivable that overspill of these or other cytokines from the healing wound into the general circulation may lead to some of the observed immune alterations.

Many of the regulatory factors present at the wound site remain incompletely characterized. Of particular interest is the presence of an immunosuppressive factor which appears between the 7th and 10th day postwounding in rats. WF and wound mononuclear cells (WMNC) recovered from 10-day-old wounds in rats inhibit the in vitro blastogenic response of normal thymic lymphocytes to the mitogens phytohemagglutinin (PHA) and concanavalin A (Table 1). In addition, both WF and WMNC inhibit in vitro allogeneic responses tested in one way mixed lymphocyte reaction (MLR) of Lewis splenocytes with inactivated ACI spleen cells by 75%–96% and 85%–98%, respectively [33]. These effects are absent before the 7th post-injury day with neither the WF nor the WMNC exhibiting immune inhibitory activity during the 1st week postwounding. Conditioned media from inhibitory WMNC also inhibit thymic lymphocyte blastogenesis [39]. Flow cytometric analysis indicates a predominance of T-suppressor lymphocytes in the WMNC preparations [39]. Further support that these cells are the source of the inhibitory factor is provided by the fact that adult thymectomy, which abrogates suppressor cell induction, leads to a marked diminution in wound inhibitory activity [40].

The action of this wound inhibitory factor appears to be specific for interleukin-2 (IL-2)-driven cellular responses. In vitro studies show that exogenous human recombinant IL-2 (rHuIL-2) failed to reverse the inhibitory action of WF on thymic lymphocyte blastogenesis. In addition, rHuIL-2 was

Table 1. Effect of wound fluid and wound cells on immune function

Wound Fluid
In vivo
   Decreases survival post sepsis
   Delays allograft rejection

In vitro
   Inhibits proliferation of thymic lymphocyte
   Inhibits proliferation of D10 and HT2 IL-2-dependent cell lines
   Inhibits allogenic mixed lymphocyte response
Wound Mononuclear cells
   Inhibit proliferation of thymic lymphocyte
   Inhibit allogenic mixed lymphocyte response

ineffective in preventing a similar inhibition of the proliferation of D10- and HT2 IL-2-dependent cell lines. This suggests that the inhibition is effected at the IL-2 receptor or post-receptor level as opposed to acting by suppressing IL-2 generation [39, 40]. Partial characterization of this wound inhibitory factor reveals it to be a protein with an approximate molecular weight of 100 000, heat stable (60 °C, 1 h) and neuraminidase sensitive, suggesting a high degree of glycosylation [35]. The inhibitory effects are not blocked by indomethacine [39] and in contrast to burn WF, WF from incisional wounds showed an insignificant increase in prostaglandin E_2 (PGE_2) [34].

Immunosuppressive activity has also been observed in postoperative human seroma fluid drained from operative wounds [41] and in burn blister fluid [42]. These "WFs" inhibited in vitro lymphocyte blastogenesis [41, 42], polymorphonuclear neutrophil (PMN) chemotaxis [41] and displayed a diminished capacity to support neutrophil phagocytosis [42, 43].

In addition to regulatory peptides a number of other substances released from damaged tissue have been shown to exhibit immune inhibitory activity. Fibrinogen degradation products cause noncytotoxic suppression of both T- and B-cell blastogenesis [44], while fibrinectin degradation peptides cause noncytotoxic depression of macrophage phagocytosis, neutrophil migration, and T-lymphocyte blastogenesis [45, 46]. Additionally, heat or protease digests of type II and type III collagen inhibit neutrophil migration but do not effect T-cell blastogenesis [47].

Thus, there is strong support for the hypothesis that overspill of the wound environment into the general circulation has a role in the induction of host posttraumatic immune suppression. Not only are a number of potent immunosuppressive factors present in the wound, but there is evidence of alteration in immune activity at sites remote from the wound. Further support for this hypothesis is provided by the fact that the appearance and degree of posttraumatic immunosuppression correlates with the extent of the initial injury. The concept that many beneficial localized cellular interactions, including normal immune activities, may have a quite different and potentially destructive effect outside the confines of their normal domain is seen in many other fields of pathophysiology. It may well be the case that in the presence of major tissue damage and the need for extensive wound repair, the processes which are normally limited to the site of healing spill into the general circulation and have multiple, possibly undesirable consequences on normal immune responsiveness.

Acknowledgements. This work was supported in part by the National Institutes of Health Grant GM38650-03.

References

1. Baker CC, Oppenheimer L, Stephens B, Lewis FR, Trunkey DD (1980) Epidemiology of Trauma Deaths. Am J Surg 140:144–150

2. Border JR, Hasset JM (1988) Multiple systems organ failure; history, pathophysiology prevention and support. In: Clowes GHA Jr (Ed) Trauma Sepsis and Shock. Decker, New York, p 335–356

3. Feller I, Tholen D, Cornell RG (1980) Improvements in burn care, 1965 to 1979. JAMA 244:2074–2078

4. Deitch EA (1988) Infection in the comprised host. Surg Clin North Am 68:181–197

5. Slade MS, Simmons RL, Yunis E, Greenberg LD (1975) Immunodepression after major surgery in normal patients. Surgery 78:363–372

6. MacLean LD, Meakins JL, Taguchi K, Duignan JP, Dhillon KS, Gordon J (1975) Host resistance in sepsis and trauma. Ann Surg 182:207–217

7. Kay GD (1957) Prolonged survival of a skin homograft in a patient with very extensive burns. Ann NY Acad Sci 64:767–774

8. Ninnemann JL, Fisher JC, Frank HA (1978) Prolonged survival of human skin allografts following thermal injury. Transplantation 25:69–72.

9. Buinauskas P, McDonald GO, Cole WH (1958) Role of operative stress on resistance of the experimental animal to inoculated cancers cells. Ann Surg 148:642–648

10. Lewis MR, Cole WH (1958) Experimental increase of lung metastases after operative trauma. Arch Surg 77:621–626

11. Constantian MB, Menzoian JO, Nimberg RB, Schmid K, Mannick JA (1977) Association of a circulating immunosuppressive peptide with operative and accidental trauma. Ann Surg 185:73–75.

12. McLoughlin GA, Wu AV, Sporoschetz I, Nimberg RB, Mannick JA (1979) Correlation between anergy and a circulating immunosuppressive factor following major surgical trauma. Ann Surg 190:297–304

13. Christou NV, Meakins JL (1983) Partial analysis and purification of polymorphonuclear neutrophil chemotactic inhibitors in serum from anergic patients. Arch Surg 118:156–160

14. Ozkam AN (1989) Serum mediators and the generation of immune suppression. In: Faist E, Ninneman J, Green D (eds) Immune consequences of Trauma, Shock and Sepsis. Springer, Berlin Heidelberg New York, p 285–291

15. Hakim AA (1977) An immunosuppressive factor from the serum of thermally traumatized patients. J Trauma 17:908–919

16. Munster AM (1976) Post-traumatic immunosuppression is due to activation of suppressor T cells. Lancet 1:1329–1330.

17. Miller CL, Baker CC (1979) Changes in lymphocyte activity after thermal injury. J Clin Invest 63:202–210.

18. Baker CC, Miller CL, Trunkey DD, Lim RC Jr (1979) Identity of mononuclear cells which compromise the resistance of trauma patients. J Surg Res 26:278–287

19. Wang BS, Heacock EH, Wu AVO, Mannick JA (1980) Generation of suppressor cells in mice after surgical trauma. J Clin Invest 66:200–209

20. Constantian MB (1978) Association of sepsis with an immunosuppresive polypeptide in the serum of burn patients. Ann Surg 188:209–215

21. O'Mahony JB, Palder SB, Wood J, McIrvine A, Roderick ML, Demling RH, Mannick JA (1984) Depression of cellular immunity after multiple trauma in the absence of sepsis. J Trauma 24:869–875

22. Ninneman JL, Fisher JC, Wachtel TL (1979) Thermal injury associated immunosuppression; occurrence and in vitro blocking effect of the post-recovery serum. J Immunol 122:1736–1741

23. Keane RM, Regan MC, Tanner WA, Bouchier-Hayes D (1988) Immunorestorative effect of obstructive jaundice after operative injury. Br J Surg 75:600

24. Stephan RN, Saizawa M, Conrad PJ, Dean RE, Getia AS, Chaudry IH (1987) Depressed antigen presentation function and membrane interleukin-1 activity of peritoneal macrophage after laparotomy. Surgery 102:147–154

25. Schonenberger GA, Burkhardt F, Kalberer F, Muller W, Stadtler K, Vogt P, Allgower M (1975) Experimental evidence for a significant impairment of host defence for gram negative organisms by a specific cutaneous toxin produced by sever thermal injury. Surg Gynecol Obstet 141:555–561

26. Barbul A, Regan MC (1990) The role of T lymphocytes in wound healing. J Trauma 30:97–100

27. Prendergrast WJ, Futrell JW (1979) Biologic determinants of tumor growth in healing wounds. Ann Surg 189:181–188

28. Baker DG, Masterson TM, Pace R, Constable WC, Wanebo H (1989) The influence of the surgical wound on local tumor recurrence. Surgery 106:525–532

29. Dolberg DS, Hollingsworth R, Hertle M, Bissell MJ (1985) Wounding and its role in RSV-mediated tumor formation. Science 230:676–678
30. Sieweke MH, Stoker AW, Bissel MJ (1989) Evaluation of the carcinogenic effect of wounding in Rous Sarcoma virus Tumorigenesis. Cancer Res 49:6419–6424
31. Fisher B, Fisher ER (1959) Experimental evidence in support of the dormant tumor cell. Science 130:918–919
32. Gunduz N, Fisher B, Saffer EA (1979) Effect of surgical removal on the growth and kinetics of residual tumor. Cancer Res 39:3861–3865
33. Barbul A, Fishel RS, Shimazu S, Damewood RB, Wasserkrug HL, Efron G (1984) Inhibition of host immunity by fluid and mononuclear cells from healing wounds. Surgery 96:315–319
34. Shimazu S (1987) Evaluation of immunosuppressive properties of fluid from healing wounds. Nippon Geka Gakkai Zasshi 88:1667–1675
35. Lazarou SA, Barbul A, Wasserkrug HL, Efron G (1989) The wound is a possible source of post traumatic immunesuppression. Arch Surg 124:1429–1431
36. Mc Irvine AJ, Wolf JHN, Collins K, Mannick JA (1983) Fatal infection in mice after injection of immunosuppressive serum fractions from surgical patients. Br J Surg 70:558–561
37. Grotendorst GR, Grontendorst CA, Gillman T (1988) Production of growth factors (PDGF and TGF-β) at the site of tissue repair. Proc Clin Biol Res 266:47–54
38. Ford HR, Hoffman RA, Wing EJ, Magee M, Mc Intyre L, Simons RL (1989) Characterization of the wound cytokines in the sponge matrix model. Arch Surg 124:1422–1428
39. Breslin RJ, Barbul A, Kupper TS, Knud-Hansen JP, Wasserkrug HL, Efron G (1988) Generation of an anti interleukin-2(IL-2) factor in healing wounds. Arch Surg 123:305–308
40. Barbul A, Damewood RB, Wasserkrug HL, Penberthy LT, Efron G (1983) Fluid and mononuclear cells from healing wounds inhibit thymocyte immune responsiveness. J Surg Res 34:505–509
41. Bridges M, Morris D, Hall JR, Deitch EA (1987) Effects of wound exudates on in vitro immune parameters. J Surg Res 43:133–135
42. Deitch EA, Smith BJ (1983) The effect of blister fluid from the thermally injured patients on normal lymphocyte transformation. J Trauma 23:106–110
43. Alexander JW, Korelitz J, Alexander NS (1976) Prevention of wound infections, a case for closed suction drainage to remove wound fluids deficient in opsonic proteins. Am J Surg 132:59–63
44. Krzystyniak PA, Stachurska J, Ryzewski J, Bykowska K, Kopec M (1978) Suppressive effects of low molecular weight fibrinogen degradation products on human and rat lymphocytes. Thromb Res 12:523–530
45. Hoyt DB, Ozkan AN, Easter DW (1988) Isolation of an immunosuppressive trauma peptide and its relationship to fibronectin. J Trauma 28:1–7
46. Easter DW, Hoyt DB, Ozkan AN (1988) Immunsuppression by a peptide from the gelatin binding domain of human fibronectin. J Surg Res 45:370–375
47. Ozkan AN, Ninnemann JL (1985) Burn associated suppressor active peptide relationship to tissue collagen. Proc Am Burn Soc 15:50

The Role of Growth Factors in the Regulation of Wound Repair

D. R. Knighton, V. D. Fiegel, and G. D. Phillips

Introduction

Wound repair involves a complex interaction between cells, biochemical mediators, extracellular matrix molecules, and the cellular microenvironment. The role of each continues to unfold as basic and clinical wound healing research advances. This review summarizes the currently known data on the regulation and acceleration of wound repair by locally acting growth factors.

Growth Factors and Repair

Wound repair is thought to be influenced by locally acting growth factors. These biomolecules, usually small polypeptides, stimulate cell proliferation, movement, and biosynthetic activity. They can act as paracrine (produced by one cell type to act on another in the local area) or autocrine (produced by a cell acting on itself) factors. To date, most of the cellular activities in wounds appear to be regulated at least in part by the presently known growth factors. This is a rapidly changing field, however, and new growth factors which could play a significant role in repair are still being found.

Locally acting growth factors can be grouped into three large categories: those which signal cells to proliferate, those which attract cells to proliferate and move, and those which alter the phenotypic state of the cell.

Mitogens which regulate cellular division have been divided (by some investigators) into two categories: "competence" and "progression" factors. In order to divide, cells must be stimulated to progress from the resting state (G0) to a state of readiness to replicate DNA and divide (G1). So-called "competence" factors appear to stimulate cells to make this transformation. Once cells enter G1, progression through the division cycle seems to require the presence of progression factors [1].

Platelet-derived growth factor (PDGF) and epidermal growth factor (EGF) act on cells in G0. Progression factors include insulin-like growth factor (IGF-1)

Department of Surgery, Box 120 UMHC, Harvard at East River Road, University of Minnesota, Minneapolis, MN 55455, USA

Host Defense Dysfunction
in Trauma, Shock and Sepsis
Eds. Faist/Meakins/Schildberg
© Springer-Verlag, Berlin Heidelberg 1993

and the other somatomedins. These factors circulate in plasma and are readily available to cells stimulated to enter G1 by the competence factors. There is also evidence that they are secreted by fibroblasts in wounds and this way act as autocrine factors.

Chemoattractants make cells move. They are divided into chemotactic factors and chemokinetic factors. Chemotactic factors work through cell surface receptors which on reaching one side of a cell in higher concentrations than the other cause the target cell to move in a given direction. Examples of chemotactic factors are C5a which is chemotactic for neutrophils and PDPG which is chemotactic for fibroblasts [2, 3]. Chemokinetic factors increase the rate of movement [4]. In the presence of albumin, neutrophils increase their random migration [5]. As noted below, some growth factors are both mitogens and chemoattractants.

The third group of growth factors are the transforming growth factors. Transforming growth factor beta (TGFβ) has many different activities [6]. In certain concentrations it inhibits fibroblast division and stimulates increased production of matrix molecules (collagen and glycosaminoglycans). It also induces the PDGF production in certain cells. Transforming growth factor alpha (TGFα) shares considerable homology with EGF, binds to the same receptor, and evokes many of the same responses as EGF [7, 8].

The growth factors presently thought to play a role in wound repair regulation include mitogens, chemoattractants, and transforming factors. Their biochemical and biological activities will be briefly summarized.

Platelet-Derived Growth Factor

PDGF is a 30000- to 32000-Da glycoprotein made up of two disulfide linked subunits [9]. Originally discovered in platelets, this competence factor has been found in monocytes, smooth muscle cells, endothelial cells, and various transformed cells [10–13]. It binds to high-affinity receptor sites, is active to the picomolar range, and is a potent mitogen for most mesenchymally derived connective tissue cells [14]. It is both a chemotactic molecule and a competence factor.

Epidermal Growth Factor

Epidermal growth factor is a 6000-Da protein made up of a single chain of 53 amino acids [15]. It binds to high-affinity receptors and is found in platelets, salivary glands, duodenal glands, and urine [16–19]. It is a competence factor for many epithelial and mesenchymal cells and stimulates epidermal regeneration after partial-thickness injuries [20].

Angiogenesis Factors

Angiogenesis is the process of new capillary formation. It is one of the most poorly understand in terms of the actual growth factor regulation since the potential list of angiogenesis factors is long and continues to grow. As presently understood, angiogenesis involves four activities; endothelial cell migration division, capillary endothelial cell enzyme production, and basement membrane matrix production. Ultrastructural studies on capillary proliferation demonstrate that capillary endothelial migration with enzyme production are the first activities seen, followed by endothelial cell proliferation [21]. An angiogenic activity is present in platelets and macrophages [22, 23]. This isolated, but not yet purified, factor has a molecular weight of 2000–14000 Da appears to be a protein, and is acid and heat stabile. This factor also causes capillary endothelial cell migration and in vivo neovascularization [24].

Fibroblast growth factors (FGF) appear to be the best candidates for the mitogen which produces endothelial cell proliferation after migration has occurred. FGF is present in acidic and basic forms. It binds to high affinity receptors and is found bound to basement membranes. The acidic form has a molecular weight of 16000 and the basic form is 18000. Both forms are heat and acid labile and are single polypeptide chains [25]. FGF is a potent mitogen for mesodermal and endothelial cells [26]. It stabilizes the phenotypic expression of cells in culture, and is purported to cause neovascularization in vivo [27, 28]. It is produced by endothelial cells and found bound to the basement membrane [29]. FGF does not have a signal peptide which allows it to be secreted by a cell, so the mechanism by which FGF leaves the cell is still unknown. There are other sources as well.

One theory which could explain the process of angiogenesis involves two and possibly three different growth factors. The chemoattractant factor from platelets or macrophages triggers the process of capillary growth by stimulating endothelial cell migration. The capillary endothelial cell must break through the basement membrane to migrate, so proteolytic enzymes must be produced [30, 31]. A very low molecular weight factor has been isolated which induces enzyme production in capillary endothelial cells and may be responsible for the increase in proteolytic enzyme production seen in stimulated capillary endothelium. FGF also stimulates production of proteolytic enzymes by capillary endothelial cells [32], As the endothelial cell migrates, it could produce FGF and/or heparinases which cause the release of membrane-bound FGF resulting in stimulation of the following cells to proliferate.

Transforming Growth Factor β

TGFβ is a 25000-Da protein made up of two chains. It is secreted from the cell as a high molecular weight precursor which is cleaved at low pH [33, 34]. It is acid and heat stable and binds to high-affinity receptors on the target cell. TGFβ

is found in many cells including platelets, macrophages, and lymphocytes [35]. It inhibits cellular proliferation, is a monocyte chemoattractant, and stimulates macrophages to produce many monokines; and it stimulates increased collagen and fibronectin production from fibroblasts and keratinocytes [36–40].

Angiogenesis Inhibitors

Neovascularization inhibition is potentially as important in wound repair as is stimulation. Presently there are three possible sources of angiogenesis inhibitors: cartilage-derived inhibitor, retinal pigment epithelium inhibitor and the combination of heparin-like molecules, and certain steroids [41–43]. The activity of epithelial cell derived inhibitors or chalones may play an important role in terminating repair. Observations made in the study of cutaneous wounds in humans show that once the growing granulation tissue is covered with dividing epithelium, no further granulation tissue growth can be stimulated with topically applied growth factors. If that new epithelium is removed, then more granulation tissue can grow until it is again covered with epithelium (Knighton, unpublished observation).

Retinal neovascularization experimentation may provide an explanation for this clinical observation. Diabetic retinopathy is successfully treated with pan retinal laser photocoagulation. When the retina is wounded with the laser, active neovascularization in the retinal vasculature is inhibited. Research in this area had identified an angiogenesis inhibitor which is made by retinal pigment epithelium [42]. It is hypothesized that injury to the retinal epithelium stimulates repair of the epithelial surface which in turn produces an inhibitor of angiogenesis which suppresses retinal neovascularization. This same process could be working in the cutaneous wound. When the growing granulation tissue is covered with new epithelium, an inhibitor of angiogenesis could be produced by the epithelium which suppresses further granulation tissue growth.

Collagen Synthesis

Collagen deposition by fibroblasts provides the molecular structure which gives tensile strength to the healing wound. The time course of collagen deposition, biochemical details of collagen production, and interplay between synthesis and lysis in wound repair are all well known. The regulatory mechanisms controlling the rate of collagen production, type of collagen produced, and proportion of collagen in the extracellular matrix are largely unknown.

The role of growth factors in wound healing collagen synthesis regulation are intimately linked to fibroblast biology. Growth factors such as PDGF which regulate fibroblast proliferation and migration affect collagen synthesis by increasing the number of fibroblasts in the wound [44]. Growth factors also affect the rate of collagen synthesis per fibroblast. TGFβ significantly increases the collagen production per cell as well as stimulating an increase in RNA levels for type I, III, and V collagen [39, 45].

The wound environment also plays an important role in collagen synthesis regulation. Collagen hydroxylation is a critical step of the triple helix molecule formation. Oxygen is required for this process to occur at normal rates. Lactate also may play a potentially pivotal role in collagen biosynthesis.

The current knowledge of wound repair regulation can be summarized by the following algorithm:

Initiation of Repair. Traumatic tissue disruption exposes plasma to connective tissue proteins which activates factor XII. The trauma creates a wound space. Activated factor XII in turn activates the clotting, kinin, complement, and plasmin cascades. The clotting cascade produces thrombin and fibrin. Thrombin stimulates platelets to release alpha granules which contain most of the growth factors needed for repair. Fibrin produces the first matrix which fills the wound space. The kinin cascade produces bradykinin which causes microvascular vasodilation at the wound edge to increase circulation in the patent capillaries. Complement activation produces C5a which brings neutrophils and monocytes into the newly formed wound space. Plasmin is produced which degrades the fibrin, starting the remodeling process and releasing fibrin degradation products which are also chemoattractants for macrophages and probably "activate" them as well [46].

Cellular Production of Locally Acting Growth Factors. Neutrophils and mono-cytes are the first cells seen in the wound space. They control bacterial contamination of the wound and clear cellular debris. Monocytes mature into wound macrophages which produce growth factors.

Platelets release their alpha granules into the wound space starting the connective tissue formation process. PDGF, platelet-derived angiogenesis factor (PDAF), TGFβ, and EGF are released. Macrophages continue to release PDGF, macrophage angiogenesis factor, TGFβ, TGFα, and lactate throughout wound repair (Fig. 1) [47]. The combination of PDGF, TGFβ, and angiogenesis factors produce granulation tissue which fills the wound space. PDGF also stimulates wound contraction. EGF, and potentially PDGF, stimulates epidermal cells to migrate and divide to cover the granulation tissue. Platelets could pay a continuing role in growth factor production throughout repair due to leakage of platelets through the loose junctions in newly formed capillaries.

Termination of Repair. As the wound heals the size of the wound space decreases as it filled with granulation tissue. One school contends that tissue growing from the wound edge completely fills the wound space and this returns the micro-environment of the space to that of "normal" vascularized connective tissue. This return may help signal the wound to stop repair since the oxygen tension will be high enough to shut off macrophage lactate and angiogenesis factor production. In addition new microvasculature produced by angiogenesis factor

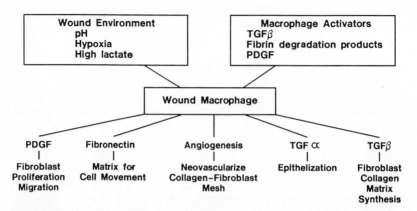

Fig 1. Schematic diagram depicting the ability of the wound macrophage to regulate the wound healing response. In response too environmental and biochemical signals, the macrophage produces various mediators of tissue repair

is initially very leaky. Plasma, red cells, and platelets continually leak through the loose junctions releasing serum mediators and platelet growth factors. When the wound space is filled, no further angiogenesis occurs and the micro-vasculature matures to form tight junctions and a basement membrane. This stops the leak of plasma and cells, and may shut off an important source of growth factors. This return of the wound space to normal connective tissue conditions tends to inhibit release of angiogenesis factors and perhaps other repair stimulators.

A second potential mechanism involves active inhibition of angiogenesis factor activity by epithelization and production of an angiogenic inhibitor.

Animal Models of Repair

To understand and interpret wound repair data, familiarity of the models used to study the subject is beneficial. Wound repair involves five major cellular responses: angiogenesis, fibroplasia, epithelization, matrix synthesis, and con-traction. Animal models have been developed which attempt to reflect and measure each of these components.

Granulation tissue formation (fibroplasia and angiogenesis) can be meas-ured by creating an artificial wound which can be removed and analyzed. Three systems are currently being used. The Schilling-Hunt wound chamber model employs a wire mesh cylinder which is implanted in the animal usually under the panniculus carnosus muscle of a rodent [48]. The easily identifiable cylinder defines the wound, aspirates or has material added by injection, and is removed.

Cellulose, collagen, or gelatin sponges are also implanted and removed for analysis [49]. The sponge has a large surface area to support tissues ingrowth. Once the granulation tissues has grown into the sponge, the sponge can be removed surgically and the tissue examined histologically, biochemically, or with immunohistochemistry. This method is excellent for harvesting wound cells since ingrowth occurs quickly.

The newest method of measuring granulation tissue formation is implantation of a small expanded tube made of polytetrafluoroethylene (PTFE) [50, 51]. Tissue grows into the tube and if the tube is left in situ long enough, tissue will fill the central space of the tube. When removed the tissue can be examined by histology, immunohistology, and biochemical analysis. This method provides an excellent analytical tool for quantitative biochemical analysis of wound tissue and matrix molecules. This is also an acceptable method to sample, for the first time in a semi-invasive manner, human granulation tissue.

Animal models for epithelization fall into two categories. Epithelial regeneration after partial-thickness wounding can be studied in many different animals by creating a partial-thickness wound surgically, by a mild burn, or suction wound. The repair of the epithelial injury is then studied by gross examination and wound area measurement, biopsy, or excision [52–54]. Epithelization over granulation tissue is much more difficult to study. Most rodents and small laboratory animals are loose skinned. This implies that their skin slides easily over the fascial covering of the muscle. When a full-thickness wound is created, these animals heal the wound primarily by contraction with a small component of epithelization. Humans are tight-skinned animals, but wounds in loose areas, especially the abdomen, neck and face do contract. When a full-thickness wound is created it must heal by epithelization of the wound bed with help from a minimal amount of wound contraction. To study this process in animals effectively, the pig is most often used [55]. Pig skin is very similar in structure and repair to human skin. The difficulty and expense of experimenting with pigs makes studies on epithelization time consuming and costly. Excellent studies by Clark have documented the chronology and morphology of full-thickness wounds in the pig [56].

Animal Studies on Growth Factors and Repair

Animal studies which demonstrate to effect of altering the locally acting growth factor environment on the repair process can be grouped into three large categories: studies which effect fibroblasts, capillary formation, and epithelization. A few examples will illustrate the type of data obtained and the difficulty determining the exact role of the growth factor tested.

The effect of PDGF on fibroblast proliferation and collagen synthesis in normal and diabetic rats was studied by Grotendorst et al. [44]. These studies used wire mesh wound cylinders implanted under the panniculus carnosus muscle of the rat as the experimental model. The investigators filled the wire cylinders with collagen into which PDGF had been incorporated and implanted them for various periods of time. The cylinders were removed and assayed for total collagen, and total amount of incorporated tritiated thymidine as a measure of the number of dividing fibroblasts in the cylinder. These studies were completed in normal rats and rats made diabetic by administration of streptozocin. Controls consisted of cylinders with collagen alone.

The investigators demonstrated that cylinders which contained PDGF had a statistically significant increase in thymidine incorporation and a significant increase in total collagen. They also demonstrated that addition of PDGF to the cylinders of diabetic rats brought the collagen level back to normal at each time point tested.

These experiments showed that a single addition of PDGF significantly alters fibroblast activity and collagen levels in experimental wounds and that a disease process such as diabetes which is known to impair wound healing can be affected by increasing the local PDGF concentration.

Angiogenesis is an important part of the repair process and facilitating angiogenesis would unquestionably affect wound healing. Experiments on capillary proliferation in vivo illustrate the effect of locally acting growth factors and also the potential problem with interpretation of the data. TGFβ has many different activities, some of which were described above. This growth factor is purported to have angiogenesis activity in vivo based on a single growth factor injection into the subcutaneous tissue of newborn mice which caused granulation tissue with a high capillary density to form [57].

Using the rabbit corneal angiogenesis assay this observation was further analysed [58]. TGFβ was delivered to the cornea in an inert slow release polymer and the effect of the growth factor on the limbal microvasculature monitored visually and histologically. This growth factor caused significant inflammatory cell migration into the cornea which was followed by intense capillary proliferation. Histology confirmed that the inflammatory infiltrate was predominantly monocytic. In vitro experimentation has demonstrated that TGFβ is a potent monocyte chemoattractant and studies show that TGFβ stimulates macrophages to produce macrophage-derived angiogenesis activity [37, 38].

Spruegel et al. utilized a modification of an in vivo wound sampling technique originally described by Goodson [50, 51]. A small PTFE tube was filled with collagen and various growth factors. The tubes were implanted subcutaneously in rats and were removed at various intervals up to 10 days. They utilized PDGF, TGFβ, basic FGF (BFGF), and EGF in the collagen matrix. They demonstrated that PDGF, TGFβ, and BFGF significantly increased the cellularity of the chambers at 10 days. The increased cellularity consisted of mononuclear leukocytes, macrophages, fibroblasts, and endothelial cells. EGF did not induce cellular accumulation or changes in DNA content. They demonstrated that the growth factors diffuse quickly from the chambers and conclude that "the responses observed at 10 days reflect a secondary process, possibly mediated by effector cells such as macrophages, lymphocytes, or granulocytes that are attracted into the chamber by each growth factor, rather than a direct effect of the factors themselves."

Pierce et al. tested the effects of PDGF and TGFβ delivered to collagen on the wound breaking strength of closed linear incisions in rats [59]. They showed a significant increase in wound breaking strength with both PDGF and TGFβ over controls and demonstrated a marked increase in inflammatory cells in the growth factor treated wounds. They also postulate that these factors work by indirectly recruiting leukocytes to the wound site.

Buckley et al. tested the effect of EGF on granulation tissue formation using subcutaneously implanted sponges [60]. The EGF was delivered using a slow-release pellet. They demonstrated a modest increase in collagen content and organization of the granulation tissue.

Davidson et al. repeated the experiments with EGF and showed similar results [61]. They tested basic FGF in the sponge model and showed that a single dose of FGF produced as great an effect as EGF in a sustained release polymer. Wound breaking strength experiments in rats were also done with basic FGF. A statistically significant increase in breaking strength was found, however the small increase in collagen content was not significant over the controls. Histologic examination showed better organization and maturation in the FGF-treated wounds.

Thompson et al. also used FGF delivered in a gelatin sponge and demonstrated enhanced granulation tissue formation into the sponge when compared with controls [62].

These animal studies consistently demonstrate enhanced granulation tissue formation when growth factors are added to various experimental models. Most observe an increased inflammatory cell response due to the growth factor presence and postulate an indirect mechanism of action involving leukocyte recruitment which in turn produce factors which sustain an elevated level of granulation tissue formation. Whether sustained release of PDGF, TGFβ, EGF, FGF or the other growth factors will have a direct effect on granulation tissue formation in vivo, independent of leukocyte recruitment, will be answered when a noninflammatory delivery system is devised.

Human Repair Models

Studying normal wound repair in humans is a more difficult problem. The fact that a surgical wound heals or fails to heal is relatively easy to determine. Simple examination of the closed wound can usually determine if it is healing or not. The effect of clinical or pharmaceutical manipulation on closed wounds is difficult to study because breaking strength is difficult to determine in human subjects. Studying nonhealing wounds, on the other hand, is relatively easy. Nonhealing wounds, or sores, can be measured, photographed, biopsied, and cultured. The repair rate can be measured over time and the effect of a therapeutic manipulation determined.

Recently, the ability to measure cellular events in human repair became available. Goodson, Hunt et al. developed a method for sampling a human wound [50]. A small tube of PTFE, a porous material used to make vascular prosthesis, is implanted into the subcutaneous tissue of the patient. This tube is approximately 1 mm in diameter. The insertion of new tissue grows into the interstices of the fabric. The tube can be removed up to ten days after insertion. The cells and matrix which have grown into the tube are removed with the tube can be analyzed in a number of different ways. Using this technique healing rates have been quantified in different patient groups. In the future, this technique could be used to measure the effect of a systemic manipulation on wound repair. Locally acting factors could also be delivered and tested by filling the tube before insertion.

Chronically Nonhealing Wounds

Chronically nonhealing human wounds provide another model to test the effect of locally acting growth factors on wound repair. The activity of the factors on the rate and character of repair can be recorded by measurement, inspection, photography, and histology of biopsy specimen.

One of the difficulties with human studies on chronic nonhealing wounds is the variability in wounds from patient to patient with the same underlying disease and the even greater variability in wounds due to different disease states. To understand this variability, a knowledge of the pathophysiology of non-healing wounds is helpful.

Wounds fail to heal, or become nonhealing sores because of 4 major factors: infection, ischemia, repeated trauma, or medication. For example, a patient with diabetes mellitus on systemic steroids due to renal transplantation, with pedal ischemia due to macro- and microvascular disease, who presents a plantar surface ulcer due to repeat trauma, has all four problems. To get his wound to heal, one must address all four problems by removing dead and infected tissue by debridement, giving the proper antibiotics to control infection, repairing the macrovascular disease to increase blood flow to the wound, use growth factors to presumably replace those not present due to steroid administration, and keep the patient off their foot and free of new injury until it heals. Many wounds are initially infected and purulent with a significant amount of necrotic tissue when the patient presents for care. As therapeutic interventions such as debridement and antibiotic administration are begun, the bacterial content of the wound may decrease and allow healing to occur. If the patient walks on the foot, the repeated trauma will cause further tissue necrosis and recurrent infection, showing down the repair process.

Chronic nonhealing wound repair is a complex and dynamic process changing over time depending on the therapeutic intervention and patient compliance with the intervention. To determine the effect of a particular intervention, such as growth factor administration, on wound repair requires careful monitoring of the state of ischemia, infection, trauma and patient compliance, along with the wound repair endpoints, including infection control, granulation tissue formation, and epithelization.

The effect of topically applied platelet growth factors in stimulating repair of chronically nonhealing cutaneous ulcers has been studied in a randomized, double-blind, placebo controlled trial. This study showed a statistically significant effect of the naturally occurring mix of growth factors from platelets on the rate of epithelization [63].

A second placebo controlled human trial using recombinant EGF on split thickness donor sites showed a small, but statistically significant effect on the rate of epithelization [20].

Conclusion

The multifactorial regulation of wound repair involves regulatory and responder cells, locally acting growth factors, and the microenvironment. Understanding this fundamental process will lead to significant advances in understanding the many diverse disease processes where wound repair plays a significant role. The ability to accelerate the wound repair rate, change the character of new tissue formed, and selectively inhibit part or all of the repair response could become a clinical reality as basic and clinical research progresses.

Acknowledgements. The authors would like to thank Ms. Lori Mercier for the editing of this manuscript.

References

1. Deuel TF (1987) Polypeptide growth factors: roles in normal and abnormal cell growth. Ann Rev Cell Biol 3:443
2. Snyderman R, Philips J, Mergenhagen SE (1970) Polymorphonuclear leukocyte chemotactic activity in rabbit serum and guinea pig serum treated with immune complexes: evidence for C5a as the major chemotactic factor. Infect Immun 1:521
3. Seppa H, Grotendorst G, Seppa S, Schiffmann E, Martin GR (1982) Platelet-derived growth factor is chemotactic for fibroblasts. J Cell Biol 92:584
4. Wilkinson PC (1988) Chemotaxis and chemokinesis: confusion about definitions. J Immunol Methods 110:143
5. Wilkinson PC, Allan RB (1978) Assay systems for measuring leukocyte locomotion: An overview. In: Gallin JI, Quie PG (eds). *Leukocyte chemotaxis methods physiology and clinical implications.* Raven, New York, p 1
6. Sporn MB, Roberts AB, Wakefield LM, de Crombrugghe B (1987) Some recent advances in the chemistry and biology of transforming growth factor-beta. J Cell Biol 105:1039
7. Massague J (1983) Epidermal growth factor-like transforming growth factor: Isolation, chemical characterization, and potentiation by other transforming factors from feline sarcoma virus transformed rat cells. J Biol Chem 258:13606

8. Derynck B, Roberts AB, Winkler ME, Chen EY, Gueddel DV (1984) Human transforming growth factor alpha: precursor structure and expression in *E. coli*. Cell 38:287
9. Raines EW, Ross R (1982) Platelet-derived growth factor: I. High yield purification and evidence for multiple forms. J Biol Chem 257:5154
10. Martinet Y, Bitterman PB, Mornex JF, Grotendorst GR, Martin GR, Crystal RG (1986) Activated human monocytes express the c-sis protocogene and release a mediator showing PDGF-like activity. Nature 319:158
11. Walker LN, Bowen-Pope DF, Ross R, Reidy MA (1986) Production of PDGF-like molecules by cultured arterial smooth muscle cells accompanies proliferation after arterial injury. Proc Natl Acad Sci USA 83:7311
12. DiCorleto PE, Bowen-Pope DF (1983) Cultured endothelial cells produce a platelet-derived growth factor-like protein. Proc Natl Acad Sci USA 80:1919
13. Deuel TF, Huang JS (1984) Platelet-derived growth factor: structure, function and roles in normal and transformed cells. J Clin Invest 74:669
14. Ross R, Raines EW, Bowen-Pope DF (1986) The biology of platelet-derived growth factor. Cell 45:155
15. Taylor JM, Mitchell WM, Cohen S (1972) Epidermal growth factor: physical and chemical properties J Biol Chem 247:5928
16. Oka Y Orth DN (1983) Human plasma epidermal growth factor/β-urogastrone is associated with blood platelets. J Clin Invest 72:249
17. Kasselberg AG, Orth DN, Gray ME, Stahlman MT (1985) Immunocytochemical localization of human epidermal growth factor/urogastrone in several human tissues. J Histochem Cytochem 33:315
18. Olsen PS, Poulsen SS, Kirkegaard P (1985) Adrenergic effects on secretion of epidermal growth factor from Brunner's glands. Gut 26:920
19. Gregory H (1975) Isolation and structure of urogastrone and its relationship to epidermal growth factor. Nature 257:325
20. Brown GL, Nanney LB, Griffen J, Cramer AB, Yancey JM, Curtsinger LJ, Holtzin L, Schulte GS, Jurkiewicz MJ, Lynch JB (1989) Enhancement of wound healing by topical treatment with epidermal growth factor. N Engl J Med 321:76–79
21. Folkman J (1984) Angiogenesis. In: Jaffe EA (ed) Biology of endothelial cells. Martinus Nijhoff, Boston, p 412
22. Knighton DR, Hunt TK, Thakral KK, Goodson WH (1982) Role of platelets and fibrin in the healing sequence. An in vivo study of angiogenesis and collagen synthesis. Ann Surg 196:379
23. Knighton DR, Hunt TK, Scheuenstuhl H, Halliday B, Werb Z, Banda MJ (1983) Oxygen tension regulates the expression of angiogenesis factor by macrophages. Science 221:1283
24. Banda MJ, Knighton DR, Hunt TK, Werb Z (1987) Isolation of a nonmitogenic angiogenesis factor from wound fluid. Proc Natl Acad Sci USA 79:7773
25. Fox GM. (1988) Fibroblast Growth Factor. In: Clark RAF Henson PM (eds) The molecular and cellular biology of wound repair. Plenum, New York, p 265
26. Gospodarowicz D, Greenberg G, Bialecki H, Zetter B (1978) Factors involved in the modulation of cell proliferation in vivo and in vitro: the role of fibroblast and epidermal growth factors in the proliferative response of mammalian cells. In Vitro 14:85
27. Vlodavsky I, Johnson LK, Greenburg G, Gospodarowicz D (1976) Vascular endothelial cells maintained in the absence of fibroblast growth factor undergo structural and functional alterations that are incompatible with their in vivo differentiated properties. J Cell Biol 83:468
28. Gospodarowicz D, Bialecki H, Thakral TK (1979) The angiogenic activity of the fibroblast and epidermal growth factor. Exp Eye Res 28:501
29. Baird A, Ling N (1987) Fibroblast growth factors are present in the extracellular matrix produced by endothelial cells in vitro: implications for a role of heparinase-like enzymes in the neovascular response. Biochem Biophys Res Commun 142:428
30. Gross JL, Moscatelli D, Rifkin DB (1983) Increased capillary endothelial cell protease activity in response to angiogenic stimuli in vitro. Proc Natl Acad Sci USA 80:2623
31. Kalebic T, Garbisa S, Glaser B, Liotta L (1983) Basement membrane collagen: degradation by migrating endothelial cells. Science 221:281
32. Moscatelli DA, Presta M, Rifkin DB (1986) Purification of a factor from human placenta which stimulates capillary endothelial cell protease production, DNA synthesis and migration. Proc Natl Acad Sci USA 83:2091
33. Pircher R, Jullien P, Lawrence DA, (1986) Beta-transforming growth factor is stored in human

blood platelets as a latent high molecular weight complex. Biochem Biophys Res Commun 136:30

34. Lawrence DA, Pircher R, Jullien P (1985) Conversion of a high molecular weight latent beta-TGF from chicken embryo fibroblasts into a low molecular weight active beta-TGF under acidic conditions. Biochem Biophys Res Commun 133:1026

35. Sporn MB, Roberts AB, Wakefield LM, de Crombrugghe B (1987) Some recent advances in the chemistry and biology of transforming growth factor-beta. J Cell Biol 105:1039

36. Moses HL, Tucker RF, Leof EB, Coffey RJ, Halper J, Shipley GD, (1985) Type beta transforming growth factor is a growth stimulator and a growth inhibitor. Cancer Cells (Cold Spring Harbor) 3:65

37. Wahl SM, Hunt DA, Wakefield LM, McCartney-Francis N, Wahl LM, Roberts AB, Sporn MB (1987) Transforming growth factor type beta induces monocyte chemotaxis and growth factor production. Proc Natl Acad Sci USA 84:5788

38. Wiseman DM, Polverini PJ, Kamp DW, Leibovich SJ (1988) Transforming growth factor-beta (TGFβ) is chemotactic for human monocytes and induces their expression of angiogenic activity. Biochem Biophys Res Commun 157:793

39. Ignotz R, Massague J (1986) Transforming growth factor-b stimulates the expression of fibronectin and collagen and their incorporation into the extracellular matrix. J Biol Chem 261:4337

40. Wikner NE, Persichitte KA, Baskin JB, Nielsen LD, Clark RAF (1988) Transforming growth factor-b stimulates the expression of fibronectin by human keratinocytes J Invest Dermatol 91:207

41. Brem H, Folkman J (1975) Inhibition of tumor angiogenesis mediated by cartilage. J Exp Med 141:427

42. Glaser BM, Campochiaro PA, Davis JL Jr, Jerdan JA (1973) Retinal pigment epithelial cells release inhibitors of neovascularization. Ophthalmology 94:354

43. Crum R, Szabo S, Folkman J (1986) A new class of steroids inhibits angiogenesis in the presence of heparin or a heparin fragment. Science 230:1375

44. Grotendorst GR, Martin GR, Pencev D, Sodek J, Harvey AK (1985) Stimulation of granulation tissue formation by platelet-derived growth factor in normal and diabetic rats. J Clin Invest 76:2323

45. Ignotz R, Endo T, Massague J (1987) Regulation of fibronectin and type I collagen mRNA levels by transforming growth factor J Biol Chem 262:6443–6446

46. Dvorak HF, Kaplan AP, Clark RAF (1988) Potential functions of the clotting system in wound repair. In: Clark RAF, Henson PM (eds) The molecular and cellular biology of wound repair. plenum, New York, p 57

47. Rappolee DA, Mark D, Banda MJ, Werb Z (1989) Wound macrophages express TGF-alpha and other growth factors in vivo: analysis by mRNA phenotyping. Science 241:708–712

48. Schilling JA, Joel W, Shurley HM (1959) Wound healing: a comparative study of the histochemical changes in granulation tissue contained in stainless steel wire mesh and polyvinyl sponge cylinders. Surgery 46:702

49. Peacock EE Jr, Madden JW (1978) Administration of beta-aminopropionitrile to human beings with urethral structures: a preliminary report. Am J Surg 136:600

50. Goodson WH III, Hunt TK (1982) Development of a new miniature method for the study of wound healing in human subjects. J Surg Res 33:394

51. Sprugel KH, McPherson JM, Clowes AW, Ross R (1987) Effects of growth factors in vivo: I. Cell ingrowth into porous subcutaneous chambers. Am J Pathol 129:601

52. Hall E, Cruickshank CND (1963) The effect of injury upon the uptake of ^{3}H thymidine by guinea pig epidermis. Exp Cell Res 31:128

53. Krawczyk WS (1971) A pattern of epidermal cell migration during wound healing. J Cell Biol 49:247

54. Pang SC, Daniels WH, Buck RC (1978) Epidermal migration during the healing of suction blisters in rat skin: a scanning and transmission electron microscopic study. Am J Anat 153:177

55. Winter GD (1972) Epidermal regeneration studied in the domestic pig. In: Maibach HI, Rovee DT (eds) Epidermal wound healing. Year Book Medical, Chicago, p 71

56. Clark RAF (1985) Cutaneous tissue repair: basic biologic considerations. J Am Acad Dermatol 13:701

57. Roberts AB, Sporn MB, Assoian RK, Smith JM, Roche NS, Wakefield LM, Heine UI, Liotta LA, Falanga V, Kehrl JH, Fauci AS (1986) Transforming growth factor type beta: rapid

induction of fibrosis and angiogenesis in vivo and stinulation of collagen formation in vitro. Proc Natl Acad Sci USA 83:4167

58. Fiegel VD, Knighton DR (1988) Transforming growth factor-beta induces indirect angiogenesis by recruiting monocytes. FASEB J 2:A1601

59. Pierce GF, Mustoe TA, Senior RM, Reed J, Griffin GL, Thomason A, Deuel TF (1988) In vivo incisional wound healing augmented by platelet-derived growth factor and recombinant c-sis gene homodimeric proteins. J Exp Med 167:974

60. Buckley A, Davidson JM, Kamerath CD, Wolt TB, Woodward SC (1985) Sustained release of epidermal growth factor accelerates wound repair. Proc Natl Acad Sci USA 82:7340

61. Davidson J, Buckley A, Woodward S, Nichols W, McGee G, Demetriou A (1988) Mechanisms of accelerated wound repair using epidermal growth factor and basic fibroblast growth factor. In:Barbul A, Pines E, Caldwell M, Hunt TK (eds) Growth factors and others aspects of wound healing: biological and clinical implications. Liss, New York, p 63

62. Thompson JA, Anderson KD, DiPiertro JM, Zwiebel JA, Zametta M, Anderson WF, Maciag T (1988) Site-directed neovessel formation in vivo. Science 241:1349

63. Knighton DR, Ciresi K, Fiegel VD, Schumerth S, Butler E, Cerra F (1990) Stimulation of repair in chronic nonhealing cutaneous ulcers: a prospectively randomized blinded trial using platelet-derived wound healing formula. Surg Gynecol Obstet 170:56–60

An Adverse Wound Environment Reduces Leukocyte Phagocytosis and Protein Synthesis

B. R. Moelleken, S. J. Mathes, A. Amerhauser, D. C. Price, and T. K. Hunt

Introduction

Little is known about the differences in behavior of leukocytes of specific types of wounds. It has been observed clinically that certain tissue types are considerably more able to resist bacterial inoculation, and some experimental evidence points to differences in leukocyte function. How is leukocyte activation affected by its immediate wound milieu, and what is it about a wound that causes a leukocyte to activate?

A wound model providing two distinct wound environments of considerably different perfusion and oxygenation is described here [1]. This study attempts to evaluate functional differences in leukocyte activation, phagocytosis, and protein synthesis by analyzing leukocytes isolated from two distinct wound types. In the first series of experiments, leukocytes were isolated from distinct wound types and analyzed in vitro, separate from the complexities of the wound environment. In a second set of experiments, peripheral (control) leukocytes were subjected to variations in pH, pO_2, and prestimulation in an effort to assess the contributions of these individual factors to the activation of leukocytes.

Methods

Wound Cylinders Cylindrical stainless steel wound cylinders measuring 4 cm in length and 1 cm in diameter were surrounded by a latissimus dorsi musculocutaneous (MC) flap on the left side of 6- to 8-week-old Yucatan miniature swine and by an identically sized random-pattern (RP) counterpart on the right side of the animal (Fig. 1). The flaps were designed with dimensions of 2.0:1 length:width so that they provided significantly different vascular milieux. The flaps were followed to 14 days in preliminary animals and documented to survive completely. Wound fluid was aspirated with a 20-gauge needle at 3 and 7 days postoperatively; these times were chosen because large numbers of neutrophils collect within this period. The wound fluid was completely aspirated

Department of Surgery, University of California 355 Nevada Street, San Francisco, CA 94110, USA

Host Defense Dysfunction
in Trauma, Shock and Sepsis
Eds. Faist/Meakins/Schildberg
© Springer-Verlag, Berlin Heidelberg 1993

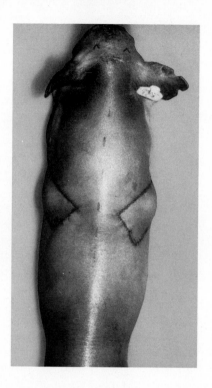

Fig. 1. Yucatan miniature swine with bilateral stainless steel wound cylinders surrounded by MC (*left*) and RP (*right*) flaps. The two flaps are of identical size (6.5 × 13.0 cm). Stainless steel mesh cylinders measure 4 cm long and 1 cm in diameter

at 3 days, so that subsequent neutrophils collecting in the chambers were comprised predominantly of new cells [2]. The wound fluid which collects is transudative in nature, with a white blood cell count of approximately $1-2 \times 10^6$ polymorphonuclear leukocytes (PMN) per cubic centimeter of wound fluid.

Wound Model and Flap Design. Dissections were carried out on Yucatan miniature swine to confirm the presence of a thoracodorsal artery and vein on the MC side and MC perforators on the contralateral RP side. The flap on the MC side measured 6.5 × 13 cm and was elevated on the thoracodorsal artery. The flap on the RP side also measured 6.5 × 13 cm. It was raised in a mirror-image fashion to the contralateral MC side. In its elevation, the latissimus dorsi muscle was left adherent to the chest wall, and the MC perforators were divided as they entered the overlying skin and subcutaneous tissue comprising the RP flap. Both flaps survived the entire experiment without necrosis of their distal tips. Barium latex injections confirmed a typical MC anatomical type, similar to that found in humans. Radiolabeled xenon injections confirmed that blood flow in the skin overlying the wound cylinders was similar to the wound surrounding them (Fig. 2).

Neutrophil Isolation For the isolation of neutrophils we used a dextran T-500 (4% in 0.85% saline) sedimentation and a discontinuous Percoll gradient by a

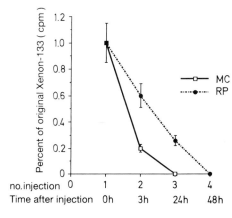

no.injection   0   1   2   3   4
Time after injection   0h   3h   24h   48h

MC: y = 0.95933 + -2.1564 *log (x) R^2 = 0.967
RP: y = 1.0338 + -1.6499 *log (x) R^2 = 0.988

Fig. 2. Washout of radiolabeled xenon from musculocutaneous (*MC*) and random pattern (*RP*) wound cylinders. Note more rapid washout from MC cylinders. Rates of washout were similar in two similar trials, one with intradermal injection into flaps overlying cylinders, the other directly into wound cylinders. In each case, washout of tracer from cylinders paralleled washout of tracer from the overlying tissue

modified (1986) method of Zimmerli et al. [3]. This procedure allowed isolation of more than 97% neutrophils which were in turn over 97% viable as determined by the trypan blue nuclear exclusion technique.

Mac-1 Expression: Surface and Total Cellular. The isolated neutrophils were stained with OKM1, a monoclonal antibody directed at the Mac-1 receptor, and an enzyme-linked immunosorbent assay (ELISA) was performed, allowing calculation of the Mac-1 receptor present on the leukocyte surface [4]. We have developed and reported a new ELISA capable of measuring Mac-1 both on whole cells (surface Mac-1) and lysed cells (total cellular Mac-1) [5]. Positive and negative controls included cell suspension alone, peroxidase-conjugated cell suspension alone, and nonspecific antibody not directed against Mac-1. For whole-cellular assays, live cells were placed directly onto ELISA plates and then treated with glutaraldehyde. For lysed cellular assays, cells were freeze-thawed three times before being applied to plates in concentrations equivalent to whole-cellular assay. Cells were placed in equal concentrations onto 96-well plates (5×10^4 cells/well) and treated with 2% glutoraldehyde in phosphate-buffered solution (PBS) to fix cells to the ELISA plate. The plates were then treated with 0.5% bovine serum albumin for 30 min at room temperature to overnight in refrigerator to bind unoccupied glutaraldehyde moieties. Cells were washed four times with PBS/Tween. Plates were treated with antibody for 1 h at 37 °C (monoclonal antibody concentration 35 mg/ml) hybridoma OKM-1 monoclonal antibody at a concentration of OKM-1 of 200 µg OKM1 per well. Wells were washed four times with PBS/Tween and subsequently incubated 90 min with peroxidase-conjugated F(ab')₂ fragments of goat anti-mouse IgG. Cells were again washed four times with PBS/Tween. Peroxidase substrate (0.1 ml) was added and incubated for 15 min. The reaction was stopped with 0.025 ml

8N H_2SO_4 and the OD read in an ELISA reader at OD 450 nm, using blank well to blank instrument. Controls included HeLa cells (negative) and P388 macrophage cell-line expressing Mac-1 constitutively (positive). For immuno-precipitation reactions, cellular isolates were radioiodinated and the membranes extracted with OKM-1 anti-Mac-1 monoclonal antibody bound to Sepharose beads. Gel electrophoresis and autoradiography demonstrated characteristic 95- and 195-kDa bands of Mac-1, very similar to those found in humans.

[^{35}S]*Methionine Incorporation to Measure Protein Synthesis.* Leukocytes isol-ated from wound fluid or blood were first incubated for 24 h in a methionine-poor medium, radioiodinated, and the membrane- and granule-associated Mac-1 extracted with OKM-1 bound to Sepharose beads. The resultant isolates were subjected to autoradiography, allowing a semiquantitative assessment of the amount of protein synthesis. This method has been described elsewhere. [6]. In both this and the previous assay, positive and negative controls were performed with cells known to be lacking in and to contain Mac-1 (HeLa and P-388 cells, respectively). Relative contributions to the CD11b and CD18 compon-ents were noted.

Phagocytosis Assay and Oxygen Determinations. *Staphylococcus aureus* (pansen-sitive strain) were cultured in tryptose-phosphate broth with 10 μci/ml [^{3}H]glycine at 35 °C for 18 h. Bacteria were centrifuged and washed in PBS twice and resuspended in 5 ml PBS. A 1 : 20 dilution of this suspension was read at 500 nm in the UV-VIS spectrophotometer and standardized. Serum (5 ml) was added to the suspension, and it was incubated at 37 °C for 30 min to opsonize the bacterial cells. Aliquots (100 μl) were counted to determine disin-tegrations per minute/colony-forming unit (dpm/CFU). Pig peripheral or wound PMN were diluted 1×10^6 cells/ml and placed into crimp-seal roller culture tubes. The tubes were sealed and gassed for 10 min under continuous flow at various oxygen concentrations. The liquid layer was mixed periodically to obtain the maximum gas interaction. Bacterial suspension (200 μl) was injected into each tube and incubated at 37 °C for 60 min. The tubes were agitated and decapped, and the contents aliquoted into 1.0 ml microfuge tubes. We added 100 μl of 100 μ/ml lysostaphin to each tube and incubated at 37 °C to digest noningested bacteria. The tubes were centrifuged in the microfuge, the supernatants aspirated, and 0.5 ml of 0.1% sodium dodecyl sulfate added to dissolve PMN/bacterial complexes. After 30 min at room temperature, the aliquots were transferred to scintillation tubes and counted in the LKM 1209 scintillation counter. CFU measurements were obtained from standard bacterial plating assays, for which each plaque on culture medium corresponded to a single viable bacterium.

Notably, although exhaust pO_2 from the sealed gas-impermeable chamber read 0, fluid pO_2 values were as high as 110 mmHg. Therefore, the pO_2 was confirmed by measuring the fluid in a calibrated blood gas analyzer.

Results

Wound Model

Anatomic dissections, barium latex injections, and radiolabeled xenon trials, both in the dermis of the flaps and in the wound cylinders were performed (Fig. 2). Measurements of pH and pO_2 (performed with standard arterial blood gas machine) on wound fluid immediately upon aspiration supported findings of a hypoxic environment in RP flap cylinders and near systemic values in the MC environment. Trials were carried out for 15 min in room air, 40% oxygen, and in 100% face-mask O_2 to see the degree to which ambient oxygen affected wound fluid oxygen content. Wound fluid from MC cylinders demonstrated large increases in pO_2 as concentrations of inspired oxygen were raised. By comparison, RP cylinders remained relatively hypoxic under hyperoxic conditions. Wound fluid pH was not affected by differences in the oxygen tension in either wound type. (Table 1).

Neutrophil Accumulation. The accumulation of neutrophils within wound cylinders has been well studied. Times of aspiration were chosen to ensure adequate neutrophils for the assays as well as a preponderance of newly arrived neutrophils. More neutrophils accumulated under RP flaps than under MC flaps [5].

Xenon Washout. Radiolabeled xenon was placed into each type of wound cylinder. Its washout was significantly faster from the MC than from the RP environment. This correlates with previous studies of dermal injections into similar wound environments.

Wound Leukocytes

Mac-1 Expression. Differences in surface Mac-1 expression have been previously reported by our laboratory and point toward early activation, probably upon entry into an adverse wound environment, of RP-associated leukocytes. Neutrophils were lysed by freeze-thawing three types, rupturing their membranes, and then subjected to an ELISA. At all time points measured, MC-

Table 1. Effect of inspired oxygen concentration on wound fluid pO_2

	pH	pO_2		
		FiO_2 0.21	FiO_2 0.41	FiO_2 1.01
Musculocutaneous	7.33	77	120	156
Random pattern	7.17	33	38	49
Peripheral	7.40	84	160	395

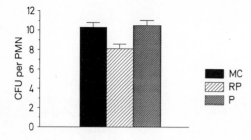

Fig. 3. Phagocytosis of tritiated bacteria. Note superior phagocytosis by MC PMN of tritiated bacteria than by RP PMN. Results expressed as organisms ingested per PMN *p* peripheral (control) leukocytes

associated neutrophils produced significantly more Mac-1 than did RP-associated neutrophils.

Bacterial Phagocytosis: MC Versus RP Flap Leukocytes Leukocytes isolated from MC wounds demonstrated superior bacterial phagocytosis of tritiated bacteria (Fig. 3; $n = 6$; $p < 0.02$).

Peripheral (Control) Leukocytes

Bacterial Phagocytosis: Prestimulation. Peripheral (control) leukocytes were tested to evaluate the effect of prestimulation. Prestimulated neutrophils were decidedly hampered in their ability to phagocytose bacteria ($n = 6$; $p < 0.05$) only 15 min after administration of phorbol myristate acetate (PMA), a maximal biologic stimulus (Fig. 4). This decrement progressed until 1 h, when neutrophils demonstrated severe decrements in function ($n = 6$; $p < 0.02$).

Bacterial Phagocytosis: pH Effect. Peripheral circulating (control) neutrophils were assayed for phagocytosis of tritiated bacteria. They were placed into RPMI medium at varying pH. Phagocytic function was adversely affected by a pH outside the physiologic range; the pH usually encountered in wound fluid

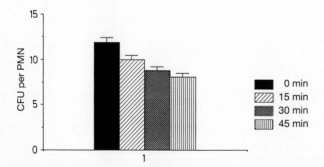

Fig. 4. Effect of prestimulation on phagocytosis of tritiated bacteria by peripheral neutrophils. Note deleterious effect on number of organisms ingested per PMN as a function of time after maximal stimulation with $10^{-8}\,M$ PMA

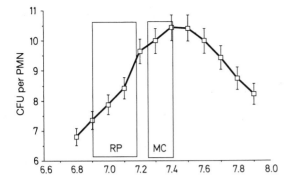

Fig. 5. Effect of pH on phagocytosis of tritiated bacteria by peripheral PMN. Note how unphysiologic pH values have a deleterious effect on phagocytosis. *Boxed areas*, pH ranges of respective flap wound cylinders

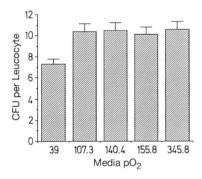

Fig. 6. Effect of pO_2 on phagocytosis of tritiated bacteria by peripheral PMN. No detrimental effect was noted until pO_2 was lowered below 40 mmHg. Results expressed as colony forming unit ingested per PMN

associated with the MC wound and RP wounds is denoted in Fig. 5 with boxes ($n = 6$; $p < 0.01$ at pH of 7.0 versus 7.4 by Student's t test).

Bacterial Phagocytosis: pO_2 Effect. Peripheral circulating (control) leukocytes in RPMI medium with controlled pO_2 demonstrated no decrement in phagocytic function until a pO_2 of 38 mmHg, when phagocytosis is markedly reduced (Fig. 6; $n = 6$; $p < 0.02$, compared to pO_2 of 107.3).

Discussion

Several cell types participate in the early inflammatory reaction and defense against foreign microorganisms seen in wound infections. It is felt that leukocytes mediate in large part the initial antibacterial properties, possibly through increased neutrophil oxidative product elaboration. Musculocutaneous flaps have demonstrated a greater resistance to bacterial inoculation in clinical and experimental settings [7, 8]. Neutrophils associated with well-oxygenated wound environments with superior blood flow and physiologic pH are associated with superior phagocytic function.

MC flaps have markedly better blood supply and oxygen delivery than conventional RP flaps [9–14]. Other investigators have found that similar numbers of neutrophils collect underneath conventional RP and MC flaps in specially designed stainless steel wound cylinders placed surgically underneath each type of flap. Yet MC flaps are superior to RP flaps in fighting infection. The intracellular killing of bacteria in the presence of muscle may therefore be greater at the individual neutrophil level [15, 16]. These data led us to believe that the anti-infective properties of the MC flap may be mediated by individual neutrophils acting at vastly different levels of bactericidal efficiency, a phenomenon which is perhaps linked to the superior blood flow and oxygenation of the muscle flap [17, 18].

Cylinder Blood Flow. Differences in tissue oxygen, pH, and blood flow between the wound environments (MC and RP) have been well characterized in this laboratory [5].

Neutrophil Isolation. Spurious activation of neutrophils occurs when they are subjected to experimental conditions found routinely in accepted isolation techniques [19]. Three precautions were taken to prevent this. Neutrophils were isolated at $0\,°C$, a temperature at which neutrophil activation is temporarily halted without subsequent damage to the neutrophils. Only endotoxin-free solutions were used as determined by the limulus assay for the presence of endotoxin, since endotoxin, a frequent contaminant of laboratory reagents, is a potent stimulant of neutrophils. All experiments requiring live neutrophils were performed expeditiously, as a permanent fall-off of neutrophil effectiveness is seen after 5–6 h in spite of unaffected Mac-1 levels. Larger numbers of neutrophils collect within RP cylinders than MC cylinders [5]. Similar findings have been noted in tumors, where poorly oxygenated regions of a mouse mammary adenocarcinoma were associated with larger amounts of PMN and other leukocytes as determined by fluorescence-activated cell sorter techniques [20]. Leukocytes have been observed to accumulate in larger numbers in adverse wounds in heart muscle, a leukotriene-dependent function [21]. Both of these studies support our finding that increased numbers of leukocytes infiltrate a hypoxic wound.

Mac-1 (CD11b/CD18) Expression. The cell surface expression of Mac-1 receptors, complement receptors, and newly recognized members of the integrin family [22] are sensitive and specific indicators of the state of activation/adaptation of the neutrophil. In this study, they were assayed by monoclonal antibodies directed against antigens in the receptor. The Mac-1 receptor is also known as the C3bi receptor, the CR-3 receptor, Mol and (perhaps most accurately) as CD11b/CD18. The Mac-1 receptor in humans is composed of an alpha subunit (170 kDa)—CD11b, which it unique to this integrin—and a beta subunit (95 kDa)—CD18, which it shares with two other integrins in the same subfamily (LFA-1, gp 150/95) [23, 24].

Functionally, the Mac-1 serves primarily as a complement receptor which binds to endothelial cell layers (hence its earlier name, complement receptor 3, or CR-3). Recently, it has been realized that another vital function of the Mac-1 may be to help the neutrophil adhere to such substances as fibronectin [25], collagen, and fibrin. Mac-1 serves as an accurate indicator of neutrophil state of activation. As the neutrophil becomes successively activated, Mac-1 located within intracellular gelatinase-containing granules (or perhaps on the membranes of lactoferrin-containing—specific—granules, a source of debate), and translocates by means of the cytoskeleton to the cell surface, where it can be measured with surface Mac-1 assays.

We have determined that M1-70 monoclonal antibody, which has previously been shown to be a blocking antibody for C3bi-mediated red blood cell rosetting, is actually a blocking antibody for Mac-1 adherence as well (unpublished data). It is therefore probable that M1-70 binds to a functional epitope on the Mac-1 glycoprotein complex. The data from the surface Mac-1 studies corroborate the findings that leukocytes activate upon entry into an adverse environment (RP cells) but not into a physiologic environment (MC leukocytes). In the 7-day maximally stimulated group, more Mac-1 was present on the surface of MC cells (Table 2; $p < 0.05$). This finding either indicates greater loss of Mac-1 at the surface of RP cells or increased production of receptor by MC cells. Protein synthesis—at least of the CD11b component of the Mac-1 glycoprotein—occurs in greater amounts in leukocytes exposed to a favorable wound environment (MC cells) than leukocytes exposed to an unfavorable environment (RP).

Mac-1 Synthesis. MC-associated neutrophils actually synthesize more Mac-1 than do cells in an unfavorable wound environment. This was suggested by our previous data reporting differences in surface Mac-1 [5] and demonstrated directly in the total Mac-1 expression and in the radioactive sulfur incorporation assays. By two independent methods, synthesis of Mac-1 was increased by 16%–20% in the well-oxygenated environment-associated leukocytes. This suggests an additional advantage of the neutrophil from a favorable wound environment: the overall synthesis of Mac-1 is increased. Only synthesis of the CD11b subunit is increased; CD18 appears to be stored constitutively in large quantities, probably because it is shared by the other integrins CD11a/CD18 and CD11c/CD18 of the same integrin subfamily. This synthesis of Mac-1 may reflect a generally improved biosynthetic capability as a result of improved

Table 2. Mac-1 expression measured from whole-cellular lysates MC cells and RP neutrophils

	3-day	3-day (PMA)	7-day	7-day (PMA)
Musculocutaneous	1.375	1.404	1.456	1.461
Random pattern	1.101	1.200	1.198	1.205
Peripheral	1.202	1.244	1.201	1.250

wound conditions (improved oxygen, nutrient delivery, less acidic conditions) or a specific ability to synthesize proteins which later become incorporated into Mac-1. It is clear, however, that cells isolated from a favorable wound milieu were more capable of synthesizing this Mac-1 subunit than cells from a hypoxic, acidic environment (RP cells).

It is known that intracellular granules, possibly [26] specific (lactoferrin-containing) granules and possibly gelatinase-containing organelles [26] house Mac-1 receptors [27], and that with activation these stores of receptor are translocated to the cell surface for subsequent expression on the cell surface [6]. This mechanism is not dependent upon new protein synthesis (not actinomycin-D inhibitable) but is dependent upon energy and an intact cytoskeleton. Yet the kinetics of this phenomenon in different wound environments are not well described. It has generally been assumed that all wounds are identical with respect to the behavior of their associated neutrophils, a finding this study refutes.

It has also generally been accepted that no Mac-1 is synthesized after a neutrophil is activated, but that Mac-1 is expressed from existing intracellular granules. Recently, however, it has been found that peripheral neutrophils synthesize Mac-1 and a number of other proteins, including FcR, MHC class I, actin, etc. [28], and that in general, primed and then stimulated leukocytes produce and express more proteins [29]. In our experiments, we have noted ^{35}S uptake in peripheral neutrophils when they are incubated overnight, which later becomes incorporated to some degree in Mac-1. The levels of Mac-1 measured in total cellular Mac-1 assays derived from lysed cells indicate that an additional 20% production of Mac-1 is occurring in MC-associated neutrophils relative to the RP counterparts.

Priming. A number of curious and sometimes paradoxical patterns of neutrophil function have been observed. Some studies have indicated that neutrophils can be primed, so that prior exposure to a stimulus results in a synergistic increase in neutrophil product expression once it is again stimulated [30, 31], compared to a modest output from a previously unstimulated neutrophil. This phenomenon has been shown to occur in wounds, in peritoneal exudate, as well as in peripheral neutrophils of burn and trauma patients. Varying degrees of activation, deactivation (chemotactic deactivation) and adaptation that neutrophils exhibit when appropriately stimulated, but no explanation on the biochemical level adequately accounts for these widely varied and seemingly paradoxical responses. [32].

These data correlate well with data published by Paty et al. [31], in which neutrophils which have entered the wound environment exhibit the phenomenon of priming, or an improved ability to respond to subsequent stimulus. In that particular study, the rabbit was used as an experimental animal. The rabbit is dissimilar from the human in that it possess a well-developed paniculus carnosus nourished by large axial perforators, not present in humans. In essence the paniculus carnosus has its own blood supply from large axial perforators rather than from MC sources (unpublished data from our laboratory showing barium latex injections to this effect). The rabbit skin, with its large percentage of muscle and a separate blood supply, may function as a MC flap. It is possible that priming reflects increased biosynthesis, explaining the later observed increase in killing capability of a mildly prestimulated neutrophil.

In Vitro pH and pO_2 Modulations. Leukocyte phagocytotic ability is decreased in unphysiologic pH and pO_2 environments. These deleterious effects on phagocytosis observed in vitro by unphysiologic pH, pO_2, and prestimulation are in the same order of magnitude as those observed in leukocytes isolated from different wounds. This suggests that altered pH, pO_2 or prestimulation alone could account for the differences in phagocytotic ability observed between MC and RP flap leukocytes.

Increased oxidative product release has been observed in reperfusion models where tissue is rendered hypoxic and then reperfused [33]. Oxidative product release, and therefore depletion of granular stores, has shown to be reduced at very low pO_2. [34] and is generally believed to be reduced in a dose-dependent fashion with decreasing oxygen tension. Low pH has been associated with other PMN defects, such as decreased migration [35]. These findings are all consistent with our findings of the defects in PMN function in adverse wound environments and the greater accumulation of neutrophils in the adverse wound environment.

Conclusions

Chronic wounds are characterized by low pH and pO_2. The wound model utilized in this study mimics this wound milieu and collects a transudative fluid rich in neutrophils.

Whole cellular Mac-1 expression (and increased Mac-1 synthesis as determined by radioactive sulphur incorporation and total cellular Mac-1 determinations) occurred in MC-associated cells. This correlates with our previous findings that superoxide anion expression, lactoferrin expression, and surface Mac-1 expression were altered in cells from an unfavorable wound environment (RP), which exhibited premature (and inappropriate) activation and degranulation compared to leukocytes from a physiologic wound environment (MC).

Peripheral (control) leukocytes, when individually subjected to the variables of low pH, low pO_2 and prestimulation with PMA, all exhibit decreases in phagocytic function similar in magnitude to those found in the poorly perfused RP wound environment. This suggests that unphysiologic pH, pO_2, or prestimulation alone can account for the differences in phagocytic function observed in vivo in the adverse wound.

It appears that the neutrophil is not predestined to degranulate in a formulaic manner but is modulated in its behavior by the wound environment that it enters. A poorly perfused wound is associated with activated leukocytes having impaired bactericidal killing reserves, phagocytic function, and protein synthesis. Control peripheral cells subjected in vitro to hypoxia, acidity, or prestimulation all demonstrate decrements in phagocytic function similar in magnitude to those observed in vivo. Unphysiologic pH and pO_2 are sufficient to explain the phenomena of premature activation and decreased phagocytosis observed in leukocytes of poorly perfused wounds.

Acknowledgments. Funding was provided through the Marion-Surgical Infection Society prize and the Paralyzed Veterans of America.

References

1. Moelleken BRW, Amerhauser A, Mathes SJ, Pytela R, Scheuenstuhl H, Breuss J, Hunt TK (1990) Adverse wound environments activate leukocytes prematurely. 10th annual meeting of the Surgical Infection Society, Cincinatti, Ohio
2. Moelleken BRW, Amerhauser A, Mathes SJ, Pytela R, Scheuenstuhl H, Breuss J, Hunt TK (1990) Adverse wound environments activate leukocytes prematurely. 10th annual meeting of the Surgical Infection Society, Cincinatti, Ohio
3. Zimmerli W, Seligmann, Gallin JI (1986) Exudation primes human and guinea pig neutrophils for subsequent responsiveness to the chemotactic peptide N-formylmethionyl-leucylphenylalanine and increases complement component Mac-1 receptor expression. J Clin Invest 77:925–933
4. Altieri DC, Edgington TS (1988) A monoclonal antibody reacting with distinct adhesion molecules defines a transition in the functional state of the receptor CD11b/CD18 (Mac-1). J Immunol 141(8):2656–2660
5. Moelleken BRW, Mathes SJ, Amerhauser A, Pytela R, Breuss J, Hunt TK (1991) An adverse wound environment activates leukocytes prematurely. Arch Surg 126(11):225–231
6. Wright DG, Gallin JI (1979) Secretory responses of human neutrophils: exocytosis of specific (secondary) granules by human neutrophils during adherence in vitro and during exudation in vivo. J Immunol 123:285–294
7. Mathes SJ, Nahai F (1982) Clinical applications for muscle and musculocutaneous flaps. St Louis, Mosby
8. Eshima I, Mathes SJ, Paty P (1990) Comparison of intracellular bacterial killing in leukocytes isolated from musculocutaneous and random pattern flaps. Plast Reconstr Surg 86(3):541–545
9. Gottrup F, Firmin R, Hunt TK, Mathes SJ (1984) The dynamic properties of tissue oxygen in healing flaps. Surgery 95(5):527–536
10. Mathes SJ, Feng LJ, Hunt TK (1983) Coverage of the infected wound. Ann Surg 198(4):420–429
11. Mathes SJ, Nahai F (1982) Clinical applications for muscle and musculocutaneous flaps. St Louis, Mosby
12. Mathes SJ, Alpert B, Chang N (1982) Use of muscle flap in chronic osteomyelitis: experimental and clinical correlation. Plast Reconstr Surg 69:815
13. Hunt TK, Twomey P, Zederfeldt B, Dunphy JE (1967) Respiratory gas tensions and pH in healing wounds. Am J Surg 114:302–307
14. Calderon W, Chang N, Mathes SJ (1986) Comparison of the effect of bacterial inoculation in musculocutaneous and fasciocutaneous flaps. Plast Reconstr Surg 77:785
15. Eshima I, Mathes SJ, Paty P (1988) Comparison of the intracellular bacterial killing activity of the leukocyte in musculocutaneous and random pattern flaps. Proc Plast Surg Res Cncl, May 19–21, pp 49–51
16. Jonsson K, Brennan SS, Mathes SJ (1988) Tissue oxygen measurements in delayed skin flaps: a reconsideration of the mechanism of the delay phenomenon. Plast Reconstr Surg 82:328
17. Jonsson K, Hunt TK, Mathes SJ (1988). Oxygen as an isolated variable influences resistance to infection. Ann Surg 208:783
18. Gottrup FR, Hunt TK, Mathes SJ (1984) Dynamic properties of tissue oxygen in healing flaps. Surgery 95:527

19. Fyfe A, Holme ER, Zoma A, Whaley K (1987) C3b receptor (CR1) expression on the polymorphonuclear leukocytes from patients with systemic lupus erythematosus. Clin Exp Immunol 67(2):300–308
20. Loeffler DA, Keng PC, Baggs RB, Lord EM (1990) Lymphocytic infiltration and cytotoxicity under hypoxic conditions in the EMT6 mouse mammary tumor. Int J Cancer 45(3):462–467
21. Gillespie MN, Kojima S, Owasoyo JO et al. (1987) Hypoxia provokes leukotriene-dependent neutrophil sequestration in perfused rabbit hearts. J Pharmacol Exp Ther 241(3):812–816
22. Pytela R (1988) Amino acid sequence of the murine Mac-1 a-1 chain reveals homology with the integrin family and an additional domain related to von Willebrand factor. EMBO J 7:1371–1378
23. Altieri DC, Morrissey JH, Edgington TS (1988) Adhesive receptor Mac-1 coordinates the activation of factor X on stimulated cells of monocytic and myeloid differentiation: an alternative initiation of the coagulation protease cascade. Proc Natl Acad Sci USA 85:7462–7466
24. Pytela R, Pierschbacher MD, Ruoslahti E (1985) Identification and isolation of a 140 kd cell surface glycoprotein with properties expected of a fibronectin receptor. Cell 40:191–198
25. Altieri DC, Bader R, Mannucci PM, Edgington TS (1988) Oligospecificity of the cellular adhesion receptor Mac-1 encompasses an inducible recognition specificity for fibrinogen. J Cell Biol 107:1893–1890
26. Petrequin PR, Todd RF, Devali LJ, Boxer LA, Curnette JT III (1987) Association between gelatinase release and increased plasma membrane expression of the Mo1 glycoprotein. Blood 69(2):605–610
27. O'Shea JJ, Brown EJ, Seligmann BE, Metcalf JA, Frank MM, Gallin JI (1985) Evidence for distinct intracellular pools of receptors for C3b and Mac-1 in human neutrophils. J Immunol 74:1280–1290
28. Jack RM, Fearon DT (1988) Selective synthesis of mRNA and proteins by human peripheral blood neutrophils. J Immunol 140(12):4286–4293
29. Hughes V, Humphreys JM, Edwards SW (1987) Protein synthesis is activated in primed neutrophils: a possible role in inflammation. Biosci Rep 7(11):881–890
30. Paty PB, Graeff R, Hunt TK, Mathes SJ (1988) Biological priming of neutrophils in subcutaneous wounds. Arch Surg 123:1509
31. Paty PB, Graeff RW, Mathes SJ, Hunt TK (1990) Superoxide production by wound neutrophils: evidence for increased activity of the NADPH oxidase. Arch Surg 125:65–69
32. Zimmerli W, Lew PD, Cohen HJ, Waldvogel FA (1984) Comparative superoxide-generating system of neutrophils from blood and peritoneal exudates. Infect Immunol 46:625–630
33. Iwai A, Itoh M, Yokohama Y et al. (1989) Role of PAF in ischemia-reperfusion injury in the rat stomach. Scand J Gastroenterol [Suppl] 162:63–66
34. Davis WB, Husney RM, Wewers MD et al. (1988) Effect of O_2 partial pressure on the myeloperoxidase pathway of neutrophils. J Appl Physiol 65(5):1995–2003
35. Rotstein OD, Fiegel VDS, Simmons RL, Knighton DR (1988) The deleterious effect of reduced pH and hypoxia on neutrophil migration in vitro. J Surg Res 45(3):298–303

Basic Fibroblast Growth Factor Inhibits the Release of Oxygen Radicals by Human Granulocytes

W. Macheiner[1], C. Oismüller[2], W. Pohl[1], and M. Micksche[1]

Introduction

Growth factors are important regulators of cell proliferation and differentiation. They are involved in the maintenance of tissue homeostasis and repair. Fibroblast growth factors (FGFs) have multiple biological activities and can stimulate a variety of processes such as mitogenesis, differentiation, chemotaxis, and angiogenesis [1]. FGFs are the most potent angiogenic factors discovered so far and they have potential for enhancement of wound healing and tissue repair. The "FGF family" consists of six proteins which are characterized by their heparin-binding properties.

Basic fibroblast growth factor (bFGF) is an ubiquitous molecule which can be isolated from a variety of normal tissues (e.g., brain, hypothalamus, retina, kidney, myocardium, endothelial cells, macrophages) as well as from specimens of malignant tumors (e.g., melanoma, chondrosarcoma, hepatoma). It is a nonsecretory factor due to a lack of a hydrophobic signal peptide sequence. bFGF is released upon requirement subsequent to cell lysis and tissue damage or by proteolytic enzymes. Release of bFGF results in the stimulation of fibroblast growth and angiogenesis which are major processes involved in wound healing [2–4].

In order to elucidate the effects of bFGF on inflammatory effector cells we investigated the influence of this factor on the respiratory burst activity (RBA) of human polymorphonuclear granulocytes (PMN).

Materials and Methods

Reagents: The following reagents were used: recombinant human bFGF (Boehringer Mannheim, FRG; formyl-methionyl-leucyl-phenylalanine (fMLP; Sigma, St. Louis, MO, USA); phorbol-myristate-acetate (PMA, Sigma); zymosan (Sigma); luminol (Sigma); Lymphoprep (Nycomed AS, Oslo, Norway); dextran 6% (Macrodex 6%, Knoll, Austria); Hank's balanced salt solution (HBSS; Flow

---

[1] Institute of Applied and Experimental Oncology, University of Vienna, Vienna, Austria
[2] Department of Anesthesia and Intensive Care Medicine, University of Vienna, Vienna, Austria

Host Defense Dysfunction
in Trauma, Shock and Sepsis
Eds. Faist/Meakins/Schildberg
© Springer-Verlag, Berlin Heidelberg 1993

Laboratories, Irvine, Scotland); polyclonal anti-bFGF antibody (British Bio-technology, GB); and suramin (Germanin; Bayer, FRG).

Cell Separation. Polymorphonuclear granulocytes (PMN) were obtained from heparinized peripheral venous blood of healthy adult volunteers. Cell isolation was performed by dextran sedimentation and density gradient (Lymphoprep) centrifugation at 600 g for 20 min at room temperature (22 °C) [5]. Remaining erythrocytes were removed by hypotonic lysis. PMN fraction was washed twice and resuspended in HBSS (5×10^6 PMN/ml). The purity of the granulocyte suspension was more than 95% as determined by Diff-Quick stains. Viability was higher than 95% tested with trypan-blue exclusion.

Respiratory Burst Activity. The RBA was determined in a chemiluminescence assay. PMN were added to a 10^{-4} M luminol solution. Subsequently the luminol-enhanced light emission was measured in a luminometer (LKB Wallac 1250) for a period of 1 h at room temperature [6]. Stimulation of RBA was done with fMLP (1μg/ml, PMA (100 ng/ml) and opsonized zymosan (50μg/ml) with or without addition of bFGF (10 ng/ml, 50 ng/ml, 100 ng/ml, 250ng/ml).

Neutralization Experiments. bFGF dilutions were preincubated with specific bFGF antibodies for 1 h at 37 °C, 5% CO_2 humidified atmosphere. After centrifugation (10 min at 700 *g*) the supernatant was added to PMN suspension and measured for RBA. Under the same conditions bFGF solutions were treated with suramin (100 μg/ml), a therapeutic agent which blocks the binding of bFGF to the receptor [7].

Results

Inhibition of RBA by bFGF. Addition of bFGF to stimulated PMN resulted in a dose-dependent inhibition of RBA. Figure 1 shows the data of four representative experiments where RBA was stimulated with fMLP. The peak values of

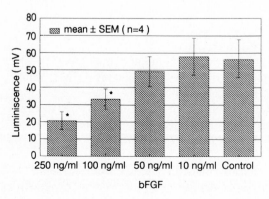

Fig. 1. Dose-dependent inhibition of respiratory burst activity (RBA) by basic fibroblast growth factor (*bFGF*). The *bars* express different doses of bFGF and the control (without bFGF); 250 and 100 ng of bFGF show a significant (*$p < 0.05$) inhibition of RBA

chemiluminescence measured 5 min after addition of fMLP are significantly ($p < 0.05$) decreased when 250 ng and 100 ng of bFGF were added to the samples. No significant inhibition of RBA was shown by 50 ng and 10 ng of bFGF in comparison to the control (without bFGF).

Similar results were obtained when RBA was stimulated with PMA or with opsonized zymosan as shown in Fig. 2.

Neutralization Experiments. In order to demonstrate the specificity of the bFGF effect on RBA of PMN we performed neutralization experiments with suramin and specific bFGF antibodies (Fig. 3). Suramin and specific antibodies could partially abrogate the inhibitory effect of bFGF on RBA. Neither with higher concentrations of antibodies and of suramin nor by changing the preincubation periods could we achieve a complete neutrilization.

Discussion

Granulocytes are potent effector cells which are able to kill bacteria by release of oxygen free radicals. They respond in vitro to a variety of stimuli such as opsonized particles (bacteria, zymosan, latex) or soluble stimuli including fMLP, PMA, and C5a by chemotaxis and/or by production of oxygen free radicals. Furthermore a variety of cytokines are able to prime PMN for respiratory burst.

Additionally granulocytes are involved in wound healing and tissue repair [2]. Thus, a homeostatis and/or a feedback mechanism must exist which regulates the activation of these cells and furthermore prevents the detrimental effects of the cytotoxic oxygen free radicals released by PMN.

In the present study we have demonstrated a dose-dependent inhibition of RBA up to 60% when bFGF was added to PMN. Both spontaneous as well as fMLP-, PMA-, and opsonized zymosan-induced RBA were significantly inhibited by bFGF. thus one might assume that bFGF released upon requirement from damaged cells is able to interface with oxygen free radical release from stimulated PMN. This could prevent damage of cells which are invading normal and/or healing tissue and could allow tissue repair.

Others have demonstrated that platelet-derived growth factor (PDGF), which is also released during wound healing and inflammatory processes, also supresses the RBA of PMN [8]. These findings and ours contribute to the notion that a hypothetical feedback loop exists (Fig. 4) in the regulation of RBA of granulocytes, providing a balance between cell damage and tissue repair. For example, endothelial cells which are very sensitive to the cytotoxic oxygen free radicals might respond by release of bFGF and/or PDGF in order to promote wound healing after tissue necrosis and cell damage caused by inflammatory processes.

The specifity of the inhibitory effect of bFGF on RBA has been substantiated by neutralization experiments using specific antibodies to bFGF. These anti-

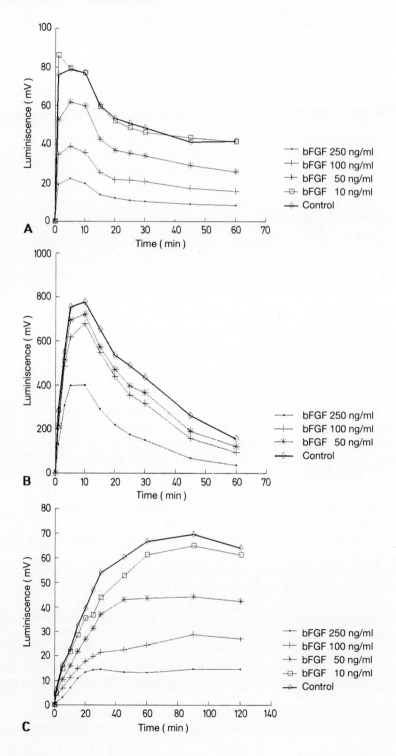

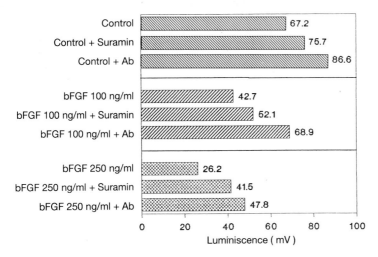

Fig. 3. Neutralization of the basic fibroblast growth factor (*bFGF*) effect on respiratory burst activity (RBA). Suramin and specific bFGF antibodies could partially abrogate the inhibitory effect of 100 ng bFGF (*middle panel*) and 250 ng bFGF (*lower panel*) on RBA. Data express the highest values of chemiluminescence measured 5 min after stimulation with fMLP

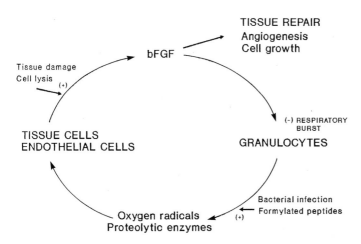

Fig. 4. A model for feedback interaction of granulocytes and tissue cells. Basic fibroblast growth factor (*bFGF*) released after tissue damage promotes angiogenesis and tissue repair and also inhibits respiratory burst activity (**RBA**) of granulocytes. Oxygen free radicals released from stimulated granulocytes cause cell lysis and tissue damage

Fig. 2 A–C. Dose-dependent inhibition of respiratory burst activity (RBA) by basic fibroblast growth factor (*bFGF*) after stimulation with fMLP (**A**), PMA (**B**) and opsonized zymosan (**C**)

bodies and suramin, which blocks the binding of bFGF to the receptor, were able to restore the RBA of PMN to a certain extent.

From this study we conclude that bFGF is able to inhibit the RBA of granulocytes and in this way promotes tissue repair and wound healing.

Acknowledgments. These studies were supported by the Anton Dreher Stiftung.

References

1. Klagsbrun M (1989) The Fibroblast Growth Factor Family: Structural and biological properties Progress in Growth Factor Research 1:207–235
2. Clark RAF (1989) Wound repair Current Opinion in Cell Biology (1989) 1:1000–1008
3. Mustoe TA, Pierce GF, Morishima C, Deuel TF (1991) Growth Factor-induced Acceleration of Tissue Repair through Direct and Inductive Activities in a Rabbit Dermal Ulcer Model Journal of Clinical Investigation 87:694–703
4. Folkman J, Klagsburn M (1987) Angiogenic Factors Science (1987) 235:442–447
5. Trautinger F, Hammerle AF, Pöschl G, Micksche M (1991) Respiratory Burst Capability of Polymorphonuclear Neutrophils and TNF-a Serum Levels in Relationship the Development of Septic Syndrome in Critically Ill Patients Journal of Leukocyte Biology 49:449–454
6. Häder M, Klausmann M, Pflüger KH, Lüben G, Seiler FR, Havemann K (1989) Granulocyte-macrophage colony stimulating factor binding sites and oxidative metabolism in human granulocytes Blut 59:486–492
7. La Rocca RV, Stein CA, Myers CE (1980) Suramin: prototype of a New Generation of Antitumor Compounds Cancer Cells 2:106–115
8. Wilson E, Laster SM, Gooding LR, Lambeth JD (1987) Platelet-derived growth factor stimulates phagocytosis and blocks agonist-induced activation of the neutrophil oxidative burst: A possible cellular mechanism to protect against oxygen radical damage Proc Natl Acad Sci USA 84:2213–2217

The Influence of Liver Regeneration on Skin Wound Healing and Lymphocyte Growth Features

N. Žarković[1], I. Stipančić[2], M. Hrženjak[1], Z. Ilić[1], S. Kiš[2], I. Vučković[2], and M. Jurin[1]

Introduction

Although intensively studied, the mechanisms controlling tissue regeneration are still not completely understood. However, substantial data show that severe trauma, particularly burns, can impair the normal function of the immune system [14, 18]. It seems that wounding can cause both local and systemic disturbances in homeostasis, which could be further manifested even as shock or multiple organ failure. Furthermore, various pathological disorders influence protein synthesis in the liver, thus causing acute-phase response [7, 26]. However, the importance of acute-phase reactants in the regulation of homeostasis, such as tissue regeneration, immune system function, and perhaps even tumor growth control, is still uncertain. However, it seems that local growth regulating factors, as well as similar humoral factors play the most important role, at least during liver regeneration [6, 20, 28]. It is also known that the immune system itself is involved in the regulation of wound healing [2, 23].

It was observed previously that tumor growth can be inhibited in partially hepatectomized animals during liver regeneration [39]. Tumor growth inhibition was caused either by certain humoral factors involved in the regulation of liver regeneration or by certain nonspecific metabolic changes resulting from partial removal of liver tissue [40]. The aim of this study was to analyze whether liver regeneration influences the intensive proliferation of nonmalignant tissue, i.e., skin wound healing, and to examine the possibility that the wounding of such induced tissue regeneration is responsible for the impaired function of the immune system.

Materials and Methods

Mice. BALB/c female animals weighing 20–23 g, 3 months old, were used in the experiment. The animals were divided into groups of ten mice each, and maintained under standard conditions with water and food given ad libitum.

---

[1] Ruder Bošković Institute, Bijenička 54, 41001 Zagreb, Croatia
[2] Military Hospital, Aleja izvidača bb, 41001 Zagreb, Croatia

Host Defense Dysfunction
in Trauma, Shock and Sepsis
Eds. Faist/Meakins/Schildberg
© Springer-Verlag, Berlin Heidelberg 1993

Partial Hepatectomy. Partial surgical removal of liver tissue (30% partial hepatectomy) was performed according to the method of Higgins and Anderson [21]. Surgery was performed on mice anesthetized by intraperitoneal injection of aqueous chloralhydrate solution (300 mg/kg).

Skin Wounds. The healing of skin wounds was induced by making two full-thickness skin defects (1%–1.5% of total body surface area each) on both sides of the dorsal midline of anesthetized mice. The wounds were measured daily for 7 consecutive days: transparent paper was gently placed above the wounds, edges were drawn, and the size of areas measured using millimeter paper.

Analysis of Murine Sera. All the animals were killed on the seventh day after surgery. Animals were anesthetized by ether and sacrificed by cutting the blood vessels of the neck using scissors. Obtained blood was then pooled according to the experimental groups. For the next 2 h the blood was held at room temperature and then centrifuged at 750 g for 15 min. The supernatant (serum) was separated from the pellet and used for further analysis. Biochemical analysis of the sera enzymes was carried out with Technicon Chem 1 Autoanalyser System (Technicon Instruments, New York). Biochemistical analysis included measurement of the concentrations of alanine aminotransferase (SGPT, ALT) [37], aspartate aminotransferase (GOT, AST) [24], alkaline phosphatase (ALP), and creatine phosphokinase (CPK) [17].

Lymphocyte Cultures. Splenic tissue as a source of lymphocytes obtained from sacrificed donors was used. All the animals were used as tissue donors, and the tissue was pooled according to the experimental groups. The organs were removed aseptically and minced under sterile conditions in cold Hanks' solution using scissors. The mash was passed through the nylon patch into a beaker and placed on ice. Five minutes later the supernatant was discarded with a syringe; the pellet was passed in the sterile test tube and washed three times on 150 g for 10 min each in Hanks' solution. The number of viable cells was determined by trypan blue exclusion, and finally adjusted to 2×10^7 cells ml. The cells were seeded into microwell plates (Nunc), 10^6 lymphocytes per culture, in RPMI 1640 medium supplemented with 10% fetal calf serum (Sigma). Lymphocytes were cultured either in medium containing 5 µg/ml concanavalin A (Con A, Sigma) mitogen or in absence of mitogen for 48 h at 37 °C with a 5% CO_2 humidified atmosphere. Afterwards, 25 µl [^{3}H]thymidine solution (methyl-[^{3}H]-thymidine, 70–85 Ci/mmol, Amersham, UK) diluted in 1:25 ratio with RPMI 1640 medium containing 10% fetal calf serum was added to the each lymphocyte culture, and the cells were further incubated for 24 h. At the end, cultures were washed over filter (Schleicher and Schuell, Dassel, FRG) using cell harvester PHD (Cambridge Technology, UK), and the intensity of incorporated [^{3}H]-thymidine determined for four culture samples per group. Statistics analysis was performed using the Mann-Whitney test.

Results and Discussion

The rate of skin wound healing observed for partially hepatectomized animals and control mice is presented in Fig. 1. Although the size of right-side wounds decreased slightly faster than the left ones, these differences were not significant. On the other hand, from the second day after surgery the size of wounds of partially hepatectomized mice were significantly larger than those measured for control mice. It is interesting that the size of wound in partially hepatectomized animals even increased during the first 4 days after surgical treatment, while at the same time the wounds of control mice healed, decreasing in size to 70%–80% of the initial wound area. After that period, the wounds seemed to heal equally in partially hepatectomized and control mice until the seventh day when the animals were killed.

It is known that the intensity of DNA, RNA and protein synthesis, as well as hepatocyte mitosis are most pronounced in the liver tissue during the first 3–4 days after partial hepatectomy [28]. However, it is still unknown what kind of liver regeneration controlling mechanism is responsible for the decrease in the dynamics of liver regeneration afterwards. There are numerous factors originating from both the liver and serum which are known as potent stimulators or inhibitors of hepatocyte mitosis in vitro and in vivo [5, 6, 30]. Some of these factors such as interleukin 1, interleukin 6, interferon-γ, and various growth factors influence the proliferation and differentiation of different kinds of cells [3, 4, 20, 30]. Thus it is possible that such factors are also responsible for the modification of skin wound healing rates observed for partially hepatectomized mice. However, most of these factors, such as tumor growth factor-beta and nerve growth factor, are known mainly as growth-stimulating factors, and it has even been shown that they can stimulate skin regeneration [29, 36].

Thus, the observed inhibition of skin wound healing during liver regeneration does not seem to be the result of the activity of such growth factors

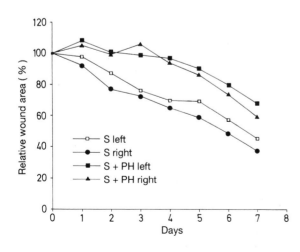

Fig. 1. Relative wound areas for left and right skin wounds of partially hepatectomized $(S + PH)$ and control (S) animals. The values are percentages of initial wound area over 7 consecutive postoperative days and were calculated as a mean value for ten mice in each group (SD = 10% –20%).*, p < 0.05, compared to controls (Mann-Whitney test)

influencing liver regeneration as well. However, the observations are completely in agreement with the already known inhibition of the growth of melanoma B16 transplanted to the hind limb of partially hepatectomized mice [40]. The explanation for the tumor growth inhibition is only speculative. Either certain factors involved in the control of liver regeneration also regulate the dynamics of skin wound healing, or the surgical trauma induces severe metabolic disturbances resulting in malnutrition, with consequental inhibiting effects on tissue regeneration [8, 22]. The second possibility seems probable since in addition to reports in the literature indicating such [10, 19], the animals in this experiment had free access to food and water, but the difference in food, and particularly water consumption, was observed between the control and operated mice (Figs. 2, 3). Moreover, the slight decrease in body weight of surgically treated mice was observed, especially in the case of partially hepatectomized mice bearing skin wounds (Fig. 4). Thus, the metabolic disturbances caused by

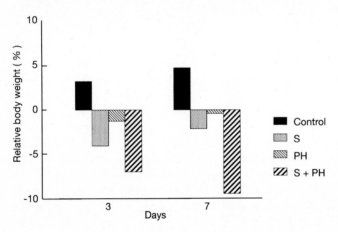

Fig. 2. The change of body weight observed for mice bearing skin wounds (*S*), partially hepatectomized animals (*PH*), and partially hepatectomized mice bearing skin wounds (*S + PH*) in comparison to the untreated control determined on the 7th day after surgery. The results are given as mean values (SD < 15%) of the relative weight change (percentage of the mice weight measured on the day of operative treatment). Each group comprised ten animals

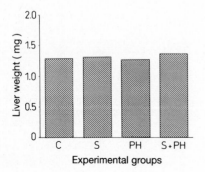

Fig. 3. Absolute liver weight values measured on the 7th day after surgery for all experimental groups. *S*, Mice bearing skin wounds; *PH*, partially hepatectomized mice; *S + PH*, partially hepatectomized animals bearing skin wounds; *C*, control. Results are presented as mean values (SD < 15%) for ten animals in each group

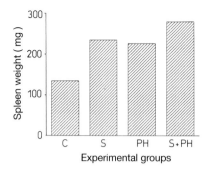

Fig. 4. Absolute spleen weight values measured on the 7th day after surgery for all experimental groups. *S*, Mice bearing skin wounds; *PH*, partially hepatectomized mice; *S + PH*, partially hepatectomized animals bearing skin wounds; *C*, control. Results are presented as mean (SD < 15%) for ten animals in each group

surgical treatment were the most obvious in the group exposed to the partial hepatectomy and skin wounding, i.e. the mice increased their food and water uptake but were losing their weight. Furthermore, although there was no difference in liver weight between the groups (Fig. 5), the splenomegaly was observed in operated animals, which was the most pronounced for partially hepatectomized mice bearing skin wounds (Fig. 6). The enlargement of the spleen is a common symptom of severe trauma, and in mice it can in part be explained as the result of nonspecific inflammation which usually accompanies the wound healing [19, 34].

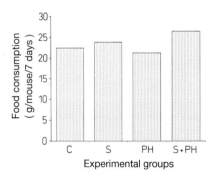

Fig. 5. Food consumption values (g/mouse) over a 7- day period for all experimental groups. *S*, mice bearing skin wounds; *PH*, partially hepatectomized mice; *S + PH*, partially hepatectomized animals bearing skin wounds; *C*, control. Results are presented as mean (SD < 15%) for ten animals in each group

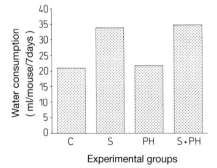

Fig. 6. Water consumption values (g/mouse) over a 7-day period for all experimental groups, *S*. Mice bearing skin wounds; *PH*, partially hepatectomized mice; *S + PH*, partially hepatectomized animals bearing skin wounds; *C*, control. Results are presented as mean (SD < 15%) for ten animals in each group

Another sign of changed metabolism in the mice exposed to trauma was obtained by analysis of the various enzyme concentrations in the murine sera. (Table 1). The concentration of ALT and AST, suggesting the liver injury, increased only slightly in partially hepatectomized mice, while a similar increase was also obtained from the sera of mice bearing skin wounds which were not exposed to partial hepatectomy at all. Increased concentration of these enzymes was more pronounced in the sera of partially hepatectomized mice bearing skin defects. The possible damage to the liver tissue may also be due to the fact that the concentration of CPK did not increase in the sear of operated mice, thus excluding the possibility that increased values of AST and ALT result from certain muscle damage [15]. However, the fact that the concentration of CPK actually decreased, particularly in the serum from partially hepatectomized mice bearing skin wounds, cannot be explained so far. Finally, since the concentration of ALP did not increase in partially hepatectomized mice, it is improbable that the liver tissue was truly damaged—at least there was no sign of cholestasis in the liver [15]. Since the other biochemical parameters which could indicate liver injury did not differ from the values obtained in normal, nonoperated mice (bilirubin, lactic dehydrogenase, etc.), just as histology did not show any sign of liver tissue damage, it can only be speculated that the observed disturbances in concentrations of different enzymes in the operated mice sera represent some kind of metabolic systemic reaction to trauma. The observed decrease of ALP in the sera of partially hepatectomized mice bearing skin wounds, just as CPK, cannot be explained yet.

It was also observed that liver regeneration, as with skin wound healing, causes a significant increase in lower density fractions of lipoproteins (low density lipoproteins, LDL and very low density lipoproteins, VLDL) in the serum [42]. Since very similar increases in LDL and VLDL concentrations were also described as the result of tumor growth [1, 37] and could be even more pronounced in partially hepatectomized tumor-bearing mice [41], it seems probable that tumor growth and liver or skin regeneration cause similar metabolic changes in the organism. However, it is uncertain whether such metabolic disturbance, as modified lipoprotein metabolism, could be responsible for the inhibition of tumor growth or skin wound healing observed for partially hepatectomized mice. On the other hand, the modified metabolism of

Table 1. Serum enzyme concentration (U/l)

Emzyme concentration (U/l)	Experimental group			
	Control	Skin wounds	Partial hepatectomy	Skin wounds + partial hepatectomy
AST	306	402	376	457
ALT	48	65	60	77
CPK	6560	6641	5135	3948
ALP	133	89	102	20

lipoproteins could probably influence the function of the immune system, since it is known that LDL and VLDL can impair the function of T lymphocytes [31]. Thus, it is possible that under the influence of the increased values of these lipoprotein fractions in the sera of operated mice the lymphocyte growth features were modified, as was observed in vitro (Table 2). The intensity of [^{3}H]thymidine incorporation into nonoperated and the surgically treated mice splenic lymphocytes in the absence of mitogen did not differ significantly. Thus, it seems that nonspecific inflammation, as an expected consequence of mechanical trauma, did not have an important role in the inhibition of wound healing or immune system function, since otherwise the spontaneous mitogenic activity of splenic lymphocytes should be observed [31]. Since there was no increase in [^{3}H] thymidine incorporation in the absence of mitogen in vitro for wounded mice lymphocytes, their weak mitogenic response to Con A cannot be explained as indirect result of postsurgical nonspecific inflammation. More likely, low mitogenic activity when cultured in presence of Con A of splenic lymphocytes obtained from mice exposed to trauma could be the symptom of immune suppression caused by trauma. Immunosuppressive effects of wounding are, well documented [16, 32], but it is still not completely understood.

However, it seems that beside the various cytokines, such as tumor necrosis factor, interleukin 1, and interleukin 6 [35], there are other factors released from wounded tissue, at least from the burned skin, which could cause immunosuppression [18, 27]. It is very uncertain whether such immunosuppressive factors are released from the tissue regenerating after mechanical trauma since such trauma does not seem to cause obvious suppression of the immune system [33]. On the other hand, increased temperature and mechanical trauma induce synthesis and release of heat-shock and stress proteins which influence both the liver metabolism and the immune system function [9, 25]. Furthermore, since some cytokines are involved not only in the regulation of the immune reactivity but also in the induction of acute phase proteins synthesis in the liver and hepatocyte growth [11, 35], it could be speculated that there are also factors involved in the control of liver regeneration which can modify the immune system function. Thus, further information is required about the activity of factors because at their possible importance not only from a scientific point of view but also for the improvement of therapy for severely injured patients.

Table 2. Blastic lymphocyte transformation

Experimental group	[^{3}H]Thymidine incorporation (cpm) N $\times$ 10^{-3}	
	Without mitogen	With Con A
Control	1.69 $\pm$ 0.71	56.97 $\pm$ 19.73
Skin wounds	2.45 $\pm$ 0.35	15.05 $\pm$ 0.92
Partial hepatectomy	1.04 $\pm$ 0.25	11.06 $\pm$ 1.68
Skin wounds + partial hepatectomy	2.01 $\pm$ 0.58	14.39 $\pm$ 3.89

References

1. Alexepopulos CG, Blatsiosis B, Avgerinos A (1987) Serum lipids and lipoprotein disorders in cancer patients. Cancer 60:3065–3070
2. Barbul A, Breslin RJ, Woodyard JP, Wasserkrug HL, Efron G (1989) The effect of in vivo T helper and T suppressor lymphocyte depletion on wound healing. Ann Surg 209:479–483
3. Barnes D (1988) Growth factors involved in repair processes: an over-view Methods Enzyme 163:707–715
4. Bryckaert MC, Lindroth M, Lonnm A, Tobelem G, Wastasen A (1988) Transforming growth factor beta decreases the proliferation of human bone marrow fibroblasts by inhibiting the platelet derived growth factor binding. Exp Cell Res 179:311–321
5. Bucher NLR, Swaffield MN (1975) Regulation of hepatic renegeration in rats by synergistic action of insulin and glucagon. Proc Natl Acad Sci USA 72:1157–1160
6. Carr BI, Hayashi I, Branum EL, Moses HL (1986) Inhibition of DNA synthesis in rat hepatocytes by platelet-derived type beta transforming growth factor. Cancer Res 46:2330–2334
7. Carr WP (1983) Acute-phase proteins. Clin Rheum Dis 9:227–239
8. Carrico TJ, Mehrhof AI, Cohen IK (1984) Biology of wound healing. Surg Clin North Am 64:721–733
9. Currie RW, White FP (1981) Trauma-induced protein in rat tissues: a physiological role of "heat shock" proteins. Science 214:72–73
10. Czaja AJ, Rizzo TA, Smith WR, et al. (1975) Acute liver disease after thermal injury. J Trauma, 15:887–894
11. Darlington GJ, Wilson DR, Lechman LB (1986) Monocyte-conditioned medium, interleukin-1, and tumor necrosis factor stimulate the acute phase response in human hepatoma cells in vitro. J Cell Biol 103:787–793
12. Deitch EA (1985) Spontaneous lymphocyte activity: an important but neglected component of the imunologic profile of the thermally injured patient. Surgery 98:587–592
13. Dickson PW, Bannister D, Schreiber G (1987) Minor burns lead to major changes in synthesis rates of plasma proteins in the liver. J Trauma 27:283–286
14. Dobke MK, Deitch EA, Harnar TJ, Baxter CR (1989) Oxidative activity of polymorphonuclear leukocytes after thermal injury. Arch Surg 124:856–859
15. Everett RM, Harrison SD Jr (1983) Clinical biochemistry. In: Foster HL, Small JD, Fox JG (eds) The mouse in biomedical research III. Academic, New York, pp 313–326
16. Gadd MA, Hansbrough JF, Hoyt DB, Ozkan N (1989) Defective T-cell surface antigen expression after mitogen stimulation. Ann Surg 209:112–118
17. German Society for Clinical Chemistry (1977) Standardization of enzyme activities in biological fluids: standard method for determination of creatine kinase activity, revised draft of 1976. J clin Chem Clin Biochem 15:255–260
18. Hansbrough JF, Peterson V, Kortz E, Piacentine J (1983) Postburn immunosuppression in an animal model: monocyte dysfunction induced by burned tissue. Surgery 93:415–423
19. Hansbrough JF, Gadd MA (1989) Temporal analysis of murine lymphocyte subpopulation by monoclonal antibodies and dual-color flow cytometry after burn and nonburn injury Surgery 106:69–80
20. Hayashi I, Carr BI (1985) DNA synthesis in rat hepatocytes: inhibition by a platelet factor and stimulation by an endogenous factor. J Cell Physiol 125:82–90
21. Higgins GM, Anderson RM (1931) Experimental pathology of the liver I: restoration of liver of white rat following partial surgical removal. Arch Pathol 12:185–202
22. Irvin TT (1978) Effects of malnutrition and hyperalimentation on wound healing Surg Gynecol Obstet 146:33–37
23. Kagan RJ, Bratescu A, Jonasson O, Matsuda T, Teodorescu M (1989) The relationship between the percentage of circulating B cells, corticosteroid levels and the other immunologic parameters in thermally injured patients. J Trauma 29:208–213
24. Karmen A (1955) Transaminase activity in human blood. Appendix: note on spectrophoto-metric assay of glutamic oxalacetic transaminase in human blood serum. J Clin Invest 34:126–133
25. Kaufmann SHE (1990) Heat shock proteins and the immune response. Immunol Today 11:129–136
26. Kushner I (1988) The actue phase response: an overview. Methods Enzymol 163:373–383

27. Lazarou SA, Barbul A, Wasserkrug HL, Efron G (1989) The wound is a possible source of posttraumatic immunosuppression. Arch Surg 124:1429–1431
28. Leong GF, Grisham JW, Hole BV, Albright ML (1964) Effect of partial hepatectomy on DNA synthesis and mitosis in heterotopic partial autografts of rat liver. Cancer Res 24:1496–1501
29. Li AKC, Koroly MJ, Schattenkerk ME, Malt RD, Young M (1980) Nerve growth factor: acceleration of the rate of wound healing in mice. Proc Natl Acad Sci USA 77:4379–4381
30. Nakamura T, Teramoto H, Tomity Y, Ichichara A (1986) Two types of growth inhibitor in rat platelets for primary cultured hepatocytes. Biochem Biophys Res Commun 134:755–763
31. Nakayasu T, Nacy M, Okano Y, McCarty B, Harmony YAK (1986) Plasma lipoproteins can suppress accessory cell function and consequently suppress lymphocyte activation. Exp Cell Res 163:103–116
32. Ninnemann JL (1982) Immunologic defences against infection: alterations following thermal injuries. J Burn Care Rehab 3:355–398
33. Richter M, Jodouin CA, Moher D, Barron P (1990) Immunologic defects following trauma: a delay in immunoglobulin sythesis by cultured B cells following traumatic accidents but not elective surgery. J Trauma 30:590–596
34. Ross R, Odland G (1968) Human wound repair II: inflammatory cells, epithelial-mesenchymal interrelations and fibrogenesis. J Cell Biol 39:152–168
35. Sehgal PB, Grieninger G, Tosato G (Eds) (1989) Regulation of the acute phase and immune responses: interleukin-6. Ann NY Acad Sci 557:1–579
36. Sporn MB, Roberts AB, Shull JH, Smith JM, Jerrold MW, Sodek J (1983) Polypeptide transforming growth factors isolated from bovine source and used for wound healing in vivo. Science 219:1329–1330
37. Steinberg D (1984) Lipoproteins and atherosclerosis: a problem in cell biology. In: Scheschter AN, Dean A, Goldberger RF (eds) The impact of protein chemistry on the biomedical sciences. Academic, Orlando, pp 251–307
38. Wroblewski F, LaDue JS (1956) Serum glutamic-pyruvic transaminase in cardiac and hepatic disease. Proc Soc Exp Biol Med 91:569–571
39. Žarković N, Jurin M, Danilović Ž (1987) Effects of regenerating tissue on tumor growth in vivo. Cell Diff 20 [Suppl]:112S
40. Žarković N, Žarković K, Jurin M, Ilić Z, Zgradić I, Danilović Ž, Gežo A (1990) Inhibition of melanoma B16 growth induced by liver regeneration. Lijec Vjesn 112:80–85
41. Žarković N, Salzer B, Pifat G (1992) The influence of liver regeneration and tumor growth on serum lipoprotein composition in mice. Period Biol 94:(in press)
42. Žarković N, Salzer B, Hrženjak M, Ilić Z, Pifat G, Stipančić I, Vučković I, Jurin M (1991) The effect of gallium arsenide laser irradiation and partial hepatectomy on murine skin wound healing and lipoprotein composition. Period Biol 93:359–361

Section 16

**Therapeutic Immunomodulatory
Approaches: Prevention**

Therapy of Secondary T-Cell Immunodeficiencies with Biological Substances and Drugs: An Update

J. W. Hadden and E. M. Hadden

Introduction

At the first meeting of this series, Meakins and Franco [1] lamented the lack of an immunopharmacologic "silver bullet" to reverse the immunosuppression observed in patients with severe trauma and burns. They pointed out that before studies of immunomodulators can be done properly, all of the variables of care must be standardized and maximized, and they particularly emphasized the opportunity for the surgeon to act as an "immunomodulator."

As an immunopharmacologist with a long history of experience in the treatment of immunodeficiency but very little experience with specific problems of trauma and burns, we would like to discuss in this contribution possible strategies to manage better these unique and particularly severe problems. Reflecting on my original paper [2], I would emphasize that the immunodeficiencies of trauma and burns have various levels of complexity and it is difficult to treat them as a single entity. They seem to have in common an acute-phase reaction which to a significant degree is glucocorticoid mediated. This acute-phase reaction is associated with leukopenia and leukocytosis, and depending on the circumstance, a number of mediators are released, including cyclooxygenase products (thromboxanes and prostaglandins) and lipoxygenase products (eicosanoids and leukotrienes), histamine and other mast cell, granulocyte, and platelet products, and complement-derived peptides. As the acute phase resolves, the situation becomes further complicated by blood and serum losses, fluid-electrolyte imbalances, protein/calorie and nutrient deficiencies, and the many consequences of sepsis. All in all, it is not a simple metabolic or immunologic circumstance. In these cascading events, a number of factors impair one or another form of body defense, and defects of granulocyte, macrophage, and lymphocyte function have been described [3-5]. It is apparent that the severity and duration of the impairments are not well explained by the mechanistic studies to date and it is not surprising that they are not easily reversed by an immunologic silver bullet.

For the purposes of this discussion, we would like to focus on the T-cell defects and discuss further the prospects for enhancing T-cell immunity in the management of the immunodeficiency associated with trauma and burns.

University of South Florida College of Medicine, Department of Internal Medicine, Division of Immunopharmacology Box 19, 12901 Bruce B. Downs Boulevard Tampa, FL 33612-4799 USA

Host Defense Dysfunction
in Trauma, Shock and Sepsis
Eds. Faist/Meakins/Schildberg
© Springer-Verlag, Berlin Heidelberg 1993

The emphasis on the restoration of cellular immune response is not to imply that other immunotherapeutic efforts are not appropriate, including (1) intravenous γ-globulin treatment for enhancing protection associated with defective B-cell function under these circumstances; (2) the use of interferon-γ or other macrophage-active agents to improve macrophage dysfunction; (3) the administration of colony stimulating factors (e.g., GM-CSF) for enhancing neutrophil number and function; and (4) antibiotics and appropriate surgical debridement to reduce the possibility of infection.

With respect to the impairment of T-cell-related immunity, it is important to note that anergy is a frequent complication of trauma and thermal injury and that its presence correlates with poor prognosis and death. Abnormalities observed include decreased overall T-cell number, impaired T-lymphoproliferative responses, and increased T suppressor cell function and reversed T4/T8 ratio. Factors which contribute to the T-cell-related defects include increase in serum glucocorticosteroids, acute phase reactants including C-reactive protein, enhanced production of prostaglandins, and possibly histamine release. The issue of histamine release was not emphasized in the prior meeting in this area, but it was noted by surgeons that they routinely treat trauma patients with cimetidine to obviate peptic ulcer development, implying a very strong histamine drive on the gastric parietal cells. It seems relevant to document elevated serum histamine levels, if they occur, since histamine is important as a possible mechanism of activation of T suppressor cells [6] and may contribute to the abnormality of T suppressor cell function. Finally, low molecular weight peptides in serum have been further implicated in immunosuppression [7]; however, their nature is unknown. The role of endotoxin and its immune dysregulating potential cannot be over emphasized.

In the previous discussion [2], were defined: the various thymic hormones thymomimetic biologicals like interleukins 1 and 2 (IL-1 and IL-2) and transfer factor, and the thymomimetic drugs of which two classes of agents were presented, one prototype being levamisole and the other isoprinosine. Comparisons of these drugs and biologicals in the manner in which they have been shown to modulate in vivo immune function of the T cell system and how they interact immunopharmacologically in the regulation of T cell ontogeny were detailed. Rather than recapitulate that discussion, we would like to update it and address somewhat more specifically the challenging issues related to immunodeficiency associated with trauma and burns. The emphasis in this discussion will be on (1) the case for countersuppression, i.e., the use of agents which interfere with the production or action of immunosuppressive influences; and (2) immunotherapeutic reconstitution of T-cell number and function using multiple agents.

The Case for Countersuppression

The initial glucocorticosteroid-dependent phase of immune suppression is physiologic in nature and although it is difficult to explain its adaptive nature, it probably poses little greater risk per se than the immune suppression routinely associated with surgery and anesthesia. Several drugs have been employed to attempt to reverse this form of suppression (see thymomimetic drugs [2]); however, none of them to our knowledge has been demonstrated to interfere specifically with steroid-mediated immune suppression. A new purine immuno-modulator detailed later in this contribution is the first to speak to this question.

The subsequent stages of suppression have been attributed to suppressor macrophages and T cells and yet uncharacterized serum suppressive factors [7, 8]. Many of the mediators associated with specific and nonspecific immune suppression have been demonstrated to impinge on the cyclic adenosine mono-phosphate (AMP) pathway [see 2] and it has been postulated that agents which interfere with these mechanisms may counter the immunosuppressive influences. Agents which either block prostglandin/cyclic AMP production, e.g., indometh-acin, or promote the cyclic guanosine monophosphate (GMP) system (e.g. thymopentin, levamisole, interleukin-2, and cimetidine) have been used in vivo and in vitro to reverse burn-induced immune dysfunction [for review see 9, 10]. Enhanced production of prostglandin by macrophages has been amply demon-strated [1], and introduction of indomethacin or similar cycloxygenase-inhibi-ting drugs can be shown to enhance the impaired lymphoproliferative responses of patients with burns [10].

Given the severity and duration of the immune suppression in these circum-stances, it is difficult to accept that suppressor macrophages are the most significant part of the story. The depletion of $CD4^+$ cells under these circum-stances is unexplained and a possible lytic mechanism independent of glucocor-ticoids needs to be defined in man. The increases in relative number of T suppressor cells and evidence for increased T suppressor cell function [8] deserves further documentation and explanation.

Increased histamine production is probably evident in patients with burns and trauma as evidenced by their propensity to peptic ulceration. Histamine is a potent inducer of T suppressor cell function via the H_2 receptor and the cyclic AMP pathway [6] and cimetidine is capable of blocking this drive mechanism. If elevated histamine levels can be demonstrated, it is, indeed, appropriate to consider H_2 blocker treatment as a therapy adjunct, not only for prevention of peptic ulcer disease, but also for immunorestoration. It is also important to note that cimetidine has immunotherapeutic potential independent of its capacity to block T suppressor cell activity, as noted in several studies [2]. Another possible approach to abrogate T suppressor function involves the use of low-dose cyclophosphamide. A single low dose of cyclophosphamide has been shown to abrogate T suppressor cell function for up to 21 days in man without otherwise being immunosuppressive [11]. This approach should be tested in animal burn and trauma models to confirm its possible efficacy and safety for man. The mechanism by which suppressor cell and factor influences act to impair the function of CD4$^+$ T lymphocytes and other immunocytes is not well understood. For the reversal of endotoxin-mediated immune dysfunction, appropriate treatment with plasma exchange, polymyxin B therapy [12], or monoclonal antibody to endotoxin [13] may prove important.

Recent work has focussed on calcium influx and protein kinase C as additional critical pathways in lymphocyte activation which may be interfered with by immunosuppressive influences such as cyclosporin A and viral immunosuppressive peptides. To the extent that these mechanisms may be involved in burns and trauma, they, like those which act via cyclic AMP, block T-lymphocyte activation including interleukin-2 (IL-2) production and IL receptor expression. Recent investigations concerning the actions of thymic hormones in relation to IL-1 in T-lymphocyte activation [14] suggest that this may be one important aspect of thymic hormone action to reverse trauma-induced immune suppression [10]. Further investigation is necessary to clarify these mechanisms.

Administration of IL-2 alone offers another way of bypassing some of these suppressive influences and it should be attempted experimentally in appropriate animal models; however, it is important to note that recombinant (r) IL-2 can promote infection through interfering with neutrophil chemotaxis [15]. Thus, its use in these circumstances should be judicious and only low doses considered. The foregoing considerations are relevant to the countersuppression issue, i.e., reversing immunosuppression of existing T lymphocytes. In these situations, immunorestoration involving T-cell lymphocyte reconstitution is a separate and important goal.

T-Lymphocyte Reconstitution

Thymic involution and T-cell depletion have been documented in animals and man under these circumstances. The following is intended as a status report on the current progress with respect to the reconstitution of the function of the cellular immune system with peptides and drugs.

Thymic Hormone and Interleukins in T-Cell Development

Various thymic hormone preparations (thymopentin, thymulin, and thymosin-α_1) have seen use in experimental and human cancer, immunodeficiency, infections, and autoimmune disorders. Only a degree of immunorestorative activity and enhanced resistance have been observed. In the context of trauma and burns, the work of Faist and coworkers [10] would indicate the appropriateness of thymopentin treatment as an immunorestorative adjunct.

Considerable controversy has arisen recently concerning the definitions of thymic hormones and doubt has been cast upon the thymus specificity and hormone nature of thymopoietin, thymosin-α_1, and thymulin. Nevertheless, three pure thymic hormone preparations have now been demonstrated to induce prothymocyte differentiation and to regulate IL-2-dependent proliferation of mature T lymphocytes [14] (E. M. Hadden and J. W. Hadden, unpublished). As noted above, many studies of dysfunction associated with burns and trauma point to defects in the triggering of lymphocytes which result in defective production of IL-2, display of IL-2 receptors and clonal expansion. Therefore, actions of these thymic hormones to augment this function may clearly relate to their capacity to participate in the reversal of these functional defects of T cells.

Based upon the experimental data available, it is not expected that these thymic hormone preparations will increase the number of T lymphocytes, particularly CD4-positive T cells, through actions to promote T-cell development via the thymus. Recent work points to interleukins as being crucial in the regulation of development of T cells [16]. Previously it was thought that thymic hormones were responsible for T-cell development; however, they appear now to be the "endocrine umbrella" under which T-cell development occurs. The language of regulation of T-cell development is clearly an interleukin language. In this language, IL-1 and IL-2 are central; in addition, IL-6 and GM-CSF, which are produced by thymic epithelial cells, participate in the process. The program involving IL-1 induction of high-affinity IL-2 receptors and the production of IL-2 leading to the clonal expansion of T lymphocytes is a central issue in the development and commitment of T cells. Thymic hormones promote this program, presumably in precursor cells and also in the proliferative expansion of mature T cells in the periphery. These studies have suggested to us that interleukins, particularly IL-1 and IL-2, may be therapeutically useful in T-cell reconstitution; we therefore studied their effects in the context of neonates and immune-suppressed adult animals. Neonatal mice (10 days of age) lack functional T cells in their spleens. After this initial period, the spleen and lymph nodes are rapidly supplied with functional T cells through thymic seeding by a regulatory process not yet understood. We attempted to speed up this process by treating neonatal mice with interleukins and thymic hormones [17]. We found that mixed interleukins (50 U IL-2 equivalents/mouse per day × 5) promoted the development of functional T cells in the neonatal spleens. rIL-1 and rIL-2 at equivalent doses alone were not active, nor was a mixture of thymic hormones (thymosin fraction V). Based upon our experiments showing IL-1 and IL-2 synergy on T-cell development [17], we presume that the mixture of IL-1 and IL-2 in this interleukin preparation accounted for the majority of the effect. These observations support our hypothesis that interleukins produced by immune activation in the periphery are important signals for the processing of T lymphocytes by the thymus.

In extending this notion, we treated aged mice (12–24 months) with a large dose of hydrocortisone to induce a "chemical thymectomy" and reduce spleen

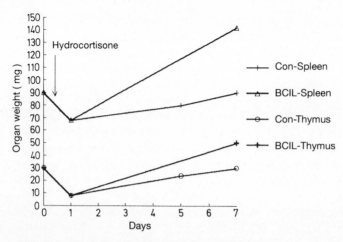

Fig. 1. Aged mice were treated with hydrocortisone (2.5 mg i.p.) on day 0, and at the nadir of T-lymphocyte depletion on day 1 daily treatment (× 5) with low-dose mixed interleukins (*BCIL*, 50 U IL-2 equivalents) was begun. On day 7 mice were sacrificed and lymphoid organ weights, cellularity, and T-lymphocyte proliferative functions to mitogens and IL-2 were assessed (*Con*, control). (From [23])

size through T-lymphocyte depletion. We treated the mice with the same protocol of interleukins and thymic hormones for 5 days, days 1–6 after hydrocortisone, and examined at 7 days the recovery of lymphoid organ weight and T-cell number and function. We observed that the mixed interleukin preparation restored thymus and spleen to above pretreatment levels (Fig. 1). Both T-cell number and function were correspondingly increased (not shown). Neither rIL-2 alone nor thymosin fraction V was active in the regard. These data further support the immunorestorative effects of mixed interleukins.

Preliminary experiments indicate that thymic hormones and interleukins are synergistic in promoting the interleukin and mitogen responsiveness of T lymphocytes of the spleen and thymus of treated mice. It seems appropriate to consider this kind of reconstitution in the context of patients with burns and trauma, particularly in conjunction with efforts to counteract suppression.

Thymomimetic Drugs

Thymomimetic drugs have been discussed in a previous publication [2]. Significant developments have taken place with respect to several of them. One of the class I thymomimetic drugs, levamisole, has been licensed by the US Food and Drug Administration for use with 5'-fluorouracil in Duke's C colon cancer, making it now available in the United States for this and certain experimental indications. Levamisole is a relatively weak thymomimetic agent with a relatively slow action, making it a low-priority agent for application in burns and trauma. Another sulfur-containing compound, diethyldithiocarbamate

(DTC-imuthiol), having a similar immunopharmacology, has recently been shown to suppress the development of infection in patients with acquired immunodeficiency syndrome (AIDS) and AIDS-related complex (ARC) in multicenter trials in the United States [18]. This agent seems to be a more active, less toxic agent than levamisole and warrants consideration in the context of reversing immunodepression in association with burns and trauma.

Of the class II purine-containing thymomimetic compounds, isoprinosine was discussed in the preceding work; evidence was presented by Faist [10] as well as others [19] to indicate some degree of reversal of immunosuppression associated with burns and trauma both in vitro and in vivo. I know of no clinical study with isoprinosine in this sector. We have recently synthesized a new purine, methylinosine monophosphate (methyl-IMP), which appears to be superior to isoprinosine with respect to many aspects of its effect on the cellular immunity.

Methyl-IMP

Methyl inosine monophosphate (methyl-IMP) is a new IMP derivative which appears to have distinct advantage over preceding immunomodulatory purines (e.g., isoprinosine or NPT 15392) in showing a more consistent activity. We therefore classify it as a "third generation" compound in our effort to produce the most effective purine immunomodulator drug. As far as its immunopharmacology has been analyzed, it has activity parallel to the precursor purines and, therefore, is classified by us as "thymomimetic" drug. In vitro, it augments lymphocyte responses to T-lymphocyte mitogens but not B-cell mitogens in both human peripheral blood lymphocytes and murine splenic lymphocytes. The action is apparent at $0.1-1$ μg/ml and increases progressively to 100 μg/ml. In more than 50 studies to date, the response is consistent and approaches a 1.5- to 2-fold increase in human and murine lymphocytes. The effect is superior to that observed with isoprinosine, inosine, or IMP itself. Methyl-IMP is able to restore depressed lymphoproliferative responses of murine lymphocytes inhibited by glucocorticoids (see Fig. 2). It restores the responses of human lymphocytes in vitro inhibited by interferon-α (100 U/ml), prostglandin (PG)E$_2$ (10^{-6} M), and also an immunosuppressive synthetic peptide derived from the P41 segment of the intramembranous portion of the GP160 of the human immunodeficiency virus (HIV). Methyl-IMP is effective at reversing immunosuppressive influences when they are mild to moderate; however, in the presence of profound inhibition, the drug effect is lost. In vitro, the effects of methyl-IMP to augment phytohemaglutinin (PHA) responses of murine lymphocytes is somewhat age dependent, with pronounced effects in young and middle-aged mice but somewhat attenuated effects in aged mice (2 years). In lymphocytes in vitro from patients with pre-AIDS (CD4 counts approximately 500), methyl-IMP restored the depressed lymphoproliferative responses to the normal range (8 patients). It had a negligible effect to restore the PHA response of lymphocytes

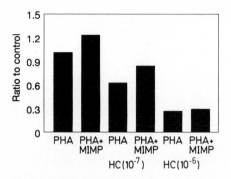

Fig. 2. Splenic lymphocytes from adult Balb/c mice were cultured in vitro in the presence of phytohemagglutinin (PHA 1.5 µg/ml). Methyl-IMP (*MIMP*) 10 µg/ml was added with PHA in the presence or absence of hydrocortisone (*HC*; 10^{-7} M and 10^{-6} M). MIMP results are expressed as a ratio to control. MIMP stimulated the PHA response in the absence of hydrocortisone, restored the suppression induced by hydrocortisone (10^{-7} M), but had no effect on the profound expression induced by hydrocortisone (10^{-6} M)

(CD4 counts approximately 40) of patients with AIDS [8]. These data indicate that methyl-IMP shows pronounced augmentive and immunorestorative activity on T-lymphocytes and suggests its appropriateness to treat individuals with T-lymphocyte impairment.

Normal mice were treated with methyl-IMP 1–100 mg/kg both intraperitoneally and orally. It augmented PHA responses and canavalin A responses of T lymphocytes from mouse spleen cells with animals treated by both routes. The effect from 1 to 100 mg/kg was progressive. Mice were immunized with sheep erythrocytes for the assessment of spleen plaque-forming (PFC) antibody-producing cells. Treatment with methyl-IMP (1–100 mg/kg) at the time of immunization resulted in augmentation, approximately 2-fold, of the number of PFC per spleen. Optimum effects were observed at 50 mg/kg with approximately equivalent effects observed down to 1 mg/kg by both the intraperitoneal and oral routes. Mice were immunized with sheep erythrocytes for the assessment of delayed-type hypersensitivity (DTH) to foot pad challenge with sheep erythrocytes. Methyl-IMP administered by both routes augmented the DTH reaction and peak response was observed at 50 mg/kg with significant effects at 1 mg/kg.

Mice were challenged with Friend leukemia virus (FLV) as a model for retrovirus infection similar to AIDS, but more rapidly lethal. Mice infected with FLV were treated with methyl-IMP from day 3 to day 13 following virus infection and surfival was monitored. Animals treated with 1, 10, and 50 mg/kg i.p. showed significant prolongation of survival. Animals treated with 1 mg/kg per day every other day and animals treated with 1 mg/kg p.o. daily showed equivalent prolongation of survival (median survival time 46 days compared to control of 39 days, $p < 0.01$). These studies indicate that methyl-IMP is effective to stimulate the proliferative responses of lymphocytes from normal donors and donors suppressed under a variety of influences, including retroviral peptide,

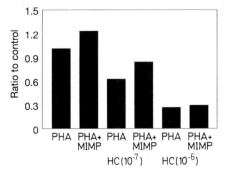

Fig. 3. Peripheral blood lymphocytes from HIV-infected humans were cultured with PHA (0.5 µg/ml) and methyl-IMP (*MIMP*, 1 µg/ml), indomethacin (*INDO*, 10^{-6} *M*), rIL-2 (4 U/ml) or their combination. Results are expressed as a ratio to control

and that this correlates with enhanced survival in a retrovirus-induced leukemia model. Insofar as methyl-IMP has been analyzed from an immunopharmacologic standpoint, the pattern of effects is directly parallel to those observed with othe thymomimetic purines; however, the magnitude and consistency of the effect is superior. Based upon the effects of isoprinosine to reverse in vitro immunosuppressive effects of trauma and burns [10] and, in vivo, to partially reverse immunosuppression associated with massive burn [19], it seems logical to test methyl-IMP in its capacity to reverse the immunologic defects associated with burns, trauma, and sepsis using lymphocytes of infected patients. If comparative positive results can be obtained, as in vivo trial would seem warranted. Based upon experimental data showing additive effects of methyl-IMP with either indomethacin or IL-2 on the PHA responses of HIV-infected individuals (see Fig. 3), it would seem possible and feasible to combine methyl-IMP with in vivo treatment using indomethacin and/or IL-2 in an effort to correct the profound immunodeficiencies associated with burns and trauma.

Other Approaches

It may also be useful to consider other more speculative but safe approaches:

Zinc Therapy. Zinc has been demonstrated to be critical for thymic function, e.g., zinc deficiency leads to thymic involution, IL-1 stimulates zinc uptake into thymus, and the thymic product thymulin requires zinc for its thymic hormone action. Zinc therapy may be important to reverse deficiency incurred in burns and trauma.

Arginine Therapy. Arginine infusion stimulates growth hormones and thymulin production [20]. Terminal arginine residues also characterize a number of immunostimulants (e.g., thymopentin, thymopoietin, tuftsin). Arginine may augment immune function by several possible mechanisms.

Prolactin/Growth Hormone Therapy. Prolactin augments T-lymphocyte proliferation under certain circumstances [21], perhaps through the stimulation of

IL-2 receptors [22]. Cyclosporin A suppresses via the prolactin receptor, and prolactin will reverse to a degree its suppressive effects. Prolactin or growth hormone may be useful in trauma and burns for immunorestoration as well as enhanced repair.

Conclusion

In conclusion, while an immunopharmacologic "silver bullet" is still not in the offing to reverse the immunosuppression associated with trauma and burns, as we learn more about the mechanisms of immune suppression in these conditions, and as we continue to perfect our immunopharmacologic agents and strategies, we should be able to offer meaningful benefit to the clinical management of these patients in the future.

References

1. Meakins JL, Franco D (1989) Immunomodulation and the surgeon. In: Faist E, Ninnemann J, Green D (eds) Immune consequences of trauma, shock and sepsis. Springer, Berlin Heidelberg New York, p 429
2. Hadden JW (1989) Therapy of secondary T-cell immunodeficiencies with biological substances and drugs. In: Faist E, Ninnemann J, Green D (eds) Immune consequences of trauma, shock and sepsis. Springer, Berlin Heidelberg New York, p 509
3. Ninneman JL (1989) The immune consequences of trauma: an overview. In: Faist E, Ninnemann J, Green D (eds) Immune consequences of trauma, shock and sepsis. Springer, Berlin Heidelberg New York, p 1
4. Olszewski WL, Grzelak I (1989) Trauma: immune deficiency, immune suppression, or just immune cell redistribution? In: Faist E, Ninnemann J, Green D (eds) Immune consequences of trauma, shock and sepsis. Springer, Berlin Heidelberg New York, p 9
5. Faist E, Ertel W, Mewes A, Alkan S, Walz A, Strasser T (1989) Trauma-induced alterations of the lymphokine cascade. In: Faist E, Ninnemann J, Green D (eds) Immune consequences of trauma, shock and sepsis. Springer, Berlin Heidelberg New York, p 78
6. Siegal JN, Schwartz A, Askenase PW, Gershon RK (1982) T-cell suppression and contra-suppression induced by histamine H_2 and H_1 receptor agonists, respectively. Proc Natl Acad Sci USA 79:5053
7. Ozkan AN (1989) Serum mediators and the generation of immune suppression. In: Faist E, Ninnemann J, Green D (eds) Immune consequences of trauma, shock and sepsis. Springer, Berlin Heidelberg New York, p 285
8. Green DR, Marcotte R, Wang N (1989) The role of inhibitory cells in burn trauma-associated immunodeficiency. In: Faist E, Ninnemann J, Green D (eds) Immune consequences of trauma, shock and sepsis. Springer, Berlin Heidelberg New York, p 55
9. Bolla K, Cappel R, Duchateau J, Faist E (1989) Immunomodulation as a potential therapeutic approach in immunodeficiencies. In: Faist E, Ninnemann J, Green D (eds) Immune consequences of trauma, shock and sepsis. Springer, Berlin Heidelberg New York, p 519
10. Faist E (1989) Perioperative immunomodulation in patients with major surgical trauma. In: Faist E, Ninnemann J, Green D (eds) Immune consequences of trauma, shock and sepsis. Springer, Berlin Heidelberg New York, p 530

11. Berd D, Maguire HC, Mastrangelo (1984) Potentiation of human cell-mediated and humoral immunity by low-dose cyclophosphamide. Cancer Res 44:5439
12. Winchurch RA, Xiao G-X, Munster AM, Adler WH, White C, Bender B (1989) Treatment of burn patients with polymyxin B: effects on lymphokine regulation. In: Faist E, Ninneman J, Green D (eds) Immune consequences of trauma, shock and sepsis. Springer, Berlin Heidelberg New York, p 458
13. Sagawa T, Abe Y, Kimura S, Hitsumoto Y, Utsumi S (1989) Mechanisms of neutralization of endotoxin by monoclonal IgG antibodies to lipopolysaccharide. In: Faist E, Ninnemann J, Green D (eds) Immune consequences of trauma, shock and sepsis. Springer, Berlin Heidelberg New York, p 495
14. Sztein MB, Serrate SA (1990) Characterization of the immunoregulatory properties of thymosin α1 on interleukin-2 production and interleukin-2 receptor expression in normal human lymphocytes. Int J Immunopharmacol 11:789
15. Klempner MS, Noring R, Mier JW, Atkins MB (1990) An acquired chemotactic defect in neutrophils from patients receiving interleukin-2 immunotherapy. N Engl J Med 5:322
16. Hadden JW, Galy A, Chen H, Wang Y, Hadden E (1989) The hormonal regulation of thymus and T lymphocyte development and function. In: Hadden JW, Masek K, Nisitco G (eds) Interactions among central nervous system, neuroendocrine and immune systems. Pythagora, Rome, p 147
17. Hadden JW, Chen H, Wang Y, Galy A, Hadden E (1989) Strategies of immune reconstitution: effects of lymphokines on murine T cell development in vitro and in vivo. Life Sci 44:v
18. Hersh EM, Abrams D, Bartlett J, Brewton G, Galpin J, Gill P, Gorter R, Gottlieb M, Jonikas JJ, Landesman S, Levine A, Marcel A, Peterson EA, Whiteside M, Zahradnik J, Negron C, Boutitie F, Caraux J, Dupuy J-M, Salmi LR (1991) A randomized double-blind, placebo-controlled multicenter study of sodium ditiocarb. JAMA (in press)
19. Singh H, Herndon DN (1989) Effect of isoprinosine on lymphocyte proliferation and natural killer cell activity following thermal injury. Immunopharmacol Immunotoxicol 11(4):631
20. Mocchegiani E, Cacciatore L, Talarico M, Lingetti M, Fabris N (1990) Recovery of low thymic hormone levels in cancer patients by lysine-arginine combination. Int J Immunopharmacol 12(4):365
21. Buckley AR, Montgomery DW, Kibler R, Putnum CW, Zukoski CF, Gout PW, Beer CT, Russell DH (1986) Prolactin stimulation of ornithine decarboxylase and mitogenesis in Nb_2 node lymphoma cells: the role of protein kinase C and calcium mobilization. Immunopharmacology 12:37
22. Mukherjee P, Mastro AM, Hymer WC (1990) Prolactin induction of interleukin-2 receptors on rat splenic lymphocytes. Endocrinology 126:88
23. Hadden E, Malec P, Hadden J (1991) Int J Immunopharmacol (in press)

Progress in Antiinfective Perioperative Immunomodulatory Therapy with Simultaneous Administration of Blocking and Enhancing Agents

E. Faist[1], A. Markewitz[2], S. Endres[3], D. Fuchs[4], L. Hültner[5], and S. Lang[1]

Introduction

Patients undergoing cardiac surgery with extracorporeal circulation (ECC) are subjected to an immediate massive impact on their host defense integrity due to the combined effect of tissue trauma, multiple blood transfusions, and a whole-body inflammationlike state, induced through the extensive contact between blood and foreign material. The resulting impairment of cell-mediated immunity (CMI) has its clinical correlate since there is enhanced susceptibility of these patients to infectious complications [1–3]. In our own institution, during the year 1990, 55% of the mortality in patients undergoing ECC was due to septic multiple organ failure.

For the reasons outlined above, it can be suggested that the major cardiac surgery patient can serve as an excellent in vivo model to investigate the efficacy of therapeutic strategies designed to counteract the impairment of immuno-mechanistics induced through severe trauma. We and others have demonstrated [4–6] that the alteration in CMI following trauma is mainly due to the disruption of intact monocyte ($M\phi$)/T-cell interaction. Within this phenomenon, we see a shift in the cell ratio in the area of mononuclear peripheral blood leukocytes (PBMC) with a considerable increase in prostaglandin E_2 (PGE_2) synthesizing $M\phi$ and a simultaneous decrease in functionally competent CD3 + and CD4 + lymphocytes. T-cell dysfunction in states of profound stress is characterized by impaired synthesis of two crucial cytokines—interleukin-2 (IL-2) and interferon-gamma (IFN-γ) [7, 8]. The inability to produce adequate amounts of IL-2, results in incomplete proliferative T-cell responses to antigenic stimuli, while a lack of IFN-γ results in inefficient $M\phi$ antigen presentation. It has been demonstrated that both defects are keystones of suppressed CMI function following trauma, with the subsequent development of sepsis [9–11].

[1] Department of Surgery, Ludwig Maximilians University, Klinikum Großhadern, 8000 Munich 70, FRG
[2] Department of Cardiac Surgery, Ludwig Maximilians University, Klinikum Großhadern, 8000 Munich 70, FRG
[3] Department of Medicine, Ludwig Maximilians University, Klinikum Innenstadt, 8000 Munich, FRG
[4] Department of Chemistry and Biochemistry, University of Innsbruck, Innsbruck, Austria
[5] Society of Radiation and Environmental Research, Institute of Experimental Hematology, 8000 Munich 70, FRG

Host Defense Dysfunction
in Trauma, Shock and Sepsis
Eds. Faist/Meakins/Schildberg
© Springer-Verlag, Berlin Heidelberg 1993

The information derived from the dissection of downregulatory mechanisms responsible for the development of injury-related immunoincompetence, provided the incentive for the development of therapeutic regimens designed to prevent a major collapse of CMI.

The use of two classes of substances seemed to be most suitable for immunoprotection and/or immunorestoration: (1) nonsteroidal antiinflammatory drugs (NSAIDS) by blocking immunoreactive PGE_2 [12], the common link of malfunction of the $M\phi$/T-cell interactive network in states of trauma and (2) the synthetic thymomimetic pentapeptide thymopentin (TP-5) with its crucial characteristics—restoration of immunobalance, T-cell activation, and acceleration of T-cell recruitment [13].

We have conducted a number of clinical trials in recent years in patients undergoing major surgery in order to scrutinize the immunoaugmenting potential of TP-5 as well as of the cyclooxygenase inhibitor indomethacin (Indo) [14]. A perioperative two-shot subcutaneous administration of 50 mg TP-5 in patients undergoing open heart surgery, resulted in a restoration of the in vitro lymphocyte proliferative responses, as well as in the delayed-type hypersensitivity (DTH) responses, compared to a placebo-treated control population. It was disillusioning to recognize, however, that T-cell receptor protection (CD3 + and CD4 +) and restoration of IL-2 synthesis could not be achieved with that treatment modality [15].

Conversely, postoperative administration of Indo in patients undergoing gastrectomy or reconstruction of the abdominal aorta, resulted in an impressive protection of T-cell receptor expression for the CD3 + , CD4 + , and IL-2 R + subpopulations. This treatment also controlled overwhelming related monocytosis. Furthermore, the preservation of the preoperative in vivo DTH immunoreactivity in contrast to untreated patients could be demonstrated [16]. However, restoration of depressed IL-2 synthesis could not be attained with Indo administration, which was in contrast to numerous in vitro experiments which showed that Indo restores depressed IL-2 production [17].

In view of the findings in these single agent studies, and based on the knowledge that trauma-induced depression of CMI represents a multimechanistic phenomenon, the protocol for a combined agent-therapeutic trial was designed. It was the objective of an extensive prospective randomized study to quantify, specify, and compare the immunorestorative potential of a combined therapy with the cyclooxygenase inhibitor Indo and the thymomimetic substance thymopentin versus single drug administration of Indo following ECC. Besides the scrutiny of cell-mediated immunomechanistics, this study was also designed to study some parameters of the "acute phase response."

The uniform reaction of the human body to a variety of damages resulting in tissue injury, e.g., infections or trauma, is known as the acute phase response. It is intended to counteract microbial invasion, to localize tissue injury, and to clear the body of debris following tissue damage and to repair damaged organs. The acute phase comprises numerous reactions including activation of the complement cascade and the cell-mediated immune system as well as fever, anorexia, or induction of the hepatocytes to synthesize proteases known as acute phase proteins [18]. Acute phase response commonly results in a complete restoration of the injured tissue. However, if the regulation of the acute phase response becomes altered, either in the case of too little activation, from which chronic inflammation would then result or when there is too much activation possibly resulting in the death of the individual. Trauma-induced dysregulation is caused by a shift in synthesis patterns of several broad spectrum inflammatory mediators, such as interleukin-1 (IL-1), interleukin -6 (IL-6), and tumor necrosis factor (TNF), together with a family of cytokines termed macrophage inflammatory proteins such as interleukin-8 (IL-8).

The immune parameters studied in vivo and in vitro included the DTH skin response to recall antigens, PBMC phenotyping, specific and nonspecific induction of lymphoproliferative responses, and the in vitro, synthesis of IL-1, IL-2, IL-6, and TNF-α. Additionally, for CMI serum markers, we evaluated the concentration of D-erythro-neopterin a sensitive indicator of Mϕ activation, as well as the concentration of IFN-γ as a marker for T-cell activation. The results indicate that simultaneous cyclooxygenase inhibition and T-cell activation can greatly enhance forward regulatory axis of cell-mediated immune mechanisms following ECC, as well as modify the acute phase response via the altered release of proinflammatory cytokines.

Materials and Methods

Patient Population. Surgical patients in the surgical wards and the intensive care unit of the Department of Cardiac Surgery of the Ludwig-Maximilians University, Klinikum Großhadern, Munich, FRG were studied. This study was approved by the Medical Ethics Committee of the Faculty of Medicine.

From 1 November 1989 until 31 October 1990, studies were conducted in 60 patients (45 men and 15 women) with an average age of 63 ± 7 years. All patients had acquired or congenital heart disease and had to undergo ECC surgery with coronary artery bypass grafting (CABG) or vavle replacement (Table 1).

Experimental Protocol. For the prospectively randomized study (Fig. 1), patients were divided into three groups: group A patients (PA; $n = 20$) were given 100 mg Indo (Confortid, Dumex, Denmark), i.v., immediately after surgery (day 0), and 50 mg three times daily until day 5 postoperatively; group B patients (PB; $n = 20$) as well as Indo therapy, also received 50 mg TP-5 (Timmunox, Cilag, FRG) subcutaneously, 2 h preoperatively and 48 h and 96 h postoperatively; group C patients (PC; $n = 20$) served as the control population, undergoing conventional intensive care unit (ICU) therapy postoperatively.

Age, underlying disease, and quality of surgical procedure were highly comparable in all three groups.

Table 1. Patient population

	Group A	Group B	Group C
Age (years)	63.45 ± 7.19	62.48 ± 6.46	64.1 ± 6.79
Male:female ratio	16:4	14:6	15:5
Preoperative ejection fraction	60.9 ± 16.9	58.3 ± 17.3	64.4 ± 13.4
Coronary heart disease	15	15	16
Number of coronary vessels compromised			
1	1	1	2
2	4	8	7
3	10	6	7
Valve disease	5	5	4
Aortic	4	5	3
Mitral	–	–	1
Both	1	–	–
Valve replacement	5	5	4
Coronary artery bypass graft	15	15	16

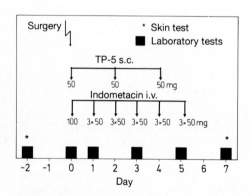

Fig. 1. Experimental protocol showing time of Indomethacin and TP-5 administration and frequency of laboratory tests

Prospective randomization

Immunologic screening of the patients was carried out twice preoperatively (immediately after admission and on the day of the operation, but was calculated as one preoperative value) as well as on days 1, 3, 5, and 7 postoperatively.

Cell Preparation and Culture. For lymphocyte studies, 50 ml peripheral blood was obtained in sterile heparinized tubes. The blood samples were diluted 1:2 in Hanks' buffered saline solution (GIBCO Laboratories, Grand Island, NY, USA) with 2% penicillin-streptomycin. PBMC isolation was carried out immediately by standard Ficoll-Hypaque density gradient centrifugation at 1500 rpm, 4 °C, for 35 min. After resuspending the cells with 15% fetal calf serum (GIBCO Laboratories), cell counts were performed with a hemocytometer, using trypan blue exclusion as a test of viability. Viability always exceeded 95%. Appropriate cell suspension concentrations were then prepared for the different assays to be carried out.

Mitogen Assay. At concentrations of 1×10^5 cells per well, PBMCs were added in triplicates to flat-bottomed, 96-well microtiter plates, and antigen cocktail (AgC) was added to the wells at a final concentration of 50 mg/l. Antigen cocktail (Behring Co, Marburg, FRG) is a mixture containing five antigens-purified protein derivative, tetanus toxoid, streptolysin, mumps, and vaccinia antigen.

The cultures were incubated at $37\,^{\circ}C$ in a 6% CO_2 incubator for 120 h. Six hours prior to harvesting, the cultures were pulsed with 18.5×10^3 Bq per well of tritiated thymidine. The cultures were harvested on glass-fiber paper with a multiple-automated sample harvester. Vials holding the filter strips and scintillation fluid were counted in a beta counter. The net count per minute of triplicate cultures were calculated as the net count for the cells with AgC minus the net count for the cells without AgC. Lymphocyte proliferation was also carried out with phytohemagglutinin (PHA) which was added to the triplicates at a final concentration of 0.5 µg/ml. These cultures were incubated for 72 h before being pulsed with thymidine.

PBMC Phenotyping. Phenotyping of Ficol-Hypaque preparations of mononuclear cells, as described elsewhere [19], was performed utilizing monoclonal antibodies to quantitate CD3+, CD4+, and CD8+ T cells (Becton Dickinson), LeuM3+ monocytes (Becton Dickinson), as well as IL-2 receptor positive (IL-2R+) cells (Biotest Diagnostics, FRG). The number of cells that were stained with the antibodies were assayed using fluorescence microscopy. The IL-2R antibody identifies the human IL-2R on mitogen- and antigen-activated T cells. Enumeration was performed following 48-h incubation of the PBMCs with 1 mg/ml PHA.

IL-2 Generation and Activity Assay. IL-2 was generated by culturing PBMC suspensions at a cell concentration of 20 PBMCs per liter in 5 ml culture tubes in the presence of highly PHA at a final concentration of 2.5 mg/l at $37\,^{\circ}C$, 6% CO_2. After 48 h, supernatants were collected and stored at $-700\,^{\circ}C$ until assayed.

The assay for the detection of IL-2 activity was a modification of the method described by Gillis et al. [20]. Briefly, frozen long-term cultures (5 days) of human T cells with concanavalin A blasts serving as IL-2-sensitive target cells were thawed, washed, and resuspended in RPMI 1640 supplemented with 2% penicillin-streptomycin and 20% pooled human serum. Supernatants to be tested for the amount of IL-2 released on stimulation with PHA were placed in 100 µl serial dilutions from 1:2 to 1:128 in 96-well, round-bottomed microtiter plates in triplicate. Next, 100 µl concanavalin A blasts were added to each well, resulting in a final concentration of 4×10^4 cells per well. The IL-2 activity of the supernatants to be tested was compared with the activity induced by the IL-2 standard solution, which contained 1 U/ml by definition (Lymphocult HP, Biotest, Offenburg, FRG). Units of IL-2 were calculated by comparison with the cell proliferation induced with the Lymphocult test solution.

Assay for IL-6. PBMC were stimulated with lipopolysaccharide (LPS) to generate IL-6 synthesis in monocytes. To generate IL-6 production in T lymphocytes, PBMCs were cultured at a cell concentration of 4×10^6 PBMC/ml in the presence of highly purified PHA at a final concentration of 2.5 µg/ml at 37 °C and 6% CO_2. After 48 h, supernatants were collected and stored at -80 °C until assayed. IL-6 was measured employing the 3-[4,5-dimethylthiazol-2-yl]-2,5-diphenyltetrazolium bormide (MTT) assay [21] as described previously [22] using a murine hybridoma cell line (7TD1) which only grows in the presence of IL-6.

Assay for IL-1β and TNF-α. IL-1 and TNF production in monocytes was generated by culturing the cell suspension at a cell concentration of 5×10^6 PBMC in 5-ml culture tubes in the presence of highly purified LPS (C-Parvum, Wellcome Inc., London, UK) at a final concentration of 1 µg/ml at 37 °C and 6% CO_2. After 24 h supernatants were collected and stored at -80 °C until assayed. IL-1 and TNF were measured using a radioimmunoassay (RIA) for human TNF and IL-1β as previously described [23, 24].

Assay for IFN-γ. Immunoradiometry was used (a gift for Centocor Inc., Malvern, PA, USA) employing a modified application [25] that allows the detection of IFN-γ in sera with sufficient sensitivity. Beads with monoclonal anti-human IFN-γ antibody were incubated with 200 µl serum at room temperature for 16 h. Then the beads were washed with 3 ml distilled water and incubated for a further 16 h with 200 µl ^{125}I-labeled tracer. With this modified procedure, more than 80% of the analyte is bound to the solid phase antibody [25]. Radioactivity was counted with a gamma counter (CliniGamma 1272; Wallac Oy, Turku, Finland). IFN-γ activity is expressed as NIH units (U) [26]. The limit of detection was 18 U/l [20].

Assay for Neopterin. Neopterin was quantified by RIA (RIAcid, Henning-Berlin, Berlin, FRG). Fifty microliters of serum were incubated with 100 µl neopterin antiserum for 1 h at room temperature and 100µl ^{125}I-labeled tracer was added followed by incubation for 1 h. Two milliliters of aqueous polyethylene glycol 6000 (PEG) solution (60 g/l) was then added. After centrifugation at $2000 \times g$ for 10 min, radioactivity was counted with the gamma counter. The detection limit was 1 nmol/l [27].

DTH Skin Testing. The DTH response to seven recall antigens was carried out 2 days prior to surgery and on day 7 postoperatively. the recall antigens (tetanus, diptheria, *Streptococcus*, old tuberculin, *Candida*, *Trichophyton*, and *Proteus mirabilis*) and a glycerin control are contained in a test system (Multitest

Mérieux, Hamburg, FRG). The antigens were applied firmly on the volar side of the forearm using a mechanical applicator. The skin test was evaluated 48 h following application. The final score consisted of the number of positive antigen reactions and the sum of the mean diameters of these reactions. A reaction smaller than 2 mm was considered negative.

Statistical Analysis. Statistical analysis was carried out using analysis of variance (ANOVA) for intergroup comparison. Student's paired t test was used for intragroup comparison. $P < .05$ was considered to be significant. The results are expressed as mean $\pm$ standard error of mean (SEM).

Results

Phenotyping Studies. A significant persistent reduction in cell surface receptor expression for the CD3+, CD4+, and IL-2R+ subpopulation following surgery compared to preoperative values was observed in PC (Fig. 2). The nadir of depression was seen in day 1 with an average range of reduction for CD3+ and CD4+ leukocytes between 20% and 30%. Indo treatment resulted in a clearly demonstrable alleviation of depressed receptor expression in PA compared to PC. In PB, following day 1 an absolute receptor protection, partially with elevations towards supranormal ranges especially for the CD4+ subpopulation was observed. On day 3 this was $114 \pm 4\%$, on day 5, $120 \pm 4\%$, and on day 7 $124 \pm 3\%$.

An adequate number of IL-2 receptor positive (CD25+) cells could be maintained with combined therapy, as well as with Indo treatment alone compared to a considerable receptor depletion in the PC group.

The baseline value of $14 \pm 0.6\%$ CD8+ cells, was elevated on day 1 in all groups, but returned to normal in PA and PB on day 7 in contrast to PC. When calculating the CD4+/CD8+ ratio on consecutive postoperative days compared to the average baseline value of 2.8 ± 0.2 for all groups, a clear gradation of values for the individual groups with crucial differences between PC versus PA and PB was observed. A striking difference appears on day 7 with a CD4+/CD8+ ratio (2.0 ± 0.1) in PC still below baseline $(p < .05)$, while there was a value (3.7 ± 0.2) for PB, expressing a significant overcorrection from baseline $(p < .05)$.

Surgery resulted in a massive initial rise of CD14+ Mϕ in all groups compared to the average baseline value of $15 \pm 0.7\%$ cells. On day 1 the number of Mϕ within the PBMC population calculated ranged between $36 \pm 2\%$ (PC), $31 \pm 2\%$ (PA), and $28 \pm 1\%$ (PB). A parallel pattern of decreasing numbers was seen on consecutive days after surgery for all groups. However, the initial significant differences in the Mϕ counts in the postoperative intergroup comparison persisted until the end of the observation period. Thus on day 5 and day 7 there was still a $+61 \pm 9\%$ and $+46 \pm 9\%$ elevation in PC, while in PA

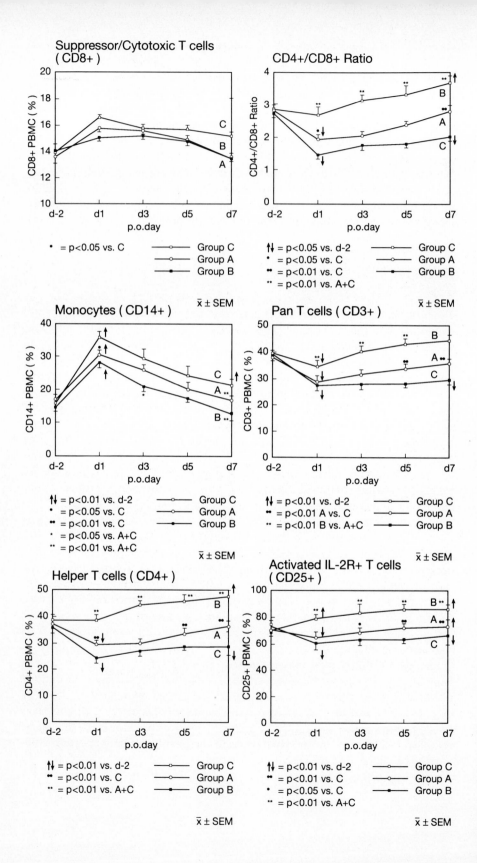

($+34 \pm 9\%$ on day 5 and $+13 \pm 7\%$ on day 7) and PB ($+29 \pm 9\%$ on day 5 and -1.5% on day 7) the counts were significantly lower.

Proliferative Responses. The preoperative average PHA-induced lymphocyte proliferation in all patient groups PC 31 892 $\pm$ 1497 CPM; PA 33 159 $\pm$ 1504 CPM; and PB, 31 548 $\pm$ 1412 CPM) was nearly identical, Moreover the AgC-induced proliferative responses were similar; PC, 17 670 $\pm$ 605 CPM; PA 18 473 $\pm$ 719 CPM; and PB,17 503 $\pm$ 396 CPM (Fig. 3).

PHA-induced proliferation in PB cultures was not depressed during the postoperative course, but showed mild elevations within the range of $+17.8\%$ (day 3) and $+23.6\%$ (day 5) compared to baseline.

In contrast, proliferation values of PC and PA cultures were significantly suppressed ($p < .05$), reaching $58.2 \pm 2.6\%$ (PC) and $74.9 \pm 2.3\%$ (PA) of baseline levels.

For PC and PA, although a gradual recovery of proliferation was seen, the responses were still significantly lower on day 7 compared to preoperative values. There was also a significant difference between the proliferative responses of PA and PC on all postoperative days.

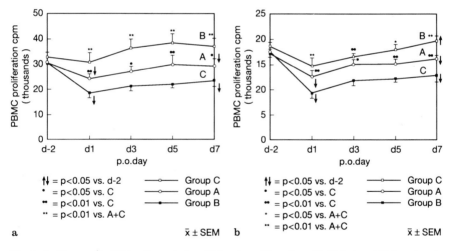

Fig. 3a,b. Nonspecific PHA mitogen induced (**a**) and specific antigen (AgC)-induced (**b**) lymphocyte blastogenesis preoperative (day -2) as well as on consecutive days following surgery for the three patient groups *A*, *B*, and *C*. *Asterisks* indicate values that are significantly different ($p < .01, p < .05$) in the intergroup and intertime (vs day -2) comparison

Fig. 2. Phenotyping of peripheral blood mononuclear cell (PBMC) subpopulations on consecutive postoperative (*p.o.*) days, for the individual patient groups *A*, *B*, and *C*. Changes in CD8 + , CD4 + / CD8 + ratio, CD14 + monocytes, CD3 + , CD4 + , and IL-2R + (CD25 +) T cells marked with the monoclonal antibody LeuM3 *Asterisks* indicate values that are significantly different ($p < .01$, $p < .05$) in intergroup and intertime (vs day -2) comparison

Compared to the average baseline values of specific antigen (AgC)-induced PBMC proliferation, a significant decreas on day 1 in all groups was observed. While PB proliferation was reduced to 84.3 ± 3.4% of baseline, PA to 67.2 ± 2.9%, and PC to 53.4 ± 3.9%, values dropped off much more substantially. There was a clear tendency towards normalization on consecutive days postsurgery in PA and PC, without reaching the baseline level by day 7, ($p < 0.05$). In contrast proliferation of PB on day 5 was already up to 103%.

IL-2 Synthesis. The preoperative values of PHA-induced IL-2 synthesis were comparable in all patient groups with 0.69 ± 0.05 U/ml (PC), 0.59 ± 0.04 U/ml (PA), and 0.60 ± 0.04 U/ml (PB), but were considerably lower, than the control value (0.80 ± 0.04 U/ml) derived from healthy human volunteers (Fig. 4).

During the postoperative course IL-2 synthesis in cell cultures of PC were massively suppressed, with lymphokine concentrations in the supernatants never above 0.27 ± 0.05 U/ml (day 3) with a nadir on day 7 (0.10 ± 0.02 U/ml). In PA cultures, a considerable impairment of IL-2 production, compared to preoperative values was observed, however, not as precipitous over all as in PC. In PA cultures, on day 7, the IL-2 production was as low as 29% (0.16 ± 0.02 U/ml) compared to preoperative values. In contrast, in PB cultures the average IL-2 production on consecutive postoperative days was never below baseline, showing even slight elevations up to +18% (0.70 ± 0.08 U/ml) on day 5. On all days there was a significant difference between the IL-2 synthesis in PB versus PA and PC.

Interleukin-1. IL-1 synthesis in LPS-stimulated cell cultures was considerably reduced in PC with a nadir on day 1 (0.28 ± 0.06 ng/ml supernatant versus 0.46 ± 0.1 ng/ml preoperatively; Fig. 5).

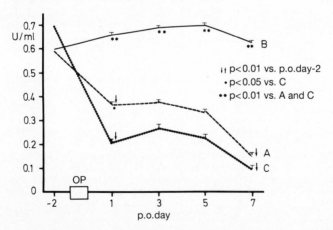

Fig. 4. PHA-induced in vitro IL-2 synthesis preoperatively (day − 2) and on various days following operative trauma for the three patient groups *A*, *B*, and *C* studied. *Horizontal bars* express the IL-2 control value (0.8 ± 0.04 U/ml) in this laboratory derived from healthy laboratory volunteers. *Asterisks* indicate values that are significantly different ($p < .01$, $p < .05$) in the intergroup and intertime (vs day − 2) comparison. *OP*, open heart surgery

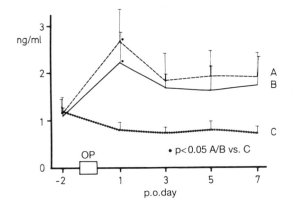

Fig. 5. Interleukin-1β synthesis on consecutive days postoperatively in groups *A*, *B*, and *C* as compared to preoperative baseline values. *Asterisks* indicate values which are significantly different in the intergroup comparison. *OP*, open heart surgery

Following the nadir on day 1 we see a slow but consistent recovery until day 7. Administration of Indo (PA) or combined therapy with TP-5 (PB) resulted in a substantial elevation of IL-1 synthesis with a peak value on day 1 of 0.75 ± 0.17 ng/ml (PA) and 0.66 ± 0.14 ng/ml (PB) versus 0.43 ± 0.12 ng/ml preoperatively. Following a slight reduction in cytokine synthesis on day 3, the cell cultures continued to synthesize elevated amounts of IL-1 up to 0.71 ± 0.17 ng/ml (PA) and 0.70 ± 0.72 ng/ml (PB) on day 7. Because of rather high SEM. of the individual data we did not see significant differences in the intragroup comparison, while we could observe a significantly higher IL-1 production on day 1 in the intergroup comparison.

Tumor Necrosis Factor. TNF synthesis in cell cultures of PC decreased from the preoperative baseline level of 0.99 ± 0.24 ng/ml to 0.54 ± 0.15 ng/ml on day 1 (Fig. 6). We saw a suppression of TNF synthesis on that level until day 5 with only a slight recovery towards a value of 0.71 ± 0.17 ng/ml on day 7. Conversely in group PA and PB we saw an immediate increase in the baseline values to 1.29 ± 0.3 ng/ml (PA) and 1.40 ± 0.3 ng/ml (PB) on day 1, compared to 0.95

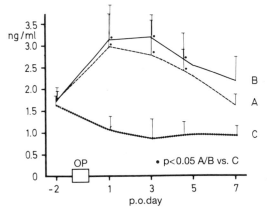

Fig. 6. Tumor necrosis factor synthesis during the first 7 postoperative days in groups *A*, *B*, and *C* after open heart surgery (*OP*). *Points* indicate values which are significantly different in the intergroup comparison

± 0.18 ng/ml (day 0). Cell cultures of PA on consecutive postoperative days were then showing a continuing decrease in TNF synthesis on consecutive days, returning to a baseline value of 0.95 ± 0.17 ng/ml on day 7. Combined therapy resulted in a peak value of 1.43 ± 0.4 ng/ml on day 3, with a slight decrease on consecutive days, but still showing elevated TNF synthesis on day 7 (1.25 ± 0.32 ng/ml).

The intergroup comparison showed significantly higher TNF synthesis for PA and PB versus PC on days 1, 3 and 5.

Interleukin-6. Results of IL-6 synthesis (Fig. 7) differed from those observed in IL-1 and TNF production. In all groups we saw a substantial increase in IL-6 synthesis following LPS challenge. The peak values were reached on day 3, 4024 ± 165 U/ml vs 2107 ± 113 U/ml preoperatively (PA), 2852 ± 842 U/ml vs 1125 ± 74 U/ml (PB), and 3508 ± 217 U/ml vs 1533 ± 63 U/ml (PC), followed by a slight decrease until day 7. At this point, however, IL-6 synthesis was still almost twofold higher when compared to preoperative baseline values in all groups:PA, 3440 ± 147 U/ml; 2207 ± 226 U/ml; and PC, 2943 ± 201 U/ml.

PBMC cultures of PC showed the highest synthesis postoperatively and those of PB the lowest augmentation of IL-6 synthesis, with PA cultures lying in between PB and PC. This result becomes even more evident when we express the augmentation rates as a percentage of the preoperative levels (Table 2).

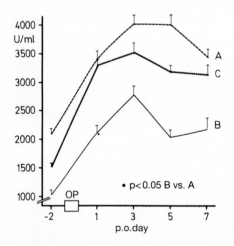

Fig. 7. Interleukin-6 synthesis in adherent (Mφ) cell cultures following stimulation with lipopolysaccharide (LPS) on consecutive postoperative days in Groups *A, B,* and *C. Points* indicate the results which are significantly different in the intergroup comparison. *OP,* open heart surgery

Table 2. Alteration of IL-6 synthesis on consecutive days following operative trauma compared to the preoperative level, expressed as a percentage

Patient group	Day 2	Day 1	Day 3	Day 5	Day 7
PC	100	216.1 ± 32.7	288.4 ± 41.2	274.9 ± 46.1	278.8 ± 40.9
PA	100	179.0 ± 24.09	249.0 ± 53.2	233.6 ± 38.8	245.2 ± 41.3
PB	100	176.0 ± 24.03	237.5 ± 48.4	209.6 ± 32.6	192.0 ± 36.8

The pattern of IL-6 synthesis following PHA stimulation, a mitogen which is primarily inducing T-cell activation (Fig. 8), was comparable to that after LPS challenge. IL-6 production increased in all groups, with a peak on day 1 for PB (1846 ± 486 U/ml versus 1608 ± 331 U/ml preoperatively), a peak on day 5 for PA (2388 ± 554 U/ml versus 1585 ± 337 U/ml) and PC (2544 ± 557 U/ml versus 1507 ± 303 U/ml). On day 7 IL-6 synthesis was still considerably elevated in PC (2356 ± 475 U/ml) and in PA (2107 ± 486 U/ml) while in PB (1770 ± 407 U/ml) it was within the preoperative range. During the whole observation period, cell cultures of controls showed the highest IL-6 values while the most modest increase in IL-6 synthesis was found in PB. The results were statistically significant between day 3 and day 5 in the intergroup comparison in B versus C.

Delayed Type Hypersensitivity Response. In PC, the operative trauma resulted in a significant depression of quantity and quality of the skin responses on day 7 compared to the preoperative scores (Fig. 9).

Thus, the average value of positive Ag-reactions (3.1 ± 0.04 = 100%) and the sum of mean diameters of the skin response (13.6 ± 1.4 = 100%) decreased to 1.9 ± 0.3 (62% of baseline) and 7.4 ± 1.3 (54% of baseline), respectively. In PA the baseline values (3.0 ± 0.3+ reactions/11.4 ± 1.4 mean diameters) dropped to 2.4 ± 0.3 (80%) and 8.5 ± 1.4 (74%), respectively. In comparison to PC, PB values on day 7 were significantly higher: $p < .05$; 3.1 ± 0.4 (100%)/ 12.4 ± 1.7 (122%) and did not fall short of their respective baseline values (3.1 ± 0.3/10.2 ± 1.2).

Serum Neopterin. The average preoperative neopterin (NPT) concentration in the patient population studied was 8.9 ± 0.9 nmol/l (Fig. 10). In PC a very rapid increase in NPT in serum was seen on day 1 (20.8 ± 3.3 nmol/l) with a peak value of 29.1 ± 3.2 nmol/l on day 3. In PA (12.8 ± 6.8 nmol/l) and PB (14.2

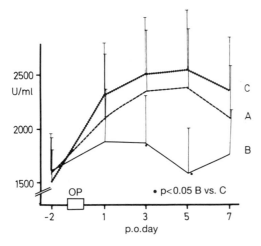

Fig. 8. Interleukin-6 synthesis in PBMC cultures following stimulation with phytohemagglutinin (PHA) in groups *A, B,* and *C. Points* indicate the results which are singnificantly different in the intergroup comparison. *OP,* open heart surgery

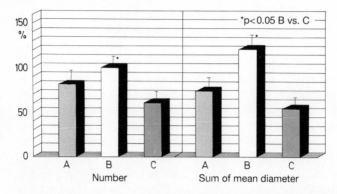

Fig. 9. Delayed type hypersensitivity (DTH) response skin testing was done preoperatively (day − 2), and on day 7 postoperatively in groups *A*, *B*, and *C*. The score of the DTH response consists of the number of positive antigen (Ag) reactions and the sum of mean diameters of the response. The different height of the individual *bars* indicates changes in the number of positive Ag reactions postoperatively. The percentages written on the bars indicate the changes in the mean diameters of response in the individual groups compared to baseline values

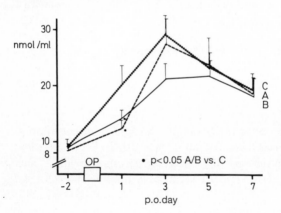

Fig. 10. Perioperative changes in serum neopterin levels (nmol/l) in the individual patient groups *A*, *B*, and *C*. *Points* denote values that are statistically different ($p < .05$) in the intergroup comparison. *OP*, open heart surgery

$\pm$ 6.6 nmol/l) there was a much more subtle increase in this monocyte activation marker. On day 3 the NPT concentration in PA (27.6 $\pm$ 4.6 nmol/l) was almost identical to the peak value of PC, while in PB a concentration of around 21 nmol/l was measured, remaining at this level until day 5.

On day 7 NPT concentrations in all patient groups declined to a level of around 19 nmol/l.

Serum IFN-γ. Serum IFN-γ concentrations in PB were rising continuously from their preoperative day 2 value of 115 $\pm$ 15 U/ml on consecutive postoperative days to 129 $\pm$ 21 U/ml on day 1, 144 $\pm$ 28 U/ml on day 3, and 143 $\pm$ 17 U/ml on day 5, finally reaching 173 $\pm$ 49 U/ml on day 7 (Fig. 11). In contrast to these findings, the IFN-γ concentrations on day 1 in PA (105 $\pm$ 15 U/ml) and PC (103 $\pm$ 13 U/ml) remained within the range of their preoperative levels, then

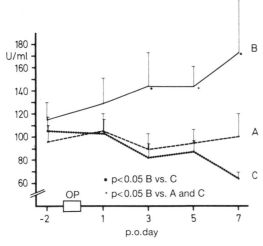

Fig. 11. Depiction of perioperative changes in serum interferon-γ levels (U/ml) in the individual patient groups A, B, and C. *Astrerisks* and *points* denote values that are statistically different ($p < .05$) in the intergroup comparison. *OP*, open heart surgery

declined in parallel on day 3 to 82 ± 13 U/ml (PC) and 90 ± 11 U/ml (PA). Until day 7 when the preoperative mediator level in PA was regained, IFN-γ concentrations in PC showed a further decline to 64 ± 5 U/ml. The difference in IFN-γ serum concentrations between PC and PB, starting on day 3, was significantly ($p < .05$).

Discussion

This study shows clearly that the combined administration of the cyclooxygenase inhibitor Indo and the thymomimetic drug TP-5 can optimally prevent the trauma-induced depression or breakdown of CMI mechanisms normally occuring in individuals following major operative and ECC injury.

While corroborating some previous data derived from single drug studies with these particular substances, this investigation, through a number of parameters, demonstrates the superiority of the immunoaugmenting effect of a combined Indo/TP-5 administration vs single drug use.

The global assessment of in vivo (DTH) immunoreactivity in PB (Indo + TP-5) postoperatively indicated no difference from the preoperative status, in contrast to a significant reduction seen in PC (no immunomodulatory treatment), while there was a 20%–25% reduction in the preoperative DTH score in PA (Indo). T-cell receptor (CD3 + , CD4 + , and IL-2R +) protection appeared to be excellent in PB during the postoperative phase, with a tendency towards overcorrection for the CD4 + and IL-2R + subpopulations on day 7, while simultaneously, under this particular regimen, the counterrregulatory activity to limit excessive monocytosis seemed to be most effective. Although Indo administration could alleviate the quantitative inbalances of PBMC subpopulations seen in PC, it could not continuously induce significant improvement as demonstrated in a recent study [16] which investigated different types of operative trauma (gastrectomy, abdominal aortic grafting).

Postoperative depression of lymphocyte blastogenesis was also counteracted most sufficiently with combined TP-5/Indo therapy, which clearly worked better than the two-shot administration of TP-5 only, as demonstrated in a previous investigation in an identical operative model [15]. In that study with Indo, the impairment of proliferative response was also significantly reduced.

In vitro IL-2 synthesis in cell cultures of PB on consecutive postoperative days did not show any suppression and the values were always on or above baseline level. To our knowledge, these findings represent the first report involving a successful intervention to preserve adequate T-cell capacity for IL-2 production in humans following trauma.

The serum levels of IFN-γ in the patient population treated with Indo/TP-5 were continuously increasing on consecutive postoperative days with an average rise of $+50\%$ above baseline between day 3 and day 7. The increased amount of IFN-γ released in PB provides evidence of the complex efficacy of T-cell activation triggered through that specific immunomodulatory treatment. IFN-γ serum levels in PA were within the baseline range on day 7, in contrast to an average reduction of 35% when compared to preoperative levels in PC on day 7.

D-erythro-neopterin, an indicator of Mϕ activation [28], rose much more rapidly in PC within the first 72 h after trauma than in PB. By day 7 postoperatively, NPT concentrations were identical in all three patient groups.

The analysis of the supernatants of LPS-stimulated PBMC cultures of PA, PB, and PC for the proinflammatory cytokines IL-1, IL-6, and TNF revealed that the cardiopulmonary bypass procedures result in a substantial activation of the acute phase response. In PC we find an upregulation of IL-6 synthesis while IL-1 and TNF production are substantially depressed during the first days after trauma.

Downregulation of IL-6 and TNF synthesis has been demonstrated in an animal model of hemorrhaged mice [29] and it was associated with an impaired antigen presentation and major histocompatibility complex (MHC) class II expression by antigen-presenting cells, which are essential for the activation of immune responses. The results corroborate the hypothesis that a depressed IL-1 and TNF synthesis might have an immunosuppressive effect. IL-1 has been reported to be downregulated in patients with major septic episodes [30].

Highly elevated IL-1 concentrations are frequently found in patients with burns or infectious episodes and one might speculate that the upregulation of IL-6 synthesis might be the result of an intracellular shifting from IL-2 production to IL-6 production [31]. The results of this clinical study show further that IL-1 and TNF synthesis in PB cultures was significantly higher when compared to PA and PC. Conversely IL-6 production in monocytes and lymphocytes could be substantially reduced through combined therapy of TP-5 and Indo when compared to single cyclooxygenase inhibition therapy or the untreated controls. In the study by Ertel et al. [29] it was demonstrated that administration of the cyclooxygenase inhibitors ibuprofen resulted in the restoration of adequate IL-1 and TNF synthesis and in parallel in a downregulation of IL-1 synthesis. As previously expressed our investigation could corroborate the effect of PGE_2 counterregulation in terms of IL-1 and TNF synthesis, however, the sole administration of Indo could not substantially decrease IL-1 synthesis. The reason for the latter remains to be elucidated. The entire body of information derived from this study provides us with striking evidence of the salutary mechanism of action induced by the Indo/TP-5 treatment.

Simultaneous PGE_2 blockade via Indo and T-cell activation via TP-5 apparently represents an ideal strategy to provide protection for the successful development of an immune response for which several levels of control are necessary. Essential steps within the forward-regulatory immune response pathway include: synthesis and release of IL-1 from $M\phi$, intact $M\phi$ function, intact T-cell receptor function, a sufficient number of functionally intact T-helper cells, IL-2 synthesis and adequate IL-2 release, as well as IL-2 sensitive responder cells with intact capacity of IL-2 receptors. Moreover, $M\phi$ participation can only be sustained via IFN-γ production by activated T cells. The downregulation of cell-mediated immune responses occurs mainly due to PGE_2, a regulatory mediator released from inhibitory monocytes which are released in large amounts following injury. One of the most prominent PGE_2 immunoregulatory activities consists of the regulation of IL-2 synthesis [32]. Mediators such as PGE_2 that are associated with both specific and nonspecific immunosuppression have been demonstrated to impinge on the prostaglandin cyclic adenosine monophosphate (AMP) pathway and it has been postulated that agents which interfere with these mechanisms may counter the immunosuppressive influences. Thus, it has been recognized that an immunopharmacological attack on T-cell disturbances in trauma should either contrasuppress the suppressor—PGE_2— by blocking cyclic AMP, or it should have immunorestorative capacities in terms of promoting the cyclic guanosine monophosphate (GMP), as for example, thymomimetic substances like TP-5 do.

Based on these reflections it appears logical that a treatment regimen that combines blocking, ideally with enhancing action, should consist of a combination of immunopotentiating agents that complement each other functionally. Maghsudi et al., in an animal model of burn injury, demonstrated that the restoration of depressed secondary immune responses to sheep red blood cells could be best accomplished through the additive effect of Indo and TP-5 [27].

Our results demonstrated that using the combination of TP-5 and Indo, all essential components within the lymphokine cascade circuit could be either protected or stabilized following ECC.

When interpreting these data however, one must stay away from oversimplification, although a dissection of the mechanisms is warranted. It will always remain difficult to demonstrate the absolute causality between a particular agent and a seemingly corresponding function. Many of the findings in this study indeed represent the result of amplification achieved through directing the therapy on two targets—the $M\phi$ and the T cell.

While excessive PGE_2-dependent monocytosis, for example, could be counteracted with Indo, as shown in a previous study [16], we noted in this present investigation that a considerable additive effect can be derived from the combination with TP-5. Most likely, it appears that TP-5 is acting by blocking off some suppressor active T-cell subpopulations [33].

The preservation of functionally intact T-cell subpopulations (CD3+ and CD4+) also clearly results from synergistic action of both agents, whereas undisturbed IL-2R expression appears to be mainly a function of cyclooxygenase inhibition [34].

The successful preservation of IL-2 under stressful conditions is evidently the consequence of the smooth interaction of several factors: the presence of adequate numbers of CD4+ cells, the induction of cyclic GMP and simultaneous shut-off of cyclic AMP, as well as the presence of IL-1 synthesizing $M\phi$— all of which are optimally conditioned via Indo/TP-5 support. Adequate production of IFN-γ from T cells depends on the presence of IL-2 in these cells. Most convincingly in this study, the preoperative serum levels of IFN-γ could only be sustained in those patients (PB) in whom the in vitro stimulation of PBMC cultures also resulted in intact IL-2 synthesis.

In a recent multicenter study with low-dose administration of IFN-γ to patients with multiple trauma, Polk and colleagues showed the mechanistic impact of this mediator on the preservation of $M\phi$ forward-immunoregulatory capacity, in terms of human leukocyte antigens-DR (HLA-DR) expression (Polk et al., this volume) following injury.

Ertel et al. in a study using their mouse model of controlled hemorrhagic shock could demonstrate that the administration of ibuprofen following hemorrhage resulted in the maintenance of IL-2 and IFN-γ synthesis in splenic lymphocytes, as well as of IL-1 in splenic $M\phi$ from C3H/HeN mice [35] following hemorrhage. In contrast, untreated hemorrhaged mice showed a massive depression of these respective functions.

The concept of strengthening the facilitory component—while simultaneously suppressing the downregulatory PGE_2-mediated component—of $M\phi$ behavior has also been advocated by Browder and coworkers [36]. In a randomized, prospective, double-blind study they investigated the effect of glucan, a macrophage stimulant, on CMI function in patients with multiple injury and found that glucan treatment resulted in a rapid rise of IL-1 serum, which was also correlated with subsequent skin test conversion of anergic patients to positive. While the use of such an immunopotentiating agent may represent an intriguing approach to immune response modification, the administration of cyclooxygenase inhibitors, however, is intended to go far beyond stimulation in its therapeutic impact. NSAIDS, by breaking down the inflammatory cycle and limiting the nondiscriminant whole-body hyperinflammation, represent in our experience the key step to avoiding the overstimulation of the $M\phi$ during the initial posttrauma phase. A number of agents, some of them acting in a self-sustaining, autoregulatory fashion like PGE_2, IL-6, complement split products, or LPS it seems, cannot turn on the deleterious suppressor mode in the Mϕ after trauma, when the rise to cyclic AMP is counteracted with an NSAID. In this study we could show that the combination of Indo and TP-5 could alleviate the steep increment of the Mϕ metabolite NPT as an indicator of a Mϕ-driven hyperimmune response [28] compared to PC. We postulate that for the intact CMI function, the potentially deleterious acute phase reaction can be downregulated with Indo/TP-5, resulting then in a significantly lower IL-6 release as shown in LPS-stimulated PBMC cultures, compared to PC.

The analysis of postoperative infectious complications within the patient population studied demonstrated a total of three cases with severe septic episodes with gram-negative bacteria in PA/PC and one case of sternal osteitis through *Staphylococcus epidermidis*. Two of the three patients with sepsis died. In PB, there were three cases of minor infectious episodes, however, all of them were only localized and not systemic infections. It is self-explanatory that the patient numbers within that specific operative model are too small to allow conclusions to be drawn with regard to clinical relevance.

In summary, this study quantified and specified with a tridimensional set of parameters the massive impact of open heart surgery under ECC [37] on CMI, including detailed information about the acute phase cytokine regulation. The scrutiny of the efficacy of different immunopotentiating substances revealed that the combined therapy with Indo and TP-5 is superior to Indo only administration. Indo/TP-5 therapy resulted in a most adequate protection of all T-cell functions tested and it alleviated postoperative monocytosis and Mϕ over-activation. We found a convincing concurrence between the results of our long-term series of in vitro mechanistic studies and the findings derived from the stimultaneous in vivo administration of blocking and enhancing agents in terms of the protection of adequate Mϕ/T-cell interaction following major operative trauma.

References

1. Van Velzken-Blad H, Dijkstra YJ, Heijnen CJ et al. (1985) Cardiopulmonary bypass and host defense functions in human beings. II. lymphocyte function. Ann Thorac Surg 39:212–217
2. Roth JA, Golub SH, Cukingnan RA et al. (1981) Cell-mediated immunity is depressed following cardiopulmonary bypass. Ann Thorac Surg 31:350–356
3. Van Oeveren W, Kazatchkine MD, Descamps-Latscha B et al. (1985) Deleterious effects of cardiopulmonary bypass. J Thorac Cardiovasc Surg 89:888–899
4. Ninnemann JL (1989) The immune consequences of trauma: an overview. In: Faist E, Ninnemann JL, Green D (eds.) The immune consequences of trauma, shock, and sepsis—mechanisms and therapeutic approaches. Springer Berlin Heidelberg New York, pp 3–8
5. Miller-Graziano CL, Szabo G, Takayama T et al. (1989) Alterations of monocyte function following major injury. In: Faist E, Ninnemann JL, Green D (eds) The immune consequences of trauma, shock, and sepsis—mechanisms and therapeutic approaches. Springer, Berlin Heidelberg New York pp 95–108
6. Faist E, Ertel W, Mewes A et al. (1989) Trauma-induced alterations of the lymphokine cascade. In: Faist E, Ninnemann JL, Green D (eds) The immune consequences of trauma, shock, and sepsis—mechanisms and therapeutic approaches. Springer, Berlin Heidelberg New York, pp 79–94

7. Wood JJ, Rodrick ML, O'Mahony JB et al. (1984) Inadequate interleukin-2 production: a fundamental immunological deficiency in patients with major burns. Ann Surg 200:311–320
8. Faist E, Mewes A, Strasser T et al. (1988) Alteration of monocyte function following major injury. Arch Surg 123:287–292
9. Rodrick ML, Wood JJ, Gribic JT et al. (1986) Defective IL-2 production in patients with severe burns and sepsis. Lymphokine Res 5 [suppl 1]:312–317
10. Polk HC, George CD, Wellhausen SR et al. (1986) A systematic study of host defense processes in badly injured patients. Ann Surg 204:282
11. Cheadle WG, Hershman MJ, Wellhausen SR et al. (1989) Role of monocyte HLA-DR expression following trauma in predicting clinical outcome. In: Faist E, Ninnemann JL, Green D (eds) The immune consequences of trauma, shock, and sepsis—mechanisms and therapeutic approaches. Springer, Berlin Heidelberg New York pp 119–122
12. Goodwin JS, Ceuppens JL (1983) Effect of nonsteroidal antiinflammatory drugs on immune function. Semin Arthritis Rheum 13:134–143
13. Goldstein G, Audhya T (1985) Thymopoietin to thymopentin: experimental studies. Surv Immunol Res 4:1–10
14. Faist E (1989) Perioperative immunomodulation in patients with major surgical trauma. In: Faist E, Ninnemann JL, Green D (eds) The immune consequences of trauma, shock, and sepsis—mechanisms and therapeutic approaches. Springer, Berlin Heidelberg New York, pp 531–549
15. Faist E, Ertel W, Salmen B et al. (1988) The immune-enhancing effect of perioperative thymopentin administration in elderly patients undergoing major surgery. Arch Surg 123:1449–1453
16. Faist E, Ertel W, Cohnert T et al. (1990) Immunoprotective effects of cyclooxygenase inhibition in patients with major surgical trauma. J Trauma 30:8–18
17. Faist E, Mewes A, Baker CC et al. (1987) Prostaglandin E_2 (PGE_2)-dependent suppression of interleukin γ (IL-2) production in patients with major trauma. J Trauma 27:837–848
18. Gordon AH, Koj A (1985) The acute phase response to injury and infection. Elsevier, Amsterdam
19. Kimball JW (1983) Introduction. Immunology 5:113
20. Gillis S, Ferm MM, Ou W et al. (1978) T-cell growth factor: parameters of production and a quantitative microassay for IL-2 activity. J Immunol 120:2027–2032
21. Mosmann T (1983) Rapid colorimetric assay for cellular growth and survival: application to proliferation and cytotoxicity assays. J Immunol Methods 65:55
22. Hültner L, Szötzs H, Welle M et al. (1989) Mouse bone marrow-derived IL-3-dependent mast cells and autonomous sublines produce IL-6. Immunology 67:408
23. Endres S, Ghorbani R, Lonnemann G et al. (1988) Measurement of immunoreactive interleukin-1β from human mononuclear cells: optimization of recovery, intrasubject consistency, and comparison with interleukin-1 alpha and tumor necrosis factor. Clin Immunol Immunopathol 49:424
24. v.D. Meer JWM, Endres S, Lonnemann G et al. (1988) Concentrations of immunoreactive human tumor necrosis factor alpha produced by human mononuclear cells in vitro. J Leukoc Biol 43:216
25. Woloszczuk W (1985) A sensitive immunoradiometric assay for gamma interferon, suitable for its measurement in serum. Clin Chem 31:1090
26. Murray HW, Hillman JK, Rubin BY et al. (1985) Patients at risk for AIDS-related opportunistic infections. Clinical manifestations and impaired gamma interferon production. N Engl J Med 313:1504–1510
27. Werner ER, Bichler A, Daxenbichler G et al. (1987) Determination of neopterin in serum and urine. Clin Chem 33:62–66
28. Fuchs D, Hausen A, Reibnegger G et al. (1988) Neopterin as a marker for activated cell-mediated immunity: application in HIV infection. Immunol Today 9:150–155
29. Ertel W, Morrison MH, Ayala A et al. (1991) Blockade of prostaglandin production increases cachectin synthesis and prevents depression of macrophage functions after hemorrhagic shock. Ann Surg 213:77–83
30. Lunger A, Graf H, Schwar P (1986) Decreased serum interleukin-1 activity and monocyte interleukin-1 production in patients with fata sepsis. Crit Care Med 14:458
31. Ertel W, Faist E, Nestle C et al. (1990) Kinetics of interleukin-2 and interleukin-6 synthesis following major mechanical trauma. J Surg Res 48:62–66

32. Wakasugi H, Bertaglio J, Tursz T et al. (1987) IL-2 receptor induction on human T-lymphocytes: role for IL-2 and monocytes. Immunology 135:321–327
33. Bolla K, Duchateau J, Cappel R (1987) Strategical aspects of immunomodulation based on the influence of thymopentin on immune responses. Immune regulation by characterized poly-peptides. Liss, New York, pp 61–68
34. Ertel W, Faist E, Salmen B et al. (1989) Influence of cyclooxygenase inhibition on interleukin-2 receptor (IL-2R) expression after major trauma. J Surg Res 5:17–23
35. Ertel W, Morrison MS, Meldrum DR et al. (1992) Ibuprofen restores cellular immunity and decrease susceptibility to sepsis following hemorrhage. J Surg Res (in press)
36. Browder W, Williams D, Pretus H et al. (1990) Beneficial effect of enhanced macrophage function in the trauma patient. Ann Surg 211(5):605–613
37. Hisatomi K, Isomura T, Kawara T et al. (1989) Changes in lymphocyte subsets, mitogen responsiveness, and interleukin-2 production after cardiac operations. J Thorac Cardiovasc Surg 98:580–591

Effect of Immunomodulation on Skin Test Reactivity Following Trauma

W. Browder[1], D. Williams[2], G. Olivero[3], P. Mao[3], A. Franchello[3], and F. Enrichens[3]

Introduction

Morbidity and mortality from sepsis continue as major problems following trauma. A primary factor in the development of sepsis following injury is depression of host immune response. Delayed hypersensitivity skin testing (DHST) can assess the overall status of immune responsiveness and, indeed, may be predictive of subsequent sepsis [1]. A reasonable approach to immune suppression posttrauma might include therapy with biologic response modifiers (BRM) to enhance immune response. Such enhancement should be reflected in improved DHST. Glucan, a potent macrophage stimulant, has been shown to be beneficial in animal models of sepsis, trauma, and wound healing [2, 3]. The present study was designed to assess the value of glucan in a prospective study of trauma patients and to evaluate its effect on DHST and the development of sepsis.

Methods

Trauma patients (ages 18–65 years) admitted to the Trauma Institute, Torino, Italy, and undergoing exploratory laparotomy or thoracotomy were entered into the prospective study protocol. Excluded were those patients with cirrhosis, renal failure, severe head injury, or reproductive potential. Patients were randomized in a double-blind fashion to receive either glucan (50 mg/m^2) or saline placebo IV daily for 7 days after operation. All patients received prophylactic antibiotics. Therapeutic antibiotic regimens were based upon clinical course and culture reports. Skin tests were applied on days 1 and 7 after trauma using the Multitest device [4]. Anergy was judged to be less than two reactions of 2 mm induration. A clinical infection was documented when the patient's temperature rose above 39 °C daily and there was evidence of major soft tissue involvement with positive bacterial cultures. Blood was collected in siliconized

[1] Department of Surgery, East Tennessee State University, Johnson City, Tennessee, USA
[2] Department of Surgery, Tulane University, New Orleans, Louisiana, USA
[3] Istituto Di Chirugia D'Urgenza, University of Torino, Torino, Italy

Host Defense Dysfunction
in Trauma, Shock and Sepsis
Eds. Faist/Meakins/Schildberg
© Springer-Verlag, Berlin Heidelberg 1993

glass tubes on days 1, 3, 5, 7, and 9 after trauma for determination of serum interleukin-1 (IL-1) levels by radioimmunoassay.

Results

Patients in both the placebo and glucan groups were similar in many respects (Table 1). There was no significant difference in either injury severity score or abdominal trauma index. While more patients in the placebo group presented with hypotension, this difference was not significant. Average transfusions were similar in the two groups.

Of the 15 patients who were anergic on day 7 posttrauma, 8 (53.3%) developed subsequent septic complications. Of the 23 reactive skin tests on day 7, only 2 (87%) developed any septic morbidity ($p < 0.01$). Of the 15 glucan-treated patients who were anergic on day 1 posttrauma, 11 (73.3%) converted to positive DHST by day 7. In contrast, only 3 (21%) of the 14 anergic placebo patients changed to positive DHST ($p < 0.02$). Overall septic morbidity was decreased in the glucan-treated group (9.5% vs 47%; $p < 0.05$). Mean serum IL-1 level on day 3 posttrauma was significantly greater in glucan patients (143.4% $\pm$ 9.3% vs 78.6% $\pm$ 11.7%, ($p < 0.05$).

Discussion

There is increasing evidence that the macrophage is a key cell in the immune response following trauma. Macrophages produce cytokines that interact with essentially all aspects of cellular and humoral immunity. Recent work has postulated the existence of two classes of macrophages in the posttrauma milieu: facilitory and inhibitory [5]. Facilitory macrophages interact with T-helper lymphocytes while inhibitory macrophages produce prostaglandin E_2 (PGE_2) which is responsible for a host of immunosuppressive events [6].

One approach to posttraumatic immunosuppression might involve the concept of selective increase and enhancement of facilitory macrophages via biologic response modifiers. Glucan, a beta-1,3-linked glucopyranose polymer,

Table 1. Risk factors for infection in trauma patients

	Placebo	Glucan
Age (years)	35.7	32.9
Injury severity score (mean and range)	23 (8–26)	26 (16–41)
Abdominal trauma index (mean and range)	15.8 (8–26)	14.4 (0–35)
BP < 90 mmHg	41% (7/17)	28.6% (6/12)
Transfusion (units)	5.3	5.0

is a potent macrophage stimulant that has been shown to be effective in a variety of experimental surgical infection models [2, 3]. Use of glucan in a murine hind limb crush injury model demonstrated a shift of macrophage function toward the facilitory state, with a resultant decrease in PGE_2 release [7].

In the present study, glucan treatment resulted in a significant increase in serum IL-1 on day 3 posttrauma. Additionally, those glucan patients who converted from anergy to a positive skin test on day 7 following trauma had a significantly increased IL-1 level when compared to glucan patients who remained anergic. The macrophage is an important factor in delayed hypersensitivity and the positive correlation between IL-1 levels and DHST reactivity further supports the concept of macrophage activation in these patients. DHST anergy in the patients in this study also correlated with the development of subsequent septic complications, as noted by previous authors [1]. However, measurement of IL-1 alone did not predict a future septic course.

In addition to reflecting the activated state of the macrophage, IL-1 may have beneficial effects following trauma. IL-1 activates lymphocytes and stimulates release of IL-2, with a resulting enhancement of lymphocyte number and function. IL-1 also initiates the acute-phase response in which hepatic synthesis of certain proteins is increased [8]. Finally, IL-1 mobilizes polymorphonuclear leukocytes from bone marrow and increases their chemotactic ability [9].

It is apparent from this prospective randomized study of trauma patients that glucan immunostimulation significantly increased conversion of DHST from anergy to positive response. Furthermore, this conversion correlated with the activated macrophage as manifest by increased IL-1 levels on day 3 posttrauma. This macrophage activation also correlated with a decreased incidence of septic complications. Based on these encouraging results, further clinical trials are indicated to more fully evaluate biologic response modifiers in trauma patients.

References

1. Christou NV (1985) Host defense mechanisms in surgical patients: a correlative study of delayed hypersensitivity skin test response, granulocyte function and sepsis. Can J Surg 28:39–49
2. Browder W, Williams DL, Sherwood E et al. (1987) Synergistic effect of non-specific immunostimulation and antibiotics in experimental peritonitis. Surgery 102:206–214
3. Browder W, Williams D, Lucore P et al. (1988) Effect of enhanced macrophage function on early wound healing. Surgery 104:224–230
4. Kniker WT, Anderson CT, Roumiantzeff M (1979) The Multitest system: a standardized approach to evaluation of delayed hypersensitivity in cell mediated immunity. Ann Allergy 43:73–79
5. Miller SE, Miller CL, Trunkey DD (1982) The immune consequences of trauma. Surg Clin North Am 62:167–181
6. Faist E, Mewes A, Baker CC et al. (1987) Prostaglandin E_2 (PGE_2) dependent suppression of interleukin alpha (IL-2) production in patients with major trauma. J Trauma 27:837–848
7. Pretus HA, Browder IW, Lucore P et al. (1989) Macrophage activation decreases macrophage prostaglandin E_2 release in experimental trauma. J Trauma 29:1152–1157

8. Dinarello CA (1984) Interleukin-1 and the pathogenesis of the acute phase response. N Engl J Med 311:1413–1418
9. Kampschmidt RF (1981) Leukocytic endogenous mediator/endogenous pyrogen. In: Pyanda MC, Canonico PG (eds) The physiologic and metabolic responses of the host to infection and inflammation. Elsevier, Amsterdam, pp 55–74

Therapeutic Use of Cytokines: Animal Models

M. L. Rodrick, N. M. Moss, D. B. Gough, P. G. Horgan, B. M. Crowley,
M. G. O'Riordain, R. G. Molloy, and J. A. Mannick

Introduction

Although many clinical studies of the effects of burn or other major traumatic injury have been carried out and have yielded important information, many questions of mechanism may not be asked in this setting for practical or ethical reasons. Animal models afford the opportunity to study these questions. This has been especially since syngeneic strains are available where all animals are essentially twins. Furthermore, the use of congenic strains allows the choice of animals different at a single genetic locus where, for example, cells may be transferred between animals and recovered later to identify homing or cellular activities in different organs of the body.

It is now clear that a major factor in the morbidity and mortality in patients who were initially resuscitated after major injury is sepsis, and that this may result from the immunosuppressive state which occurs in these patients after a few days. Major changes in the secretion of cytokines involved in the immune response have been reported in patients and in animal models of trauma and have been discussed elsewhere in this book. For this reason, therapy with cytokines would seem to have great potential. Although the cells involved in the immune response make very small amounts of these cytokines and the process of isolating them is tedious and expensive, early clinical trials of interleukin-2 and interferon were carried out with material isolated from cultured stimulated human cells.

The advent of molecular biological methods of cloning of cells, and isolation and insertion of genes into fast-growing bacteria such as *Escherichia coli* have allowed production of large quantities of cytokines, allowing their use in clinical and experimental models of disease.

The purpose of this manuscript is to discuss the animal models of major trauma which have been and are presently being used to assess not only the mechanisms involved in the immunosuppression following major injury but also the therapeutic use of cytokines in these models and their potential for use in the clinical setting.

Dept of Surgery, Brigham and Women's Hospital, Harvard Medical School, Boston, MA, USA

Host Defense Dysfunction
in Trauma, Shock and Sepsis
Eds. Faist/Meakins/Schildberg
© Springer-Verlag, Berlin Heidelberg 1993

Animals Models

Models of trauma including burn injury, amputation, laparotomy, and hemorrhage have been developed primarily in mice, guinea pigs, and rats (Table 1). Most of these models also include a later or concomitant infectious challenge. All procedures are carried out under anesthesia with permission of animal experimentation committees of the institutions where the research was done under guidelines established by the US Public Health Service.

Thermal Injury

Walker and Mason in 1968 [1] described a standardized animal model of thermal injury which has been used extensively in this field. Mice are anesthetized, the dorsum clipped and the animals placed in a mold which allows a standardized percentage of body surface to be exposed. The thermal injury is a scald of the exposed skin by exposure to water heated to $85\,°\text{--}90\,°$ C for 8–9 s. The animals are dried, resuscitated with intraperitoneal saline, and allowed to recover. This results in a full-thickness third-degree burn injury, and no analgesia is required. The burn injury alone results in between 0 and 20% mortality. Kupper et al. [2] described a model of burn injury and showed that when suppressor T cells from burned mice were adoptively transferred to normal syngeneic mice, they became unable to overcome the challenge of peritonitis caused by cecal ligation and puncture (CLP).

In our laboratory, the work of Moss et al. [3] showed that normal 7- to 8-week-old A/J mice subjected to a 30% scald injury were susceptible to septic death from CLP in this same model only after they had become maximally immunosuppressed, i.e., after 7–10 days. Mortality in burn + CLP mice was > 80% when the CLP was performed 7–10 days after burn. These studies showed that there was suppression of the T cell response to phytohemagglutinin (PHA) and significantly suppressed secretion of interleukin-2 (IL-2) by concanavalin A-stimulated splenocytes.

Table 1. Animal models of trauma

Injury	Infection
Thermal injury	Cecal ligation and puncture
	Topical application of bacteria
Hemorrhagic shock + resuscitation	Subcutaneous inoculum
Laparotomy	Intraperitoneal and subcutaneous inoculum
Splenectomy	Aerosol infection
Surgically simulated infection	Inoculum or infected suture
Radiation	Natural infection

Silver et al. [4] have used a model of thermal injury in mice in which BDF1 mice were subjected to a 15% full-thickness scald injury followed immediately by placement of a solution containing varying concentrations of *Pseudomonas aeruginosa* on the burn wound. This model resulted in a mortality of about 80% in animals receiving burn plus infectious challenge in 5 days. Hershman et al. [5] have utilized a model resulting in a 30% full-thickness scald burn injury. They followed the injury with infectious challenge by topical application of either *P. aeruginosa* or *Klebsiella pneumoniae.*.

All models of thermal injury result in 0–20% mortality and only result in mortality after septic challenge in addition to burn injury. Controls are normal untreated animals, sham-burned animals, and sham-infected animals.

A model of radiation injury in mice has been used extensively by Neta and Oppenheim [6]. In this model mice are subjected to total body irradiation and if untreated will succumb due to natural sepsis some days later.

Trauma

Models of trauma have included amputation of a limb [7], in which immuno-suppression was observed. Hershman et al. [8] used a model in which mice were first infected intraperitoneally with *E. coli* and underwent surgical laparotomy. Finally, the mice were secondarily infected 5 days later intramuscularly with *K. pneumoniae*. Infection with *E. coli* plus laparotomy resulted in about 20% mortality. Mortality of 63% was observed in mice after *E. coli* plus laparotomy plus *K. pneumoniae*.

Models of shock due to hemorrhage have been described. Livingston and Malangoni [9] described a model in which female adult Sprague-Dawley rats were subjected to hemorrhagic shock by bleeding at 45 mm Hg for 45 min and then resuscitating with shed blood and saline. Animals were then subjected to septic challenge by subcutaneous inoculation of 10^8 *Staphylococcus aureus*. In this model the parameter assessed was not survival *S. aureus*-induced abscess number and diameter and weight.

Hamawy et al. [10] have used a model of surgical trauma in which male Sprague-Dawley rats were subjected to end-to-side portacaval anastomosis by a nonsuture method using Teflon tubing or a portacaval anastomosis and splenectomy or a sham laparotomy procedure. This procedure resulted in hepatic dysfunction, decreasing the ability of the body to clear a septic challenge which was given by administration of *P. aeruginosa*. Hebert et al. [11] have used a model of surgical trauma in which male CD-1 mice were splenectomized, then exposed to type III *S. pneumoniae* by aerosol exposure. These procedures resulted in an 80% mortality in untreated mice.

Surgically simulated wound infection has been used as a model by Hershman et al. [12]. They infected sutures in vitro by culture in the presence of *K. pneumoniae* and inserted lengths of this suture into the thighs of mice. This resulted in a 75% mortality in 5 days. The infection model was associated with a

Table 2. Use of cytokines in trauma models

IL-1	
Hamawy et al. [10]	Improved blood bacteria clearance following infection after portacaval anastomosis and splenectomy
Silver et al. [4]	Improved survival in mice after burn and infection with as little as 1 ng twice daily for 7 days
Neta et al. [14]	Improved survival in radioprotection model even after radiation
Crowley et al. [15]	Did not improve survival in burn/CLP model at doses of 10 ng–2 µg
O'Riordain et al. [16]	Improved survival in burn/CLP model when combined with indomethacin
IL-2	
Gough et al. [19]	Improved survival in burn/CLP model given after burn and before infection
Horgen et al. [20]	Improved survival in burn/CLP model at very low dose if combined with cyclooxygenase inhibitor
IFN-γ	
Hershman et al.	Improved survival after infection + laparotomy
Hershman et al.	Improved survival after burn injury + infection with *K. pneumoniae*, not *P. aeruginosa*
Malangoni et al. [23]	Decreased abscess formation after infection in hemorrhagic shock when combined with cefoxitin
IL-6	
Neta et al. [14]	Did not improve survival when used alone in lethal radiation model, but synergized with IL-1 to improve survival
TNF	
Livingston et al. [24]	Decreased abscess formation after infection with hemorrhagic shock when combined with cefoxitin
Hershman et al. [12]	Protected against surgically simulated wound infection
G-CSF	
Hebert et al. [11]	Protected against pneumococcal infection in a non-neutrophenic splenectomy model
O'Reilly	Improved survival in burn/sepsis model
GM-CSF	
Molloy et al. [31]	Improved survival in burn/CLP model

decrease in interferon-γ (IFN-γ) and tumor necrosis (TNF) secretion by in vitro cultured splenocytes. Shock may also be induced by infection with Gram-negative bacteria or endotoxin (lipopolysaccharide; LPS) from these bacteria [13]. In this model it was shown that TNF plays a central role in mediating the pathophysiologic changes that occur during endotoxic shock.

Therapy of Animal models with Cytokines

Attempts to increase survival or decrease infection in the models described above have been made using several cytokines. Most of these molecules have been recombinantly derived. It should be noted that the recombinant molecules are not the same as natural cytokines as most of them—having been produced in bacteria—are not glycosylated. Furthermore, these molecules have been associated with dose-limiting toxicities in clinical trials in cancer patients. Thus, a goal of clinical therapy with cytokiens will be to use the lowest dose possible that has clinical efficacy or to use combinations of cytokines and/or other drugs which may lower the dose of cytokine needed.

Interleukin-1 (IL-1)

Partially purified IL-1 was found to improve host immunity in the model of portacaval anastomosis and splenectomy described by Hamawy et al. [10]. Three to four weeks after operation the rats were found to have decreased ability to clear infection with *P. aeruginosa*. Animals which were treated with partially purified human IL-1 20 h before infection were found to have a significantly improved blood clearance of bacteria. Recombinant human IL-1 has been used by Silver et al. [4] in burn wound sepsis model in mice. IL-1 was administered subcutaneously immediately after burn injury and septic challenge. A single injection immediately after burn/sepsis of 100 ng/ mouse resulted in a better survival (60%) than a higher (1000 ng) dose (40%), compared to 0% survival in mice receiving saline after burn and sepsis. Furthermore, animals that received 7 days of therapy with 1 ng IL-1 twice daily also had significantly improved survival (70% compared to saline-treated 20%).

Neta and her colleagues have used IL-1 extensively in a model of radioprotection (reviewed in [6]). When IL-1 was injected either before or within 3 h after radiation, survival was significantly improved, and this was found to correlate with increased production of the hemopoietic colony stimulating factors. Suboptimal doses of IL-1 were found to synergize with either granulocyte–macrophage colony-stimulating factor (GM-CSF) or granulocyte CSF (G-CSF) to confer optimal radioprotection [14]. Crowley et al. [15], in work done in the burn/CLP model described above [3], found that recombinant human IL-1 in doses of 10 ng–2 µg/day for 7 days after thermal injury did not improve survival. However, O'Riordain et al. [16] found improved survival in this model when IL-1 was combined with therapy with the cyclooxygenase inhibitor indomethacin.

Interleukin-2 (IL-2)

Decreased T cell function and significant and prolonged decrease of IL-2 secretion by these cells has been found following injury in humans and in mouse models [3, 17, 18]. Using the burn/CLP model, Gough et al. [19] tested doses of recombinant human IL-2 given intraperitoneally (i.p.) for 6 days after thermal injury and before CLP on day 10 from 250 units to 250 000 units/day.

Improved survival was found to be optimal at a dose of 16 000 units/day for 6 days. Improved T cell function was found at a dose of 250 units, but survival, although improved, failed to reach significance. Horgan et al. [20] combined the dose of IL-2 of 250 units/day with a dose of indomethacin of 1 µg/mouse per day and achieved significantly improved survival and immune response in the burn/CLP model.

Tumor Necrosis Factor α (TNF-α)

Defective antigen presentation and monocyte expression of immune response antigens have been reported following injury [21, 22] and suggest that there are defects in monocyte/macrophage (MM) function as well as T cell function. TNF-α is another product, like IL-1, produced primarily by MM. Malangoni et al. [23] tested the effect of TNF-α therapy in a model of hemorrhagic shock and resuscitation (described in [9]) followed by infection with *E. coli* and *Bacteroides fragilis*. They found that recombinant human TNF-α alone (7500 units/dose), inoculated 30 min before and for 3 days after septic challenge, did not have effect on abscess formation. However, combination of TNF with the antibiotic cefoxitin significantly decreased abscess formation. Livingston et al. [24], using the same model, found that TNF plus cefoxitin also decreased abscess formation caused by the Gram-positive organism *S. aureus*. Hershman et al. [12] showed that recombinant human TNF (7500 units daily for 5 days prior to infection) was protective against *K. pneumoniae* infections in mice in the simulated wound infection model described above. Treatment at 1 h after and for 7 days after bacterial challenge resulted in significantly improved survival from day 6 onward after infection, with final survival of about 70%, compared with only a 15% survival in the control infected mice. The dose of TNF equivalent to 6 µg/kg is well below the dose shown to have toxic effects in rats (600 µg/kg).

Interferon γ (IFN-γ)

Suzuki and Pollard [25, 26], using a mouse model of thermal injury, showed that endogenous interferon production is reduced following thermal injury. Hershman et al. [5] used murine IFN-γ therapy in a burn/infection model described above. IFN-γ was administered daily at a dose of 7500 units for 5 days prior to 30% body surface burn injury and topical bacterial challenge. Mice which were infected with *K. pneumoniae* and treated with IFN-γ had significantly better survival over controls. However, mice infected with *P. aeruginosa* did not show improved survival with IFN-γ therapy. Improved survival was associated with maintenance of macrophage Ia antigen expression.

Hershman et al. [8] have also studied the therapeutic benefit of IFN-γ in a mouse model of trauma described above. Mice were treated with 7500 units IFN-γ, subcutaneously, postlaparotomy and daily for 5 days until the second bacterial challenge. Mice treated with IFN-γ survived significantly longer than vehicle controls. Again, Ia antigen expression was maintained in IFN-γ treated mice. Hershman et al. [12] studied the therapeutic effect of IFN-γ in a model of surgically simulated wound infection. Treatment with IFN-γ for 5 days prior to infection in this model did not improve survival significantly, although a modest but significant effect was found when IFN-γ was given therapeutically 1 hr after challenge continuing for 7 days [27]. Malangoni et al. [23], in the hemorrhagic shock model [9] in rats, found that recombinant rat IFN-γ alone did not decrease Gram-negative infection but when combined with cefoxitin reduced abscess formation and size.

Interleukin-6 (IL-6)

Dinarello and Neta [28] investigated the ability of recombinant IL-1 and IL-6 to improve survival in a lethal radiation model in mice. They found that, unlike IL-1, IL-6 did not result in improved survival. In fact, such treatment given 20 h before radiation resulted in reduced survival. However, IL-6 was able to augment the effects of IL-1. IL-1 induced circulating CSF and IL-6 did not, suggesting that this induction of the CSFs plays an important role for the effectiveness of cytokine therapy in this model.

Granulocyte Colony Stimulating Factor (G-CSF)

Silver et al. [29] used the mouse model [4] of thermal injury and sepsis to test the efficacy of recombinant human G-CSF. G-CSF significantly improved survival when 100 ng was administered twice daily for 7 days. Even better survival was found when G-CSF therapy at the same dose was combined with a single dose of the antibiotic gentamicin at 6 mg/kg immediately after injury. Hebert et al. [11], using the model of splenectomy plus infection, found that G-CSF at a dose of 100 ng/mouse, administered 2 weeks after surgery and for 3 days commencing 24 h after exposure to infection, significantly improved survival (70%) compared with vehicle control splenectomized infected mice (20%). Furthermore, significantly fewer bacteria were recovered from the lungs and lymph nodes in the G-CSF treated animals.

Granulocyte–Macrophage Colony Stimulating Factor (GM-CSF)

GM-CSF is a species-specific cytokine, so all work done with this cytokine in murine models must be done with murine GM-CSF. Although not in a model of trauma-induced increased susceptibility to infection, recombinant murine GM-CSF has been shown to protect neonatal rats against septic death due to *S. aureus* by Frenck et al. [30]. Similar to other studies with cytokines, it was found that very large and very small doses were not as effective as moderate ones. For example, the efficacy of doses was 30pg/g > 300 > 3000 > 10 000 > 0.3. Recently, Molloy et al. [31] in our burn/CLP model in A/J mice [3] showed that recombinant mouse GM-CSF significantly improves survival when injected either intraperitoneally or subcutaneously once per day at 200 ng/mouse from days 5 to 10 after burn and before septic challenge on day 10.

Conclusions

The experimental models and use of cytokines in those models we have described suggest that there is a potential for use numerous cytokines in therapy of the infectious complications of major injury. Therapy with the cytokines in cancer has used very large doses, but these cytokines have dose-limiting toxicities not acceptable in the compromised burn or trauma patient. Results presented here have suggested that smaller doses of cytokines may be better than larger ones, and we may reduce the quantity of these molecules needed by combination with antibiotics, modulation of the cyclooxygenase pathway by combination with inhibitors such as ibuprofen, and/or taking advantage of synergy between two or more cytokines.

References

1. Walker HL, Mason AD Jr (1968) A standard animal burn. J Trauma 19:1049–1051
2. Kupper TS, Baker CC, Ferguson TA, Green DR (1985) A burn-induced Ly-2 suppressor T cell lowers resistance in bacterial infection. J Surg Res 38:606–612
3. Moss NM, Gough DB, Jordan AL, Grbic JT, Wood JJ, Rodrick ML, Mannick JA (1988) Temporal correlation of impaired immune response after thermal injury with susceptibility to infection in a murine model. Surgery 104:882–887
4. Silver GM, Gamelli RL, O'Reilly M, Hebert JC (1990) The effect of interleukin 1α on survival in a murine model of burn wound sepsis. Arch Surg 125:922–925
5. Hershman MJ, Sonnenfeld G, Logan WA, Pietsch JD, Wellhausen SR, Polk HC Jr (1988) Effect of interferon-γ treatment on the course of a burn wound infection. J Interferon Res 8:367–373
6. Neta R, Oppenheim JJ (1988) Cytokines in therapy of radiation injury. Blood 72:1093–1095
7. Wang BS, Heacock EH, Mannick JA (1982) Characterization of suppressor cells generated in mice after surgical trauma. Clin Immunol Immunopathol 24:161–170
8. Hershman MJ, Polk HC Jr, Pietsch JD, Shields RE, Wellhausen SR, Sonnenfeld G (1988) Modulation of infection by gamma interferon treatment following trauma. Infect Immun 56:2412–2416
9. Livingston DH, Malangoni MA (1989) An experimental study of susceptibility to infection after hemorrhagic shock. Surg Gynecol Obstet 168:138–142
10. Hamawy KJ, Yamazaki K, Georgieff M, Dinarello CA, Moldawer LL, Blackburn GL, Bistrian BR (1986) Improvements in host immunity by partially purified interleukin 1 in rats with portacaval anastomosis and splenectomy JPEN J Parenter Enteral Nutr 10:146–150
11. Hebert JC, O'Reilly M, Gamelli RL (1990) Protective effect of recombinant human granulocyte colony-stimulating factor against pneumococcal infections in splenectomized mice. Arch Surg 125:1075–1078
12. Hershman MJ, Pietsch JD, Trachtenberg L, Mooney THR, Shields RE, Sonnenfeld G (1989) Protective effects of recombinant human tumour necrosis factor α and interferon γ against surgically simulated wound infection in mice. Br J Surg 76:1282–1286
13. Mathison JC, Wolfson E, Ulevitch RJ (1988) Participation of tumor necrosis factor in the mediation of gram negative bacterial lipopolysaccharide-induced injury in rabbits. J Clin Invest 81:1925–1937

14. Neta R, Oppenheim JJ, Douches SD (1988) Interdependence of the radioprotective effects of human recombinant interleukin 1 alpha, tumor necrosis factor alpha, granulocyte colony-stimulating factor, and murine recombinant granulocyte-macrophage colony-stimulating factor. J Immunol 140:108–111
15. Crowley BM, Ellwanger K, Collins K, Mannick JA, Rodrick ML (1989) Can interleukin-1 improve the immune deficiency associated with thermal injury? Surg Forum 40:70–72
16. O'Riordain MG, Collins KH, Saporoschetz IB, Mannick JA, Rodrick ML (1991) Modulation of macrophage hyperactivity improves survival in a burn/sepsis model. Surgical Infection Society Meeting, Boca Raton
17. Wood JJ, Rodrick ML, O'Mahony JB, Palder SB, Saporoschetz I, d'Eon P, Mannick JA (1984) Inadequate interleukin 2 production: a fundamental immunological deficiency in patients with major burns. Ann Surg 200:311–320
18. Rodrick ML, Wood JJ, O'Mahony JB, Davis CF, Demling RH, Moss NM, Saporoschetz I, Jordan A, d'Eon P, Mannick JA (1986) Mechanisms of immunosuppression associated with severe non-thermal traumatic injuries in man. Production of interleukin 1 and 2. J Clin Immunol 6:310–318
19. Gough DB, Moss NM, Jordan A (1988) Recombinant interleukin-2 (rIL-2) improves immune response and host resistance to septic challenge in thermally injured mice. Surgery 104:292
20. Horgan PG, Mannick JA, Dubravec DB, Rodrick ML (1990) Effect of low dose recombinant interleukin 2 plus indomethacin on mortality after sepsis in a murine burn model. Br J Surg 77:401–404
21. Ayala A, Perrin MM, Chaudry IH (1990) Defective macrophage antigen presentation following haemorrhage is associated with the loss of MHC class II (Ia) antigen. Immunology 70:33–39
22. Polk HC Jr, George CD, Wellhausen SR, Cost K, Davidson PR, Regan MP, Borzotta AP (1986) A systematic study of host defense processes in badly injured patients. Ann Surg 204:282
23. Malangoni MA, Livingston DH, Sonnenfeld G, Polk HC Jr (1990) Interferon gamma and tumor necrosis factor alpha. Use in gram-negative infection after shock. Arch Surg 125:444–446
24. Livingston DH, Malangoni MA, Sonnenfeld G (1989) Immune enhancement by tumor necrosis factor-alpha improves antibiotic efficacy after hemorrhagic shock. J Trauma 29:967–971
25. Suzuki F, Pollard RB (1982) Alterations of interferon production in a mouse model of thermal injury. J Immunol 129:1806–1810
26. Suzuki F, Pollard RB (1982) Mechanism for the suppression of γ-interferon responsiveness in mice after thermal injury. J Immunol 129:1811–1815
27. Hershman MJ, Polk HC Jr, Pietsch JD, Juftinec D, Sonnenfeld G (1988) Modulation of Klebsiella pneumoniae infection of mice by interferon-gamma. Clin Exp Immunol 72:406–409
28. Dinarello CA, Neta R (1989) An overview on interleukin-1 as a therapeutic agent. Biotherapy 1:245–254
29. Silver GM, Gamelli RL, O'Reilly M (1989) The beneficial effect of granulocyte colony-stimulating factor (G-CSF) in combination with gentamicin on survival after Pseudomonas burn wound infection. Surgery 106:452–456
30. Frenck RW, Sarman G, Harper TE, Buescher ES (1990) The ability of recombinant murine granulocyte-macrophage colony-stimulating factor to protect neonatal rats from septic death due to Staphylococcus aureus. J Infect Dis 162:109–114
31. Molloy RG, Nestor M, Mannick JA, Rodrick M (1991) GM-CSF: a therapeutic role in the prevention of mortality after burn sepsis. FASEB J (in press)

The Rationale for Gamma-Interferon Administration in Trauma Patients*

H. C. Polk, Jr., S. Galandiuk, G. Sonnenfeld, and W. G. Cheadle

Introduction

The search for a method of immunostimulation is certainly an old one and probably even antedates this century. Clearly, individuals familiar with the clinical situation of infection in man viewed a stimulation of normal host defenses as a potent therapeutic option; indeed, it may even be that Wright's obsession with this concept may have played a role in binding Fleming to the potential therapeutic value of penicillin. Notwithstanding the same, after nearly 50 years of antimicrobial chemotherapy, it is long past time to reassess whether or not stimulation of innate host defenses, or correction of fundamental host defense abnormalities, can play a significant role in the care of the patient who is extremely likely to develop infection or has become infected. For much of the last decade, a variety of surgeons have examined the specific and nonspecific effects of a potent array of immunostimulants, ranging from lipopolysaccharide itself to increasingly well-defined components thereof, and to even more primitive "witches' brew" kinds of materials. Philosophically, it is interesting to view the shift from the idea of general and nonspecific immunostimulation to the definition of specific defects that occur in some surgical patients and the conceptual shift of therapy toward immunoreconstitution. We had been frustrated by the inability to get certain promising agents to the bedside for properly stratified clinical trials. Everyone recognizes the enormous costs involved in such an undertaking, but the failure to be able to take agents, such as muramyl dipeptide, and put them in definitive trials, basically eliminated a promising clinical outlet.

Clinical Survey

We then turned back to the bedside in our well-known Trauma Surgery Unit at the University of Louisville to attempt to define in a prospective sense any

* A substantial portion of this work has been supported by a variety of fellowships and specifically by initial laboratory and subsequent clinical trial funds provided by Genentech, Inc., San Francisco, California, USA.
Departments of Surgery and Microbiology, and the Price Institute of Surgical Research, University of Louisville School of Medicine, Louisville, Kentucky, USA

putative abnormalities that might be truly responsible for and/or closely associated with the propensity of some badly hurt trauma victims to develop infection. The initial study was clearly a geographic and descriptive survey attempting to identify which, if any, of currently measurable host defense abnormalities might be most closely associated with clinically relevant poor outcomes due to infection [1]. We entered this study convinced that the null hypothesis would be true and were surprised to identify an important role of the capacity of monocytes to present class II antigens on their surface for processing [2]. Clearly this an important event in host defense responses to infection, but it was a surprise to us that it stood as an apparent independent variable which has now been confirmed in multiple other studies and the work of Faist and associates [3] in consistent fashion.

In separate extensive studies in man, Cheadle and associates [4] sequentially:

1. Defined the normal distribution of HLA-DR antigen expression on the surface of circulating monocytes in healthy volunteers
2. Showed that volunteers with a history of chronic and/or recurrent infection tended to display lower values
3. Demonstrated no influence on values in the face of immunosuppressive therapy in transplant recipients or acute alcohol intoxication
4. Found a stray association with and possible predictive value for monocyte expression of HLA-DR in patients who developed infection after a variety of elective operations and other severe nonsurgical infections
5. Suggested that monocyte antigen expression may, in terms of unusually high or low values, be an inherited trait

Having identified this apparent significant association and its possible predictive value, we were then obviously tantalized by the idea of whether this abnormality could be returned to normal ranges by any form of safe and tolerable therapy. Obviously, therapy would best apply in an individual who bore several characteristics, i.e., badly hurt and with sufficient bacterial contamination to be likely to develop an infection that would cause clinical morbidity or, in some cases, be associated with death.

Potential Correction

The thread of therapy depended on two key observations. The first was the recognition by others that endogenous gamma-interferon production was often impaired in individuals after trauma and burns. The second was our demonstration that in vitro incubation with gamma-interferon of monocytes harvested from badly hurt trauma victims rapidly returned those values to normal [5-7]. These data obviously suggested that one might be able to use such as agent in a corrective fashion early on in the course of injury. We then, through the primary efforts of Michael Hershman, were able to develop a sequence of models of clinical infection that were worthy of further testing. The infected thigh suture has long been a model in our laboratory that has reproduced virtually all the parameters of clinical surgical would infection [8]. Clearly, in a large number of animals, there was some modest benefit shown by administration of gamma-interferon prior to challenge, but this was significantly attenuated as the agent was given longer and longer after bacterial challenge (Fig. 1) [9, 10]. Furthermore, gamma-interferon was shown to be effective in a seeded burn model and also provided some significant protection in an elaborate set of experiments in which shock was followed by subsequent bacterial contamination, reoperation, and general anesthesia (Fig. 2) [11, 12]. Having consistently found in dozens of experiments a variable but regularly positive degree of protection associated with gamma-interferon prophylaxis and/or therapy, it was more than obvious that we needed to once again address the challenge of constructing a meaningful clinical trail.

It was abundantly clear that gamma-interferon was a safe agent for administration in man by virtue of the many patients with neoplastic disease who had safely received the material [13]. Separate studies have also established its

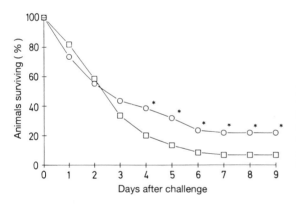

Fig. 1. Survival of mice treated with placebo (*squares*) or gamma-interferon 7500 U/day for 7 days (*circles*), beginning 1 h after IM challenge with 10^3 *Klebsiella pneumoniae.* *Statistically significant. (With permission from [9])

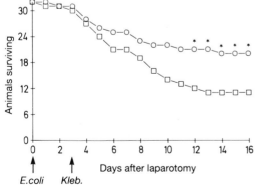

Fig. 2. Survival of mice treated with placebo (*squares*) of gamma-interferon 7500 U/day for 3 days (*circles*) following an initial challenge of intraperitoneal *E. coli* and laparotomy, and a second challenge of IM *K. pneumoniae* (*Kleb.*) *Statistically significant. (With permission [12])

clinical efficacy in children with chronic granulomatous disease [14]. Further-more, we had been able to stratify our trauma patients into groups clinically aligned as: (1) alive, well, and free of infection; (2) infected survivors; and (3) those who died, usually of a progressive infection [15, 16]. Interestingly, by using a combination of injury severity score, a simple scale of bacterial contamination, and an early monocyte HLA-DR antigen presentation sample from the flow cytometer, we were able to stratify patients in a significant way (Figs. 3 and 4). In preparation for a clinical trial, a pilot trial was undertaken in 15 consecutive badly hurt patients, after appropriate Human Studies Committee approval, that confirmed the clinical safety of the agent in question. Furthermore, it was also quite clear that there was a reasonably broad dosage range from 0.01 µg/day to 0.1 µg/day that would be clinically acceptable. Data from that trial still leaves ambivalent as to what is the proper time of termination of gamma-interferon therapy in such high risk patients. Figure 5 illustrates the effect of 0.05 µg/day treatment for 10 days in five patients from the pilot study. When compared with

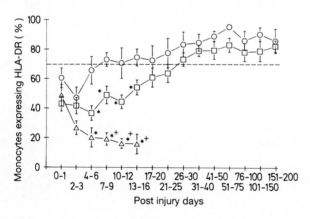

Fig. 3. Percent of circulating monocytes that expressed HLA-DR antigen in patients following severe injury; patients with uneventful recovery (*circles*), patients who developed major sepsis (*squares*), and patients who died (*triangles*). *Error bars* refer to standard error of the mean. *Statistically significant difference from uneventful recovery group; +statistically significant differ-ence from major sepsis group. (With permission from [16])

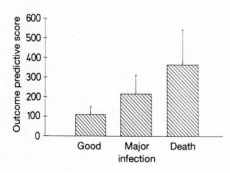

Fig. 4. Outcome predictive score in patients ac-cording to clinical outcome. Score based on percentage LD_{50}, degree of contamination, and percentage MO2-DR. (With permission from [15]

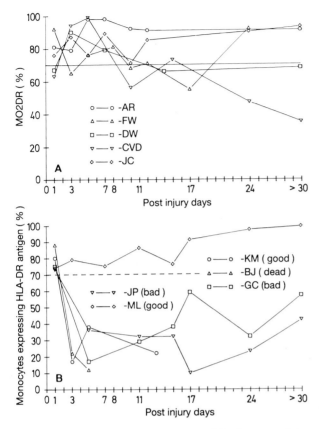

Fig. 5. A Percentage MO2-DR in patients following severe injury receiving 0.05 µg/day gamma-interferon **B** Percentage MO2-DR in patients following severe injury. Patients matched to patients in **A** with respect to initial MO2-DR and percentage LD_{50}. Note the tendency of the gamma-interferon-treated patients in **A** to exceed 70% and the tendency of the matched patients from historical controls in **B** to display values well below that. The single patient in the normal range in **B** recovered without infection.

five patients matched for LD_{50} and day 1 MO2-DR, the quick return of low MO2-DR values to normal is apparent. Clearly, we chose to go with 7 days therapy empirically, and another clinical trial has been launched which is examining a group of patients who are not necessarily bacterially contaminated and continued for 3 weeks or the full duration of hospitalization, whichever is shorter. The laboratory data from that clinical trial now indicate that a sustained increase in monocyte HLA-DR antigen expression is produced by gamma-interferon therapy, but that it rapidly decreases with the cessation of therapy. "How long is the ideal course?" may be difficult to define clinically. Fever was thought to be a clinical complication of gamma-interferon therapy but was only slightly more prevalent in the treatment arm of the study than in the other (approximately 70% versus 50%).

Having completed the trial with the accession of 212 patients in primarily three university trauma centers, we can attest to the drug's safety and are awaiting the formal unblinding of the study to speak to its efficacy. The impact of gamma-interferon therapy can, however, be rated in at least two ways:

1. A sustained increase in percent of monocyte expression HLA-DR as well as mean fluorescent intensity in patients receiving gamma-interferon, which precipitously declined to the same level as seen in the placebo patients 48 after cessation of therapy.
2. Monocytes drawn from patients receiving gamma-interferon were capable of further stimulation in terms of HLA-DR expression lipopolysaccharide.

Furthermore, the association between very low early monocyte HLA-DR expression and ultimate severe infection was confirmed for both placebo and gamma-interferon-treated patients.

Irrespective of the effectiveness of gamma-interferon in this clinical trial, we believe that some kind of agent, in addition to careful surgical technique, full resuscitation, continuing meticulous intensive care, and judicious systemic antibiotic therapy, may make a long-term difference in the frequency of life-threatening infection in at least some subsets of surgical patients. Such efforts are exemplified by the recent modest success of human monoclonal antibody against endotoxin in clinical trials [17] and the additive effect of an endotoxin filter to a full range of other therapies in a mouse model of surgical infection [18].

References

1. Polk HC Jr, George CD, Wellhausen SR et al. (1986) A systematic study of host defense processes in badly injured patients. Ann Surg 204:282–299
2. Unanue ER (1984) Antigen-presenting function of the macrophage. Annu Rev Immunol 2:395–428
3. Faist E, Kupper TS, Baker CC, Chaudry IH, Dwyer J, Baue AE (1986) Depression of cellular immunity after major trauma: its association with post-traumatic complications and its reversal with immunomodulation. Arch Surg 121:1000–1005
4. Cheadle WG, Hershman MJ, Wellhausen SR, Polk HC Jr (1991) HLA-DR antigen expression on peripheral blood monocytes correlates with surgical infection. Am J Surg 161:639–645
5. Faist E, Mewes A, Strasser G (1988) Aleration of monocyte function following major injury. Arch Surg 123:287–292
6. Livingston DH, Appel SA, Wellhausen SR, Sonnenfeld G, Polk HC Jr (1988) Depressed interferon gamma production and monocyte HLA-DR expression after severe injury. Arch Surg 123:1309–1312
7. Hershman MJ, Appel SA, Wellhausen SR, Polk HC Jr (1989) Interferon-gamma increases HLA-DR expression on monocytes in severely injured patients. Clin Exp Immunol 77:67–70
8. Reuben DP, Fagelman K, McCoy MT, Polk HC Jr (1977) Enhancement of nonspecific host defenses against local bacterial challenge. Surg Forum 28:44–45
9. Hershman MJ, Polk HC Jr, Peitsch JD, Kuftinec D, Sonnefeld G (1988) Modulation of *Klebsiella pneumoniae* infection of mice by interferon-gamma. Clin Exp Immunol 72:406–409
10. Hershman MJ, Sonnenfeld G, Mays BW, Fleming F, Trachtenberg LS, Polk HC Jr (1988) Effects of interferon-gamma treatment on surgically simulated wound infection in mice. Microb Pathog 4:165–168

11. Hershman MJ, Sonnenfeld G, Logan WA, Pietsch JD, Wellhausen SR, Polk HC Jr (1988) Effect of interferon-gamma treatment of the course of a burn wound infection. J Interferon Res 8:367–373
12. Hershman MJ, Polk HC Jr, Pietsch JD, Shields RE, Wellhausen SR, Sonnenfeld G (1988) Modulation of infection by gamma interferon treatment following trauma. Infect Immun 56:2412–2416
13. Jaffe HS, Sherwin SA (1986) The early clinical trials of recombinant human interferon-gamma In: Friedman RM, Merigan T, Sreevalsan T (eds) Interferons as cell growth inhibitors and antitumor factors. Liss, New York, pp 509–522
14. Ezekowitz RAB, Dinaver MC, Jaffe HS et al. (1988) Partial correction of the phagocyte defect in patients with linked chronic granulomatous disease by subcutaneous interferon gamma. N Engl J Med 319:146–151
15. Hershman MJ, Cheadle WG, Kuftinec D, Polk HC Jr, George CD (1988) An outcome predictive score for sepsis and death following injury. Injury 19:263–266
16. Hershman MJ, Cheadle WG, Wellhausen SR, Davidson PF, Polk HC Jr (1990) Monocyte HLA-DR antigen expression characterizes clinical outcome in the trauma patient. Br J Surg 77:204–207
17. Ziegler EJ, Fisher CJ Jr, Sprung CL et al. (1991) Treatment of gram-negative bacteria and septic shock with HA-IA human monoclonal antibody endotoxin. N Engl J Med 324:429–436
18. Cheadle WG, Hanasawa K, Gallinaro RN, Nimmonwudipong T, Kodama M, Polk HC Jr (1991) Endotoxin filtration and immune stimulation improve survival from gram negative sepsis. Surgery 110:785–792

Immunomodulators of the Thermal Injury Response

J. M. Mlakar[1] and J. P. Waymack[2]

Infection remains the most common cause of postburn mortality in burn victims who survive the initial cardiopulmonary insult [35]. Infection is promoted by the loss of skin's epithelial barrier and by a generalized postburn immunosuppression due to release of immunoactive agents from the burn wound [15]. Burn injury leads to suppression of nearly all aspects of the immune system [29]. Postburn serum levels of immunoglobulins, fibronectin, and complement are reduced, resulting in a diminished capacity for opsonization. Chemotaxis, phagocytosis, and the killing function of neutrophils, monocytes, and macrophages are impaired. Burn injury results in reductions in lymphocyte blastogenic response, cytotoxic ability, interleukin-2 (IL-2) production, and CD4/CD8 (helper/suppressor) cell ratio. Efforts at correcting this postburn immunosuppression using immunomodulators are increasingly being investigated [11, 17].

Endotoxins are heat stable, high-molecular-weight lipopolysaccharides (LPS) which are components of the cell wall of most gram-negative bacilli. Postburn serum concentrations of endotoxin are proportional to the extent of injury with peak levels commonly occurring at 3–4 days after injury [49]. Endotoxins are felt to play a major role in the immunosuppression of thermal injury.

Polymyxin B is a cationic polypeptide antimicrobial agent known to bind endotoxin via its lipid A moiety both in vitro and in vivo [21]. Polymyxin B administered systemically to burned mice increases lymphocyte blastogenesis and antibody production [8]. Low-dose intravenous polymyxin B has been shown to reduce serum endotoxin levels in burn patients [33]. Intravenous polymyxin B can maintain a normal CD4/CD8 ratio and can preserve lymphocyte responsiveness to mumps and candida antigens in burn patients [31, 51]. Polymyxin B therapy has been associated with decreased levels of serum IL-6 in the burn patients. In vivo polymyxin B treatment enhances in vitro lymphocyte recognition of antigens and response to stimulation with IL-2 [6].

Corynebacterium parvum 936B when administered as a killed vaccine is an unusually potent stimulator of the recticuloendothelial system. It was originally investigated for its tumoricidal properties. Its cell wall appears to be responsible for a variety of immunomodulatory properties. Much of the nonspecific immune

[1] Shriners Burns Institute, Galveston, TX, 77550 USA
[2] University of Texas Medical Branch, Galveston, TX, 77550 USA

Host Defense Dysfunction
in Trauma, Shock and Sepsis
Eds. Faist/Meakins/Schildberg
© Springer-Verlag, Berlin Heidelberg 1993

stimulation following *C. parvum* administration is presumed to be macrophage mediated. *C. parvum* has been shown to activate complement, increase bone marrow macrophage colony production, stimulate interferon production by lymphocytes, and attract monocytes and neutrophiles. Many of *C. parvum*'s actions are T-cell independent, as evidenced by an enhanced rate of clearance of *Listeria* bacteremia during treatment of infected nude mice. However, *C. parvum* vaccine has been demonstrated to decrease delayed hypersensitivity, reduce in vitro T-lymphocyte mitogenic responses, and reduce graft vs host reactions in experimental models [3].

C. parvum has been shown to improve survival in burned animal models [37]. Interestingly, the *C. parvum* effect may be somewhat species-specific. Burned dogs had an increased rate of survival in response to treatment [37], while in a similar model burned guinea pigs did not [44]. In man, clinical trials on burned patients showed an 80% reduction in the number of bacteremic episodes in *C. parvum*-treated groups [1]. However, its bacterial nature and complexity have limited the wide-spread use of *C. parvum* in man.

Glucan is a polysaccharide molecule derived from the inner cell wall of *Saccharomyces cerevisiae*. In animal models, glucan increases host resistance to viral, bacterial, fungal, and parasitic infections. It enhances reticuloendothelial function and increases production of both IL-1 and colony-stimulating factor (CSF) [3]. Unfortunately, glucan toxicity is a frequent occurrence, sometimes producing severe side effects [3]. This has prevented widespread use of glucan in human trials.

Immunoglobulin infusion for correcting postburn immunosuppression through passive immunization remains somewhat controversial. Serum immunoglobulins are known to be depressed following burn injury [30]. This appears due to an increased rate of utilization of immunoglobulins rather than a decreased rate of synthesis. Indeed, the serum half-life of immunoglobulin is markedly reduced in burn patients. It has been shown to vary from 47 h on postburn day 3 to 154 h on postburn week 3, compared to 21 days in unburned controls.

Alexander and Fisher reported a reduced mortality from *Pseudomonas* infection in burned mice treated with an anti-*Pseudomonas* vaccine (from 14.7% to 3.1%), which was further reduced to 0 with concominant use of γ-globulin [2]. Holder et al. also reported that intravenous γ-globulin given prior to *Pseudomonas aeruginosa* challenge in burned mice increased survival rates [19].

There have been a number of clinical trials of immune globulin in burn patients. Shirani et al. [36] documented that γ-globulin infusion could return depressed serum levels of immunoglobulin to normal, but did not offer proof of clinical efficacy. Stone et al. [39] reported that globulin infusions in burn patients failed to decrease the incidence of infections, sepsis, or mortality. Munster et al. [32], in a randomized trial of immune globulin in burn patients, also found no effect on mortality rates, mortality secondary to sepsis, incidence of positive blood cultures, or number of positive wound biopsies. Sequential analysis of immune function in these patients failed to demonstrate any effect of the γ-globulin therapy on neutrophil chemotaxic index, lymphocyte function, or CD4/CD8 ratio. There was a significant decrease in the number of poly-microbial bacteremias, the mean blood endotoxin levels, and the cytomegalo-virus titers in the immunoglobulin-treated group. Hansbrough et al. [18], in a similar study, noted in earlier return to normal of serum immunoglobulin G (IgG) levels in the treated group. There were no differences in mortality or morbidity between groups. Opsonic capacity of the patient's serum remained defective in both groups for up to 15 days after injury despite earlier correction of the serum IgG levels in the treated group. Finally, Waymack et al. [42], in a randomized trial of 50 adult and pediatric burn patients with greater than 20% total body surface area (TBSA) burn, failed to find any differences in infection rates or mortality with IgG infusions.

Fibronectin is a circulating nonspecific opsonin which is thought to particip-ate in some phases of bacterial and particulate matter opsonization and phagocytosis. Serum fibronectin levels drop acutely following burn injury [24]. Serum fibronectin levels are also decreased during septic episodes [9]. Infusion of cryoprecipitate can replete serum fibronectin levels, and increase serum opsonization activity [34]. However, Lanser et al. [24] were unable to docu-ment clinical improvement in patients administered fibronectin extracts, and a trial of purified fibronectin replacement in septic patients failed to improve survival rates over controls [26].

Tuftsin is a tetrapeptide of the sequence L-Thr-L-Lys-L-Pro-L-Arg which is derived from the highly conserved CH2 domain on all classes of human immunoglobulin. Its major immunomodulating effects appear to be stimulation of macrophage functions and enhancement of phagocytosis by neutrophils [3]. Tuftsin has been shown to have a variety of potential beneficial immunothera-peutic effects, including increased antibody-dependent cell-mediated cyto-toxicity (ADCC), enhancement of chemotaxis of neutrophils and monocytes, and augmentation of neutrophil and natural killer (NK) cell cytotoxicity [3]. Mice given tuftsin have been documented to have increased survival rates in multiple septic models. The clinical use of tuftsin has been disappointing, and has failed to demonstrate any immunologic response when given to trauma patients [7].

Thymosin is a hormone derived from the thymus which has a major role in the maturation process of T cells. Although its action as an immunomodulator is less than that of its analog thymopoietin, thymosin improves postburn blastogenic response when added to in vitro lymphocyte cultures [20].

Thymopoietin was originally isolated from bovine thymus extracts during research on myesthenia gravis. In vivo and in vitro studies have shown that thymopoietin stimulates the maturation of precursor T lymphocytes (pro-thymocytes), and can enhance the activation of mature T cells [3]. Although its serum half-life is only 30 s [40], the immunologic effects from a single dose remain detectable for at least 2 weeks [25].

Thymopentin (TP-5) is a pentapeptide that contains the active site of the thymopoietin molecule [3]. TP-5 has been shown to alter multiple components of the immune system including neutrophil, macrophage, and lymphocyte functions [46]. TP-5 restores diminished cell-mediated immunity [45] and increases survival of burned infected guinea pigs [38]. TP-5 has also been demonstrated to improve survival in bacterial peritonitis models [44]. When given systemically TP-5 can improve granulocyte cytotoxicity, but when tested in in vitro it impairs granulocyte cytotoxicity [43]. This probably indicates the need for an initial TP-5–T lymphocyte interaction for subsequent generation of a TP-5 granulocyte effect. Finally, TP-5 can correct impaired antibody-cell response to sheep erythrocytes in splenocytes obtained from burned guinea pigs [27].

TP-5 has documented efficacy as an immunomodulator in a number of human studies. Renal failure patients have an enhanced response to hepatitis B vaccination after TP-5 therapy [53]. TP-5 administration has been reported to reduce clinical symptoms in patients with chronic recurrent viral infections [46]. Impairments in T lymphocyte function from aging or thymectomy can be reversed with TP-5. Faist et al. found that perioperative TP-5 significantly increases cell-mediated immunity and restored lymphocyte blastogenic response in coronary artery bypass patients [12]. However, in a randomized trial of critically burned patients, TP-5 failed to alter mortality or the rate of infectious complications [47]. In that study TP-5 did reduce the incidence of silver-sulfadazine-associated leukopenia by 67%.

Indomethacin is a cyclooxygenase inhibitor which decreases production of the arachidonic acid metabolites including prostaglandin E (PGE). Indomethacin administration has been reported to increase survival [52], to increase the helper to suppressor cell ratio and to improve cell-mediated immunity in septic burned mice [50]. Addition to indomethacin to in vitro cultures of lymphocytes obtained from trauma patients reversed the posttrauma impairment of blastogenesis.

Patients undergoing major surgery have been reported to have a decreased rate of early opportunistic infections when treated with perioperative indomethacin [13]. In that study patients treated with indomethacin maintained cell-mediated immunity at preoperative levels, and had a decreased postoperative monocytosis [13]. In vitro testing showed that the indomethacin group had a higher lymphocyte proliferation capacity and an apparent protective effect for $CD3^+$, $CD4^+$, and IL-2R T cell receptors.

There are other animal data indicating that the use of cyclooxygenase inhibitors may have adverse effects in burn patients. Ibuprofen has been shown to decrease survival rates in septic burned rat models [41]. This may be due to the importance of PGE in downregulating tumor necrosis factor (TNF) production in response to endotoxin exposure [48]. It is likely that more specific antagonists of arachidonic acid metabolites other than PGE, such as thromboxane, may ultimately be found to be beneficial in burn patients.

The H_2-receptor blockers cimetidine and ranitidine have been shown to augment lymphocyte activity following burn injury [14], presumably, by blocking H_2 receptors on suppressor T lymphocytes. Murine burn studies have demonstrated an increased survival in cimetidine-treated groups given a septic challenge [52]. Pretreatment with cimetidine prevented the trauma-induced reduction in the $LY1^+/LY2^+$ ratio and decreased mortality from septic challenges [16]. Finally, treatment with low-dose (2 or 10 mg/kg per day) but not high-dose cimetidine (20 or 50 mg/kg per day) restored cell-mediated immunity following burn injury, but did not reverse suppression of mitogen-induced blastogenesis [5]. Although H_2-blockers would seem to offer reasonable immunomodulation in a clinical setting, an effective dose–response curve has not been established in man.

Levamisole is an anthelmintic agent that potentiates immune responses both in vivo and in vitro in immunocompromised hosts, but has little effect on normal hosts [3]. In vitro, levamisole increases phagocytosis by neutrophils and macrophages, increases the migration, chemokinesis, and chemotaxis of neutrophils, and may increase interferon production. Its mechanism of action is not yet clear. In a double-blind study, levamisole was able to decrease septic complications in high-risk, anergic or relatively anergic patients [28].

IL-1 is a macrophage/monocyte product with a variety of immune responses. IL-1 increases chemotaxis of monocytes and neutrophils, and augments neutrophil phagocytosis and bactericidal functions [3]. IL-1 is a potent stimulator the production of IL-2. In vitro studies in burned mice found IL-1 able to prevent early immunosuppression by restoring the ability to respond to antigen [23]. However, when administered in vivo, IL-1 inhibited antigen recognition [22].

IL-2 is produced by T lymphocytes, and is primarily associated with the T-cell proliferation and development [3]. IL-2 plays a role in the control of cytotoxicity of T cells and NK cells. IL-2 also induces the release of interferon by T cells and NK cells. Use of recombinant IL-2 in burned guinea pigs increased survival rates [4]. IL-2 has been shown in burn patients to restore lymphocyte function in vitro [4]. Finally, IL-2 increases IgM synthesis in cultures of leukocytes obtained from trauma patients [10].

In summary, immunomodulators are increasingly being tested for their ability to correct the burn-induced immunosuppression. A number of such immunomodulators have been successful in correcting the immunosuppression in multiply burned animal models and in nonburn clinical trials. However to date, none have been successful in clinical burn trials.

References

1. Alexander JW (1984) Cellular immune dysfunction in severe burns and major trauma. In: Alexander JW, Munster AM, Pruitt BA (eds) *Applied immunology: severe burns and major trauma*. Berkeley West, Berkeley, pp 2–5
2. Alexander JW, Fisher MW (1974) Immunization against *Pseudomonas* injection after thermal injury. J Infect Dis 130:S152
3. Alexander JW, Babcock FG, Waymack JP (1987) Immunotherapeutic approaches to the prevention and treatment of infection in the surgical patient. In: Howard RJ, Simmons RL (eds) *Surgical infectious diseases*. Norwalk, Appleton and Lange, pp 307–317
4. Antonacci AC, Calvano SE, Reaves LE, Prajapati A, Bockman R, Welte K, Mertelsmann R,

Gupta S, Good RA, Shires GT (1984) Autologuous and allogeneic mixed-lymphocyte responses following thermal injury in man: the immunoregulatory effects of interleukin-1, interleukin-2, and a prostaglandin inhibitor WY-18251. Clin Immunol Immunopathol 30:304–320

5. Bender EM, Hansbrough JF, Zapata-Sirvent R, Sullivan J, Claman HN (1985) Restoration of immunity in burned mice by cimetidine. J Trauma 25:131–137

6. Bender BS, Winchurch RA, Thupari JN, Proust JJ, Adler WH, Munster AM (1988) Depressed natural killer cell function in thermally injured adults: successful in vivo and in vitro immunomodulation and the role of endotoxin. Clin Exp Immunol 71:120–125

7. Carroll J, Fuks L, Catone E (1982) The effect of tuftsin on human monocyte cytotoxicity. J Biol Response Mod 1:245

8. Chiccone TG, Munster AM, Birmingham W (1983) Successful immunomodulation in burned animals and humans with homeopathic doses of polymyxin B. J Burn Care Rehabil 4:153

9. Deitch EA, Gelder F, McDonald JC (1984) Sequential prospective analysis of the nonspecific host defense system after thermal injury. Arch Surg 119:83–89

10. Ertel W, Faist E, Nestle C, Schuebel I, Storck M, Schildberg FW (1989) Dynamics of immunoglobulin synthesis after major trauma: influence of recombinant lymphokines. Arch Surg 124:1437–1442

11. Faist E, Kupper TS, Baker CC, Chaudry IH, Dwyer J, Baue AE (1986) Depression of cellular immunity after major injury. Its association with post-traumatic complications and its reversal with immunomodulation. Arch Surg 121:1000–1005

12. Faist E, Ertel W, Salmen B, Weiler A, Ressel C, Bolla K, Heberer G (1988) The immune-enhancing effect of perioperative thymopentin administration in elderly patients undergoing major surgery. Arch Surg 123:1449–1453

13. Faist E, Ertel W, Cohnert T, Huber P, Inthorn D, Heberer G (1990) Immunoprotective effects of cyclooxygenase inhibition in patients with major surgical trauma. J Trauma 30:8–17

14. Griswold DE, Alessi S, Badger AM, Poste G, Hanna N (1984) Inhibition of T suppressor cell expression by histamine type 2 (H_2) receptor antagonists. J Immunol 132:3054–3057

15. Hansbrough JF, Zapata-Sirvent R, Peterson V, Wang X, Bender E, Claman H, Boswick J (1984) Characterization of the immunosuppressive effect of burned tissue in an animal model. J Surg Res 37:383–393

16. Hansbrough JF, Zapata-Sirvent RL, Shackford SR, Hoyt D, Carter WH (1986) Immunomodulating drugs increase resistance against sepsis in traumatized mice. J Trauma 26:625–630

17. Hansbrough JF, Zapata-Sirvent RL, Peterson VM (1987) Immunomodulation following burn injury. Surg Clin North Am 67:69–92

18. Hansbrough JF, Miller LM, Field TO Jr, Gadd MA (1988) High dose intravenous immunoglobulin therapy in burn patients: pharmokinetics and effects on microbial opsonization and phagocytosis. Pediatr Infect Dis J 7:S49–S56

19. Holder IA, Naglich JG (1984) Experimental studies of the pathogenesis of infections due to *Pseudomonas aeruginosa*. Treatment with intravenous globulin. Am J Med 76:161–167

20. Ishizawa S, Sakai H, Sarles HE, Larson DL, Daniels JC (1978) Effect of thymosin on T-lymphocyte functions in patients with acute thermal burns. J Trauma 18:48–52

21. Jacobs DM, Morrison DC (1977) Inhibition of the mitogenic response to lipopolysaccharride (LPS) in mouse spleen cells by polymyxin B. J Immunol 118:21–27

22. Kupper TS, Green DR (1985) In vivo exposure to IL-1 or ETAF causes a loss of antigen presenting cell function. Br J Rheumatol 24:98–101

23. Kupper TS, Green DR, Durum SK, Baker CC (1985) Defective antigen presentation to a cloned IT helper cell by macrophages from burned mice can be restored with interleukin-I. Surgery 98:199–206

24. Lanser ME, Saba TM (1983) Correction of serum opsonic defects after burn and sepsis by opsonic fibronectin administration. Arch Surg 118:338–342

25. Lau CY, Goldstein G (1980) Functional effects of thymopoietin 32–36 (TP-5) on cytotoxic lymphocyte precursor units (CLP-U): I. Enhancement of splenic CLP-U in vitro and in vivo after suboptimal antigenic stimulation. J Immunol 124:1861–1865

26. Lundsgoard-Housen P, Doran JE, Rubli E, Papp E, Morgenthaler JJ, Spath P (1985) Purified fibronectin administration to patients with severe abdominal infections: A controlled clinical trial. Ann Surg 202:745–759

27. Maghsudi M, Miller CL (1984) The immunomodulating effect of TP-5 and indomethacin in burn-induced hypoimmunity. J Surg Res 35:133–138

28. Meakins JL, Christou NV, Shizgal HM, Macleen LD (1978) Theurapeutic approaches to anergy in surgical patients: surgery and levamisole. Ann Surg 190:285–296

29. Moran K, Munster AM (1987) Alternations of host defense mechanisms in burned patients. Surg Clin North Am 67:47–56
30. Munster AM, Hoagland HC, Pruitt BA Jr (1970) The effect of thermal injury on serum immunoglobulins. Ann Surg 172:965–969
31. Munster AM, Winchurch RA, Thupari JN, Ernst CB (1986) Reversal of postburn immunosuppression with low-dose polymyxin B. J Trauma 26:995–998
32. Munster AM, Moran KT, Thupari J, Allo M, Winchurch RA (1987) Prophylactic intravenous immunoglobulin replacement in high-risk burn patients. J Burn Care Rehabil 8:376–380
33. Munster AM, Xiao G-X, Guo Y, Wong LA, Winchurch RA (1989) Control of endotoxemia in burn patients by use of polymyxin B. J Burn Care Rehabil 10:327–330
34. Saba TM, Blumenstock FA, Shah DM, Kaplan JE, Cho E, Scovill W, Stratton H, Newell J, Gottlieb M, Sedransk N et al. (1984) Reversal of fibronectin and opsonization deficiency in patients. A controlled study. Ann Surg 199:87–96
35. Sevitt S (1979) A review of the complications of burns, their origin and importance for illness and death. J Trauma 19:358–369
36. Shirani KZ, Vaughan GM, McManus AT, Amy BW, McManus WF, Pruitt BA Jr, Mason AD Jr (1984) Replacement therapy with modified immune-globulin G in burn patients: preliminary kinetic studies. Am J Med 76:175–180
37. Stinnett JD, Alexander JW, Morris MJ, Dreffer RL, Craycraft TK, Anderson PE, Ogle CK, MacMillan BG (1981) Improved survival in severely burned animals using intravenous *Corynebacterium parvum* vaccine postinjury. Surgery 89:237–242
38. Stinnett JD, Loose L, Miskell P, Tenney CL, Gonce SJ, Alexander JW (1983) Synthetic immunomodulators for prevention of fatal infections in a burned guinea pig model. Ann Surg 198:53–57
39. Stone HH, Graber CD, Martin JD Jr, Kolb L (1965) Evaluation of gamma globulin for prophylaxis against burn sepsis. Surgery 58:810–814
40. Tischio JP, Patrick JE, Weintroub HS, Chasin M, Goldstein G (1979) Short in vitro half-life of thymopoietin (32–36) penta-peptide in human plasma. Int J Pept Protein Res 14:479–484
41. Waymack JP (1989) The effect of ibuprofen on postburn metabolic and immunologic function. J Surg Res 46:172–176
42. Waymack JP, Jenkins ME, Alexander JW, Warden GD, Miller AC, Carey M, Ogle CK, Kopcha RG (1979) A prospective trial of prophylactic intravenous immune globulin for the prevention of infections in severely burned patients. Burns 15:71–76
43. Waymack JP, Gonce S, Miskell P, Alexander JW (1984) Mechanisms of action of two new immunomudulators. Arch Surg 120:43–48
44. Waymack JP, Miskell P, Gonce S, Alexander JW (1984) Immunomodulators in the treatment of peritonitis in burned malnourished animals. Surg 96:308–314
45. Waymack JP, Metz J, Garnett D, Sax H, Alexander JW (1985) Effect of immunomodulators on macrophage function in burned animals. Surg Forum 36:110–112
46. Waymack JP, Alexander JW (1986) Immunostimulation by TP-5 in immunocompromised patients and animals—current status of investigation. Comp immunol Microbiol Infect Dis 9:225–232
47. Waymack JP, Jenkins M, Warden GD, Solomkin J, Law E Jr, Hummel R, Miller A, Alexander JW (1987) A prospective study of thymopentin in severely burned patients. Surg Gynecol Obstet 164:423–430
48. Waymack JP, Moldawer LL, Lowry SF, Guzman RF, Okerberg CV, Mason AD Jr, Pruitt BA Jr (1990) Effect of prostaglandin E in multiple experimental models. IV. Effect of resistance to endotoxin and tumor necrosis factor shock. J Surg Res 49:328–332
49. Winchurch RA, Thupari JN, Munster AM (1987) Endotoxemia in burn patients: levels of circulating endotoxins are related to burn size. Surgery 102:808–812
50. Zapata-Sirvent RL, Hansbrough JF (1985) Postburn immunosuppression in an animal model: III. Maintenance of normal splenic helper and suppressor lymphocyte subpopulations by immunomodulating drugs. Surgery 97:721–727
51. Zapata-Sirvent R, Hansbrough JF, Bartle EJ (1986) Prevention of posttraumatic alterations in lymphocyte subpopulations in mice by immunomodulating drugs. Arch Surg 121:116–122
52. Zapata-Sirvent RL, Hansbrough JF, Bender EM, Bartle EJ, Mansour A, Carter WH (1986) Postburn immunosuppression in an animal model: IV. Improved resistance to septic challenge with immunomodulating drugs. Surgery 99:53–58
53. Zaruba K, Rastorfer M, Grob PJ, Joller JH, Bolla K (1983) Thymopentin as adjuvant in nonresponders or hyporesponders to hepatitis B vaccination. Lancet 2:1245

Section 17

Endotoxin Neutralization with IV-Immunoglobulins and Monoclonal Antiendotoxin Antibodies

Antiendotoxic Therapy with Polyclonal and Polyvalent Immunoglobulins: In Vitro and In Vivo Studies

D. Berger, S. Schleich, M. Seidelmann, and H. G. Beger

Introduction

Today endotoxins or lipopolysaccharides are accepted as representing the main pathogenetic mediators of gram-negative bacteria [1]. In a variety of diseases endotoxin was found circulating in the blood stream [2–6]. Ever since the mediator principle of septic disease has been generally accepted endotoxin has been seen as the primary trigger molecule of different mediator systems, at least in gram-negative sepsis [7, 8]. Recently, some excellent studies have been published demonstrating a correlation between endotoxin plasma levels and the course of sepsis that supports this interpretation [9, 10]. Thus, from a clinical point of view an adjuvant therapy seems desirable.

One approach to neutralizing circulating endotoxin is the intravenous administration of immunoglobulins. Many clinical studies dealing with the benefit of the immunoglobulin substitution are available [11–14]. The results, however, have been quite inconsistent, so the general use of immunoglobulins cannot be recommended. Most often the inconsistency of the results is explained by insufficient doses or belated administration. Furthermore, the administration of polyclonal and polyvalent immunoglobulins seems not to be a specific therapy, because of the lack of high antibody titers against the variety of pathogens.

Because of the trigger function of endotoxin, the therapeutical use of immunoglobulins should be considered from a new point of view. More specific antiendotoxin therapy is needed, and not only sepsis therapy. Experimental data have revealed the antiendotoxic efficacy of monoclonal and monospecific antibodies [15, 16]. In clinical situations monospecificity is obviously worthless. On the other hand, monoclonal antibodies can be obtained after immunization with mutants of the lipopolysaccharide molecule lacking the O-specific chain [17]. Using this method, a cross-reactivity between different endotoxin preparations seems to be possible and has even been established in animal experiments. However, monoclonal antibodies cannot be obtained for routine clinical use. In contrast, some polyclonal and polyvalent immunoglobulin

---

* The study was supported by a grant of the Deutsche Forschungs gemeinschaft, Be 1189/2–1.
Department of General Surgery, University of Ulm, Steinhoevelstrasse 9, 7900 Ulm, FRG

Host Defense Dysfunction
in Trauma, Shock and Sepsis
Eds. Faist/Meakins/Schildberg
© Springer-Verlag, Berlin Heidelberg 1993

preparations are commercially available and recommended for sepsis therapy, and occasionally for antiendotoxin therapy, according to the manufacturers. The aim of the present study was to establish an experimental basis for antiendotoxin therapy. First of all, the influence of two pure immunoglobulin G (IgG) preparations and one IgM-enriched immunoglobulin preparation on endotoxicity was tested in the *Limulus* amebocyte lysate (LAL) test. Furthermore, the collaboration of immunoglobulins and plasma was studied in this system. In two animal models of endotoxic (and septic) shock the attempt was made to reproduce in vitro results in vivo.

Materials and Methods

The LAL was obtained from Byk-Sangtec GmbH (Dietzenbach, FRG). The endotoxin standard for setting up the standard curve was provided along with the lysate. The standard is adapted to the EC5 Standard of the US Food and Drug Administration. The chromogenic substrate was purchased from LPS (Dietzenbach, FRG). The LAL test was performed as a two-step and endpoint determination in microtiter plates (Greiner, Nürtingen, FRG). The immunoglobulin preparations were obtained from Biotest Pharma GmbH (Dreieich, FRG; IgM-enriched preparations) and Cutter Tropon (Cologne, FRG; pure IgG preparations).

The following solutions were used:

- Solution A: lysate, dissolved in pyrogen-free water, according to the recommendations of the manufacturer
- Solution B: chromogenic substrate, 10 μmol in 6.6 ml of pyrogen-free water
- Solution C: buffer, 0.5 mol/l tris/HCl, pH 9.0, 0.2 mol/l in NaCl
- Solution D: acetic acid, 20%

In order to determine the endotoxin content of aqueous solutions the following steps were performed: 50 μl of the sample was incubated with 50 μl of solution A for 25 min at 37 °C. Subsequently, 100 μl of solution B, which was diluted 1:2 with solution C, was added. A further incubation for 3 min at 37 °C was then performed. The chromogenic reaction was stopped by the addition of 200 μl of solution D. The released chromogen *p*-nitroaniline was quantified at 405 nm in a spectrophotometer (SLT, Salzburg, Austria). The endotoxin contents of unknown samples were determined according to a standard curve which was set up in parallel. The standard endotoxin concentrations were solubilized in pyrogen-free isotonic sodium chloride solution; the immunoglobulin preparations were also diluted with the same medium, according to the protein concentrations given in "Results."

In order to determine the endotoxin content of plasma samples, the incubation between solution A and sample was prolonged to 35 min at 37 °C. The further steps of the chromogenic reaction did not have to be changed. The plasma samples were inactivated by a 1:10 dilution with isotonic sodium chloride, and heated for 10 min at 75 °C before being analyzed in the LAL test.

Two animal models of endotoxic and septic shock were established, using male Wistar rats with a body weight of about 250 g. Both models were anaesthetized with ketamine hydrochloride (Ketanest), and in addition, a catheter was implanted in the common carotid artery in order to determine the mean arterial pressure. An endotoxic shock was produced by the intravenous application of neostigmine at a concentration of 0.01 mg/kg bodyweight, followed by an intravenous injection of endotoxin (*Escherichia coli* 0111:B4) at a concentration of 10 mg/kg bodyweight 5 min later. The immunoglobulin preparation was given at the same time as the endotoxin preparation; in a second series the immunoglobulin preparation was also applied 15 min after the administration of endotoxin. The model of septic shock primarily consisted in a cecal perforation. After median laparotomy a 1.5-cm incision of the caecum was made and the ascending colon was ligated 0.5 cm from the ileocecal region. Before the laparotomy a catheter was again implanted in the common carotid artery. After having closed the abdomen, the immunoglobulin preparation was given intravenously; in a second set of experiments the immunoglobulin preparation was also given 15 min after having closed the abdomen.

Results

Influence of the Immunoglobulins on Endotoxicity

For these experiments a standard curve of the LAL test was set up in a protein-free isotonic sodium chloride solution. Simultaneously, a standard curve was also set up in the presence of different concentrations of the IgM-enriched immunoglobulin preparations. Endotoxin and the immunoglobulins were incubated for 20 min at 24 °C before being introduced in the LAL test. The samples were not inactivated before being tested. Blank values were also determined from endotoxin-free samples which contained immunoglobulins at the different concentrations. These blank values were about 10%–20% higher than the protein- and endotoxin-free blank. The addition of albumin up to a concentration of 5 mg/ml produced no difference in the change of extinction compared to the standard protein-free curve.

Figure 1 shows the change of extinction on the ordinate, and the endotoxin concentration on the abscissa. Obviously, the addition of low immunoglobulin concentrations led to an enhanced change of extinction, i.e., enhanced endotoxicity in the LAL test. This increase can be seen at an immunoglobulin concentration of 0.5 and also at 1 mg/ml. At an immunoglobulin concentration of 2 mg/ml no endotoxin can be detected any more up to a concentration of 0.2 endotoxin units (EU)/ml. As shown in Fig. 2, the changes of extinction of the

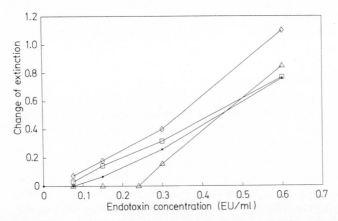

Fig. 1. Endotoxin neutralization by IgM-enriched immunoglobulins. The *ordinate* depicts the change of extinction; on the *abscissa*, the endotoxin concentration is shown in EU/ml. A standard curve was set up in a protein-free isotonic sodium chloride (NaCl) solution; furthermore, standard curves were also set up in the presence of various amounts of IgM-enriched immunoglobulin preparation. No inactivation of the samples was performed before they were tested in the LAL test. △, IgM 2 mg/ml; □, IgM 1 mg/ml; ◇, IgM 0.5 mg/ml; ■, standard curve in protein-free NaCl solution

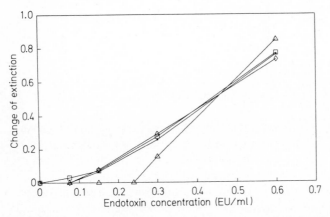

Fig. 2. Endotoxin neutralization by pure IgG immunoglobulin preparations. As in Fig. 1, except that 2 mg/ml of two pure IgG and the IgM-enriched immunoglobulin preparations were added to isotonic sodium chloride solution. □, IgG 1; ◇, IgG 2; △, IgM; ■, standard curve in protein-free Isotonic NaCl

standard curves obtained in the presence of 2 mg of pure IgG preparations do not differ from the protein-free ones.

Influence of Immunoglobulins and Plasma on Endotoxicity

In the first experiments at least, the IgM-enriched immunoglobulin preparation revealed an endotoxin-neutralizing effect at low endotoxin and high protein concentrations; on the other hand, at lower protein and higher endotoxin concentrations an enhancement of endotoxicity was observed. So a further question arose: Do endogenous plasma proteins combined with immunoglobulins have any influence on endotoxicity? In order to demonstrate or exclude such an effect, pyrogen-free, thrombocyte-poor plasma was obtained from healthy volunteers (150 IU heparin/10 ml blood). The samples were stored for a maximum of 4 weeks at –20 °C. In the following experiments a standard curve was set up in the presence of pyrogen-free plasma. The standard endotoxin concentrations were added to plasma, the samples were diluted 1:10 with isotonic sodium chloride, and, in addition, primarily pyrogen-free plasma was supplemented with endotoxin at concentrations of 0.6 and 1.2 EU/ml, simultaneously with the immunoglobulin preparations at a concentration of 2 mg/ml. After various incubation times and temperatures the samples were diluted and heat inactivated in the manner described given above and analyzed by means of the LAL test. In order to exclude an unspecific effect of plasma without exogenously added immunoglobulins, blank values were also determined, consisting of plasma samples containing endotoxin at the different concentrations without immunoglobulins and plasma samples without endotoxin but containing immunoglobulins. These blanks were incubated for the various times and temperatures before being tested. These studies showed a maximum endogenous endotoxin inactivation of 10% after 60 min at 37 °C. This endogenous activation, which was established for each incubation temperature and time point, was subtracted from the values obtained after the addition of immunoglobulins.

In Fig. 3, the time and temperature dependence of the inactivation reaction after the addition of 2 mg of the IgM-enriched immunoglobulin preparation is

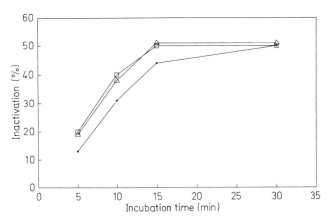

Fig. 3. Endotoxin inactivation by plasma and the IgM-enriched Ig preparation. As described in "Methods" and "Results," endotoxin was added to primarily pyrogen-free plasma at a concentration of 0.6 EU/ml, as IgM-enriched immunoglobulin preparation at a concentration of 2 mg/ml. The different incubation times are given on the *abscissa; the ordinate* shows the percent of inactivation, i.e., the reciprocal value of the endotoxin recovery. Before the samples were tested in the LAL test, they were inactivated after dilution 1:10 with isotonic sodium chloride solution by heating for 10 min at 75 °C. Different incubation temperatures were also tested. ■, 4 °C; □, 24 °C; △, 37 °C

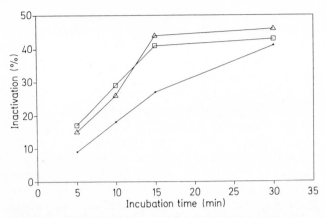

Fig. 4. Endotoxin inactivation by plasma and the IgM-enriched immunoglobulin preparation. The experimental setting is as given in Fig. 3, except that the concentration of the exogenously added endotoxin was 1.2 EU/ml

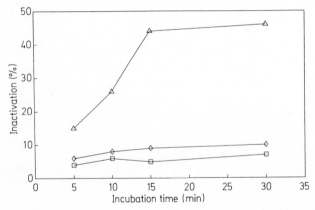

Fig. 5. Endotoxin inactivation by plasma and pure IgG immunoglobulin preparations. The effects of pure IgG immunoglobulin preparations were tested as in the experiments shown in Figs. 3 and 4. The concentration of the immunoglobulin was 2 mg/ml. Because of the lack of any temperature dependence of the inactivation reaction, only the results obtained after an incubation at 37 °C are depicted. □, IgG 1; ◇, IgG 2; △, IgM. The experiments in Figs. 1–5 were repeated eight times, and the mean values are depicted. Standard deviations are not given in order to retain clarity. The standard deviations were under 10% throughout all experiments

depicted. Obviously, after 30 min about 50%–55% of the 0.6 EU/ml in the plasma were no longer recovered. There is no striking temperature dependence of the detoxification reaction. However, after incubation temperatures of 24 °C and 37 °C, maximal inactivation is achieved after only 15 min. As shown in Fig. 4, in these experiments 1.2 EU were added to 1 ml of plasma, together with 2 mg of an IgM-enriched immunoglobulin preparation; once again the maximal inactivation is achieved after 15 min (at least incubation temperatures of 24 °C and 37 °C). After being incubated at 4 °C, the inactivation process needs more time; the maximal inactivation was observed after 30 min. The absolute value is slightly lower, as shown in Fig. 3; it amounted to about 40%–45%.

Again, the addition of the two pure IgG immunoglobulin preparations did not reveal a significant effect on the endotoxin recovery, as depicted in Fig. 5. 1.2 EU and 2 mg of the IgG preparations were added to 1 ml of plasma, and the samples were incubated at 37 °C for the times given on the abscissa. Only about 5%–10% of the endotoxin, exogenously added, was no longer recovered, i.e., inactivated. This inactivation is much lower than that obtained after the addition of the IgM-enriched immunoglobulin. We also tested various temperatures but the results after the addition of the IgG preparations are not different from those shown in Fig. 5.

Influence of the IgM-Enriched Immunoglobulin Preparation on the Arterial Hypotension in Endotoxic Shock

As described in "Methods," an endotoxic shock was produced in male Wistar rats by the intravenous administration of neostigmine at a concentration of 0.01 mg/kg body weight, followed by an intravenous injection (*E. coli* 0111:B4, 10 mg/kg body weight, 5 min later). As shown in Fig. 6, neostigmine without endotoxin was not able to change the course of the mean arterial pressure, compared with that of the control animals. After the intravenous administration of endotoxin a rapid drop of the mean arterial pressure was observed, and none of the six animals lived longer than 100 min. Administering cristalloids or colloids did not inhibit the hypotensive reaction. The addition of 50 mg of the

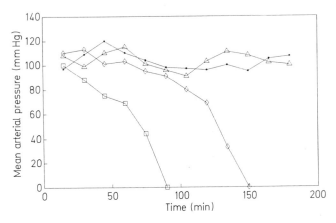

Fig. 6. Influence of the IgM-enriched immunoglobulin preparation on the endotoxin-induced hypotension. The experimental conditions are described in detail in "Methods." The *ordinate* shows the mean arterial pressure in mmHg; on the *abscissa*, the observation period in min is depicted. The experiments were completed after 180 min. Each group consisted of six animals; the median values are given. ■, sham operation; □, untreated control group; △, therapy group; ◇, delayed therapy

IgM-enriched immunoglobulin preparation per kilogram of body weight, together with endotoxin, completely inhibited the drop of the mean arterial pressure in all six animals which were tested in this assay. All the animals lived longer than the 180 min that the experiment lasted. The time course of arterial pressure did not differ from that in control animals. An important point is that endotoxin and the immunoglobulins were not incubated before being administered intravenously. The immunoglobulin preparation was given immediately after the administration of endotoxin. In a further set of experiments (again with six animals) the immunoglobulin preparation was given 15 min after endotoxin. In this system endotoxin-induced hypotension can be seen, but administration of the immunoglobulin preparation delayed the hemodynamic response. The median survival time was 130 min ($p < 0.01$), compared with the nontherapy group, Wilcoxon test). Thus in this model the hemodynamic situation can be dramatically influenced by the IgM-enriched immunoglobulin preparation.

Influence of the IgM-Enriched Immunoglobulin Preparation on Sepsis-Induced Hypotension

The details of this animal model, which primarily consists of a combination of cecal perforation and mechancial ileus, is described in detail in "Methods." As demonstrated in Fig. 7, the untreated animals developed a rapid hypotension and all animals died after 150 min. The median survival time amounted to 135 min. High-volume resuscitation with either cristalloid or colloid infusions did

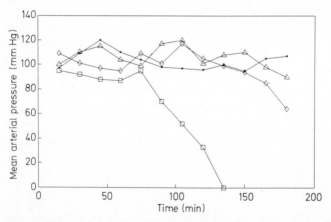

Fig. 7. Influence of the IgM-enriched immunoglobulin preparation on sepsis-induced hypotension. This experiment is also described in "Methods," and the observation period is again 180 min. Each group consisted of six animals, of which the median values are depicted. The median values correspond exactly to the arithmetic mean and the standard deviations are below 20%, so that a statistical significance could be calculated for both therapy groups, as was the case for the experiments shown in Fig. 6. ■, sham operation; □, untreated control group; △, therapy group; ◇, delayed therapy

not inhibit the fatal outcome. Sham-operated animals showed no drop in arterial pressure over 180 min. The same holds for those animals treated with 50 mg IgM-enriched immunoglobulin preparation given immediately after the closure of the laparotomy. Even giving immunoglobulins 15 min after the onset of peritonitis drastically delayed the beginning of the hemodynamic reaction. In neither of the groups treated did an animal die during the 180 min, and only in the delayed therapy group was a small drop in arterial pressure observed at the end of the observation period; however, no statistical significance could be ascertained.

Discussion

As outlined in the "Introduction," endotoxins play an important role in the pathogenesis of gram-negative sepsis. The present study was undertaken in order to clarify possible antiendotoxic properties of different commercially available immunoglobulin preparations suitable for intravenous use. The IgM-enriched immunoglobulin preparation obviously enhances endotoxicity in the absence of any other proteins, at least at high endotoxin concentrations. We would like to explain this effect in terms of a disaggregating capacity. Endotoxins are known to form large complexes in aqueous solutions [18]. Probably the IgM fraction interacts with these complexes; this leads to a disaggregation followed by an increase in the change of extinction compared to the protein-free standard curve in Fig. 1. Using monoclonal antibodies (MAB), Sagawa et al. demonstrated a change of the sedimentation behavior after incubation of lipopolysaccharide (LPS) with MAB, according to their specific epitopes [19]. These authors postulated that an interaction of antibodies with the natural micellic structure is a prerequisite for rapid clearance of the complexes. Our simple experiments, in which immunoglobulin and endotoxins were incubated in an isotonic sodium chloride solution, support this view. A similar pattern, namely, the enhancement of endotoxicity, was recently described for transferrin, a major endotoxin-binding protein of human plasma [20]. The relatively small amount of neutralized endotoxin at higher IgM concentrations could be explained by a small amount of specific antibodies. However, the more probable explanation is a further unspecific interaction between IgM and endotoxin, which is primarily disaggregated, leading to a masking of the LAL-stimulating region of the LPS molecule. Pure IgG preparations did not exhibit any effect on endotoxicity in this assay. Also, since the amount of detoxified endotoxin was quite low after the addition of IgG to plasma, a significant interaction between endotoxin and these immunoglobulin preparations seems to be ruled out.

On the other hand, endotoxin is actually detoxified by plasma which is supplemented with 2 mg of the IgM-enriched immunoglobulin preparation per milliliter. Combined with the former experiments this should lead one to postulate that the endotoxin detoxification process takes place as a multistep procedure, as Ulevitch proposed some years ago [21]. At first the endotoxin complexes have to be destroyed or disaggregated; this is followed by a possibly more specific binding to other plasma proteins which mask the pathogenic region of the LPS. So, after incubation of endotoxin and plasma supplemented with IgM a real inactivation was observed, although the pure effect of the immunoglobulins is the opposite one.

The fact that only the IgM-enriched immunoglobulin preparation exhibits an interaction with endotoxin seems to be astonishing. However, it should be taken into account that in previous studies also demonstrating the antiendo-toxic property of IgG, usually hyperimmune globulin or even monospecific and monoclonal antibodies were used [15, 16, 22, 23]. Unfortunately, the efficacy of these immunoglobulin preparations was restricted by the endotoxin preparation used for immunization. On the other hand, IgG was obtained after immunization with endotoxins lacking the O-specific chain [17]. The antibodies were believed to be cross-reactive with various endotoxins from various bacterial strains because of the more conservative core structure of LPS molecule [24] compared to the O-specific chain. Some years ago, however, it was demonstrated that antibodies against lipid A did not cross-react with the intact LPS molecule [25]. These studies were recently confirmed by Pollack et al. in a very elegant manner [26], showing that there is almost no cross-reaction between antibodies directed to the core or lipid A region of endotoxin and the whole LPS molecule. Thus, the demonstrated interaction in our experiments between endotoxin and IgM also seems to be an unspecific one.

Teng et al. [27] produced monoclonal antibodies against endotoxin of E. coli J5. This antibody preparation consisting of pure IgM also exhibits strong antiendotoxic properties in vivo, as confirmed by various endotoxin preparations. McCabe et al. [28] used polyclonal antibodies and endotoxin of E. coli J5 and found that only the IgM fraction is protective in vivo. The IgG fraction did not exhibit any significant effect. In both studies the effects of the immunoglobulins are not restricted to that endotoxin which was used as the primary antigen. In contrast with our study, only the IgM-enriched preparation was able to interact with endotoxin. In a recently published study Shimatsoto et al. demonstrated the inhibition of endotoxin-induced tumor necrosis factor release in murine monocytes [29] by a commercially available IgG preparation. However, they also showed that this inhibition was caused by a direct effect of the immunoglobulins on monocytes and not by an interaction between the immunoglobulins and endotoxin. For this reason, an antiendotoxic therapy is not possible with pure IgG preparations.

In contrast to this, the previously cited studies, together with the demonstrated results obtained in the LAL test, indicate that IgM is able to interact with endotoxin. Even though this interaction is unspecific, this unspecific interaction is also important in vivo. The endotoxin-induced hypotension can be inhibited by the IgM-enriched immunoglobulin preparation, at least when endotoxin and immunoglobulins are given simultaneously. Even after delayed administration of immunoglobulins a significant effect of survival time and onset of hypotension was obvious. The studies by Teng et al. and McCabe et al. [27, 28] had already shown a similar effect. Even in the model of septic shock where an early and dramatic drop in arterial pressure is characteristic, the benefit of immunoglobulin therapy could be demonstrated. These in vivo results lead to the conclusion that the effect of IgM on endotoxicity is not only restricted to in vitro conditions.

In summary, the data presented should rule out the adjuvant therapy of gram-negative sepsis with pure IgG preparations because of the lack of any interaction with endotoxin. The therapeutic use of IgM-enriched immunoglobulin preparations is favored. Our results should justify the clinical use of IgM during endotoxemia, at least in clinical trials. However, it should be taken into account that it has been necessary to begin therapy before the deleterious effects of the activated mediator cascades are fully developed. Otherwise, in these prognostically poor cases, the use of IgM might inactivate circulating endotoxin, but irreversible multiple organ failure would nevertheless lead to death. If these preconditions are considered, clinical studies should also reveal the benefit of the immunoglobulin therapy of gram-negative sepsis.

Acknowledgements. These results were presented in part at the fifth European Congress of Intensive Care Medicine, Amsterdam, The Netherlands, 5–8 June 1990, and have won the Young investigator's award for D. Berger.

References

1. Brade H, Brade L, Schade U, Zähringer U, Holst O, Kuhn HM, Rozalski A, Röhrscheidt E, Rietschel E (1988) Structure, endotoxicity, immunogenicity, and antigenicity of bacterial lipopolysaccharides (endotoxins, O-antigens). In: Levin J, Büller HR, ten Cate JW, van Deventer SJH, Struck A (eds) Bacterial endotoxins. Pathophysiological effects, clinical significance and pharmacological control, New York, pp 17–45
2. Aoki K (1978) A study of endotoxemia in ulcerative colitis and Crohn's disease: II. An experimental study. Acta Med Okayama 32:207–216
3. Beger HG, Gögler H, Kraas E, Bittner R (1981) Endotoxin bei bakterieller Peritonitis. Chirurg 52:81–88
4. Klein K, Fuchs GJ, Kulapongs P, Mertz G, Suskind RM, Olsen RE (1988) Endotoxemia in protein-energy malnutrition. J Pediatr Gastroenterol Nutr 7:225–228
5. Rocke DA, Gaffin SL, Wells MT, Koen Y, Brock-Utine JG (1987) Endotoxemia associated with cardiopulmonary bypass. J Thorac Cardiovasc Surg 93:832–837
6. Rudbach JA, Johnson AG (1964) Restoration of endotoxin activity following alteration by plasma. Nature 202:811–812
7. Schottmüller H (1914) Wesen und Behandlung der Sepsis. Verh Dtsch Ges Inn Med 31:257–280
8. Neugebauer E, Lorenz W, Schirren J, Dietrich A (1989) Mediators in the pathogenesis of septic shock-state of the art. In: Reinhart K, Eyrich K (eds) Sepsis—an interdisciplinary challenge. Springer, Berlin Heidelberg New York, pp 205–215
9. Pearson FC, Dubczak J, Weary M, Bruszer G, Donohue G (1985) Detection of endotoxin in plasma of patients with gram-negative bacterial sepsis by the limulus amebocyte lysate test. J Clin Microbiol 21:865–868
10. van Deventer SJ, ten Cate JW, Tytgat GN (1988) Intestinal endotoxemia. Clinical significance. Gastroenterology 94:825–831.

11. Grundmann R, Hornung M (1988) Immunoglobulin therapy in patients with endotoxemia and postoperative sepsis—a prospective randomized study. Prog Clin Biol Res 272:339–349
12. Calandra TH, Glauser MP, Schellekens J, Verhoeff J (1988) Treatment of gram-negative septic shock with human IgG antibody to escherichia coli J5: a prospective, double-blind, randomized study. J Infect Dis 158:312–319
13. Ziegler EJ, McCutchan JA, Fierer J, Glauser MP, Sadoff JC, Douglas H, Braude AI (1982) Treatment of gram-negative bacteremia and shock with human antiserum to a mutant *Escherichia coli*. N Engl J Med 307:1225–1230
14. Jesdinsky HJ, Tempel G, Castrup HJ, Seifert J (1987) Cooperative group of additional immunoglobulin therapy in severe bacterial infections: results of a multicentre randomized controlled trial in fibrinopurulent peritonitis. Klin Wochenschr 65:1132–1138
15. Salles MF, Mandine E, Zalisz R, Guenounou M, Smets P (1989) Protective effects of murine monoclonal antibodies in experimental septicemia: *E. coli* antibodies protect against different serotypes of *E. coli*. J Infect Dis 159:641–647
16. Shnyra AA, Kalantarov GF, Vlasik TN, Trakht IN, Majatnikov A Ju, Tabachnik AL, Borovikov DV, Golubykh VL (1990) Monoclonal antibody to lipid A prevents the development of haemodynamic disorders in endotoxemia. Adv Exp Med Biol 256:681–684
17. Kaijser B, Ahlstedt S (1977) Protective capacity of antibodies against *Escherichia coli* O and K antigens. Infect Immun 17:286–289
18. Galanos C, Lüderitz O (1975) Electrodialysis of lipopolysaccharides and their conversion to uniform salt forms. Eur J Biochem 54:603–610
19. Sagawa T, Abe Y, Kimura S, Hitsumoto Y, Utsumi S (1989) Mechanisms of neutralization of endotoxin by monoclonal antibodies to lipopolysaccharide. In: Faist E, Ninnemann J, Green D (eds) Immune consequences of trauma, shock and sepsis. Mechanisms and therapeutic approaches. Berlin Heidelberg New York, pp 495–500
20. Berger D, Winter M, Beger HG (1990) Influence of human transferrin and group-specific protein on endotoxicity in vivo. Clin Chim Acta 189:1–6
21. Ulevitch RJ, Johnston AR, Weinstein DB (1981) New function for high density lipopolysaccharides. Isolation and characterization of a bacterial lipopolysaccharide-high density lipoprotein complex formed in rabbit plasma. J Clin Invest 67:827–837
22. Nelles MJ, Niswander CA (1984) Mouse monoclonal antibodies reactive with 35 lipopolysaccharide exhibit extensive serological cross-reactivity with a variety of gram-negative bacteria. Infect Immun 46:677–681
23. Dunn DL, Ewald DC, Chandan N, Cerra FB (1986) Immunotherapy of gram-negative bacterial sepsis. A single murine monoclonal antibody provides cross-genera protection. Arch Surg 121:58–62
24. Galanos C, Lüderitz O, Rietschel E Th, Westphal O (1977) Newer aspects of the chemistry and biology of bacterial lipopolysaccharides, with special reference to their lipid A component. In: Goodwin TW (ed) International review of biochemistry. Biochemistry of lipids II, vol 14. University Park Press, Baltimore, pp 239–335
25. Nolan JP, Vladutiu AO, Moreno DM, Cohen SA, Camara DS (1982) Immunoradiometric assay of lipid A: a test for detecting and quantitating endotoxins of various origins. J Immunol Methods 55:63–72
26. Pollack M, Chia JKS, Koles NL, Miller M, Guelde G (1989) Specificity and cross-reactivity of monoclonal antibodies reactive with the core and lipid A regions of bacterial lipololysaccharides. J Infect Dis 159:168–188
27. Teng NNH, Kaplan HS, Hebert JM, Moore C, Douglas H, Wunderlich A, Braude I (1985) Protection against gram-negative bacteremia and endotoxemia with human monoclonal IgM antibodies. Proc Natl Acad Sci USA 82:1790–1794
28. McCabe WR, DeMaria A, Berberich H, Johns MA (1988) Immunization with rough mutants of Salmonella minnesota: protective activity of IgM and IgG antibody to the R595 (Re chemotype) mutant. J Infect Dis 158:291–300
29. Shimozato T, Iwata M, Tamura N (1990) Suppression of tumor necrosis factor alpha production by a human immunoglobulin preparation for intravenous use. Infect Immun 58:1384–1390

The Use of Polyvalent Immunoglobulin G in Patients with Sepsis and Multiple Organ Failure

G. Pilz and K. Werdan

Among critically ill patients admitted to intensive care units, septic multiple organ failure (MOF) and shock are major causes of death, with fatality rates in the case of septic shock in the range of 40%–90% [24]. This unvaryingly high sepsis mortality, despite advances in antibiotic treatment, provides the rationale for the investigation of supplementary sepsis treatment regimens as an attempt to improve the poor outcome of septic patients.

Rationales for Supplemental Sepsis Treatment Using Immunoglobulins

One therapeutic approach—in addition to antibiotics and supportive management of MOF—is the administration of immunoglobulins (Ig) to provide the patient with higher titers of antibodies against bacterial endo- and exotoxins and/or with opsonic activity [5, 10, 16, 30]. Furthermore, Ig can synergize with β-lactam antibiotics, owing to their content of antilactamase antibodies [7] and to their ability to sensitize gramnegative bacteria by disorganizing their outer membranes [8]. In vitro results [23, 34] as well as animal experiments [6, 16, 25] have shown the protective effect of intravenous Ig preparations against various infections. The results of clinical studies, however, do not yet allow firm conclusions regarding the effectiveness of Ig treatment in sepsis [1, 35].

Results of Controlled Clinical Trials with Intravenous Ig in Patients with Sepsis and MOF

Within the last decade, several placebo-controlled clinical trials have studied the role of supplementary Ig therapy in intensive care patients. These trials enrolled between 24 and 329 patients with a dosage range of 0.6–1.6 g Ig/kg body weight, divided into at least two doses on consecutive days. With these Ig dosages, a significant increase in at least IgG levels can be achieved, lasting for several

Department of Medicine I, Grosshadern University Hospital, University of Munich, Marchioninistrasse 15, 8000 Munich 70, FRG

Host Defense Dysfunction
in Trauma, Shock and Sepsis
Eds. Faist/Meakins/Schildberg
© Springer-Verlag, Berlin Heidelberg 1993

Table 1. Supplementary immunoglobulin therapy and prophylaxis in sepsis: mortality rates in placebo-controlled clinical trials

Patients	n	Immuno-globulin	Verum n	%	Mortality Placebo n	%	Significance	References
Polytrauma	150	IgG P	23/76	30	15/74	20	NS	Glinz et al. (1985) [14]
Intensive care	104	IgGMA T	22/50	44	22/54	41	NS	Just et al. (1986) [18]
Purulent peritonitis	288	IgG, IgGMA T	66/145	46	58/143	41	NS	Jesdinsky et al. (1987) [17]
Severe sepsis	24	IgG T	7/12	58	9/12	75	NS	De Simone et al. (1988) [9]
Severe sepsis	50	IgGMA T	6/25	24	11/25	44		Vogel (1988)[a] [33]
Medical/surgical	54	IgGMA T	5/27	19	18/27	67	$p < 0.01$	Schedel (1988)[a] [31]
Burn injury	60	P-IgG P	9/30	30	9/30	30	NS	Stuttmann et al. (1989) [32]
Severe trauma or major surgery	40	IgG P	2/15	13	4/17	24	NS	Mao et al. (1989) [22]
Pseudomonas pneumonia	45	P-IgG T	0/25	0	3/20	15	NS	Class and Schjaorer (1989) [4]
Intensive care	97	IgG P	3/49	6	5/48	10	NS	Lehmkuhl and Pichlmayr (1991) [20]
Abdominal surgery	220	IgG P	15/108	14	22/112	20	NS	Baumgartner (1991) [2]
Surgical (sepsis score ≥ 20)	62	IgG T	11/29	38	22/33	67	$p < 0.05$	Dominioni et al. (1991) [11]

IgG Immunoglobulin G; IgGMA, Immunoglobulin GMA; PIgG *Pseudomonas* immunoglobulin G; T, Therapy; P, Prophylaxis.

[a] Abstract/preliminary report.

[b] 8 patients omitted due to early (48 h) death (verum 5; placebo 3).

days [11]. So far, 5S and 7S Ig, IgG, and IgGMA preparations as well as *Pseudomonas* Ig have come into use (see Table 1). Beneficial effects of Ig treatment were documented with respect to: (1) a reduction in the number of local infections in surgical patients (prophylactic measure; $n = 150$ [12]); (2) a lowered rate of pneumonia in polytraumatized patients (prophylactic measure; $n = 150$ [14]); (3) a reduction in time of mechanical ventilation and of treatment in the intensive care unit in patients with infectious complications after surgery, trauma, or intoxication ($n = 104$ [18]); (4) a lowering of the occurrence of infections in patients after severe abdominal operations (prophylaxis; $n = 329$ [2]); (5) a depression of fever, elevation of complement fractions C3 and C4, less positive blood cultures, and less clinically overt sepsis in patients with severe trauma or surgery (prophylaxis; $n = 40$ [22]).

However, with regard to the unequivocal endpoint of all sepsis treatment trials—the reduction in mortality—the results of the presently available trials are in most cases disappointing (Table 1). Excluding two preliminary reports where complete data are not yet available [31, 33], only one study [11] with 62 surgical patients has demonstrated a reduction in mortality from 67% to 38% with supplementary IgG (Table 1). The inclusion criterion in this trial was a sepsis score of 20 or greater, showing the severity of postoperative sepsis in these patients, mainly after abdominal surgery. In all other studies listed in Table 1, no benefit regarding prognosis could be demonstrated, either with IgG or Ig GMA, given either prophylactically in surgical and medical patients at high risk for sepsis or therapeutically in cases of assumed or proven sepsis.

Reflecting on these disappointing trial data, one must keep in mind that "the results of the presently available trials are subject to criticism owing to problems in study designs, such as nonblinded evaluation of outcome, weak micro-biological documentation of infections, analysis of the results in subgroups made 'a posteriori,' or unreported death rates" [1]. To document a reduction in mortality by 1/3 with a therapeutic measure, about 800 patients must be included in a placebo-controlled trial, assuming a mortality in the placebo group of 30% [21]. Taking into account these data, representative of sepsis mortality (Table 1), no controlled trial has yet been published which ultimately proves or disproves a beneficial effect of intravenous polyvalent Ig as supplementary treatment in sepsis and MOF.

Criteria for "Response to Therapy" in Patients with Sepsis and MOF Treated with Supplementary IgG

Rationale for an Observational Study

Besides placebo-controlled treatment trials—the "gold standard" approach—some information can also be gained from observational studies, documenting the effects seen in close time relationship with supplementary Ig treatment in septic patients. The following questions, answers to which might be useful in subsequent controlled randomized studies, can be addressed: (1) Can any beneficial effects be recorded during treatment, and what is the maximum achievable response? (2) Are there any differences between patient groups that should lead to inclusion or exclusion of subgroups in future studies? (3) What is the impact of baseline sepsis and MOF severity on the response to treatment? (4) Which organ systems show an improvement and should particularly be monitored further? (5) Can any "responses criterion" be defined, in close time relationship to the Ig treatment, which is correlated with a higher probability of survival?

Supplementary Intravenous IgG Treatment in 163 Patients with Sepsis and Septic Shock: An Observational Study as a Prerequisite for a Placebo-Controlled Clinical Trial [27]

163 intensive care unit patients with a total of 173 septic episodes treated with IgG were enrolled in an observational study in 18 hospitals/departments from 1988 to 1990 (for contributors see Appendix). The entry criteria were as follows: (1) clinical suspicion of sepsis or septic shock; (2) deterioration or failure to improve of the patients's condition despite antibiotic therapy, leading to additional treatment with IgG based on clinical judgement. There was no restriction regarding the antibiotic regimen or intensive care supportive measures such as ventilation, parenteral nutrition, volume replacement, and vasopressor use.

Patients' data are given in Table 2. There a high percentage of overt septic shock and respiratory failure requiring artificial ventilation. Positive blood cultures were obtained in 28%, 2/3 having gram-negative and 1/3 gram-positive bacteria. Quantitative evaluation using the sepsis score of Elebute and Stoner [13] documented the septic state, the mean score of 19. 89% of all patients had at least 12 points, a value validated in surgical patients as being strongly suggestive of a septic state [15]. Disease severity with regard to MOF was characterized by the APACHE II score [19] with a mean value of 24. In a subgroup of 66 patients, complete hemodynamic monitoring data were available (Table 3), demonstrating a hyperdynamic shock state with vasodilation, severely decreased systemic vascular resistance (SVR), hypercirculation, a high cardiac index (CI). Myocardial depression was documented by a reduced left ventricular stroke work index (LVSWI). All patients were sufficiently volume treated (mean right atrial pressure 13 mm Hg).

Deterioration of the clinical course despite adequate antibiotic therapy prompted supplementary treatment with intravenous IgG on two consecutive days. In the case of *Pseudomonas* sepsis (*n* = 50 septic episodes), a *Pseudomonas* IgG (Psomaglobin) was given, 8 ml/kg body weight on day 0 and 4 ml/kg body weight on day 1. In all other cases (*n* = 123 septic episodes), a polyvalent IgG (Polyglobin N) was given, 12 ml/kg body weight on day 0 and 6 ml/kg body

Table 2. Supplementary intravenous immunoglobulin G treatment in 163 patients with sepsis and septic shock: characteristics of the observational study population [27]

Patients (*n*)	163
Treatment episodes (1)	173
Medical (%)	30
Surgical (%)	70
Age (years)	49.7
Sex (female/male)	25%/75%
Mortality (%)	41
Septic shock (%)	68
Respiratory failure (artificial ventilation) (%)	83
White blood cell count > 12 or < 3.5 g/l (%)	69
Thrombopenia < 100 g/l (%)	36
Positive blood culture (%)	28
Elebute sepsis score[a]	19 ± 1
Patients with Elebute score > 12 (%)	89
APACHE II score[a]	24 ± 1

[a]Mean ± SEM

Table 3. Supplementary intravenous immunoglobulin G Treatment in patients with sepsis and septic shock: baseline hemodynamics ($n = 66$) [27]

Systemic vascular resistance (SVR) (DYN CM^{-5} S)	571 ± 23
Cardiac index (CI) (L/MIN M^2 BSA)	4.7 ± 0.2
Left ventricular stroke work index (LVSWI) (G × M/M^2 BSA)	40 ± 2
Right atrial pressure (mmHg)	13 ± 1

Mean ± SEM

weight on day 1. No serious side effects attributable to the Ig treatment were observed. Antibiotic treatment was continued unchanged in the majority of the cases.

The deterioration of the patients' courses prior to the onset of Ig therapy (day − 1 to 0) was evident in both a further SVR decrease and APACHE II score increase (MOF disease severity; Fig. 1). After starting Ig therapy on day 0, a marked rise in the low SVR was observed in about half of the patients. In these "hemodynamic responders," a concurrent fall in the APACHE II score values occurred, indicating MOF improvement. The other half of the patients—the "nonresponders"—did not improve, either in vascular or dysfunction or in MOF (Fig. 1).

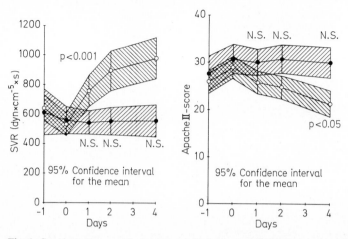

Fig. 1. Supplementary sepsis treatment with immunoglobulin (intravenous IgG) and intravenous *Pseudomonas* IgG) on day 0 and day 1: "Responders" (○) and "Non-responders" (○) with respect to changes in systemic vascular resistance (SVR) and APACHE II score. Data are for patients treated at Department of Medicine I, Grosshadern University Hospital, Munich (see Appendix)

Based on these results, "responder criteria" have been determined, demonstrating improvement of either MOF severity (decrease of APACHE II score of at least 4 points from day 0 to day 4) or the cardiovascular impairment (increase in SVR of at least 160 units lasting longer than 24 h [26].

The APACHE II score responder criterion was also applied to the total of 173 septic episodes in the observational study of intravenous IgG [27] in septic patients (Fig. 2, right): similarly to in the hemodynamically monitored subgroup shown in Fig. 1, in the whole study group about half of the patients (44% of all septic episodes) improved in MOF in a close time relationship to the Ig therapy (fall in APACHE II score of at least 4 points on day 4; Fig. 2, right). The prognosis of these "responders" was significantly better than of the non-responders: mortality rates were 24% vs 55% (Table 4).

This APACHE II score responder criterion was applicable (Table 2) in all patient subgroups: medical as well as surgical patients with non-*Pseudomonas* vs *Pseudomonas* sepsis [28], patients with a higher or lower degree of MOF (APACHE II ≥ 24 vs < 24), and patients with either positive or negative blood cultures. In all subgroups tested, the mortality rate was only about half as high in responders as in nonresponders (Table 4).

One might argue that this fall in APACHE II score in close time relationship with Ig treatment solely reflects the natural course of the disease, without any linkage to the Ig treatment. This argument, of course, cannot be ruled out. However, the response rate after starting supplementary Ig therapy was 30% higher than the response rate after initiating antibiotic treatment in another study population with comparable severity of disease (Fig. 2). Thus, the decrease in APACHE II score in the Ig-treated responders is consistent with an improve-

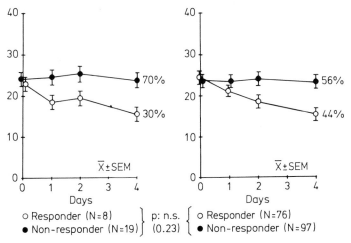

Fig. 2. APACHE II score response to new onset sepsis treatment. *Left*, After initiating antibiotic treatment, APACHE II scoring (*ordinate*) was monitored in 27 patients with sepsis and MOF for the next 4 days. 30% of the patients fulfilled the APACHE II score "responder criterion" (see text). *Right*, APACHE II scoring in 163 septic patients with 173 septic episodes, supplementally treated with IgG (day 0 and 1) and *Pseundomonas* IgG (days 0 and 1) [27]. Antibiotic treatment was continued; the mean period since the onset of or last substantial change in the antibiotic regimen was 2.6 ± 0.3 days. In 44% of all episodes, the APACHE II score responders criterion (see text) was fulfilled

Table 4. Supplementary intravenous immunoglobulin G treatment in 163 patients with sepsis and septic shock: subgroup analysis [27]

| | *n* | Response rate % | Mortality (%) | | |
			Responders	Non responders	*p*
Total	163	44	24	55	0.0001
i.v. IgG	123	42	25	59	0.0003
Pseudomonas gG	50	48	21	42	n.s.
Medicial patients	52	44	35	59	n.s.
Surgical patients	121	44	19	53	0.003
With septic shock	118	42	26	62	0.003
Without septic shock	55	47	19	38	n.s.
Severe MOF (APACHE II $\geq$ 24)	85	44	38	69	0.009
Moderate MOF (APACHE II $<$ 24)	88	44	10	41	0.003
Positive blood cultures	48	52	16	61	0.004
Negative blood cultures	125	41	27	53	0.009

Responder, decrease in APACHE II score of at least 4 points from day 0 to day 4; MOF; the multiple organ failure. n.s., not significant ($p \geq 0.05$). In the case of Total *n* reflects the number of patients; in all other cases, *n* reflects septic episodes

Table 5. Supplementary intravenous immunoglobulin G Treatment in patients with sepsis and septic shock: "organ response" in responders [27]

	Day 0	Day 4
Cardiovascular function		
Mean arterial pressure (mmHg)	74	86*
Heart rate (min^{-1})	121	101*
Vasopressor requirement	3.1	2.1*
CNS function		
Glasgow coma score	7.9	10.4*
Respiratory function		
FIO$_2$	0.48	0.35*
AaDO$_2$ (mmHg)	191	96*
Body temperature ($^\circ$C)	39.1	38.0*
Hematology/hemostaseology		$\varnothing$
Liver function		$\varnothing$
Renal function		$\varnothing$

In all patients with a decrease in APACHE II score of at least 4 from day 0 (Ig therapy day 0 and 1) to day 4 ("responders"), changes in clinical and laboratory parameters have been calculated for day 0 and day 4. For further details see [27].
$\varnothing$, No significant changes encountered.
*$p < 0.05$, change between days 0 and 4.

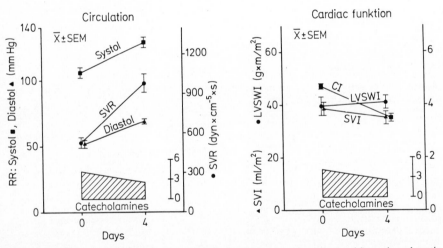

Fig. 3. Supplementary intravenous immunoglobulin G treatment in patients with sepsis and septic shock: effect on cardiovascular parameters in "responders" ($n = 22$) (same study population as described in the legend of Fig. 1). SVR, systemic vascular resistance; SVI, stroke volume index; LVSWI, left ventricular stroke work index; CI, cardiac index

ment in MOF during the acute treatment period; this could be documented for cardiovascular, cerebral, and respiratory function (Table 5). In contrast, no significant change in any of the variables tested could be found in the non-responder group. Regarding cardiovascular improvement in the responder patients, there was a recovery only in the vascular tone (increase in SVR; Fig. 3), while myocardial depression was not improved by the Ig treatment (no significant increase of the low LVSWI; Fig. 3).

Pretreatment analysis of a variety of patient parameters presently does not allow identification of subsequent treatment responders and nonresponders [27].

Conclusions

Evaluation of every sepsis therapy is hampered by the complexitiy of the clinical picture of sepsis and the sepsis syndrome [3]. In our opinion, acute changes in the promptly available APACHE II score during treatment reflect, and may even quantitate, the immediate response to sepsis therapy [26, 29]. Scoring systems validated for either sepsis or MOF severity may also serve as inclusion criteria for placebo-controlled treatment trials, since they allow quantification of the optimal range of the determinants of an adequate study design, depending on (1) overall mortality, (2) response rate to therapy, and (3) reduction of mortality in responders [27].

The observational study described has markedly influenced a placebo-controlled IgG trial, meanwhile started in patients with sepsis (planned enrollment of 800 patients); (1) according to the response rates, all patient subgroups tested (Table 4) should benefit equally from the Ig treatment and therefore should be included into the study; (2) with score-based inclusion criteria (APACHE II score 20–35; Elebute sepsis score 12–27), we attempt optimize the study design determinants with respect to a maximum benefit (response and mortality reduction in responders [27].

Is it still worthwhile to plan and carry out a placebo-controlled trial with Ig, after the recent publication of the excellent results in sepsis treatment described with the monoclonal endotoxin antibody HA-1A [36]? In our opinion it still is, since the significant reduction in mortality by HA-1A was achieved only in a subgroup of 37% of all patients, namely in those with culture proven gram-negative bacteremia. However, regarding the total population of septic patients included in this trial, no significant reduction in mortality has been observed [36].

In the case of polyvalent Ig, the data published so far neither prove nor disprove the assumption that Ig may improve prognosis in septic patients, because of the relatively small population sizes as well the already mentioned problems encountered with study designs. Therefore, according to Baumgartner [1], "additional data from well designed studies are needed to investigate the cost-effectiveness of prophylactic or therapeutic IVIG administration to critically ill patients." The results obtained in the observational study presented may be helpful in this respect.

Appendix: List of Contributors

Drs. E. Reuschel-Janetschek, R. Hettich, R. Haberl, U. Nattermann, and G. Pilz, Dept. of Medicine I, Grosshadern University Hospital, Munich (56 IgG treatment cases [IgG], 22 controls [c]); Dr. G. Neeser, Dept. of Anesthesiology, Central Hospital, Augsburg (44 IgG); Dr. I. Class, Dept. of Anaesthesiology, Marienhospital, Stuttgart (18 IgG, 5 C); Prof. Dr. U. Schweigart, Drs. M. Drescher and R.-R. Fink, Dept. of Medicine II, Technical University Hospital, Munich (10 IgG); Dr. A. Brähler, Dept. of Anesthesiology, St.-Marien-Hospital, Siegen (10 IgG); Dr. J. Cremer, Dept. of Thoracic Surgery, University Hospital, Hanover (6 IgG); Drs. E. Müller and M. Knoch, Dept. of Anesthesiology, University Hospital, Marburg (6 IgG); Dr. H. Prießnitz, Dept. of Anesthesiology, Siloah Hospital, Hanover (4 IgG); Drs. T. Haferlach and M. Appelt, Dept. of Medicine II, University Hospital, Kiel (4 IgG); Dr. L. Dvorak-Lansloot, Dept. of Surgery, Nordstadt Hospital, Hanover (3 IgG); Dr. H. Meyer, Dept. of Surgery, Oststadt Hospital, Hanover (3 IgG); Dr. R. Brobeil, Dept. of Surgery, County Hospital, Lahr (2 IgG); Dr. K. Weber-Fink, Dept. of Anesthesiology, City Hospital, Landshut (2 IgG); Dr. M. Arning, Dept. of Oncology, University Hospital, Düsseldorf (1 IgG); Dr. N. Ernst, Dept. of Medicine I, Hospital Bad Oeynhausen (1 IgG); Dr. U. Knorr, Dept. of Medicine, City Hospital, Landshut (1 IgG); Dr. U. Weiß, Dept. of Anesthesiology, University Hospital, Hanover (1 IgG); Dr. K. Zwack, Dept. of Medicine III, Central Hospital, Augsburg (1 IgG); all in Germany.

References

1. Baumgartner JD (1990) Arguments for the administration of immunoglobulins in critically-ill patients. In: Peter K, Lawin P, Bein T, Briegel J (eds) Intensivmedizin, vol 76. Thieme, Stuttgart, pp 152–157
2. Baumgartner JD (1991) Prophylactic study of standard intravenous immunoglobulin and core LPS immunoglobulin in high-risk post surgical patients. Abstract SY 81 2nd International congress on the immune consequences of trauma, shock and sepsis—mechanisms and therapeutic approaches, Munich, 6–9 March. Demeter Gräfelfing, p 26
3. Bone RC, Fisher CJ, Clemmer TP, Slotman GJ, Metz CA, Balk RA, and the Methylprednisolone Severe Sepsis Study Group (1989) Sepsis syndrome: a valid clinical entity. Crit Care Med 17:389–393
4. Class I, Schorer R (1989) Adjuvant therapy with Pseudomonas hyperimmune globulin. Anasth Intensivther Notfallmed 24:167–171
5. Collins MS, Roby RE (1984) Protective activity of an intravenous immune globulin (human) enriched in antibody against lipopolysaccharide antigens of Pseudomonas aeruginosa. Am J Med 76, Suppl 3A:168–174
6. Collins MS, Hector RF, Roby RE, Edwards AA, Ladehoff DK, Dorsey JH (1987) Prophylaxis of Gram-negative and Gram-positive infections in rodents with three intravenous immunoglobulins and therapy of experimental polymicrobial burn wound sepsis with Pseudomonas immunoglobulin and Ciprofloxacin. Infection 15:60–68
7. Dalhoff A (1984) Synergy between acylureidopenicillins and immunoglobulin G in experimental animals. Am J Med 76:91–100

8. Dalhoff A (1985) In vitro and in vivo effect of immunoglobulin G on the integrity of bacterial membranes. Infection 13, Suppl 2:S185–191
9. De Simone C, Delogu G, Corbetta G (1988) Intravenous immunoglobulins in association with antibiotics: a therapeutic trial in septic intensive care unit patients. Crit Care Med 16:23–26
10. Dickgießer N, Kustermann B (1986) IgG antibodies against toxic shock syndrome toxin-1 (TSST-1) in human immunoglobulins. Klin Wochenschr 64:633–635
11. Dominioni L, Dionigi R, Zanello M, Chiaranda, M, Dionigi R, Acquarolo A, Ballabio A, Sguotti C (1991) Effects of high-dose IgG on survival of surgical patients with sepsis scores of 20 or greater. Arch Surg 126:236–240
12. Duswald KH, Müller K, Seifert J, Ring J (1980) Wirksamkeit von i.v. Gammaglobulin gegen bakterielle Infektionen chirurgischer Patienten—Ergebnisse einer kontrollierten, randomisierten klinischen Studie. Münch Med Wochenschr 122:832–836
13. Elebute EA, Stoner HB (1983) The grading of sepsis. Br J Surg 70:29–31
14. Glinz W, Grob, PJ, Nydegger UE, Ricklin T, Stamm F, Stoffel D, Lasance A (1985) Polyvalent immunoglobulins for prophylaxis of bacterial infections in patients following multiple trauma—a randomized, placebo-controlled study. Intensive Care Med 11:288–294
15. Grundmann R, Kipping N, Wesoly C (1988) Der "Sepsisscore" von Elebute und Stoner zur Definition der postoperativen Sepsis auf der Intensivstation. Intensiv Med 25:268–273
16. Hill HR, Bathras JM (1986) Protective and opsonic activities of a native, pH 4.25 intravenous immunoglobulin G preparation against common bacterial pathogens. Rev Infect Dis 8, Suppl 4:S396–S400
17. Jesdinsky HJ, Tempel G, Castrup HJ, Seifert J (1987) Cooperative group of additional immunoglobulin therapy in severe bacterial infections: results of a multicenter randomized controlled trial in cases of diffuse fibrinopurulent peritonitis. Klin Wochenschr 65:1132–1138
18. Just HM, Metzger M, Vogel W, Pelka RB (1986) Therapeutic effects of immunoglobulin in intensive care patients with severe infections. Klin Wochenschr 64:245–256
19. Knaus WA, Draper EA, Wagner DP, Zimmerman JE (1985) APACHE II: A severity of disease classification system. Crit Care Med 13:818–829
20. Lehmkuhl P, Pichlmayr I (1991) Sepsis-Therapie mit 5-S-Immunglobulinen. In: Deutsch E, Gadner H, Graninger W, Kleinberger G, Lenz K, Ritz R, Schuster HP, Zaunschirm HA (eds) Infektionen auf Intensivstationen. Springer, Vienna New York, pp 127–137 (Inensivmedizinisches Seminar, vol. 3)
21. Machin D, Campbell MJ (1987) Statistical tables for the design of clinical trials. Blackwell, Oxford
22. Mao P, Enrichens F, Olivero G, Festa T, Benedetto G, Sciascia C, Visetti E, Mauri A, Olivero S (1989) Early administration of intravenous immunoglobulins in the prevention of surgical and post-traumatic sepsis: a double blind randomized clinical trial. Surg Res Comm 5:93–98
23. Müller U, Werdan K (1990) Pseudomonas exotoxin A inhibits protein biosynthesis in neonatal rat heart muscle cells and modifies the inotropic state of these cells. J Mol Cell Cardiol 22: Suppl 3:26
24. Parker MM, Parrillo JE (1983) Septic shock: hemodynamics and pathogenesis. JAMA 250:3324–3327
25. Pennington JE, Pier GB (1987) Pseudomonas aeruginosa immunoglobulin in experimental pneumonia. Infection 15, Suppl 2:S47–S49
26. Pilz G, Werdan K (1990) Cardiovascular parameters and scoring systems in the evaluation of response to therapy in sepsis and septic shock. Infection 18:253–262
27. Pilz G, Kääb S, Neeser G, Class I, Schweigart U, Brähler A, Bujdoso O, Neumann R, Werdan K (1991) Supplemental immunoglobulin (ivIgG) treatment in 163 patients with sepsis and septic shock—an observational study as a prerequisite for placebo-controlled clinical trials. Infection 19:216–227
28. Pilz G, Class I, Boekstegers P, Pfeifer A, Müller U, Werdan K (1991) Pseudomonas immunoglobulin therapy in patients with Pseudomonas sepsis and septic shock. Antibiot Chemother 44:120–135
29. Pilz G, Gurniak T, Bujdoso O, Werdan K (1991) A BASIC program for calculation of APACHE II and Elebute scores and sepsis evaluation in intensive care medicine. Comput Biol Med 21:143–159
30. Pollack M (1983) Antibody activity against Pseudomonas aeruginosa in immune globulins prepared for intravenous use in humans. J Infect Dis 147:1090–1098
31. Schedel I (1988) Ein IgM angereichertes Immunglobulinpräparat in der Behandlung von Sepsis und septischem Schock—eine knotrollierte randomisierte Studie. In: Deicher H, Schoeppe W

(eds) Klinisch angewandte Immunologie—Sepsistherapie mit IgM-angereichertem Immunglobulin. Springer, Berlin Heidelberg New York pp 16–29

32. Stuttmann R, Hartert M, Coleman JE, Kill H, Germann G, Doehn M Prophylactic administration of Pseudomonas immunoglobulin to burn patients. Intensiv Med 26 [Suppl. 1]:130–137

33. Vogel F (1988) Bewertung der intravenösen IgM-Therapie bei schweren nosokomialen Infektionen (Ergebnis einer kontrollierten randomisierten Studie). In: Deicher H, Schoeppe W (eds) Klinisch angewandte Immunologie—Sepsistherapie mit IgM-angereichertem Immunglobulin. Springer, Berlin Heidelberg New York pp 30–41

34. Werdan K, Melnitzki SM, Pilz G, Kapsner T (1989) The cultured rat heart cell: a model to study direct cardiotoxic effects of Pseudomonas endo- and exotoxins. In: Schlag G, Redl H (eds) Progress in clinical and biological research 2nd Vienna Shock Forum, vol 308. Liss, New York, pp. 247–251

35. Yap PL (1987) The use of intravenous immunoglobulin for the treatment of infection: an overview. J Infect 15, Suppl 1:21–28

36. Ziegler EJ, Fisher CJ, Sprung CL, Straube RC, Sadoff JC, Forlke GE, Wortel CH, Fink MP, Dellinger RP, Teng NNH, Allen IE, Berger HJ, Knatterud GL, LoBuglio AF, Smith CR, and the HA-1A, Sepsis Study Group (1991) Treatment of Gram-negative bacteremia and septic shock with HA-1A human monoclonal antibody against endotoxin—a randomized, double-blind, placebo-controlled trial. N Engl J Med 324:429–436

Clinical Effects of Immunoglobulin Administration in Patients with Major Burn Injury

A. M. Munster

Depletion of serum immunoglobulins following burns, particularly of immunoglobulin G (IgG), has been well documented for over 20 years [1–3]. This deficiency has been associated with the incidence of septic complications [3–4]. The markedly reduced serum level is probably due principally to leakage and catabolism, rather than an intrinsic failure of immunoglobulin production. Immunoglobulin M (IgM) concentration is diminished far less than the levels of either IgG or immunoglobulin A (IgA) [3], IgM being a larger molecule. IgG production in cultured lymphocytes from burn patients is normal or supernormal [5], and although IgM production, requiring helper T-cell-derived factors for B cell differentiation, is deficient [6], this deficiency is more than compensated for by the large size and relative lack of leakage of the molecule. Because patients with major burns often have serum IgG concentrations as low as 300 mg% following admission, a level clearly associated with the risk of septic complications, and since IgG concentration returns to normal without specific therapy within 10–14 days of injury, there has been a great deal of interest in the administration of immunoglobulin products to burn patients within the first 2 weeks of injury in an effort to restore normal serum concentration.

γ-Globulin replacement in burn patients was attempted as early as 1964 [7]. The passive administration of immunoglobulin is theoretically attractive because of the success of active vaccination programs in restoring antibody titers in the serum (this subject is extensively overviewed in [8]). The failure of active vaccination as a universal prophylactic against sepsis in burns is not due to a lack of adequate antibody levels, but rather to the constantly changing colonizing flora of patients and the specificity of the invading organism, necessitating a large array of specific vaccines to prevent infection by even simplest species. To be effective, the administration of immunoglobulin to burn patients should result in reduced morbidity and mortality from septic complications, preferably correlated with a demonstrable improvement of in vitro parameters physiologically associated with a biologic function of immunoglobulins. To study these possibilities, we initiated a prospective randomized trial of IgG administration in burn patients.

Baltimore Regional Burn Center, Francis Scott Key Medical Center and the Department of Surgery, Johns Hopkins University, Baltimore, Maryland, USA

Host Defense Dysfunction
in Trauma, Shock and Sepsis
Eds. Faist/Meakins/Schildberg
© Springer-Verlag, Berlin Heidelberg 1993

Materials and Methods

Twenty patients admitted to the Baltimore Regional Burn Center participated in our study. Patients were randomized by a prearranged system into study patients or controls, with ten patients assigned to each group. Prior to the commencement of therapy, blood was drawn for in vitro immunological measurements and for plasma endotoxin assay. Study patients then received intravenous IgG (Sandoglobulin) in a dose of 500 mg/kg infused intravenously at 7-day intervals. If a patient underwent excisional surgery of the burn wound, he or she received IgG again on postoperative day 1 and the 7-day cycle was begun at that point. Therapy was continued until death or wound closure. Control patients received 6% intravenous albumin infusion timed identically to the study patients. The IgG/albumin solutions were prepared by a research pharmacist and supplied blinded.

The following measurements were carried out. Patients were closely observed for clinical signs of sepsis, the details of which have been previously published in detail [9]. Quantitative wound cultures were carried out at regular intervals, and death accompanied by a wound culture of over 10^5 organisms per gram tissue and one or more clinical criteria of sepsis was classified as a "septic death."

Total IgG and subset IgG1, IgG2, IgG3, and IgG4 concentrations were measured 15 min prior to an infusion and at 1 h, 24 h, and 96 h postinfusion as well as daily to determine globulin kinetics. Neutrophil chemotactic index was measured against the standard laboratory *Staphylococcus aureus* and *Escherichia coli*; bactericidal ability was measured by standard techniques. In vitro lymphocyte responsiveness to the antigens *Candida*, streptokinase-streptodornase, mumps antigen, and purified protein derivative (PPD) were measured, a one-way mixed lymphocyte reaction was assayed, and T4 and T8 lymphocyte subsets were assayed. Cytomegalovirus (CMV) antibody assay was measured by a latex agglutination scan, and plasma endotoxin was measured by the chromogenic *Limulus* amoebocyte lysate. Details of these tests have been previously published [9].

Results

The clinical and bacteriological outcome of this study is illustrated in Table 1.

There was no significant difference between the IgG group and the albumin control group in the number of deaths, septic deaths, positive blood cultures, positive wound cultures, urine infections, or intravenous line infections.

Kinetic studies showed that the return of total IgG as well as all subsets to within the normal range was immediate after the first administration of immunoglobulin. In treated patients, IgG and all subset levels remained in the

Table 1. Clinical and bacteriological results

	IgG group (n = 10)	Albumin control group (n = 10)
Male/female	10/0	8/2
Mean (range) age (years)	53.8 (1–85)	41.5 (19–77)
Mean (range) burn size (%)	38.1 (12–78)	36.4 (12–85)
Inhalation injury	8	8
Deaths	3	5
Septic deaths	2	4
Mean number of positive cultures per patient		
Blood	1.7	1.6
Wound (10^5/g)	1.5	1.8
Urine	0.6	0.7
IV line	1.2	1.5
Total number of patients with polymicrobic sepsis		
Blood	0	3
Wound	3	3
Sputum	0	0
Urine	3	4
IV line	1	2

normal range from the second day of therapy onwards to the end of the study, while controls showed the previously documented deficiencies and return to the normal range within approximately 10 days. Control patients demonstrated an average CMV titer of between 1 in 16 and 1 in 32, with no change in the 2-week period after onset of therapy, while the IgG group demonstrated a statistically significant rise in the CMV titers from an average of 1 in 16 to an average of 1 in 128 during the treatment period. These changes parallel the titers of the G1 and G3 subset, which are specific to CMV.

Assays of neutrophil function showed the expected diminution of chemotactic index and neutrophil bactericidal index in burn patients as compared to controls, but there were no statistically significant differences between the indices of IgG-treated patients and albumin controls for either chemotaxis, bactericidal index for *S. aureus*, or bactericidal index for *E. coli*. Assays of lymphocyte function similarly showed no significant differences between the IgG group and the albumin group either within 24 h of admission for 2 weeks following therapy.

Intravenous immunoglobulin was markedly effective in reducing plasma endotoxin concentration. Endotoxemia in burn patients is related to burn size. [10]. In our control patients within 24 h of admission the average endotoxin concentration in the plasma was between 20 and 30 pg/ml, rising to between 40 and 50 pg/ml by postburn day 4. By contrast, the endotoxin concentration in IgG-treated patients never rose higher than 10 pg/ml and remained at low levels throughout the study. Interestingly, albumin-treated patients also showed a slight diminution in plasma endotoxin concentration.

Discussion

Our findings are essentially in agreement with those of other workers in the area. Waymack et al. analyzed 50 patients prospectively following 5 weeks of therapy and reported no differences in morbidity or mortality as a result of therapy [11]. Hansborough et al. reported improved neutrophil opsonization and phagocytosis in treated patients, but no difference in outcome [12]. Burleson et al. reported no effect of therapy on the number of total, helper, or suppressor T-cells, some improvement in IgM secretion in pokeweed mitogen (PWM)-stimulated patients, but no alteration in IgG production [13].

Although the complete lack of signification responsiveness in in vivo and in vitro results is disappointing, it is not altogether unexpected. It is clear that immunoglobulin deficiency in burn patients is only part of the immunosuppressive spectrum, the etiology of which has been widely studied and continues to be controversial. Since the association between immunoglobulin, particularly IgG, in deficiency and septic complications is strong, IgG replacement still has a potential future as adjunct therapy to other biologic or immunological methods of supporting the host defense of the burn patient, probably not justifying the complete omission of burns and trauma from the recent Immunoglobulin Consensus Conference of the National Institutes of Health [14]. Whether this method of support will take the form of biologic response modifiers, stimulation, or blockade of the inflammatory reaction, or pharmacologic intervention, remains yet to be defined.

References

1. Arturson G, Hogman CF, Johansson SGO et al. (1969) Changes in immunoglobulin levels in severely burned patients. Lancet I:546
2. Daniels JC, Larson DL, Abston S et al. (1974) Serum protein profiles in thermal burns. J Trauma 14:137
3. Munster AM, Hoagland HC, Pruitt BA Jr (1970) The effect of thermal injury on serum immunoglobulins. Ann Surg 172:965
4. Hershman MJ, Cheadle WG, George CD, Cost KM, Appel SH, Davidson PF, Polk HC (1988) The response of immunoglobulins to infection after thermal and nonthermal injury. Am Surg 54:408
5. Shorr RM, Ershler WB, Gamelli RL (1984) Immunoglobulin production in burned patients. J Trauma 24:319
6. Teodorczyk-Injeyan JA, Sparkes BG, Peters WJ (1989) Regulation of IgM production in thermally injured patients. Burns Incl Therm Inj 15:241
7. Kefalides NA, Aranaja B et al. (1964) Evaluation of antibiotic prophylaxis and gamma-globulin, plasma, albumin and saline soaks in severe burns. Ann Surg 159:496
8. Munster AM (1987) Immunization therapy in burn patients. In: Boswick JA Jr (ed) art and science of burn care. Aspen, Rockville
9. Munster AM, Moran KT, Thupari J, Allo M, Winchurch RA (1987) Prophylactic intravenous immunoglobulin replacement in high-risk burn patients. J Burn Care Rehab 8:376
10. Winchurch RA, Thupari JN, Munster AM (1987) Endotoxemia in burn patients: levels of circulating endotoxins are related to burn size. Surgery 102:808

11. Waymack JP, Jenkins ME, Alexander JW et al. (1989) A prospective trial of prophylactic intravenous immune globulin for the prevention of infections in severely burned patients. Burns Incl Therm Inj 15:71
12. Hansborough JF, Miller LM, Field TO Jr et al. (1988) High dose intravenous immunoglobulin therapy in burn patients: pharmacokinetics and effects on microbial opsomization and phago-cytosis. Pediatr Infect Dis J 7:549
13. Burleson DG, Mason AD, McManus AT, Pruitt BA Jr (1988) Lymphocyte phenotype and function changes in burn patients after intravenous IgG therapy. Arch Surg 123:1379
14. Office of Medical Applications of Research, NIH (1990) JAMA 264:3189

Treatment of Gram-Negative Septic Toxic Diseases with an Immunoglobulin Preparation Containing IgG, IgM and IgA: A Prospective Randomized Clinical Trial

I. Schedel, U. Dreikhausen, B. Nentwig, M. Höckenschneider, D. Rauthmann, S. Balikcioglu, R. Coldewey, and H. Deicher

Introduction

Endotoxin may play a major role in the pathogenesis of multiorgan failure in the context of the toxic process in septicemia induced by gram-negative pathogens [1–5]. The hypothesis which has led to this prospective clinical study consisted in the idea of inhibiting the effects of the endotoxin and the development of multiorgan failure by neutralizing and/or eliminating endotoxin as early as possible, and thereby attempting to attain a positive effect on the clinical course of these diseases. Previous animal experimental and clinical investigations have indicated that such an effect is possible ([6–15]; B. J. Appelmelk, personal communication).

Methods

Determination of Serum Endotoxin Activity. The endotoxin assays were carried out using the Coatest Endotoxin Kit (Kabi Vitrum, Stockholm, Sweden) in a modification of our own as described in detail elsewhere [16]. For control of specificity in the limulus amebocyte lysate (LAL) test in a subgroup of patients an enzyme-linked immunosorbant assay (ELISA) system, using self-prepared monoclonal antibody preparations to lipid A was applied. This method has been described elsewhere [17].

Semiquantitative Determination of Antibodies Against Endotoxin Determinants. To detect antibodies against lipid A and core polysaccharide, an ELISA was used and performed as described earlier [17, 18].

Clinical trial

Patients population and Patient Selection Criteria. Patients enrolled in this study were admitted to the Medical School Hospital Hanover, FRG, and had to fulfill the following criteria:

Host Defense Dysfunction
in Trauma, Shock and Sepsis
Eds. Faist/Meakins/Schildberg
© Springer-Verlag, Berlin Heidelberg 1993

- Inclusion of the patients in the study within 24 h after the onset of the symptoms according to the list of additional criteria below
- Detection of endotoxemia (endotoxin determination > 12.5 pg/ml)
- Declaration of consent

In addition at least five of the following criteria were to be fulfilled for inclusion in the study:
- Clinical indications of the focus of septicemia
- Fever higher than 38.5 °C
- Thrombopenia of < 100 000/l or a fall in thrombocyte count by > 30% in 24 h
- Shift to the left in the blood count (> 5% stab cells of total white blood cell count)
- Granulocytopenia (< 1500 but of more than 600 cells/l
- Pulmonary congestion (auscultation and radiological examination)
- Disseminated intravascular clotting (DIC)
- Hypotension (systolic blood pressure < 100 mmHg)
- Tachycardia (> 120/min)
- Oliguria

The detection of endotoxemia was regarded as obligatory for the inclusion of patients in the study, but the demonstration of a positive blood culture was not. Patients who fulfilled any of the following criteria were excluded from the study:
- More than 75 years old
- Pregnant
- Life expectancy estimated to be below 1 week owing to other underlying diseases
- Septic disease already present for more than 24 h on the basis of clinical criteria

Fresh blood and/or blood products such as fresh frozen plasma were administered at the discretion of the physician in accordance with the clinical requirements. Hemodialysis and hemofiltration were carried out in accordance with clinical requirements. The antibiotic therapy was carried out in accordance with the guidelines in the study by the Paul Ehrlich Society (August 1985 Protocol).

Study Design. Patients who fulfilled the inclusion criteria were assigned by a group of three persons who were not involved in the clinical care of the patients using a randomization list to group A (with immunoglobulin therapy) or group B (without immunoglobulin therapy). In addition to the therapy administered on the basis of clinical requirements, group A received immunoglobulin treatment. Group B received all kinds of therapy (antibiotics, shock therapy, etc.), according to clinical necessities, but no immunoglobulin administration.

Deaths definitively due to causes other than the bacterial infection, (e.g., pulmonary embolism, heart failure), were documented but not evaluated as mortality secondary to septic disease (see above).

Immunoglobulin Preparation. A human immunoglobulin preparation containing 5% total protein for intravenous infusion (Pentaglobin, Biotest, Dreieich, FRG) was used. The preparation was shown to contain 38 g/l IgG, 6 g/l IgM, and 6 g/l IgA [10]. Besides a broad spectrum of antibodies with specificities to different bacterial determinants, this preparation also contains IgG-, IgA- and IgM-antibodies against endotoxic determinants of the core, as well as of the lipid A region [10]. Additionally, antibody titers against *Escherichia coli* J5 of the IgG-, IgM- and IgA-type were found in this immunoglobulin preparation by Appelmelk and coworkers using specific ELISA (B. J. Appelmelk, personal communication).

Administration Schedule. Group A: The patients randomized in this group received the immunoglobulin preparation in the following dosage: On the first day, 600 ml i.v. over more than 8 h. On the second and the third day, 300 ml i.v. each day over more than 8 h, 24 h after the previous dose.

Criteria for Discontinuation of the Study. The study was discontinued after the evaluation of the data from 55 patients although the envisaged number of patients had not been reached, since the difference between the therapy and control group with regard to lethality was evidently statistically significant in favor of the therapy group at this time.

Statistical Evaluation. The clinical course of the randomized group of patients was evaluated by multivariable evaluation of clinical and laboratory data. In addition, lethality was used as a test criterion. The Student's *t* test, the U test, the generalized log-rank-test, the generalized Wilcoxon (Breslow) test, and Kaplan-Meier survival curves were used as statistical test systems.

Results

During a 33-month period, 860 patients were checked for inclusion in this study. Of these 860 patients 69 were found to fulfill the criteria and were allocated randomly to the two groups in the study. Fourteen patients had to be excluded from the final evaluation. Nine patients did not receive the adequate dosage of immunoglobulins and five patients ultimately failed to meet the criteria for admission to this study.

The demographic data of the patients taken initially are summarized in Table 1. The randomization groups did not differ statistically significantly with regard to the demographic criteria or the clinical and laboratory data.

Altogether, 55 patients were included in the analysis of the prospective clinical investigation: 29 men and 26 women. Twenty-seven patients were allocated randomly to the group receiving immunoglobulin therapy and 28 patients to the group without immunoglobulin therapy. Thirty-eight patients

Table 1. Demographic data of the groups of patients investigated

	With IG treatment	Without IG treatment	Total
Total number:	27	28	55
Male	15	14	29
Female	12	14	26
Age (years)			
Average	46 ± 16	37 ± 18	41.5 ± 17
Median (range)	47(20–73)	38(7–71)	41
Body weight (kg)	64.61 ± 15.6	58.1 ± 17.2	61.4 ± 16.5
Height (cm)	167 ± 9.47	167.8 ± 16.35	167.7 ± 12.7
Source:			
Medical Division	20	18	38
Surgical Division	7	10	17

Table 2. Sources of gram-negative infections in the groups of patients investigated

Source[a]	No. of patients in treatment groups	
	IG preparation ($n = 27$)	Without IG preparation ($n = 28$)
Pneumonia	10	8
Urinary tract infection	3	1
Upper respiratory tract infection	1	
Peritonitis	1	2
Intra-abdominal abscess	6	4
Burn	2	3
Phlebits		2
Perirectal abscess	1	
Cholangitis	1	2
Wound infection		1
Arthritis	2	1
Cerebral abscess	1	

[a] More than one condition often existed in the same patient.

came from the Medical Division and 17 patients from the Abdominal Surgery Division, Hanover Medical University.

The clinical diagnoses, underlying diseases, and the concomitant diseases of the patients included in the investigations are shown in Tables 2 and 3. The randomized groups are homogenous and comparable with regard to the parameters evaluated (no statistically significant differences in the application of the chi-square test). The randomized groups were also found to be comparable regarding the parameters evaluated by the Apache II scoring system (Fig. 1) [19].

The mortality showed significant differences between the randomized groups. The group of patients with immunoglobulin therapy had a lower mortality (in the overall observation period) than the patient group not treated with immunoglobulin preparation (Table 4). The mortality data after the

Table 3. Underlying conditions in the groups of patients investigated

Underlying condition[a]	No. of patients in treatment groups	
	IG preparation ($n = 27$)	Without IG preparation ($n = 28$)
Neoplasm	9	10
Hematologic	7	9
Nonhematologic	2	1
Thrombopenia	2	
Hepatobiliary disease	1	3
Trauma or burn	2	4
Chronic inflammatory bowel disease	4	2
Alcoholism	1	
Chronic lung disease	1	
Cardiac failure		2
Chronic renal failure	4	3
Acute renal failure	2	
Hemodialysis	1	1
Chronic infection	2	1

[a] More than one condition often existed in the same patient.

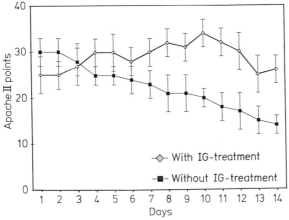

Fig. 1. Development of severity of septic disease as assessed by the APACHE II score system. On days 7–14 $p < 0.01$. Mean $\pm$ 2SD

inclusion of 50 and 55 patients are given in Fig. 2. The study was discontinued after the assessment of statistically significant differences in the mortality rate after the inclusion and evaluation of 50 and 55 patients. One patient within the group of immunoglobulin-treated patients died from pulmonary embolism 28 days after inclusion without any sign of septic disease. In the group of 14 patients excluded from the final evaluation seven patients received immunoglobulin treatment. In this group no patient died, whereas in the group of seven patients who did not receive immunoglobulin treatment two patients died.

Table 4. Mortality of the patients involved in the study

Treatment	No. of patients		
	Dead	Alive	Total
[a]A. With IG treatment	1	26	27
[a]B. Without IG treatment	9	19	28
Total number of patients	10	45	55

[a] General chi-square test $p < 0.01$

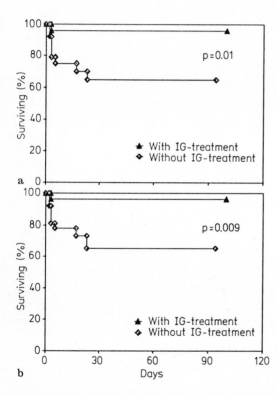

Fig. 2 a,b. Survival of the groups of patients investigated after the inclusion of **a** 50 and **b** 55 patients (Kaplan-Meier plots, Wilcoxon chi-square test)

Inclusion of these 14 patients in the overall evaluation would not have modified the results.

A statistically relevant decrease in the Apache II score beyond the fifth day after inclusion was observed (Fig. 1). These changes were mainly due to body temperature, leukocyte counts, mean aterial pressure, and heart rate in patients treated with immunoglobulin preparation, in contrast to the patients not treated with immunoglobulin preparation ($p < 0.05$, chi-square test). However, results of the evaluation of body temperature, or heart rate, or systolic and diastolic arterial pressure as single parameters showed no statistically significant differences between the randomization groups.

The results of positive blood cultures are summarized as follows:

- *Pseudomonas aeruginosa*   15
- *E. Coli*   12
- *Enterobacter*   8
- *Proteus*   6
- *Klebsiella pneumoniae*   5
- *Serratia marcescens*   2
- *Citrobacter freundii*   8
- *Morganella morganii*   1

More than one microorganism was identified in 8 patients.

Positive blood cultures with gram-negative bacteria were found to correlate with positive LAL tests in 86% (correlation coefficient *r*). Considering all positive blood cultures, the correlation with positive LAL tests was found in

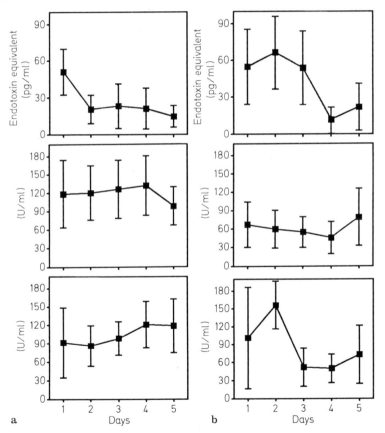

Fig 3. Endotoxin and LPS antibody results in the randomized groups of patients **a** with immunoglobulin treatment (*n* = 27) and **b** without (*n* = 28). (Means, standard deviations, results of the LAL test between days 1 and 2 in the group with Ig treatment and between days 1 and 5 in the group without Ig treatment are statistically different; *p* < 0.01, chi-square test)

92%. No correlation with positive LAL tests was to be found with local detection of bacteria (sputum, wound smears. etc.).

The results of measurements of endotoxin by means of the LAL test revealed a statistically significant decrease in LAL reactivity in the course of the first 24 h of the observation period in the patient population treated with immunoglobulin (Fig. 3, chi-square test: $p < 0.01$). A corresponding decline in the untreated patient population was only to be found after 4 days (Fig. 3).

The determinations of plasma endotoxin levels during the first 24 h after the inclusion of the patients in the study showed significantly lower values in the group of patients who stayed alive throughout the observation period than in the group of patients who did not survive (Fig. 4). In addition, the measurement of IgG antibodies against lipid A and lipopolysaccharide (LPS-RE determinants) revealed a statistically decreased binding activity ($p < 0.05$, U test) in the sera of patients who did not survive the septic episode, which was obtained during the first 24 h after inclusion in the study (Fig. 5). Side effects of

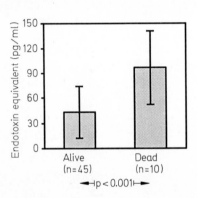

Fig. 4. Plasma endotoxin results during the first 24 h after inclusion of the patients in the study (mean, standard deviations)

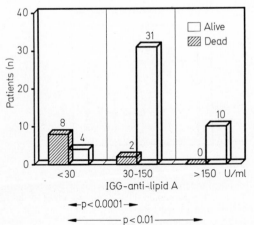

Fig. 5. Results of serum IgG-antibodies to Lipid A during the first 24 h after inclusion of the patients in the study (mean, standard deviations)

the immunoglobulin preparation used, which would have necessitated the discontinuation of the therapy, were not observed.

Discussion

The results of this study demonstrate that passive administration of the polyclonal IgG-, IgM- and IgA-containing human immunoglobulin preparation used in this trial is well tolerated in patients with septic toxic disease and leads to a statistically significant reduction in mortality.

The effect of immunoglobulin preparations containing antibodies to different determinants of the endotoxin molecule of gram-negative bacteria in patients with septic shock was investigated by different groups [12–15, 20]. The rationale for the use of antibodies against determinants of endotoxin in septic toxic disease is to neutralize endotoxin in the patient's circulation in order to prevent the harmful consequences provoked by the lipid A component of the endotoxin molecule. Although antibiotics are required to clear bacteremia, they are unable to prevent the toxic effects of endotoxins and may even promote its release from bacteria. Therefore, strategies for intervention in gram-negative shock have focussed, in particular, on the application of antibodies against LPS and on its core determinants. Clinical studies have demonstrated that sera from volunteers hyperimmunized with E. coli J5 may be effective in the treatment of gram-negative bacteremia and shock [14, 21–25]. However, some investigators have been unable to reproduce the results of others. Furthermore, it could not be established that the clinical effects observed are really due to antibodies to LPS core determinants [15, 24].

A new investigation by McCabe et al. showed that after vaccination with Salmonella minnesota R595 [15] protection against bacteria and bacterial-toxic effects could be detected in the serum IgM fraction, but not in the IgG fraction of human or sera This may have been the cause of the divergent results of clinical investigations using immunoglobulin preparations containing different classes of immunoglobulin.

For our clinical study, an immunoglobulin preparation was used which contained IgM and IgA, as well as IgG. The results of this study cannot show conclusively whether the significant acceleration in the fall in LAL activity in the patient's sera, which was observed under immunoglobulin substitution in the patients treated with immunoglobulin as compared to the control group, was an effect induced by the IgG or the IgM fraction of the immunoglobulin preparation used, even if specific antibodies against endotoxic determinants (both of the IgM and IgG type) could be detected in this preparation [10].

Even though the significantly accelerated fall in LAL reactivity could be demonstrated in the patients receiving the immunoglobulin preparation when compared to the untreated patient group, it cannot be established definitely on the basis of these data whether specific antibodies against LPS determinants are really responsible for the clinical effects observed, and above all for the significantly more favorable mortality in the patient population treated with immunoglobulin. On the other hand, there is no consistent evidence that antibodies of other specificity than those to LPS determinants (i.e., anti-idiotypic antibodies to the hypervariable region of antibodies to LPS determinants) may be responsible for the observed effects. Preliminary studies in our laboratory did not reveal any binding activity of the immunoglobulin preparation used in this study to LPS-specific antibodies prepared from the patients' sera nor to a spectrum of mouse monoclonal antibody preparations to different LPS determinants (unpublished results).

In our investigation, the immunoglobulin preparations were administered on the basis of the hypothesis that the deleterious consequences of septic toxic diseases can be minimized by endotoxin neutralization at as early a time as possible before the onset of the physiological and biological consequences of endotoxemia. Administration of the immunoglobulin preparation at as early a stage as possible in the course of the septic toxic episode was attempted under the conditions of our clinical investigations. Conversely, use of immunoglobulin preparations in the late phases of septic toxic diseases, after the occurrence of multiorgan failure, appears not to be justified. The efficacy of an immunoglobulin substitution continued over a period longer than 3 days; a repetition of the substitution after a few days may appear promising on the basis of our investigations. For further clarification of the mechanisms involved and in order to optimize the effect of immunoglobulin treatment in septic toxic diseases prospective clinical trials should be carried out.

References

1. Lode HJ, Wagner F, Mnller M et al. (1988) Epidemiologie, Klinik und Prognose der Sepsis bei 691 Patienten. In: Reinhart K, Eyrich K (eds) Sepsis. Springer, Berlin Heidelberg New York, pp 8–13
2. Rietschel E, Zhringer U, Wollenweber H, Miragliotta W, Musehold J, Lnderitz T, Schade U (1984) Bacterial Endotoxins. Chemical structure and biologic activity. Am J Emerg Med 2:60
3. Michie HR, Spriggs DR, Manogue KR, Sherman ML, Revhaug A, O'Dwyer ST, Arthur K, Dinarello CA, Cerami A, Wolff SM, Kufe DW, Wilmore DW (1988) Tumor necrosis factor and endotoxin induce similar metabolic responses in human beings. Surgery 104:280
4. Mathison JC, Wolfson E, Ulevitch RJ (1988) Participation of tumor necrosis factor in the mediation of gram-negative bacterial lipopolysaccharide-induced injury in rabbits. J Clin Invest 81:1925
5. Ziegler EJ (1988) Tumor necrosis factor in humans. N Engl J Med 318:1533
6. Michie HR, Manogue KR, Spriggs DR, Revhaug A, O'Dwyer S, Dinarello CA, Cerami A, Wolff SM, Wilmore DW (1988) Detection of circulating tumor necrosis factor after endotoxin administration. N Engl J Med 318:1481
7. Lüderitz O, Galanos C, Rietschel ET (1982) Endotoxins of gram-negative bacteria. Pharmacol Ther 15:383
8. Komuro T, Galanos C (1988) Analysis of salmonella lipopolysaccharides by sodium deoxycholate-polyacrylamide gel electrophoresis. J Chromatogr 450:381
9. Galanos C, Freudenberg MA, Jay FA, Nerkar D, Veleva K, Brade H, Strittmatter W (1984) Immunogenic properties of lipid A. Rev Infect Dis 6:546

10. Stephan W, Dichtelmnller H, Schedel I (1985) Eigenschaften und Wirksamkeit eines humanen Immunglobulin M-Preparates fnr die intravenöse Anwendung. Arzneimittelforschung/Drug Res 35:933
11. Ziegler EJ (1988) Protective antibody to endotoxin core: the emperor's new clothes. J Infect Dis 158:286
12. Kirkland TN, Ziegler EJ, Tobias P, Ward DC, Michalek SM, McGhee JR, Macher I, Urayama K, Appelmelk BJ (1988) Inhibition of lipopolysaccharide activation of 70Z/3 cells by anti-lipopolysaccharide antibodies. J Immunol 141:3208
13. Pohlson EC, Suehiro A, Ziegler EJ, Suehiro G, McNamara JJ (1988) Antiserum to endotoxin in hemorrhagic shock. J Surg Res 45:467
14. Ziegler EJ, McCutchan JA, Fierer J, Glauser MP, Sadoff J, Douglas H, Braude AI (1982) Treatment of gram-negative bacteremia and shock with human antiserum to a mutant of *Escherichia coli*. N Engl J Med 307:1225
15. McCabe WR, DeMaria AJr, Berberich H, Johns M (1988) Immunization with rough mutants of *Salmonella minnesota*: protective activity of IgM and IgG antibody to the R595 (Re chemotype) mutant. J Infect Dis 158:291
16. Schedel T (1988) An IgM-enriched immunoglobulin preparation for treatment of sepsis and septic shock: a controlled randomized study. In: Deicher H, Schoeppe W (eds) Klinisch angewandte Immunologie. Springer, Berlin Heidelberg New York, pp 3–13
17. Stoll C, Schedel I, Peest D (1985) Serum antibodies against common antigens of bacterial lipopolysaccharides in healthy adults and in patients with multiple myeloma. Infection 13:115
18. Schedel I, Dreikhausen U., Nentwig B, Höckenschnieder M, Rauthmann D, Balikcioglu S, Coldewey R, Deicher H (1991) Treatment of gram-negative septic toxic diseases with an immunoglobulin preparation containing IgG, IgM and IgA: a prospective randomized clinical trial. Crit Care Med 19:1104–1113
19. Knaus WA, Drader EA, Douglas PW, Wagner DP, Zimmerman JE (1985) APACHE II: a severity of disease classification system. Crit Care Med 13:818
20. Calandra T, Glauser MP Schellekens J, Verhoef J (1988) Treatment of gram-negative septic shock with human IgG antibody to *Escherichia coli* J5: a prospective, double-blind, randomized trial. J Infect Dis 158:312
21. Teng NNH, Kaplan HS, Hebert JM, Moore C, Douglas H, Wunderlich A, Braude AI (1985) Protection against gram-negative bacteremia and endotoxemia with human monoclonal IgM antibodies. Proc Natl Acad Sci USA 82:1790
22. Greisman SE, Johnston CA (1988) Failure of antisera to J5 and R595 rough mutants to reduce endotoxemic lethality. J Infect Dis 157:54
23. Baumgartner JD, Glauser MP, McCutchan JA, Ziegler EJ, van Melle G, Klauber MR, Vogt M, Muehlen E, Leuthy R, Chiolero R, Geroulanos S (1985) Prevention of gram-negative shock and death in surgical patients by antibody to endotoxin core glycolipid. Lancet 2:59
24. DeMaria A, Johns MA, Berberich H, McCabe WR (1988) Immunization with rough mutants of *Salmonella minnesota*: initial studies in human subjects. J Infect Dis 158:301
25. McCabe WR, Kreger BE, Johns M (1972) Type-specific and cross-reactive antibodies in gram-negative bacteremia. N Engl J Med 287:261

Immunotherapeutic Strategies for Passive Immunization Against *Pseudomonas aeruginosa*

L. Saravolatz[1], J. Kilborn,[1] and J. Pennington[2]

The advances of medical technology have resulted in a population of patients at increased risk of serious infections from opportunistic pathogens. Despite the availability of major new antimicrobial agents with in vitro activity, *Pseudomonas aeruginosa* has emerged as the most common cause of hospital-acquired pneumonia with a mortality of 50%–100%. A recent publication of bacteremia from 1984 to 1987 revealed a mortality of 51.1% at the time of discharge [1]. This mortality is approximately twofold higher than with other gram-negative pathogens or with gram-positive bacterial infections.

Considerable interest has developed in the immunotherapy of infectious diseases and especially of *P. aeruginosa*. Data from experimental studies have supported active immunization with lipopolysaccharide (LPS) *P. aeruginosa* antigens as effective against pneumonias. Unfortunately, seriously ill hospitalized patients may either have a blunted immunologic response or may not be able to afford the delay in developing antibody to the bacterial pathogen causing their infection. Therefore, the need for providing a rapid transfer of protective antibodies has prompted the development of a hyperimmune globulin as an adjunct to antimicrobial chemotherapy.

Rationale for Passive Immunization

The rationale for passive immunization against *P. aeruginosa* is based on limitations of active vaccination against *P. aeruginosa*. Firstly, the occurrence of *P. aeruginosa* serious infections, especially pneumonia or bacteremia, frequently occurs within the first week of hospitalization. The optimal immune response after active immunization usually requires 10 –14 days. Secondly, *P. aeruginosa* infection accounts for only 10%–15% of all nosocomial infections [2]. Finally, most active immunizations with *P. aeruginosa* vaccines contain LPS which is associated with serious side effects. Thus, the benefit in using a potentially hazardous vaccine would be limited to a relatively small number of patients at risk.

[1] Henry Ford Hospital, Detroit, MI, USA
[2] Cutter Laboratories, Berkeley, CA, USA

Host Defense Dysfunction
in Trauma, Shock and Sepsis
Eds. Faist/Meakins/Schildberg
© Springer-Verlag, Berlin Heidelberg 1993

Passive immunotherapy against *P. aeruginosa* offers the advantage of providing a rapid and safe method of administering type-specific antibodies to patients with proven *P. aeruginosa* infections. One problem the clinicians encounter in initiating immunotherapy is how to rapidly identify *P. aeruginosa* infection. Unfortunately, the current diagnostic modalities require 48–72 h to confirm a gram-negative isolate as *P. aeruginosa*. The delay in diagnosis may be responsible for suboptimal use of antibody therapy.

An additional critical consideration for passive immunotherapy against *P. aeruginosa* is the identification of the antigen target that is most important for protective effect by antibodies. Several studies have demonstrated a superior protection against *P. aeruginosa* infection by antibodies directed against LPS when compared to antibodies against outer membrane protein and exotoxin A [3].

In Vitro and In Vivo Experimental Observations

In vitro observations have demonstrated enhanced phagocytic uptake and killing of opsonized *P. aeruginosa* [4]. Also, animal experiments have demonstrated both prophylactic and therapeutic efficacy of serotype-specific antibodies against *P. aeruginosa* [5–7].

Polyclonal Antibodies

The level of natural *P. aeruginosa* antibodies in plasma is relatively low. Thus, human plasma-derived intravenous immunoglobulin (IGIV) preparations (polyclonal antibodies) have been prepared with enhanced antibody titers against *P. aeruginosa*. This has been done by preimmunizing human volunteers with *P. aeruginosa* polyvalent vaccine or by screening plasma donors for naturally high *P. aeruginosa* antibodies.

Preparations of hyperimmune *P. aeruginosa* IGIV preparations have been evaluated in several studies. A study by Alexander and Fisher in burn patients suggested that hyperimmune globulin to *P. aeruginosa* was an effective adjunctive measure for the treatment of life-threatening infections [8]. Animal studies have demonstrated that in *P. aeruginosa* pneumonia, the survival rate improved from 0% to 43% with *P. aeruginosa* hyperimmune IgG antibody. Furthermore, when combined with antimicrobial chemotherapy, survival rose to 86% [9].

Monoclonal Antibodies

In view of the limited supply of human plasma-derived polyclonal *P. aeruginosa* hyperimmune antibody, monoclonal antibodies (mAbs) are seen as an attractive alternative. Murine anti-LPS mAb has demonstrated in vivo protection against *P. aeruginosa* [10–12]. In additional studies, a mAb preparation provided protection at a protein dosage that was 100-fold less than required for a polyclonal preparation [10].

Recently, human mAbs against *P. aeruginosa* have been developed. A cocktail of five human IgM mAbs directed against *P. aeruginosa* serotypes (1, 2, 3/7, 4 and 6 of the Fisher Devlin Gnabasik typing scheme) were combined with a human IgG mAb against exotoxin A. This polyvalent preparation was administered to 20 patients to evaluate safety and pharmacokinetics. The first 12 patients (phase 1-A) were at high risk of developing *P. aeruginosa* infection but were not presently infected. The next eight patients (phase 1-B) included patients with *P. aeruginosa* pneumonia and/or bacteremia. All patients provided written informed consent. A dose escalation was administered starting at 0.3 ml/kg body weight, which provided 0.75 mg total IgM protein and 0.048 mg IgG protein per kilogram body weight. Three patients received each scheduled dose before increasing the dosages twofold to 0.6 and 1.2 ml/kg. In addition, three patients received two doses of 1.2 ml/kg 24 h apart. Patients were evaluated clinically for adverse reactions for up to 48 h after the infusions. Routine hematology, chemistry, and urinalysis were followed at 3, 24, and 48 h, and 7 days after infusion. Sera were collected for pharmacokinetic analysis, anti-mAb immune response, and anti-Epstein-Barr virus (EBV) immune response and opsono-phagocytic assays.

Clinical and laboratory parameters revealed the infusion was well tolerated. The laboratory changes revealed a rise in platelet count during the week following infusion in six patients. These rises were felt to be secondary to thrombocytosis after surgical procedures. Two patients had transient rises in their serum glutamine pyruvate transaminase during the 2-week period after PsmAb infusions. These changes were felt to be secondary to medications and ischemic liver injury. No patient developed antibody against individual *P. aeruginosa* mAbs in the polyvalent preparation.

A dose response was noted for each mAb in the polyvalent preparation (Fig. 1). The $t_{1/2,s}$ for noninfected patients ranged from 52 to 99 and for infected patients from 34 to 58 h.

Specific immunotypes of each of the *P. aeruginosa* strains included in the cocktail of PsmAb were used for the opsonophagocytic assays. These assays evaluated the reduction in colony-forming units for each IgM mAb using pre- and postinfusion serum specimens. All immunotypes, except for immunotype 2, resulted in 1 $\log_{10}$ increase in the killing of the homologous immunotype bacteria.

In the eight patients who were infected, two with pneumonia died. *P. aeruginosa* was felt to have contributed to the fatal outcome. In all eight cases, the clinical isolate of *P. aeruginosa* was typeable and present in the PsmAb polyvalent preparation. The number of patients treated in this clinical evaluation is too small to draw conclusions about the efficacy of the mAb preparation.

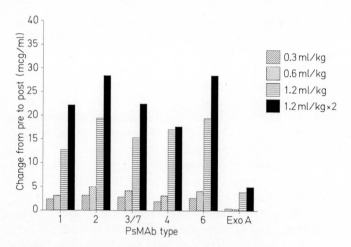

Fig. 1. Dose effect of PsmAb on pre-vs postantibody concentrations

This study has demonstrated that PsmAb can be given as a dose escalation to 1.2 ml/kg body weight without any adverse clinical signs or symptoms. Asymptomatic platelet rises occurred in patients and was probably related to the bone marrow's physiologic response to surgery and blood loss. Pharmacokinetic analysis revealed a dose-related elevation of all six immunotypes after infusions. The $t_{1/2}$ of each specific mAb was long enough to assure concentrations above the proposed effective level ($> 4\mu$ gm/ml) would last for at least 2 days or longer. If the patient is not responding to the initial therapy, a repeat infusion might be considered in 3–5 days.

In conclusion, this study suggests that PsmAb is well tolerated and should be considered for future trials in evaluating the efficacy of monoclonal immunotherapy in the treatment of life-threatening *P. aeruginosa* infections.

References

1. Roberts FJ, Geere IW, Coldman A (1991) A Three-year Study of Positive Blood Cultures with Emphasis on Prognosis. Rev Infect Dis 13:34–46
2. Anonymous (1984) Nosocomial infection surveillance: CDC morbidity and mortality weekly report, vol 35, pp. 17ss–29ss
3. Pennington JE (1990) *Pseudomonas aeruginosa* vaccines and immunotherapy. Infect Dis Clin North Am 4/2:259–270
4. Collins MS, Roby RE (1984) Protective activity of an intravenous immune globulin (human) enriched in antibody against lipopolysaccharide antigens of *Pseudomonas aeruginosa*. Am J Med 76: 168–174
5. Pennington JE (1979) Lipopolysaccharide Pseudomonas vaccine: efficacy against pulmonary infection with *Pseudomonas aeruginosa*. J Infect Dis 140:73–80
6. Pennington JE, Peir GB, Small GJ (1986) Efficacy of intravenous immune globulin for treatment of experimental *Pseudomonas aeruginosa*. J Crit Care 1:4–10

7. Young LS (1972) Human immunity to *Pseudomonas aeruginosa* II. Relationship between heat-stable opsonins and type-specific lipopolysaccharides. J Infect Dis 126:277–287
8. Alexander JW, Fisher MW (1974) Immunization against *Pseudomonas* in infection after thermal injury. J Infect Dis 130 [Suppl] :S152–S158
9. Pennington JE, Small GJ (1987) Passive immune therapy for experimental *Pseudomonas aeruginosa* pneumonia in the neutropenic host. J Infect Dis 155:973–978
10. Pennington JE, Small GJ, Lostrom ME et al. (1986) Polyclonal and monoclonal antibody therapy for experimental *Pseudomonas aeruginosa* pneumonia. Infect Immun 54:239–244
11. Sadoff JC, Wright DC, Futrovsky S et al. (1986) Characterization of mouse monoclonal antibodies directed against *Pseudomonas aeruginosa* lipopolysaccharides. Antibiot Chemother 36:134–146
12. Sawada S, Suzuki M, Kawamura T et al. (1984) Protection against infection with *Pseudomonas aeruginosa* by passive transfer of monoclonal antibodies to lipopolysaccharides and outer membrane proteins. J Infect Dis 150:570–576

Binding Characteristics of the Antiendotoxin Antibody Xomen-E5 to Bacterial Whole-Cell Antigens

K. J. Gorelick[1], D. M. Wood[2], J. B. Parent[2], E. Lim[2], K. D. Knebel[2], D. M. Fishwild[2], D. T. Reardan[2], P. W. Trown[2], and P. J. Conlon[2]

Introduction

Sepsis is a common, life-threatening complication of infection with gram-negative bacteria. While the pathophysiology of gram-negative sepsis has not been fully elucidated, a significant portion of the clinical syndrome can probably be attributed to the activation by endotoxin of a cascade of secondary mediators. These mediators initiate a series of complicated events, including systemic response to infection (fever or hypothermia, tachycardia, tachypnea) and dysfunction or failure of critical organ systems including the kidney, lung, brain, liver, and cardiovascular and coagulation systems [1].

Endotoxin is a ubiquitous constituent of the cell walls of gram-negative bacteria. It is a lipopolysaccharide (LPS) consisting of a nontoxic, immunogenic polysaccharide (O-specific side chain) which is unique to each strain of gram-negative bacteria, and an oligosaccharide core linked via 2-keto-3-deoxyoctanoic acid (KDO) to a common lipid A structure. The core region, especially the inner core, is highly conserved across bacterial species [2]. Animal studies have demonstrated that the lipid A portion of the inner core is the pathogenic moiety of LPS and that it is responsible for the release of many of the mediators, including tumor necrosis factor (TNF), interleukin-1α (IL-1α), and interleukin-1β (IL-1β), thought to be involved in the pathogenesis of gram-negative sepsis [2–4].

Ever since the early observation [5] that survival from gram-negative sepsis was associated with the presence of elevated titers of anti-endotoxin antibodies, therapeutic administration of such antibodies has been investigated as a possible means to reduce mortality from this disease. Clinical trials using polyclonal antisera [6, 7] have had mixed results. One difficulty in using polyclonal antibodies is that it is not clear which antibodies present in the sera are actually the most useful. The development of antiendotoxin monoclonal antibodes, like Xomen-E5 (E5) [8], has been one approach to obviate this problem.

Antibodies that recognize epitopes located on the O-specific side chain, or type-specific antibodies, have been shown to reduce mortality of animals infected with the bacterial strain that had been used for immunization, but not

[1] Department of Critical Care, XOMA Corporation, Berkeley, CA, USA
[2] Department of Pre-Clinical Research, XOMA Corporation, Berkeley, CA, USA

Host Defense Dysfunction
in Trauma, Shock and Sepsis
Eds. Faist/Meakins/Schildberg
© Springer-Verlag, Berlin Heidelberg 1993

mortality of animals infected with other organisms [9]. This lack of broad-spectrum reactivity severely limits the usefulness of type-specific antibodies in clinical practice.

Another therapeutic approach has been to make monoclonal antibodies which react with antigens shared by all gram-negative organisms, such as lipid A. To that end, E5 was developed from mice immunized against the J5 mutant of *Escherichia coli* O111:B4. This rough Rc mutant lacks O-specific side chains and outer core and has increased expression of the inner core and lipid A. In this paper we discuss some of the in vitro binding characteristics of E5 to a variety of gram-negative bacteria.

Materials and Methods

Monoclonal Antibodies. Murine immunoglobulin (IgM) monoclonal anitbody (mAb) Xomen-E5 (E5) was produced by immunization of BALB/c mice with heat-killed *E. coli* J5 cells [8]. E5, a murine IgM isotype control antibody (B55, reactive with a peptide portion of milk fat globulin) and the anti-*Pseudomonas aeruginosa* Fisher type 2 specific anitbody, designated OP2 (which is similar to OP1, described by Stoll et al. [9]), were produced and purified to homogeneity from either ascites fluid (E5) or tissue culture supernatants (B55 and OP2). All samples were found to have less than 5 endotoxin units (EU)/mg protein in the *Limulus* amebocyte lysate assay (QCL-1000, Whittaker Bioproducts Inc., Walkersville, MD, USA).

Bacterial Isolates. Rough mutant strains and clinical isolates were provided by Dr. Lowell Young, Kuzell Institute for Arthritis and Infectious Diseases, San Francisco, CA, USA.

Nitrocellulose Immunodot Enzyme-Linked Immunoabsorbent Assay. Boiled bacterial cells were diluted to approximately 2.5×10^8 cells/ml in Dulbecco's phosphate-buffered saline, pH 7.4 (D-PBS). Approximately 0.5-µl dots were formed on nitrocellulose strips and air-dried 10 min before blocking with 0.3 ml of 1% gelatin in D-PBS (D-PBS/gel) in 24-well culture plates. After three washes in D-PBS, 0.3 ml of 5 µg/ml antibody in D-PBS (either E5 or the isotype control antibody, B55) was then incubated with the strips for 30 min at room temperature (RT). Following three washes, 0.3 ml of a 1:300 dilution of horseradish peroxidase-conjugated goat anti-mouse IgM (µ-chain-specific, Zymed Laboratories Inc., San Francisco, CA, USA; HRP-GAMIgM) in D-PBS was added and incubated for 30 min at RT. The strips were then washed four times, and the amount of bound antibody determined using a 4-chloro-naphthol (4-CN) substrate solution made by mixing 25 ml D-PBS, 5 ml 4-CN (3 mg/ml) in methanol, and 10 µl 30% hydrogen peroxide. The resulting reaction intensity was scored visually on duplicate samples from no reactivity (−) to maximum reactivity (+ + +).

Microtiter EIA. Antigens (at about 5×10^6 cells/ml in D-PBS) were dispensed in 100-μl aliquots into microtiter plates and incubated overnight at 37 °C in the presence of 25 μg/ml DNase I to minimize bacterial aggregation. Following a wash with D-PBS containing 0.05% Tween 20 (D-PBS/T), the wells were blocked with 300 μl D-PBS/gel for 2 h at 37 °C. Wells were then washed with D-PBS/T, 50-μl aliquots of E5 or the isotype control (at 10 μl/ml in D-PBS/T) were added, and the plates incubated for 1 h at 37 °C. Following five washes in D-PBS/T, 50 μl/well of a 1:1000 dilution of HRP-GAMIgM in D-PBS/T was added, and the plates incubated for 1 h at RT. The plates were then washed five times in D-PBS/T and the amount of bound antibody determined by adding 100 μl/well substrate solution. A 20 mg/ml stock solution of 2-2'-azino-di-[3-ethylbenzthiazoline sulfonate (6)] diammonium salt (ABTS, Boehringer Mannheim Biochemicals, Indianapolis, IN, USA) substrate in 0.1 M citrate buffer, pH 4.5, was diluted 1:50 in citrate buffer and 1 μl 30% hydrogen peroxide was added per milliliter of substrate solution immediately prior to use. Absorbance at 405 nm (OD 405) was then recorded using an automated plate reader (V_{max}, Molecular Devices Corp., Menlo Park, CA, USA). Results are expressed as the mean of triplicate samples ± standard error of the mean.

Flow Cytometry Analysis. In order to reduce background noise, all buffers were filtered through 0.1- or 0.22-μm filters twice prior to use. *E. coli* J5 bacteria were grown in trypticase soy broth, harvested in early log phase by centrifugation (20 min at $600 \times g$), and washed three times with D-PBS. Bacterial suspensions were washed twice in normal saline containing 1% bovine serum albumin (NSBSA) and resuspended to 1×10^8 colony-forming units (CFU) in 1 ml NSBSA. To each sample was added 10 μg/ml of the appropriate antibody (either E5, B55, or OP2) and the samples incubated for 1 h at 37 °C. After the

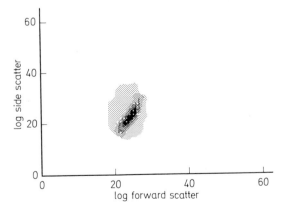

Fig. 1. Light scatter profile of *Escherichia coli* J5 cells as analyzed by flow cytometry

incubation, the samples were washed twice with NSBSA and 10 µg/ml of the goat anti-mouse IgM fluorescein isothiocyanate (FITC, µ-chain-specific, Caltag, San Francisco, CA, USA) was added to all tubes. The samples were then incubated for 30 min on ice, washed twice with NSBSA, and fixed with 1% formaldehyde in D-PBS.

Samples were analysed on a FACScan (Becton Dickinson, San Jose, CA, USA) using log amplification of both forward and side scatter. A region of the single cell scatter was gated to eliminate interfering signals (Fig. 1). The fluorescence was detected using 488-nm laser excitation and a 530/30-nm bandpass filter and log amplification. Approximately 20 000 events in the gated region were collected and analyzed.

Table 1. Binding of antibodies to boiled whole-cell antigens from bacteria in the immunodot EIA

Organism	Antibody binding	
Gram-positive	E5	B55
Staphylococcus aureus	−	−
Gram-negative		
Salmonella minnesota		
wild-type	+	−
R595 (Re)	+ + +	−
Escherichia coli		
O4:K12	+	−
O7:K7:H4	+	−
CDC 008	−	−
O14:K7	+ +	−
O14:H31 4310-65	+	−
O18	+ +	−
O55:B5	+	−
O55:B6	+ +	−
O85:H9	+ +	−
J5 (Rc)	+ +	−
Shigella boydii	+ +	−
Klebsiella caroli	+	−
Enterobacter cloacae	+ +	−
Serratia marcescens	+	−
Proteus mirabilis	+	−
Proteus vulgaris	+	−
Pseudomonas aeruginosa		
Fisher type 2 #3632	−	−
PAC 557	+ +	−
PAC 605	+ +	−
Pseudomonas maltophilia	+ +	−
Acinetobacter calcoaceticus	−	−
Citrobacter freundi	+	−
Providencia stuartii	+	−

EIA, enzyme-linked immunoabsorbent assay; E5, Xomen-E5

Results

The binding of E5 and the isotype control antibody B55 to boiled whole-cell antigen preparations in immunodot enzyme-linked immunoabsorbent assay (EIA) is shown in Table 1. As can be seen, E5 bound to varying degrees to 22 of the 25 gram-negative organisms tested, including 11/13 clinical isolates representing Enterobacteriaceae, Pseudomonadaceae, and other gram-negative bacterial families. In addition, E5 did not react to the one gram-positive strain tested in the immunodot format, nor was B55 reactive to any of the antigens tested.

The observation that E5 recognizes antigen(s) common to gram-negative but not gram-positive organisms was confirmed and extended using the microtiter EIA format. As seen in Table 2, E5 reacted to isolates from representatives of *Salmonella*, *Escherichia*, and *Pseudomonas* species to a greater extent than with the isotype control antibody. In addition, E5 did not react to the gram-positive strains tested.

The ability of E5 to bind to live bacteria was then studied, using fluorescein-conjugated antibodies and flow cytometric analysis similar to that recently reported by Evans et al. [10]. As seen in Fig. 2, E5 binds to live *E. coli* J5 bacteria. This binding of E5 to the live bacteria was uniform in that the majority of cells bound with a similar intensity. Moreover, no significant reactivity was

Table 2. EIA reactivity of bacterial whole-cell antigens to E5 or the isotope control antibody B55

Strain	OD_{405} nm		
	E5	B55	E5-B55
Gram-negative			
Escherichia coli J5 (Rc)	0.701	0.094	0.607
Salmonella minnesota R595 (Re)	0.671	0.068	0.603
Pseudomonas aeruginosa			
PAC 605	0.627	0.186	0.441
Fisher type 1	0.131	0.084	0.046
Fisher type 2(#3632)	0.217	0.111	0.106
Fisher type 3	0.882	0.09	0.792
Gram-positive			
Staphylococcus aureus			
Smith	0.123	0.185	0.000
#82	0.095	0.067	0.028
Streptococcus pneumoniae	0.082	0.093	0.000

Boiled bacterial whole cells were diluted to approximately 5×10^8 cells/ml in D-PBS and 100-µl aliquots were added to Immulon 1 plates. After incubation, the plates were washed, blocked, and the binding of each antibody determined as described in "Materials and Methods." Values represent the mean of triplicate samples.

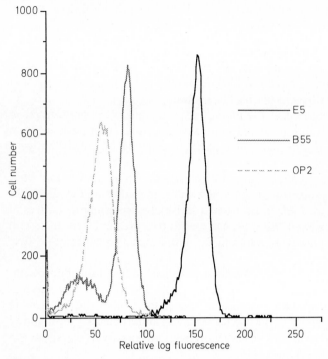

Fig. 2. *E. coli* J5 cells were grown overnight in trypticase soy broth, washed, resuspended to 1×10^8 bacteria/ml, and incubated with 10 µg/ml of either E5 (——), the isotype control B55 (······), or a *Pseudomonas aeruginosa* O-side chain specifc antibody, OP2 (   ). Following washing and counterstaining with a fluorescein-conjugated goat anti-mouse IgM antibody, the fluorescence intensity was analyzed using a FACScan (Becton-Dickinson, Calif, USA)

seen with isotype control antibody, B55, nor with OP2 (an IgM antibody specific for *Pseudomonas aeruginosa* Fisher type 2 LPS). As expected, the type-specific antibody OP2 did react to live *P. aeruginosa* bacteria (data not shown).

Discussion

We have shown that the E5 antibody reacts specifically to most gram-negative organisms by several different in vitro assays. This broad reactivity is consistent with the notion that E5 recognizes an epitope shared by many of the gram-negative bacteria. Further investigations by our laboratory [11, 12] and others [8, 13] have confirmed that E5 reacts to the lipid A portion of the LPS molecule. Using a variety of assays, (including EIA, radioimmunoassay, and antigen competition), we have found that E5 is reactive to a majority of LPS isolated from smooth and rough organisms, as well as most lipid A forms tested.

These results support and extend those observations published by Young and his colleagues [8, 13] who showed that E5 was an anti-lipid A antibody which provided protection against a variety of gram-negative organisms in murine animal model systems of sepsis. Indeed, recent clinical trials using this antiendotoxin antibody have shown that Xomen-E5 can significantly reduce the mortality from gram-negative sepsis whether or not bacteremia is present [14], and that the effects of E5 therapy are especially striking among those patients with multiple organ failure [15, 16]. Further investigations are underway to support and extend our observations that the antiendotoxin antibody E5 has wide application in the treatment of gram-negative sepsis.

References

 1. Bone RC, Fisher LT, Clemmer TP et al. (1989) Sepsis syndrome: a valid clinical entity. Crit Care Med 17:389–393
 2. Lüderitz O, Tanamoto K, Galanos C et al. (1984) Lipopolysaccharides: structural principles and biologic activities. Rev Infect Dis 6:428–431
 3. Andersson JF, Melchers C, Galancos C et al. (1973) The mitogenic effects of lipopolysaccharide on bone marrow derived mouse lymphocytes. J Exp Med 39:943–950
 4. Galanos C, Lüderitz O, Rietschel ET et al. (1985) Synthetic and natural *Escherichia coli* free lipid A express identical endotoxic activities. Eur J Biochem 148:1–5
 5. McCabe WR, Kreger BE, Johns M (1972) Type-specific and cross-reactive anti-bodies in Gram-negative bacteremia. N Engl J Med 287:261–267
 6. Ziegler EJ, McCutchan JA, Fierer J et al. (1982) Treatment of Gram-negative bacteremia and shock with human antiserum to a mutant *Escherichia coli*. N Engl J Med 307:1225–1230
 7. Calandra T, Glauser MP, Schellekens J et al. (1988) Treatment of Gram-negative septic shock with human IgG antibody to *Escherichia coli* J5: a prospective, double-blind, randomized trial. J Infect Dis 158:312–319
 8. Young LS (1984) Functional activity of monoclonal antibodies against lipopolysaccharide (LPS) antigens of Gram negative bacilli. Clin Res (abstract) 32/2:518A
 9. Stoll BJ, Pollack M, Young LS et al. (1986) Functionally active monoclonal antibody that recognizes an epitope on the O side chain of *Pseudomonas aeruginosa* immunotype-1 lipopoly-saccharide. Infect Immun 53:656–662
10. Evans ME, Pollack M, Hardegen NJ et al. (1990) Fluorescence-activated cell sorter analysis of binding by lipopolysaccharide-specific monoclonal antibodies to Gram-negative bacteria. J Infect Dis 162:148–155
11. Wood D, Parent JB, Gazzano-Santoro H (1992) Reactivity of monoclonal antibody E5® with endotoxin. I. Binding to lipid A and rough lipopolysaccharides. Circ Shock (in press)
12. Parent JB et al. (1992) Reactivity of monoclonal antibody E5® with endotoxin. II. Binding to short- and long-chain smooth lipopolysaccharides. Circ Shock (in press)
13. Young LS, Gascon R, Alam S et al. (1989) Monoclonal antibodies for treatment of Gram-negative infections. Rev Infect Dis 11/Suppl 7:S1564–S1571
14. Gorelick K, Scannon PJ, Hannigan J et al. (1990) Randomized placebo-controlled study of E5 monoclonal antiendotoxin antibody. In: Larrick JW, Borrebaeck CK (eds) Therapeutic mono-clonal antibodies. Stockton, New York, pp 253–261
15. MacIntyre NR, Schein RM, Hannigan JF et al. (1990) E5 antibody enhances resolution of multi-organ failure in Gram-negative sepsis. Chest (abstract) 98/2 Suppl:135S
16. MacIntyre NR, Emmanuel G, Wedel NI et al. (1991) E5 antibody improves outcome from multi-organ failure in survivors of Gram-negative sepsis. Crit Care Med (abstract) 19/4 Suppl:S14

Immunotherapy with Human Antiendotoxin Antibodies in the Treatment of Gram-Negative Sepsis: Practical Considerations

C. H. Wortel

Gram-negative sepsis is an increasingly common disease, with a high mortality rate [1]. Endotoxin, present in the outer membrane of all gram-negative bacteria, is an important trigger in the development of the septic syndrome [2]. Recently, a multicenter, double-blind, placebo-controlled trial showed a significant reduction in mortality in gram-negative bacteremic patients who were treated with the human antiendotoxin monoclonal immunoglobulin M (IgM) antibody HA-1A (Centoxin) [3].

Antiendotoxin therapy should be most effective in endotoxemic patients. Furthermore, there is strong evidence that the pathophysiologic effects of endotoxin are due to the induction of tumor necrosis factor (TNF) release from host defense cells [4, 5]. Reducing the amount of circulating TNF could be one of the mechanisms by which the antiendotoxin antibody HA-1A influences the pathophysiology of gram-negative sepsis in humans.

These hypotheses were tested in a controlled prospective study in which 90 consecutive patients with suspected gram-negative sepsis were enrolled [6, 7]. In 82 patients, serial blood samples for detection of endotoxin could be assessed. Endotoxemia was present in 27 of 82 patients, which in 33% of the total study population. Forty-one patients were treated with placebo and 41 received 100 mg HA-1A in a single intravenous dose. The presence of gram-negative infections and gram-negative bacteremia was well matched between the two groups. Treatment with HA-1A reduced the 28-day mortality in all patients from 61% (25/41 placebo-treated patients) to 34% [14/41 HA-1A-treated patients ($p < 0.01$)]. THe observed treatment effect was mainly attributable to the reduction seen in endotoxemic patients. The mortality was 73% in the placebo-treated patients versus 31% in the HA-1A-treated patients ($p = 0.02$). In nonendotoxemic patients, the mortality decreased from 57% in the placebo-treated patients to 39% in the HA-1A-treated patients ($p = 0.13$). In the 24-h period following treatment, HA-1A caused a significant decrease in serum levels of TNF. The median change was -12 ng/l in the HA-1A-treated patients versus 0 ng/l in the placebo-treated patients ($p = 0.04$). Interestingly, this phe-

Infectious Disease Clinical Research, Centocor Inc., 200 Great Valley Parkway Malvern, Pennsylvania 19355-1307 USA and Baylor College of Medicine, Department of Critical Care, Ben Taub Hospital, 1504 Taub Loop, Houston, Texas 77030, USA

Host Defense Dysfunction
in Trauma, Shock and Sepsis
Eds. Faist/Meakins/Schildberg
© Springer-Verlag, Berlin Heidelberg 1993

nomenon was already apparent 1 h after administration of HA-1A. The ability of HA-1A to decrease serum TNF levels has been confirmed in another study in which higher dosages of HA-1A were given.

These studies show that HA-1A is highly effective in patients with endotoxemia or a high incidence of endotoxemia, such as gram-negative bacteremic patients. The observed decrease in circulating TNF levels supports the concept that the beneficial effects of HA-1A in gram-negative sepsis may be caused by interference with endotoxin-induced activation of host defense cells.

Now that a clear benefit of therapy with the human antiendotoxin has been established, the challenge of selecting the appropriate patients becomes an important issue. Unfortunately, our ability to make a timely diagnosis of gram-negative bacteremia is limited. Chromogenic modifications of the Limulus method for detection of endotoxin in blood have resulted in increased assay sensitivity and permitted a more accurate diagnosis of endotoxemia [8, 9]. Furthermore, this assay provides a rapid assessment of endotoxin levels in blood, providing results within 3 h. However, the clinical usefulness of this assay is currently limited. A sensitivity of 3 ng/l is needed to detect endotoxemia in nonmeningococcal septic patients. A concomitant high frequency of false positives due to contamination with exogenous endotoxin is observed unless appropriate procedures are rigorously followed. Since endotoxemia may be an intermittent phenomenon, one can only rely on a (true) positive test result. In case of a negative result, multiple samples over time will have to be obtained. Endogenous mediators implicated in the pathogenesis of sepsis could possibly be used for identifying septic patients. To evaluate patients for antiendotoxin therapy, the use of mediators instead of endotoxin would possibly delay administration of the treatment, since the mediators appear as a result of the endotoxemic insult [10]. Furthermore, the mediators are common to many forms of "systemic immune response syndrome", such as both gram-negative- and gram-positive sepsis, fungal or parasitic sepsis, pancreatitis, and anaphylactic shock [11, 12]. Therefore, it would be impossible to make a distinction between the various forms of sepsis, using mediator levels. For future trials involving antimediator antibodies both the TNF and interleukin-6 (IL-6) assays are thought to be of value. TNF assays still require a substantial amount of time, preventing a prospective selection of patients on the basis of their TNF levels. Faster radioimmuno assays have been developed, but at present it is still unclear whether these assays detect the same epitopes as the older assays that have been found useful in predicting mortality. Therefore these new assays need to be clinically validated. IL-6 levels provide the most accurate prediction of mortality in the septic patient [13–15]. However, elevated levels are found following all sorts of disturbance of the hemostasis of the organism. For instance, IL-6 levels are elevated following surgery and may reflect the magnitude of the surgical trauma [16, 17]. Therefore, IL-6 levels could not be used to determine whether a patient is septic during the postoperative period. At present, none of the assays available are capable of selecting patients for antiendotoxin antibody therapy in a clinical setting.

Nonetheless, a logical approach to decision making in administering HA-1A can be developed. The decision is based on the severity of the systemic response to infection and the likelihood of gram-negative organism etiology. First, a systemic response to infection should be present, (e.g., fever or hypothermia, tachycardia, or tachypnea), combined with evidence of systemic organ dysfunction, (e.g., hypotension, arterial hypoxemia, metabolic acidosis, oliguria, thrombocytopenia, or acute hepatic failure). Second, a high likelihood of a gram-negative organism etiology of the systemic response should be present. Typically, one would expect such a high likelihood of gram-negative etiology in patients with pyelonephritis, nosocomial pneumonia, peritonitis complicating a ruptured bowel or abdominal surgery, wound or soft-tissue infection complicating abdominal surgery, and septic shock without evidence of a source of infection. Patients who meet these criteria are candidates for HA-1A therapy. Gramstains, an old but undervalued test, could enhance our diagnostic abilities. HA-1A should be administered as soon as possible after establishing the criteria as outlined above. This is a matter of importance, since 20% of the patients who are not in shock at the time they meet the criteria will establish shock within 12 h; a condition which is associated with a much higher mortality [3].

Advances in biotechnology during the last decade have led to the development of specific products that modify the biological effects of exogenous and endogenous molecules. HA-1A is the first human monoclonal antiendotoxin antibody proven effective in man. It will prove to be an important addition to our armamentarium against gram-negative sepsis and will further increase our understanding of the pathophysiology of this disease.

References

1. Bone R, Fisher C, Clemmer T, Slotman G, Metz C, Balk R, Methylprednisolone Severe Sepsis Study Group (1989) Sepsis syndrome: a valid clinical entity. Crit Care Med 17:389–393
2. Hamill RJ, Maki DG (1986) Endotoxin shock in man caused by gram-negative bacilli. Etiology, clinical features, diagnosis, natural history and prevention. In: Proctor RA (ed) Handbook of endotoxin, vol. 4. Elsevier, Amsterdam, pp 55–126
3. Ziegler EJ, Fisher CJ, Sprung CL, Straube RC, Sadoff JC, Foulke GE et al. (1991) Treatment of gram-negative bacteremia and septic shock with HA-1A human monoclonal antibody against endotoxin. A randomized, double-blind, placebo-controlled clinical trial. N Engl J Med 324:429–436
4. Tracey K, Vlassara H, Cerami A (1989) Cachectin/tumor necrosis factor. Lancet I:1122–1126
5. Beutler B, Cerami A (1987) Cahectin: more than a tumor necrosis factor. N Engl J Med 316:379–385
6. Wortel CH, Sprung CL, van Deventer SJH, Lubbers MJ, ten Cate JW (1990) Anti-endotoxin treatment with HA-1A: possible mechanism of beneficial effects in patients with gram-negative septicemia. Proceedings of the international congress for infectious diseases, Montreal, p 206
7. Wortel CH, von der Mohlen MAM, van Deventer SJH, Sprung CL, Jastremski M, Lubbers MJ et al. (1992) Effectiveness of a human monoclonal anti-endotoxin antibody (HA-1A) in gram-negative sepsis: relationship to endotoxin and cytokine levels (to be published)
8. Sturk A, van Deventer SJH, Wortel CH, Levels JHM, ten Cate JW, Buller HR et al. (1990) Detection and clinical relevance of human endotoxemia. Z Med Lab Diagn 31:147–158
9. Sturk A, ten Cate JW (1985) Endotoxin testing revisited. Eur J Clin Microbiol 4:382–385

10. Michie HR, Manogue KR, Spriggs DR et al (1988) Detection of circulating tumor necrosis factor after endotoxin administration. N Engl J Med 318:1481–1486
11. Meager A (1990) Cytokines. Open University Press, Buckingham
12. Kern P, Hemmer CJ, van Damme J, Gruss HJ, Dietrich M (1989) Elevated tumor necrosis factor alpha and interleukin-6 serum levels as markers for complicated *Plasmodium falciparum* malaria. Am J Med 87:139–143
13. Hack CE, de Groot ER, Felt-Bersma RJF et al. (1989) Increased plasma levels of interleukin-6 in sepsis. Blood 74:1704–1710
14. Wortel CH, van Deventer SJH, Buller HR et al. (1990) Relationship between IL-6 level and the efficacy of HA-1A, a human monoclonal, anti-endotoxin antibody. 30th interscience conference of antimicrobial agents and chemotherapy, Atlanta, p 239
15. Wortel CH, Ziegler EJ, van Deventer SJH (1991) Therapy of gram-negative sepsis in man with anti-endotoxin antibodies: a review. Prog Clin Biol Res 367:161–178
16. Wortel CH, van Deventer SJH, Verbeek CPR et al (1990) Interleukin-6 mediates host defense responses induced by abdominal surgery. Circ Shock 31:254
17. Wortel CH, van Deventer SJH, von der Mohlen MAM et al. (1990) Both abdominal and plastic surgery induce systemic interleukin-6 release. Circ Shock 31:255

The Use of Antibody Specificity and Affinity in Determining the Protectiveness of Human Monoclonal Antibodies Against Fatal Infections with Nosocomial Gram-Negative Bacteria

U. Bruderer, A. B. Lang, B. Byl, A. Crusiaux, J. Deviere

Introduction

Passive immunization with human monoclonal antibodies (mAb) may become a feasible alternative to the classical treatment of fatal infections with antibiotic-resistant gram-negative bacteria. However, the search for and the generation of therapeutically active human mAb depends upon an improvement in the understanding of the immunological basis of protection.

Here, in an attempt to define binding properties associated with protective potential, we analyzed lipopolysaccharide (LPS)-specific mAb for their fine specificities, affinities, and the capacities to protect against lethal bacterial infection.

Materials and Methods

Antigens. Growth of bacteria and the isolation of LPS has been described [1].

Monoclonal Antibodies. A17H193, 2-8AH79, and 109PAN have been described [2–4].

Polyclonal Antibodies. The standard IVIG preparation Globuman Berna i.v., lot no. 040287 was prepared in the Swiss Serum and Vaccine Institute, Berne, Switzerland. The standard IVIG Sandoglobulin, lot no. 83622060 was purchased from Sandoz-Wander Pharma AG, Berne, Switzerland. The hyper-immune IVIG Nosocuman, lot no. 170490 was prepared in the Swiss Serum and Vaccine Institute, Berne, Switzerland from the blood of donors immunized with a polyvalent PS-ToxA conjugate vaccine [5].

Protection Assay. The protective capacity of antibody preparations was tested using a murine burn wound model [6]. Fold protection was determined by dividing the lethal dose value for 50% of the group (LD_{50}) of immunized mice by that of nonimmunized control mice.

Swiss Serum & Vaccine Institute, POB, 3001 Berne, Switzerland

Host Defense Dysfunction
in Trauma, Shock and Sepsis
Eds. Faist/Meakins/Schildberg
© Springer-Verlag, Berlin Heidelberg 1993

Determination of Antibody Specificity and Affinity. The molar concentration of inhibitor resulting in 50% inhibition of the antibody binding was determined as described [7]. The apparent affinity constants (aK_a) were determined by the Nieto et al. method [8]. Calculations of the molar concentrations were based on the assumed molecular weight of 10000 for LPS as described by Schwartzer et al. [9].

Results

From a panel of LPS-specific mAb, we selected three examples of the fine specificities generally occurring (Table 1). 109PAN recognizes an epitope in the core/lipid A moiety, which is conserved among all the tested *Pseudomonas aeruginosa* serotypes. 2-8AH79 is specific for a determinant in the O chain which is restricted to four of the nine serotypes tested. A17H193 binds a serotype-specific O-chain determinant.

109PAN exhibits no detectable protective activity against infection with bacteria of any of the nine serotypes (Table 1). The remaining two human mAb protect against infections with bacteria of two (2-8AH79) or one serotype (A17H193).

All three mAb exhibit comparable affinities for the LPS of the *P. aeruginosa* PA220 strain (Table 2). But only A17H193 confers protection against the challenge with PA220 bacteria (Table 2). These results suggest that the non-protectiveness of 2-8AH79 and 109PAN is due to differences in the fine specificity rather than the affinity.

Table 3 shows that a polyclonal hyperimmune IVIG preparation (Nosocuman) exhibits significantly higher affinity for LPS than two standard IVIG preparations (Sandoglobulin, Globuman). Whereas 10 µg Nosocuman/mouse results in complete protection against a lethal dose of bacteria, even 1000 µg Sandoglobulin or Globuman/mouse confers no more than partial protection.

Table 1. In vitro and in vivo properties of LPS-specific antibodies

	Pseudomonas aeruginosa								
	Fisher serotypes							Habs serotypes	
mAb	1	2	3	4	5	6	7	3	4
109PAN	+	+	+	+	+	+	+	+	+
2-8AH79	+	−	✚	✚	−	+	−	−	−
A17H193	✚	−	−	−	−	−	−	−	−

LPS, lipopolysaccharide; mAb, monoclonal antibody; +, recognition of LPS of the corresponding serotype by enzyme-linked immunosorbant assay (ELISA) and western blot; ✚, recognition of LPS of the corresponding serotype by ELISA and western blot and protection in vivo against lethal challenge with bacteria of the corresponding serotype; −, no binding, no protection.

Table 2. Affinity and protective capacity of LPS-specific antibodies

mAb	aK_a ($\times 10^6 M^{-1}$)[a]	Protection[b]
A17H193	56	+
2-8AH79	59	−
109PAN	29	−

LPS, lipopolysaccharide; mAb, monoclonal antibody; [a]Affinity against the LPS of the *P. aeruginosa* strain PA220.
[b] Protection against a lethal challenge with bacteria of the strain PA220.

Table 3. Influence of affinity in the protective capacities of polyclonal preparations

Preparation[b]	aK_a ($\times 10^6 M^{-1}$)[c]	Protection[a] 10	100	1000
Sandoglobulin	0.25	0	20	60
Globuman	0.27	0	10	80
Nosocuman	5.9	100	100	100

[a] Percentage of mice surviving a challenge of 2.5×10^4 PA220 bacteria 20 h after the application of 10, 100, or 1000 µg antibodies/mouse.
[b] Globuman, Sandoglobulin: standard IVIG preparations; Nosocuman: hyperimmune IVIG preparation.
[c] Average affinities of the corresponding preparations for PA220 LPS

Discussion

Our results reveal that only antibodies specific for the O-chain moiety of LPS confer significant protection in a murine burn-wound sepsis model. However, specificity for the O chain of LPS is necessary but not sufficient. Protective capacity seems to be restricted to a small population of antibodies with high affinity for particular epitopes of the O chain. Within polyclonal O-chain-specific antibody populations, we show a strong correlation between affinity and protectivity (Table 3). From these results it seems that the protective capacity of antibodies with affinities above 10^6 is at least 100-fold higher than that of antibodies with affinities below 10^6.

Our results suggest that LPS-specific human mAb differ enormously in their potential to protect against fatal bacterial infections. Consequently, we focus our interests on determining those human mAb exhibiting high protection. At present, we have selected a panel of highly protective human mAb with high affinity for a significant portion of the clinically relevant serotypes of *P. aeruginosa*, *Escherichia coli*, and *Klebsiella pneumoniae*.

References

1. Cryz SL Jr, Pitt TL, Fürer E, Germanier R (1984) Role of lipopolysaccharide in virulence of *Pseudomonas aeruginosa.* Infect Immun 44:508
2. Lang AB, Fürer E, Larrick JW, Cryz SJ Jr (1989) Isolation and characterization of a human monoclonal antibody that recognizes epitopes shared by *Pseudomonas aeruginosa* immunotypes 1, 3, 4, and 6 lipopolysaccharides. Infect Immun 57:3851
3. Lang AB, Fürer E, Senyk G, Larrick JW, Cryz SJ Jr (1990) Systematic generation of antigen-specific human monoclonal antibodies with therapeutical activities using active immunization. Hum Antibod Hybridomas 1:96
4. Lang AB, Bruderer U, Larrick JW, Cryz SL Jr (1990) Immunoprotective capacities of human and murine monoclonal antibodies recognizing serotype specific and common determinants of gram-negative bacteria. In: Borrebaeck C, Larrick JW (eds) Therapeutic monoclonal antibodies. Stockton, New York
5. Cryz SL Jr, Lang AB, Sadoff JC, Germanier R, Fürer E (1987) Vaccine Potential of *Pseudomonas aeruginosa* O-Polysaccharide-Toxin A conjugates. Infect Immun 55:1547
6. Cryz SJ Jr, Fürer E, Germanier R (1983) Protection against *Pseudomonas aeruginosa* infection in a murine burn wound sepsis model by passive transfer of antitoxin A, antielastase, and antilipopolysaccharide. Infect Immun 39:1072
7. Bruderer U, Fürer E, Cryz SL Jr, Lang AB (1980) Qualitative analysis of antibody binding. An in vitro assay for the evaluation and development of vaccines. J Immunol Methods 133:263
8. Nieto A, Gaya A, Jansa M, Vives J (1984) Direct measurement of antibody affinity distribution of hapten-inhibition enzyme immunoassay. Mol Immunol 21:537
9. Schwartzer TA, Alcid DV, Numsuwan V, Glocke DJ (1989) Immunochemical specificity of human antibodies to lipopolysaccharide from the J5 rough mutant of *Escherichia coli* O11:B4. J Infect Dis 259:35

Section 18

**Interventional Strategies
in the Therapy of Septic Shock**

Potential Benefits of Platelet Activating Factor Receptor Antagonists in Endotoxemia/Sepsis

J. R. Fletcher[1], J. A. Moore[2], A. G. DiSimone[2], N. Abumerad[2], P. Williams[2], J. Pollard[1], J. Collins[1], and E. Graves[1]

Introduction

Endotoxemia/sepsis in animals and man is a complex entity that consists of a focus of infection and an inflammatory phase with a release of potent mediators that produce variable responses in the host. The relative degree of tissue/organ injury in these instances is dependent on the severity of insult and the state of the organ function.

The seminal mechanisms that are evident in endotoxemia/sepsis are unknown. Recently, platelet activating factor (PAF) has been implicated as a potential candidate for a central role in endotoxemia/sepsis [1]. The concept is supported by the observations that (a) exogenous PAF induces shock-like states in many animal species [2, 3], (b) PAF is synthesized/released in endotoxemia [4, 5, 6, 7], (c) PAF is increased in clinical sepsis [8], and (d) specific PAF receptor antagonists attenuate many of the pathophysiological events in endotoxemia and improve the survival [1, 9, 10]. All of the above suggest that PAF may have a role in endotoxemia/sepsis.

Previous reports from our laboratory have focused on the relationship of the eicosanoids to the circulatory dysfunction in endotoxemia/sepsis [1]. That the eicosanoids are significant participants in the pathophysiology of endotoxemia/sepsis is generally accepted by investigators in this field [11, 12]. Of particular interest are the observations that suggest that endotoxin, the eicosanoids, and PAF produce similar effects in animals: systemic hypotension, capillary permeability, pulmonary hypertension, organ failure, and death. Recent data that indicate there exists an intimate relationship between PAF and the eicosanoids in vivo [13] stimulated a series of studies addressing the issue in endotoxemia.

In this report, the results of the three most recent studies will be presented.

[1] Department of Surgery, University of South Alabama, Mobile, AL, USA
[2] Department of Surgery, Vanderbilt University, Nashville, TN, USA

Host Defense Dysfunction
in Trauma, Shock and Sepsis
Eds. Faist/Meakins/Schildberg
© Springer-Verlag, Berlin Heidelberg 1993

Materials and Methods

Rodent Endotoxemia

Male Sprague-Dawley rats (250–300 g, Charles River Laboratories) were stabilized from 2 to 4 days prior to experimentation. They were maintained in a 12-h light-dark sequence and allowed water and antibiotic-free chow ad libitum. On the day of the experiment animals were placed in individual cages. Each animal was lightly anesthetized with a halothane-oxygen mixture and had anterior neck incision followed by insertion of catheters (PE50) into the left carotid artery and left jugular vein. Catheters were flushed with heparinized saline, tunneled to the dorsal neck of the rat, and secured. The jugular vein catheter was utilized for injections of saline or pharmacological agents. Rats were allowed to recover from the effects of anesthesia for at least 1 h before baseline parameters were measured. At the completion of the experiments, animals were sacrificed.

Canine Endotoxemia

Adult male mongrel dogs (17–22 kg) were stabilized in large cages for at least 7 days prior to study. On the day before the experiments, dogs were anesthetized with Surital 25 mg/kg. Following intubation and ventilation, a Swan-Ganz catheter was inserted into the pulmonary artery via the right jugular vein utilizing pressure monitoring. From the same neck incision, a silicone catheter was placed in the right carotid artery and advanced into the aorta. The catheters were tunneled subcutaneously to the dorsum of the neck and secured. Catheters were placed in a pocketed vest designed to protect them. Animals were extubated, allowed to recover from anesthesia, and returned to their cages. They were given food and water ad libitum until 24 h before the experiment, then they had only free access to water. Surgical procedures were performed using sterile techniques.

Blood samples were collected in heparinized syringes and immediately placed on ice. The blood was immediately aliquoted for determination of arterial blood gases, hematocrit, hemoglobin, and plasma bicarbonate determination on an acid-base analyzer (Radiometer, ABL-30, Copenhagen, Denmark). *Escherichia coli* endotoxin (055:B5, Difco Laboratories, Detroit, MI, USA) was reconstituted in saline (10 mg/ml) on the day of the experiment. BN52021 was generously supplied by Dr. Pierre Braquet, Institut Henri Beaufour, Le Plessis Robinson, France, and reconstituted in phosphate-buffered saline on the day of the experiment (10 mg/ml).

Experimental Design

Rodent Endotoxemia

All experiments were performed in an Association for Accreditation for Laboratory Animal Care (AALAC) approved facility and according to the National Institutes of Health (NIH) guidelines for animal use. Rats for hemodynamic and eicosanoid measurements were studied in individual cages. Indwelling catheters were flushed with sterile heparinized saline. There was a 30-min ($-$ 30 to 0 min) basal period and a 2-h (0–120 min) experimental period during which hemodynamic measurements were recorded continuously. These consisted of measurements of heart rate (HR) and mean arterial pressure (MAP). At time (t) 0, the animals received an i.v. bolus injection of endotoxin. In studies where the effect of PAF antagonists were examined, the antagonists were given at specified time points prior to 0 min.

For the survival studies, male rates were randomized into two groups. Group I ($n = 10$) and group II ($n = 13$) received $E.$ $coli$ endotoxin (20 mg/kg) i.p. at time 0. Group I animals received diluent (0.5 ml) for the PAF receptor antagonist BN52021 administered subcutaneously at $-$ 30 min, whereas group II animals received BN52021 (25 mg/kg) administered subcutaneously at $-$ 30 min. The animals had free access to food and water. Survival was determined at 24, 48, and 72 h. Permanent survival was determined at 72 h and is reported in percent.

The animals for hemodynamic and eicosanoid measurements were randomized into two groups following catheter insertion: group III ($n = 5$) received the diluent of BN52021 i.v. at $-$ 30 min and then $E.$ $coli$ endotoxin (20 mg/kg) i.v. at 0 min, whereas group IV ($n = 5$) received BN52021 (25 mg/kg) i.v. $-$ 30 min and then $E.$ $coli$ endotoxin (20 mg/kg) i.v. at 0 min. Blood samples for eicosanoid analysis were collected in heparinized tubes containing indomethacin (100 μg), the blood was centrifuged, and the plasma was removed and stored at $-$ 80 °C until assayed. For each milliliter of blood removed, 1 ml 0.9% saline was returned to the animal via the arterial catheter. Following completion of the experiment, animals were sacrificed.

For the studies that compared the effects of PAF receptor antagonist to the effects of a cyclooxygenase inhibitor on eicosanoid synthesis/release the above rat model for hemodynamic events was used. Rats were randomized into four groups: group I ($n = 7$), $E.$ $coli$ endotoxin (12 mg/kg) alone; group II ($n = 7$), $E.$ $coli$ endotoxin/PAF receptor antagonist (BN52021, 25 mg/kg i.v., $-$ 30 min); group III ($n = 8$), $E.coli$ endotoxin/cyclooxygenase inhibitor (Ibuprofen 30 mg/kg i.v., $-$ 40 min and $+$ 240 min); group IV ($n = 4$), PAF receptor antagonist alone (BN52021, 25 mg/kg, i.v.).

The selection of doses of endotoxin was determined with dose-response studies in our laboratory. Control studies in animals not given endotoxin were performed in rats with the following groups: (1) anesthesia alone ($n = 4$); (2)

anesthesia plus incision and ligation of vessels ($n = 5$); (3) anesthesia, incision, catheter placement, and vehicle administration (saline) for the endotoxin studies ($n = 5$); and (4) the diluent for the BN52021 studies ($n = 5$). None of the perturbations had any significant effect on either the hemodynamic or eicosanoid changes and hence were not included.

Data analysis was accomplished by ANOVA for repeated measures and least squares regression for significance between the groups. Differences in survival were determined by the chi-square method. A p value of < 0.05 was considered significant.

Canine Endotoxemia

All experiments were performed in an AALAC-approved facility and according to the NIH guidelines for animal use. The dogs were studied in a body support (sling) and allowed to stand during the experiment. Indwelling catheters were flushed with sterile heparinized saline. A 30-min basal period (-30 to 0 min) during which hemodynamic measurements were recorded continuously. Hemodynamic measurements included HR, MAP, mean pulmonary arterial pressure (PAP), pulmonary capillary wedge pressure (PCWP), central venous pressure (CVP), and cardiac output (CO). Each CO value was determined as the average of two consecutive measurements. Systemic vascular resistance (SVR) and pulmonary vascular resistance (PVR) were calculated from the data [SVR$-$(MAP $-$ CVP)/CO and PVR $-$ (PAP $-$ PCWP)/CO)] and expressed in arbitrary units. At time 0, each animal received a bolus injection of endotoxin (1 mg/kg, i.v.).

Blood samples were obtained at time 0, then at 2, 60, 120, and 240 min after endotoxin administration. Hemodynamic parameters were determined at the same time as the blood sampling. Animals were randomized into two groups: group I, endotoxin-vehicle ($n = 10$), received a lethal dose for 100% of the group (LD$_{100}$ dose) of E. coli endotoxin (1 mg/kg) i.v. at time 0; group II, endotoxin-BN52021 ($n = 10$), received BN52021 (5 mg/kg) i.v. 30 min before and 240 min after E. coli endotoxin administration. All animals received initial volumes of saline (0.9% w/v) to standardize the PCWP to 6 Torr before the experiment. During the 4-h experiment, 400 ml balanced salt solution was administered, and at the end of 4 h an additional 400 ml was given over 30 min. The catheters were removed and the animals were returned to their individual cages. They were given free access to food and water. Survival was determined at 24, 48, and 72 h. Only five animals in each group were used to determine survival, as dictated by our animal-use committee.

For hemodynamic measurements of both rats and dogs, the catheters were connected to a Gould Brush physiograph (RS2300) via a PE23 transducer (Statham, Oxnard, CA, USA). Cardiac outputs of the dogs were calculated with an Edwards computer (Model 9320) using a thermodilution method. Levels of thromboxane (TxB_2) and prostaglandin $E_2(PGE_2)$ were measured in plasma specimens collected at baseline, then at 5, 30, 60, and 120 min after endotoxin administration in coincident with hemodynamic measurements. Analyses were performed by radioimmunoassay. Cross-reactivity of the antibodies is less than 3% with other eicosanoid metabolites. Radiolabeled TxB_2, 6-keto-PGF_1, and PGE_2 were obtained from New England Nuclear (Boston, MA, USA). Authentic eicosanoids TxB_2, PGI_2, and PGE_2 were generously supplied by Dr. John Pike (Upjohn Co., Kalamazoo, MI, USA). *E. coli* endotoxin (055:B5, Difco Laboratories, Detroit, MI, USA) was reconstituted in saline (10 mg/ml) on the day of the experiment. The PAF receptor antagonist BN52021 was supplied by Dr. Pierre Braquet, Institut Henri Beaufour, Le Plessis Robinson, France. BN52021 was diluted in a phosphate solution (pH 7.3) on the day of the experiment (10 mg/ml).

The survival data were analyzed using a chi-square test. For the other parameters, the two treatments were compared using a repeated-measures ANOVA. Between treatment groups, the values were compared to each time point using a least squares regression analysis test. A probability of $p < 0.05$ was considered significant.

Results

The Effects of the PAF receptor antagonist BN52021 on the hemodynamic events, eicosanoid release, and survival in *rat endotoxemia* were as follows:

1. The PAF receptor antagonist did not attenuate the early systemic hypotension induced by endotoxin (88 ± 3, 90 ± 8 Torr), but did attenuate the 4-h hypotension (74 ± 7 vs 100 ± 4 Torr).
2. PAF receptor antagonism attenuated thromboxane (TxB_2) synthesis/release for all time points after endotoxin except at 120 min, when TxB_2 values 734 ± 93 pg/ml were significantly ($p < 0.05$) different from the baseline values (368 ± 88) pg/ml). PGE_2 values were significantly increased after endotoxin, similar to TxB_2 values. PAF receptor antagonism attenuated PGE_2 synthesis/release.
3. PAF receptor antagonism improved survival from 20% (2/10) in the endotoxin alone group to 85% (11/13) in the PAF receptor antagonist group ($p < 0.01$).

The effects of the PAF receptor antagonist BN52021 on the hemodynamic events. eicosanoid release, and survival in *lethal canine endotoxemia* were as follows:

1. Endotoxin alone increased the HR (baseline 116 ± 6 bpm vs 149 ± 8 bpm at 240 min); produced systemic hypotension (baseline 123 ± 5 Torr vs 54 ± 5

Torr at 2 min); decreased the CO (baseline 3.01 ± 31 l/min vs 1.26 ± 0.2 l/min at 2 min); and increased PVR (baseline 3.2 ± 0.6 units vs 13 ± 3 units at 2 min). PAF receptor antagonism attenuated the increase in HR, but had minimal effect on the other parameters.

2. PAF receptor antagonism minimally attenuated the metabolic acidosis and had little effect on hematocrit, PCO_2, PaO_2, and white blood cell (WBC) and platelet counts.

3. Endotoxin alone significantly ($p < 0.05$) enhanced release of all eicosanoids (TxB_2, PGE_2, 6-keto-PGF_1): TxB_2 baseline 0.26 ± 0.04 ng/ml versus 2.64 ± 0.96 ng/ml at 240 min ($p < 0.05$); PGE_2 baseline 0.20 ± 0.10 ng/ml versus 0.79 ± 0.35 ng/ml at 240 min (0.79 ± 0.35); 6-keto-PAF_1 baseline 0.140 ± 0.05 ng/ml versus peak of 2.07 ± 0.84 ng/ml at 60 min ($p < 0.05$). Administration of PAF receptor antagonist attenuated the increases in TxB_2 at 60, 120, and 240 min but had minimal effect on PGE_2 and 6-keto $PGF_{1\alpha}$ values.

4. There was a significant ($p < 0.01$) increase in permanent survival with PAF receptor antagonist pretreatment 100% (5 of 5) versus 0% (0 of 5) in canine endotoxemia.

The effects of the PAF receptor antagonist BN52021 on the eicosanoid release and hemodynamic events when compared with a cyclooxygenase inhibitor in *severe rat endotoxemia* were as follows:

1. PAF receptor antagonist did not attenuate the early systemic hypotension (80 ± 6 vs 84 ± 4 Torr) induced by endotoxin whereas cyclooxygenase pretreatment did (80 ± 6 vs 109 ± 5 Torr). Both PAF receptor antagonism and cyclooxygenase inhibition attenuated ($p < 0.05$) the hypotension at 2 h and beyond: endotoxin alone 72 ± 13 Torr; endotoxin + BN52021 105 ± 8 Torr; endotoxin + ibuprofen 112 ± 4 Torr.

2. PAF receptor antagonist alone significantly ($p < 0.02$) increased TxB_2: baseline 65 ± 15 pg/ml vs 126 ± 13 pg/ml at 5 min. PAF receptor antagonist significantly increased synthesis/release of PGE_2: baseline 79 ± 42 pg/ml vs 140 ± 28 pg/ml at 5 min. Ibuprofen alone increased TxB_2: baseline 65 ± 15 pg/ml vs 124 ± 36 pg/ml at 5 min.

3. With PAF receptor antagonism, endotoxin increased TxB_2 values 2.6 times (baseline 289 ± 132 pg/ml vs 764 ± 153 pg/ml at 4 h), compared with a 20-fold increase with endotoxin alone (base 68 ± 25 pg/ml vs 1460 ± 80 pg/ml at 4 h). PAF receptor antagonism had minimal effect on PGI_2 release by endotoxin, but the effects of PAF receptor antagonism on PGE_2 values were significantly greater (endotoxin alone baseline 99 ± 28 pg/ml vs 486 ± 70 pg/ml at 4 h; endotoxin + BN52021 baseline 144 ± 28 pg/ml vs 274 ± 39 pg/ml at 4 h, twice the baseline value).The PAF receptor antagonist attenuated the PGE values to less than one half the stimulation that endotoxin produced.

4. Ibuprofen attenuated the synthesis and release of all the cyclooxygenase products more effectively than did the PAF receptor antagonist.

Discussion

The results of these preliminary studies support the notion that PAF has a substantive role in the pathophysiology of severe endotoxemia. Further, these studies indicate that PAF receptor antagonists attenuate eicosanoid release in endotoxemia and that an intimate relationship exists between PAF and the eicosanoids in endotoxemia. Indeed, these studies imply that the early systemic hypotension of endotoxemia is not related to the effects of PAF but more likely reflects eicosanoid actions.

That PAF is a significant mediator in endotoxemia/sepsis is supported by others who have reported similar findings to those in the present study [14–17]. The existence of the intimate relationship between the eicosanoids and PAF in endotoxemia was first reported by us in 1990 [1]. The second study in canine endotoxemia suggests the original observation has merit [10]. Others have reported that exogenous PAF infusion is associated with increased plasma values of TxB_2 and 6-keto-PGF_{1a} [14]. PAF effects on coronary blood flow have been related to TxB_2 release [15]. Pulmonary hypertension and increased vascular permeability in the lung induced by exogenous PAF are, in part, due to a cyclooxygenase-dependent mechanism [16]. The injection of PAF into an isolated gastric perfusion model demonstrated an increase in eicosanoid release. PAF receptor antagonism attenuated the vasoconstriction and the eicosanoid release [17]. The present studies of endotoxemia provide additional evidence that the relationship between PAF and the eicosanoids is important.

The exact steps involved in this interaction are speculative. It could be that endotoxin activates the cell membrane phospholipase A_2 which cleaves the lyso-PAF and arachidonic acid. The arachidonic acid which is released accounts for a certain percentage of the cyclooxygenase end-products observed. The lyso-PAF is converted to active PAF which then further stimulates arachidonic acid release and a greater percentage of the cyclooxygenase products. The data from our studies is endotoxemia suggest that PAF effects amplify cyclooxygenase end-product synthesis/release. Additional, more detailed studies are needed to clarify this complicated system.

References

1. Fletcher JR, DiSimone AG, Earnest MA (1990) Platelet activating factor receptor antagonist improves survival and attenuates eicosanoid release in severe endotoxemia. Ann Surg 211:312–316
2. Halonen M, Palmer TD, Lohman IC et al. (1980) Respiratory and circulatory alterations induced by acetyl glyceryl ether phosphorylcholine, a mediator of IgE anaphylaxis in the rabbit. Am Rev Respir Dis 122:915–924
3. Bessin P, Bonnet J, Apfel D et al. (1983) Acute circulatory collapse caused by platelet activating factor (PAF-ACETHER) in dogs. Eur J Pharmacol 86:403–413
4. Gonzalez-Crussi F, Hseuh W (1987) Large cell lymphoma. Diagnostic difficulties and case study. Am J Pathol 112:127–135

5. Hseuh W, Gonzalez-Crussi F, Arroyave JL (1987) Platelet activating factor. an endogenous mediator for bowel necrosis in endotoxemia. FASEB J 1:403–405
6. Doebber TW, Wu MS, Robbins JC et al (1985) Platelet activating factor involvement in endotoxin-induced hypotension in rats, studies with PAF receptor antagonist kadsurenone. Biochem Biophys Res Commun (1985) 127:799–808
7. Chang SW, Feddersen CO, Henson PM et al. (1987) Platelet activating factor mediates hemodynamic changes and lung injury in endotoxemia-treated rats. J Clin Invest 79:1498–1509
8. Inanea P, Gomez-Cambronera J, Pascual et al. (1985) Synthesis of PAF acether and blood volume changes in gram negative sepsis. Immunopharmacology 9:45–52
9. Adnot S, Lelfort, Braquet P, Vargaftig BB (1986) Interference of the PAF-acether antagonist BN52021 with endotoxin-induced hypotension in the guinea pig. Prostaglandins 32:791–802
10. Moore JM, Earnest MA, DiSimone et al. (1985) A PAF receptor antagonist, BN25021, attenuates thromboxane release and improves survival in lethal canine endotoxemia. Circ Shock 35:53–59, 1991
11. Traber DL (1987) Endotoxin: the causative factor of mediator release during sepsis. Prog Clin Biol Res 236A:377–392
12. Coker SJ, Hughes B, Parratt JR et al. (1983) Br J Pharmacol 78:561–570
13. Haroldsen PE, Voelkl NF, Henson JE et al. (1987) J Clin Invest 79:1869–1877
14. Bessin P, Bonnet J, Apfel D et al. (1986) Eur J Pharmacol 86:403–413
15. Ezra D, Fluerstein G, Ramwell PW et al. Adv Prostaglandin Thromboxane Leukotreine Res 13:14–21
16. Burhop KE, VanDerZee H, Bizios R et al. Am Rev Respir Dis 134:548–554
17. Dembina-Kiec A, Peskar BA, Meuller MK et al. (1989) Prostaglandins 37:69–91

Phospholipase A_2: A New Target for Monoclonal Antibody Therapy in Sepsis

K. F. Scott, G. M. Smith, J. A. Green, C. Salom, C. Gabelish, D. Cairns, A. Tseng, P. Mackie, R. Buchta, K. Ho, R. Lee, and I. A. Rajkovic

Monoclonal antibody therapy in sepsis has focussed on intervention at very early stages in the pathogenesis, aiming to neutralise the potent effects of molecules such as endotoxin and tumour necrosis factor (TNF). While antibodies directed to these molecules show efficacy in the treatment of shock, it would be of considerable advantage to identify targets for intervention at later stages in the pathology. One such target is phospholipase A_2 (PLA_2), since this enzyme is proinflammatory (Vadas and Pruzanski 1986), and the activity in serum is associated with the onset and severity of septic shock in humans (Vadas 1984; Vadas et al. 1988).

Animal model experiments have shown that administration of endotoxin to rabbits results in an elevation of circulating PLA_2 (Vadas and Hay 1983). Also, infusion of PLA_2 into rabbits can generate the hypotension characteristic of septic shock (Vadas and Hay 1983). This hypotension is likely to result from the release of arachidonic acid from cell membranes by PLA_2 and its subsequent metabolism to potent vasoactive prostanoid mediators such as leukotrienes and prostaglandins. Taken together, these data suggest that the PLA_2 activity associated with sepsis is a reasonable target for intervention to prevent the hypodynamic effects of bacterial infection. The identity of the PLA_2 activity associated with sepsis is unknown. These studies have aimed to identify this phospholipase and to develop reagents capable of neutralising the activity.

Materials and Methods

The PLA_2cDNA (Seilhamer et al. 1989) and an inactive PLA_2 mutein (generated by site-directed mutagenesis of His_{48} to Gln_{48}) were expressed in Chinese hamster ovary cells under the control of a heavy metal inducible promoter. Cell lines were grown in serum-containing medium and transferred to serum-free medium at time of induction. Viable cell numbers were determined using a trypan blue exclusion assay in triplicate flasks at time of seeding, at induction and 72 h after induction. Cell numbers are expressed as means $\pm$ SE. PLA_2 expression in media was demonstrated by western blot analysis using

Garvan Institute of Medical Research, 384 Victoria Street, Darlinghurst NSW 2010, Australia

Host Defense Dysfunction
in Trauma, Shock and Sepsis
Eds. Faist/Meakins/Schildberg
© Springer-Verlag, Berlin Heidelberg 1993

peptide antisera (data not shown) and a PLA_2 activity assay as described (Green et al. 1991).

Patients with sepsis were chosen based on the following criteria: core temperature < 35.6 or $> 38.9\,°C$, tachycardia, WCC < 3500 or > 15000 per mm^3, altered sensorium, rigors, documented site of infection. Septic shock was diagnosed as systemic blood pressure < 90 mm Hg supine. The capture ELISA was used as described (Smith et al. 1992) on a range of plasma dilutions. Plasma PLA_2 activity was determined at $1/100$ dilution using a mixed-micelle assay and ^{14}C-labelled phosphotidylethanolamine as substrate essentially as described (Green et al. 1991). All data points are the means of triplicate analyses. Affinity purification was carried out using standard methodologies and elution conditions (Green et al. 1991). Amino terminal sequence analysis was done on a 477A automated sequencer (Applied Biosystems). Inhibition assays were done with 1 h preincubation of antibody (in molar excess at 100 µg/ml) with varying dilutions of plasma prior to the addition of substrate. Assays were performed in triplicate.

Results and Discussion

A cDNA sequence isolated from a peritoneal exudate library (Seilhamer et al. 1989) was cloned behind a heavy metal inducible promoter and used to generate stable transfectants in Chinese hamster ovary cells. The cDNA was also mutated in vitro using standard site-directed mutagenesis to generate a mutein construct which, on transfection, produced inactive but conformationally indistinguishable PLA_2. As shown in Fig. 1, induction of these constructs in serum-free

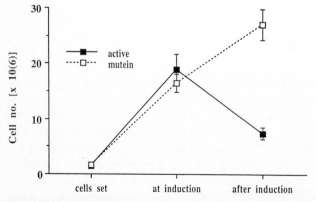

Fig. 1. Cytotoxicity of PLA_2 expression. Viable cell counts were made of Chinese hamster ovary cells transfected with cDNA constructs expressing either active or inactive PLA_2. Cell counts were measured by trypan blue exclusion at time of cell seeding, at time of induction with heavy metals or 72 h after induction. Cell numbers are means of three experiments plus or minus standard errors

media resulted in a dramatic decrease in cell viability of the line producing active PLA$_2$ while there was no effect on the viability of the line expressing inactive PLA$_2$. Further, addition of active PLA$_2$-conditioned medium to Chinese hamster ovary cells resulted in a loss of viability of these cells relative to addition of equivalent amounts of mutein-conditioned medium (data not shown). These data indicate that this PLA$_2$ is toxic to mammalian cells in culture when expressed internally or added externally.

Purified recombinant PLA$_2$ was used to generate high-affinity monoclonal antibodies, and these antibodies were used to establish a specific-capture enzyme-linked immunosorbent assay (ELISA) capable of detecting PLA$_2$ in plasma. This ELISA was used to quantitate PLA$_2$ levels in patients with sepsis, post-operative trauma and in normal subjects. As shown in Fig 2, PLA$_2$ activity is significantly elevated in patients with sepsis relative to those with trauma or normal subjects. This activity elevation correlates with an elevation of circulating PLA$_2$ as measured by ELISA. Patients who later progressed to shock in general had higher levels of circulating PLA$_2$. These data confirm the previous observation of PLA$_2$ levels in association with sepsis (Vadas 1984) and demonstrate that the increase in activity is due to a dramatic elevation in the level of circulating enzyme.

The antibodies were also used to purify PLA$_2$ from patients with sepsis. As shown in Fig. 3, affinity purification, followed by amino-terminal protein sequence analysis showed that this protein is essentially identical to that isolated from synovial fluid of patients with active rheumatoid arthritis (Seilhamer et al. 1989) and that isolated from placenta (Lai and Wada 1988). The enzyme has only 30% homology with human pancreatic PLA$_2$ (Verkeij et al. 1983).

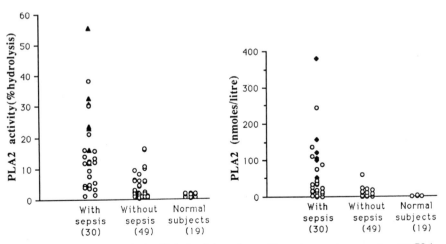

Fig. 2. Quantitation of circulating PLA$_2$ levels in patients with sepsis or post-surgery trauma. PLA$_2$ activity and concentration were determined using an in vitro activity assay and a newly developed capture ELISA. *Closed symbols*, patients who progressed to septic shock after blood samples were taken

```
                              1           10          20
SEPTIC SHOCK PLA₂             NLVNF HRMIK-LTTGKEAALSYGFY

SYNOVIAL FLUID PLA₂           NLVNF HRMIK-LTTGKEAALSYGFY

PLACENTAL PLA₂               NLVNF HRMIK-LTT

PANCREATIC PLA₂              AVWQF RKMIKCVIPGSDPFLEYNNY
```

Fig. 3. Identification of the circulatory PLA_2 associated with sepsis. Amino-terminal sequence analysis was carried out on affinity-purified PLA_2 isolated from a pooled sample of plasma from patients with sepsis. The sequence is compared with that isolated from rheumatoid synovial fluid (Seilhamer et al. 1989), placenta (Lai and Wada 1988) and pancreas (Verkeij et al. 1983)

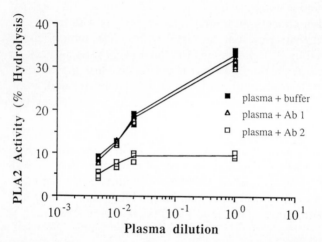

Fig. 4. Inhibition of PLA_2 activity in septic plasma by neutralising monoclonal antibodies. PLA_2 activity was determined using an in vitro activity assay. *Ab1*, Non-inhibitory murine monoclonal; *Ab2*, inhibitory murine monoclonal. Both monoclonal antibodies show cross-reactivity with recombinant PLA_2 in an ELISA (data not shown)

The monoclonal antibodies were also screened for their ability to neutralise recombinant PLA_2 in vitro. A number of antibodies were identified which showed up to 90% inhibition of activity under these conditions (data not shown). One of these antibodies was chosen to establish whether the antibodies could inhibit PLA_2 activity in the plasma of a patient with sepsis. As shown in Fig. 4. This antibody is capable of neutralising the activity of PLA_2 in plasma while a second PLA_2-specific antibody has no effect on the activity. The antibody can clearly bind to and inhibit the activity of circulating PLA_2 in the presence of plasma components.

Given the timing of the onset of PLA_2 elevation in the baboon shock model (Buchta et al., this volume) after the transient elevation in TNF and prior to the hypodynamic and tissue damage phase of the model, its previous clinical association with the severity of shock in humans (Vadas et al. 1988), and the known toxicity of phospholipases (Vadas and Pruzanski, 1986), the data presented here suggest strongly that this enzyme is a reasonable target for intervention with monoclonal antibody therapy directed at the later inflammatory events in the pathogenesis of shock.

Acknowledgement. This work was supported by an Australian Government Discretionary Grant (# 5209).

References

Green JA, Smith GM, Buchta R, Lee R, Ho KY, Rajkovic IA, Scott KF (1991) The circulating phospholipase A$_2$ activity associated with sepsis is indistinguishable from that associated with rheumatoid arthritis. Inflammation 15:355–367

Lai C, Wada K (1988) Phospholipase A$_2$ from synovial fluid: purification and structural homology to the placental enzyme. Biochem Biophys Res Commun 157:488–493

Seilhamer JJ, Pruzanski W, Vadas P, Plant S, Miller J, Kloss J, Johnsan L (1989) Cloning and recombinant expression of phospholipase A$_2$ present in rheumatoid arthritic synovial fluid. J Biol Chem 264:5335–5338

Smith GM, Ward RL, McGuigan L, Rajkovic IA, Scott KF (1992) Measurement of human phospholipase A$_2$ in arthritis plasma using a newly developed sandwich ELISA. Br J Rheumatol 31:175–178

Vadas P (1984) Plasma phospholipase A$_2$ levels correlate with the hemodynamic and pulmonary changes in gram-negative septic shock in man. J Lab Clin Med 104:873–881

Vadas P, Hay JB (1983) Involvement of circulating phospholipase A$_2$ in the pathogenesis of the hemodynamic changes in endotoxin shock. Can J Physiol Pharmacol 61:561–566

Vadas P, Pruzanski W (1986) Role of secretory phospholipase A$_2$ in the pathobiology of disease. Lab Invest 55:391–404

Vadas P, Pruzanski W, Stefanski E (1988) Pathogenesis of hypotension in septic shock: correlation of circulatory phospholipase A$_2$ levels with circulatory collapse, Crit Care Med 16:1–7

Verkeij HM, Westerman J, Sternby B, de Haas G (1983) The complete primary structure of phospholipase A$_2$ from human pancreas. Biochim Biophys Acta 747:93–99

Administration of Antiadhesion Molecules: A Feasible Approach?

R. K. Winn, S. R. Sharar, W. J. Mileski, C. L. Rice, and J. M. Harlan

Introduction

Trauma is the leading cause of death in individuals between the ages of 1 and 44 years and constitutes a major health problem worldwide. In 1980 there were 160 000 trauma deaths in the United States [1]. Of these deaths 50% occurred at the scene of the injury, 25% within the first 24 h as a result of their initial injuries, and the final 25% between 2 days and several weeks after injury. The usual cause of late death in these multiply injured patients is the multiple organ failure syndrome (MOFS). The cause of MOFS is unknown, but affected organs include the central nervous system, lung, gastrointestinal tract, heart, kidney, liver, and coagulation system [2]. Patients suffering from MOF appear to have massive activation of the inflammatory system due to tissue trauma and/or subsequent sepsis, although generalized inflammation results from a nonseptic cause in 50%–60% of MOFS cases [3]. If the underlying cause of MOFS can be determined, late deaths in trauma patients may be preventable.

Neutrophils play a key role in host defense following bacterial invasion, but also are capable of causing host-tissue destruction as a consequence of widespread activation. These cells contain an arsenal of proteases and reactive oxygen products used to kill bacteria within phagosomes. However, when these products are released into the circulation they may cause endothelial injury. The abundance of antiproteases and antioxidants circulating in blood suggests that neutrophil-mediated vascular injury must result from local effects at the endothelium. Neutrophil adherence to endothelial cells forms a protected microenvironment for such a local effect. Activated neutrophils have been shown to cause injury to endothelial cells in vitro and it appears that neutrophil adherence to the endothelial cell is required to produce injury [4].

Neutrophils have been implicated in organ injury, particularly in causing damage to the lung. Heflin and Brigham [5] have examined lipopolysaccharide (LPS) infusions in experimental animals and showed an increased vascular permeability that was prevented by neutrophil depletion. Increased lung permeability following combined administration of LPS and one of the neutrophil stimulants, zymosan-activated plasma or formylated peptide (fMLP), also was

Departments of Anesthesiology, Surgery, Medicine, and Physiology-Biophysics, University of Washington, Harborview Medical Center, Seattle, WA 98104, USA

Host Defense Dysfunction
in Trauma, Shock and Sepsis
Eds. Faist/Meakins/Schildberg
© Springer-Verlag, Berlin Heidelberg 1993

shown to be neutrophil dependent [6]. These results suggest that neutrophils are responsible for lung injury, but they have not been reproduced by other investigators using similar protocols [7, 8]. Conclusions reached in all of these studies suffer from a serious defect in that protocols rely on neutrophil depletion by chemical means. Neutrophil depletion was not complete, nor was it clear what direct effect the chemical agents used for depletion had on the vascular wall. Neutrophils have also been implicated in hepatic and myocardial injury due to sepsis [9, 10]. The injurious effects of neutrophils may be exacerbated by neutrophil plugging of microvascular beds, thereby disturbing microcirculatory flow and/or causing diffuse endothelial injury.

These observations have led to clinical trials using drugs that modulate neutrophil function to produce an anti-inflammatory effect. Anisodamine has been shown to result in decreased neutrophil aggregation and in one study was shown to improve survival during sepsis [11]. Corticosteroids are also known to be anti-inflammatory, acting to stabilize lysosomal membranes and to inhibit neutrophil aggregation. They have been shown to be effective in the treatment of septic shock in animals [12]. Corticosteroids, in conjunction with antibiotics, have been used similarly in man, but beneficial effects have not been demonstrated, especially if administered late in the course of septic shock [13].

Any attempt to eliminate the neutrophil's role in sepsis must be tempered with an understanding of its significant role in host defense against bacterial invasion. Neutrophils may cause tissue injury as a result of overstimulation but their removal might be outweighed by detrimental effects of impaired host defense. However, temporary removal of neutrophils from the circulation might be effective in preventing some of the adverse effects of an overstimulated inflammatory system while still allowing a return of normal host defense.

A small group of patients have been identified that suffer from the syndrome of leukocyte adherence deficiency (LAD) [14]. Neutrophils from these patients are normal in that they are able to degranulate and undergo an oxidative burst. However, they are defective in their ability to adhere to surfaces following stimulation. The primary mechanism of neutrophil adhesion involves the cell membrane glycoprotein adherence complex designated CD11/CD18. The LAD patients' neutrophil adherence abnormality results from a congenital lack of functional CD11/CD18. This complex contains three heterodimers consisting of three distinct heavy α-chains (CD11a, CD11b, CD11c) noncovalently linked to a common light β-chain (CD18). These heterodimers are commonly referred to as LFA-1, MAC-1 and p150/95, respectively.

Monoclonal antibodies (MAbs) have been produced that recognize these molecules in the CD11/CD18 glycoprotein complex. Use of the anti-CD18 MAb designated 60.3 has been effective in vitro in preventing endothelial cell injury that resulted from activating neutrophils with phorbol ester and subsequently exposing them to endothelial cell cultures [4]. In that study there were no differences between neutrophils saturated with MAb 60.3 and neutrophils from LAD patients. The MAb 60.3 provided significant protection against endothelial injury compared with saline treatment. This MAb has also been shown to prevent neutrophil emigration into tissue in response to LPS-soaked sponges in rabbits [15]. The half-life of MAb 60.3 is dose dependent and is approximately 18 h at a dose that is effective in preventing emigration into the sponges. Thus, these antibodies may be effective in transiently preventing neutrophil-mediated injury without producing the equivalent harm of LAD syndrome.

We have used MAb 60.3 in a number of settings to prevent tissue injury. These included hemorrhagic shock in rabbits [16, 17] and primates [18], ischemia-reperfusion injury of the rabbit ear [19] and severe cold injury (W. J. Mileski et al., unpublished). These experiments have been described briefly elsewhere in this volume. Results from these experiments suggest that treatment with antiadhesion molecules may provide a clinically relevant method of treating patients at risk for inflammatory microvascular injury.

This paper will review two of the limited number of experiments investigating the safety of MAb 60.3, examining protocols of abdominal sepsis following appendiceal devascularization and subcutaneous bacterial inoculation. In addition, we will describe some preliminary work examining the effectiveness of MAb 60.3 in preventing injury as a result of peritonitis.

Experimental Models of Sepsis and MAb 60.3

Rabbit Peritonitis [20]. Abdominal sepsis was induced in rabbits by devascularizing their appendix and ligating it at the base [21]. This preparation results in a necrotic appendix and abdominal bacterial colonization that leads to leukocyte emigration into the peritoneum. Animals were returned to their cages overnight with free access to food and water, and after 18 to 19 h an appendectomy was performed. Ten animals were treated with saline and ten were treated with MAb 60.3 at the time of the devascularization, and again at the time of the appendectomy. Animals were studied for 10 days. Bacterial cultures and neutrophil counts in the peritoneal fluid were obtained at the time of the appendectomy. Survival and infectious complications were assessed to evaluate the safety of transient exposure to anti-CD18 antibody. All surviving animals were killed at 10 days with an overdose of pentobarbital and necropsies performed to assess intra-abdominal abscesses and wound infections.

Bacterial cultures from the peritoneal fluid were obtained by placing peritoneal fluid directly onto TSA blood agar plates. These were incubated at 37 °C for 72 h and the presence, absence, and types of colonies were determined. Anaerobic cultures were not performed.

Survival was not different between the saline- and MAb-treated groups (see Fig. 1). Half of the animals died in each group, and there was no difference in the timing of death. Infectious complications were similar between the two groups as defined by the number of wound infections plus the number of abdominal abscesses. There were a total of four infectious complications in the saline-treated animals (one wound infection and three abdominal abscesses) and six

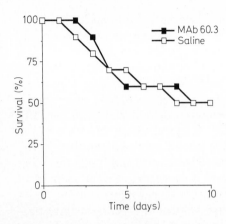

Fig. 1. Comparative survival curves are shown for rabbits with experimental peritonitis. Mortality was equal between the two groups. Experimental protocol is described in text. (Adapted from [21])

in the MAb 60.3-treated group (four wound infections and two abdominal abscesses). The peritoneal bacterial cultures were positive in all animals in both groups. There were significantly more neutrophils in the peritoneal fluid of the saline-treated animals ($22.7 \pm 6.1 \times 10^6$ cells/ml) compared with the MAb 60.3-treated animals ($8.7 \pm 3.3 \times 10^6$ cells/ml).

Apparently, bacterial infections in the antibody-treated animals were limited by the small number of neutrophils that migrated into the peritoneal space during deterioration of the appendix, as well as by other host defense mechanisms. The appearance of neutrophils despite CD18 blockade suggests that there was a non-CD18 mechanism of emigration in this setting. We have reported such a pathway in rabbits following instillation of *Streptococcus pneumoniae* into the lung [22] and under certain conditions in the peritoneum [23]. In the case of the peritoneum, the presence of macrophages appears to be necessary to initiate the non-CD18 pathway.

Rabbit Soft Tissue Infection [24]. Standard clinical laboratory *Staphylococcus aureus* bacterial colonies (ATCC 25923) were cultured on TSA blood agar plates 1 day prior to study. On the day of study bacteria were suspended in sterile saline at concentrations of approximately 10^6, 10^7, 10^8 or 10^9 colony forming units (CFU) per ml. The backs of rabbits were shaved under light ketamine sedation and two 1-ml injections of each of the bacterial solutions were administered subcutaneously to each rabbit. The inoculations were performed within 30 min of bacterial harvest and suspension. In preliminary experiments designed to determine a dose/response relationship, 11 rabbits were treated prior to bacterial inoculation with cefazolin (20 mg/kg and every 8 h for the subsequent 72 h) and either saline placebo ($n = 5$) or MAb 60.3 ($n = 6$). Abscesses were not observed in either group at inoculation sites of 10^6 or 10^7 CFU during observation for up to 6 days. However, at higher inocula abscesses formed in both groups.

Additional animals were then divided into two groups of eight and again received either MAb 60.3 or saline prior to inoculation. Each rabbit was given two subcutaneous bacterial injections of 10^8 CFU and two injections of 10^9 CFU. Cefazolin was administered prior to bacterial inoculation and every 8 h for the next 72 h. Animals were killed at 7 days by ketamine overdose, the skin dissected free, and the surface area of the abscesses determined by photographic projection and planimetry. The abscesses in both groups were predominately flat and therefore, the calculated surface area was a two-dimensional area defined by the border of the abscess.

Abscess incidence (as a percent of the total number of injection sites) is shown in Fig. 2. There were significantly more abscesses formed in the MAb 60.3-treated group at 10^8 CFU compared with the saline-treated group. At 10^9 CFU nearly all of the injection sites in both groups resulted in abscess formation, with a 75% incidence in the saline-treated group and 100% in the antibody-treated group. The abscesses in the saline-treated rabbits were slightly raised, pustular, and well encapsulated within the subcutaneous tissue. In contrast, the abscesses in the antibody-treated group were gangrenous, poorly encapsulated, displayed irregular borders, and covered a larger area than the controls. Abscess surface areas are shown in Fig. 3, with the area measuring nearly 20 times greater at inoculation sites of 10^9 CFU in the MAb 60.3-treated group compared with the saline group. The following calculations, assuming the contour of the abscesses had been perfectly round, were made for ease of comparison. To achieve the observed difference in abscess area at 10^9 CFU, abscess diameter in the saline-treated rabbits would be approximately 1.19 cm and in the antibody-treated rabbits approximately 5.14 cm. Significantly larger abscesses were observed in antibody-treated animals at both the 10^8 and 10^9 CFU inoculation sites.

Light microscopic evaluation of the abscesses revealed a typical abscess at days 1 and 2 in the saline-treated animals, with neutrophil infiltration and accumulated cellular debris. At day 7 the lesions were rimmed with granulation tissue suggesting that the reparative process had begun. In sharp contrast, abscesses in the MAb 60.3-treated group at days 1 and 2 consisted almost entirely of bacteria that were proliferating along the subcutaneous plane between skeletal muscle and dermis. There were no neutrophils associated with these lesions although an occasional macrophage was found.

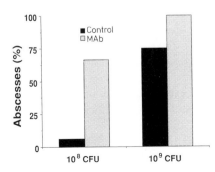

Fig. 2. Incidence of subcutaneous abscess formation in rabbits after inoculation with S. aureus is shown as a function of inoculum concentration. Incidence is shown as percentage × 100 (where percentageenumber of inoculation sites with abscess-/total number of inoculation sites). Rabbits pretreated with monoclonal antibody (MAb) 60.3 are compared to those receiving saline placebo. CFU, colony forming units. (Adapted from [24])

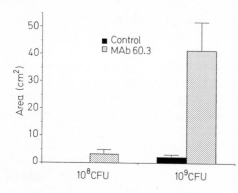

Fig. 3. Subcutaneous abscess surface area 7 days after inoculation with *S. aureus* is shown as a function of inoculum concentration. Rabbits pretreated with monoclonal antibody (*MAb*) 60.3 are compared to those receiving saline placebo. (*CFU*, colony forming units.) (Adapted from [24])

These observations confirmed prior work showing that neutrophil emigration in response to bacterial stimulation in the systemic circulation is CD18-dependent [23]. In rabbits, subcutaneous inoculation with 10^9 CFU *S. aureus* produced a syndrome similar to that seen in LAD patients. Specifically, uncontrolled soft-tissue infections developed that, if allowed to progress, most likely would have led to death. However, the response to lower bacterial doses revealed that rabbits were able to overcome a transient loss of neutrophil function and prevent extension of soft tissue infection. The half-life of MAb 60.3 is known to be dose dependent, and at the dose of 2 mg/kg used in these experiments, is approximately 18 h [15]. Based on these data the antibody concentration necessary to block neutrophil adherence was present for 24–36 h. The ultimate elimination of bacteria following subcutaneous injection was probably aided by the eventual emigration of neutrophils, although delayed, into bacterial inoculation sites.

Results from the peritonitis study and the soft-tissue abscess study appear at first glance to be contradictory, since the latter suggests an adverse effect of MAb 60.3 treatment. The apparent contradiction may be explained by different mechanisms of neutrophil emigration. We have previously shown that neutrophil emigration into the peritoneum in response to *S. pneumoniae* can be CD18 independent if there are a significant number of macrophages present at the site of inflammation [23]. Macrophages may participate directly in host defense in the peritoneum, or they may release monokines that initiate neutrophil migration into the peritoneum by a non-CD18 mechanism. In addition, there were neutrophils in the peritoneum at the time of the appendectomy even in the presence of the anti-CD18 MAb 60.3. These neutrophils may have been able to perform some of their host defense function by injesting and killing bacteria.

Treatment of Rabbit Peritonitis. Preliminary experiments in our laboratory have investigated the potential beneficial effects of anti-CD18 therapy in sepsis. Induction of peritonitis was similar to that described above. In these experiments sepsis was induced by devascularizing the appendix, leaving it in situ for 19 h, and then performing an appendectomy. Rabbits were treated with either saline or mAb 60.3 and the antibotic cefazolin. Treatment was given at the time of the appendectomy and every 12 h for 72 h. Weight loss was monitored daily for 10 days. The rabbits were assumed to be irreversibly septic if they lost more than 20% of their body weight and they were killed. Sixty percent of the saline-treated rabbits were either killed or died during the observation period, whereas 10% of the MAb 60.3-treated group died. Results from this group of experiments suggest that antiadhesion therapy will be effective in the treatment of peritonitis.

Summary

Patients with LAD suffer recurrent soft-tissue infections that can progress to death if they are not aggressively treated with bacteriocidal antibiotics. In the most severe cases treatment may require transfusion of functional leukocytes to control infections. On the other hand, anti-CD18 MAbs have been shown to provide protection against ischemia-reperfusion injuries. The efficacy of these MAbs, particularly in hemorrhagic shock, has led to speculation that they may provide protection against MOFS for severely injured trauma victims. One of the major questions that must be answered before this proposed therapy can be examined clinically is whether brief inhibition of neutrophil adherence can result in a septic syndrome similar to the LAD patient.

The experiments examining mortality in abdominal sepsis suggest that MAb 60.3 does not render rabbits more susceptible to infection. The MAb 60.3-treated animals had more neutrophils in the peritoneal space as compared with the number that are normally there, and these cells could provide effective host defence against bacteria released by the necrotic appendix. Conversely, soft-tissue infections were more severe in MAb-treated animals at the injection sites of 10^8 and 10^9 CFU S. aureus. These are not clinically relevant concentrations of bacteria, however, and thus, may not be of physiologic significance in trauma patients. However, trauma patients that are candidates for use of antiadhesion therapy may be somewhat immunosuppressed as a result of their injuries and may be more susceptible to infection. Considerable investigation needs to be completed before the patient population most likely to safely benefit from antiadhesion therapy can be defined.

References

1. Committee on Trauma Research (1985) Injury in America. A continuing public health problem. National Academy, Washington DC
2. Nuytinck HKS, Offermans XJMW, Kubat K, Goris RJA (1988) Whole-body inflammation in trauma patients; an autopsy study. Arch Surg 123:1519–1524
3. Goris RJA, te Boekhorst TPA, Nuytinck JKS, Gimbrere JSF (1985) Multiple-organ failure. Generalized autodestructive inflammation? Arch Surg 120:1109–1115

4. Diener AM, Beatty PG, Ochs HD, Harlan JM (1985) The role of neutrophil membrane glycoprotein 150 (GP150) in neutrophil-mediated endothelial cell injury in vitro. J Immunol 135:537–543
5. Heflin AC, Brigham KL (1981) Prevention by granulocyte depletion of increased vascular permeability of sheep lung following endotoxemia. J Clin Invest 68:1253–1260
6. Worthen GS, Haslett C, Rees AJ, Gumbay RS, Henson JE, Henson PM (1987) Neutrophil-mediated pulmonary vascular injury. Am Rev Respir Dis 136:19–28
7. Pingleton WW, Coalson JJ, Guenter A (1975) Significance of leukocytes in endotoxic shock. Exp Mol Pathol 22:183–194
8. Winn R, Maunder R, Chi E, Harlan J (1987) Neutrophil depletion does not prevent lung edema after endotoxin infusion in goats. J Appl Physiol 62:116–121
9. Asher EF, Garrison RN, Ratcliffe DJ, Fry DE (1983) Endotoxin, cellular function, and nutrient blood flow. Arch Surg 118:441–445
10. Manson NH, Hess ML (1983) Interaction of oxygen free radicals and cardiac sarcoplasmic reticulum: proposed role in the pathogenesis of endotoxin shock. Circ Shock 10:205–213
11. Rui-Juan X, Hammerschmidt DE, Coppo PA, Jacob HS (1982) Anisodamine inhibits thromboxane synthesis, granulocyte aggregation, and platelet aggregation: a possible mechanism for its efficacy in bacteremic shock. JAMA 247:1458–1460
12. Schumer W (1976) Steroids in the treatment of clinical septic shock. Ann Surg 184:333–341
13. Hinshaw L, Peduzzi P, Young E et al. (1987) Effect of high-dose glucocorticoid therapy on mortality in patients with clinical signs of systemic sepsis. N Engl J Med 317:659–665
14. Harlan JM, Schwartz BR, Wallis WJ, Pohlman TH (1987) The role of neutrophil membrane proteins in neutrophil emigration. In: Movat HZ (ed) Leukocyte emigration and its sequelae. Karger, Basel, pp 94–104
15. Price TH, Beatty PG, Corpuz SR (1987) In vivo inhibition of neutrophil function in the rabbit using monoclonal antibody to CD18. J Immunol 139:4174–4177
16. Vedder NB, Winn RK, Rice CL, Chi E, Arfors K, Harlan JM (1988) A monoclonal antibody to the adherence promoting leukocyte glycoprotein CD18 reduces organ injury and improves survival from hemorrhagic shock and resuscitation in rabbits. J Clin Invest 81:939–944
17. Vedder NB, Fouty BW, Winn RK, Harlan JM, Rice CL (1989) Role of neutrophils in generalized reperfusion injury associated with resuscitation from shock. Surgery 106:509–516
18. Mileski WJ, Winn RK, Vedder NB, Pohlman TH, Harlan JM, Rice CL (1990) Inhibition of CD18-dependent neutrophil adherence reduces organ injury after hemorrhagic shock in primates. Surgery 108:206–212
19. Vedder NB, Winn RK, Rice CL, Chi EY, Arfors KE, Harlan JM (1990) Inhibition of leukocyte adherence by anti-CD18 monoclonal antibody attenuates reperfusion injury in the rabbit ear. Proc Natl Acad Sci USA 87:2643–2646
20. Mileski WJ, Winn RK, Harlan JM, Rice CL (1991) Transient inhibition of neutrophil adherence with the anti-CD18 monoclonal antibody (MAb 60.3) does not increase mortality in abdominal sepsis. Surgery (in press)
21. Freischlag J, Backstrom B, Kelly D, Keehn G, Busutil RW (1986) Comparison of blood and peritoneal PMN activity in rabbits with and without peritonitis. J Surg Res 40:145–151
22. Doerschuk CM, Winn RK, Coxson HO, Harlan JM (1990) CD18-dependent and -independent mechanisms of neutrophil emigration in the pulmonary and systemic microcirculation of rabbits. J Immunol 144:2327–2333
23. Mileski W, Harlan J, Rice C, Winn R (1990) Streptococcus pneumoniae-stimulated macrophages induce neutrophils to emigrate by a CD18-independent mechanism of adherence. Circ Shock 31:259–267
24. Sharar SR, Winn RK, Murry CE, Harlan JM, Rice CL (1991) A CD18 monoclonal antibody increases the incidence and severity of subcutaneous abscess formation after high dose S. aureus injection in rabbits. Surgery 110:213–220

Local Administration of Interleukin-2 Protects Mice from Lethal Intra-Abdominal Bacterial Sepsis

R. Richards[1] and D. R. Green[2]

Introduction

Bacterial sepsis is one of the major challenges facing clinicians who treat critically ill and injured patients. This is especially true in those cases in which the immune response is impaired, such as following trauma or major surgery [1], and approximately 75% of late deaths following trauma are attributable to systemic sepsis [2]. The progression from sepsis to multiple organ failure and death is complex and depends on a number of factors. Among these factors are a variety of specific and nonspecific host defense mechanisms, including phago-cytosis, complement activation, and specific antibody production. In recent years, it has also become clear that specific cell-mediated responses also play important roles in the control of bacterial infection, and it is therefore possible that such responses influence the outcome of sepsis. *Pseudomonas aeruginosa* is an important cause of morbidity and mortality in severely compromised patients, and it is therefore under intense study. Animal models of infection with this organism have required extensive pretreatment with cyclophosphamide [3], very large numbers of bacteria [4, 5], or full-thickness burn [6, 7] in order to produce susceptibility to sepsis.

Barium sulfate is known to increase the mortality of peritonitis in the clinical setting [8] and has been found to suppress delayed-type hypersensitivity (DTH) when administered intraperitoneally [9]. We took advantage of these observations to devise a model of *P. aeruginosa* infection in which low doses of bacteria are lethal to normal animals. By implanting a mixture of bacteria and barium sulfate contained in a capsule, intra-abdominal abscess formation was induced with lethal sepsis occurring over the course of the next 4 days (unpublished observations). During the course of our studies on intra-abdominal abscess formation in mice we observed that immune animals displayed differences in the nature of the cellular infiltrate into the bacterial abscess. In these studies, animals were immunized with killed *P. aeruginosa* bacteria or with bacterial pili, following which the animals were induced to abscess formation by intra-peritoneal exposure to bacteria plus barium sulfate. Histological examination of

[1] Department of Plastic Surgery, University of Alberta, Edmonton, Alberta, Canada T6G 2H7
[2] Department of Immunology, University of Alberta, Edmonton, Alberta Canada

Host Defense Dysfunction
in Trauma, Shock and Sepsis
Eds. Faist/Meakins/Schildberg
© Springer-Verlag, Berlin Heidelberg 1993

the abscesses revealed that while naive animals showed cellular infiltrates composed predominantly of neutrophils, the infiltrates into abscesses in immune mice contained a high percentage of macrophages and lymphocytes (unpublished observations).

We therefore asked whether growth factors known to be involved in such responses might influence the outcome of the bacterial sepsis resulting from this procedure. Here we report that local administration of low doses of T cell derived lymphokines, including interleukin-2 (IL-2), dramatically protected animals from lethal sepsis in this model. This protection was dependent upon the presence of T cells in the treated animals. Further, in a preliminary study, such local administration of lymphokine was also effective in protecting animals from lethal sepsis induced by cecal ligation and puncture. These results may suggest new approaches to the control of sepsis.

Materials and Methods

Animals. C57B1/6, BALB/c, and BALB/c nu/nu mice, 8–12 weeks of age, were bred and housed in the Animal Facility at the University of Alberta. All groups were age and sex matched in each experiment.

Bacteria. P. aeruginosa strain PAK was kindly provided by Dr. W. Paranchych (Department of Microbiology, University of Alberta) and was maintained on tryptic soy broth agar (Difco) and subcultured weekly. Inocula were prepared by adding the contents of a 10-μl loop to 10 ml L-broth followed by incubation at 37 °C for 18 h.

Experimental Infection. We added 100 mg/ml of barium sulfate to the diluted inoculum, and 0.1 ml suspension was placed in a #4 gelatin capsule (Parke-Davis). The capsule was surgically implanted into the peritoneal cavity of anesthetized mice. Following recovery, animals were housed and observed twice a day. Titration experiments established that 10^5 bacteria induced an average mortality of 80% ($n = 25$) in this system. Cecal ligation and puncture was performed as previously described [10, 11], using a 23-guage needle.

Lymphokine. Recombinant human IL-2 (rIL-2) was the generous gift of Dr. Warner Greene (Duke University). T cell growth factor (TCGF) was produced by culture of rat spleen cells with 2 μg/ml concanavalin A(con A) [12]. Alternatively, EL-4 lymphoma cells were cultured with 10 ng/ml phorbol myristate acetate (PMA) and supernatants dialyzed (EL-4 LK) [13]. As a control, unactivated EL-4 supernatants (which contain no IL-2) were employed. Approximate IL-2 U/ml were calculated for the TCGF and activated EL-4 supernatants using the IL-2 responsive cell line CTL-L [12]. In all cases, each injection contained 300–400 U IL-2 per mouse.

Splenic T Cells. Spleens from BALB/c $+/+$ were dissociated and Ig$^+$ cells were removed by passage over a T cellpass column (Biotex, Edmonton). Viable cells were counted using a hemocytometer.

Results and Discussion

Groups of C57B1/6 mice were implanted with capsules containing barium sulfate plus 10^5 *P. aeruginosa* bacteria to induce abscesses and lethal bacterial sepsis. This dose of bacteria had been found to induce approximately 80% mortality in a number of trials (data not shown). On days -3, -2, and -1 prior to this challenge, each animal was pretreated with daily intraperitoneal injections of lymphokines (equivalent to 300–400 U IL-2 per injection). As shown in Fig. 1a, pretreatment with control supernatants failed to protect the animals, while treatment with lymphokine-containing, PMA-activated EL-4 cells (EL-4 LK) or con A- activated rat spleen cells (TCGF) produced significant protection. Protection was also afforded by treatment with rIL-2; however, the animals protected by this treatment displayed more pronounced signs of distress (fur ruffling, lethargy) than did the other lymphokine-treated mice (results not shown). In other experiments (not shown) lymphokines were administered either intraperitoneally or intravenously. Protection was observed only following intraperitoneal treatment.

In another study, animals were implanted with 10^5 bacteria plus barium sulfate, following which each animal received a single injection of activated EL-4 supernatants or rIL-2. In both cases, significant protection was observed (Fig. 1b). Thus, local administration of lymphokine can afford protection even after septic challenge. However, in other experiments (not shown) this posttreatment often showed variable results.

IL-2 is the product of type 1 helper T cells (Th1), and it is these cells that direct DTH responses [14]. Histologic examination of the abscesses from the

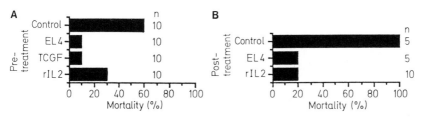

Fig. 1a,b Local administration of lymphokines protects mice from lethal intra-abdominal sepsis. **a** Animals were injected daily, intraperitoneally with activated EL-4 supernatants (EL4 LK), TCGF, or rIL-2 (300–400 U or equivalent in each case), for 3 days. Control animals received supernatants from unactivated EL-4 cells. Capsules containing barium sulfate plus 10^5 *P. aeruginosa* were then surgically implanted into the peritoneum and the animals were observed over the next several days. Reported mortality is for 7 days, although all deaths occurred by 72 h. **b** As in (a) except that animals received only one dose of lymphokine, following the septic challenge lymphokine-protected animals revealed an infiltrate containing macrophages and lymphocytes (not shown), a response reminiscent of DTH. Therefore, in order to determine whether T lymphocytes are required for the protective effect of IL-2 administration, the following experiments was performed. Congenitally athymic BALB/c nu/nu mice were challenged with bacteria and barium sulfate as above. One group of mice was injected daily with 300 U rIL2 for 3 days prior to bacterial challenge. Another group was injected intra-peritoneally with a T cell enriched population of spleen cells from normal BALB/c + / + mice 3 days before challenge. The final group received T cells on day − 3 and daily injections of rIL2 (days − 3, − 2, and − 1). Results are shown in Fig. 2. Animals treated with both T cells and IL-2 were protected from lethal sepsis, while all of the animals in the other groups succumbed. Thus, the protective effects of IL-2 in this system is dependent upon the presence of T cells.

While these results suggest that lymphokines, especially IL-2, can protect animals from lethal bacterial sepsis, it was possible that this was an effect limited to our model system. We therefore examined the effects of locally administered lymphokines on lethal sepsis in the cecal ligation and puncture model [10, 11]. Mice were pretreated with three daily intra-peritoneally injections of supernatants from activated EL-4 cells, following which sepsis was induced by

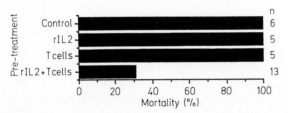

Fig. 2. The protective effect of local administration of IL-2 depends upon the presence of T cells in the host. Congenitally athymic BALB/c nu/nu mice injected intra-peritoneally, with rIL-2 (300 U/injection, days − 3. − 2, − 1), with splenic T cells from BALB/c + / + mice (3×10^6/mouse, day − 3), or both rIL-2 and T cells, and were challenged with barium sulfate and *P. aeruginosa* on day 0. Animals were observed for 7 days

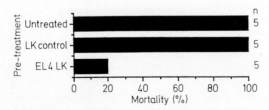

Fig. 3. Local administration of lymphokines protects animals from lethal sepsis induced by cecal ligation and puncture. Animals were injected intraperitoneally with supernatants from activated EL4 cells (EL4 LK) or control supernatants from unactivated cells (LK control) daily for 3 days. All animals were then subjected to cecal ligation and puncture as described [11] using a 23-guage needle. Animals were observed daily for 7 days

puncture of the ligated cecum with a 23-gauge needle. As shown in Fig. 3, this procedure produced lethal sepsis in untreated mice and in animals treated with a control (unactivated) EL-4 supernatant. Animals treated by local administration of lymphokine prior to challenge were protected. Thus, the protection afforded by this treatment is not restricted to *Pseudomonas*, nor to the barium sulfate model.

Workers in several laboratories have shown that administration of IL-2 can protect animals from bacterial sepsis involving *Escherichia coli* [15–17] or *Klebsiella pneumoniae* [18]. In these studies, much higher doses of IL-2 (5000–45 000 U/mouse) than used in our studies were used to give protection from lethal sepsis. However, in these models mice were challenged with very large numbers of bacteria ($> 10^8$ versus 10^5 in our studies), and untreated animals rapidly succumbed to lethal sepsis (< 24 h versus 24–72 h in our studies). As in our studies, the route of administration of IL-2 was important; protection from intraperitoneal challenge was seen only upon intraperitoneal administration of lymphokine [15].

Our results suggest that local administration of relatively low doses of lymphokines can provide protection from lethal peritoneal sepsis. While IL-2 can mediate this effect, it is likely that other lymphokines may contribute, since infected animals treated with crude supernatants appeared healthier than those treated with recombinant IL-2 (results not shown). Similarly, in a rat model of intraperitoneal sepsis, supernatants from human mixed lymphocyte cultures were found to protect animals more efficiently than do equivalent doses of rIL-2 (M. McPhee, personal communication). It is tempting to suggest that local administration of IL-2 (plus other undefined lymphokines) may provide a novel avenue to immunotherapy for bacterial sepsis.

*Acknowledgments.*This work was supported by grants to DRG from the Canadian Foundation of Ilietis and Colitis and from the Medical Research Council of Canada.

References

1. Miller SE, Miller CL, Trunkey DD (1982) The immune consequences of trauma. Surg Clin North Am 62:167
2. Baker CC (1989) Macrophage- T cell interactions in surgical sepsis. In: Faist E, Ninnemann J, Green DR (eds) Immune consequences of trauma shock and sepsis. Springer, Berlin Heidelberg New York, p 63
3. Cryz SJ, Furer E, Germanier T (1983) Simple model for the study of *Pseudomonas aeruginosa* infections in leukopenic mice. Infect. Immun. 39:1067.
4. Grogan JB (1975) *Pseudomonas aeruginosa* infection in mice after treatment with cyclophosphamide. Arch Surg 110:1473
5. Ozaki Y, Ohashi T, Minami A, Nakamura S (1987) Enhanced resistance of mice to bacterial infection induced by recombinant human interleukin-1α. Infect Immun 55:1436
6. McRipley RJ, Garrison DW (1964) Increased susceptibility of burned rats to *Pseudomonas aeruginosa*. Proc Soc Exp Biol Med 111:336.
7. Stieritz DD, Holder IA (1975) Experimental studies of the pathogenesis of infections due to *Pseudomonas aeruginosa*: description of a burned mouse model. J Inf Dis 131:688–691

8. Grobmeyer AJ, Kerlan RA, Peterson CM, Dragstedt LR (1984) Barium peritonitis Am Surg 50:116.
9. Bohnen JMA, Christou NV, Meakins JL (1987) Suppression of delayed cutaneous hypersensitivity and inflammatory cell delivery by sterile barium peritonitis. J Surg Res 43:430.
10. Wichterman KA, Baue AE, Chaudry IH (1980) Sepsis and septic shock—a review of laboratory models and a proposal. J. Surg Res 29:189.
11. Baker CC, Chaudry IH, Gaines HO, Baue AE (1983) Evaluation of factors affecting mortality following sepsis in a murine cecal ligation and puncture model. Surgery 94:331.
12. Coligan JE, Kruisbeek AM, Margulies DH, Shevach EM, Strober W (1991) Current protocols in immunology. Wiley, New York
13. Farrar JJ, Fuller-Bonar J, Simon PL, Hilfiker ML, Stadler BM, Farrar WL (1980) Thymoma production of T cell growth factor (interleukin 2). J Immunol 125:2555.
14. Mosmann TR, Coffman RL (1989) TH1 and TH2 cells: Different patterns of lymphokine secretion lead to different functional properties. Ann Rev Immunol 7:145.
15. Chong KT (1987) Prophylactic administration of interleukin-2 protects mice from lethal challenge with gram-negative bacteria. Infect Immun 55:668
16. Weyand C, Goronzy J, Fathman CG, O'Hanley P (1987) Administration in vivo of recombinant interleukin 2 protects mice against septic death. J Clin Invest 79:1756.
17. Goronzy J, Weyand C, Quan J, Fathman CG, O'Hanley P (1989) Enhanced cell-mediated protection against fatal *Escherichia coli* septicemia induced by treatment with recombinant IL-2 J Immunol 142:1134.
18. Iizawa Y, Nakao M, Kondo M, Yamazaki T (1990) Protective effect of recombinant human interleukin-2 against lethal infection caused by *Klebsiella pneumoniae*. Microbiol Immunol 34:185.

Murine Intraabdominal Abscess:
Immune Modulation with Interferon-γ

S. Galandiuk, S. Appel, J. D. Pietsch, W. G. Cheadle, and H. C. Polk Jr.

Introduction

Investigations in our laboratory have focused on changes in major histocompatibility complex (MHC) antigen expression on monocytes occurring in association with injury and clinical infection [1]. Expression of class II MHC antigens on the surface of monocytes appears to be essential for antigen recognition and T-cell proliferation [2].

Clinical studies have shown decreased MHC antigen expression (HLA-DR) following severe injury and/or operation in humans [3, 4]. Endogenous interferon-γ production in severely injured patients has also been shown to be reduced [3, 5]. Several in vitro studies have shown that such decreased MHC antigen expression can be restored to normal values by incubation with interferon-γ [6]. Animal experimental studies also suggest that interferon-γ, used either as prophylaxis or therapy, may result in increased survival in a variety of mild bacterial challenges [7–10]. We wished to evaluate the effect of interferon-γ therapy in a murine model of severe bacterial challenge.

In order to assess whether changes in MHC antigen expression on monocytes of peripheral blood are representative of cellular changes at the site of infection, we examined MHC antigen expression in monocytes of peripheral blood, peritoneal fluid, cells of abscess wall, and pus. In addition to this, we also examined opsonic capacity, phagocytic ability, and complement receptor expression of leukocytes in these various compartments.

Methods

A cecal ligation and puncture (CLP) model in outbred CD-1 mice (Charles Rivers Laboratories, Wilmington, MA, USA) was used [11].

After a 48-h acclimatization period, animals were divided into two groups: 20 animals underwent standard CLP and received 7500 U interferon-γ per day beginning 1 h after CLP and daily for 5 days thereafter, and another group of 20 animals underwent CLP alone. Survival was assessed daily for 7 days. In a

Department of Surgery, University of Louisville, Louisville, KY 40292, USA

Host Defense Dysfunction
in Trauma, Shock and Sepsis
Eds. Faist/Meakins/Schildberg
© Springer-Verlag, Berlin Heidelberg 1993

second experiment, 80 animals were divided into two groups: (1) control mice that underwent a standard CLP and (2) mice that underwent CLP with interferon-γ administered for 5 days beginning 1 h after CLP. Three animals from each group were sacrificed on postoperative days 1, 2, 4, 7, 10, and 28. Blood was collected from the retroorbital plexus after brief ether anesthesia, and peritoneal exudate cells (PEC) harvested after lavage of the peritoneal cavity with 5 ml RPMI culture medium. Pus was drained and diluted with RPMI. The abscess wall was minced using fine scissors, and likewise diluted to 1 ml.

Flow Cytometry. Specimens were analyzed using a FACScan flow cytometer. Leukocytes were analyzed by forward and 90° scatter of the laser beam to optically distinguish cell types. Once the analysis area was determined, the cellular uptake of fluorescent dye was measured by red or green fluorescence detectors as appropriate.

Opsonic Capacity. In order to quantitate the amount of opsonic material present in various compartments, 20 l of heat-killed Texas red-labelled *S. taphylococcus aureus*, corresponding to 10^9 bacteria, was then added to 200 l of diluted serum, PEC supernatant, pus supernatant, or abscess wall supernatant, and incubated for 30 min at 37 °C. Human neutrophils were then isolated from blood of a healthy volunteer. One milliliter of the neutrophil cell suspension was then added to the opsonized *S. aureus*, and incubated for 30 min at 37 °C. Neutrophils were fixed in 1% paraformaldehyde and examined by flow cytometry. Pooled mouse serum was used as a control in each assay.

Phagocytosis Assay. Heat-killed Texas red-labelled *S. aureus* were opsonized by incubation with pooled mouse serum for 30 min at 37 °C. Twenty liters of *S. aureus* were then added to either blood, PEC, cells from abscess wall, or pus. Control samples of cells without added *S. aureus* were obtained for each specimen. Cell solutions were incubated at 37 °C, lysed, washed, fixed, and then analyzed flow cytometrically to determine the density (mean channel fluorescence) of red dye in phagocytic cells. The ratio of this mean channel fluorescence to the mean channel of fluorescence of pure Texas red-labelled bacteria was obtained and used to compare the relative phagocytic capability of polymorphonuclear neutrophils (PMNs), monocytes, and macrophages from different compartments.

Ia Staining. The percentage of cells in the monocyte and PMN region expressing Ia were determined by flow cytometry after 40 µl of each specimen had been stained using 3µl of fluorescein isothiocyanate (FITC)-conjugated 043p anti-rat-Ia monoclonal antibody.

Anti-MAC-1 Staining. Cells were counterstained with 3µl FITC-labelled anti-rat immunoglobulin G (IgG) after preliminary staining with the monoclonal antibody anti-MAC-1 (M1/70), and then analyzed using flow cytometry. Anti-

MAC-1 binds to the CR3 receptor for C3bi, which is expressed on macrophages, monocytes, PMNs, and natural killer cells [12].

Results

Mortality. Interferon-γ treatment in this model was associated with a 70% 7-day mortality, compared to 40% observed with CLP alone (Fig. 1).

Opsonic Capacity. The highest opsonic capacity in both treated and untreated groups was observed in PEC supernatant. In untreated animals, opsonic capacity at first decreased, followed by an increase at 7 days. In treated animals, opsonic capacity continued to drop for the entire time period studied (Fig. 2).

Phagocytosis. Interferon-treated animals had increased phagocytosis in all compartments compared to untreated animals. As with untreated animals, pus cells had at least double the phagocytic ability of peripheral blood phagocytes at most time periods measured. Both pus cell and PEC phagocytic capability of treated animals increased after day 7 (Fig 3).

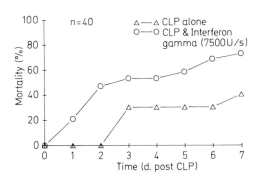

Fig. 1. Mortality following CLP alone (△) versus CLP and treatment with 7500 U interferon-γ per day for 5 days (○)

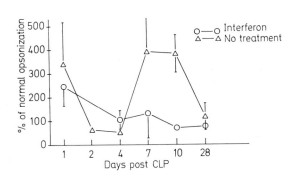

Fig. 2. Opsonic capacity of PEC supernatant over time, following CLP alone versus CLP and treatment with 7500 U interferon-γ per day for 5 days

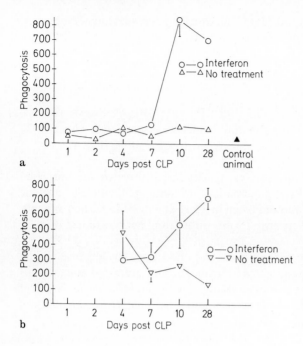

a

b

Fig. 3a,b. Phagocytic capability of **a** PEC and **b** pus cells over time following CLP alone versus CLP and treatment with 7500 U inter-feron-γ per day for 5 days

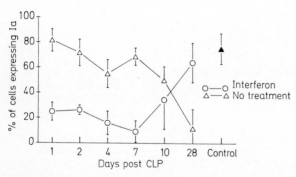

Fig. 4. Percentage of PEC monocytes/macrophages expressing Ia over time following CLP alone versus CLP and treatment with 7500 U interferon-γ per day for 5 days

Ia Antigen Expression. Monocyte Ia antigen expression in interferon-treated animals showed an initial decrease, followed by a rise in PEC Ia, not seen in untreated animals (Fig. 4). Ia in all other compartments remained markedly depressed compared to untreated animals.

Anti-MAC-1. In pus, complement receptor expression decreased markedly over time in untreated animals, while increasing steadily in interferon-treated animals (Fig. 5). No significant change was seen in other compartments.

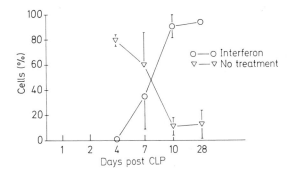

Fig. 5. Percentage of pus monocytes/macrophages staining with MAC-1 over time following CLP alone versus CLP and treatment with 7500 U interferon-γ per day for 5 days

Discussion

This study was undertaken to determine the effect of interferon administration on survival in a model of severe infection resulting in intraabdominal abscess formation and the degree to which cells in various physiologic compartments respond to exogenous interferon administration.

Several animal experimental studies have shown that prophylactic or therapeutic administration of interferon-γ results in increased survival in a variety of models of moderate bacterial challenge. In man, both in vitro and in vivo studies have shown that interferon-γ administration results in increased MO_2DR expression on monocytes. Since expression of HLA-DR on monocytes is felt to be necessary for processing of foreign antigens, this is presumably beneficial. In our model of severe surgical infection with intra-abdominal abscess formation, such interferon administration did not result in either increased survival or increased Ia expression. PEC Ia did, however, begin to rise after day 7 in treated animals. Changes in the amount of opsonic material present within peritoneal fluid suggest that complement is depleted after abdominal operation, then produced in increasing amounts. In treated animals, this increase in opsonic capacity was absent. The increase in complement receptor expression on pus cells of treated animals over time may correlate with the late increase in phagocytic ability noted in pus cells of treated animals. It may be that beneficial effects of interferon-γ treatment are only evident after the first 7 days of infection. We are not aware of any prior study defining the phagocytic ability of leukocytes in abscesses over time and comparing this with that of leukocytes in peripheral blood and peritoneal exudate. Although interferon-γ has been shown to have a beneficial effect when used prophylactically or therapeutically in less severe models of infection, clearly in this situation, interferon-γ administration had an adverse effect. This may have been different had interferon been administered *prior* to bacterial challenge, as was done in most of the other studies.

Further studies will be needed to determine whether changes in the dosage and timing of administration will alter the adverse effect seen on survival, despite the improvement in immunologic parameters described above.

References

1. Polk HC Jr, George CD, Wellhausen SR, Cost K, Davidson PR, Regan MP, Borzotta AR (1986) A systematic study of host defense processes in badly injured patients. Ann Surg 204:282–299
2. Unanue ER (1984) Antigen-presenting function of the macrophage. Annu Rev Immunol 2:395–428
3. Faist E, Mewes A, Strasser G, Walz A, Alkan S, Baker C, Ertel W, Heberer G (1988) Alteration of monocyte function following major injury. Arch Surg 123:287–292
4. Hershman MJ, Cheadle WG, Wellhausen SR, Davidson PR, Polk HC Jr (1990) Monocyte HLA-DR antigen expression characterizes clinical outcome in the trauma patient. Br J Surg 77:204–207
5. Livingston DH, Appel SA, Wellhausen SR, Sonnenfeld G, Polk HC Jr (1988) Depressed interferon gamma production and monocyte HLA-DR expression after severe injury. Arch Surg 123:1309–1312
6. Hershman MJ, Appel SA, Wellhausen SR, Polk HC Jr (1989) Interferongamma increases HLA-DR expression on monocytes in severely injured patients. Clin Exp Immunol 77:67–70
7. Hershman MJ, Polk HC Jr., Peitsch JD, Kuftinec D, Sonnenfeld G (1988) Modulation of *Klebsiella pneumoniae* infection of mice by interferon-gamma. Clin Exp Immunol 72:406–409
8. Hershman MJ, Sonnenfeld G, Mays BW, Fleming F, Trachtenberg LS. Polk HC Jr (1988) Effects of interferon-gamma treatment on surgically simulated wound infection in mice. Microb Pathog 4:165–168
9. Hershman MJ, Sonnenfeld G, Logan WA, Pietsch JD, Wellhausen SR, Polk HC Jr (1988) Effect of interferon-gamma treatment of the course of a burn wound infection. J. Interferon Res 8:367–373
10. Hershman MJ, Polk HC Jr, Pietsch JD, Shields RE, Wellhausen SR, Sonnenfeld G (1988) Modulation of infection by gamma interferon treatment following trauma. Infect Immun 56:2412–2416
11. Baker CC, Chaudry IH, Gaines HO, Baue AE (1983) Evaluation of factors affecting mortality rate after sepsis in a murine cecal ligation and puncture model. Surgery 94:331–335
12. Beller DI, Springer TA, Schreiber RD (1982) Anti-Mac-1 selectively inhibits the mouse and human type three complement receptor. J Exp Med 156:1000–1009

Acute Resuscitation and Antioxidant Therapy*

B. E. Hedlund and P. E. Hallaway

Introduction

The following discussion is divided into two parts. The first deals with the role of iron in the genesis of tissue injury occurring during regional or global ischemia and subsequent reperfusion. The second pertains to current practices of fluid replacement and how antioxidant therapies can be incorporated into acute fluid resuscitation regimens following severe burn and trauma.

The appearance of increased levels of plasma iron subsequent to global hypoperfusion has been described in several papers published in the mid-1950s by Mazur and coworkers [1–3]. In one of these reports [1], the authors demonstrated that iron, in quantities sufficient to completely saturate the available transferrin binding capacity, was released during hemorrhagic shock. At the time of these studies, superoxide and superoxide dismutase had not yet been discovered, and Mazur proposed that uric acid could directly reduce and liberate iron from ferritin [1]. A few years after Mazur's studies, Janoff and coworkers [4] observed similar increases in plasma iron following hypovolemic, but not septic, shock.

In the more than 30 years since Mazur's germinal study of the role of xanthine oxidase, ferritin, and iron in the context of tissue hypoperfusion, our knowledge of the biochemical mechanisms leading to microvascular dysfunction following severe ischemic insults has gradually expanded. The concept of reperfusion injury is now well defined and the critical role of reactive, oxygen-derived radicals in the genesis of this type of vascular injury is fully documented. In addition, there is a general recognition that iron may be an important component of this process, because of its ability to act as a catalyst in Haber-Weiss and Fenton-type reactions leading to the formation of the highly reactive hydroxyl radical.

* Supported by NIH grant R44 DK37207
Biomedical Frontiers, Inc, Minneapolis, MN 55414, USA

Host Defense Dysfunction
in Trauma, Shock and Sepsis
Eds. Faist/Meakins/Schildberg
© Springer-Verlag, Berlin Heidelberg 1993

Role of Iron in Reperfusion Injury

Our understanding of the importance of "free," catalytically active iron as a causative agent in tissue injury or organ dysfunction secondary to ischemia and reperfusion derives from preclinical studies in which iron chelators have afforded protection. In most of these studies, the evidence for the involvement of iron is indirect. Thus, if a compound neutralizes iron and protects against tissue injury, iron is presumably involved in the reactions leading to the observed injury. Other explanations for this protection, such as direct scavenging of free radicals, have been proposed but are unlikely. Recently, Halliwell [5] concluded that the protective effect of deferoxamine (DFO; Desferal, CIBA-Geigy) in animal models of human disease is due largely to its ability to inhibit iron-dependent free radical reactions. Furthermore, several investigators have shown that the iron-saturated form of DFO, ferrioxamine, is no longer efficacious in these models, thereby implicating iron chelation as the protective mechanism.

Despite the impressive number of papers indicating that DFO protects against reperfusion injury, relatively few provide evidence of actual release of iron in the context of ischemia/reperfusion. Some of the more significant studies dealing with this topic will be discussed in the following section.

Paller and coworkers [6–8] have demonstrated that DFO and other antioxidants protect against both heme protein- and warm ischemia-induced renal dysfunction in the rat. Importantly, these investigators [8] also reported a tenfold increase in the urinary iron concentration during reperfusion following a 60-min period of ischemia. Several studies have demonstrated that injury to the mucosa of the stomach and intestine following ischemia and reperfusion is caused, in part, by oxygen radicals. Smith et al. [9] demonstrated that DFO provided impressive protection against mucosal leak in a hemorrhage model in the rat. Similarly, Hernandez and coworkers [10] have contributed further evidence that iron is a critical component in the genesis of reperfusion injury using a feline model of intestinal ischemia. The authors demonstrated that DFO and apotransferrin afforded considerable protection against the mucosal leak occurring after 60 min of incomplete ischemia (10%–15% of normal arterial blood flow). The protective effect of apotransferrin, an iron-binding protein with a molecular weight of 80000, suggests that the protective agent does not need to penetrate cells to be effective. Robinson and Hedlund [11] noted a significant increase in the plasma iron concentration in rats exposed to 90 min of total intestinal ischemia. This released iron may decrease the intrinsic antioxidant potential of the plasma by lowering the effective iron-binding capacity. Infusion of additional apotransferrin, as in the case of the Hernandez study, enhances the plasma antioxidant potential in an animal exposed to a severe ischemic insult.

An early study implicating iron in the pathophysiology of the severely ischemic myocardium was conducted by Holt and collaborators [12]. These workers demonstrated increased levels of low molecular weight iron compounds in homogenates of myocardial tissue exposed to 2 h of ischemia "in vivo," Bolli et al. [13], using intravenous pretreatment, and Farber et al. [14], using intraatrial infusion of DFO, showed significant attenuation of postischemic ventricular dysfunction of the canine stunned myocardium, a model associated with reversible myocardial injury. In more severe models of myocardial ischemia, Lesnefsky et al. [15] and Reddy et al. [16] documented reduction in infarct size when DFO was given prior to the ischemic insult.

Bolli et al. [17, 18] have demonstrated that both the hydroxyl radical scavenger mercaptopropionylglycine and DFO, given immediately prior to reperfusion protect the stunned myocardium, while administration of these agents 1 min after the initiation of reperfusion fails to afford protection.

Although DFO has provided impressive protection in several animal models of myocardial ischemia, it has several drawbacks when given intravenously. Most notable are its rapid excretion and the significant hypotension associated with intravenous infusion of the drug [13, 19, 20, 21]. A new form of DFO, lacking the hypotensive effect but retaining the powerful iron binding properties, has been prepared by the covalent attachment of the drug to biocompatible polymers such as dextran and hydroxyethyl starch [21]. In a study of the hemodynamic effects of slow intra-atrial infusion of DFO in conscious dogs, Forder et al. [20] noted significant hypotension and, more importantly, alteration in segmental shortening of the myocardium in animals receiving the native drug. In contrast, animals receiving the polymer-DFO conjugate at equivalent doses showed no adverse hemodynamic or cardiac effects. Maruyama et al. [19] have recently shown that these high molecular weight forms of DFO provide improved return of segmental shortening in a canine stunned myocardium model, whereas native DFO provides no benefit.

In summary, release of iron has been demonstrated to occur from the ischemic myocardium, kidney and intestine. Furthermore, it has been clearly established that deferoxamine (DFO) affords considerable protection against tissue injury mediated by iron and free radical or organ dysfunction in several relevant preclinical models.

Experimental global ischemia can be acheived by two distinctly different approaches. The first involves cardiac arrest, in which the brain is the primary target organ for ischemic injury. The second involves hemorrhage leading to global hypoperfusion, in which the gut, liver, kidney and lung become target organs for injury. Systemic oxidant-mediated damage has been well documented and a variety of antioxidants have been tested in both models. These studies cannot be reviewed in detail in this brief communication. This discussion will be limited to the role of iron in the observed pathophysiology and the use of iron chelators as therapeutic agents.

The involvement of iron in brain injury following cardiac arrest has been studied by two groups, with initial results reported in 1985 [22, 23]. Babbs [22] and Kompala and Babbs [24] noted improved survival in DFO-treated rats following cardiac arrest. White and coworkers [23] clearly demonstrated iron-mediated lipid peroxidation in dogs exposed to a cerebral ischemia. The same group has also shown that brain injury occurring after an ischemic insult is due, in part, to iron and iron-mediated reactions involving oxygen and lipid radicals [25–27]. However, evidence that iron chelation therapy, or any other approach aimed at oxygen radical scavenging, improves neurological outcome in a relevant preclinical model is less impressive. In one model of stroke, iron chelation therapy failed to demonstrate any effect [28]. The rather universal lack of neurological efficacy obtained by iron chelator treatment may be due to intrinsic problems associated with systemic delivery of DFO, the iron chelator used in these studies. In order to achieve maximal efficacy, relatively high concentrations of the drug must be delivered to the ischemic brain. Intravenous administration of DFO is associated with significant hypotension which may further aggravate the ischemic injury.

In summary, injury to the brain occurring secondary to ischemia and reperfusion is due, in part, to iron-catalyzed reactions leading to lipid peroxidation. As in the case of the myocardium, kidney, and intestine, iron delocalization has been demonstrated to occur in the ischemic brain. Iron chelation therapy decreases lipid peroxidation in the brain and appears to attenuate morphological signs of cellular injury. Inclusion of iron chelators and other antioxidants in the resuscitation protocol has only marginally attenuated neurological dysfunction in preclinical models reported to date.

Preclinical studies of hypovolemic shock in which an iron chelator has been tested as part of resuscitative therapy are less common in the literature. One study deserves mention in this context. Sanan and collaborators [29] demonstrated that intramuscular injection of DFO (25 mg/kg) improved survival and decreased liver pathology in animals exposed to severe hemorrhagic shock. The authors conclude that "the salutory effects of desferrioxamine may be due to inhibition of iron catalyzed free-radical production. . ." In addition, delivery of the pharmacological agent during the hypotensive period was superior to administration at the time of fluid therapy. Sanan et al. confirmed earlier studies [1, 4] documenting systemic release of iron in the course of a severe hypotensive insult. In this type of hypovolemic global ischemia it seems likely that a major fraction of iron appearing in the vascular compartment originates from the ischemic liver.

Three conclusions can be drawn from the multitude of studies discussed above. First, iron is an important component in the genesis of tissue injury following ischemia and reperfusion. Second, systemic or targeted delivery of the potent iron chelator DFO, reduces "reperfusion injury." Third, the earlier the therapeutic agent is administered, the better the protection. Of particular relevance to the treatment of shock and trauma is that therapeutic intervention with the chelator/radical scavenger should take place as early as possible during resuscitative procedures.

Incorporation of Antioxidants in Acute Resuscitation

Since iron chelation, and in particular, the clinically used chelator DFO, provide considerable protection against tissue injury caused by ischemia and reperfusion, one would expect this drug to be incorporated into clinical medicine in situations involving reperfusion injury as part of the overall pathophysiology. Although a limited number of reports describe the use of DFO, as a component of cardioplegic solutions [30, 31] or in the context of cardiac transplantation [32], the drug has not been generally incorporated into clinical practice. The primary reasons for the limited use of DFO as a means for reducing reperfusion injury are its short vascular half-life and its tendency to produce hypotension.

In most situations of severe hypovolemic shock/trauma, the first therapeutic intervention normally involves fluid therapy using crystalloid or colloid solutions. Whenever blood is available, either whole blood or red cells suspended in crystalloid is administered to provide oxygen carrying capacity. By initially providing crystalloid solution to a hypovolemic patient some degree of tissue oxygenation is achieved, but the opportunity to combine oxygenation with antioxidant therapy is lost. Crystalloid and colloid solutions have no antioxidant capacity. Red cells in crystalloids lack the primary antioxidants found in human plasma, namely, apotransferrin and ceruloplasmin.

Based on accumulated knowledge from a large number of studies of reperfusion injury it seems abundantly clear that principles learned from individual organs can be applied to acute resuscitation of the globally hypoperfused victim of shock, burn, and trauma. Incorporation of anti-oxidant therapy at the time of fluid resuscitation will provide protection against iron-mediated free radical reactions that occur at reperfusion. By reducing "resuscitation-induced" microvascular injury, one can reasonably hypothesize that the severity of additional sequelae of shock and trauma, such as degree of microvascular leak, magnitude of neutrophil margination into hypoperfused tissue, and overall post shock inflammatory response can be significantly attenuated.

What are the candidates for a therapeutic agent to provide antioxidant protection at the time of initial resuscitation? Although this discussion has focused on the critical role of iron in the context of reperfusion injury, there is abundant evidence that enzymatic radical scavengers may prove highly efficacious in this context. Thus, superoxide dismutase, catalase and synthetic mimics thereof could, in principle, be administered at the time of resuscitation. The usefulness of superoxide dismutase and catalase is diminished by two factors. The vascular half-time of these proteins is relatively short and it seems likely that incorporating these proteins into resuscitation fluids would be relatively expensive. The normally occurring iron binding protein transferrin and the ferrioxidase ceruloplasmin both represent powerful antioxidants. Transferrin and ceruloplasmin have not been extensively used in models of reperfusion injury. The relatively low iron binding capacity of transferrin, two sites per molecule, would necessitate infusing as much as 10 g in a normal adult to increase plasma iron binding capacity by a factor of two. Synthetic, high molecular weight, iron chelators may provide compounds with a much higher iron binding capacity. One example of such a "synthetic transferrin", obtained by covalent attachment of DFO to colloids, has been described by Hallaway et al. [21]. These compounds contain 10–20 times as many iron binding sites as tranferrin on a per weight basis. Furthermore, attachment of the chelator to the colloid dramatically reduces the toxicity of DFO. Results obtained with this novel high molecular weight chelator suggest significant efficacy in a number of relevant models [19, 33–36]. Of importance to fluid therapy in the context of resuscitation following hypovolemic and/or traumatic injury is that the iron chelator-colloid conjugate can be incorporated into conventional colloid therapy, thereby simultaneously achieving combined volume replacement and antioxidant therapy.

References

1. Mazur A, Baez S, Shorr E (1955) The mechanism of iron release from ferritin as related to its biological properties. J Biol Chem 213:147–160
2. Green S, Mazur A (1957) Relation of uric acid metabolism to release of iron from hepatic ferritin. J Biol Chem 219:653–668
3. Mazur A, Green S, Saha A, Carleton A (1958) Mechanism of release of ferritin iron in vivo by xanthine oxidase. J Clin Invest 37:1809–1817
4. Janoff A, Zweifach BW, Shapiro LR (1960) Levels of plasma-bound iron in experimental shock in the rabbit and dog. Am J Physiol 198:1161–1165
5. Halliwell B (1989) Protection against tissue damage in vivo by desferrioxamine: what is its mechanism of action? Free Radic Biol Med 7:645–651
6. Paller MS, Hoidal JR, Ferris TF (1984) Oxygen free radicals in ischemic acute renal failure in the rat. J Clin Invest 74:1156–1162
7. Paller MS (1988) Hemoglobin- and myoglobin-induced acute renal failure in rats: role of iron in nephrotoxicity. Am J Physiol 255 (Renal Fluid Electrolyte Physiol 24): F539–F544
8. Paller MS, Hedlund BE (1988) Role of iron in post-ischemic renal injury in the rat. Kidney Int 34:474–480
9. Smith SM, Grisham MB, Manci EA et al. (1987) Gastric mucosal injury in the rat: role of iron and xanthine oxidase Gastroenterology 91:950–956
10. Hernandez LA, Grisham MB, Granger DN (1987) A role for iron in oxidant-mediated ischemic injury to intestinal microvasculature. Am J Physiol 253 (Gastrointest Liver Physiol 16):G49–G53
11. Robinson E, Hedlund B (1989) Role of iron in ischemia and reperfusion (abstract). Circ Shock 27:367
12. Holt S, Gunderson M, Joyce K et al. (1987) Myocardial tissue iron delocalization and evidence for lipid peroxidation after two hours of ischemia. Ann Emerg Med 15:1155–1159
13. Bolli R, Patel BS, Zhu WY et al. (1988) The iron chelator DFO attenuates post-ischemic dysfunction. Am J Physiol 253 (Heart and Circ Physiol) H1372–H1380
14. Farber NE, Vercellotti GM, Jacob HS et al. (1988) Evidence for a role of iron-catalyzed oxidants in functional and metabolic stunning in the canine heart. Circ Res 63:351–360
15. Lesnefsky EJ, Repine JE, Horwitz LD (1990) DFO pretreatment reduces canine infarct size and oxidative injury. J Pharmacol Exp Therap 253:1103–1109
16. Reddy BR, Kloner RA, Przyklenk K (1989) Early treatment with DFO limits myocardial ischemic/reperfusion injury. Free Radic Biol Med 7:45–52
17. Bolli R, Jeroudi MO, Patel BS et al. (1989) Marked reduction of free radical generation and contractile dysfunction by antioxidant therapy begun at the time of reperfusion. Circ Res 65:607–622
18. Bolli R, Patel BS, Jeroudi MO et al. (1990) Iron mediated radical reactions upon reperfusion contribute to myocardial "stunning". Am J Physiol 259 (Heart Circ Physiol 28):H1901–H1911
19. Maruyama M, Pieper GM, Kalyanaraman B et al. (1991) Effects of hydroxyethyl starch conjugated DFO on myocardial functional recovery following coronary occlusion and reperfusion in dogs. J Cardiovasc Pharmacol 17:166–175
20. Forder JR, McClanahan TB, Gallagher KP et al. (1990) Hemodynamic effects of intraatrial administration of DFO or DFO-pentafraction conjugate to conscious dogs. J Cardiovasc Pharmacol 16:742–749

21. Hallaway PE, Eaton JW, Panter SS, Hedlund BE (1989) Modulation of DFO toxicity and clearance by covalent attachment to biocompatible polymers. Proc Nat Acad Sci USA 86:10108–10112
22. Babbs CF (1985) Role of iron ions in the genesis of reperfusion injury following successful cardiopulmonary resuscitation: preliminary data and a biochemical hypothesis. Ann Emerg Med 14:777–783
23. White BC, Krause GS, Aust SD (1985) Postischemic tissue injury by iron-mediated free radical lipid peroxidation. Ann Emerg Med 14:804–809
24. Kompala CF, Babbs CF (1986) Effect of DFO on late deaths following CPR in rats. Ann Emerg Med 15:405–407
25. Krause GS, Joyce KM, Nayini NR et al. (1985) Cardiac arrest and resuscitation. Brain iron delocalization during reperfusion. Ann Emerg Med 14:1037–1043
26. Komar JS, Nayini NR, Bialick HA et al. (1986) Brain iron delocalization and lipid peroxidation following cardiac arrest. Ann Emerg Med 15:384–389
27. Krause GS, Nayini NR, White BC et al. (1987) Natural course of iron delocalization and lipid peroxidation during the first eight hours following a 15-minute cardiac arrest in dogs. Ann Emerg Med 16:1200–1205
28. Fleischer JE, Lanier WL, Milde JH, Michenfelder JD (1987) Failure of DFO, an iron chelator, to improve neurologic outcome following complete cerebral ischemia in dogs. Stroke 18:124–127
29. Sanan S, Sharma G, Malhotra R et al. (1989) Protection by desferrioxamine against histopathological changes of the liver in the post-oligaemic phase of clinical hemorrhagic shock in dogs: correlation with improved survival rate and recovery. Free Radic Res Commun 6:29–38
30. Menasché P, Pasquier C, Bellucci S et al. (1988) DFO reduces neutrophil-mediated free radical production during cardiopulmonary bypass in man. J Thorac Cardiovasc Surg 96:582–589
31. Illes RW, Silverman NA, Krukenkamp IB et al. (1989) Amelioration of postischemic stunning by DFO-blood cardioplegia. Circulation 80, Suppl 3:30–35
32. Menasché P, Grousset C, Mouas C, Piwnica A (1990) A promising approach for improving the recovery of heart transplants. Prevention of free radical injury through iron chelation by DFO. J Thorac Cardiovasc Surg 100:13–21
33. Mahoney JR, Hallaway PE, Hedlund BE, Eaton JW (1989) Acute iron poisoning rescue with macromolecular chelators. J Clin Invest 84:1362–1366
34. Demling RH, Lalonde C, Knox J et al. (1991) Fluid resuscitation with DFO prevents systemic burn induced oxidant injury. J Trauma 31:538–544
35. Drugas GT, Paidas CN, Yahanda AM et al (1991) Conjugated DFO attenuates hepatic microvascular injury following ischemia-reperfusion. Circ Shock 34:278–283
36. Jacobs DM, Julsrud JM, Bubrick MP (1991) Iron chelation with a DFO conjugate in hemorrhagic shock. J Surg Res 51:484–490

Clinical Indications for the Administration of Oxygen Radical Scavengers*

J. Hill[1], T. Lindsay[1], C. R. Valeri[2], D. Shepro[3], and H. B. Hechtman[1]

Introduction

The role of oxygen free radicals (OFRs) as mediators of tissue injury has been the subject of extensive research during the last 20 years. The ubiquity of free radicals in biological systems has led to great optimism about the potential benefits of their pharmacological manipulation. Despite the wealth of information in animal models of injury, the assessment of OFR scavengers in human disease has only just begun.

Source of OFRs

Two important sources of OFRs are tissue xanthine oxidase (XO) and neutrophil reduced nicotinamide adenine dinucleotide phosphate (NADPH) oxidase. During tissue ischemia the intracellular enzyme xanthine dehydrogenase (XD) is converted to XO, which results in the enzyme using oxygen rather than nicotinamide adenine dinucleotide (NAD) as an oxidant. At the same time during ischemia, cellular adenosine triphosphate (ATP) is converted to hypoxanthine. When oxygen is reintroduced to tissues on reperfusion, XO catalyzes the conversion of hypoxanthine to urate and in so doing reduces molecular oxygen to superoxide (O_2^-) and hydrogen peroxide (H_2O_2).

The second important source of OFRs in tissue injury is the polymorphonuclear leukocyte. Phagocytic leukocytes contain NADPH oxidase which reduces molecular oxygen to superoxide. Activated neutrophils also secrete myeloperoxidase, an enzyme which catalyzes the formation of hypochlorous acid from hydrogen peroxide and chloride ions (Fig. 1).

Hydrogen peroxide can be produced directly by XO, or indirectly through the spontaneous dismutation of O_2^-, in addition to the H_2O_2 produced by

* Supported in part by the National Institutes of Health, grants GM 24891-11, GM 35141-03, HL 16714-13; the U.S. Navy Office of Naval Research, contract no. N00014-88-C-0118; the Brigham Surgical Group, Inc.; and the Trauma Research Foundation

[1] Departments of Surgery and Pathology, Brigham and Women's Hospital, 75 Francis St., Boston, MA 02115. USA and the Harvard Medical School, Cambridge, MA 02138, USA

[2] Naval Blood Research Laboratory, Boston, Massachusetts

[3] Biological Science Center, Boston University, Boston, MA 02215, USA

Host Defense Dysfunction
in Trauma, Shock and Sepsis
Eds. Faist/Meakins/Schildberg
© Springer-Verlag, Berlin Heidelberg 1993

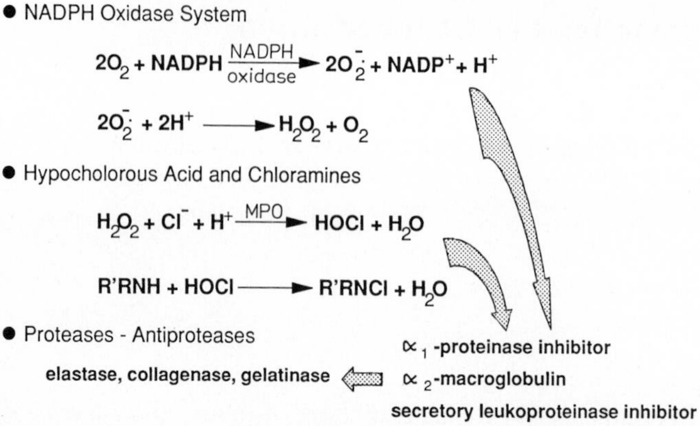

● NADPH Oxidase System

$$2O_2 + NADPH \xrightarrow[\text{oxidase}]{\text{NADPH}} 2O_2^- + NADP^+ + H^+$$

$$2O_2^- + 2H^+ \longrightarrow H_2O_2 + O_2$$

● Hypocholorous Acid and Chloramines

$$H_2O_2 + Cl^- + H^+ \xrightarrow{MPO} HOCl + H_2O$$

$$R'RNH + HOCl \longrightarrow R'RNCl + H_2O$$

● Proteases - Antiproteases α_1-proteinase inhibitor

   elastase, collagenase, gelatinase ⟸ α_2-macroglobulin

                                   secretory leukoproteinase inhibitor

Fig. 1. Tissue destruction by neutrophils

neutrophils. Further sources of free radicals are those produced during cyclo- and lipoxygenation. Superoxide is also formed during the autooxidation of many substances of biological importance, including epinephrine, thiols, and hemoglobin. The spontaneous dismutation of O_2^- proceeds rapidly in aqueous solution, so the production of O_2^- is always accompanied by production of H_2O_2. The dismutation of superoxide is greatly accelerated by the enzyme superoxide dismutase.

O_2^- and H_2O_2 react in the presence of transition metals such as iron or copper, in the Haber-Weiss reaction, to produce the reactive hydroxyl radical (OH·). For the reaction to proceed, not only must iron (or copper) be present, but these metals cannot be complexed. Fe(citrate), Fe(ADP), Fe(ATP) and a number of other potential physiological chelates prevent the production of OH·. Iron in plasma and extracellular fluids is almost exclusively bound to protein and therefore not available as a catalyst. Other potential sources of iron are transferrin, hemoglobin, other heme proteins, and ferritin. Neither transferrin nor the heme compounds generate OH·.

However, ferritin iron can be mobilized by O_2^- generated during ischemia/-reperfusion (I/R) injury and this may lead to OH· production. Evidence of the importance of iron in intestinal I/R injury is the observation that either desferoxamine (an iron chelator) or apotransferrin (an iron binding protein) provide protection against the increased microvascular permeability produced by I/R. When desferoxamine and apotransferrin were iron loaded their protective effects were lost [1].

Neutrophils release two iron proteins, lactoferrin and myeloperoxidase, neither of which is able to catalyze production of OH·. At present, it is unclear whether the neutrophil has a source of catalytic iron. Further, there is no firm evidence that neutrophil-induced tissue damage is due to OH·.

Evidence for OFR-Mediated Tissue Injury

Evidence for the involvement of free radicals in tissue damage is based on the following observations. Firstly, the measurement of free radicals in tissues following injury. Secondly, that conversion of XD to XO and ATP to hypoxanthine conversion occur in ischemic tissue. Thirdly, that amelioration of injury can be achieved with both OFR and XO inhibitors. Finally, tissue injury can be reproduced by the introduction of OFRs.

OFRs can be measured directly by electron paramagnetic resonance spectroscopy combined with spin-trapping techniques, but these techniques are difficult and none of them are absolutely specific at distinguishing the different radicals. It is not yet possible to directly measure the concentrations of OFRs in vivo. Indirect measurements using assays of malondialdehyde and conjugated dienes are commonly used. These techniques measure end products of lipid peroxidation. The results are frequently used as an index of free radical generation.

Unfortunately, lipid peroxidation occurs in any in vivo situation involving cell injury or death and therefore does not provide conclusive evidence that OFRs are produced or responsible for the observed injury. Indeed, direct OFR measurements do not provide conclusive evidence regarding their relationship to cellular injury. Finally, some regions defy measurement such as OFRs released in the microenvironment formed by neutrophils adherent to endothelium.

Pharmacological data is the principal argument for the involvement of OFRs in tissue injury. Unfortunately, the mechanism of action of OFR scavengers is not necessarily specific. Allopurinol and oxypurinol probably have direct free radical scavenging properties as well as inhibiting XO. Further, oxypurinol will scavenge neutrophil-derived hypochlorous acid. We have shown that allopurinol will inhibit neutrophil diapedesis in response to leukotrienes; clearly not a XO-mediated event. Superoxide dismutase (SOD), dimethylthioruea (DMTU), dimethylsulfoxide (DMSO), and mannitol all inhibit thromboxane and leukotriene synthesis in addition to scavenging free radicals [2]. Indeed, Kaufman, et al. have demonstrated that SOD and DMTU inhibited thromboxane synthesis by ADP-stimulated platelets in a dose-dependent manner [3] (Fig. 2). Further confusing interpretation is the observation that DMSO reduces neutrophil chemotaxis and SOD and catalase prevent neutrophil infiltration. This has led to the hypothesis that OFRs may act directly or indirectly as chemoattractants [4].

Although tissue injury can be produced by injection of OFR-generating systems directly into the circulation, experiments using this technique are not modeled after pathologic events as most OFRs are produced within tissues. Further, not all investigators have been able to generate tissue injury with OFR systems. McCord, et al. were unable to produce an edematous lesion by the intradermal injection of XO and purine [5]. Thus, despite the enormous amount

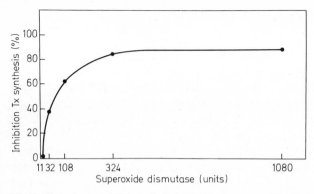

Fig. 2. Thromboxane (*TX*) synthesis inhibition by superoxide dismutase

of data that has been collected, the relationship between OFR generation and tissue injury remains unclear.

Natural Antioxidant Defences

The O_2^- produced within living cells is efficiently scavenged by the intracellular enzyme SOD. There are at least three SOD isoenzymes in mammals: CuZn-SOD in the cytosol of cells; Mn-SOD in the mitochondrial matrix; and extracellular SOD. As O_2^- is directly toxic to cells, SOD is an important naturally occurring free radical scavenger in mammalian cells and bacteria. H_2O_2 produced within living cells is also scavenged by the intracellular enzymes catalase and glutathione peroxidase.

Many investigators have attributed the combined toxicity of O_2^- and H_2O_2 to the production of the hydroxyl radical. No known enzymes regulate the concentration of this agent. However, there are scavengers, both water and lipid soluble, that effectively neutralize the hydroxyl radical. Vitamin E, a mixture of four lipid-soluble phenols called tocopherols, is believed to owe its biological effects to its antioxidant activity. Further, α-tocopherol is the most active of the four in trapping peroxy radicals. Vitamin E is incorporated into membranes and protects the polyunsaturated fatty acids from peroxidation. Ascorbic acid also protects against lipid peroxidation, probably by maintaining vitamin E in a reduced state. Carotenoids are another oxidant defence. However, their mechanism of action is poorly understood. Although the ability of vitamins C, E, and the carotenoids to function as antioxidants is known, the importance of their homeostatic action remains speculative.

Inhibitors of Potential Clinical Value

The antiinflammatory activity of SOD was discovered more than two decades ago. Since then, other OFR scavengers including catalase, DMSO, DMTU, mannitol, N-acetyl-L-cysteine, reduced glutathione, and desferroxamine have been described. Inhibition of free radical synthesis largely relates to antagonism of XO. This is done competitively by allopurinol and oxypurinol. XD to XO conversion can be inhibited by Trasylol and Ca^{2+} channel blockers which prevent protease and phospholipase A_2 activation. Using one or more of these agents, OFR inhibition has been demonstrated to prevent tissue injury in a large variety of experimental models, most often involving I/R or complement activation. OFR inhibition can ameliorate local tissue damage associated with reperfusion of ischemic tissue in the heart, brain, intestine, kidney, skeletal muscle, lung, and liver as well as the remote lung injury following lower torso ischemia. In the setting of presumed complement activation, OFR inhibition has been shown to be of benefit in burns, pancreatitis, and sepsis. Animal models of arthritis, gastric ulcer, and liver disease can also be benefitted with these agents.

The ubiquitous nature of OFRs in biological systems might suggest that their inhibition might prove to be a universal panacea. This is not the case. Although conflicting reports may reflect different dosages, methods of administration, or interspecies variations in tissue XO levels, some doubt exists as to the role of OFRs and their mechanism of tissue injury as well as the mechanism of action of OFR inhibitors. Thus, some studies of myocardial and renal I/R injury have not demonstrated a benefit with OFR inhibition. During myocardial ischemia, hypoxic myocytes show an oxygen-dependent Ca^{2+} uptake which is unaffected by OFR scavengers. Further, OFR scavengers have not proven to be of benefit in experimental endotoxemia induced lung injury. Endotoxin is thought to lead to complement fragment C5a release with resultant neutrophil activation and oxygen radical generation. Although OFRs can be measured following endotoxin administration, the lung injury and hemodynamic changes associated with endotoxemia are unaffected by treatment with SOD, catalase, or DMTU. It is unclear why the early endotoxin-induced hemodynamic changes, granulocytopenia, and increased permeability of the alveolar-capillary membrane may be attenuated with catalase. Some reports indicate improved survival using OFR scavengers in rats following endotoxin administration while others do not. Thus, in certain experimental injuries, OFR scavengers are at best only partially effective.

In most clinical situations an injurious event such as ischemia cannot be predicted, e.g., myocardial infarction. If OFR scavengers are to be of benefit clinically, it should be possible to administer the drug at the time of reperfusion or later. Several studies have shown that this is possible. If the ischemia can be predicted, as in organs harvested for transplantation, OFR scavengers can be used during the ischemic period. Both modified Collins solution (containing mannitol) and University of Wisconsin solution (containing allopurinol and glutathione) are used effectively for organ preservation in man. It may be possible to improve the results by supplementation with additional OFR scavengers at the time of reperfusion.

Studies in Man

In comparison with the huge number of animal reports, there are relatively few studies in man. The hydroxyl radical scavenger mannitol has been used effectively to prevent the reperfusion pulmonary injury which follows abdominal aortic aneurysm surgery. In this setting its mechanism of action is unclear since there is inhibition of the eicosanoids [6]. Secondly, in a large clinical trial bovine SOD was shown to reduce early renal failure in patients receiving cold-ischemia preserved kidneys, but this reduction did not achieve significance [7]. Thirdly, a small clinical trial in France has shown a potential benefit of bovine copper zinc SOD in the treatment of Crohn's disease [8]. The use of bovine-derived SOD was generally safe and well tolerated, although one patient in the Crohn's study suffered an anaphylactic reaction to the drug. Finally, it is now thought that several drugs that have enjoyed extensive clinical use may act through OFR inhibition, such as gold therapy in arthritis and desferroxamine in hemochromatosis.

There has been considerable interest in the development of a recombinant human SOD (rHSOD). To date there have been few completed trials in man using this drug. A trial of the drug in patients undergoing percutaneous transluminal angioplasty for myocardial infarction did not demonstrate improved patency rates or improved myocardial function when treated with rHSOD [9]. The results of further trials of rHSOD in patients with rheumatoid arthritis, ulcerative colitis, myocardial infarction, and renal transplantation are awaited.

Therapeutic Limitations

Both SOD and catalase (CAT) are high-molecular-weight proteins (33 000 and 240 000 respectively) which makes delivery into cells difficult. In many studies pretreatment with both SOD and CAT over several hours has been necessary in order to achieve a therapeutic effect. Liposomal encapsulation of SOD has been used to improve delivery and lengthen the half-life from 6 min to 5 h. Linking SOD and CAT to polyethylene glycol also increases the half-life up to 35 h without reducing efficacy. Unfortunately, rHSOD also has a short half-life and a bolus injection followed by a continuous infusion is required to achieve satisfactory tissue levels.

The different isoenzymes of SOD have different efficacies. Extracellular SOD, which is associated with vessel endothelium in addition to being present in plasma, is more effective than CuZn-SOD in inhibiting microvascular permeability in ischemia. These aspects of OFR research have received little attention, but may have important implications for treatment in man.

Conclusion

There are as yet no clear indications for the use of oxygen radical scavengers in man. The results of ongoing clinical trials with rHSOD are awaited with interest. Whilst the results of these studies may provide a clearer picture of their potential benefit in man, precisely how the drugs work remains to be determined.

References

1. Hernandez LS, Grisham MB, Granger DN (1987) A role for iron in oxidant-mediated ischemic injury to intestinal microvasculature. Am J Physiol 253:G49–53
2. Michael LH, Zhang Z, Hartley CJ, Bolli R, Taylor AA, Entman ML (1990) Thromboxane B_2 in cardiac lymph: effect of superoxide dismutase and catalase during myocardial ischemia and reperfusion. Circ Res 66:1040–1044
3. Kaufman RP, Klausner JM, Anner H, Feingold H, Kobzik L, Valeri CR, Shepro D, Hechtman HB (1988) Inhibition of thromboxane synthesis by free radical scavengers. J Trauma 28:458–464
4. Petrone WF, English DK, Wong K, McCord JM (1980) Free radicals and inflammation: superoxide-dependent activation of neutrophil chemotactic factor in plasma. Proc Natl Acad Sci USA 77:1159–1163
5. McCord JM, Wong K, Stokes SH, Petrone WF, English D (1980) Superoxide and inflammation: a mechanism for the anti-inflammatory activity of superoxide dismutase. Acta Physiol Scand [Suppl] 492:25–30
6. Paterson IS, Klausner JM, Goldman G, Pugatch R, Feingold H, Allen P, Mannick JA, Valeri CR, Shepro D, Hechtman, HB (1989) Pulmonary edema following aneurysm surgery is modified by mannitol. Ann Surg 210:796–801
7. Schneeberger H, Illner WD, Abendroth D, Bulkley G, Rutili F, Williams M, Thiel M, Land W (1989) First clinical experiences with superoxide dismutase in kidney transplantation—results of a double blind randomized study. Transplant Proc 21:1245–1246
8. Emerit J, Pelletier S, Tosoni-Verlignue D, Mollet M (1989) Phase II trial of copper zinc superoxide dismutase (CuAnSOD) in treatment of Crohn's disease. Free Radic Biol Med 7:145–149
9. Werns S, Brinker J, Gruber J, Rothbaum D, Heuser R, George B, Burwell L, Kereiakes D, Mancini GBJ, Flaherty J (1989) A randomized, double-blind trial of recombinant human superoxide dismutase (SOD) in patients undergoing PTCA for acute MI. Circulation [Suppl] 80:113

First Experiences with Recombinant Human Superoxide Dismutase Therapy in Polytraumatized Patients

I. Marzi[1], V. Bühren[1], A. Schüttler[2], and O. Trentz[1]

Introduction

The important role of oxygen-derived free radicals in the development of tissue and organ injury after ischemia has been demonstrated in a variety of experimental studies over the past decade [1, 11, 18, 32]. Postischemic reperfusion injury was most likely due to the generation of oxygen-derived free radicals via the xanthine oxidase mechanism early during reperfusion [18]. Furthermore, activation and adhesion of leukocytes during the later time course of reperfusion was found as a second step resulting in postischemic tissue injury due to the local release of free radicals [8, 19, 20]. Free radical mediated tissue injury after trauma and local or remote tissue injury by activated leukocytes have been suggested as early events contributing to the adult respiratory distress syndrome (ARDS) or multiple organ failure syndrome (MOF) [4, 15, 17, 23]. During the development of ARDS or MOF, interactions of oxygen free radicals with other inflammatory mediators such as complement, endotoxin, cytokines, eicosanoids, and others seems likely [17, 21, 31].

Since severe trauma regularly involves shock, hypotension, and tissue injury, the aim of our study was to evaluate the effect of an oxygen radical scavenger given after trauma in regard to the reduction of organ failure. The availability of quantitative amounts of recombinant human superoxide dismutase (rHSOD) permitted this first clinical trial with the aims of: (a) assessing the safety of high-dosage therapy with rHSOD in severely traumatized patients, and (b) evaluating prophylactic and therapeutic effects of rHSOD in preventing or reducing MOF after polytrauma.

Study Protocol

Patients. A total of 24 patients were enrolled consecutively in a prospective, randomized, placebo-controlled, single-blinded, parallel pilot study. The inclusion criteria were: (a) age between 18 and 64 years; (b) injury severity score equal

---

[1] Department of Trauma Surgery, University of Saarland, 6650 Homburg/Saar, FRG
[2] Grünenthal Research Center, 5100 Aachen, FRG

Host Defense Dysfunction
in Trauma, Shock and Sepsis
Eds. Faist/Meakins/Schildberg
© Springer-Verlag, Berlin Heidelberg 1993

or higher 27 [9]; (c) maximal 48 h elapsed after trauma; (d) informed consent. Exclusion criteria were: (a) positive skin test prior therapy; (b) administration of corticoids or aprotinin; (c) isolated brain injury. Patients of the verum (SOD) group and those in the placebo group were comparable in respect to age (31.8 $\pm$ 11.1 versus 32.0 $\pm$ 12.9), sex (male/female ratio: 8/4 and 9/3), and Injury Severity Score (36.2 $\pm$ 10.6 versus 33.3 $\pm$ 4.3). No positive skin test prior to the start of therapy was observed.

Treatment Protocol. Patients of the SOD group received a continuous intravenous infusion of 3000 mg/day rHSOD (Grünenthal, Aachen, FRG) during the first 5 days of the study. Patients of the placebo group received carrier (sucrose) for the same time period intravenously.

Clinical Evaluation. The investigational therapy was monitored in respect to drug-related side effects during the time course of the study. The efficacy of the regimen was clinically evaluated by determining the MOF scores of patients during the 5 days treatment period and the subsequent 9-day observation period, as proposed by Goris et al. [7].

Laboratory Evaluation. Three times daily on days 1 and 2 and thereafter once daily, blood samples were collected, and parameters were either immediately determined or plasma was frozen at $-70\,°C$ for later measurements. Inflammatory mediators presented here were: C-reactive protein (particle enhanced nephelometry using latex CRP reagent; Behringwerke, Marburg, FRG), polymorphonuclear leukocyte elastase (PMN elastase IMAC, Merck, Darmstadt, FRG), and phospholipase A_2 (PLA_2, bioassay using [^{14}C] oleate-labeled *Escherichia coli* according to Vadas et al. [29].

Results

Clinical Results. No observable drug-related side effects were noted during the time course of the study, indicating safety of the drug in the dosage given to severely polytraumatized patients. MOF scores decreased in parallel in both groups during the first 5 days of the study. Up to day 13, the mean MOF score of the SOD group was consistently lower than that in the placebo group. However, there was no statistical significance of this consistent tendency in the overall MOF score (Fig. 1). Assessment of the MOF score subgroups indicated a lower cardiovascular organ failure score in the SOD group. For example, dopamine was required up to 10 $\mu g\,kg^{-1}\,min^{-1}$ to keep the mean arterial blood pressure higher than 100 mmHg (grade 1) on day 7 (and 14) in 11 (6) patients of the placebo group and 5 (1) patients of the SOD group ($p < 0.05$). Three patients died during the study period. One patient of the placebo group died due to MOF, and two patients of the SOD group died of acute intracranial hemo-

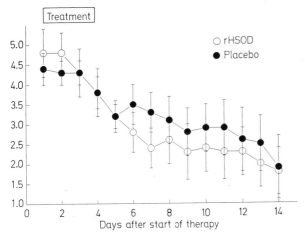

Fig. 1. Multiple organ failure score after polytrauma according to Goris et al. [7]. Data expressed as mean ± SEM

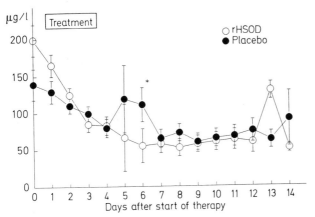

Fig. 2. PMN elastase after trauma. Values are expressed as mean ± SEM. *,$p < 0.05$ using Student's *t* test

rrhage and septic syndrome after spontaneous perforation of the sigma. The median length of the intensive care treatment of the surviving patients was 30 days in the placebo and 21 days in the SOD group.

Inflammatory Mediators. PMN elastase decreased continuously in both groups during the treatment period (Fig. 2). In the placebo group a second increase was noted on days 5 and 6 which was not observed in the SOD group (Fig. 2; $p < 0.05$). CRP was elevated in both groups during the first 4 days. Thereafter, CRP values in the placebo group rose up to day 7 whereas in the SOD group CRP values decreased from day 5 on and remained in at a constant range during the following days (Fig. 3). PLA_2 rose continuously in both groups during the

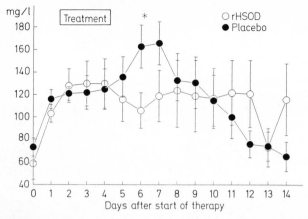

Fig. 3. C-reactive protein after trauma. Data expressed as mean ± SEM. *,$p < 0.05$ using Student's
t test

first 4 days of the study (e.g., placebo group day 1, 20.9 ± 2.1; day 3, 30.5 ± 4.2;
SOD group day 1, 23.0 ± 4.5; day 3, 27.5 ± 3.8 × 10^3 U/ml). In the placebo
group, PLA$_2$ rose further to 39.3 ± 4.9 × 10^3 U /ml on day 7, whereas PLA$_2$ was
significantly reduced in the SOD group (28.4 ± 5.0 × 10^3 U/ml; $p < 0.05$).

Discussion

No drug-related side effects were noted in the patients receiving rHSOD in the
given dosage, with plasma concentrations ranging between 12.4 and 40.4 µg/ml.
This indicates that the applied therapy reached a 350- to 1000-fold increase in
normal plasma concentrations [16] and was safe in this group of severely
traumatized patients. This is consistent with observations of previous studies
using lower doses of rHSOD during kidney transplantation [24] and in phase 1
studies [3].

The clinical results of this study reveal an attenuation of organ injury at the
end of the 1st week after trauma as indicated by the MOF scores. The significant
improvement in the cardiovascular MOF score together with the substantial
decrease of requirement for intensive care therapy indicates a beneficial effect of
r-HSOD after trauma in clinical practice. The improvement in the cardiovascular MOF score expressed itself mainly in a lower requirement for catecholamines, for example, dopamine, dobutrex, or arterenol.

PMN elastase, reflecting the release of proteases by activated leukocytes
[13], decreased continuously in both groups during the first 4 days after trauma.
This reflects most likely the repair of primary tissue injury, in part involving
activated phagocytosing leukocytes. The secondary increase in the placebo
group on days 5 and 6, however, may indicate a second activation of leukocytes
during the posttraumatic inflammatory process, a mechanism suggested by

results of experimental and clinical studies in sepsis and endotoxemia [15, 25, 26, 30]. The decreased PMN elastase values in the SOD group reveal an attenuation of this secondary activation of leukocytes by rHSOD given during the first 5 days. An attenuated inflammatory response after trauma was supported by lower CRP values after the rHSOD therapy (Fig. 3), CRP is a well-accepted unspecific marker of inflammation [22] and is additionally one of the proteins synthetized in hepatocytes as part of the acute-phase reaction (APR) [12, 14]. The APR after an appropriate stimulus, for example, trauma, is largely regulated by interleukines, mainly interleukin-6 [2, 12]. Indeed, interleukin-6 plasma levels, determined in this study by the B9 bioassay [399], were significantly reduced during the early period after trauma, particularly on days 2 and 3 [6]. The attenuation of the late phase of the inflammatory response in the rHSOD treated patients was also indicated by the decrease in PLA_2 plasma levels, in contrast to the further rise in the placebo group. PLA_2, another inflammatory marker and key enzyme of the eicosanoid and platelet-activating factor metabolism [28], therefore seems to be reduced by rHSOD treatment [27].

Further understanding of the mechanisms involved in reduction of the inflammatory response after trauma may be possible when all parameters of this study are determined, including complement, tumor necrosis factor-alpha, endotoxin, lipid peroxidation products, and xanthine oxidase (Marzi et al., in preparation). However, it may be likely that reduction in an early free radical mediated tissue injury results in a decrease in a systemic whole body inflammatory response. Alternative mechanisms such as prevention of microvascular vasoconstriction due to neutralization of the vasodilatatory-acting, endothelium-derived relaxing factor by oxygen radicals [10], thus decreasing hypoxic injury, may also account for the beneficial effect of SOD. Validation of the beneficial clinical effect and attenuation of the inflammatory reaction after trauma by rHSOD as observed in this pilot study, however, requires further evaluation in a far more extensive number of trauma patients.

References

1. Adkinson D, Höllwarth ME, Benoit JN, Parks DA, McCord JM, Granger ND (1986) Role of free radicals in ischemia-reperfusion injury to the liver. Acta Physiol Scand [Suppl] 548:101–107
2. Baumann H, Gauldie J (1990) Regulation of hepatic acute phase plasma protein genes by hepatocyte stimulating factors and other mediators in inflammation. Mol Biol Med 7:147–159
3. Brater DC, Voelker JR, Black PK, Odlund B (1989) Effects of recombinant human superoxide dismutase (r-HSOD) on renal and cardiac function in normal men. Clin Res 37:527 A
4. Carrico CJ, Meakins JL, Marshall JC, Fry D, Maier RV (1986) Multiple-organ-failure syndrome. Arch Surg 121:196–208
5. Castell JV, Gomez-Lechon MJ, David T, Andus T, Geiger T, Trullenque R, Fabra R, Heinrich PC (1989) Interleukin-6 is the major regulator of acute phase protein synthesis in adult human hepatocytes. FEBS Lett 242:237–239
6. Flohé S, Marzi I, Schüttler A, Heinrich PC, Bühren V (1991) Influence of rh-superoxide

dismutase on interleukin-6 plasma levels in polytraumatized patients. (abstract). Circ Shock 34:149

7. Goris RJA, Te Boekhorst TPA, Nuytinck IKS, Gimbrere ISF (1985) Multiple organ failure. Arch Surg 120:1109–1115

8. Granger DN (1988) Role of xanthine oxidase and granulocytes in ischemia-reperfusion injury. Am J Physiol 255:H1269–H1275

9. Greenspan L, McLellan BA, Greig RN (1985) Abbreviated injury scale and injury severity score: a scoring chart. J Trauma 25(1):60–64

10. Gryglewski RJ, Palmer RMJ, Moncada S (1986) Superoxide anion is involved in the breakdown of endothelium-derived vascular relaxing factor. Nature 320:454–456

11. Halliwell B (1987) Oxidants and human disease: some new concepts. FASEB J 1:358–364

12. Heinrich PC, Castell JV, Andus T (1990) Interleukin-6 and the acute phase response. Biochem J 265:621–636

13. Jochum M, Fritz H, Nast-Kolb D, Inthorn D (1990) Granulozyten-Elastase als prognostischer Parameter. Dtsch Aerztebl 87(19):B-1106–B-1110

14. Kushner I, Feldmann G (1979) Control of the acute phase response: demonstration of C-reactive protein synthesis and secretion by hepatocytes during acute inflammation in the rabbit. J Exp Med 466–477

15. Mallik AA, Ishizaka A, Stephens KE, Hatherill JR, Tazelaar HD, Raffin TA (1989) Multiple organ damage caused by tumor necrosis factor and prevented by prior neutrophil depletion. Chest 95:1114–1120

16. Marklund S (1980) Distribution of CuZn superoxide dismutase and Mn superoxide dismutase in human tissues and extracellular fluids. Acta Physiol Scand [Suppl] 492:19–23

17. Matuschak GM, Rinaldo JE (1988) Organ interactions in the adult respiratory distress syndrome during sepsis. Role of the liver in host defense. Chest 94:400–406

18. McCord JM (1985) Oxygen-derived free radicals in postischemic tissue injury. N Engl J Med 312:159–163

19. O'Neill PG, Charlat ML, Michael LH, Roberts R, Bolli R (1989) Influence of neutrophil depletion on myocardial function and flow after reversible ischemia. Am J Physiol 256:H341–H351

20. Otamiri T (1989) Oxygen radicals, lipid peroxidation, and neutrophil infiltration after small-intestinal ischemia and reperfusion. Surgery 105:593–597

21. Parsons PE, Worthen GS, Moore EE, Tate RM, Henson PM (1989) The association of circulating endotoxin with the development of the adult respiratory distress syndrome. Am Rev Respir Dis 140:294–301

22. Pepys MB (1981) C-reactive protein fifty years on. Lancet 21:653–653

23. Petty TL (1988) ARDS: refinement of concept and redefinition. Am Rev Respir Dis 138:724

24. Schneeberger H, Schleibner S, Schilling M, Illner WD, Abendroth D, Hancke E, Jänicke U, Land W (1990) Prevention of acute renal failure after kidney transplantation by treatment with rh-sod: interim analysis of a double-blind placebo-controlled trial. Transplant Proc 22:2224–2225

25. Simons RK, Maier R, Lennard ES (1987) Neutrophil function in a rat model of endotoxin-induced lung injury. Arch Surg 122:197–203

26. Swank DW, Moore SB (1989) Roles of the neutrophil and other mediators in adult respiratory distress syndrome. Mayo Clin Proc 64:1118–1132

27. Tikku R, Marzi I, Dike J, Trentz O, Bühren V (1991) Circulating phospholipase A2 and C-reactive protein after polytrauma — effect of superoxide dismutase. Acta Chir Austriaca 23:2–4

28. Vadas P, Pruzanski W (1984) Role of extracellular phospholipase A2 in inflammation. In: Otterness R, Capetola R, Wong S (eds) Advances in inflammation research, vol 7. Raven, New York, pp 51–59

29. Vadas P, Stefanski E, Pruzanski W (1985) Characterization of extracellular phospholipase A_2 in rheumatoid synovial fluids. Life Sci 36:579–587

30. Warren JS, Ward PA (1986) Review: oxidative injury to the vascular endothelium. Am J Med Sci 29:97–103

31. Zilow G, Sturm JA, Rother U, Kirschfink M (1990) Complement activation and the prognostic value of C3a in patients at risk of adult respiratory distress syndrome. Clin Exp Immunol 79:151–157

32. Zweier JL (1988) Measurement of superoxide-derived free radicals in the reperfused heart. J Biol Chem 263:1353–1357

Subject Index